Primer on the Rheumatic Diseases

THIRTEENTH EDITION

Primer on the Rheumatic Diseases

THIRTEENTH EDITION

Edited by

JOHN H. KLIPPEL, MD

John H. Stone, MD, MPH

Leslie J. Crofford, MD

Patience H. White, MD, MA

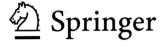 Springer

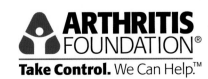

John H. Klippel, MD
President and CEO
Arthritis Foundation
Atlanta, GA, USA

Leslie J. Crofford, MD
Gloria W. Singletary Professor of
   Internal Medicine
Chief, Division of Rheumatology &
   Women's Health
University of Kentucky
Lexington, KY, USA

John H. Stone, MD, MPH
Associate Physician
Massachusetts General Hospital
Deputy Editor for Rheumatology
UpToDate
Boston, MA, USA

Patience H. White, MD, MA
Chief Public Health Officer
Arthritis Foundation
Atlanta, GA, USA

Library of Congress Control Number: 2007925709

ISBN: 978-0-387-35664-8   e-ISBN: 978-0-68566-3

Printed on acid-free paper

9 8 7 6 5

springer.com

The 13th edition of the *Primer on the Rheumatic Diseases* is an extraordinary handbook for clinical care. The *Primer* will educate trainees, update established clinicians, and help health care providers from all walks of the profession provide better care for patients with arthritis and rheumatic diseases.

In achieving these purposes, the *Primer* continues a tradition of excellence dating back more than 70 years. The *Primer* and its precursors have served as a major learning tool for medical students, house officers, fellows, and allied health professionals since 1934, when the early publications of the American Committee for the Control of Rheumatism included the *Primer on Rheumatism: Chronic Arthritis* in 1934. Since that work, which consisted of a 52-page brochure, the *Primer* has evolved into a reference guide of nearly 90 chapters and 4 appendices.

The *Primer* is designed to provide up-to-date information about the major clinical syndromes seen by primary care physicians, rheumatologists, orthopedic surgeons, as well as physician assistants, nurse practitioners, physical and occupational therapists, and allied health professionals whose expertise contributes to patient care. Emphasis on the evaluation of the patient, the physical examination including musculoskeletal signs and symptoms, laboratory and imaging evaluations, and current and novel therapeutic approaches are essential for all who work in this field. Arthritis and other rheumatic diseases, which affect more than 46 million Americans (including 300,000 children), remain a leading cause of disability and the most common chronic illness in the United States.

I congratulate the editors on their superb work. In addition, the multiple contributors—many of whom are members of the American College of Rheumatology—should be thanked for their scholarly contributions to the *Primer*. Rheumatology has never been more exciting than it is today, and there is no doubt that the 13th edition of the *Primer* reflects this. I join clinicians and patients alike in thanking the Arthritis Foundation for the continuing achievements of this book.

MICHAEL E. WEINBLATT, MD
Professor of Medicine
Harvard Medical School
Brigham and Women's Hospital
Boston, MA, USA

Students, residents, and fellows interested in learning about the rheumatic diseases are faced with the daunting challenge of trying to integrate learning about a multitude of fascinating and diverse clinical disorders with an ever-expanding and complex body of basic science.

This need encapsulates the principal rationale for the major changes in the 13th edition of *The Primer on the Rheumatic Diseases*. Although the first part of all recent editions of *The Primer* have summarized succinctly the physiology of tissues and cells that mediate inflammation and musculoskeletal disease, preparation of the new edition resulted in the identification of two major problems with this "tried-and-true" formula. First, for readers who really wished to understand the molecular basis of rheumatic disease to the depth that would facilitate laboratory research and improve patient care, the initial chapters no longer provided sufficient detail. Second, for readers seeking an introduction or update within the clinical realm of rheumatic disorders, the first part of *The Primer* bore virtually no relation to the diseases described so engagingly in the rest of the book. In short, in this era of increasing integration between the basic and clinical sciences, the preliminary *Primer* chapters were at risk for becoming simply the pages thumbed through quickly to get to the good stuff.

Therefore, in the 13th edition, the clinical descriptions that *The Primer* has always done best have been augmented by including the clinically relevant basic science components in the same sections. Thus, for each major rheumatic disease—for example, rheumatoid arthritis, osteoarthritis, systemic lupus erythematosus, and idiopathic inflammatory myopathies—the chapter describing the clinical and epidemiological features is accompanied by another chapter devoted to "Pathology and Pathogenesis." This second chapter incorporates the appropriate (and updated) elements from previous *Primer* chapters entitled "Synovium," "Articular Cartilage," "The Complement System," and "Muscle" that are essential to understanding a particular disease today.

Moreover, this fundamental change in the contents is only the beginning of the improvements to the 13th edition. Other changes include:

- New chapters on "Clinical Immunology" and "Applied Genetics" designed to heighten the translational nature of the book.
- Color figures that are particularly important for depicting cutaneous findings and histopathology.
- An expanded chapter on the cutaneous manifestations of disease, emphasizing the types of disorders rheumatologists often see in consultation.
- A section devoted entirely to juvenile inflammatory arthritis, with individual chapters on "Clinical Features," "Pathology and Pathogenesis," "Treatment and Assessment," and "Special Considerations."
- Separate chapters on ankylosing spondylitis and the reactive and enteropathic arthropathies, once lumped together (with psoriatic arthritis) as "seronegative spondyloarthopathies."

- A tripling of the text devoted to psoriatic arthritis, an acknowledgement of the substantial treatment advances in that disorder.
- Individual chapters (and more than doubling of the text) to the metabolic and inflammatory myopathies, once included in the same chapter.
- Reorganization of the vasculitis section along more rational and all-inclusive lines, with a chapter entitled "ANCA-Associated Vasculitis" that addresses together Wegener's granulomatosis, microscopic polyangiitis, and the Churg-Strauss syndrome, disorders with striking similarities but important contrasts.
- Now entering its eighth decade, *The Primer* has rejected strongly the notion that "If it ain't broke, don't fix it." In view of the recent remarkable strides in understanding and treating rheumatic disease, students, trainees, and practicing clinicians all need a standard textbook that can change with the times and reflect these advances. *The Primer* continues to fill that need. Read, learn, and enjoy.

John H. Klippel, MD
John H. Stone, MD, MPH
Leslie J. Crofford, MD
Patience H. White, MD, MA

CONTENTS

Roy D. Altman, MD
Professor, Deparment of Medicine/Rheumatology and Immunology, University of California, Los Angeles, Los Angeles, CA, USA

Erin L. Arnold, MD
Partner/Rheumatologist, Illinois Bone and Joint Institute, The Center for Arthritis and Osteoporosis, Morton Grove, IL, USA

William J. Arnold, MD
Partner/Rheumatologist, Illinois Bone and Joint Institute, The Center for Arthritis and Osteoporosis, Morton Grove, IL, USA

Alan N. Baer, MD
Associate Professor, Department of Medicine, Chief, Section of Rheumatology, University at Buffalo, State University of New York, Buffalo, NY, USA

W. Timothy Ballard, MD
Director, Joint Replacement Center, Department of Orthopaedics, Memorial Hospital, Chattanooga, TN, USA

Joan M. Bathon, MD
Professor, Department of Medicine, Director, Johns Hopkins Arthritis Center, Johns Hopkins University School of Medicine, Baltimore, MD, USA

Thomas D. Beardmore, MD, FACP, FACR
Chief, Department of Rheumatology, Rancho Los Amigos National Rehabilitation Center, Downey, CA; Professor, Department of Medicine, Keck School of Medicine, The University of Southern California, Los Angeles, CA, USA

Francis Berenbaum, MD, PhD
Professor, Department of Rheumatology, Saint-Antoine Hospital; University Pierre & Marie Curie, Paris, France

Joseph J. Biundo, Jr., MD
Clinical Professor, Department of Medicine, Tulane University School of Medicine, Kenner, LA, USA

Linda K. Bockenstedt, MD
Professor, Department of Internal Medicine, Yale University School of Medicine, New Haven, CT, USA

David Borenstein, MD
Clinical Professor of Medicine, The George Washington University Medical Center; Arthritis and Rheumatism Associates, Washington, DC, USA

Teresa J. Brady, PhD
Senior Behavioral Scientist, Arthritis Program, Centers for Disease Control and Prevention, Atlanta, GA, USA

Juergen Braun, MD
Professor, Department of Rheumatology, Rheumazentrum Ruhrgebiet, Herne, Germany

Maya H. Buch, MBchB, MRCP
Clinical Lecturer and Research Fellow, University of Michigan Scleroderma Program, University of Michigan Health System, Ann Arbor, MI, USA; Academic Unit of Musculoskeletal Disease, University of Leeds, UK

Joseph A. Buckwalter, MS, MD
Professor and Head, Orthopedic Surgery, Department of Orthopaedics and Rehabilitation, University of Iowa, Iowa City, IA, USA

Gerd-Rüdiger Burmester, MD
Professor, Department of Rheumatology and Clinical Immunology, Charité University Hospital, Berlin, Germany

Frank Buttgereit, MD
Professor, Department of Rheumatology and Clinical Immunology, Charité University Hospital, Berlin, Germany

Jill P. Buyon, MD
Professor, Department of Medicine, Division of Rheumatology, New York University School of Medicine, New York, NY; Director, Lupus Clinic, New York University Hospital for Joint Diseases, New York, NY, USA

Leonard H. Calabrese, DO
Professor, Department of Rheumatic and Immunologic Diseases, Cleveland Clinic Lerner College of Medicine of Case Western Reserve University, Cleveland Clinic Foundation, Cleveland, OH, USA

Kenneth T. Calamia, MD
Associate Professor, Department of Medicine, Division of Rheumatology, Mayo Clinic College of Medicine, Jacksonville, FL, USA

Jeffrey P. Callen, MD
Professor, Department of Medicine (Dermatology); Chief, Division of Dermatology, University of Louisville School of Medicine, Louisville, KY, USA

Juan J. Canoso, MD, FACP, MACR
Attending, American British Cowdray Medical Center, Mexico City, Mexico

Rowland W. Chang, MD, MPH
Professor of Preventive Medicine, Medicine, and Physical Medicine and Rehabilitation; Director, Program in Public Health, Northwestern University, Feinberg School of Medicine, Chicago, IL, USA

Edward S. Chen, MD
Assistant Professor, Department of Medicine, Division of Pulmonary and Critical Care Medicine, Johns Hopkins University School of Medicine, Baltimore, MD, USA

Lan X. Chen, MD, PhD
Clinical Assistant Professor, Department of Medicine/ Rheumatology, University of Pennsylvania, Philadelphia, PA, USA

Hyon K. Choi, MD, MPH, DrPH, FRCPC
Associate Professor of Medicine and Mary Pack Arthritis Society Chair in Rheumatology, Department of Medicine, Division of Rheumatology, The University of British Columbia, Vancouver, British Columbia, Canada

Daniel J. Clauw, MD
Professor, Department of Internal Medicine, Division of Rheumatology, University of Michigan, Ann Arbor, MI, USA

Andrew J. Cooper, MD
Resident, Department of Orthopaedic Surgery, University of Miami, Miami, FL, USA

Leslie J. Crofford, MD
Gloria W. Singletary Professor of Internal Medicine, Chief, Division of Rheumatology & Women's Health, University of Kentucky, Lexington, KY, USA

Dina Dadabhoy, MD
Clinical Lecturer, Department of Internal Medicine, Division of Rheumatology, University of Michigan, Ann Arbor, MI, USA

Troy Daniels, DDS, MS
Professor, Schools of Dentistry and Medicine, University of California, San Francisco, San Francisco, CA, USA

John C. Davis, Jr., MD, MPH
Associate Professor, Department of Medicine, Division of Rheumatology, University of California San Francisco, San Francisco, CA, USA

William J. Didie, MD
Fellow, Musculoskeletal Imaging, Department of Radiology, Johns Hopkins University, Baltimore, MD, USA

Paul Dieppe, MD
Professor, Department of Social Medicine, University of Bristol, Bristol, UK

N. Lawrence Edwards, MD
Professor and Vice Chairman, Department of Medicine, University of Florida, Gainesville, FL, USA

Hani S. El-Gabalawy, MD, FRCPC
Professor, Department of Medicine, Arthritis Centre, University of Manitoba, Winnipeg, Manitoba, Canada

Kevin Elias, MD
Howard Hughes Medical Institute-National Institute of Health Research Scholar, Lymphocyte Cell Biology Section, National Institute of Arthritis, Musculoskeletal, and Skin Diseases, Bethesda, MD, USA

John M. Esdaile, MD, MPH
Scientific Director, Arthritis Research Centre of Canada; Professor, University of British Columbia, Vancouver, British Columbia, Canada

Adel G. Fam, MD, FRCP(C), FACP
Emeritus Professor of Medicine, Department of Medicine, Division of Rheumatology, Sunnybrook & Women's College Health Sciences Centre, University of Toronto, Toronto, Ontario, Canada

Laura M. Fayad, MD
Assistant Professor, The Russell H. Morgan Department of Radiology and Radiological Science, Johns Hopkins University School of Medicine, Baltimore, MD, USA

Gary S. Firestein, MD
Professor, Department of Medicine, Chief, Division of Rheumatology, Allergy and Immunology, University of California San Diego, School of Medicine, La Jolla, CA, USA

Kenneth H. Fye, MD
Clinical Professor, Department of Medicine, University of California, San Francisco, San Francisco, CA, USA

Dafna D. Gladman, MD, FRCPC
Professor, Department of Medicine/Rheumatology, University of Toronto; Senior Scientist, Toronto Western Research Institute; Director, Psoriatic Arthritis Program, University Health Network, Toronto, Canada

Duncan A. Gordon, MD, FRCPC, MACR
Professor, Department of Medicine, University of Toronto; Rheumatologist, University Health Network, Toronto Western Hospital, Toronto, Ontario, Canada

Jörg J. Goronzy, MD
Co-Director, Department of Medicine, Kathleen B. and Mason I. Lowance Center for Human Immunology, Emory University School of Medicine, Atlanta, GA, USA

Philip J. Hashkes, MD, MSc
Head, Section of Pediatric Rheumatology, Department of Rheumatic Diseases, Cleveland Clinic Foundation, Cleveland, OH, USA

George Ho, Jr., MD
Professor, Department of Internal Medicine, Division of Rheumatology, Brody School of Medicine at East Carolina University, Greenville, NC, USA

William A. Horton, MD
Director, Research Center/Molecular and Medical Genetics, Shriners Hospital for Children; Professor, Oregon Health and Science University, Portland, OR, USA

Robert D. Inman, MD
Professor, Department of Medicine, Division of Rheumatology, University of Toronto, Toronto Western Hospital, Toronto, Ontario, Canada

Preeti Jaggi, MD
Assistant Professor, Department of Infectious Diseases, Department of Pediatrics, Ohio State University, Columbus, OH, USA

Amy H. Kao, MD, MPH
Assistant Professor, Department of Medicine, Division of Rheumatology and Clinical Immunology, University of Pittsburgh School of Medicine, Pittsburgh, PA, USA

Daniel L. Kastner, MD, PhD
Chief, Genetics and Genomics Branch; Clinical Director and Director of Translational Research, National Institute of Arthritis and Musculoskeletal and Skin Diseases, Bethesda, MD, USA

Jonathan Kay, MD
Associate Clinical Professor, Department of Medicine, Harvard Medical School; Director of Clinical Trials, Rheumatology Unit, Massachusetts General Hospital, Boston, MA, USA

James Kelley, PhD
Postdoctoral Fellow, Department of Medicine, Division of Clinical Immunology and Rheumatology, University of Alabama at Birmingham, Birmingham, AL, USA

Robert P. Kimberly, MD
Howard L. Holley Professor of Medicine and Director, Division of Clinical Immunology and Rheumatology, Senior Associate Dean for Research, Department of Medicine, University of Alabama at Birmingham, Birmingham, AL, USA

John H. Klippel, MD
President and CEO, Arthritis Foundation, Atlanta, GA, USA

Denise Kruszewski, MS
Graduate Student/Research Assistant, Department of Psychology, Arizona State University, Tempe, AZ, USA

Ronald M. Laxer, MD, FRCPC
Vice President, Education and Quality, The Hospital for Sick Children; Professor, Department of Pediatrics and Medicine, The University of Toronto, Toronto, Ontario, Canada

Carol B. Lindsley, MD
Professor, Department of Pediatrics, Director of Pediatric Rheumatology, University of Kansas Medical Center, Kansas City, KS, USA

Geoffrey Littlejohn, MD, MPH, MBBS[Hon], FRACP, FRCP(Edin)
Director of Rheumatology and Associate Professor of Medicine, Department of Medicine, Monash University at Monash Medical Centre, Melbourne, Australia

Daniel J. Lovell, MD, MPH
Joseph Levinson Professor of Pediatrics, Division of Rheumatology, Cincinnati Children's Hospital Medical Center, Cincinnati, OH, USA

Harvinder S. Luthra, MD
John Finn Professor of Medicine, Department of Rheumatology, Mayo Clinic College of Medicine, Rochester, MN, USA

Susan Manzi, MD, MPH
Associate Professor, Department of Medicine, Division of Rheumatology and Clinical Immunology, University of Pittsburgh School of Medicine, University of Pittsburgh Graduate School of Public Health, Pittsburgh, PA, USA

David Marker, BS
Medical Student, Rubin Institute for Advanced Orthopedics, Sinai Hospital of Baltimore, Baltimore, MD, USA

Manuel Martinez-Lavin, MD
Chief, Department of Rheumatology, National Institute of Cardiology, Mexico, DF, Mexico

Maureen D. Mayes, MD, MPH
Professor, Department of Internal Medicine, Division of Rheumatology and Immunogenetics, University of Texas-Houston Medical School, Houston, TX, USA

Geraldine McCarthy, MD, FRCPI
Associate Professor/Consultant Rheumatologist, Division of Rheumatology, Department of Medicine, University College Dublin, Dublin/Mater Misericordiae University Hospital, Dublin, Ireland

Philip J. Mease, MD
Head, Seattle Rheumatology Associates; Chief, Division of Rheumatology Research, Swedish Medical Center; Clinical Professor, University of Washington School of Medicine, Seattle, WA, USA

Peter A. Merkel, MD, MPH
Associate Professor, Department of Medicine, Section of Rheumatology, Boston University School of Medicine, Boston, MA, USA

Frederick W. Miller, MD, PhD
Chief, Environmental Autoimmunity Group, Office of Clinical Research, National Institute of Environmental Health Sciences, National Institutes of Health, Bethesda, MD, USA

Michael A. Mont, MD
Director, Rubin Institute for Advanced Orthopedics, Sinai Hospital of Baltimore, Baltimore, MD, USA

Kerstin Morehead, MD
Assistant Clinical Professor, Department of Medicine, Division of Rheumatology, University of California, San Francisco, San Francisco, CA, USA

Barry L. Myones, MD
Associate Professor, Pediatric Rheumatology Center, Baylor College of Medicine/Texas Children's Hospital, Houston, TX, USA

Chester V. Oddis, MD
Professor, Department of Medicine, Division of Rheumatology and Clinical Immunology, University of Pittsburgh School of Medicine, Pittsburgh, PA, USA

Alyce M. Oliver, MD, PhD
Fellow in Rheumatology, Department of Medicine, Division of Rheumatology and Immunology, Duke University Medical Center, Durham, NC, USA

John J. O'Shea, MD
Scientific Director, National Institute of Arthritis and Musculoskeletal and Skin Diseases; Chief, Molecular Immunology and Inflammation Branch; Chief, Lymphocyte Cell Biology Section, National Institutes of Health, Bethesda, MD, USA

Michelle Petri, MD, MPH
Professor, Department of Medicine, Johns Hopkins University School of Medicine, Baltimore, MD, USA

David S. Pisetsky, MD, PhD
Chief, Department of Medicine, Division of Rheumatology and Immunology, Duke University School of Medicine, Durham, NC, USA

Reed Edwin Pyeritz, MD, PhD
Professor, Department of Medicine and Genetics, Hospital of the University of Pennsylvania, Philadelphia, PA, USA

James D. Reeves, MD
Resident, Department of Orthopaedic Surgery, University of Miami, Miami, FL, USA

Lisa G. Rider, MD
Deputy Chief, Environmental Autoimmunity Group, Office of Clinical Research, National Institute of Environmental Health Sciences, National Institutes of Health, Clinical Research Center, Bethesda, MD, USA

Christopher Ritchlin, MD
Associate Professor, Department of Medicine, Division of Allergy, Immunology and Rheumatology, University of Rochester Medical Center, Rochester, NY, USA

David B. Robinson, MD, MSc, FRCPC
Associate Professor, Department of Medicine, Arthritis Centre, University of Manitoba, Winnipeg, Manitoba, Canada

Ann K. Rosenthal, MD
Professor, Department of Medicine, Division of Rheumatology, Medical College of Wisconsin/Zablocki VA Medical Center, Milwaukee, WI, USA

Keith T. Rott, MD, PhD
Assistant Professor, Department of Medicine, Division of Rheumatology, Emory University School of Medicine, Atlanta, GA, USA

John G. Ryan, MB, MRCPI
Clinical Fellow, Genetics and Genomics Branch, National Institute of Arthritis and Musculoskeletal and Skin Diseases, National Institutes of Health, Bethesda, MD, USA

Kenneth G. Saag, MD, MSc
Associate Professor, Director, Center for Education and Research on Therapeutics of Musculoskeletal Disorders, Division of Clinical Immunology and Rheumatology, University of Alabama at Birmingham, Birmingham, AL, USA

Carlo Salvarani, MD
Director, Division of Rheumatology, Hospital S. Maria Nuova, Reggio Emilia, Italy

Philip Sambrook, MD, FRACP
Professor, Department of Rheumatology, University of Sydney, Sydney, NSW Australia

Pasha Sarraf, MD, PhD
Fellow, Department of Medicine, Division of Rheumatology, Allergy and Immunology, Massachusetts General Hospital, Boston, MA, USA

H. Ralph Schumacher, MD
Professor, Department of Medicine/Rheumatology, University of Pennsylvania; VA Medical Center, Philadelphia, PA, USA

William W. Scott, Jr., MD
Associate Professor, The Russell H. Morgan Department of Radiology and Radiological Science, Johns Hopkins University School of Medicine, Baltimore, MD, USA

Sean P. Scully, MD, PhD
Professor, Department of Orthopaedics, Miller School of Medicine, University of Miami, Miami, FL, USA

James R. Seibold, MD
Professor, Department of Internal Medicine/Rheumatology, Director, University of Michigan Scleroderma Program, University of Michigan Health System, Ann Arbor, MI, USA

Philip Seo, MD, MHS
Co-Director, Johns Hopkins Vasculitis Center, Division of Rheumatology, Johns Hopkins University School of Medicine, Baltimore, MD, USA

Thorsten M. Seyler, MD
Center for Joint Preservation and Reconstruction, Rubin Institute for Advanced Orthopedics, Sinai Hospital of Baltimore, Baltimore, MD, USA

Leena Sharma, MD
Professor, Department of Internal Medicine, Division of Rheumatology, Feinberg School of Medicine at Northwestern University, Chicago, IL, USA

Stanford Shulman, MD
Chief, Department of Infectious Diseases; Professor, Department of Pediatrics, Northwestern University Feinberg School of Medicine/The Children's Memorial Hospital, Chicago, IL, USA

Richard Siegel, MD, PhD
Principal Investigator, Immunoregulation Group, National Institute of Arthritis and Musculoskeletal and Skin Diseases, National Institutes of Health, Bethesda, MD, USA

Robert F. Spiera, MD
Adjunct Clinical Instructor, Department of Medicine/ Rheumatology, Mount Sinai School of Medicine, New York, NY, USA

E. William St. Clair, MD
Professor, Department of Medicine, Division of Rheumatology and Immunology, Duke University Medical Center, Durham, NC, USA

John H. Stone, MD, MPH
Associate Physician, Massachusetts General Hospital; Deputy Editor for Rheumatology, UpToDate, Boston, MA, USA

Christopher V. Tehlirian, MD
Post-Doctoral Fellow, Department of Medicine, Division of Clinical and Molecular Rheumatology, Johns Hopkins University School of Medicine, Baltimore, MD, USA

Robert A. Terkeltaub, MD
Chief, Rheumatology Section, Department of Medicine, Veterans Affairs Medical Center San Diego; Professor, Department of Medicine, University of California San Diego School of Medicine, San Diego, CA, USA

Désirée Van der Heijde, MD, PhD
Professor, Department of Rheumatology, University Hospital Maastricht, The Netherlands

John Varga, MD
Gallagher Professor of Medicine, Department of Medicine, Division of Rheumatology, Northwestern University Feinberg School of Medicine, Chicago, IL, USA

Jean-Marc Waldburger, MD, PhD
Post-Doctoral Scholar, Department of Medicine, Division of Rheumatology, Allergy, and Immunology, University of California San Diego School of Medicine, La Jolla, CA, USA

Nelson B. Watts, MD
Professor, Department of Internal Medicine, University of Cincinnati College of Medicine, Cincinnati, OH, USA

Sterling West, MD
Professor, Department of Rheumatology, University of Colorado Health Sciences Center, Denver, CO, USA

Cornelia M. Weyand, MD
Co-Director, Kathleen B. and Mason I. Lowance Center for Human Immunology, Department of Medicine, Emory University School of Medicine, Atlanta, GA, USA

Patience H. White, MD, MA
Chief Public Health Officer, Arthritis Foundation, Atlanta, GA, USA

John B. Winfield, MD
Smith Distinguished Professor of Medicine Emeritus, Department of Medicine, University of North Carolina, Chapel Hill, NC, USA

Patricia Woo, BSc, MBBS, PhD, MRCP, FRCP, CBE
Professor, Department of Immunology and Molecular Pathology, University College London, London, UK

Robert L. Wortmann, MD, FACP, FACR
Professor and C. S. Lewis, Jr., MD Chair of Medicine, Department of Internal Medicine, The University of Oklahoma College of Medicine, Tulsa, OK, USA

Steven R. Ytterberg, MD
Associate Professor, Department of Medicine, Division of Rheumatology, Mayo Clinic College of Medicine, Rochester, MN, USA

Alex Zautra, PhD
Foundation Professor, Department of Psychology, Arizona State University, Tempe, AZ, USA

CHAPTER 1

Public Health and Arthritis: A Growing Imperative

PATIENCE H. WHITE, MD, MA
ROWLAND W. CHANG, MD, MPH

- Forty-six million people have doctor-diagnosed arthritis and by 2030 it is projected to be 67 million, or 25% of the US population.
- Arthritis is the number one cause of disability and costs the United States an estimated 128 billion annually.

- Public health focuses on the assessment and reduction of health burden in the population.
- Three types of prevention strategies can be applied to arthritis.

The Merriam-Webster Dictionary defines public health as "the art and science dealing with the protection and improvement of community health by organized community effort and including preventive medicine and sanitary and social science." Until the mid-20th century, the field of public health was primarily concerned with the prevention and control of infectious diseases. More recently, public health scientists and practitioners have also been engaged in the prevention and control of chronic diseases. In the mid-19th century, when the therapeutic armamentarium of physicians was limited, the relationship between the fields of public health and medicine was very close. Indeed, most public health professionals were physicians. However, as biomedical science led to more and more diagnostic and therapeutic strategies for physicians in the 20th century, and as separate schools of medicine and public health were established in American universities, the fields have developed different approaches to solving health problems. Medicine has been primarily concerned with the diagnosis and the palliative and curative treatments of disease and the health of the individual patient. Public health has been primarily concerned with the prevention and control of disease and the health of the population. The goal of this chapter is to illustrate the magnitude of the arthritis public health problem in the United States and to describe potential public health approaches to mitigate this problem. In order to more clearly describe public health perspective, science, and intervention, contrasts will be made with the medical approach, but this should not be interpreted to mean that one approach is superior to the other. In fact, it is likely that arthritis patient–physician encounters will be more effective when arthritis public health efforts are successful and vice versa. It is this synergy for which both fields should be striving.

RATIONALE FOR ARTHRITIS PUBLIC HEALTH INITIATIVE

Arthritis and other rheumatic conditions are the leading cause of disability in the United States (1), making it a major public health problem. Arthritis is one of the most common chronic diseases in the United States. Forty-six million Americans, or one out of every five adults, has doctor-diagnosed arthritis, and 300,000 children have arthritis (http://www.cdc.gov/arthritis/). Between 2003 and 2004, an estimated 19 million US adults reported arthritis-attributable activity limitation and 8 million reported arthritis affected their work (2). Arthritis is a large clinical burden, with 36 million ambulatory visits and 750,000 hospitalizations (3,4). In 2030, due to the aging of the population and the growing epidemic of obesity, the prevalence of self-reported, doctor-diagnosed arthritis is projected to increase to nearly 67 million (25% of the adult population) and 25 million (9.3% of the adult population) will report arthritis-attributable activity limitations (Table 1-1) (5).

In the future, this arthritis-related clinical and health care system burden will require a planned

TABLE 1-1. ESTIMATED US POPULATION AND PROJECTED PREVALENCE OF DOCTOR-DIAGNOSED ARTHRITIS AND ACTIVITY LIMITATION FOR ADULTS AGES 18 AND OLDER IN THE UNITED STATES.

YEAR	ESTIMATED US POPULATION IN THOUSANDS	PROJECTED PREVALENCE OF DOCTOR-DIAGNOSED ARTHRITIS IN THOUSANDS	PROJECTED PREVALENCE OF ARTHRITIS-ATTRIBUTABLE ACTIVITY LIMITATIONS IN THOUSANDS
2005	216,096	47,838	17,610
2015	238,154	55,725	20,601
2030	267,856	66,969	25,043

SOURCE: Hootman JM, Helmick CG, Arthritis Rheum 2006;54:226–229, by permission of *Arthritis and Rheumatism.*

coordinated approach with increased need for more arthritis specialists, increased need for training of primary care providers in arthritis management, and increased availability of public health interventions to improve quality of life through lifestyle changes and disease self-management.

THE MEDICAL MODEL COMPARED WITH THE PUBLIC HEALTH MODEL

There are several differences between medicine and public health, but perhaps the most important difference is that of perspective. Medicine focuses on the *diagnosis and treatment of individuals*, whereas public health focuses on the *assessment and the reduction of health burden in the population*. The diagnostic tools of the physician includes history, physical examination, and a vast array of diagnostic tests including blood tests, imaging, and tissue sampling, all performed on the individual patient. Medical treatment includes pharmaceuticals, surgery, and rehabilitation. The assessment tools of the public health professional include surveys and disease registries for defined populations (local, state, and/or national). Public health intervention includes community health education and programs and advocacy for public policy reform. Medical research programs emphasize basic science, drilling down to individual abnormalities at the molecular and genomic level, whereas public health research programs emphasize epidemiology and the social sciences, searching out risk factors that pertain to a large proportion of the population. While medical science has undeniably improved the individual treatment of some forms of arthritis (e.g., rheumatoid arthritis), still much more needs to be done to deal with the coming increases in arthritis prevalence and

arthritis-related disability associated with the aging of the US population. This is perhaps the most important reason to embrace an arthritis public health initiative: to have a greater impact on the health of the population.

PUBLIC HEALTH'S EMPHASIS ON PREVENTION AND HOW IT RELATES TO ARTHRITIS

Traditionally, public health has been concerned with the prevention of disease and the prevention of disease consequences (e.g., death and disability). Three types of prevention have been described: primary, secondary, and tertiary. Primary prevention is the prevention of the disease itself. In the infectious disease realm, this is made possible by the identification of the etiologic microorganism and the development of a vaccine that will protect the host from developing the infection even when the host is exposed to the microorganism. Primary prevention of a chronic disease requires the identification of an etiologic factor associated with the disease and the successful intervention (lifestyle change and/or pharmacologic treatment) on the risk factor. For example, the reduction of weight by dietary and physical activity intervention has been successful in the primary prevention of diabetes, and the pharmacologic treatment of hypertension has proven effective in the prevention of coronary artery disease. An example of a primary arthritis prevention trial showed that a vaccine for the spirochete associated with Lyme disease reduced the risk for this disease in endemic areas (6). While several etiologic factors associated with knee osteoarthritis (most notably obesity) have been identified, no trials have been performed to inform public health practice regarding the primary prevention of this condition, although data will hopefully be available in the coming years.

Secondary prevention involves the detection of disease in its preclinical (i.e., asymptomatic) phase to allow for early treatment and the prevention of important consequences, such as death or disability. For example, mammography has been shown to prevent breast cancer–related death by detecting breast cancer before clinical signs and symptoms develop such that early treatment can be initiated. Similarly, screening for osteoporosis with dual-energy x-ray absorptiometry (DXA) scanning has been shown to reduce fracture rates and subsequent disability by allowing for early detection and treatment of this common condition. Secondary prevention of rheumatoid arthritis is likely to be successful because of effective medical treatment that limits joint destruction and arthritis-related disability. Studies have shown that the earlier the treatment, the less the ultimate destruction and disability. The challenge here is to identify a suitable screening test.

Tertiary prevention involves the treatment of clinical disease in order to prevent important consequences, such as death or disability. Thus, tertiary prevention is typically in the realm of medicine. However, public health and public policy efforts to make medical, surgical, and rehabilitation treatment more effective and more accessible are common public health tertiary prevention interventions.

ARTHRITIS PUBLIC HEALTH ACCOMPLISHMENTS

The Arthritis Foundation has focused its public health activities by promoting the health of people with and at risk for arthritis through its leadership and involvement in the National Arthritis Act, the National Arthritis Action Plan, the arthritis section of Healthy People 2010, and the National Committee on Quality Assurance (NCQA) to develop an arthritis-related Health Plan Employer Data and Information Set (HEDIS) measure (2003).

National Arthritis Act

In 1974, the Arthritis Foundation joined in a partnership that pushed the US Congress to pass the National Arthritis Act, which initiated an expanded response to arthritis through research, training, public education, and treatment. The National Arthritis Act called for a long-term strategy to address arthritis in the United States.

TABLE 1-2.   THE NATIONAL ARTHRITIS ACTION PLAN.

The overarching aims of the NAAP are:
- Increase public awareness of arthritis as the leading cause of disability and an important public health problem.
- Prevent arthritis whenever possible.
- Promote early diagnosis and appropriate management for people with arthritis to ensure the maximum number of years of healthy life.
- Minimize preventable pain and disability due to arthritis.
- Support people with arthritis in developing and accessing the resources they need to cope with their disease.
- Ensure that people with arthritis receive the family, peer, and community support they need.

The aims of the NAAP will be achieved through three major types of activities:
- Surveillance, epidemiology, and prevention research
- Communication and education
- Programs, policies, and systems

National Arthritis Action Plan

The National Arthritis Action Plan (NAAP) brought together over 40 partners to create a blueprint for population-oriented efforts to combat arthritis. The NAAP emphasizes four public health values: prevention, the use and expansion of the science base, social equity, and building partnerships. The NAAP is now widely utilized by other public health and professional organizations as a model program for population-oriented efforts to combat a chronic disease (see Table 1-2 for the aims and activities of NAAP). In 2000, the federal government funded the Arthritis Program at the Centers for Disease Control (CDC) that provides the infrastructure for the program at the CDC, implementation of the arthritis public health plan through the establishment of arthritis programs in state health departments (see http://www.cdc.gov/arthritis/), limited investigator-initiated grant program, and a peer-reviewed grant to the Arthritis Foundation. With this funding, the CDC Arthritis Program and the Arthritis Foundation have created effective public education and awareness activities in both English and Spanish and have developed evidence-based programs for people with arthritis, including an arthritis-specific self-help course, an exercise program, and a water exercise program (see the Life Improvement Series descriptions at http://www.arthritis.org).

The Arthritis Group at the Center for Disease Control have developed arthritis data collection plans through the Behavioral Risk Factor Surveillance System (BRFSS), the National Health Interview Survey

(NHIS), and the National Health and Nutrition Examination Survey (NHANES), and it has published an annual arthritis data report during Arthritis Month in May.

Healthy People 2010

Healthy People 2010 is the nation's public health plan that was created in consultation with the nation's health constituencies by the Department of Health and Human Services. Healthy People 2010 has two goals: (1) increase quality and years of life and (2) eliminate health disparities. Healthy People 2010 contains a separate chapter on Arthritis and Other Rheumatic Conditions, including osteoporosis and back pain. The overall goal of this section of Healthy People 2010 is to "prevent illness and disability related to arthritis and other rheumatic conditions, osteoporosis, and chronic back conditions" (www.healthypeople.gov).

The general Healthy People 2010 arthritis objectives are to:

- Reduce the mean level of joint pain among adults with doctor-diagnosed arthritis.
- Reduce the proportion of adults with doctor-diagnosed arthritis who experience a limitation in activity due to arthritis or joint symptoms.
- Reduce the proportion of adults with doctor-diagnosed arthritis who have difficulty in performing two or more personal care activities, thereby preserving independence.
- Increase health care provider counseling for persons with doctor-diagnosed arthritis.
- Increase health care provider counseling about weight loss among persons with doctor-diagnosed arthritis.
- Increase health care provider counseling for physical activity or exercise for persons with doctor-diagnosed arthritis.
- Reduce the impact of doctor-diagnosed arthritis on employment.
- Increase the employment rate among adults with doctor-diagnosed arthritis in the working-aged population.
- Decrease the effect of doctor-diagnosed arthritis on paid work.
- Eliminate racial differences in the rate of total knee replacements.
- Increase the proportion of adults who have seen a health care provider for their chronic joint symptoms.
- Increase the proportion of persons with doctor-diagnosed arthritis who have had effective, evidence-based arthritis education as an integral part of the management of their condition.

Quality of Care Measures for People with Arthritis

The Arthritis Foundation Quality Indicators Project (AFQUIP) created indicators for treatment of rheumatoid arthritis and osteoarthritis, and for analgesics and pain use (7).

These were used by the National Committee for Quality Assurance (NCQA) to develop a HEDIS measure for disease-modifying antirheumatic drugs (http://www.ncqa.org). The osteoarthritis indicators have been used by the American Medical Association (AMA) Physician Consortium for Performance Improvement.

Through a focus on public health goals, several organizations are cooperating and collaborating to lessen disability in the aging population, decrease health disparities, and increase physical activity and reduce calorie intake in order to mitigate the epidemic of obesity and its serious impacts on health. The Arthritis Foundation and the CDC are actively forming partnerships with state public health departments, federal government agencies such as the National Institute of Arthritis and Musculoskeletal and Skin Diseases at the National Institutes of Health, the Agency for Orthopedic Surgery, community health organizations, volunteer health organizations, other volunteer organizations such as Research! America, and professional organizations such as the American College of Rheumatology and the American Academy of Healthcare Research and Quality to move this agenda forward.

REFERENCES

1. Centers for Disease Control and Prevention. Prevalence of disabilities and associated health conditions among adults: United States 1999. Morb Mortal Wkly Rep 2001;50:120–125.
2. Centers for Disease Control and Prevention. Racial/ethnic differences in the prevalence and impact of doctor diagnosed arthritis: United States, 2002. Morb Mortal Wkly Rep 2005;54:119–121.
3. Hootman JM, Helmick CG, Schappert SM. Magnitude and characteristics of arthritis and other rheumatic conditions on ambulatory medical visits, United States 1997. Arthritis Rheum 2002;47:571–581.
4. Lethbridge-Cejku M, Helmick CG, Popovic JR. Hospitalizations for arthritis and other rheumatic conditions: data from the 1997 National Hospital Discharge Survey. Med Care 2003;41:1367–1373.

5. Hootman JM, Helmick CG. Projections of US prevalence of arthritis and associated activity limitations. Arthritis Rheum 2006;54:226–229.

6. Steere AC, Sikand VK, Meurice F, et al. Vaccination against Lyme disease with recombinant Borrelia burgdorferi outer-surface lipoprotein A with adjuvant. Lyme Disease Vaccine Study Group. N Engl J Med 1998;339: 209–215.

7. MacLean CH, Saag KG, Solomon DH, Morton SC, Sampsel S, Klippel JH. Measuring quality in arthritis care: methods for developing the Arthritis Foundation's quality indicator set. Arthritis Rheum 2004;51:193–202.

1

Evaluation of the Patient
A. History and Physical Examination

DAVID B. ROBINSON, MD, MSC, FRCPC
HANI S. EL-GABALAWY, MD, FRCPC

- The patient history and physical examination form the basis of diagnosis and monitoring the course of rheumatic and musculoskeletal diseases.
- Attention is focused on signs and symptoms of both joint and extra-articular features.

- The joint examination must include pattern, range of motion, signs of inflammation, stability, weakness, and deformity.

Musculoskeletal complaints are among the most common problems in clinical medicine. It is therefore important that all physicians are able to conduct a basic screening evaluation that identifies the presence of pathology or dysfunction of musculoskeletal structures.

RHEUMATOLOGICAL HISTORY

A thoughtful and detailed history plays a critical role in determining the nature of the complaint and helps to focus the clinical evaluation (1). The history should be structured to answer specific questions.

Questions for the Clinician to Address

1. Is the problem regional or generalized, symmetric or asymmetric, peripheral or central?
2. Is it an acute, subacute, or chronic problem? Is it progressive?
3. Do the symptoms suggest inflammation or damage to musculoskeletal structures?
4. Is there evidence of a systemic process? Are there associated extra-articular features?
5. Is there an underlying medical disorder which may predispose to a specific rheumatologic problem?
6. Has there been functional loss and disability?
7. Is there a family history of a similar or related problem?

Location and Symmetry

The location of a musculoskeletal problem is often the most important clue in identifying the specific cause. Musculoskeletal problems can broadly be categorized as regional or generalized, although there is often considerable overlap between these two categories. Regional syndromes typically affect a single joint or periarticular structure, or an entire extremity or body region. A regional pain syndrome can be on a referred basis, and have little to do with the area where the pain is experienced. Joints both immediately above and below the painful area should be routinely examined for pathology.

Specific arthropathies have a predilection for involving specific joint areas (2). Involvement of the wrists and the proximal small joints of the hands and feet is an important feature of rheumatoid arthritis (RA). In contrast, psoriatic arthritis (PsA) often involves the distal joints of the hands and feet. An acutely painful and swollen great toe is most likely caused by a gouty attack. An important aspect of the articular pattern of involvement is symmetry. Rheumatoid arthritis tends to involve joint groups symmetrically, whereas the seronegative spondyloarthropathies and osteoarthritis (OA) tend to be asymmetrical in their articular patterns.

Onset and Chronology

The mode of onset and evolution of musculoskeletal symptoms over time is very helpful in establishing a diagnosis. For most chronic arthropathies such as RA, the onset is typically subacute, occurring over weeks to months rather than hours to days. Attacks of gout and septic arthritis, on the other hand, have an acute onset, reaching a crescendo within hours. The pain of fibromyalgia is often reported as being present for years with episodic exacerbations. A temporally associated traumatic event or history of repetitive use of a joint can be a particularly good clue to diagnosing a regional musculoskeletal syndrome.

Inflammation and Weakness

Articular pain and swelling can be on an inflammatory or non-inflammatory basis. When intra-articular inflammation is present, the process involves the synovial membrane, and is termed *synovitis*. The swelling is usually due to accumulation of fluid in the articular cavity and/or infiltration and enlargement of the synovium. Pain and swelling associated with the presence of synovitis often occur at rest, whereas in degenerative disorders such as OA, these symptoms become more evident with joint use. In the presence of synovitis, the patient may also complain of difficulty moving the joints after a period of immobility, a symptom referred to as *stiffness*. In inflammatory disorders such as RA, this stiffness is most evident in the early morning. Indeed, the duration of morning stiffness, typically established by asking the patient, "How long does it take you before you are moving as well as you are going to move for the day?" is a semiquantitative measure of the degree of articular inflammation.

Complaints of limitation in joint motion, deformity, and joint instability are usually caused by damage to articular and periarticular structures. The patient should be carefully questioned to establish the circumstances around which these symptoms were initiated, and the types of movements that aggravate them.

Patients with musculoskeletal pathology often complain of muscle weakness. This feeling of weakness may be associated with pain, stiffness, and, in some cases, parasthesia or other neurological symptoms. Generalized weakness may be in response to pain from articular or periarticular inflammation, as in the case of RA and polymyalgia rheumatica. Alternatively, weakness may be caused by a primary neuropathic or myopathic process. In the case of myopathies, the weakness is typically symmetrical and involves proximal muscles most severely, whereas neuropathies more commonly affect the distal musculature.

Systemic and Extra-Articular Features

Constitutional symptoms of fatigue, weight loss, anorexia, and low grade fever can be associated with any systemic inflammatory process, and their presence is an important diagnostic clue. In addition, systemic rheumatic diseases are commonly associated with nonarticular features that are of value in diagnosis. For example, a history of recent genitourinary symptoms in association with lower extremity asymmetric oligoarthritis is highly suggestive of reactive arthritis, whereas this same articular pattern in association with recurrent abdominal pain and bloody diarrhea is more suggestive of the arthropathy of inflammatory bowel disease. It is thus important that the clinician perform a complete review of systems and directly question the patient regarding the presence of specific symptoms, such as rashes or skin changes, photosensitivity, Raynaud's phenomenon, mouth ulcers, and dryness in the eyes and mouth.

Functional Losses

Questioning regarding functional loss is essential for understanding the impact of a musculoskeletal disorder and, in turn, developing a plan of management. The questioning should span the spectrum of activities, from simple activities of daily living such as dressing and grooming to more physically demanding activities such as sports. In some cases, the functional loss may be quite severe, impairing basic activities such as stair climbing and gripping, while in others it may be quite subtle, detectable only as a reduction in strenuous activities such as jogging.

Family History

A number of rheumatic diseases have a strong genetic basis. Disorders such as ankylosing spondylitis are much more common in HLA-B27–positive families than in the general population. Questioning regarding family history should not be restricted only to ascertaining whether other family members have a similar arthritis, but should be as complete as possible regarding autoimmune diseases, many of which (e.g., RA, thyroid disease, and diabetes) tend to cluster in families.

PRINCIPLES OF RHEUMATOLOGICAL EXAMINATION

Evaluation of musculoskeletal complaints involves examination of the joints and their soft tissue support structures, the bony skeleton, and the muscle groups that move the skeletal structures (3). The joints, bones, and muscles can be directly accessible to examination, as in the extremities, or they may be inaccessible to direct examination, as in the case of the spine and hip joints.

All joint areas should be inspected from multiple angles to assess for deformity (sometimes seen as loss of symmetry with the contralateral side), muscular atrophy, swelling, erythema, or surgical scars. Extremity joints should be palpated for warmth using the dorsum of the hand. Superficial joints are normally slightly cooler than the surrounding soft tissue. The joint line and major bony and soft tissue structures should be palpated for tenderness.

Functional joint motion should be tested both by having the patient actively move the joint to its extremes and by having the examiner passively move the joint through its range. Tenderness elicited by gentle stress on the joint at its end range of motion (stress tenderness) is characteristic of joint pathology and may be absent in pain syndromes such as fibromyalgia. Loss of range of motion is seen both with acute articular inflammation and with chronic arthritis and damage. Joints should be assessed for the presence of swelling. The cardinal signs of articular inflammation are warmth, joint line tenderness, pain on motion (particularly at the extremes of the range of motion), and intra-articular swelling or effusion.

Deformity caused by loss of alignment is a consequence of destructive arthropathies such as RA. The damage is commonly associated with loosening of the soft tissue support structures surrounding the joints. In some cases, the joint may not exhibit any obvious deformity, but may be unstable when put through its range of motion or is mechanically stressed.

A key part of the musculoskeletal evaluation involves examination of the ligaments, tendons, menisci, and muscles. These structures may be the primary source of the pathology, or may be involved secondary to the articular pathology. Examination of individual muscle groups requires a basic knowledge of the origin, insertion, and primary action of each muscle. Atrophy and weakness of the muscles surrounding a particular joint is an important indicator of chronic articular pathology.

A Screening Musculoskeletal Exam

The GALS (Gait, Arms, Leg, Spine) system has been devised to screen rapidly for musculoskeletal disease (4). Initially, the patient is asked three basic questions: "Have you any pain or stiffness in your muscles, joints, or back?"; "Can you dress yourself completely without any difficulty?"; "Can you walk up and down stairs without any difficulty?". Depending on the answers to the questions, further questioning is undertaken to explore specific areas.

The examiner then systematically inspects the patient's gait, arms, legs, and spine, first with the patient standing still and then responding to instructions (Table 2A-1). Abnormalities detected on this screening are followed up with a more detailed regional or generalized musculoskeletal examination.

TABLE 2A-1. MAIN FEATURES OF THE GAIT, ARMS, LEG, SPINE (GALS) SCREENING INSPECTION.

POSITION/ACTIVITY	NORMAL FINDINGS
Gait	Symmetry, smoothness of movement; normal stride length; normal heel strike, stance, toe-off, swing through; able to turn quickly
Inspection from behind	Straight spine, normal symmetric paraspinal muscles, normal shoulder and gluteal muscle bulk, level iliac crests, no popliteal cysts, no popliteal swelling, no hindfoot swelling/deformity
Inspection from the side	Normal cervical and lumbar lordosis, normal thoracic kyphosis
"Touch your toes."	Normal lumbar spine (and hip) flexion
Inspection from the front	
Arms	
"Place your hands behind your head, elbows out."	Normal glenohumeral, sternoclavicular, and acromioclavicular joint movement
"Place your hands by your side, elbows straight."	Full elbow extension
"Place your hands in front, palms down."	No wrist/finger swelling or deformity, able to fully exend fingers
"Turn your hands over."	Normal supination/pronation, normal palms
"Make a fist."	Normal grip power
"Place the tip of each finger on the tip of the thumb."	Normal fine precision, pinch
Legs	Normal quadriceps bulk/symmetry, no knee swelling or deformity, no forefoot/midfoot deformity, normal arches, no abnormal callous formation
Spine	
"Place your ear on your shoulder."	Normal cervical lateral flexion

SOURCE: Modified from Doherty et al., Ann Rheum Dis 1992;51:1165–1169, with permission of *Annals of Rheumatic Diseases*.

EXAMINATION OF SPECIFIC JOINT AREAS

The Hand and Wrist

A number of generalized arthropathies have distinctive patterns of hand involvement, and the recognition of these patterns is highly valuable diagnostically. Examination of the hands should be initiated with the patient sitting comfortably with the hands open and the palms facing down. In this position, the examiner can inspect the alignment of the digits relative to the wrist and forearm. Atrophy of the intrinsic muscles of the hands can readily be appreciated as a hollowing out of the spaces between the metacarpals. The nails should be inspected for evidence of onycolysis or pitting suggestive of psoriasis. Redness and telangiectasia of the nail fold capillaries can by detected on close inspection, and is often indicative of a connective tissue disease such as systemic lupus erythematosus (SLE), scleroderma, or dermatomyositis. Tightening of the skin around the digits, or sclerodactyly, is typical of scleroderma and is usually both visible and palpable. The pulp of the digits should be examined for the presence of digital ulcers, also seen most commonly in scleroderma.

Articular swelling of the distal interphalangeal (DIP) and proximal interphalangeal (PIP) joints can represent bony osteophytes as in the case of Heberden's and Bouchard's nodes in the DIP and PIP joints, respectively, or can represent an intra-articular effusion associated with synovitis in the joint. Palpation will help in differentiating these. Swelling and redness of an entire digit, termed *dactylitis*, is highly suggestive of a spondylarthropathy such as psoriatic arthritis or reactive arthritis.

Swelling of the metacarpophalangeal (MCP) joints can be visually appreciated as a fullness in the valleys normally found between the knuckles (heads of the metacarpal bones). In cases of RA where the MCP synovitis has been longstanding, it is often associated with ulnar subluxation of the extensor tendons, resulting in the ulnar drift of the digits that is typical of this diagnosis. Swelling on the dorsum of the wrist area can result from synovitis of the wrist or tenosynovitis of the extensor tendons. Getting the patients to gently wiggle the fingers helps differentiate these two findings in that the swelling will tend to move with the tendons if it is a result of tenosynovitis. Inspection of the palmar aspect of the hands is important for identifying atrophy of the thenar or hypothenar eminences, which can result either from disuse due to articular involvement of the wrist or, in the case of the thenar eminence, carpal tunnel syndrome.

Global function of the hand should be evaluated by asking the patient to make a full fist and to fully extend and spread out the digits. Pincer function of the thumb and fingers should be tested. The grip strength can be estimated by having the patient squeeze two of the examiner's fingers. Individual hand joints should be palpated to determine the presence of joint line tenderness and effusion, these being the most important indicators of synovitis. The technique for palpating the DIP and PIP joints is similar. The thumb and index finder of one hand palpates in the vertical plane, while the thumb and index finder of the other hand palpates in the horizontal plane (Figure 2A-1). Alternating gentle pressure between the two planes will displace small amounts of synovial fluid back and forth, allowing the examiner to detect effusions in these small joints. Likewise, tenderness suggestive of synovitis can be elicited by this technique. The technique for palpating the MCP joints is somewhat modified because of the inability to directly palpate these joints from the horizontal plane. The thumbs are used to palpate the dorsolateral aspects of the joint, while the index fingers palpate the palmar aspect.

Palpation of the wrist involves a similar technique to that used for the MCPs. The thumbs are used to palpate the dorsum of the joint, while the index fingers palpate the volar aspect (Figure 2A-2). Synovial thickening and tenderness suggestive of wrist joint synovitis can usually be palpated on the dorsum of the joint. Particular attention should be paid to swelling and tenderness in the area just distal to the ulnar styloid, where the extensor and flexor carpi ulnaris tendons are directly palpable. This area is very commonly involved in early RA. Pain and tenderness confined to the radial aspect of the wrist are most commonly due to either OA of the first carpo-

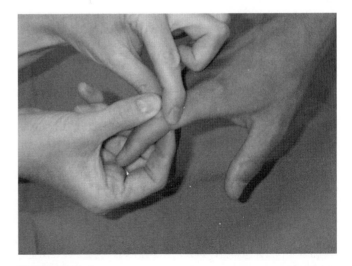

FIGURE 2A-1

Technique for examining the small joints of the hands and feet. The thumb and index finger of the examiner's hands are used to gently ballot small amounts of intra-articular fluid back and forth to elicit evidence of joint line tenderness.

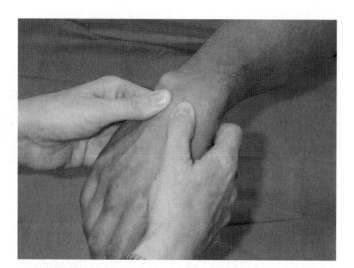

FIGURE 2A-2

The dorsum of the wrist joint is palpated for tenderness and swelling using the examiner's thumbs. The wrist should be examined in slight flexion to allow the joint line of the radiocarpal, intercarpal, and carpometacarpal joints to be optimally palpated.

metacarpal joint, or to DeQuervain's tenosynovitis. All the joints of the hand and wrist should be evaluated for stress tenderness.

The Elbow

Flexion and extension of the forearm occur exclusively at the elbow joint and involve the hinge type of articulation between the proximal ulna and distal humerus. In examining the elbow, a number of surface landmarks need to be identified. These are the olecranon process, the medial and lateral epicondyles of the humerus, and the radial head. A triangular recess is formed in the lateral aspect of the joint between the olecranon process, the lateral epicondyle, and the radial head. This recess is the point where the synovial cavity of the elbow is most accessible to inspection and palpation.

Examination of the elbow should be undertaken with the patient sitting comfortably and the entire arm being well supported in order to eliminate muscle tension. Initially the joint should be inspected with forearm flexed to 90°. Particular attention should be paid to the lateral recess described above. Obvious bulging in this area is highly suggestive of an effusion and synovitis. In contrast, swelling directly over the olecranon process is more suggestive of olecranon bursitis. Any process that causes true synovitis of the elbow is typically associated with a reduction in the range of motion of the joint, both in flexion–extension and in supination–pronation. Having the patient extend the forearm as much as possible will detect the presence of a flexion contracture, this being an almost invariant feature of elbow synovi-

tis. With this maneuver, the bulge in the lateral recess will tend to enlarge, becoming more tense due the reduction in the internal dimension of the elbow in the position of extension.

The synovial cavity and joint line can best be palpated for swelling and tenderness in the area of the lateral recess. This is also the site where arthrocentensis of the elbow is performed. It should be noted that pain in the lateral aspect of the elbow area is a common clinical problem, and is usually due to lateral epicondylitis or tennis elbow rather than elbow joint pathology. Tenderness directly palpable over the lateral epicondyle and with stressing the wrist and finger extensors is suggestive of this diagnosis.

The Shoulder

Proper examination of the shoulder should always begin with appropriate visualization of the entire shoulder girdle area, both from the front and the back. This includes the sternoclavicular, glenohumeral, and acromioclavicular joints as well as the scapulothoracic articulation. Comparison should be made with the contralateral shoulder. Any asymmetry between the two sides should be noted. For example, patients with rotator cuff tears often hold the affected shoulder higher than the other side. Atrophy of the shoulder girdle musculature is an important sign of chronic glenohumeral joint pathology, as occurs in RA. This is most evident as squaring of the shoulder due to deltoid atrophy and scooping out of the upper scapular area due to supraspinatus atrophy. Effusions in the shoulder joint are visible anteriorly just medial to the area of the bicipital groove, and if large enough are also evident laterally below the acromion. It should be noted that large amounts of fluid can accumulate in the glenohumeral joint space without much visible evidence due to considerable redundancy in the joint capsule.

After inspecting the shoulder area in the resting position, the patient is asked to demonstrate the active range of motion of the shoulder. Abduction is observed as the patient moves both outstretched arms from their side in the lateral plane until the palms meet overhead. The movement is evaluated for discomfort, symmetry, and fluid scapulohumeral coordination. Patients with shoulder pathology will usually move the arm forward somewhat in order to complete the maneuver. External rotation can then be tested by having the patient attempt to touch the back of their head with the palm of the hand from the fully abducted position. If abduction is abnormal, active flexion should be tested by having the patient lift the outstretched arm from their side directly up in front of them. Active internal rotation and extension is observed by having the patient reach behind their back and attempt to have their fingertips touch the highest point possible on their scapula.

Palpation should include the entire shoulder girdle area. The sternoclavicular joint is palpated, then the fingers are walked laterally over the clavicle to the acromioclavicular joint, which is palpated for tenderness and swelling. The subacromial space, containing the supraspinatus tendon and subacromial bursa, lies directly below the acromion. Immediately below the acromioclavicular joint, the coracoid process should be identified. The short head of the biceps inserts on this process. The long head of the biceps can be palpated lateral to this in the bicipital groove. The anterior aspect of the glenohumeral joint can be palpated between the coracoid process and the long head of the biceps and follows the contour on the rounded anterior aspect of the humeral head. Shoulder synovitis can be palpated in this area as joint line tenderness and/or boggy effusion.

Passive range of shoulder motion is then evaluated. The most informative parts of the range of motion are internal/external rotation and abduction. When testing these movements it is very important to immobilize the scapula to prevent rotation at the scapulothoracic area. In this way, glenohumeral motion can be isolated and appropriately evaluated. One effective technique to achieve this is to firmly press down on the top of the shoulder area with the palm of one hand, while the other hand moves the arm through the range of motion (Figure 2A-3). Internal/external rotation should be tested with the arm by the patient's side and with the arm abducted to 90°. Examination of the patient in the supine position may aid in relaxing musculature in patients who are unable to fully relax during this maneuver.

A large number of special maneuvers have been described that suggest specific clinical syndromes in the

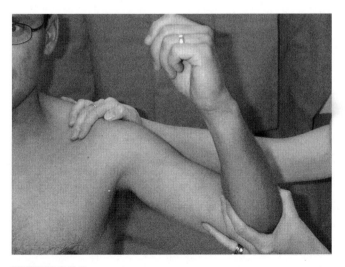

FIGURE 2A-3

Glenohumeral joint motion is best examined with the elbow flexed to 90° and the upper arm in partial abduction. Internal and external rotation of the shoulder are then examined in this position. Care should be taken to immobilize the scapula using a technique such as that shown.

shoulder. The predictive value of these maneuvers is modest (5). Forced supination of the hand with the elbow flexed at 90° will cause pain in the area of the long head of the biceps in patients with bicipital tendinitis. Impingement of the subacromial bursa or supraspinatus tendon is suggested by pain with forced internal rotation and flexion of the glenohumeral joint from a position of 90° flexion with the elbow flexed at 90°. Supraspinatus tendinitis can be detected by having the patient position their outstretched arm at 90° of abduction while maximally internally rotating the glenohumeral joint such that the thumb is pointing downward. The examiner then asks the patient to resist attempts to push the arm down. In patients with superspinatus tendinitis, the maneuver will be associated with pain, and may result in the patient suddenly dropping the arm.

The Hip

Pain resulting from hip arthritis is typically experienced in the groin or, less commonly, the buttock. It tends to radiate down the anteromedial aspect of the thigh, occasionally down to the knee. Pain in the lateral trochanteric area is most often indicative of bursitis involving the trochanteric bursa.

Because the hip joint cannot be directly examined, the examiner needs to glean important diagnostic clues from observing the patient's gait, buttock and thigh musculature, and from evaluating passive range of motion of the hip joint. As with all load bearing joints, evaluation of functional joint motion needs to be assessed under load with the patient walking and standing. Subtle hip pathology may be detected by having the patient perform a squat. The patient with true hip disease often walks with a coxalgic gait, tending to quickly swing the pelvis forward on the affected side in order to avoid weight bearing on the hip affected by arthritis. If the hip arthritis is prolonged and severe, the buttock musculature tends to atrophy, as does the thigh musculature. In severe cases, the abductor muscles are unable to hold the pelvis in a horizontal position when the patient is asked to stand only on the affected hip. This forms the basis of the Trendelenburg test, where the patient's pelvis tends to sag down on the contralateral side when the patient is asked to hold their entire weight on the affected leg.

With the patient in the supine position, passive range of motion should initially be screened by log rolling the entire extended leg. The leg is then flexed maximally to assess completeness of this motion. With the knee flexed to 90° and the hip flexed to 90°, internal and external rotation of the hip are then tested. Care should be taken that the hip movements are isolated, and that the patient's pelvis is not rotating to compensate for lost range of motion. Pain and loss of motion on internal rotation are particularly sensitive indicators of hip pathology. Flexion contracture of the hip tends to accompany longstanding severe hip arthritis.

The Sacroiliac Joint

Palpation of the sacroiliac (SI) joint is undertaken with the patient lying flat on their abdomen. With the palm of the examiner's hand held around the iliac crest, the thumb tends to fall directly over the joint which extends down below the dimples in the posterior pelvic area. To elicit tenderness in the SI joint, direct pressure is applied with the thumb in this area. In addition to direct palpation, the examiner can perform other maneuvers to further establish the presence of sacroiliitis. Direct pressure over the sacrum will produce pain in an inflamed SI joint. Gaenslen's maneuver is performed by having the patient hyperextend their leg over the edge of the examining table, thereby stressing the ipsilateral SI joint.

The Spine

The spine should be examined initially with the patient standing and the entire spine well visualized. The normal curvature of the spine, lumbar lordosis, thoracic kyphosis, and cervical lordosis should be evaluated by observing the patient from the both the back and the side, and any loss or accentuation of these curves noted. If scoliosis is noted with the patient standing upright, they should be asked to bend forward and flex the spine to evaluate the effects of this movement on the scoliosis. True scoliosis will be present irrespective of the state of spinal flexion, while a functional scoliosis due to leg length discrepancy will tend to decrease with spinal flexion. The level of the iliac crests relative to the spine should also be evaluated by observing the patient from the back, and the examiner sitting with their eyes at approximately the level of the iliac crests. A tilted pelvis can be due to compensation for a primary scoliosis in the spine or, alternatively, due to a leg length discrepancy.

The range of motion of the entire spine should be examined in segments. The lumbar spine is assessed by having the patient attempt to touch their toes and then extend their back. Lateral flexion is assessed by having the patient reach their fingertips as far as possible down the lateral aspect of their leg. Lateral rotation, which involves both the lumbar and thoracic spine, is tested by having the patient turn their upper body with the examiner holding the pelvis stable.

The Schober test is performed to specifically assess movement in the lumbar spine. With the patient standing, a distance of 10 cm is measured up the lumbar spine from the lumbosacral junction at the level of the sacral dimples. Marks are placed at both ends of this 10 cm segment. The patient is then asked to flex forward as far as possible, attempting to touch their toes. With this motion, the marks identifying this 10 cm segment normally expand to 15 cm or more, indicative of distraction between the vertebrae. While reduction in this measurement is not specific for any particular pathology, it can be used over time to follow disorders with progressive loss of motion, such as ankylosing spondylitis.

Patients presenting with symptoms suggestive of a lumbar radiculopathy, such as pain and parasthesia shooting down the leg, need to undergo an examination of the lumbosacral area and a detailed neurological examination of the leg. Maneuvers that put traction on the lumbar spinal roots are used to provide further evidence of a radiculopathy. The most commonly used of these maneuvers is the straight leg raising test, where the patient lies in the supine position and the leg is passively raised by the examiner with the knee fully extended. A positive test requires that the patient experience pain and parasthesia shooting down the leg to the level of the foot.

Cervical range of motion begins with the patient upright and the examiner in front. The patient is asked to flex, extend, laterally flex (patient attempts to touch their ear to their shoulder), and laterally rotate (patient attempts to touch their chin to their shoulder) their head. Movements should be evaluated for symmetry, fullness of motion, and discomfort. Gentle passive range of motion may be attempted with the patient supine. Spinous processes and surrounding musculature should be palpated for spasm or tenderness. It should be noted that pain in the neck area often radiates down the arm, up the occiput, or down to the scapular area. The pain may be aggravated by particular parts of the range of motion.

The Knee

Examination of the knee starts with inspection of the patient's gait and with the patient standing. When inspecting from the front, attention should first be paid to the areas above and below the knee. Atrophy of the quadriceps usually indicates chronic knee pathology. Swelling due to synovial fluid accumulation or synovial infiltration and thickening is most readily appreciated in the suprapatellar bursa. When a large effusion is present, it can be seen to also cause bulging of both the lateral and medial compartments of the knee. Inspection of the knee from the back with the patient standing up is the best way to evaluate the alignment of the femur relative to the tibia. Varus deformities of the knee causing a bow-legged appearance most commonly result from OA preferentially involving the medial compartment. Valgus deformities, causing a knock-knee appearance are more commonly associated with RA. Posterior inspection is also important for detecting popliteal or Baker's cysts, which can be large enough to track down the calf.

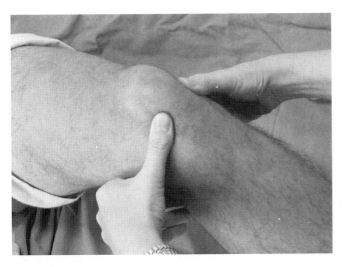

FIGURE 2A-4

The joint line of the knee is palpated on the medial and lateral aspects for tenderness suggestive of synovitis. Stability of the cruciate ligaments can also be assessed in this position. Using the bulge sign or patellar tap sign, an effusion can be detected in the knee with the joint fully extended (see text for details).

After inspecting the patient in the standing position, the knee is evaluated with the patient in the supine position, and the joint fully extended. Flexion contractures should be noted. Loss of normal contours may suggest swelling. The knee should be palpated for warmth. Bony and soft tissue landmarks should be palpated for tenderness, including the anserine bursa—a common nonarticular source of knee pain. The medial and lateral joint line are palpated for tenderness with the knee in partial flexion (Figure 2A-4).

Detection of synovial fluid in the knee is an important diagnostic clue. Large amounts of fluid cause distention of the joint in the suprapatellar area, as well as the medial and lateral compartment. The fluid can be confirmed by firmly pushing the swelling in the suprapatellar area down into the main compartment of the knee with the palm of one hand. While maintaining pressure over the suprapatellar area, the examiner's other hand is used to either ballot the fluid back and forth between the medial and lateral compartments of the knee, or alternatively to perform the patellar tap by pushing the patella up and down against the femoral condyles. Small amounts of fluid in the knee may be detected using the bulge sign. The medial aspect of the knee is stroked from the inferior aspect towards the suprapatellar area in order to move the fluid into the lateral compartment. The lateral aspect of the knee is then stroked in a similar manner while the medial compartment is observed for the return of the fluid bulge.

While firmly supporting the joint with one hand (or by holding the foot in the examiner's armpit area), varus and valgus stress are gently applied to the joint to test the medial and collateral ligaments. The cruciate ligaments are tested using the drawer sign, where anteroposterior stress is placed on the upper tibia with the knee in flexion. Instability of the ligaments will result in the tibia moving back and forth relative to the femur, much as a drawer would if pushed back and forth.

The Ankle and Hindfoot

The ankle and hindfoot should be examined as a unit, because arthropathies often involve several structures in this area. Valgus deformities of the ankle and hindfoot can best be seen by inspecting the area from behind with the patient standing. Swelling in the ankle area eliminates the normal contours associated with the malleoli.

The joint line of the ankle is palpated anteriorly (Figure 2A-5). Boggy swelling and tenderness in this area are typical of ankle synovitis. Tenderness and swelling posteriorly at the insertion of the Achilles tendon usually indicates enthesitis, although this can also result from bursitis of the retrocalcaneal bursa. Tenderness in the heel region can indicate plantar fasciitis, another enthesitis associated with spondylarthropathies but also common in overuse injuries and arch abnormalities.

The ankle and hindfoot unit should be put through the range of motion, isolating parts of the range associated with specific joints. The ankle proper, or talotibial joint, is only capable of dorsi and plantar flexion. Pain and limitation in this part of the range is associated with ankle synovitis. The subtalar joint, separating the talus and the calcaneus, can be tested by rocking the calcaneus laterally from side to side with one hand, while

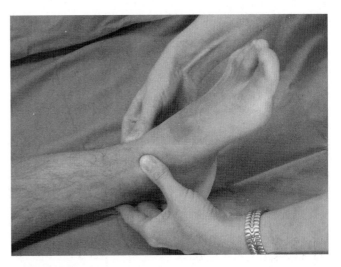

FIGURE 2A-5

Palpation for tenderness and swelling in the ankle is undertaken medial and lateral to the extensor tendons on the anterior part of the joint below the malleoli.

holding the talus stable with the other. Talonavicular motion is tested by stabilizing the talus and calcaneus and rotating the midfoot.

The Midfoot and Forefoot

Observation of the patient in the standing position will reveal abnormalities in the longitudinal arch and the anterior part of the foot. Pes planus (flat foot, collapsed arch) or pes cavus (high arch) will be most evident with the patient standing. Hallux valgus deformities causing bunions are some of the most commonly observed problems in the joints.

Swelling of the metatarsophalangeal joints (MTPJ) causes a visible spreading of the toes referred to as the daylight sign. Direct pressure over each of the metatarsophalangeal joints will confirm the presence of tenderness and swelling. In cases of advanced RA, subluxation of the MTPJ results in a hammer toe deformity, which can cause skin breakdown on the dorsum of the toes from constant rubbing against the footwear. Inflammation of the interphalangeal joints of the toes is more common with spondylarthropathies. In some cases the entire digit becomes swollen and inflamed, a process termed *dactylitis* and referred to as a sausage digit. Examining the plantar aspect of the forefoot is important for identifying areas of callus formation. These tend to occur in conjunction with subluxation of the MTPJ, where the metatarsal head can be directly palpated subcutaneously.

REFERENCES

1. Dieppe P, Sergent J. History. In: Klippel J, Dieppe P, eds. Rheumatology. Mosby, London 1998:1.1–1.6.
2. Hubscher O. Pattern recognition in arthritis. In: Klippel J, Dieppe P, eds. Rheumatology. Mosby, London 1998:3.1–3.6.
3. Grahame R. Examination of the patients. In: Klippel J, Dieppe P, eds. Rheumatology. Mosby, London 1998:2.1–2.16.
4. Doherty M, Dacre J, Dieppe P, Snaith M. The GALS locomotor screen. Ann Rheum Dis 1992;51:1165–1169.
5. Calis M, Acgun K, Birtane M, Karacan I, Calis H, Fikret T. Diagnostic values of clinical diagnostic tests in subacromial impingement syndrome. Ann Rheum Dis 2000;59: 44–47.

Evaluation of the Patient
B. Laboratory Assessment

KERSTIN MOREHEAD, MD

■ Laboratory testing is often valuable for screening for disease, confirming diagnoses, establishing disease stage, determining prognosis, gauging disease activity, and following responses to therapy.

■ The erythrocyte sedimentation rate (ESR) and C-reactive protein (CRP) frequently correlate well with disease activity in inflammatory disorders.

■ Rheumatoid factor (RF) and anti-cyclic citrullinated peptide (anti-CCP) anti-bodies are helpful in diagnosing rheumatoid arthritis. The specificity of RF for rheumatoid arthritis is poor.

■ Antinuclear antibodies (ANA) are found in many patients with rheumatic diseases and in essentially all patients with systemic lupus erythematosus (SLE) and systemic sclerosis. Under the proper clinical conditions, the finding of a positive ANA assay is an indication for additional investigations directed at identifying the precise autoantibody leading to the ANA pattern.

■ Among others, anti-Ro, -La, -Sm, and -RNP antibodies may all result in a positive ANA. These autoantibodies are associated with a range of different rheumatic diseases.

■ Positive immunofluorescence assays for antineutrophil cytoplasmic antibodies (ANCA) should be confirmed by enzyme immunoassays for antibodies directed specifically against two antigens: proteinase-3 and myeloperoxidase.

■ Decreased serum complement levels usually indicate a disease process mediated by immune complex deposition within tissues.

Laboratory testing is an important part of the evaluation for many patients with possible rheumatic diseases. As the understanding of rheumatic disease progresses, new biomarkers are developed and the utility of existing ones is refined. Laboratory tests can be valuable guides for screening, confirming diagnosis, establishing disease stage, and prognosis, as well as for following disease activity and response to treatment. Because no single test can provide absolute certainty about diagnosis, prognosis, or state of disease activity, however, results must be interpreted in the context of the broader clinical picture. Sensitivity, specificity, positive and negative predictive values, and likelihood ratios all warrant careful consideration when interpreting the utility of any test. Although laboratory testing has grown substantially as an aid to clinical diagnosis and management over the past several decades, treatment decisions are rarely based on the result of a single test alone. In addition to appreciating the strengths and shortcomings of testing approaches, the clinician must also be aware of the variability that often exists between different assay methods and individual laboratories. In general, the most useful tests are those that are ordered to answer well-defined questions.

ERYTHROCYTE SEDIMENTATION RATE

Inflammatory stress alters hepatic synthesis of plasma proteins. As a result, fibrinogen and immunoglobulin levels increase during the acute phase response. When red blood cells (RBCs) interact with these proteins, they form clusters that sediment at a faster rate than individual RBCs. In chronic states of inflammation, decreased serum albumin and hematocrit levels also lead to increased rates of erythrocyte sedimentation.

Method (Westergren)

Whole serum is anticoagulated with sodium citrate and allowed to stand. After 1 hour, the distance in millimeters between the top of the tube and the erythrocyte sediment is measured. The test is sensitive to handling and temperature (1). Normal values are not adjusted for age or gender in most laboratories, yet these characteristics have well-known (if erratic) influences on the erythrocyte sedimentation rate (ESR). The ESR generally increases with age and is somewhat higher in women.

The upper limits of normal for a man is equal to the age divided by 2; for a woman, add 10 to the age and divide by 2 (2).

Interpretation

The ESR is sensitive for most types of inflammation, but cannot distinguish if the underlying cause is infectious, inflammatory, or paraneoplastic (3). A normal value may help to rule out inflammatory disease, but an increased ESR, especially if the increase is only moderate, can be confusing. In addition, the normalization of a high ESR often lags behind the resolution of inflammation, making it less than ideal for monitoring disease activity. Along with normal elevation due to age and gender, the ESR can be increased by any condition that raises serum fibrinogen, such as diabetes, end-stage renal disease, and pregnancy. Conversely, the ESR can be lowered by congestive heart failure, sickled erythrocytes, and the presence of cryoglobulins.

C-REACTIVE PROTEIN

The c-reactive protein (CRP) is an acute phase protein synthesized in response to tissue injury. Serum CRP levels change more quickly than the ESR; with sufficient stimulus, the CRP can increase within 4 to 6 hours and normalize within a week (4). The CRP is often measured simultaneously with (and sometimes in place of) the ESR as a general measure of inflammation. Although CRP and ESR values tend to correspond with each other, some patients' disease processes appear to correlate better with one measure or the other.

Method

Specific antibodies to CRP allow direct quantification by a variety of means. Nephelometry uses antibodies to bind target proteins and then measures the scatter of light by antigen–antibody complexes. The enzyme-linked immunosorbant assay (ELISA) uses coated plates to form antigen–antibody complexes. These complexes are detected by addition of secondary antibodies labeled with an enzyme that, when mixed with a substrate, produces color that is measured by spectrophotometry. Because the CRP is a stable serum protein and its measurement is not affected by other serum components, it tends to be less variable than the ESR. The CRP is affected by age and gender, as is the ESR (5). In general, levels <0.2 mg/dL are considered normal and levels >1 mg/dL are deemed consistent with inflammation, but there is considerable laboratory-to-laboratory variation.

Interpretation

Because a certain degree of injury is required before CRP is synthesized, a normal or indeterminate value does not exclude an inflammatory process. Moreover, other disease processes, including heart disease, infection, and malignancy, can lead to CRP elevations, as can obesity, diabetes, and cigarette smoking.

RHEUMATOID FACTOR

Rheumatoid factor (RF) is an autoantibody that binds to the Fc region of human IgG. IgM is the most common RF isotype, but IgG and IgA RF may also be detected in the serum (6).

Method

The latex fixation test measures only RF IgM by precipitating the antibody with IgG-coated latex particles mixed with serial dilutions of serum. Titers greater than 1:20 are positive. Nephelometry and ELISA are able to detect all three isotypes.

Interpretation

In established rheumatoid arthritis (RA), RF has a sensitivity on the order of 70%. In early RA the sensitivity is somewhat lower, approximately 50%, as some patients seroconvert only after having clinical disease for weeks or months. A positive RF assay, far from specific for RA, can be found in many other autoimmune diseases, mixed essential cryoglobulinemia (see cryoglobulinemia, below), chronic infections, sarcoidosis, malignancy, and a small percentage of healthy people. The IgA isotype has been linked to erosive disease and to rheumatoid vasculitis, but its precise clinical utility remains unclear. Higher titers of RF are associated with more severe disease, but as a longitudinal measure of disease activity RF fares poorly. CRP values may be more reliable for monitoring disease activity (7).

ANTI-CYCLIC CITRULLINATED PEPTIDE ANTIBODIES

Anti-cyclic citrullinated peptide antibodies (ANTI-CCP) are autoantibodies directed against the amino acids formed by the posttranslational modification of arginine. Some investigators believe anti-CCP antibodies have a role in the pathogenesis of RA (8).

Method

IgG anti-CCP are measured by ELISA using synthetic citrullinated peptides. Reference ranges vary (9).

Interpretation

Anti-cyclic citrullinated peptide antibodies have a sensitivity for RA that is similar to that of RF, but anti-CCP antibodies are much more specific. These test characteristics lend considerable usefulness to anti-CCP antibodies in the setting of seronegative patients suspected of having RA, patients with other forms of connective tissue disease who are RF positive, and patients with hepatitis C or other infections that are often associated with RF positivity. Anti-CCP antibodies are often detectable in early RA and, in some cases, antedate the onset of inflammatory synovitis. Although anti-CCP antibodies may be a better predictor of erosive disease than is RF, they do not correlate with extra-articular disease. A positive anti-CCP combined with a positive RF IgM correlates strongly with radiographic progression. Anti-CCP levels are not useful in the longitudinal monitoring of disease activity (10).

ANTINUCLEAR ANTIBODIES

Antinuclear antibodies (ANA) are a diverse group of autoantibodies that react with antigens in the cell nucleus. Different patterns reflect different nuclear components including nucleic acid, histones, and centromeres (Table 2B-1).

Method

Hep-2 cells (a human tumor cell line) are incubated with serial dilutions of serum. Using immunofluorescence microscopy, labeled antihuman IgG is used as a stain. The result reflects the highest serum dilution that is positive for staining and the pattern of the stain.

Interpretation

Aninuclear antibody assays are nearly universally positive in SLE, to the extent that ANA-negative lupus is virtually nonexistent. Patients with systemic sclerosis (scleroderma) and many other connective tissue diseases are also ANA positive with a very high frequency, often in high titers. Depending on the exact technique used, up to 30% of healthy people may have a positive titer (11). The prevalence of positive ANAs increases in women and older people. A positive ANA is not specific for SLE or autoimmune disease, especially if it is transient or in low titer.

Specific Autoantibodies

Autoantibodies directed against individual antigens have increased specificity for particular diseases. Some of these autoantibodies also predict disease severity (Table 2B-2) (12). These are ordered separately from the ANA test.

ANTINEUTROPHIL CYTOPLASMIC ANTIBODY

Antineutrophil cytoplasmic antibodies (ANCA) are autoantibodies that react with the cytoplasmic granules of neutrophils. Two general staining patterns, cytoplasmic (C-ANCA) or perinuclear (P-ANCA) can be detected by immunofluorescence. In forms of systemic

TABLE 2B-1. ANTINUCLEAR ANTIBODY PATTERNS.

PATTERN	NUCLEAR ANTIGEN	CLINICAL ASSOCIATIONS
Homogenous	Double-stranded DNA	Systemic lupus erythematosus
Diffuse	Histone	Drug reaction Systemic lupus erythematosus
	Topoisomerase I	Systemic sclerosis
Speckled	Extractable nuclear antigens (Sm, RNP)	Mixed connective tissue disease Systemic lupus erythematosus
	Ro-SSA/La-SSB	Sjögren's syndrome
	Other	Poly/dermatomyositis Various autoimmune diseases Infection Neoplasia
Nucleolar	RNA-associated antigens	Systemic sclerosis
Peripheral	Double-stranded DNA	Systemic lupus erythematosus
Centromere	Centromere	Limited systemic sclerosis

TABLE 2B-2. AUTOANTIBODIES IN RHEUMATIC DISEASES.

TYPE	DESCRIPTION	CLINICAL ASSOCIATION
Anti-dsDNA	Antibodies to double-stranded DNA	High specificity for SLE Often correlates with more active, more severe disease ELISA test is very sensitive and can be positive in other diseases, normal people
Anti-histone	Five major types exist	SLE, drug-induced SLE, other autoimmune disease SLE patients will likely be positive for other autoantibodies as well
Anti-ENA	Sm (Smith) RNP (ribonucleoprotein) RNA–protein complexes	High specificity for SLE Mixed connective tissue disease Higher prevalence in African American and Asian patients
Anti-SSA (Ro)	Ribonucleoproteins	SLE (especially subacute cutaneous lupus), neonatal lupus, Sjögren's syndrome
Anti-SSB (La)	Ribonucleoproteins	Sjögren's syndrome, SLE, neonatal SLE
Anti-centromere	Antibody to centromere/kinetochore region of chromosome	Limited scleroderma High rate of pulmonary hypertension Primary biliary sclerosis
Anti-Scl 70	Antibodies to DNA topoisomerase 1	Diffuse scleroderma Risk of pulmonary fibrosis
Anti-Jo-1	Antibody to histidyl tRNA synthetase	Poly/dermatomyositis Patients tend to have interstitial lung disease, Raynaud's phenomenon, mechanic's hands, arthritis Typically resistant to treatment
Anti-SRP	Antibody to signal recognition protein	Cardiomyopathy Poor prognosis
Anti-PM-Scl	Antibody to nucleolar granular component	Polymyositis/scleroderma overlap syndrome
Anti-Mi-2	Antibodies to a nucleolar antigen of unknown function	Dermatomyositis Favorable prognosis

vasculitis, such as Wegener's granulomatosis, microscopic polyangiitis, and the Churg–Strauss syndrome, these patterns reflect autoantibodies to two lyzosomal granule enzymes: serine protease-3 (PR3) and myeloperoxidase (MPO), respectively. Upon immunofluorescence testing of sera, many patients with other forms of inflammatory disease (e.g., SLE, autoimmune hepatitis, inflammatory bowel disease) have positive ANCA assays. ELISA testing in such patients, however, reveals antibody specificities for antigens other than PR3 and MPO. ANCA directed against PR3 and MPO are termed PR3-ANCA and MPO-ANCA, respectively.

Method

To identify C- and P-ANCA patterns of immunofluorescence, ethanol- or formalin-fixed human neutrophils are coated with the patient's serum and stained with labeled anti-IgG. Formalin fixation is preferred because the presence of antinuclear antibodies may cause a false-positive P-ANCA pattern on ethanol-fixed cells.

One common laboratory approach is to screen with ethanol-fixed cells and to perform assays on formalin-fixed cells if immunofluorescence is observed on screening. Increasingly reliable ELISA assays for the detection of both PR3 and MPO have been available since the early 1990s. For optimal clinical utility, any positive immunofluorescence assay should be confirmed by the performance of anti-PR3 and -MPO ELISAs.

Interpretation

The combination of C-ANCA and PR3-ANCA has a high positive predictive value for ANCA-associated vasculitis, particularly Wegener's granulomatosis. Similarly, the combination of P-ANCA and MPO-ANCA has a high positive predictive value for microscopic polyangiitis. (For further discussion of the role of ANCA assays in these diseases and in the Churg–Strauss syndrome, please see Chapter 21C.)

The more active and extensive the vasculitis, the more likely are ANCA assays to be positive. ANCA titers often normalize with treatment but do not always do so, even if clinical remissions are achieved. Some data suggest that a persistent rise in ANCA titer or return of ANCA positivity heralds an increased risk of recurrent disease, but neither persistently positive ANCA tests nor rising ANCA titers provide reliable information about the timing of a disease flare. Treatment decisions in ANCA-associated vasculitis are never based entirely ANCA assay result. Moreover, positive ANCA tests may be caused by infection, drugs (particularly thyroid medications such as propylthiouracil), and, as noted, other autoimmune diseases. Thus, under most clinical circumstances, tissue biopsy remains the gold standard for diagnosis (13).

COMPLEMENT

The complement cascade is a tightly regulated complex of proenzymes, regulatory proteins, and cell-surface receptors that mediate and augment both of complement the humoral and cellular immune response. Activation by antigen–immune complexes, bacterial surface proteins, and polysaccharides begins a fixed sequence of reactions that lead to increased vascular permeability, chemotaxis, cell lysis, antigen–immune complex clearance, and opsonization. The classical pathway (C1, C4, C2), the alternative pathway (factors B, D, and properdin), and the mannose-binding lectin pathway all share the final step of cleaving C3. The released product (C3b) then induces formation of the terminal membrane attack complex (C5–C9) (14).

Method

Serum levels of individual components such as C3 and C4 are measured by ELISA and nephelometry. The plasma total hemolytic complement assay, or CH50, assesses the functional integrity of the classical pathway. Serum is diluted and added to sheep antibody–coated RBCs. The value reported is the reciprocal of the highest dilution able to lyse 50% of the RBCs.

Interpretation

Decreased serum levels of individual components, especially C3 and C4, correlate with the increased consumption observed in active immune complex mediated disease, for example, SLE. In contrast, most inflammatory disorders that are not associated with immune complex deposition demonstrate elevated levels of complement because these proteins are acute phase reactants. Hypocomplementemia, though useful in narrowing the differential diagnosis, is generally not specific for any particular disease. C4 levels that are disproportionately low compared to those of C3 may

indicate the presence of cryoglobulins. Unfortunately, the correlations between changes in complement levels and disease activity are poor. In addition, hypocomplementemia may also be secondary to nonrheumatic diseases, notably subacute bacterial endocarditis and poststreptococcal glomerulonephritis (15). Low or undetectable CH50 may indicate a deficiency of one or more complement components. Patients with genetic deficiencies of early complement components (C1–C4) are at increased risk for developing immune-complex diseases (16), particularly some forms of SLE.

CRYOGLOBULINS

Cryoglobulins are immunoglobulins that precipitate reversibly at cold temperatures. In a variety of diseases, cryoglobulins often bind with complement proteins and other peptides to form immune complexes. Based on their composition, cryoglobulins are classified into three types. Type I cryoglobulins are monoclonal immunoglobulins, frequently of the IgM isotype. Type II cryoglobulins are a mixture of polyclonal IgGs and monoclonal IgM. Type III cryoglobulins are a combination of polyclonal IgGs and polyclonal IgMs. In both type II and type III cryoglobulinemia, the IgM component has RF activity (i.e., it binds to the Fc portion of IgG), accounting for the fact that essentially all patients with these disorders are RF positive (often creating confusion in diagnosis with RA) (17).

Method

For proper collection of cryoglobulins, careful attention to detail and preparation in advance are required. Whole blood must be drawn and maintained at body temperature until it coagulates. The sample is then centrifuged and the clot removed. The remaining serum is allowed to stand at 4°C for up to several days until precipitation is observed. The sample is spun again and the cryocrit is measure in a calibrated tube. Isotype and clonality are established by various immunochemical techniques.

Interpretation

Cryoglobulins are not specific for any one disease. Type I cryoglobulins do not activate the complement cascade and are therefore associated with normal complement levels. They are linked to lymphoproliferative disorders, malignancies, and hyperviscosity syndromes, and often associated with sludging in the small vasculature of the extremities, eye, or brain. Type II and type III cryoglobulins, able to bind complement, are associated with hepatitis C virus infections and a syndrome of small vessel vasculitis (see Chapter 21D) (18).

REFERENCES

1. Sox HC Jr, Liang MH. The erythrocyte sedimentation rate: guidelines for rational use. Ann Intern Med 1986; 104:515–523.

2. Miller A, Green M, Robinson D. Simple rule for calculating normal erythrocyte sedimentation rate. BMJ 1983; 286:266.

3. Bridgen M. The erythrocyte sedimentation rate. Still a helpful test when used judiciously. Postgrad Med 1998; 103:257–262.

4. Morley JJ, Kushner I. Serum C-reactive protein levels in disease. Ann N Y Acad Sci 1982;389:406–418.

5. Wener MH, Daum PR, McQuillan GM. The influence of age, sex and race on the upper limit of serum C-reactive protein concentration. J Rheumatol 2000;27:2351–2359.

6. Johsson T, Valdimarsson H. Is measurement of rheumatoid factor isotypes clinically useful? Ann Rheum Dis 1993;52:161–164.

7. Witherington RH, Teitsson I, Valdimarsson H, et al. Prospective study of early rheumatoid arthritis. II Association of rheumatoid factor isotypes with fluctuations in disease activity. Ann Rheum Dis 1984;43:679–685.

8. Vossenaar ER, Smeets TJ, Kraan MC, et al. The presence of citrullinated proteins is not specific for rheumatoid arthritis. Arthritis Rheum 2004;50:3485–3494.

9. Zendman AJW, Van Venroij, Pruijn GJM. Use and significance of anti-CCP autoantibodies in rheumatoid arthritis. Rheumatology 2006;45:20–25.

10. Niewold TB, Harrison MJ, Paget SA. Anti-CCP antibody testing as a diagnostic and prognostic tool in rheumatoid arthritis. QJM 2007;100:193–201.

11. Tan E, Feltkamp TE, Smolen JS, et al. Range of antinuclear antibodies in "healthy" individuals. Arthritis Rheum 1997;40:1612–1618.

12. Lyon R, Sonali N. Effective use of autoantibody tests in the diagnosis of systemic lupus erythematosis. Ann N Y Acad Sci 2005;1050:217–228.

13. Bartunkova J, Tesar V, Sediva A. Diagnostic and pathogenic role of antineutrophil cytoplasmic autoantibodies. Rheumatology (Oxford) 2003;106;73–82.

14. Walport MJ. Advances in immunology: complement. N Engl J Med 2001;344:1058–1066, 1140–1144.

15. Egner W. The use of laboratory tests in the diagnosis of SLE. J Clin Pathol 2000;53:424–432.

16. Ratnoff WD. Inherited deficiencies of complement in rheuamtologic diseases. Rheum Clin North Am 1996;22:1–21.

17. Brouet JC, Clauvel JP, Danon F, et al. Biological and clinical significance of cryoglobulins: a report of 86 cases. Am J Med 1974;57:775–788.

18. Ferri C, Zignego AL, Pileri SA. Cryoglobulins. J Clin Pathol 2002;55:4–13.

Evaluation of the Patient
C. Arthrocentesis, Synovial Fluid Analysis, and Synovial Biopsy

KENNETH H. FYE, MD

- When the diagnosis of an inflammatory arthropathy is unclear, synovial fluid should be evaluated for the three Cs: cell count, culture, and crystals.
- Removal of infected synovial fluid is often a critical adjunct to antibiotics in the treatment of a septic joint.
- Careful preparation, appropriate assistance, and planning of the approach to the joint enhance the likelihood of success in performing arthrocentesis.
- Synovial fluid neutrophil counts in excess of 100,000/mm^3 spells an infection until proven

otherwise, and should be treated empirically with antibiotics until the results of culture are available.
- Microcrystalline disorders (gout and pseudogout) occasionally lead to synovial fluid neutrophil counts >100,000/mm^3.
- Examination of synovial fluid under polarized microscopy is the only way of securing the diagnosis of a microcrystalline disease.

Despite the development of increasingly sophisticated serologic tests and imaging techniques, synovial fluid (SF) analysis remains one of the most important diagnostic tools in rheumatology (1). Normal SF lubricates the joint and, along with blood vessels in subchondral bone, supplies nutrients to the avascular articular cartilage. The majority of SF constituents originate in the subsynovial vasculature, diffusing through the synovium into the joint space. However, certain important macromolecules, such as hyaluronic acid and lubricin, are synthesized and secreted by synoviocytes (which line the joint). Plasma proteins not found in SF include prothrombin, fibrinogen, factor V, factor VII, antithrombin, large globulins, and some complement components (2).

Synovial fluid protein concentrations reflect the interplay between plasma concentration, synovial fluid blood flow, endothelial cell permeability, and lymphatic drainage. There are few cells in normal SF. In arthritis, invading inflammatory cells produce additional proteins and release activated cytokines into SF. Elevated intra-articular pressure due to increased amounts of SF leads to diminished perfusion of synovial microvasculature, disrupting the process of diffusion that supplies synovial nutrients (3). In addition, offending substance such as microorganisms, foreign bodies, or abnormal crystals,

may be present. Analyzing SF may yield information invaluable in making the diagnosis, determining prognosis, and formulating appropriate therapy in patients with arthritis (4).

ARTHROCENTESIS

Indications

An acute, inflammatory, monarticular arthritis should be considered either infectious or crystal-induced until proven otherwise. Arthrocentesis is the only method of identifying infection or crystal-induced disease unequivocally. Because acute bacterial infections can lead rapidly to joint and bone destruction, arthrocentesis must be performed immediately if there is any suspicion of infection. If preliminary analysis of the SF is compatible with infection—that is, the white blood cell (WBC) count is markedly elevated but no crystals are identified—antibiotic therapy should be initiated pending definitive culture results. SF analysis can confirm the presence of crystal-induced arthritis and enable the clinician to identify the culprit crystal precisely. If a polarized microscope is used, the sensitivity of SF analysis for identifying a crystal-induced arthropathy is 80% to 90%

(4). Trauma can sometimes result in an acute monarticular arthropathy. Analysis of joint fluid is the only way to distinguish posttraumatic hemarthrosis from posttraumatic arthritis with bland synovial fluid.

Arthrocentesis can also be useful in the evaluation of chronic or polyarticular arthropathies. SF analysis enables the clinician to differentiate inflammatory and noninflammatory arthritides. The procedure is often essential in distinguishing chronic crystal-induced arthritide such as polyarticular gout or calcium pyrophosphate dehydrate deposition disease from other arthropathies, such as rheumatoid arthritis (RA). Although chronic mycobacterial or fungal infections can sometimes be identified in SF, synovial biopsy is frequently necessary to distinguish indolent infections from other unusual chronic inflammatory processes, such as pigmented villonodular synovitis. Because people with chronic inflammatory arthropathies (e.g., RA) have an increased susceptibility to infection, acute monarticular arthritis in a patient whose disease is otherwise well controlled is an indication for a diagnostic arthrocentesis.

The cellular and humoral components of inflammatory SF can damage articular and periarticular tissues (5). The activated enzymes in septic SF are highly destructive to cartilage. Thus, in a septic joint, repeated arthrocentesis may be necessary to minimize the accumulation of purulent material (6). If purulent SF reaccumulates despite repeated arthrocenteses, surgical arthroscopy with drain placement should be performed to ensure adequate drainage of the infected joint. For joints that are noninfected but inflamed, drainage of as much SF as possible removes inflammatory cells and other mediators, decreases intra-articular pressure, and reduces the likelihood of articular damage (7). Removal of inflamed fluid also increases the efficacy of intra-articular corticosteroids. Finally, blood in a joint, such as may occur in hemophilia, can lead quickly to adhesions that inhibit joint mobility. When clinically indicated, therefore, therapeutic arthrocentesis may be prudent in a patient with hemarthrosis. When contemplating such a procedure in a hemophiliac, careful consideration should be given to approaches to maximize hemostasis (e.g., the use of clotting factor VIII concentrate; see Chapter 25A) and prevent additional intra-articular bleeding as a result of the procedure.

Techniques
Sterile Procedures

Infections caused by arthrocentesis are very rare. Nevertheless, preventive measures to minimize the likelihood of postarthrocentesis infection are prudent. Betadine or povidone–iodine should be applied to the aspiration site and allowed to dry. Alcohol should then be used to swab the area to prevent an iodine burn. Although it is wise to wear gloves during any procedure involving exposure to potentially infected body fluids, sterile gloves are generally not necessary. Sterile gloves should be used if the clinician anticipates having to palpate the target anatomy *after* preparation of the arthrocentesis site using antiseptic technique.

Local Anesthesia

Local anesthesia with 1% lidocaine without epinephrine significantly reduces discomfort associated with the procedure. One-quarter to 1 cc of lidocaine is usually sufficient, depending on the joint being anesthetized. A 25- or 27-gauge needle should be used to infiltrate the skin, subcutaneous tissue, and pericapsular tissue. Larger caliber needles are more uncomfortable and can lead to local trauma. Although many clinicians apply ethyl chloride to the skin before injecting the anesthesia, others believe this practice is cumbersome and results in no clinically significant additional anesthesia.

After the periarticular tissues have been anesthetized, a 20- or 22-gauge needle can be used to aspirate small- to medium-sized joints. An 18- or 19-gauge needle should be used for aspirating large joints or joints suspected of infections, intra-articular blood, or viscous, loculated fluid. Small syringes are easier to manipulate and provide greater suction than large syringes, but must be changed frequently when aspirating large joints with copious amounts of SF. When using a large syringe to aspirate a significant amount of fluid, the suction in the syringe should be broken before use and the plunger drawn. Excessive negative pressure can suck synovial tissue into the needle and prevent an adequate joint aspiration. A Kelly clamp can stabilize the hub of the needle while removing a full syringe.

Typical landmarks are often obscured around a swollen joint. Therefore, after a thorough physical examination and before sterilizing and anesthetizing the skin, it is often helpful to mark the approach with a ballpoint pen. If landmarks are still obscure, use sterile gloves to maintain a clean field while using palpation to identify an aspiration site for the target joint. Many joints, such as the knee, ankle, and shoulder, are amenable to both medial or lateral approaches.

In contrast to joint injection, aspiration is performed most easily when a joint is in a position of maximum intra-articular pressure. For example, injection of the knee is best done with the knee in 90° flexion while the patient is seated at an examining table with the foot dangling. This position allows gravity to open the joint space, offering easy access to the intra-articular space from either side of the infrapatellar tendon. However, this position decreases intra-articular pressure, thereby decreasing the likelihood of a successful aspiration. Conversely, therefore, the optimal positioning of the

TABLE 2C-1. ANATOMIC APPROACH TO ASPIRATION.

JOINT	POSITION OF JOINT	LOCATION OF APPROACH
Knee	Extended	Medial or lateral under the patella
Shoulder	Neutral adduction, external rotation	Anterior: inferolateral to coracoid Posterior: under the acromion
Ankle	Plantar flexion	Anteromedial: medial to extensor hallucis longus Anterolateral: lateral to extensor digiti minimi
Subtalar	Dorsiflexion to 90°	Inferior to tip of lateral malleolus
Wrist	Midposition	Dorsal into radiocarpal joint
First carpometacarpal	Thumb abducted and flexed	Proximal to base of metacarpal
Metacarpophalangeal or interphalangeal	Finger slightly flexed	Just under extensor mechanism dorsomedial or dorsolateral
Metatarsophalangeal or interphalangeal	Toes slightly flexed	Dorsomedial or dorsolateral
Elbow	Flexed to 90°	Lateral in triangle formed by lateral epicondyle, radial head, and olecranon process

patient for aspiration of the knee is lying supine with the knee fully extended, thereby maximizing intra-articular pressure. Although most joints can be aspirated without radiologic assistance, some joints, such as the hips, sacroiliac joints, or zygoapophyseal joints, should be aspirated using computed tomography guidance. Aspirations should generally not be done through areas of infection, ulceration, or tumor, or obvious vascular structures. Table 2C-1 lists suggestions for optimal anatomic approaches for aspirating or injecting specific joints.

If corticosteroids are to be injected after aspiration is complete, the drug should be prepared in a separate syringe ahead of time so that the aspirating needle already in the joint can be used for the injection. If difficulties arise during the procedure, the needle should not be manipulated aggressively because of the risk of damaging the cartilage, capsule, or periarticular supporting structures. If bone is encountered, slight withdrawal of the needle followed by redirection and another attempt at aspiration is indicated. In unsuccessful aspiration attempts, the needle may be outside the joint space, blocked by synovium or SF debris, or too small for the degree of SF viscosity.

SYNOVIAL FLUID ANALYSIS

The four general classes of SF, defined by differences in gross examination, total and differential WBC count, the presence or absence of blood, and the results of culture are shown in Table 2C-2. SF characteristics of arthritic conditions can be extremely variable and may change with therapy. Therefore, the classes of SF are

TABLE 2C-2. CLASSES OF SYNOVIAL FLUID.

	CLASS I (NONINFLAMMATORY)	CLASS II (INFLAMMATORY)	CLASS III (SEPTIC)	CLASS IV (HEMORRHAGIC)
Color	Clear/yellow	Yellow/white	Yellow/white	Red
Clarity	Transparent	Translucent/opaque	Opaque	Opaque
Viscosity	High	Variable	Low	NA
Mucin clot	Firm	Variable	Friable	NA
WBC count	<2,000	2,000–100,000	>100,000	NA
Differential	<25% PMNs	>50% PMNs	>95% PMNs	NA
Culture	Negative	Negative	Positive	Variable

ABBREVIATIONS: PMN, polymorphonuclear leukocytes; NA, not applicable.

parallel to its long pole when the long pole of the crystal is parallel to the slow axis of the red compensator, an addition pattern of slow-plus-slow vibration will result in a blue color. By convention, a birefringent crystal that is blue when the long pole is parallel to the slow axis of vibration of the red compensator is considered to be positively birefringent. Calcium pyrophosphate dehydrate crystals, for example, are positively birefringent. Birefringence can be strong, meaning the birefringent crystal is bright and easy to see, or weak, meaning the birefringent crystal is muted and difficult to detect.

Crystals are identified by a combination of shape and birefringence characteristics. Monosodium urate crystals are needle shaped and have strong, negative birefringence (see Figure 12A-7). In contrast, calcium pyrophosphate dehydrate crystals are short and rhomboid, and show weak, positive birefringence. Calcium oxalate crystals, which can be seen in primary oxalosis or in chronic renal failure, are rod or tetrahedron shaped and positively birefringent. Cholesterol crystals are flat and boxlike, tend to stack up, and often have notched corners. Spherules with birefringence in the shape of a Maltese cross generally represent lipid. However, it has been suggested that some forms of urate or apatite may take this shape (15,16). Hydroxyapatite is usually difficult to recognize in SF, partly because it is not birefringent. However, sometimes it forms clumps large enough to be seen when stained with alizarin red S. Finally, glucocorticoid crystals injected into the joint as a therapeutic measure are birefringent and may be misinterpreted by the unwary observer.

The presence of intracellular crystals is virtually diagnostic of a crystal-induced arthropathy. However, a superimposed infection must be excluded even if crystals are identified. In addition, a patient may have more than one crystal-induced disorder. For example, up to 15% of patients with gout also have calcium pyrophosphate dihydrate deposition disease. It is important to make that determination, because it will affect therapy. A patient with chronic gout may require only ongoing hypouricemic therapy (and perhaps prophylactic colchicine). In contrast, a patient with both gout and calcium pyrophosphate dihydrate deposition disease may require continued nonsteroidal anti-inflammatory therapy in addition to ongoing hypouricemic therapy.

Attempts to aspirate inflammatory joints are not always successful. For example, aspiration of an inflamed first metatarsophalangeal joint is difficult. However, if the clinician keeps negative pressure on the syringe as the needle is withdrawn from articular or periarticular tissues, there is almost always enough interstitial fluid in the needle to allow adequate polarized-light examination for crystals. Simply remove the needle from the syringe, fill the syringe with air, reattach the needle, and use the air to blow the fluid in the needle onto a slide. This is a particularly valuable technique when looking for monosodium urate crystals in podagra.

Culture

An inflammatory monarticular arthritis should be considered infectious until proven otherwise. In most bacterial infections, Gram stain and culture and sensitivity yield valuable diagnostic information and are crucial components of analysis. Generally, SF need only be collected in a sterile culture tube and transported to the laboratory for routine analysis. Unfortunately, some important infectious agents are difficult to culture, so negative Gram stains and cultures do not necessarily preclude an infection. For example, SF cultures are negative in more than two-thirds of people with gonococcal arthritis, even if chocolate agar is used as the culture medium. In addition, tuberculosis is often difficult to culture from SF, and special techniques and culture media are required for anaerobic or fungal pathogens. Sometimes mycobacterial (17) or fungal (18) infections can be detected only on synovial biopsy material. Because bacterial infections can lead rapidly to joint destruction, early antibiotic therapy is essential. Antibiotic therapy should be initiated based on the results of WBC count, WBC differential, and Gram stain, and adjusted later if necessary, based on the results of culture and sensitivity.

SYNOVIAL BIOPSY

Arthroscopy has greatly facilitated the clinician's ability to obtain synovial tissue for analysis. At one time, synovial tissue could only be obtained by open arthrotomy or blind needle biopsy (19). Advances in the technology of arthroscopy have led to the development of small, flexible instruments that allow direct visualization and biopsy of synovium (20). In certain clinical settings, synovial biopsy can add significant diagnostic information.

The granulomatous diseases are frequently difficult to diagnose by SF analysis alone. SF acid-fast smears and cultures are negative in a significant number of patients with tuberculosis. The diagnosis of tuberculous arthritis is often based on histologic demonstration of caseating granulomata and acid-fast stain or culture evidence of *Mycobacterium tuberculosis* in synovial tissue. Atypical mycobacterial and fungal arthropathies can be indolent, inflammatory, oligoarticular infections that cannot be diagnosed without obtaining synovial tissue for histologic and microbiologic analysis (18). In patients without pulmonary involvement, the diagnosis of sarcoid arthropathy may rest on the demonstration of noncaseating granulomata in synovial tissue.

Malignant infiltrations of the synovium can be seen in synovial sarcomas, lymphomas, metastatic disease, and leukemias. The diagnosis of synovial osteochondromatosis can be made based on the presence of foci of osteometaplasia or chondrometaplasia on synovial biopsy. Sometimes cytologic examination of SF reveals a malignancy. However, the diagnosis of a malignant arthropathy is generally based upon histologic demonstration of malignant cells in synovial tissue. Therefore, synovial biopsy is indicated if there is a suspicion of articular malignancy.

The diagnosis of some infiltrative nonmalignant processes depends on the histologic or microscopic evaluation of synovial material. A diagnosis of amyloid arthropathy can be made if apple green birefringence is observed in Congo red–stained synovial biopsy material examined under polarized light. Hemochromatosis is characterized by the deposition of golden brown hemosiderin in synovial lining cells. Hydroxyapatite deposits in synovial tissue appear as clumps of material that stain with alizarin red S and have a typical appearance on electron micrography. The synovium of patients with multicentric reticulohistiocytosis is filled with multinucleated giant cells and histiocytes with a granular ground-glass appearance. The SF from patients with ochronosis has a ground-pepper appearance due to pigmented debris. The synovial biopsy from these patients contains shards of ochronotic pigment that is diagnostic. In Whipple's disease, foamy macrophages containing periodic acid-Schiff (PAS)–positive material can be seen on synovial biopsy. Pigmented villonodular synovitis is defined by the presence of giant cells, foamy cells, and hemosiderin deposits in synovial tissue.

The ease of direct biopsy of target tissues that has resulted from advances in arthroscopic techniques has not changed the clinical indications for synovial biopsy. Biopsy should be done only if the diagnosis cannot be made using traditional, less invasive procedures.

REFERENCES

1. Swan A, Amer H, Dieppe P. The value of synovial fluid assays in the diagnosis of joint disease: a literature survey. Ann Rheum Dis 2002;61:493–498.
2. Gatter RA, Schumacher HR Jr. A practical handbook of joint fluid analysis, 2nd ed. Philadelphia: Lea & Febiger; 1991.
3. Gaffney K, Williams RB, Jolliffe VA, Blake DR. Intra-articular pressure changes in rheumatoid and normal peripheral joints. Ann Rheum Dis 1995;54:670–673.
4. Shmerling RH. Synovial fluid analysis. A critical appraisal. Rheum Dis Clin North Am 1994;20:503–512.
5. Chapman PT, Yarwood H, Harrison AA, et al. Endothelial activation in monosodium urate monohydrate crystal-induced inflammation. Arthritis Rheum 1997;40: 955–965.
6. Sack KE. Joint aspiration and injection: a how-to guide. J Musculoskel Med 1999;16:419–427.
7. Zuber TJ. Knee joint aspiration and injection. Am Fam Physician 2002;66:1497–1507.
8. Pasqual E, Jovani V. Synovial fluid analysis. Best Pract Res Clin Rheumatol 2005;19:371–386.
9. Dorwart BB, Schumacher HR. Joint effusions, chondrocalcinosis and other rheumatic manifestations in hypothyroidism. A clinicopathologic study. Am J Med 1975; 59:780–790.
10. Krey PR, Bailen DA. Synovial fluid leukocytosis. A study of extremes. Am J Med 1979;67:436–442.
11. Trampuz A, Hanssen AD, Osmon DR, et al. Synovial fluid leukocyte count and differential for the diagnosis of prosthetic knee infection. Am J Med 2004;117:556–562.
12. Kerolus G, Clayburne G, Schumacher HR. Is it mandatory to examine synovial fluids promptly after arthrocentesis? Arthritis Rheum 1989;32:271–278.
13. Gordon C, Swan A, Dieppe A. Detection of crystals in synovial fluid by light microscopy: sensitivity and reliability. Ann Rheum Dis 1989;48:737–742.
14. Joseph J, McGrath H. Gout or "pseudogout": how to differentiate crystal-induced arthropathies. Geriatrics 1995; 50:33–39.
15. McCarty DJ, Halverson PB, Carrera GF, Brewer BJ, Kozin F. "Milwaukee shoulder"—association of microspheroids containing hydroxyapatite crystals, active collagenase, and neutral protease with rotator cuff defects. Arthritis Rheum 1981;24:464–473.
16. Beaudet F, de Medicis R, Magny P, Lussier A. Acute apatite podagra with negatively birefringent spherulites in the synovial fluid. J Rheumatol 1993;20:1975–1978.
17. Sequeira W, Co H, Block JA. Osteoarticular tuberculosis: current diagnosis and treatment. Am J Ther 2000;7:393–398.
18. Kohli R, Hadley S. Fungal arthritis and osteomyelitis. Infect Dis Clin North Am 2005;19:831–851.
19. Schumacher HR, Kulka JP. Needle biopsy of the synovial membrane—experience with the Parker-Pearson technic. N Engl J Med 1972;286:416–419.
20. Gerlag D, Tak PP. Synovial biopsy. Best Pract Res Clin Rheumatol 2005;19:387–400.

Evaluation of the Patient
D. Imaging of Rheumatologic Diseases

WILLIAM W. SCOTT, JR., MD
WILLIAM J. DIDIE, MD
LAURA M. FAYAD, MD

- Conventional radiographs are the initial imaging agent of choice for most rheumatic conditions. For most forms of arthritis, no additional imaging studies are required.
- Trabecular bone and small bone erosions are visualized well by conventional radiography.
- Weight-bearing views of the knees are important in the evaluation of significant knee osteoarthritis.
- Computed tomography (CT) is superior to conventional radiographs in the assessment of certain joint conditions, including many cases of tarsal coalition, sacroiliitis, osteonecrosis, and sternoclavicular joint disease.

- High resolution CT of the lungs is an essential adjunct to the evaluation of many inflammatory rheumatic diseases, for example, systemic sclerosis, systemic vasculitis, and other disorders associated with signs of interstitial lung disease.
- Magnetic resonance imaging (MRI), which has superior imaging capabilities of soft tissue and bone marrow lesions, is the study of choice for a host of musculoskeletal diagnoses, including meniscal tears of the knee, spinal disc herniations, osteonecrosis, osteomyelitis, skeletal neoplasms, and others.
- Bone densitometry plays a crucial role in the diagnosis and treatment of osteopenia and osteoporosis.

Imaging techniques may aid in making diagnoses, permit objective assessments of disease severity and response to treatment, and promote new understandings of disease processes. Imaging modalities that are valuable in rheumatology include conventional radiography, computed tomography (CT), magnetic resonance imaging (MRI), ultrasound, radionuclide imaging, arthrography, bone densitometry, and angiography.

A basic knowledge of the merits and limitations of these techniques is essential in selecting the most appropriate and cost-effective imaging. In the discussion to follow, *high spatial resolution* will indicate excellent ability of an imaging modality to demonstrate fine bone detail and to detect small calcifications. *High contrast resolution* will indicate excellent ability to distinguish different soft tissue structures. Techniques such as conventional radiography have good spatial resolution. MRI generally has best contrast resolution among current imaging techniques. This chapter reviews the basic imaging techniques with regard to their spatial and contrast resolution (which determine the degree to

which individual structures are visualized), radiation dose to the patient, availability, and specific uses in assessing musculoskeletal signs and symptoms.

CONVENTIONAL RADIOGRAPHY

Conventional radiographs are the starting point for most imaging evaluations in rheumatic disorders, even when studies such as MRI are expected to follow. The cost is low and spatial resolution is very high, permitting good visualization of trabecular detail and tiny bone erosions. When necessary, resolution can be enhanced further by magnification techniques and film–screen combinations optimized for detail. However, contrast resolution is poor compared to that obtainable with CT and MRI. This limitation is especially noticeable when trying to evaluate soft tissues. Although plain radiography is a useful tool to assess the effect of a soft tissue mass on nearby bone and to detect calcification within soft tissue, other techniques should be employed if optimal soft tissue imaging is required.

Examination of peripheral structures, such as the hands and feet, delivers a low radiation dose to the patient. Serial studies of the extremities can be performed without concern about excessive radiation exposure. Studies of central structures, however, such as the lumbar spine and pelvis, expose patients to high radiation doses. Close proximity to the gonads and to bone marrow increases the potentially detrimental effects to the patient. Whenever possible, the pelvic region of pregnant or potentially pregnant women should not be exposed to x-rays, and radiation to children should be minimized stringently. When such studies are necessary in these patients, radiation physicists can calculate the minimum radiation dose required for the imaging study. These same basic principles apply to all other x-ray imaging techniques.

Conventional radiography is widely available and convenient. Moreover, a vast fund of knowledge about plain radiographic findings in various rheumatic diseases is available (Figures 2D-1–2D-3). In many cases, simple, low cost imaging may provide all the information necessary to make clinical decisions. If the plain radiograph of the shoulder shows upward subluxation of the humeral head so that it contacts the undersurface of the acromion, one can be quite certain that the rotator cuff is torn with atrophic musculature, and likely very difficult to repair (Figure 2D-4). This may argue against a decision to undertake surgery. If surgery is contemplated, however, then MRI can confirm the large size of the rotator cuff tendon tear, the extent of muscle

atrophy, and evaluate the state of the biceps tendon and articular cartilage in such cases.

Knee radiographs are useful in cases of advanced arthritis, when they may demonstrate complete loss of knee joint cartilage and bone-on-bone contact. This marks the end point for useful arthroscopic and medical treatment of knee arthritis and time to consider joint replacement. Weight-bearing views are necessary because hyaline cartilage loss is deduced from the degree of apposition of the bony surfaces. In this regard, the flexed posterior–anterior (PA) standing radiograph is often more useful than an anterior–posterior (AP) view in full extension, as the flexed view images the portion of the articular surface subject to the greatest wear (Figure 2D-5). However, for earlier stages of arthritis, MRI is important for detection of small focal articular cartilage defects that may potentially be treated with recently developed surgical techniques.

DIGITAL RADIOGRAPHY

Computed radiography uses a photosensitive phosphor plate to create a digital image, rather than the analog image of conventional radiography. At present, computed radiography images are utilized at most centers. The resolution is adequate for many routine joint evaluations and can be improved by magnification, if necessary for special tasks. The radiation dose is approximately the same as for conventional radiography. Soft tissue is better visualized than on conventional radiographs.

Direct radiography is a technique whereby digital images are created at the time of x-ray exposure. The advantages of digital images, whether digitized conventional radiographs, computed radiography, or direct radiography, include the ability to manipulate images electronically and to display images simultaneously in several remote areas. Image manipulation permits technically excellent final images to be obtained under adverse circumstances. For this reason, computed radiography is currently popular in emergency departments and intensive care units, locations where it is often difficult to obtain optimal radiographic exposures. The ability to manipulate digital data is also useful to researchers wishing to make automated measurements on radiographs and to clinicians wishing to send images via the Internet.

The resolution of computed radiography can be improved and conventional high resolution radiographs can be converted into digital format. CT, MRI, and ultrasound images are also acquired in digital form, and are easily transported and manipulated. Digital imaging, now widely utilized, has the advantages of rapid transmission, cost-effective storage, and easy retrieval.

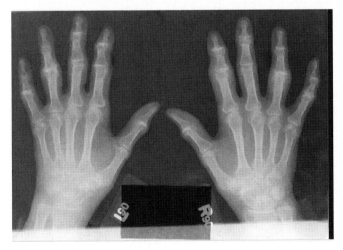

FIGURE 2D-1

Typical radiographic findings in osteoarthritis of the hand showing asymmetric joint narrowing with osteophyte formation. The distal interphalangeal joints, proximal interphalangeal joints, and first carpometacarpal joint are most commonly involved.

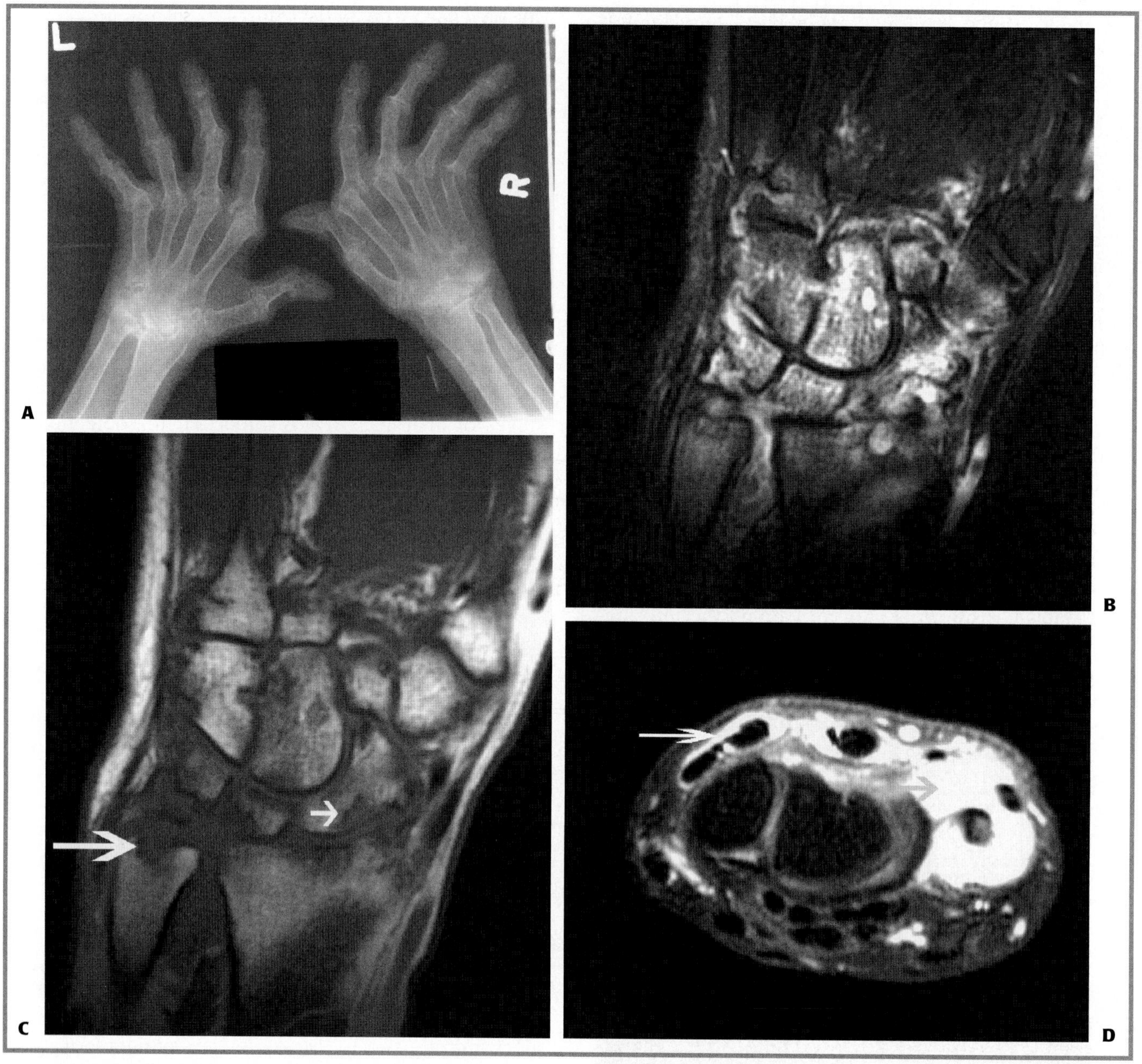

FIGURE 2D-2

(A) Severe rheumatoid arthritis in an elderly woman showing erosive changes and marked cartilage narrowing of wrist, intercarpal, metacarpophalangeal, and proximal interphalangeal joints. The joints involved are typical for rheumatoid arthritis. Alignment abnormalities with ulnar deviation of the metacarpals and osteoporosis are also typical. (B) Coronal short time inversion recovery (STIR) image of the wrist in a different patient showing multiple osseous erosions and synovial thickening, characteristic findings of rheumatoid arthritis. (C) T1 weighted coronal image showing more extensive erosions (*arrows*) with areas of synovial thickening. (D) Axial postcontrast fat-saturated image depicting tenosynovitis, with fluid distention of the tendon sheaths (*arrow*).

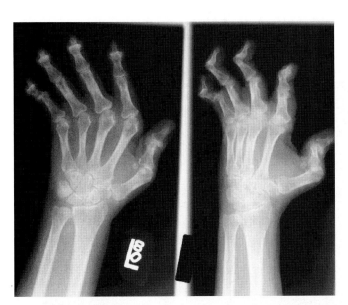

FIGURE 2D-3

A 57-year-old woman with systemic lupus erythematosus (SLE) shows striking alignment abnormalities without erosions as well as periarticular osteoporosis. Similar changes are seen in the arthropathy associated with rheumatic fever (Jaccoud's arthropathy). The cartilage destruction and synovial proliferation of rheumatoid arthritis is lacking. Early in the disorder, the alignment abnormalities can be corrected by passive positioning.

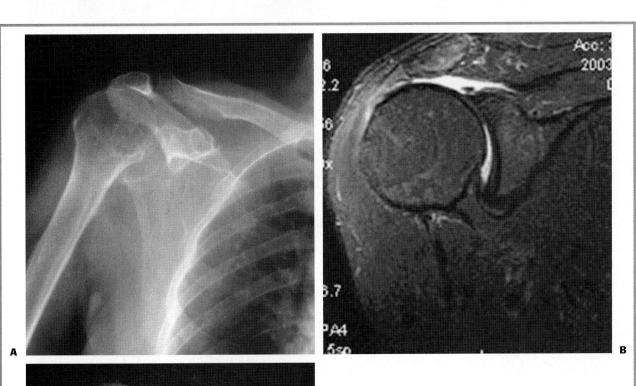

A

B

C

FIGURE 2D-4

(A) An 80-year-old woman with weakness and pain in the right shoulder. Radiograph shows superior subluxation of the humeral head and markedly decreased space between humeral head and acromion. (B) Oblique–coronal STIR MRI image shows similar decreased distance between the acromion and humeral head, as well as a complete rotator cuff tendon tear. (C) Sagittal oblique T1 weighted image demonstrating a significant degree of atrophy of the supraspinatus, infraspinatus, and subscapularis muscles. MRI findings could have been predicted from the plain radiograph and the clinical history. However, in this case the MRI provides an accurate estimation of the size of the rotator cuff tear, as well as commonly associated findings such as the status of the long head of the biceps tendon and articular cartilage. These soft tissue abnormalities cannot be assessed by plain radiography.

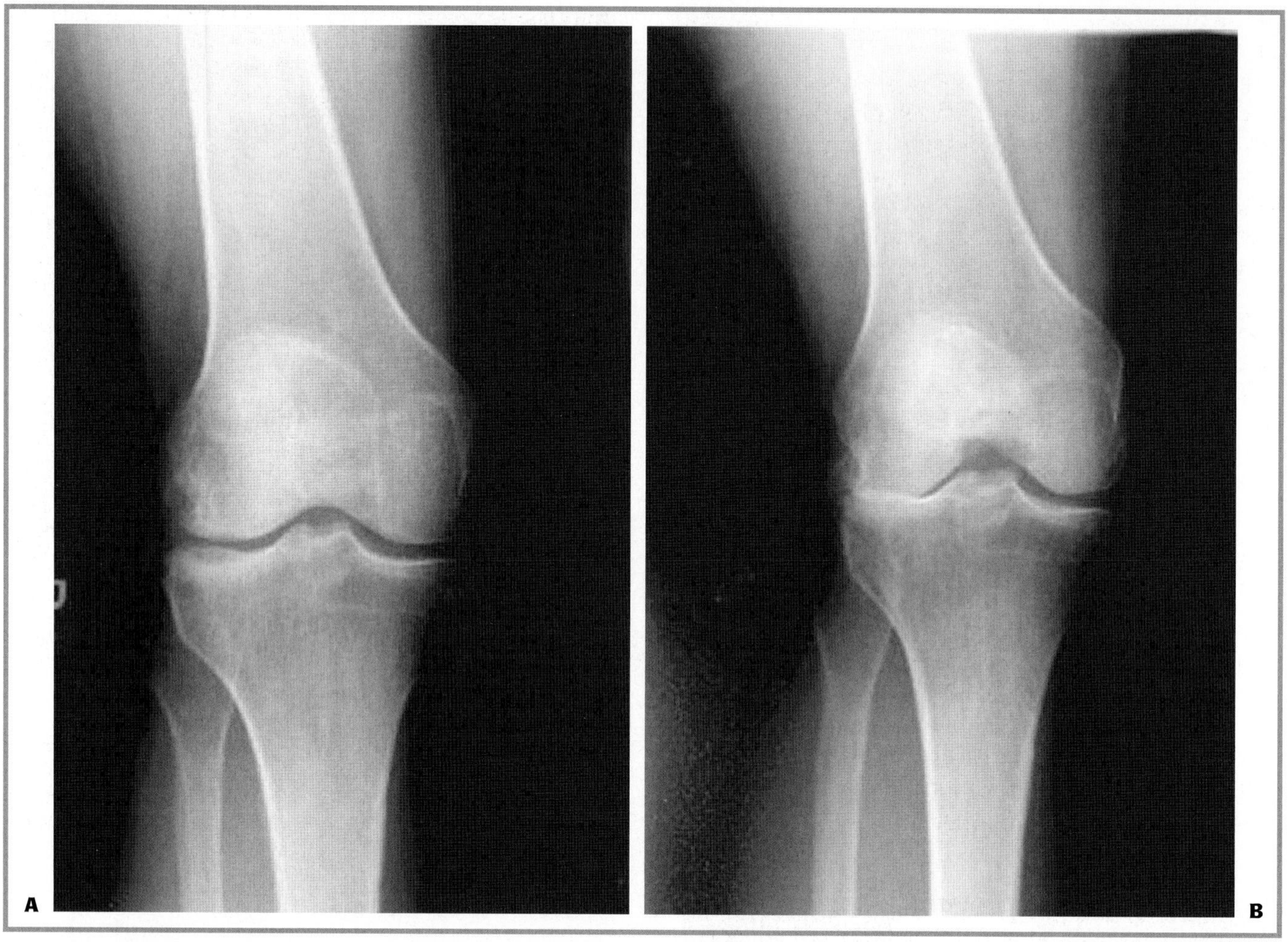

FIGURE 2D-5

(A, B) Standing anteroposterior (A) and standing flexed posteroanterior (B) views of the right knee. In (A), no significant narrowing of the joint is identified although osteophytes and subchondral sclerosis, indicative of osteoarthritis, are evident. In (B), however, the standing flexed view demonstrates complete articular cartilage loss in the lateral compartment.

COMPUTED TOMOGRAPHY

Compared with radiography, CT offers superior contrast resolution, but spatial resolution of CT remains inferior. CT is especially useful in specific locations difficult to evaluate by radiography, such as the sacrum. Although relatively expensive, CT is less costly than MRI. With the advent of multidetector technology capable of producing CT datasets with isotropic resolution, the spatial resolution of CT is comparable or superior to that of MRI, but its contrast resolution is inferior. Consequently, CT is not as sensitive as MRI for defining bone marrow or soft tissue abnormalities.

Computed tomography is an excellent technique for evaluating degenerative disc disease of the spine and possible disc herniations in older patients, in whom radiation dose is less critical than in young patients. CT

myelography and CT with intravenous contrast enhancement are used to evaluate disc disease and other spinal processes. In general, MRI is preferred over CT for investigating disc disease (following plain radiography). For cases in which MRI is contraindicated, CT is an acceptable alternative and may be useful in circumstances where additional information about osteophytes is important. Elsewhere in the musculoskeletal system, CT is useful for evaluating structures in areas of complex anatomy where overlying structures obscure the view on conventional radiographs. Examples include tarsal coalitions not visible on plain radiographs (Figure 2D-6) (1); sacroiliitis, especially that of infectious origin (Figure 2D-7); and articular collapse of the femoral head following osteonecrosis, indicating the need for joint replacement rather than a core procedure. The sternoclavicular joint, which is notoriously difficult to see on conventional radiography, is quite visible with CT.

The radiation dose from CT is relatively high compared with a single plain radiograph of the same region, but the radiation doses between these imaging techniques are comparable when several conventional radiographic views of the same area are required.

If the correct initial data are obtained by appropriately adjusting the thickness of the collimation used and the thickness of the reconstructed slice width, images can be reconstructed satisfactorily in any plane, especially with the advent of advanced multidetector technology capable of isotropic resolution datasets. In addition to multiplanar reconstructions, three-dimensional images can be obtained, which may aid in evaluating abnormalities of the pelvis and other areas of complex anatomy. Using multidetector technology, including multiplanar reformatting, better images of joints affected by respiratory motion, such as the shoulder, can be acquired rapidly during a single breath, minimizing motion artifact.

High resolution (thin cut) CT of the lung may reveal details of disease not seen on thicker CT slices of the thorax. Thin cut CT scans have the additional advantage of not requiring intravenous contrast—often a concern in patients with rheumatic disease who have tenuous renal status. The interstitial lung disease that

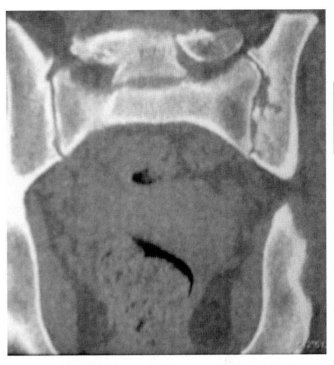

FIGURE 2D-7

Woman with left hip and back pain. Plain radiographs demonstrated no abnormalities. CT scan shows marked erosion and widening of the left sacroiliac joint, consistent with sacroiliitis. Note relative osteopenia on the adjacent sacral side, indicating hyperemia.

occurs in many patients with a variety of rheumatic conditions (systemic sclerosis, rheumatoid arthritis, inflammatory myopathy, microscopic polyangiitis) is characterized well by high resolution CT. The demonstration of "ground glass" infiltrates connotes an active process that may respond to treatment, but unfortunately this finding does not distinguish between infection, inflammation, and other conditions (2).

Multidetector spiral CT is now used increasingly as a means of excluding pulmonary emboli, a complication to which many patients with rheumatic disorders (systemic lupus erythematosus, primary antiphospholipid antibody syndrome, Wegener's granulomatosis) are susceptible. For pulmonary thromboembolism detection, the chest is scanned rapidly following a bolus intravenous injection of contrast medium, timed so that the pulmonary arteries are opacified to optimal effect.

MAGNETIC RESONANCE IMAGING

Because of its ability to image soft tissue structures not visible on conventional radiographs, MRI has brought significant advances to musculoskeletal imaging. The

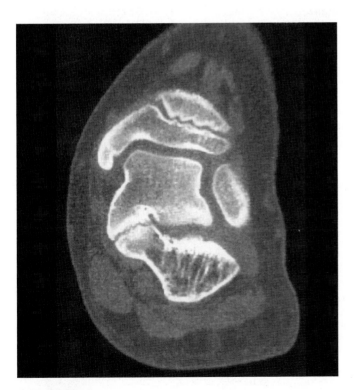

FIGURE 2D-6

A 50-year-old woman with suspected tarsal coalition. CT scan shows the non-osseous talocalcaneal coalition between the sustentaculum of the calcaneus and the talus above.

technique derives structural information from the density of protons in tissue and the relationship of these protons to their immediate surroundings.

Magnetic resonance imaging involves changing the strength and timing of magnetic field gradients, as well as altering radiofrequency pulses and sampling the emitted energy. By altering these factors appropriately, varying amounts of T1 and T2 weighting are imparted to the images. T1 reflects the time constant for spins to align themselves with the main magnetic field of the equipment and T2 reflects the time constant for loss of coherence among spins, resulting in decay of the component of magnetization perpendicular to the main magnetic field. These relaxation times are different in different tissues, permitting optimal imaging of different tissues by selection of an appropriate mix of T1 and T2 weighting.

As a result, MRI highlights different types of tissue and metabolic states. Altering these parameters can produce radically different images of the same anatomic site. CT images, which basically map the density of tissues in a manner similar to conventional radiographs, are intuitively easier to grasp than are MR images.

Magnetic resonance imaging is more expensive than most other imaging approaches, largely because of the cost of equipment and the time required to perform the studies. In the future, more attention will probably be given to tailored, limited imaging sequences, which potentially could lower the cost. Newer, faster imaging sequences continue to be developed, which may reduce the time and cost of MRI, as well as provide dynamic studies of joint motion.

Magnetic resonance imaging is free of the hazards of ionizing radiation, a major advantage in examining central portions of the body. The technique does pose some unique potential hazards, however. For example, the strong magnetic field can move metal objects such as surgically implanted vascular clips and foreign metal in the eyes, cause pacemaker malfunction, heat metal objects, and draw metal objects into the magnet. Metallic objects in the vicinity of the magnetic field can also compromise the quality of MRI images. Because of these risks and the adverse effect on imaging quality, operators must screen patients and visitors carefully. Patients suffering from claustrophobia may be unable to tolerate the procedure, which is performed with the patient positioned in a hollow tube. More open configurations for the magnet can circumvent this problem, but the quality of images produced by these devices varies. MRI c̄ gadolinium is contraindicated in patients with significant renal dysfunction, because of the risk of inducing nephrogenic systemic fibrosis (3). Finally, because MRI instruments can be noisy, hearing protection should be provided for the patient.

Spatial resolution using the latest MRI equipment is similar to spiral CT, but contrast resolution in soft tissues as well as bone marrow is superior among imaging modalities. Intra-articular soft tissue structures, such as the menisci and cruciate ligaments of the knee, are demonstrated clearly by MRI (Figure 2D-8). In fact, tiny ligamentous structures in the wrist or ankle can be assessed quite readily (4). The synovium can be imaged, especially using intravenous gadolinium. Joint effusions, popliteal cysts, ganglion cysts, meniscal cysts, and bursi-

FIGURE 2D-8

(A) Sagittal proton density images of the knee, depicting vertical tear of the posterior horn of the medial meniscus. (B) Sagittal proton density images of the knee. Bucket-handle tear of the medial meniscus, with "double Posterior Cruciate Ligament sign."

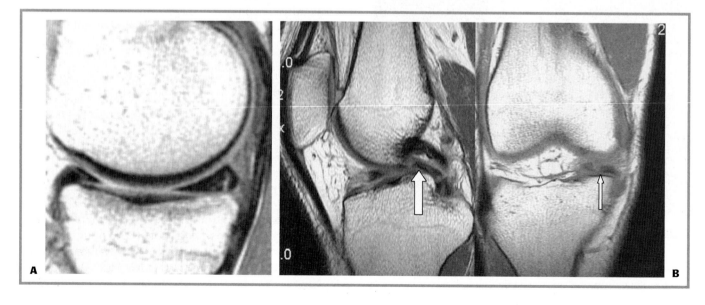

tis can be imaged clearly (Figure 2D-9), and the integrity of tendons assessed accurately as well (5). One limitation of MRI is in the detection of calcifications, which present as signal voids and are therefore not as well seen by MRI as by radiographic images. For example, chondrocalcinosis, important to the diagnosis of calcium pyrophosphate dehydrate deposition disease (CPPD), is demonstrated more reliably by plain radiography (Figure 2D-10). Otherwise, MRI remains the modality of choice for evaluating potential internal joint derangements.

Magnetic resonance imaging has specific utility in the assessment of:

- **Imaging Cartilage.** MRI has a negative predictive value close to 100% for the presence of meniscal tears in the knee. MRI is also a sensitive method for diagnosing labral tears of the shoulder and triangulofibrocartilage tears in the wrist.

  Alterations in articular hyaline cartilage are visible on MRI. Although direct observation with arthroscopy is more sensitive to small superficial changes, refinements are being made that improve the ability of MRI to detect small articular cartilage defects (6). With recent improvements in therapy for cartilage defects, MRI provides a useful noninvasive method for quantifying cartilage loss as well as evaluating the success of surgical repair. In addition, MRI is the study of choice for evaluating osteochondritis dissecans when information is needed about whether the osteochondral fragment is loose or detached.

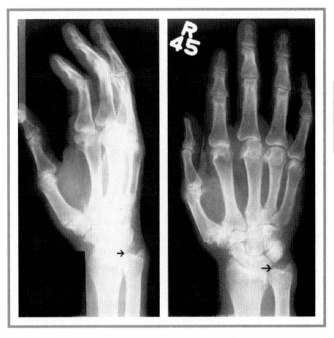

FIGURE 2D-10

Chondrocalcinosis in the hand: 58-year-old man with chondrocalcinosis in triangular fibrocartilage and lunotriquetral ligaments (*arrows*). Note MCP joint degenerative changes, a typical location for CPPD arthropathy. First carpometacarpal (CMC) joint also shows moderate degenerative change.

Recent studies have suggested that MRI may have a role in assessing responses to therapy in arthritis. For example, in rheumatoid arthritis, MRI can quantify the volume of enhancing inflammatory tissue (7). In ankylosing spondylitis, MRI may be used to assess changes over time in spinal inflammation (8). MRI has been established as the most sensitive modality for the detection of bony erosions (Figure 2D-11) (9), although its specificity for early erosive changes has been reported to be low. Healthy subjects can occasionally demonstrate imaging findings suggestive of mild synovitis or erosions, indistinguishable from early rheumatoid arthritis (10). Finally, as bone marrow edema and synovitis can precede frank erosions, MRI may have a predictive role, and thus affect patient management early in the disease course (11).

- **Detecting Bony Abnormalities.** MRI is extremely sensitive to subtle bony abnormalities. In fact, microfractures due to trauma or stress—often referred to as "bone bruises"—were essentially unknown before MRI. Now, recognizing their presence is quite important. The pattern of bone bruises is also closely related to ligamentous injuries (12). Similarly, much of the pain accompanying some acute meniscal tears may be caused by associated bone marrow edema. When the edema subsides, the pain disappears, despite the persistent meniscal tear. This finding

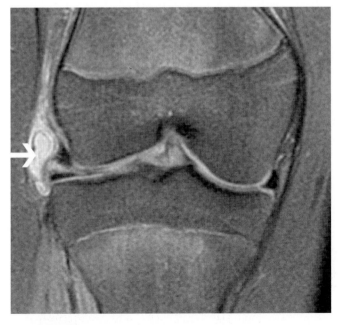

FIGURE 2D-9

Adolescent with knee pain. Coronal proton density fat-saturated image shows horizontal cleavage tear of the lateral meniscus, with associated parameniscal cyst (*arrow*).

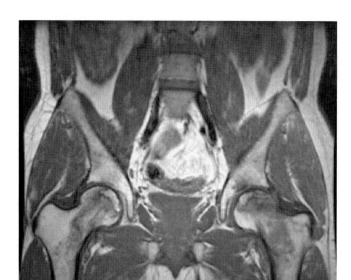

FIGURE 2D-11

MRI images of a patient treated with corticosteroids. T1 weighted image of hips demonstrates characteristic serpentine foci of low signal intensity within the femoral heads bilaterally, consistent with osteonecrosis.

could have important implications for therapy. One should possibly wait for the edema to resolve before attempting surgical intervention to repair or remove the meniscus. In some cases intervention might be unnecessary. MRI studies of the knee in older people often reveal asymptomatic meniscal tears. These individuals may have had pain at the time of the tear which resolved with the edema and did not cause them long-term disability.

- **Diagnosing Osteonecrosis.** MRI is the study of choice for diagnosing osteonecrosis (Figure 2D-11). Early in the course of disease, plain radiographs show no abnormalities.
- **Evaluating Musculoskeletal Neoplasms.** MRI is also the best method for evaluating the extent of a musculoskeletal neoplasm. Plain radiographs are still the mainstay for detecting bone neoplasms.
- **Identifying Bone Infections.** MRI is highly sensitive to the presence of bone infection because of alterations in the marrow signal. Osteomyelitis cannot be detected on radiography until approximately 30% to 40% bone destruction has occurred. Thus, MRI is the study of choice for the early detection of osteomyelitis (13). Small studies have shown variable results for MRI in differentiating osteomyelitis and neuropathic arthropathy, which is very difficult with other imaging techniques.

- **Diagnosing Disc Herniation.** Following plain radiography, MRI is an excellent study of the spine and its contents in cases of suspected disc herniation, particularly in young patients, because it does not employ ionizing radiation.
- **Localizing Muscle Abnormalities, Including Inflammation-Associated Edema in Inflammatory Muscle Disease.** MRI is indicated in the assessment of muscle abnormalities for detection of potential tears and contusions. The activity of different muscles during joint motion can also be studied by noting signal changes that occur with muscle activity. In inflammatory myopathies (polymyositis, dermatomyositis, inclusion body myositis), MRI demonstrates characteristic (albeit not diagnostic) edema, and may be useful in identifying sites to biopsy and following disease activity.

SCINTIGRAPHIC TECHNIQUES

Scintigraphy following intravenous administration of agents such as 99m technetium methylene diphosphonate (^{99m}Tc MDP) for bone scans, ^{99m}Tc sulphur colloid for bone marrow scans, 67 gallium citrate (^{67}Ga citrate), and leukocytes labeled with 111 indium [^{111}In-labeled white blood cells (WBCs)] are useful for evaluating a variety of musculoskeletal disorders (Figure 2D-12). These studies, similar in cost to CT, deliver a radiation dose similar to a CT scan of the abdomen. Scintigraphy is quite sensitive for detecting many disease processes, and has the advantage of imaging the entire body at once. The technique is nonspecific, however, because a number of processes may cause radionuclide accumulation. When areas of increased uptake are detected, additional studies such as radiography are often necessary to define the type of abnormality further. In clinical situations where the presence of skeletal disease is uncertain, a bone scan can be useful in excluding disease.

Localization of Scintigraphic Imaging Agents

99m Technetium methylene diphosphonate, the most commonly used radionuclide, accumulates in areas of bone formation, calcium deposition, and high blood flow. ^{99m}TC sulphur colloid localizes in the reticuloendothelial system (liver, spleen, and bone marrow). ^{67}Gallium citrate accumulates in inflammatory and certain neoplastic processes, and ^{111}In-labeled WBCs localize in inflammatory sites, especially acute inflammatory processes.

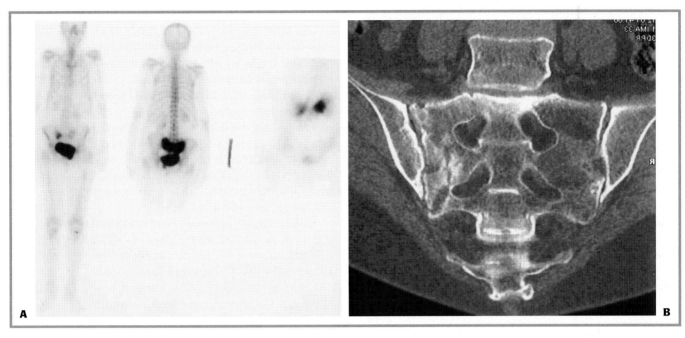

FIGURE 2D-12

(A) An 82-year-old woman with a history of breast cancer and recent onset of lower back pain. Metastases were suspected. ^{99m}Tc MDP bone scan shows increased uptake in the sacrum and right pubic ramus, typical of insufficiency fractures rather than metastatic cancer. (B) Computed tomography scan in the same 82-year-old woman. This test demonstrates the linear nature of the healing fracture in the sacrum, adjacent to the right sacroiliac joint, lending specificity to the diagnosis suggested by the radionuclide scan.

Using Radionuclide Imaging to Diagnose Osteomyelitis

The ^{99m}Tc MDP triple-phase bone scan is commonly used for early detection of osteomyelitis. Images are obtained in the early vascular phase (during bolus injection of the radionuclide), intermediate blood pool phase (5 minutes postinjection), and late bone phase (3 hours postinjection). A fourth phase (24 hours postinjection) can be added to accentuate areas of increased bone uptake, during which time soft tissue background is decreased, although delayed imaging is not widely used because of its inconvenience. If necessary, the specificity of scanning can be increased by also using ^{67}gallium citrate or ^{111}In-labeled WBCs. The ^{111}In-labeled WBC scan is especially useful when osteomyelitis is suspected to be superimposed on a healing fracture or surgical incision because uptake of ^{99m}Tc MDP is increased at these sites even in the absence of infections. ^{111}In-labeled WBC scans may also be useful in diagnosing osteomyelitis of the foot in people with diabetes. In suspected osteomyelitis of the hematopoietic bone marrow, the combination of ^{99m}Tc MDP and ^{111}In-labeled WBC appears to be an effective diagnostic technique. Spatial localization of bone scans can be improved with single-photon emission computed tomography (SPECT), and radiographs of scan-positive areas can be used to increase specificity.

Other Uses of Radionuclide Imaging

Bone scans are a reasonable alternative for early detection of osteonecrosis if MRI is not available. Bone scans can also detect stress injuries such as shin splints, tendon avulsions, insufficiency fractures, and stress fractures, which sometimes mimic arthritis symptome (Figure 2D-12).

ULTRASOUND

Ultrasound provides unique information by creating images based on the location of acoustic interfaces in tissue. It is relatively inexpensive, widely available, and free of the hazards of ionizing radiation. Spatial resolution is similar to CT and MRI, but this depends on the transducer. However, resolution is limited by the depth of tissue being studied; resolution is much higher for superficial structures.

One limitation of ultrasound is dependence on the operator. It is not always possible for one investigator to reproduce the results of another. Furthermore, because ultrasound has no cross-sectional orientation, it may be difficult for individuals who were not actually present during the study to interpret the images later.

In some centers, ultrasound has proved accurate in detecting rotator cuff tears. It is also excellent for assessing fluid collections, such as joint effusions, popliteal cysts, and ganglion cysts, and can therefore be used to guide aspiration of fluid. Superficially located tendons, such as the Achilles tendon and patellar tendon, can be studied for tears.

Ultrasound is excellent for differentiating thrombophlebitis from pseudothrombophlebitis. With real-time compression ultrasonography, venous thrombosis and popliteal cysts can be identified.

Ultrasound, similar to MRI, has been shown to be much more sensitive than radiography in detection of erosions in rheumatoid arthritis (14). With amplitude color Doppler (ACD), it can demonstrate synovial hyperemia in active disease. The technique requires a skilled operator and is more effective in the examination of the metacarpophalangeal (MCP) and interphalangeal (IP) joints than the intercarpal joints, but is relatively inexpensive and convenient. It avoids the potentially uncomfortable positioning that may be necessary with MRI.

Finally, although ultrasound has been reported to be useful in the diagnosis of temporal arthritis, there is an absence of blinded studies confirming its utility for this purpose.

ARTHROGRAPHY

Arthrography involves injecting a contrast agent into the joint followed by radiography. In conventional arthrography, the joint cavity is filled with an iodine-containing contrast medium and sometimes air. The cost is less than that of CT or MRI, and the procedure can be performed wherever fluoroscopy is available. The possibility of introducing bacteria into a joint or encountering reactions to the local anesthetic or contrast medium must be considered, but these complications are very rare.

One of the major reasons for developing arthrography was to examine structures within the joint, such as the menisci of the knee, which were not visible on conventional radiographs. Now these structures can be imaged noninvasively by MRI. However, certain important roles remain for arthrography.

Conventional arthrography, using iodine-containing contrast medium either alone or combined with air, accurately detects full-thickness rotator cuff tears (Figure 2D-13). CT scanning can be added to the air–contrast arthrogram (CT arthrography), providing an excellent study of the glenoid labrum that can be an alternative to MRI in selected patients (15).

Knee arthrography can confirm the diagnosis of a popliteal cyst, and permits injection of corticosteroids at the same time. It is an alternative for evaluating the menisci in patients who are claustrophobic or whose size precludes MRI examination (Figure 2D-14).

Wrist arthrography is excellent for evaluating the integrity of the triangular fibrocartilage, ligaments between the scaphoid and lunate, and ligaments between the lunate and triquetrum (16). Some clinicians prefer arthrography to MRI in this situation.

FIGURE 2D-13

(A) Single contrast arthrogram of a normal shoulder. (B) Single contrast shoulder arthrogram of a 66-year-old man with a painful shoulder and history of injury in distant past. Contrast media fills not only the shoulder joint [as in Figure 2D-11(A)] but has filled the subdeltoid–subacromial bursa superiorly, a finding diagnostic of full-thickness rotator cuff tear.

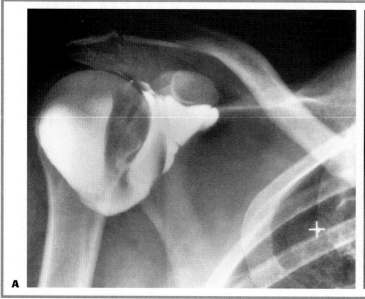
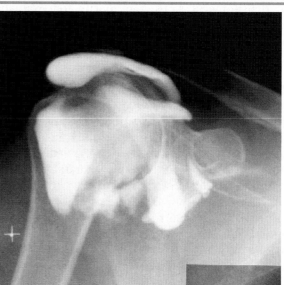

A

B

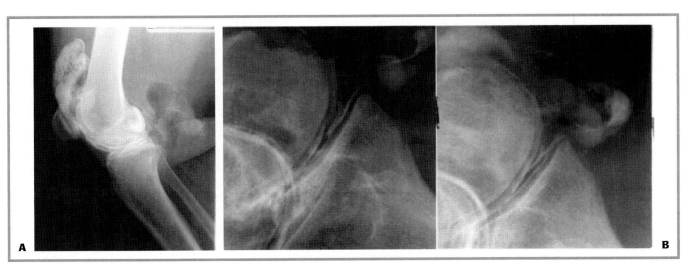

FIGURE 2D-14

(A, B) A 40-year-old woman, too large to fit in the MRI scanner, was suspected of having a popliteal cyst. Double contrast arthrogram demonstrated popliteal cyst and also a torn medial meniscus. Ultrasonography would have been an appropriate alternative approach to making this diagnosis.

Magnetic resonance arthrography is performed by distending a joint with a dilute solution of a gadolinium-containing contrast medium. This technique, not widely studied, probably increases the diagnostic accuracy of glenoid and acetabular labral tears, as well as rotator cuff tears (17).

BONE DENSITOMETRY

Bone densitometry is used primarily for evaluating osteoporosis. Two precise, accurate, and widely available techniques are dual-energy x-ray absorptiometry (DXA) and quantitative computed tomography (QCT) (18).

Dual-energy x-ray absorptiometry scans with a narrow x-ray beam that alternates energy (kilovoltage peak; KVP). A sensitive receptor detects the fraction of the x-ray beam that traverses the body at each point along the scan path. Because the absorption characteristics of bone and soft tissue vary at different x-ray energies, the amount of radiation absorbed by bone can be calculated. From this, the amount of bone in the path of the x-ray beam at any point along the scan is determined.

Dual-energy x-ray absorptiometry is relatively inexpensive and delivers very little radiation to the patient. It is thus a good choice for studies that must be repeated. Any part of the body can be studied. Standard values are available for lumbar spine and proximal femur, which are the most widely studied.

Quantitative computed tomography scans several lumbar vertebrae while simultaneously scanning a phantom containing different concentrations of bone-equivalent material. A standard curve is constructed from the concentration values versus CT attenuation, and then the bone density at any location scanned is determined from the standard curve. The cost of this study is moderate and the radiation dose fairly low, although not as low as that for DXA. One purported advantage of this technique is that trabecular bone in the middle of the vertebrae can be evaluated because overlying cortical bone and posterior elements of the vertebrae are not measured. Trabecular bone, which has tremendous surface area, is more rapidly affected during bone loss than is cortical bone.

ANGIOGRAPHY

Angiography is useful in the primary diagnosis of rheumatologic disorders with vascular components. In polyarteritis nodosa, for example, demonstration of multiple small aneurysms in medium-sized arteries may be diagnostic. Similarly, in Takayasu's arteritis, the long, smooth tapering of involved vessels—most often the subclavian arteries—is highly characteristic. Aortography with central aortic pressure measurement is also important in patients with Takayasu's disease, whose blood pressures in the arms and sometimes even the legs are not accurate because of proximal arterial narrowing. In Buerger's disease, angiography reveals "corkscrew" collaterals at the levels of the hands and wrists.

IMAGE-GUIDED ASPIRATION AND INJECTIONS

Examination of joint fluid often plays an important part in the diagnosis of arthritic conditions such as septic arthritis, gout, and pseudogout. In most cases, the rheumatologist has no difficulty in obtaining fluid using external landmarks for needle placement. In more difficult cases, aspiration using imaging guidance may prove useful. The source of the specimen can be documented by contrast injection and radiography.

Using imaging guidance to be certain of needle tip position, injection of specific joints with local anesthetic can prove whether or not the joint is responsible for the patient's pain. The injection of glucocorticosteroids for longer term relief can be directed in a similar fashion for greater precision in administration.

IMAGING DECISIONS

Almost all imaging should begin with plain radiography, which is frequently all that is required. If additional diagnostic information is required to make clinical decisions, MRI is frequently the second imaging study. In many cases, MRI findings must be correlated with plain films because MRI does not easily demonstrate soft tissue calcifications or subtle cortical abnormalities of bone.

Recent MRI studies show that many individuals have anatomic abnormalities that are unrelated to symptoms (19). Therefore, imaging findings must be correlated with the clinical presentation. Imaging studies should not be obtained unless they have the potential to answer clinically significant questions. In the absence of clear clinical questions, imaging studies may raise more questions than they answer.

Finally, it is critically important for the clinician to work closely with the radiologist to decide exactly what information is needed from an imaging study, and then to select the technique that will supply that information. MRI provides such a wealth of information about so many structures that an exhaustive MRI study may be appropriate in a very puzzling joint condition. In other cases, a tailored, abbreviated MRI or a simpler imaging procedure may provide the specific diagnostic information in less time for less money.

REFERENCES

1. Wechsler RJ, Karasick D, Schweitzer. Computed tomography of talocalcaneal coalition: imaging techniques. Skeletal Radiol 1992;21:353–359.
2. Lee JS, June-GI I, Ahn JM, Kim YM, Han MC. Fibrosing alveolitis: prognostic implication of ground glass attenuation of high-resolution CT. Radiology 1992;184:451–454.
3. Kuo PH, Kanal E, Abu-Alfa AK, Cowper SE. Gadolinium-based MR contrast agents and nephrogenic systemic fibrosis. Radiology 2007;242:647–649.
4. Schweitzer ME, Brahme SK, Hodler J, et al. Chronic wrist pain: spin-echo and short tau inversion recovery MR imaging and conventional and MR arthrography. Radiology 1992;182:205–211.
5. Schweitzer ME, Caccese R, Karasick D, Wapner KL, Mitchell DG. Posterior tibial tendon tears: utility of secondary signs for MR imaging diagnosis. Radiology 1993;188:655–659.
6. McCauley TR, Disler DG. MR imaging of articular cartilage. Radiology 1998;209:629–640.
7. Argyropoulou MI, Glatzouni A, Voulgari PV, et al. Magnetic resonance imaging quantification of hand synovitis in patients with rheumatoid arthritis treated with infliximab. Joint Bone Spine 2005;72:557–561.
8. Sieper J, Baraliakos X, Listing J, et al. Persistent reduction of spinal inflammation as assessed by magnetic resonance imaging in patients with ankylosing spondylitis after 2 yrs of treatment with the anti-tumour necrosis factor agent infliximab. Rheumatology 2005;44:1525–1530.
9. Hoving JL, Buchbinder R, Hall S, et al. A comparison of magnetic resonance imaging, sonography, and radiography of the hand in patients with early rheumatoid arthritis. J Rheumatol 2004;31:663–675.
10. Ejbjerg B, Narvestad E, Rostrup E, et al. Magnetic resonance imaging of wrist and finger joints in healthy subjects occasionally shows changes resembling erosions and synovitis as seen in rheumatoid arthritis. Arthritis Rheum 2004;50:1097–1106.
11. Benton N, Stewart N, Crabbe J, et al. MRI of the wrist in early rheumatoid arthritis can be used to predict functional outcome at 6 years. Ann Rheum Dis 2004;63:555–561.
12. Mair SD, Schlegel TF, Gill TJ, Hawkins RJ, Steadman JR. Incidence and location of bone bruises after acute posterior cruciate ligament injury. Am J Sports Med 2004;32:1681–1687.
13. Aloui N, Nessib N, Jalel C. Acute osteomyelitis in children: early MRI diagnosis. J Radiol 2004;85:403–408.
14. Wakefield RJ, Gibbon WW, Conaghan PG, et al. The value of sonography in the detection of bone erosions in patients with rheumatoid arthritis: a comparison with conventional radiography. Arthritis Rheum 2000;43:2762–2770.
15. Stiles RG, Otte MT. Imaging of the shoulder. Radiology 1993;188:603–613.
16. Metz VM, Mann FA, Gilula LA. Three-compartment wrist arthrography: correlation of pain site with location of uni- and bidirectional communications. AJR Am J Roentgenol 1993;160:819–822.

17. Palmer WE, Brown JH, Rosenthal DI. Labral-ligamentous complex of the shoulder: evaluation with MR arthrography. Radiology 1994;190:645–651.
18. Guglielmi G, Grimston SK, Fischer KC, Pacifici R. Osteoporosis: diagnosis with lateral and posteroanterior dual x-ray absorptiometry compared with quantitative CT. Radiology 1994;192:845–850.
19. Jensen MC, Brant-Zawadski MN, Obuchowski N, et al. Magnetic resonance imaging of the lumbar spine in people without back pain. N Engl J Med 1994;331:69–73.

2

Musculoskeletal Signs and Symptoms
A. Monarticular Joint Disease

H. Ralph Schumacher, MD
Lan X. Chen, MD, PhD

■ Pain or swelling of a single joint merits prompt evaluation to rule out infectious causes and to identify patients in need of urgent and aggressive care.

■ The underlying causes of monarthritis are divided into two groups: inflammatory diseases and mechanical or infiltrative disorders.

■ Analyzing synovial fluid is a helpful way to delineate the cause of monarthritis.

Pain or swelling of a single joint merits prompt evaluation to identify patients in need of urgent and aggressive care (1). Although there are many minor and easily managed causes of monarthritis, infectious arthritis with its risk of prolonged morbidity (and even mortality, if untreated) requires that this very serious problem always be considered. The underlying causes of monarthritis are divided into two groups: inflammatory diseases (Table 3A-1) and mechanical or infiltrative disorders (Table 3A-2). Triage into one of these categories is the first step in the differential diagnosis of monarthritis.

DIAGNOSIS OF MONARTICULAR JOINT DISEASE

History

It is important to determine the course and duration of symptoms, although patients frequently have difficulty establishing the exact time of onset, duration, and the rate of evolution. Acute problems or sudden onset of monarthritis often require immediate evaluation and therapy. The course of symptoms may provide critical information. Bacterial infection tends to increase in severity until treated. Viral monarthritis often resolves spontaneously. Fungal or tuberculous (TB) arthritis can be chronic and can elude diagnosis for years (2). Osteo-

arthritic symptoms wax and wane with physical activity. Morning stiffness lasting more than an hour suggests an inflammatory disease.

A history of previous episodes provides support for a crystalline or other noninfectious cause, such as palindromic rheumatism (3). Patients with established rheumatoid arthritis (RA) who develop a dramatic monarthritis should always be evaluated for superimposed septic arthritis or crystal-associated disease (4). Patients with antecedent joint disease or surgery should raise the clinician's concern about infection. In patients with a prosthesis in the involved joint, loosening of the implant should also be investigated.

Monarticular arthritis is occasionally the first symptom of polyarticular disease, such as reactive arthritis, inflammatory bowel disease, psoriatic arthritis, or RA. A history of fever, chills, tick bites, sexual risk factors, travel outside the country, and intravenous drug use (5) can contribute clues to infectious causes. Symptoms such as rash, diarrhea, urethritis, or uveitis might suggest reactive arthritis. Weight loss can suggest malignancy or other serious systemic disease.

A history of trauma suggests fracture or an internal derangement, but minor trauma can also precipitate acute gout or psoriatic arthritis, or can introduce infection. Occupations involving repetitive use of the joint favor osteoarthritis. Concurrent illnesses and medication use may also provide important clues; in addition, they can affect test results and influence the choice or

TABLE 3A-1. SOME INFLAMMATORY CAUSES OF MONARTHRITIS.

Crystal-induced arthritis
   Monosodium urate (gout)
   Calcium pyrophosphate dihydrate
   Hydroxyapatite
   Calcium oxalate
   Liquid lipid microspherules

Infectious arthritis
   Bacteria
   Fungi
   Lyme disease or disease due to other spirochetes
   Mycobacteria
   Virus (HIV, hepatitis B, others)

Systemic diseases presenting with monarticular involvement
   Psoriatic arthritis
   Reactive arthritis
   Rheumatoid arthritis
   Systemic lupus erythematosus

outcome of therapy. Because some monarticular diseases are inherited, family history can be helpful.

PHYSICAL EXAMINATION

The clinician must first distinguish arthritis, which involves the articular space, from problems in periarticular areas, such as bursitis, tendinitis, osteomyelitis, or cellulitis. In arthritis, the swelling and tenderness tend to surround the joint. If normal joint motion is retained, true arthritis is unlikely. Painful limitation of passive motion of the joint in all planes usually indicates joint involvement. Pain limited to one movement or tenderness on only one side of the joint suggests a periarticular problem.

In any patient with acute monarthritis, it is important to look for extra-articular signs that might provide clues to specific causes. For example, mouth ulcers may occur in Behcet's syndrome, reactive arthritis, and systemic lupus erythematosus (SLE). Small patches of psoriasis may be found in the anal crease or behind the ears. The keratoderma blennorrhagicum of reactive arthritis can be subtle and often affects only the feet. Erythema nodosum may occur in sarcoidosis and inflammatory bowel disease. Skin ulcerations can be a source of infection.

SYNOVIAL FLUID ANALYSIS

Arthrocentesis should be performed in almost every patient with monarthritis, and it is obligatory if infection is suspected. Virtually all the important information from synovial fluid analysis is obtained through the gross examination, total leukocyte and differential count, cultures, Gram staining, and examination of a wet preparation for crystals and other microscopic abnormalities (6). All these studies can be performed with only 1 to 2 mL of synovial fluid. Even a few drops may be adequate for culture, Gram staining, and wet preparations. Cloudy synovial fluid is likely to be caused by inflammatory arthritis and is confirmed by a leukocyte count (see also Chapter 7C).

Normally, synovial fluid contains fewer than 200 leukocytes/mm^3, most of which are mononuclear cells. In general, the leukocyte count and the suspicion of infection should rise at the same rate—the higher the count, the greater the suspicion. Effusions with more than 100,000 leukocytes/mm^3 are considered septic until proved otherwise. However, leukocyte counts vary widely in both sterile and septic inflammatory arthritis. Synovial fluid should be cultured if there is any suggestion of infection. Special stains and cultures for mycobacteria and fungi are sometimes appropriate.

Careful examination for crystals in synovial fluid can establish a diagnosis early and avoid unnecessary hospital admissions for the treatment of suspected infectious arthritis. A tentative diagnosis can be made by standard light microscopy. Monosodium urate crystals are needle or rod shaped, and calcium pyrophosphate dihydrate (CPPD) crystals are usually short rods, squares, or rhomboids. Polarized light examination can confirm the nature of these crystals. Individual apatite crystals, which cause acute monarthritis or periarthritis, are visible only on electron microscopy. However, masses of these crystals look like shiny, nonbirefringent

TABLE 3A-2. SOME NON-INFLAMMATORY CAUSES OF MONARTHRITIS.

Amyloidosis

Osteonecrosis

Benign tumor
   Osteochondroma
   Osteoid osteoma
   Pigmented villonodular synovitis

Fracture

Hemarthrosis

Internal derangement

Malignancy

Osteoarthritis

Foreign bodies

clumps that resemble cell debris. Special stains such as alizarin red S can confirm that these clumps are masses of calcium crystals.

The presence of crystals does not exclude infection, however, especially because antecedent joint disease such as gout may coexist with or predispose to septic arthritis (7). Large fat droplets in synovial fluid suggest a fracture involving the bone marrow space. Small lipid droplets may also indicate fracture or pancreatic fat necrosis.

LABORATORY TESTS

Synovial fluid cultures may be negative in some infectious arthritis. This is especially true for gonococcal arthritis, as only about 25% of patients have positive synovial fluid cultures. For this reason, cultures and Gram stains of blood, skin lesions or ulcers, cervical or urethral swabs, urine, or any other possible sources of microorganisms should be ordered in suspected infectious arthritis. Tests for human immunodeficiency virus (HIV) antibodies and Lyme antibodies may also be appropriate. However, no single serologic test can establish the cause of any arthritis. For example, rheumatoid factor can be positive in many diseases besides RA, including sarcoidosis and subacute bacterial endocarditis. Similarly, an elevated serum uric acid does not mean a patient has gout, and normal urate levels can be seen during the acute phase of gouty arthritis.

RADIOGRAPHS

Radiologic findings are typically unremarkable in most patients with acute inflammatory arthritis, other than showing soft tissue swelling. However, x-ray studies can help exclude some causes and can provide a useful baseline for future comparisons. Radiographs of the involved joint may show fractures, tumors, or signs of antecedent chronic disease such as osteoarthritis. Chondrocalcinosis in the involved joint suggests, but does not prove, that the arthritis is caused by CPPD crystals. X-rays or ultrasound can show calcific peri-arthritis. Magnetic resonance imaging (MRI), although often overused, can localize an infectious or inflammatory process to the joint, its surrounding tissue, or bone (8). MRI can also identify meniscal tears and ligament damage.

SYNOVIAL BIOPSY

Needle biopsy of the synovial membrane or a biopsy obtained during arthroscopy may be critical in patients with monarthropathy that remains undiagnosed (9). A culture of synovial tissue may be more informative than a synovial fluid culture in certain settings, such as when gonococcal or mycobacterial disease is suspected or when no fluid is available for culture. Biopsies can identify infiltrative diseases, such as amyloidosis, sarcoidosis, pigmented villonodular synovitis, or tumor. The polymerase chain reaction and immunoelectron microscopy may help identify DNA sequences from many organisms including mycobacteria (10), *Borrelia burgdorferi*, *Neisseria gonorrhoeae*, chlamydia, and ureaplasma (11).

INITIAL TREATMENT

Management decisions often must be made before all test results are available. For example, a patient with synovial fluid indicating a highly inflammatory process, a negative Gram stain, and no obvious cause or source of infection requires antibiotic coverage while testing proceeds. Try to obtain several cultures before initiating treatment.

Suspected crystal-induced arthritis in a patient whose course is uncomplicated can be treated with full doses of nonsteroidal anti-inflammatory drugs (NSAIDs) with tapering as the inflammation subsides. Oral corticosteroids or occasionally colchicine are also effective in gout and pseudogout. NSAIDs are an acceptable initial symptomatic treatment in other unexplained inflammatory arthritis. Acetaminophen may be used during the evaluation of non-inflammatory arthritis. However, because NSAIDs and acetaminophen can mask fever patterns and delay diagnosis, propoxyphene or codeine might be preferred in some instances. Acutely swollen joints can safely be rested, but should not be casted unless a fracture is proved.

SPECIFIC TYPES OF MONARTHRITIS

Infection

Between 80% and 90% of nongonococcal bacterial infections are monarticular. Most joint infections develop from hematogenous spread. The discovery of a primary site of infection can be an important clue to the infectious agent involved. By far the most common agents are Gram-positive aerobes (approximately 80%) (12), with *Staphylococcus aureus* accounting for 60%. Gram-negative bacteria account for about 18% of infections, and anaerobes are increasingly common causes as a result of parenteral drug use and the rising number of immunocompromised hosts. Anaerobic infections are also more common in patients who have wounds of an extremity or gastrointestinal cancers.

N. gonorrhoeae remains a common cause of septic arthritis. It is often preceded by a migratory tendinitis or arthritis. Mycobacterial infection may cause monoarthritis or may involve several joints. The disease is more likely to be chronic, but acute mycobacterial arthritis has been reported and may even cause podagra (13). *[gout]* Atypical mycobacterial infections can involve the synovium and should be considered in the differential diagnosis, especially in immunocompromised hosts and in patients whose joints have been injected frequently with corticosteroids. Fungal arthritis is usually indolent, but cases of acute monarthritis due to blastomycosis or Candida species have been reported. Acute monarthritis associated with herpes simplex virus, Coxsackie B, HIV, parvovirus, and other viruses has also been described (14).

The joint symptoms of Lyme disease range from intermittent arthralgias to chronic monarthritis (most often in the knee) to oligoarthritis. Monarthritis can also rarely be caused by other spirochetes, such as *Treponema pallidum*.

Crystal-Induced Arthritis

Gout, which is caused by monosodium urate crystals, is the most common type of inflammatory monarthritis. Typically, gout initially involves one first metatarsophalangeal (MTP) joint, ankle, midfoot, or knee. However, acute attacks of gout can occur in any joint. Later attacks may be monarticular or polyarticular. Accompanying fever, although less common with monarticular than with polyarticular gout, can mimic infection.

Calcium pyrophosphate dihydrate crystals can cause monarthritis that is clinically indistinguishable from gout and thus is often called pseudogout. Pseudogout is most common in the knee and wrist, but it has been reported in a variety of other joints, including the first MTP joint. Among other crystals known to cause acute monarthritis are apatites, calcium oxalate, and liquid lipid crystals. Apatites have also been recognized as a cause of goutlike podagra.

Osteoarthritis, Osteonecrosis, Trauma, and Foreign Body Reactions

Although osteoarthritis is primarily a chronic and slowly progressive disease, it may present with suddenly worsening pain, swelling, and even erosions in a single joint (15). New pain in the knee is often due to an effusion as a result of overuse or minor trauma. Spontaneous osteonecrosis, especially of the knee, is seen in elderly patients and can lead to pain in a single joint with or without effusion. Trauma to a joint leading to internal derangement, hemarthrosis, or fracture can also lead to

monarticular disease. Penetrating injuries from thorns, wood fragments, or other foreign materials can cause monarthritis (16).

Hemarthrosis

The most common causes of hemarthrosis, or bleeding into a joint, are clotting abnormalities due to anticoagulant therapy or congenital disorders such as hemophilia. Hemarthrosis can also result from scurvy. Fracture of the joint should always be considered in patients with hemarthrosis, especially if the synovial fluid is bloody and contains fat.

Systemic Rheumatic Diseases

Many systemic diseases may present as acute monarticular arthritis, but this is decidedly uncommon and should not be emphasized in the differential diagnosis. RA, SLE, arthritis of inflammatory bowel disease, psoriatic arthritis, Behçet's disease, and reactive arthritis can all begin as acute monarthritis. Other causes include sarcoidosis, serum sickness, hepatitis, sickle cell disease, hyperlipidemias, and malignancies. Persistence in evaluating patients for underlying systemic diseases can sometimes lead to an early diagnosis of systemic disease.

In a substantial number of patients with synovial fluid findings indicative of inflammatory arthritis, the cause cannot be determined. Many of these patients have transient monarthritis with no recurrences (17). Guidelines for the initial evaluation of patients with acute musculoskeletal symptoms have been published and include aspects of evaluation of monarthropathy (see Appendix II) (18).

REFERENCES

1. Baker DG, Schumacher HR. Acute monarthritis. N Engl J Med 1993;329:1013–1020.
2. Pinals Robert S. Sarah's knee: a famous actress with chronic, inflammatory monoarthritis. J Clin Rheumatol 2004;10:13–15.
3. Schumacher HR. Palindromic onset of rheumatoid arthritis: clinical, synovial fluid, and biopsy studies. Arthritis Rheum 1982;25:366–369.
4. VanLinhoudt D, Schumacher HR. Acute monosynovitis or oligoarthritis in patients with quiescent rheumatoid arthritis. J Clin Rheumatol 1995;1:46–53.
5. Ross JJ, Shamsuddin H. Sternoclavicular septic arthritis: review of 180 cases. Medicine (Baltimore) 2004;83:139–148.
6. Gatter RA, Schumacher HR, eds. A practical handbook of synovial fluid analysis. Philadelphia: Lea & Febiger; 1991:14–23.
7. Yu KH, Luo SF, Liou LB, et al. Concomitant septic and gouty arthritis: an analysis of 30 cases. Rheumatology (Oxford) 2003;42:1062–1066.

8. Hoving JL, Buchbinder R, Hall S, et al. A comparison of magnetic resonance imaging, sonography, and radiography of the hand in patients with early rheumatoid arthritis. J Rheumatol 2004;31:663–675.

9. Schumacher HR, Kulka JP. Needle biopsy of the synovial membrane: experience with the Parker-Pearson technic. N Engl J Med 1972;286:416–419.

10. van der Heijden IM, Wilbrink B, Schouls LM, et al. Detection of mycobacteria in joint samples from patients with arthritis using genus specific PCR and sequence analysis. Rheumatology 1999;38:547–553.

11. Rahman MU, Cheema S, Schumacher HR, Hudson AP. Molecular evidence for the presence of chlamydia in the synovium of patients with Reiter's syndrome. Arthritis Rheum 1992;35:521–529.

12. Goldenberg DL, Reed JI. Bacterial arthritis. N Engl J Med 1985;312:764–771.

13. Boulware DW, Lopez M, Gum OB. Tuberculosis podagra. J Rheumatol 1985;12:1022–1024.

14. Rivier G, Gerster JC, Terrier P, Cheseaux JJ. Parvovirus B19 associated monarthritis in a 5 year old boy. J Rheumatol 1995;22:766–777.

15. Punzi L, Ramonda R, Sfriso P. Erosive osteoarthritis. Best Pract Res Clin Rheumatol 2004;18:739–758.

16. Stevens KJ, Theologis T, McNally EG. Imaging of plant thorn synovitis. Skeletal Radiol 2000;29:605–608.

17. Schumacher HR, Habre W, Meador R, Hsia EC. Predictive factors in early arthritis: long-term follow-up. Semin Arthritis Rheum 2004;33:264–272.

18. American College of Rheumatology Ad Hoc Committee on Clinical Guidelines. Guidelines for the initial evaluation of the adult patient with acute musculoskeletal symptoms. Arthritis Rheum 1996;39: 1–8.

Musculoskeletal Signs and Symptoms
B. Polyarticular Joint Disease

STERLING WEST, MD

- Polyarticular joint pain can be caused by problems within the joint, around the joint (such as tendons and adjacent bone), and from psychogenic factors.
- The two most important diagnostic tools in the evaluation of a patient with polyarticular joint complaints are a thorough history and physical examination.
- Onset and course of symptoms, pattern of joint involvement, and pain characteristics separate inflammatory from non-inflammatory causes.

Polyarticular joint pain can be caused by problems within the joint (arthritis), from adjacent bone (periostitis, osteonecrosis), from surrounding soft tissues (bursa, tendon, muscle, nerve), or from psychogenic factors (depression). Arthritis generally causes diffuse joint pain that is aggravated by movement. The purpose of this chapter is to discuss the diagnostic approach and differential diagnosis of acute and chronic polyarthritis. The two most important diagnostic tools in the evaluation of a patient with polyarticular joint complaints is a thorough history and skillful physical examination (1–4). Laboratory and radiographic studies or, rarely, tissue biopsy can support or confirm the diagnostic impression formulated after the initial examination. Following a correct diagnosis, more effective therapy can be prescribed and prognosis discussed.

CLASSIFICATION OF POLYARTICULAR JOINT DISEASE

There are two main categories of polyarticular joint disease: inflammatory (Table 3B-1) and non-inflammatory (Table 3B-2). Both groups can be further subdivided by characteristic mode of presentation (acute vs. chronic) and pattern of joint involvement (polyarticular vs. oligoarticular; symmetric vs. asymmetric; with or without axial involvement). Recognition of the pattern of joint involvement is a key to the diagnosis of polyarthritis. However, it is important to understand that all patients will not fit the expected patterns, and atypical presentations frequently occur.

Despite the lengthy list of diseases that cause polyarthritis, a few disorders explain most cases. In one study of over 200 patients with early inflammatory synovitis, 60% were diagnosed with either rheumatoid arthritis (RA) or a spondyloarthropathy at presentation or during the following year (5). In another study of 566 patients with early arthritis followed for 2 years, 30% were diagnosed with RA and 46% were given another diagnosis (crystalline-induced arthritis, sarcoidosis, reactive arthritis, and psoriatic arthritis) (6). Among patients with a non-inflammatory polyarthritis, osteoarthritis is overwhelmingly the most common diagnosis.

DIAGNOSTIC APPROACH
History

The history and physical examination are critical in narrowing the differential diagnosis in a patient presenting with polyarthritis. The evaluation should focus on the time course of the joint symptoms and whether or not inflammatory signs are present. Additionally, the number and distribution of joint involvement and the presence of any extra-articular manifestations are critical components to consider.

TABLE 3B-1. CLASSIFICATION OF POLYARTICULAR INFLAMMATORY JOINT DISEASE.

SYMMETRIC POLYARTICULAR	ASYMMETRIC OLIGOARTICULAR

Infectious arthritis
  Viral
  Parvovirus
  Hepatitis B and C
  Others: HIV, EBV, rubella
	Infectious arthritis
	  Gonococcal/meningococcal
	  Lyme disease (late phase)
	  Fungal and mycobacterial
	  Bacterial endocarditis
	  Whipple's disease

Postinfectious or reactive arthritic
  Rheumatic fever
  Poststreptococcal arthritis (PSA)
	Postinfectious or reactive arthritic
	  Rheumatic fever
	  Poststreptococcal arthritis
	  Reactive arthritis
	  (Enteric, urogenital)

Palindromic rheumatism	Enteropathic arthritis of IBD
Juvenile idiopathic arthritis (Polyarticular)	Juvenile idiopathic arthritis (Pauciarticular)
Rheumatoid arthritis	Undifferentiated spondyloarthritis
Psoriatic arthritis	Psoriatic arthritis

Systemic rheumatic disease
  Systemic lupus erythematosus
  Sjögren's syndrome
  Systemic sclerosis
  Poly/dermatomyositis
  Mixed connective tissue disease
  Still's disease (juvenile, adult)
  Relapsing seronegative symmetrical synovitis
    with pitting edema (RS3PE)
  Polymyalgia rheumatica
  Systemic vasculitis
  Relapsing polychondritis
	Systemic rheumatic disease
	  Relapsing polychondritis
	  Behçet's disease
	Crystal-induced
	  Gout
	  Pseudogout (calcium pyrophosphate
	    deposition disease)
	  Basic calcium phosphate
	Other systemic illnesses
	  Familial Mediterranean fever
	  Carcinomatous
	  Pancreatic disease–associated arthritis
	  Hyperlipoproteinemia
	  Sarcoidosis (chronic)
	  Multicentric reticulohistiocytosis

Other systemic illnesses
  Celiac disease
  Sarcoidosis (acute type)
  Acute leukemia (children)	

Peripheral arthritis with axial involvement
  Ankylosing spondylitis
  Enteropathic arthritis associated with
    inflammatory bowel disease (IBD)
  Psoriatic arthritis
  Reactive arthritis (enteric, urogenital)
  SAPHO (synovitis, acne, pustulosis, hyperostosis,
    osteitis)
  Whipple's disease	

Time Course of Joint Symptoms

Polyarticular joint symptoms may have an acute or insidious onset. Acute polyarthritis, especially when accompanied by fever, is always due to an inflammatory disease and requires immediate evaluation to rule out infection or crystalline arthritis (7,8). Alternatively, there are both inflammatory and non-inflammatory causes of polyarthritis with an insidious onset. Variations, however, may occur, and a disorder that typically has an insidious onset may have an acute onset in some patients.

Pattern of Joint Involvement

Particular attention should be given to the pattern of joint involvement, which can be additive, migratory, or intermittent. The *additive* pattern is most common but least specific. It refers to recruitment of new joints while previously involved joints remain involved

TABLE 3B-2. CLASSIFICATION OF NON-INFLAMMATORY POLYARTICULAR JOINT DISEASE.

SYMMETRIC POLYARTICULAR	ASYMMETRIC OLIGOARTICULAR

Osteoarthritis
  Primary generalized
  Erosive
	Osteoarthritis
	  Localized

Crystal-induced
  CPPD (pseudo-RA type)
  Basic calcium phosphate
	Crystal-induced
	  CPPD (pseudo-OA type)
	  Hematologic
	  Hemoglobinopathies
	  Hemophilia

Hereditary metabolic
  Hemochromatosis
  Wilson's disease
  Gaucher's disease
	Peripheral arthritis with axial
	  involvement

Endocrine
  Myxedematous arthropathy
	Osteoarthritis
	  Diffuse idiopathic skeletal
	  hyperostosis (DISH)
	  Ochronosis

Hematologic
  Amyloid arthropathy
  Hemoglobinopathies
	Spondyloepiphyseal dysplasia

Hypertrophic osteoarthropathy	

Pain Characteristics

Inflammatory joint pain involves the joints diffusely and is present at rest and with normal use. Nocturnal pain may interfere with sleep. This joint pain is associated with prolonged stiffness for greater than 30 to 60 minutes, which is worse in the morning or after inactivity (gelling). Fatigue is common, may be severe, and typically occurs by early afternoon after stiffness has improved. Patients with non-inflammatory joint pain have pain with activity that is relieved by rest. Although they may have stiffness or gelling after inactivity, it typically lasts less than 15 minutes, and systemic fatigue is not common.

Number and Distribution of Joint Involvement

Polyarthritis refers to involvement of five or more joints. The joint distribution typically is symmetric, although distribution may go through an initial asymmetric phase. A wide variety of inflammatory disorders may present as acute or chronic polyarthritis and may be recognized by their presenting pattern of arthritis. The most common identifiable cause of a self-limited disorder causing acute symmetric polyarthritis involving the small joints of the hands and wrists is parvovirus-associated arthritis. The most common cause of a chronic inflammatory polyarthritis that involves small and large joints bilaterally and symmetrically in the upper and lower extremities is RA. The metacarpophalangeal (MCP) joints and proximal interphalangeal (PIP) joints of the fingers, metatarsophalangeal (MTP) joints of the feet, and wrists are commonly affected, while the distal interphalangeal (DIP) joints, lumbar spine, and sacroiliac joints are spared. Inflammatory arthritis in an RA pattern but also involving the DIP joints of the fingers should always suggest psoriatic arthritis or multicentric reticulohistiocytosis. Any patient with inflammatory arthritis involving both ankles predominantly should be evaluated for acute sarcoid arthropathy.

A number of non-inflammatory disorders may cause a chronic polyarthritis. The most common of these is primary generalized osteoarthritis, which typically involves the DIPs, PIPs, and first carpometacarpal (CMC) joint of the fingers, hips, knees, and first MTP. Hemochromatosis and calcium pyrophosphate disease (CPPD) should be considered in a patient with chronic non-inflammatory polyarthritis involving the MCPs, wrists, shoulders, and ankles, which are joints not typically involved with osteoarthritis.

Oligoarticular arthritis refers to arthritis at two to four separate joints. The joint distribution is typically asymmetric. The most common causes of an acute or

and is commonly seen in RA and other systemic rheumatic diseases. A *migratory* pattern refers to symptoms being present in certain joints for a few days and then remit, only to reappear in other joints. This pattern is most characteristic of rheumatic fever, the early phases of Neisserial infection and Lyme disease, and acute childhood leukemia. An *intermittent* pattern is typified by repetitive attacks of acute polyarthritis with complete remission between attacks. A prolonged period of observation may be necessary to establish this pattern. Palindromic rheumatism, crystal-induced diseases, familial Mediterranean fever, and Whipple's disease can intermittently affect joints for a few to several days at a time, followed by asymptomatic periods of varying length over a number of years. RA, relapsing seronegative symmetrical synovitis with pitting edema (RS3PE syndrome), systemic lupus erythematosus (SLE), sarcoidosis, and Still's disease can also appear episodically, particularly early in their disease course. The seronegative spondyloarthropathies may have an intermittent course, but the articular symptoms in these diseases last for weeks (not days) at a time before resolving. The self-limited nature of these intermittent arthritides are a valuable discriminating feature used to narrow the differential diagnosis.

chronic inflammatory oligoarticular arthritis are the seronegative spondyloarthropathies. An asymmetric oligoarthritis involving scattered DIP and PIP finger joints characterizes psoriatic arthritis. The lower extremity inflammatory oligoarthritis involving knees and ankles asymmetrically is typical of an HLA-B27–associated reactive arthritis or an enteropathic arthritis due to inflammatory bowel disease (IBD). Dactylitis due to inflammation of the small joints of the toes and enthesitis due to inflammation at sites of ligament/tendon insertion into bone are frequently seen in reactive arthritis. Some diseases, such as septic arthritis and crystalline disease, that characteristically present as a monoarticular inflammatory arthritis may have an oligoarticular onset. The most common cause of a non-inflammatory asymmetric oligoarthritis is osteoarthritis.

Axial involvement of the spine in a patient presenting with peripheral polyarthritis is an important clue to the diagnosis. Up to 25% of patients with ankylosing spondylitis may present with hip or knee oligoarthritis, but eventually all will have evidence of inflammatory sacroiliitis and spondylitis characterized by night pain and prolonged morning stiffness that improves with exercise. Patients with psoriatic arthritis, reactive arthritis, or enteropathic arthritis associated with IBD can have evidence of inflammatory sacroiliitis/spondylitis in 25% of cases. Apart from the sacroiliac joints and spine, centrally located joints, such as the sternoclavicular and manubriosternal joints, and chest wall can also be involved. The most common non-inflammatory cause of polyarthritis affecting both peripheral joints and the spine simultaneously is osteoarthritis.

Associated Extra-Articular Symptoms and Medical Conditions

The presence of past or current extra-articular manifestations may provide important clues to the etiology of polyarticular arthritis (Table 3B-3). Fever suggests a subset of illness including infection (viral, bacterial), postinfectious (rheumatic fever, reactive arthritis), systemic rheumatic diseases (RA, SLE, Still's disease, vasculitis, IBD), crystal-induced diseases (gout, pseudogout), and miscellaneous diseases (malignancy, sarcoidosis, mucocutaneous disorders) (7). Night sweats and weight loss may also be important. Rashes such as psoriatic plaques, erythema migrans (Lyme disease), erythema nodosum (IBD, sarcoidosis), erythema marginatum (rheumatic fever), and butterfly malar rash (SLE), among others, can be particularly useful in the diagnosis. Other potentially important diagnostic clues are a history of Raynaud's disease, serositis, oral ulcers (IBD, Behçet's disease), or involvement of the lungs, heart, kidney, or liver (Table 3B-3). Other important associated symptoms include a history of diarrhea, abdominal pain, urethral discharge, low back pain, and uveitis, which may indicate a reactive arthritis or other spondyloarthropathy.

A review of a patient's concomitant medical conditions, medications, travel, and social history is important. Certain disorders, like renal insufficiency, obesity, and alcoholism, or use of medications such as diuretics and cyclosporine, among others, are associated with gouty arthritis, while hyperparathyroidism and hemochromatosis are associated with chondrocalcinosis and pseudogout. The sexual history should be elicited to help exclude reactive arthritis, gonococcal arthritis, and human immunodeficiency virus (HIV) exposures. A history of blood transfusions or intravenous drug use puts patients at risk for hepatitis B, hepatitis C, HIV, or septic arthritis. The use of certain medications, such as procainamide, hydralazine, and minocycline, can cause drug-induced lupus. Travel history or a history of a tick bite in an endemic area may indicate Lyme disease. Frequent exposure to children may predispose to parvovirus infection and rheumatic fever. Tobacco abuse may indicate lung cancer in a patient with hypertrophic osteoarthropathy.

Demographics and Family History

The sex, age, and ethnicity of the patient may help narrow the differential in a patient with polyarthritis. Juvenile idiopathic arthritis occurs in children under age 16 years. Young adult women are the most likely group to develop disseminated gonococcal arthritis, parvovirus, rubella arthritis, and SLE, and rarely develop gout unless they have an underlying metabolic disorder. Young adult men are more likely to develop ankylosing spondylitis, reactive arthritis, HIV- and hepatitis C-related arthritis. RA and osteoarthritis of the fingers are most frequently seen in middle-aged women, whereas gout and hemochromatosis are more common in middle-aged men. Individuals 55 to 60 years of age are more likely to have primary generalized osteoarthritis, CPPD disease, and polymyalgia rheumatica. African Americans have a high prevalence of SLE and sarcoidosis, while Asians have more gout. Caucasians are more likely to develop a seronegative spondyloarthropathy, polymyalgia rheumatica, hemochromatosis, and celiac disease. Certain regions of the world have a higher prevalence of specific diseases, such as Lyme disease in southern New England, the mid-Atlantic states, upper Midwest, and northern California. Rheumatic fever is more likely to occur in various South American and Asian nations, while Behçet's disease is more frequent in Japan and the eastern Mediterranean. Family history is important but can be difficult to obtain accurately. It may be especially important in a patient with oligo- or polyarthritis who has a family history of gout, pseudogout, psoriasis, ankylosing spondylitis, rheumatoid arthritis, or SLE.

TABLE 3B-3. SYSTEMIC AND ORGAN INVOLVEMENT ASSOCIATED WITH POLYARTHROPATHY.

DISORDER	Fever	Lungs	Eye	Gastrointestinal system or liver	Heart	Kidney
Amyloidosis	–	–	–	✓	✓	✓
Bacterial arthritis	✓	–	–	–	–	–
Bacterial endocarditis	✓	–	–	–	✓	✓
Behçet's disease	–	–	✓	–	–	–
Crystal-induced arthritis	✓	–	–	–	–	–
Erythema nodosum	✓	–	✓	–	–	–
Familial Mediterranean fever	✓	✓	–	✓	–	–
Hemochromatosis	–	–	–	✓	✓	–
Hypertrophic osteoarthropathy	–	✓	–	–	–	–
Inflammatory bowel disease	✓	–	✓	✓	–	–
Juvenile idiopathic arthritis	–	–	✓	–	✓	–
Leukemia	✓	–	✓	–	–	–
Lyme disease	✓	–	–	–	✓	–
Polymyositis/dermatomyositis	–	✓	–	–	✓	–
Reactive arthritis	✓	–	✓	✓	–	–
Relapsing polychondritis	✓	✓	✓	–	✓	–
Rheumatic fever	✓	✓	–	–	✓	–
Rheumatoid arthritis	–	✓	✓	–	✓	–
Sarcoidosis	✓	✓	✓	–	✓	–
Seronegative spondyloarthropathy	–	–	✓	✓	✓	–
Sjögren's syndrome	–	✓	✓	–	–	–
Still's disease	✓	✓	✓	–	✓	–
Systemic lupus erythematosus	✓	✓	–	✓	✓	✓
Systemic sclerosis	–	✓	–	✓	✓	✓
Systemic vasculitis	✓	✓	✓	✓	✓	✓
Viral arthritis	✓	–	–	–	–	–
Whipple's disease	✓	✓	✓	✓	✓	–

Physical Examination

The physical examination should be used to verify the presence of historical features as well as additional findings the patient may have not reported. Vital signs can help determine the severity of the illness with fever being most important. Other findings on general examination that suggest a systemic disorder include lymph-adenopathy, parotid enlargement, oral and genital ulcers, eye disease (conjunctivitis, uveitis, scleritis, keratoconjunctivitis sicca, funduscopic abnormalities), heart murmurs (subacute bacterial endocarditis [SBE], rheumatic fever), bruits, pericardial or pleural friction rubs, fine inspiratory rales due to interstitial lung disease, hepatosplenomegaly, muscle weakness (polymyositis), and any neurologic abnormalities (vasculitis). Particular attention should be given to the skin and nails, looking for characteristic rashes or nodules (rheumatoid, tophi, or, rarely, xanthomas or amyloid masses).

In addition to symptomatic joints, all 66 joint areas should be examined. Particular attention should be given to the spine examination to rule out an underlying axial arthritis. Upon examination of the symptomatic joints, the presence or absence of synovitis should be documented. The detection of synovitis limits the differential diagnosis to an inflammatory arthritis and is characterized by diffuse involvement of the joint with tenderness, soft tissue swelling, warmth over the joint, and possibly a joint effusion. Significant erythema should suggest an infectious or crystalline arthropathy. Active and passive range of motion will be limited in all planes. Crepitus may be heard or felt as the joint is put through a range of motion. Fine crepitus can arise from synovitis, while more medium crepitus can arise from grating of roughened cartilage surfaces or from bone rubbing against bone. The examination of symptomatic joints in patients with a non-inflammatory arthritis typically shows diffuse involvement with tenderness, bony enlargement or spurs, minimal if any warmth, and no erythema. An effusion, particularly in the knee, may be demonstrated. Range of motion is limited, both passively and actively, in all planes, and medium or coarse crepitus may be felt.

The musculoskeletal examination may reveal other characteristic findings to help narrow the diagnostic possibilities. Tenosynovitis causes tenderness and swelling along the track of the tendon between joints; it is a characteristic feature of RA, gout, reactive arthritis, and gonococcal arthritis, being distinctly uncommon in other causes of polyarthritis. Diffuse bilateral hand edema can be seen in the RS3PE syndrome, mixed connective tissue disease, scleroderma, polymyalgia rheumatica, RA, and, rarely, psoriatic arthritis. Diffuse swelling of all fingers is seen in hypertrophic osteoarthropathy and thyroid acropachy. Painful thickening of the palmar area of the hands with contractures of the fingers may occur in association with neoplastic conditions such as ovarian cancer.

Laboratory Studies

A limited number of laboratory tests are helpful in the evaluation of polyarthritis. A complete blood count, biochemical tests of renal and liver function, and a urinalysis may help to identify patients with a systemic illness. Serum uric acid levels are usually elevated in gout but can be normal, particularly in patients with a polyarticular onset. Additional tests should be ordered, depending on the clinical suspicion. For example, iron studies should be ordered in a patient suspected of having hemochromatosis who has osteoarthritis affecting atypical joints, while an HLA-B27 test may be useful in a patient with a suspected undifferentiated spondyloarthropathy.

An elevated erythrocyte sedimentation rate (ESR) and C-reactive protein (CRP) are not specific but are elevated in over 90% of patients with an inflammatory cause for their polyarthritis. Unfortunately, patients with non-inflammatory arthritides may have an elevated ESR/CRP because of another problem such as diabetes, dysproteinemia, or occult malignancy. Specific antibody tests can identify exposure to potential pathogens such as Group A streptococcus (antistreptolysin O antibody), parvovirus B19, hepatitis B and C, Epstein–Barr virus, and *Borrelia burgdorferi* (Lyme disease) and should be ordered when these diseases are suspected clinically.

Autoantibodies, including rheumatoid factor and antinuclear antibodies (ANA), can be seen in a variety of diseases. Rheumatoid factor should be ordered in patients suspected to have RA but can also be present in high titers in patients with other diseases which can cause a polyarthritis resembling RA, such as SLE, subacute bacterial endocarditis, and hepatitis C. The ANA test has high sensitivity but low specificity for SLE. A negative ANA rules out SLE whereas a positive ANA with specific antibodies to double-stranded DNA or Smith (Sm) are virtually diagnostic of SLE in a patient with polyarthritis.

Synovial fluid should be obtained for total white blood cell count, crystal examination, and cultures when the diagnosis remains uncertain after history, physical examination, and standard laboratory tests. Synovial fluid is only diagnostic in patients with infections, gout, and pseudogout. Otherwise, synovial fluid analysis can only classify the polyarthritis as inflammatory (>2000 WBC/mm^3) or non-inflammatory based on the synovial fluid WBC count.

Radiographic Studies

In an appropriate clinical setting, plain radiographs may be supportive of a particular diagnosis. The findings of chondrocalcinosis and osteoarthritic changes suggest, but do not prove, these diagnoses without corresponding synovial fluid analysis. In acute polyarthritis, radiographs lack specificity and usually only show soft tissue swelling and intra-articular fluid. In chronic inflammatory polyarthritis, marginal joint erosions are seen earliest in the small joints of the hands, wrists, and feet in patients with RA. Chronic gout can also cause erosions with an overhanging edge that typically involve small peripheral joints such as the first MTP joint. Radiographs of the axial skeleton may show sacroiliitis early in the course of ankylosing spondylitis or other seronegative spondyloarthropathies. Syndesmophytes are seen in more longstanding disease. Magnetic resonance imaging is more sensitive than plain radiographs in demonstrating erosions early in the course of RA or sacroiliitis in patients with a recent onset of a seronegative spondyloarthropathy.

Tissue Biopsy

Rarely will a diagnosis of polyarthritis depend on a biopsy of synovium or other tissues. However, tissue biopsy may be helpful in establishing a diagnosis of Whipple's disease, Lyme disease, sarcoidosis, amyloidosis, hemochromatosis, leukemia, and multicentric reticulohistiocytosis.

DIFFERENTIAL DIAGNOSIS

In addition to polyarthritis, there are several other disorders that need to be considered in the patient presenting with polyarticular pain. These patients may complain of joint pain, but the joint examination will be normal with full passive range of motion and no evidence of synovitis. The most common disorder causing polyarticular symptoms is fibromyalgia manifested as diffuse pain, characteristic tender points in periarticular areas, and normal joint examination, laboratories, and radiographs. Another important cause of diffuse pain is depression. Patients with psychogenic factors contributing to their joint pain typically have pain that does not change with rest and activity and may have severe fatigue. Their joint examination, however, will be normal. A common cause of oligoarticular pain is multiple areas of tendinitis or bursitis. This manifests as localized joint pain in specific areas that may cause limitation of active range of motion in only one plane with preserved passive range of motion. Other less common but important disorders causing polyarticular pain include muscle disorders, neuropathies, hypothyroidism, primary bone diseases (osteomalacia, Paget's disease, osteonecrosis, stress fractures), myeloma, metastatic cancer, vasculitis, vaso-occlusive diseases (emboli), and malingering.

SPECIFIC DISEASES CAUSING POLYARTHRITIS

The preceding discussion emphasizes that the key to the correct diagnosis of polyarticular pain is an accurate history and physical examination supported by laboratory and radiographic tests. What follows is an abbreviated discussion of the most common diseases causing certain patterns of polyarthritis. Notably, several of these diseases may have more than one presentation, may change their articular pattern over time, or may have an atypical course.

Acute Inflammatory Polyarthritis

Viral Arthritis

A common cause of acute inflammatory polyarthritis is *parvovirus B19–associated arthritis*. It occurs most commonly in young women with frequent exposure to young children. This self-limited polyarthritis resembles acute RA with morning stiffness and symmetric involvement of the hands and wrists, often lasting for weeks. The typical viral exanthem may be absent. The diagnosis is confirmed serologically. A similar arthritis can be seen with *hepatitis B*, *HIV*, *Epstein–Barr virus (EBV)*, and *rubella*. Hepatitis B–associated arthritis precedes other signs of hepatitis and is often accompanied by an urticarial rash. Acute HIV and EBV can resemble SLE with fever, rash, polyarthritis, hematologic abnormalities, and a positive ANA.

Rheumatic Fever

Acute rheumatic fever in children typically presents with fever and a migratory arthritis that involves several joints simultaneously but persists in each joint for only a few days. In adults, the arthritis is typically less acute, additive, of longer duration, and has been termed *post-streptococcal reactive arthritis*. Large joints of the lower extremities are most commonly involved. Carditis, erythema marginatum, and chorea, which can occur in childhood, are rare in adults. Streptococcal pharyngitis is commonly asymptomatic. Therefore, serologic evidence should be sought in all patients with polyarthritis and fever. The fever usually fluctuates without returning to normal for a week or more. In children, the fever and arthritis respond well to high dose aspirin therapy, while in adults the response is less dramatic.

Rheumatic Diseases

Adult and juvenile *rheumatoid arthritis* and *psoriatic arthritis* can present as acute polyarthritis but typically have a more insidious onset. Both children and adults can develop *Still's disease*, which is characterized by high spiking fevers, polyarthritis, pericarditis, an evanescent truncal rash, neutrophilic leukocytosis, and the absence of a rheumatoid factor and ANA. The fever characteristically spikes up to 104°F once or twice a day and returns to normal or below normal between fever spikes. The synovitis may be intermittent initially, but a persistent polyarthritis develops in most patients.

Systemic lupus erythematosus may present with acute polyarthritis that can be additive, migratory, or intermittent and may occur with fever. Characteristic rashes, other extra-articular manifestations, and a positive ANA support the diagnosis. *Relapsing seronegative symmetrical synovitis with pitting edema* (RS3PE) is associated with marked joint stiffness and symmetric polysynovitis involving the hands and feet. The onset is abrupt. Profound pitting edema of the hands may lead to carpal tunnel syndrome, and large joints can be involved. It is typically seen in patients over the age of 60 and is more common in men. Patients with *polymyalgia rheumatica* can have a similar presentation.

Other Systemic Illnesses

Acute leukemia in children may cause recurrent acute episodes of arthritis and bone pain. *Acute sarcoid arthritis* usually is accompanied by fever, erythema nodosum, and hilar adenopathy. Marked periarticular swelling and erythema in both ankles is characteristic of this disease.

Acute Inflammatory Oligoarthritis
Infectious Arthritis

Bacterial septic arthritis usually presents as a monoarthritis, but in 10% to 20% of adults can involve two or more large joints. Risk factors for this presentation include immunosuppression, intravenous drug use, and preexisting joint disease such as RA. In contrast, *gonococcal and meningococcal arthritis* frequently involve more than one joint and may present with a migratory pattern. Vesiculopustular skin lesions on the extremities may provide an important diagnostic clue. Tenosynovitis frequently is found in the wrist and ankle extensor tendon sheaths. Synovial fluid cultures are usually sterile early in the course, but blood cultures may be diagnostic. *Fungal and mycobacterial* infections typically cause a chronic monarthritis but in immunosuppressed patients can rarely cause an acute oligoarticular arthritis. *Bacterial endocarditis* may present with fever, back pain, and arthralgias. A minority of the patients have large joint oligoarticular arthritis, usually of the lower extremities. Synovial fluid cultures are sterile, and rheumatoid factor may be positive. Endocarditis should be suspected in anyone with a heart murmur and fever. Blood cultures will be confirmatory.

Crystalline Arthritis

Crystal-induced arthritis is generally monoarticular but may present as an acute oligoarticular arthritis, often with fever. Typically, joint pain comes on suddenly and reaches a maximum intensity within hours. The joints are warm and erythematous, and swelling extends to the soft tissues well beyond the joint. *Gouty arthritis* usually affects the feet, especially the first MTP joint, and tophi

may be present. *Pseudogout* as a presentation of CPPD favors the wrist and knee, and occurs primarily in elderly patients. In each disease, demonstration of appropriate crystals in the synovial fluid confirms the diagnosis. Radiographs may show typical erosions in chronic gout or chondrocalcinosis in CPPD disease.

Rheumatic Diseases

Reactive arthritis due to prior enteric or genitourinary infection may present with fever and an acute sterile lower extremity oligoarticular arthritis. Dactylitis, inflammatory back pain, and extra-articular manifestations of conjunctivitis, uveitis, oral ulcers, or characteristic rashes support the diagnosis. A similar large joint oligoarticular arthritis may occur in patients with active *inflammatory bowel disease*. It usually remits when the bowel disease is suppressed. Palindromic *rheumatism* causes recurrent attacks of acute synovitis in one to five joints at a time with irregular, symptom-free intervals between attacks. The pattern of joints involved tends to be the same in an individual patient. Attacks are sudden and pain intense, often reaching a peak within a few hours. In some patients, this presentation may be the earliest manifestation of RA or SLE, particularly if they have positive serologies.

Other Systemic Diseases

Familial Mediterranean fever is characterized by irregular attacks lasting 1 to 3 days of fever, abdominal pain, and arthritis with onset in childhood. Arthritic attacks typically involve one or more lower extremity joints. Although pain is severe, joint erythema and warmth are notably absent. *Carcinomatous polyarthritis* is a seronegative, lower extremity large joint arthritis with an explosive onset that occurs in close temporal relationship with the diagnosis of a malignancy. The arthritis improves with treatment of the underlying cancer. Episodic arthritis and periarthritis have been described in some types of *hyperlipoproteinemia*.

Chronic Inflammatory Polyarthritis

Patients with inflammatory polyarthritis and oligoarticular arthritis of less than 3 months duration are the most difficult to classify accurately. The most important factor is to identify patients who are likely to have persistent arthritis that might cause joint injury. Recently, a prediction model based upon data from over 500 patients with early arthritis demonstrated that a combination of clinical, laboratory, and radiographic data could predict which patients were at risk for developing persistent and/or erosive disease (6). The seven most important features included: (1) symptoms lasting over 12 weeks;

(2) morning stiffness lasting over 1 hour; (3) demonstrable synovitis in three or more joint areas; (4) pain with metatarsal compression; (5) positive rheumatoid factor; (6) positive anti-cyclic citrullinated protein (CCP) antibodies; and (7) erosions on radiographs of the hands or feet. Not surprisingly most of these patients have or will develop RA. However, many patients with early inflammatory polyarthritis have only a couple of these features yet will manifest a persistent arthritis that defies classification. Two recent studies have emphasized that 25% to 30% of patients presenting with early synovitis continue to have an undifferentiated polyarthritis even after 1 to 2 years of follow-up (6,9). This is an important group, as up to 42% have progressive disease that will need therapy (9).

The remainder of this section will discuss causes of chronic inflammatory polyarthritis that can be classified.

Rheumatoid Arthritis

Adult and juvenile *rheumatoid arthrtis* is the most common cause of a chronic inflammatory polyarthritis. Approximately 30% to 40% of patients presenting to an early polyarthritis clinic have RA (5,6). Patients classically present with a symmetric polyarthritis that usually affects MCPs, PIPs, wrists, and MTPs. Other patients may have an additive pattern with an oligoarticular onset. Prolonged morning stiffness upon awakening and gelling after periods of inactivity are common. Proliferative synovitis of symptomatic joints may lead to deformities and erosions on radiographs. Extra-articular manifestations include subcutaneous nodules (25%), pleural effusions, episcleritis, and vasculitis, among others. Rheumatoid factor is positive in 70% to 85% of patients, while anti-CCP is positive in only 50% to 60% of patients, but is more specific (95%).

Psoriatic Arthritis

Psoriatic arthritis can have several presentations. The typical onset is as an oligoarticular arthritis that may evolve into a symmetric small and large joint polyarthritis resembling RA. The involvement of the DIP joints, presence of psoriatic plaques, and the absence of rheumatoid factor support the diagnosis.

Systemic Rheumatic Disease

Systemic lupus erythematosus frequently presents as a symmetric polyarthritis that may be confused with RA if other extra-articular manifestations have not yet appeared. The arthritis may be migratory or intermittent and extremely painful. Synovial proliferation is not as evident as with RA but can lead to RA-like deformities. Notably, articular erosions are not present on radiographs, even in patients with a deforming arthritis. *Drug-induced lupus* presents with a symmetric polyarthritis associated with systemic manifestations such as fever and serositis. Other systemic rheumatic diseases can have an inflammatory polyarthritis, including *mixed connective tissue disease* and *systemic sclerosis*. Patients with these diseases will also have Raynaud's disease and skin thickening. Patients with *polymyositis* and *dermatomyositis* may have a polyarthritis accompanied by proximal muscle weakness and/or a characteristic rash.

Other Systemic Illnesses

Hepatitis C viral infection may be associated with a chronic polyarthritis resembling RA. These patients may have a high titer rheumatoid factor but negative anti-CCP antibodies and no erosions on radiographs. Cryoblobulinemia, hypocomplementemia, and vasculitis may be seen. Any patient with polyarthritis and elevated liver-associated enzymes should be evaluated for hepatitis C infection. *Multicentric reticulohistiocytosis* can also cause a destructive arthritis that mimics RA. Involvement of the DIP joints and the presence of periungual nodules should help define the diagnosis.

Chronic Inflammatory Oligoarticular Arthritis with or Without Axial Involvement

Seronegative Spondyloarthropathies

This group includes ankylosing spondylitis, psoriatic arthritis, reactive arthritis, and enteropathic arthritis related to IBD. These diseases are the most common cause of an asymmetric oligoarticular inflammatory arthritis. Dactylitis and enthesopathy are common findings. The sacroiliac joints and spine are frequently involved. *Ankylosing spondylitis* may present with peripheral arthritis (25%), typically of the hips, shoulders, and knees. Some may also develop an acute anterior uveitis, while all will eventually have inflammatory low back pain and stiffness leading to bilateral sacroiliitis and possibly syndesmophytes on radiographs. This disease occurs primarily in Caucasian males less than age 40 and has a strong association with HLA-B27. *Psoriatic arthritis* most commonly presents with an oligoarticular upper extremity arthritis with DIP involvement, while *reactive arthritis* and *enteropathic arthritis associated with IBD* cause a lower extremity oligoarticular arthritis involving knees, ankles, and toes. Sacroiliitis can be present in 25% and characteristically is unilateral or asymmetric on radiographs.

Musculoskeletal Signs and Symptoms
C. Neck and Back Pain

DAVID BORENSTEIN, MD

- Low back pain is one of the most common symptoms, being second only to the common cold.
- The role of the physician is to separate mechanical from systemic causes of neck and low back pain.

- For most people with low back pain, radiographs and laboratory tests are not necessary.

Low back and neck pain are second only to the common cold as the most common affliction of mankind. Approximately 10% to 20% of the US population has back or neck pain each year (1). Low back pain is the fifth most common reason for visiting a physician, according to a US National Ambulatory Care Survey (2).

The symptom of axial skeleton pain is associated with a wide variety of mechanical and systemic disorders (Table 3C-1) (3). Mechanical disorders of the axial skeleton are caused by overuse (muscle strain), trauma, or physical deformity of an anatomic structure (herniated intervertebral disc). Systemic disorders that cause spine pain are associated with constitutional symptoms, disease in other organ systems, and inflammatory or infiltrative disease of the axial skeleton. Mechanical disorders cause the vast majority of low back or neck pain episodes. Characteristically, mechanical disorders are exacerbated by certain physical activities and are relieved by others, and most of these disorders resolve over a short period of time. More than 50% of all patients will improve after 1 week, and up to 90% may improve by 8 weeks. However, a recurrence of spinal pain occurs in up to 75% of people over the next year. Back pain will persist for 1 year and longer in 10% of the spinal pain population (4).

INITIAL EVALUATION

In the initial evaluation of patients with spinal pain, the physician *must* separate individuals with mechanical disorders from those with systemic illnesses. The patient's symptoms and physical signs help differentiate mechanical from systemic causes of axial pain. The initial diagnostic evaluation includes a history and physical examination with complete evaluation of the musculoskeletal system, including palpation of the axial skeleton and assessment of range of motion and alignment of the spine. Neurologic examination to detect evidence of spinal cord, spinal root, or peripheral nerve dysfunction is essential. In most patients, radiographic and laboratory tests are not necessary. Plain radiographs and erythrocyte sedimentation rate (ESR) are most informative in patients who are 50 years or older, who have a previous history of cancer, or who have constitutional symptoms (5).

The initial evaluation should eliminate the presence of cauda equina syndrome and cervical myelopathy, which are rare conditions that require emergency interventions. *Cauda equina compression* is characterized by low back pain, bilateral motor weakness of the lower extremities, bilateral sciatica, saddle anesthesia, and bladder or bowel incontinence. The common causes of cauda equina compression include central herniation of an intervertebral disc, epidural abscess or hematoma, or tumor masses. In the cervical spine, myelopathy with long tract signs (e.g., spasticity, clonus, positive Babinski's sign, incontinence) indicate compression of the spinal cord. The common causes of myelopathy include disc herniation and osteophytic overgrowth. If cauda equina syndrome or cervical myelopathy is suspected, radiographic evaluation is mandatory. Magnetic resonance imaging (MRI) is the most sensitive radiographic technique for visualizing

TABLE 3C-1. DISORDERS AFFECTING THE LOW BACK AND/OR NECK.

Mechanical
Muscle strain
Herniated intervertebral disc
Osteoarthritis
Spinal stenosis
Spinal stenosis with myelopathy[a]
Spondylolysis/spondylolisthesis[b]
Adult scoliosis[b]
Whiplash[a]

Rheumatologic
Ankylosing spondylitis
Reactive arthritis
Psoriatic arthritis
Osteochondroma
Enteropathic arthritis
Rheumatoid arthritis[a]
Diffuse idiopathic skeletal hyperostosis
Vertebral osteochondritis[b]
Polymyalgia rheumatica
Fibromyalgia
Behçet's syndrome[b]
Whipple's disease[b]
Hidradenitis suppurativa[b]
Osteitis condensans ilii[b]
Behcet's syndrome[b]
Whipple's disease[b]

Endocrinologic/Metabolic
Osteoporosis[b]
Osteomalacia[b]
Parathyroid disease[b]
Microcrystalline disease
Ochronosis[b]
Fluorosis[b]
Heritable genetic disorders

Neurologic/Psychiatric
Neuropathic arthropathy[b]
Neuropathies
Tumors
Vasculitis
Compression
Psychogenic rheumatism
Depression
Malingering

Miscellaneous
Paget's disease
Vertebral sarcoidosis
Subacute bacterial endocarditis[b]
Retroperitoneal fibrosis[b]

Infectious
Vertebral osteomyelitis
Meningitis[a]
Discitis
Pyogenic sacroiliitis[b]
Herpes zoster
Lyme disease

Neoplastic/Infiltrative
Benign tumors
    Osteoid osteoma
    Osteoblastoma
    Giant cell tumor
    Aneurysmal bone cyst
    Hemangioma
    Eosinophilic granuloma
    Gaucher's disease[b]
    Sacroiliac lipoma[b]
Malignant tumors
    Skeletal metastases
    Multiple myeloma
    Chondrosarcoma
    Chordoma
    Lymphoma[b]
Intraspinal lesions
    Metastases
Meningioma
    Vascular malformations
    Gliomas
    Syringomyelia[a]

Hematologic
Hemoglobinopathies[b]
    Myelofibrosis[b]
    Mastocytosis[b]

Referred Pain
Vascular
    Abdominal aorta[b]
    Carotid[a]
    Thoracic aorta[a]
Gastrointestinal
    Pancreas
    Gallbladder
Intestine
    Esophagus[a]
Genitourinary
Kidney
    Ureter
    Bladder
    Uterus
    Ovary
    Prostate

SOURCE: Modified from Borenstein DG, Wiesel SW, Boden SD. Low back and neck pain: comprehensive diagnosis and management. Philadelphia: Saunders; 2004.
[a] Neck predominant.
[b] Low back predominant.

the spine. If the clinician's suspicion is confirmed, surgical decompression of the compromised neural elements is indicated with best results with surgery within 48 hours of onset of symptoms (6).

SYSTEMIC DISORDERS

The majority of people with spinal pain and systemic illnesses can be identified by the presence of one or more of the following: fever or weight loss; pain with recumbency; prolonged morning stiffness; localized bone pain; or visceral pain.

Fever and Weight Loss

In people with a history of fever or weight loss, spinal pain frequently is caused by an infection or tumor (7). Vertebral osteomyelitis causes pain that is slowly progressive, may be either intermittent or constant, is present at rest, and is exacerbated by motion. Tumor pain progresses more rapidly. Plain radiographs generally are not helpful unless more than 30% of the bone calcium has been lost in the area of the lesion. Bone scintigraphy is a sensitive but nonspecific test for bone lesions. Areas of bony involvement and soft tissue extension are identified best by computed tomography (CT) or MRI, respectively.

Pain with Recumbency

Tumors, benign or malignant, of the spinal column or spinal cord are the prime concern in patients with nocturnal pain or pain with recumbency (8). Compression of neural elements by expanding masses and associated inflammation accounts for the pain. Physical examination demonstrates localized tenderness, and if the spinal cord or roots are compressed, neurologic dysfunction. MRI is the most sensitive method to detect bony abnormalities, spinal cord or root compromise, and soft tissue extension of neoplastic lesions.

Morning Stiffness

Morning stiffness lasting an hour or less is a common symptom of mechanical spinal disorders. In contrast, morning stiffness of the lumbar or cervical spine lasting several hours is a common symptom of seronegative spondyloarthropathy. Bilateral sacroiliac pain is associated with ankylosing spondylitis and enteropathic arthritis, while reactive arthritis and psoriatic spondylitis may have unilateral sacroiliac pain, or spondylitis without sacroiliitis. Women with spondyloarthropathy may have neck pain and stiffness with minimal low back pain. On physical examination, these patients demon-

strate stiffness in all planes of spinal motion. Plain radiographs of the lumbosacral spine are helpful for identifying early changes, loss of lumbar lordosis, joint erosions in the lower one third of the sacroiliac joints, and squaring of vertebral bodies. More costly radiographic tests are not necessary to identify skeletal abnormalities in patients with spondylitis.

Localized Bone Pain

Spinal pain localized to the midline over osseous structures is associated with disorders that fracture or expand bone. Any systemic process that increases mineral loss from bone (osteoporosis), causes bone necrosis (hemoglobinopathy), or replaces bone cells with inflammatory or neoplastic cells (multiple myeloma) weakens vertebral bone to the point that fractures may occur spontaneously or with minimal trauma. Patients with acute fractures experience sudden onset of pain. Bone pain may be the initial manifestation of the underlying disorder. On physical examination, palpation of the affected area produces pain. Plain radiographs may reveal alterations but do not show microfractures. Scintigraphy can detect increased bone activity soon after a fracture occurs, and a CT scan may identify the abnormality. However, locating the lesion is not sufficient to define the specific cause of the bony changes. Laboratory tests including ESR, serum chemistries, and complete blood count are most helpful in differentiating between metabolic and neoplastic disorders that cause localized bone pain.

Visceral Pain

Abnormalities in organs that share segmental innervation with part of the axial skeleton can cause referred back pain. Viscerogenic pain may arise as a result of vascular, gastrointestinal, or genitourinary disorders. The duration and sequence of back pain follows the periodicity of the diseased organ. Colicky pain is associated with spasm in a hollow structure, such as the ureter, colon, or gallbladder. Throbbing pain occurs with vascular lesions. Exertional pain that radiates into the left arm in a C7 distribution may be associated with angina and coronary artery disease. Back pain that coincides with a woman's menstrual cycle may be related to endometriosis.

Physical examination of the abdomen may reveal tenderness over the diseased organ. Laboratory tests are useful to document the presence of an abnormality in the genitourinary (hematuria) or gastrointestinal (amylase) systems. Radiographic tests are helpful for diagnosing some visceral disorders. For example, a CT of the aorta can show abdominal aneurysm and a barium swallow test can reveal esophageal diverticulum.

MECHANICAL DISORDERS OF THE LUMBOSACRAL SPINE

Mechanical disorders are the most common causes of low back pain. They include muscle strain, herniated nucleus pulposus, osteoarthritis, spinal stenosis, spondylolisthesis, and adult scoliosis. The clinical characteristics of these disorders are listed in Table 3C-2.

Back Strain

Back strain is preceded by some traumatic event that can range from coughing or sneezing to lifting an object heavier than can be supported by the muscles and ligaments of the lumbosacral spine (9). The typical history of muscle strain is acute back pain that radiates up the ipsilateral paraspinous muscles, across the lumbar area, and sometimes caudally to the buttocks without radiation to the thigh. Physical examination reveals limited range of motion in the lumbar area, with paraspinous muscle contraction. No neurologic abnormalities are present.

The Agency for Health Care Policy and Research published an evidence-based review of the effective therapies for acute low back pain in 1994 (Table 3C-3) (10). Therapy that combines controlled physical activity with nonsteroidal anti-inflammatory drugs (NSAIDs) and muscle relaxants can help resolve acute low back pain (11).

Lumbar Disc Herniation

Intervertebral disc herniation causes nerve impingement and inflammation that results in radicular pain (sciatica). Herniation occurs with sudden movement, and frequently is associated with heavy lifting. Sciatica is exacerbated by activities that increase intradiscal pressure, such as sitting, bending, or Valsalva's maneuver. On physical examination, any movement that creates tension in the affected nerve, such as the straight-leg raising test, elicits radicular pain. Neurologic examination may reveal sensory deficit, asymmetry of reflexes, or motor weakness corresponding to the damaged spinal nerve root and degree of impingement (Table 3C-4). An MRI is the best technique to identify the location

TABLE 3C-2. MECHANICAL LOW BACK PAIN.

	SPINAL STENOSIS	BACK STRAIN	HERNIATED NUCLEUS PULPOSUS	OSTEOARTHRITIS
Age at onset	>60	20–40	30–50	>50
Pain Pattern				
Location	Back	Back/leg	Back	Leg
Onset	Acute	Acute	Insidious	Insidious
Upright	I	D	I	I
Sitting	D	I	D	D
Bending	I	I	D	D
SLR test	–	+	–	+(exertion)
Plain x-ray	–	–	+	+
CT/myelogram	–	+	+/–	+
MRI	–	+	+/–	+

	SPONDYLOLISTHESIS	ADULT SCOLIOSIS
Age at onset	20–30	20–40
Pain Pattern		
Location	Back	Back
Onset	Insidious	Insidious
Upright	I	I
Sitting	D	D
Bending	I	I
SLR	–	–
Plain x-ray	+	+
CT/myelogram	+	–
MRI	+/–	+/–

ABBREVIATIONS: I, increase; D, decrease; SLR, straight leg raising test.

TABLE 3C-3.   AHCPR GUIDELINE FOR ACUTE LOW BACK PAIN TREATMENT.

Patient Education
* Natural history of rapid recovery and recurrence
* Safe and effective methods of symptom control
* Activity modifications
* Limit recurrences
* Special investigations required when systemic disorders suspected
* Risks of common diagnostic tests
* Treatment recommendations for persistent symptoms

Medications
* Acetaminophen
* NSAIDs: decision based on comorbidities, toxicities, cost, patient preferences

Physical Treatments
* Spinal manipulation in the first month in the absence of radiculopathy (efficacy short term)

Activity Modification
* Bed rest no more than 4 days
* Gradual return to normal activities
* Low-impact aerobic exercise

SOURCE: From Agency for Health Care Policy and Research. Acute low back problems in adults, clinical practice guideline. Rockville, MD: Agency for Health Care Policy and Research; 1994. Publication no. 95-0642.

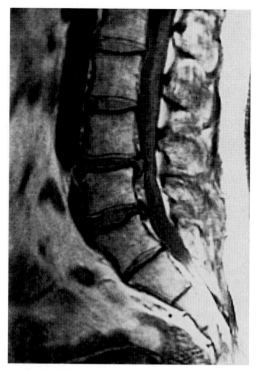

FIGURE 3C-1

Magnetic resonance scan sagittal view of a 45-year-old man with right leg radicular pain. The scan reveals herniated discs at the L3 to L4 and L4 to L5 levels.

of disc herniation and nerve impingement, but is significant only when correlated with clinical symptoms (Figures 3C-1 and 3C-2) (12). Large disc fragments that enhance with gadolinium during MRI examination are more likely to resorb spontaneously without the need for surgical excision (13). Electromyography (EMG) and nerve conduction tests may document abnormal nerve function after impingement has been present for 8 weeks or longer.

Therapy for disc herniation includes controlled physical activity, NSAIDs, and epidural corticosteroid injection. For most patients, radicular pain resolves in a 12-week period. Only 5% or fewer of patients with a herniated disc require surgical decompression (14).

Lumbosacral Spondylosis

Osteoarthritis of the lumbosacral spine may cause localized low back pain. As the intervertebral disc degenerates, intersegmental instability and approximation of the vertebral bodies shift the compressive forces across the zygapophyseal joints. The transition of these facet joints from nonweight-bearing to weight-bearing joints leads to zygapophyseal osteoarthritis (lumbosacral spondylosis). As a result, patients develop lumbar pain that increases at the end of the day and radiates across the low back. The disorder may progress, causing increased

TABLE 3C-4.   RADICULAR SYMPTOMS AND SIGNS.

	PAIN DISTRIBUTION	SENSORY LOSS	MOTOR LOSS	REFLEX LOSS
Lumbar				
4	Anterior thigh to medial leg	Medial leg to medial malleolus	Anterior tibialis	Patellar
5	Lateral leg to dorsum of foot	Lateral leg to dorsum of foot	Extensor hallucis longus	(Posterior tibial)
S1	Lateral foot	Lateral foot sole	Peroneus longus and brevis	Achilles
Cervical				
5	Neck to outer shoulder, arm	Shoulder	Deltoid	Biceps, supinator
6	Outer arm to thumb, index finger	Thumb, index fingers	Biceps, wrist extensors	Biceps, supinator
7	Outer arm to middle finger	Index, middle fingers	Triceps	Triceps
8	Inner arm to ring, little fingers	Ring, little fingers	Hand muscles	None

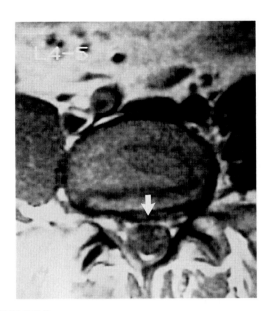

FIGURE 3C-2

Magnetic resonance scan axial view of L4 to L5 disc space demonstrating an extruded herniated disc (*white arrow*).

narrowing of the spinal canal that results in spinal stenosis and compression of neural elements (spinal stenosis). The clinical manifestation of spinal stenosis is neurogenic claudication. Physical examination reveals that pain worsens with extension of the spine, and no neurologic deficits are present. Pain radiates into the posterior thigh and is exacerbated by ipsilateral bending to the side with the osteoarthritic joints (facet syndrome). Oblique views of the lumbar spine demonstrate facet joint narrowing, periarticular sclerosis, and osteophytes (Figure 3C-3). These findings have significance only with clinical correlation with historical and physical factors (15).

Lumbar Spinal Stenosis

Spinal stenosis is secondary to the growth of osteophytes, redundancy of the ligamentum flavum, and posterior bulging of the intervertebral discs. Lumbar stenosis may be located in the center of the canal, the lateral recess, or the intervertebral foramen, and may occur at single or multiple levels. The pattern of radiation depends on the location of nerve compression. With central canal stenosis, pain in one or both legs occurs with walking. Unlike vascular claudication, leg pain appears after walking variable distances. Individuals with vascular claudication must stop walking to gain relief of pain, whereas those with neurogenic claudication must sit or flex forward, which increases *room* in the spinal canal and restores blood flow to the spinal roots to decrease pain.

Lateral stenosis causes unilateral leg pain with standing. Stenosis of the intervertebral foramen causes leg

pain that is persistent, regardless of the patient's position. The physical examination may be unrevealing unless the patient exercises to the point of developing symptoms. Sensory, motor, and reflex examination during the episode of pain reveals abnormal function that reverses when the pain disappears. Motor weakness is present in one third of patients, and one half have reflex abnormalities. Plain radiographs of the lumbar spine may demonstrate degenerative disc disease with zygapophyseal joint narrowing, even in patients who are asymptomatic. Thus, radiographic alterations are significant only if the patient has corresponding symptoms. A CT scan can identify the presence of zygapophyseal joint disease, trefoil configuration of the spinal canal, and reduced dimensions of the canal. An MRI can document the location of neural compression (see Figure 3C-1).

Prescribing NSAIDs and teaching patients appropriate spinal biomechanics are the initial therapies for osteoarthritis and spinal stenosis (16). Facet joint injections should be considered when conservative medical therapy does not provide enough relief. People with spinal stenosis may benefit from epidural corticosteroid injections given every 2 to 3 months. Surgical decompression is reserved for patients who are totally incapacitated by pain. Most people with spinal stenosis do not require surgery. In patients of any age who have no serious comorbid illness, the first decompression

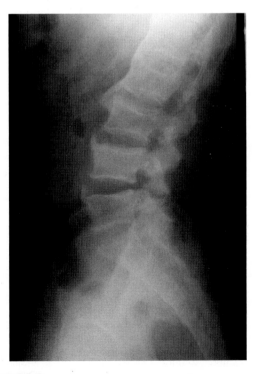

FIGURE 3C-3

Lateral radiograph of the lumbar spine demonstrating traction osteophytes at the superior endplate of L5 and L4.

operation for spinal stenosis has the greatest chance for an excellent outcome.

Spondylolisthesis

Spondylolisthesis is the anterior displacement of a vertebral body in relation to the underlying vertebra. Spondylolisthesis usually is secondary to degeneration of intervertebral discs and reorientation of the plane of motion of the zygapophyseal joints. The process also may occur as a developmental abnormality with separation of the pars interarticularis (spondylolysis) (17). People with spondylolisthesis complain of low back pain that is exacerbated with standing and is relieved with rest. Individuals with severe subluxation also have leg pain. Physical examination reveals increased lordosis with a "step off." The neurologic examination reveals no abnormality. Plain radiographs are adequate to demonstrate the lytic lesions in the pars interarticularis, and lateral x-rays demonstrate the degree of subluxation. An MRI can detect the entrapment and direct impingement of spinal nerve roots associated with this disorder.

Treatment of spondylolisthesis includes flexion strengthening exercises, NSAIDs, and orthopedic corsets. Fusion surgery is useful for patients with greater than grade II slippage and persistent symptoms of neural compression.

Scoliosis

Scoliosis, a lateral curvature of the spine in excess of 10°, most commonly begins to develop in adolescent girls (18). In the lumbar spine, a curve greater than 40° generally leads to a constant rate of progression of 1° per year. Patients complain of increasing back pain that is relieved with bed rest. Neurologic examination reveals findings of nerve compression in more severely affected patients. Plain radiographs allow the clinician to measure the degree of scoliosis by Cobb's method.

In people with scoliosis of 40° or less, exercises, braces, and NSAIDs are effective in reducing pain and maintaining function. Surgical fusion and placement of Harrington rods are reserved for patients with progressive scoliosis who are at increased risk for pulmonary compromise (19).

MECHANICAL DISORDERS OF THE CERVICAL SPINE

Mechanical disorders of the cervical spine are less common than lumbar spine disorders, tend to be less disabling, and result in fewer physician consultations (Table 3C-5).

TABLE 3C-5.   MECHANICAL NECK PAIN.

	NECK STRAIN	HERNIATED NUCLEUS PULPOSUS	OSTEOARTHRITIS	MYELOPATHY	WHIPLASH
Age at onset (years)	20–40	30–50	>50	>60	30–40
Pain Pattern					
Location	Neck	Neck/arm	Neck	Arm/leg	Neck
Onset	Acute	Acute	Insidious	Insidious	Acute
Flexion	I	I	D	D	I
Extension	D	I/D	I	I	I
Plain x-ray	–	–	+	+	–
CT/myelogram	–	+	+/–	+	–
MRI	–	+	+/–	+	–

ABBREVIATIONS: I, increase; D, decrease.

Neck Strain

Neck strain causes pain in the middle or lower part of the posterior aspect of the neck. The area of pain may be unilateral or bilateral and may cover a diffuse area. Pain may radiate toward the head and shoulder, sparing the arms. Neck strain, which rarely is associated with a specific trauma, typically is triggered by sleeping in an awkward position, turning the head rapidly, or sneezing. Physical examination reveals local tenderness in the paracervical muscles, with decreased range of motion and loss of cervical lordosis (20). Muscles most commonly affected include the sternocleidomastoid and the trapezius. No abnormalities are found on shoulder or neurologic examination, laboratory tests, or radiographic studies.

Treatment of neck strain includes controlled physical activity, limited use of cervical orthoses, NSAIDs, and muscle relaxants. Injections of anesthetic and corticosteroid are helpful to decrease local muscle pain, and isometric exercises should be prescribed to maintain strength in the neck. Modifications in the body mechanics while the patient is at work may help prevent recurrences.

Cervical Disc Herniation

Intervertebral disc herniation in the cervical spine causes radicular pain (brachialgia) that radiates from the shoulder to the forearm to the hand (21). The pain may be so severe that the use of the arm is limited. Neck pain is minimal or absent. Cervical herniation occurs with sudden exertion and frequently is associated with heavy lifting. Physical examination reveals increased radicular pain with any maneuver that narrows the intervertebral foramen and places tension on the affected nerve. Spurling's sign (compression, extension, and lateral flexion of the cervical spine) causes radicular pain. Neurologic examination may reveal sensory deficit, reflex asymmetry, or motor weakness corresponding to the damaged spinal nerve root and degree of impingement (Table 3C-3). An MRI is the best tool to identify the location of disc herniation and nerve impingement. An EMG and nerve conduction tests may document abnormal nerve function.

Therapy includes controlled physical activity, cervical orthoses, NSAIDs, and cervical traction. The pain typically subsides within 3 months; only 20% or fewer of patients require surgical decompression.

Cervical Spondylosis

Osteoarthritis of the cervical spine produces a clinical syndrome similar to that in the lumbosacral spine. As the disc degenerates and the articular structures are brought closer together, the cervical spine becomes unstable. Increased instability results in osteophyte formation in the uncovertebral and zygapophyseal joints, and local synovial inflammation (cervical spondylosis). Neck pain is diffuse and may radiate to the shoulders, suboccipital areas, interscapular muscles, or anterior chest. Involvement of the sympathetic nervous system may cause blurred vision, vertigo, or tinnitus. Physical examination of most patients reveals little, other than midline tenderness. Plain radiographs of the cervical spine are adequate to show the intervertebral narrowing and facet joint sclerosis (Figure 3C-3). The presence of abnormalities is not necessarily associated with clinical symptoms.

Conservative therapy is effective for cervical spondylosis. NSAIDs and local injections may diminish neck and referred pain. The appropriate amount of immobilization is controversial, however. The use of cervical orthoses may increase neck stiffness and pain. Patient education should stress the importance of balancing the need to restrict neck movement with a cervical collar and to maintain neck flexibility with range-of-motion exercises. Most people with cervical spondylosis have a relapsing course, with recurrent exacerbations of acute neck pain.

Myelopathy

The most serious sequelae of cervical spondylosis is myelopathy. This disorder occurs as a consequence of spinal cord compression by osteophytes, ligamentum flavum, or intervertebral disc (spinal stenosis). Cervical spondylotic myelopathy is the most common cause of spinal cord dysfunction in individuals older than 55 years (22). With disc degeneration, osteophytes develop posteriorly and project into the spinal canal, compressing the cord and its vascular supply. Symptoms may occur with or without movement. The size of the spinal canal is the important static component. Stenosis is associated with an anteroposterior diameter of 10 mm or less. Dynamic stenosis, which is secondary to instability, causes compression of the spinal cord with flexion or extension of the neck. Protruding structures that are located anterior to the spinal cord can compress the posterior and lateral columns. Compression of the anterior spinal artery in the lower cervical spine is another mechanism of spinal cord injury (23). Neck pain is mentioned by only one third of people with myelopathy.

Clinical symptoms include a history of peculiar sensations in the hands, associated with weakness and uncoordination. In the lower extremities, this disorder can cause gait disturbances, spasticity, leg weakness, and spontaneous leg movements. Older patients may describe leg stiffness, foot shuffling, and a fear of falling. Incontinence is a late manifestation. Physical examination reveals weakness of the appendages in association with spasticity and fasciculations. Sensory deficits include decreased dermatomal sensation and loss of proprioception. Hyperreflexia, clonus, and positive Babinski's sign are present in the lower extremities. Plain radiographs reveal advanced degenerative disease with narrowed disc spaces, osteophytes, facet joint sclerosis, and cervical instability. An MRI is the most useful method to detect the extent of spinal cord compression and the effects of compression on the integrity of the cord. Combined CT/myelogram imaging is useful for distinguishing protruding discs from osteophytes.

Although some patients improve with conservative therapy, progressive myelopathy requires surgery to prevent further cord compression and vascular compromise. Surgical intervention works best before severe neurologic deficits are present.

Whiplash

Cervical hyperextension injuries of the neck are associated with rear-collision motor vehicle accidents. Impact from the rear causes acceleration–deceleration injury to the soft tissue structures in the neck. Paracervical muscles (sternocleidomastoid, longus coli) are stretched or torn, and the sympathetic ganglia may be damaged, resulting in Horner's syndrome (ptosis, meiosis, anhydrosis), nausea, or dizziness. Cervical intervertebral disc injuries may occur.

The symptoms of stiffness and pain with motion are first noticed 12 to 24 hours after the accident. Headache is a common complaint. Patients may have difficulty swallowing or chewing, and may have paresthesias in the arms. Physical examination reveals decreased range of neck motion and persistent paracervical muscle contraction. Neurologic examination is unremarkable, and radiographs do not show soft tissue abnormalities other than loss of cervical lordosis.

Treatment of whiplash includes the use of cervical collars for minimal periods of time (24). Mild analgesics, NSAIDs, and muscle relaxants are prescribed to encourage motion of the neck. Most patients improve after about 4 weeks of therapy. Patients with persistent symptoms for greater than 6 months rarely experience significant improvement. The mechanism of chronic pain in whiplash patients remains to be determined (25).

REFERENCES

1. Andersson GBJ. The epidemiology of spinal disorders. In: Frymoyer JW, ed. The adult spine: principles and practice, 2nd ed. New York: Raven Press; 1977:93–133.
2. Hart LG, Deyo RA, Cherkin DC. Physician office visits for low back pain. Frequency, clinical evaluation, and treatment patterns from a U.S. national survey. Spine 1995;20:11–19.
3. Borenstein DG, Wiesel SW, Boden SD. Low back and neck pain: comprehensive diagnosis and management, 3rd ed. Philadelphia: Saunders; 2004.
4. van den Hoogen HJM, Koes BW, Deville W, van Eijk JTM, Bouter LM. The prognosis of low back pain in general practice. Spine 1997;22:1515–1521.
5. Deyo RA, Rainville J, Kent DL. What can the history and physical examination tell us about low back pain? JAMA 1992;268:760–765.
6. Kohles SS, Kohles DA, Karp AP, et al. Time-dependent surgical outcomes following cauda equina syndrome diagnosis: comments on a meta-analysis. Spine 2000;25: 1515–1522.
7. Tsiodras S, Falagas ME. Clinical assessment and medical treatment of spine infections. Clin Orthop 2006;444: 38–50.
8. Nicholas JJ, Christy WE. Spinal pain made worse by recumbency: a clue to spinal cord tumors. Arch Phys Med Rehabil 1986;67:598–600.
9. Cooper RG. Understanding paraspinal muscle dysfunction in low back pain: a way forward? Ann Rheum Dis 1993;52:413–415.
10. Agency for Health Care Policy and Research. Acute low back problems in adults, clinical practice guideline. Rockville, MD: Agency for Health Care Policy and Research; 1994. Publication no. 95-0642.
11. Nordin M, Balague F, Cedraschi C. Nonspecific lower-back pain. Clin Orthop 2006;443:156–167.
12. Boos N, Semmer N, Elfering A, et al. Natural history of individuals with asymptomatic disc abnormalities in magnetic resonance imaging: predictors of low back pain-related medical consultation and work incapacity. Spine 2000;25:1484–1492.
13. Komori H, Okawa A, Haro H, Muneta I, Yamamoto H, Shinomiya K. Contrast-enhanced magnetic resonance imaging in conservative management of lumbar disc herniation. Spine 1998;23:67–73.
14. Awad JN, Moskovich R. Lumbar disc herniations: surgical versus nonsurgical treatment. Clin Orthop 2006;443: 183–197.
15. Boden SD. The use of radiographic imaging studies in the evaluation of patients who have degenerative disorders of the lumbar spine. J Bone Joint Surg Am 1996;78: 114–124.
16. Atlas SJ, Delitto A. Spinal stenosis: surgical versus nonsurgical treatment. Clin Orthop 2006;443:198–207.
17. Hammerberg KW. New concepts on the pathogenesis and classification of spondylolisthesis. Spine 2005;30(Suppl 6): S4–S11.
18. Perennou D, Marcelli C, Herisson C, Simon L. Adult lumbar scoliosis: epidemiologic aspects in a low-back pain population. Spine 1994;19:123–128.
19. Rizzi PE, Winter RB, Lonstein FE, Denis F, Perra JH. Adult spinal deformity and respiratory failure. Surgical results in 35 patients. Spine 1997;22:2517–2531.
20. Helliwell PS, Evans PF, Wright Y. The straight cervical spine: does it indicate muscle spasm? J Bone Joint Surg Br 1994;76:103–106.
21. Carette S, Fehlings MG. Cervical radiculopathy. N Engl J Med 2005;353:392–399.

22. Bernhardt M, Hynes RA, Blume HW, White AA III. Cervical spondylotic myelopathy. J Bone Joint Surg Am 1993;75:119–128.

23. Fehlings MG, Skaf G. A review of the pathophysiology of cervical spondylotic myelopathy with insights for potential novel mechanisms drawn from traumatic spinal cord injury. Spine 1998;24:2730–2737.

24. Spitzer WO, Skovron ML, Salmi LR, et al. Scientific monograph of the Quebec Task Force on Whiplash-Associated Disorders: redefining "whiplash" and its management. Spine 1995;20:1S–73S.

25. Freeman MD, Croft AC, Rossignol AM, Weaver DS, Reiser M. A review and methodologic critique of the literature refuting whiplash syndrome. Spine 1999;24:86–96.

3

Musculoskeletal Signs and Symptoms
D. Regional Rheumatic Pain Syndromes

JOSEPH J. BIUNDO, JR., MD

- Regional rheumatic pain syndromes typically result from injuries related to a specific activity or event.
- Injuries leading to regional rheumatic pain syndromes may be caused by a single episode or be the result of repetitive overuse. In either case, abnormal body position or mechanics is usually present.
- This chapter reviews 62 different regional rheumatic pain syndromes, involving the shoulder, elbow, wrist and hand, hip, knee, and ankle and foot.

- Although medications may be useful in the treatment of regional pain syndromes, a more comprehensive management approach that takes into consideration the etiology of the complaint—often leading to activity modification—is a critical part of effective therapy.
- Nonsteroidal anti-inflammatory drugs are prescribed frequently for these conditions.
- Local injections and physical therapy also can be useful components of treatment.

The regional rheumatic pain syndromes, because of their prevalence, complexity, and lack of diagnostic laboratory tests, present a challenge to the clinician. Yet success in diagnosis and treatment is most gratifying. The conditions discussed in this chapter include disorders involving muscles, tendons, entheses, joints, cartilage, ligaments, fascia, bone, and nerve. A working knowledge of regional anatomy and an approach utilizing a regional differential diagnosis helps lead to specific diagnoses and problem-focused therapies (1).

A precise history is needed to identify the conditions present; more than one syndrome can occur concomitantly. A complete neuromusculoskeletal examination should be performed emphasizing careful palpation, passive range of motion (ROM), and active ROM alone and, sometimes, with resistance.

CAUSATIVE FACTORS

Many syndromes of the neuromusculoskeletal system are the result of injury from a specific activity or event, ranging from one episode to repetitive overuse, espe-

cially when abnormal body position or mechanics is present. Tendons become less flexible and elastic with aging, making them more susceptible to injury. Also with aging and with disuse atrophy, the muscles become weaker and exhibit less endurance and bulk, resulting in a decreased muscle absorption of mechanical forces otherwise transmitted to joints, tendons, ligaments, and entheses. A musculotendinous unit shortened from lack of stretching is more prone to injury. Tendon syndromes are basically overuse injuries. Tendinitis may occur when the tendon repeatedly bears more load than it can withstand. This may result from excessive high loads across normal tendons, or from normal loads across degenerated tendons.

Any site of tendinitis may result in a calcific tendinitis, which usually produces more inflammation with pain and swelling. The calcification may be detected by plain x-ray. Magnetic resonance imaging (MRI) and ultrasonography are helpful in confirming a diagnosis of tendinitis. Even though the term *tendinitis* is used throughout this chapter, the term *tendinosis* might be more appropriate, as these conditions exhibit degenerative changes and few inflammatory cells (2). Tendinopathy is also an acceptable terminology. Tenosynovitis and peritendinitis refer to an inflammatory response of the tenosynovium or peritenon. In addition to the overuse, degenerative and inflammatory causes, there appears to be a genetic predisposition to certain regional syndromes, resulting from variations in anatomy and abnormal biomechanics. Unfortunately, causative factor(s) often are not identified.

GENERAL CONCEPTS OF MANAGEMENT

Drug Therapy

Oral medications, including nonsteroidal anti-inflammatory drugs (NSAIDs) and analgesics, play a role in management of regional musculoskeletal disorders. The NSAIDs help reduce inflammation and pain. For additional pain relief, analgesics such as acetaminophen, or tramadol, and propoxyphen alone or in combination with acetaminophen can be added. Tricyclic antidepressants, such as amitriptyline, may also be useful in chronic pain and neurogenic or myofascial pain.

Comprehensive management of these regional syndromes should be undertaken rather than relying on oral medications alone. The causative aspects should be evaluated, and activity modification advised, as needed. Local injections and physical therapy also can be useful components of treatment and will be described below. Some guidelines for the management of these conditions are provided in Table 3D-1.

Intralesional Injections

After specific diagnosis of a regional rheumatic pain syndrome, local injection with lidocaine, corticosteroids, or both is often of benefit (3). In fact, the immediate pain relief from a properly directed injection into a tendon sheath, bursa, enthesis, or nerve area for a specific problem further validates the diagnosis. Injection of an area of nonspecific muscle tenderness with a corticosteroid preparation should be discouraged.

Basic principles of intralesional injections include aseptic technique and use of small needles (25-gauge 5/8″ or 1½″ or a 22-gauge 1½″). The use of separate syringes for lidocaine and corticosteroid avoids mixing of the two substances, and permits infiltration of lidocaine beginning intracutaneously with a small wheal and continuing to the site of the lesion. This method makes the injection relatively painless. When the needle reaches the desired site, the syringe is changed with the needle left in place, and the corticosteroid is then injected. This technique helps avoid possible subcutaneous and skin atrophy secondary to corticosteroid use. When injecting a tendon sheath, the needle should be placed parallel to the tendon fibers and not into the tendon itself. Using a more water-soluble corticosteroid may lessen the possibility of corticosteroid-induced tendon weakness or postinjection flare in some patients.

Physical Therapy

The goals of therapeutic exercise are to increase flexibility by stretching, increase muscle strength by resistive exercises, and improve muscle endurance by some repetitive regimen. The physician should become knowledgeable about exercise prescriptions for the various conditions (4). For example, older women tend to have tight calf muscles, which predispose to calf cramps, Achilles tendon problems, or other ankle and foot disorders. Tight quadriceps, hamstring, and iliopsoas muscles are related to problems in the low back, hip, and knee regions. Exercise to stretch these muscles can be taught by the physician. Instruction for quadriceps strengthening, especially by straight leg raising from the sitting position, and for pelvic tilt exercise can be given in the office (5). Heat or cold modalities provide pain relief and muscle relaxation and serve as a prelude to an exercise regimen. They are of doubtful benefit when used alone over an extended period.

TABLE 3D-1. GUIDELINES FOR MANAGEMENT OF REGIONAL RHEUMATIC PAIN SYNDROMES.

1. Exclude systemic disease and infection by appropriate methods. Diagnostic aspiration is mandatory in suspected septic bursitis. Gram's stain and culture of bursal fluid provide prompt diagnosis of a septic bursitis.
2. Teach the patient to recognize and avoid aggravating factors that cause recurrence.
3. Instruct the patient in self-help therapy, including the daily performance of mobilizing exercises.
4. Provide an explanation of the cause of pain, thus alleviating concern for a crippling disease. When the regional rheumatic pain syndrome overlies another rheumatic problem, the clinician must explain the contribution each disorder plays in the symptom complex and then help the patient deal with each one.
5. Provide relief from pain with safe analgesics, counterirritants (heat, ice, vapocoolant sprays), and, if appropriate, intralesional injection of a local anesthetic or anesthetic with depository corticosteroid agent.
6. Provide the patient with an idea of the duration of therapy necessary to restore order to the musculoskeletal system.
7. Symptomatic relief often corroborates the diagnosis.

DISORDERS OF THE SHOULDER REGION

Rotator Cuff Tendinitis

Rotator cuff tendinitis, or impingement syndrome, is the most common cause of shoulder pain. Tendinitis (and not bursitis) is the primary cause of pain, but secondary involvement of the subacromial bursa occurs in some cases (Table 3D-2). The condition may be acute or chronic and may or may not be associated with calcific deposits within the tendon. The key finding is pain in the rotator cuff on active abduction, especially between 60° and 120°, and sometimes when lowering the arm. In more severe cases, however, pain may begin on initial abduction and continue throughout the ROM. In acute tendinitis, pain comes on more abruptly and may be excruciating. Such cases tend to occur in younger patients and are more likely to have calcific deposits in the supraspinatus tendon insertion (Figure 3D-1). The deposits are best seen on roentgenogram in external rotation,

appearing round or oval and several centimeters in length. These deposits may resolve spontaneously over a period of time. A true subacromial bursitis may also be present when calcific material ruptures into the bursa.

The more typical chronic rotator cuff tendinitis manifests as an ache in the shoulder, usually over the lateral deltoid, and occurs on various movements, especially on abduction and internal rotation. Other symptoms include difficulty in dressing oneself and night pain due to difficulty in positioning the shoulders. Tenderness on palpation and some loss of motion may be evident on examination. The initial movement to detect rotator cuff tendinitis is to determine whether pain is present on active abduction of the arm in the horizontal position. Passive abduction is then carried out. Usually less pain is present on passive abduction than active abduction. Conversely, pain may be increased on active abduction against resistance. The impingement sign is nearly always positive. This maneuver is performed by the examiner using one hand to raise the patient's arm in forced flexion while the other hand prevents scapular rotation (6). A positive sign occurs if pain develops at

TABLE 3D-2. REGIONAL RHEUMATIC SYNDROMES.

Shoulder
1. Rotator cuff tendinitis
2. Rotator cuff tear, complete and incomplete
3. Proximal bicipital tendinitis
4. Tear of proximal bicipital tendon
5. Adhesive capsulitis (frozen shoulder)
6. Suprascapular neuropathy
7. Long thoracic nerve paralysis
8. Brachial plexopathy
9. Thoracic outlet syndrome

Elbow
1. Olecranon bursitis
2. Lateral epicondylitis (tennis elbow)
3. Medial epicondylitis (golfer's elbow)
4. Distal biceps tendinopathy
5. Distal biceps rupture, complete and incomplete
6. Cubital bursitis
7. Triceps tendinitis
8. Triceps tendon rupture
9. Ulnar nerve entrapment

Wrist and hand
1. Ganglion
2. de Quervain's tenosynovitis
3. Intersection syndrome
4. Tenosynovitis of the wrist
5. Pronator teres syndrome
6. Anterior interosseous nerve syndrome
7. Radial nerve palsy
8. Posterior interosseous nerve syndrome
9. Superficial radial neuropathy (cheiralgia paresthetica)
10. Carpal tunnel syndrome
11. Ulnar nerve entrapment at the wrist
12. Volar flexor tenosynovitis
13. Dupuytren's contracture

Hip
1. Trochanteric bursitis
2. Iliopsoas bursitis (iliopectineal)
3. Ischial bursitis (ischiogluteal)
4. Piriformis syndrome
5. Meralgia paresthetica
6. Coccydynia

Knee
1. Popliteal cysts (Baker's cysts)
2. Anserine bursitis
3. Prepatellar bursitis
4. Medial plica syndrome
5. Popliteal tendinitis
6. Pellegrini–Stieda syndrome
7. Patellar tendinitis
8. Quadriceps tendon and patellar tendon rupture
9. Peroneal nerve palsy
10. Patellofemoral pain syndrome

Ankle and foot
1. Achilles tendinitis
2. Achilles tendon rupture
3. Subcutaneous Achilles bursitis
4. Retrocalcaneal bursitis
5. Plantar fasciitis
6. Posterior tibialis tendinitis
7. Posterior tibialis tendon rupture
8. Peroneal tendon dislocation and tendinitis
9. Bunionette
10. Hammer toe
11. Metatarsalgia
12. Pes planus
13. Pes cavus
14. Morton's neuroma
15. Tarsal tunnel syndrome

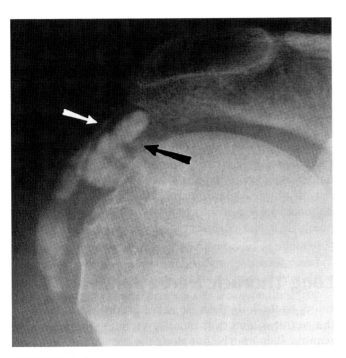

FIGURE 3D-1

Right shoulder of a 44-year-old man illustrating massive calcareous deposits in the supraspinatus tendon (*white arrow*) and subdeltoid bursa (*black arrow*).

or before 180° of forward flexion. Another useful test to confirm rotator cuff disease is the *impingement test*, performed by injecting 2 to 5 mL of 2% lidocaine into the subacromial bursa. Pain relief on abduction following the injection denotes a positive impingement test. The same test can be used in another way to determine whether apparent shoulder weakness is due to pain. Once pain is eliminated with the injection, the arm is retested for weakness. If the weakness is still present, the result is again considered positive.

The causes of rotator cuff tendinitis are multifactorial, but relative overuse, especially from overhead activity causing impingement of the rotator cuff, is commonly implicated. Compression of the rotator cuff occurs above by the edge and undersurface of the anterior third of the acromion and the coracohumeral ligament and below by the humeral head. There is also age-related decrease in vascularity and degeneration of the cuff tendons and reduction of strength of the cuff muscles due to aging or decline in use. Osteophytes on the inferior portion of the acromioclavicular joint or acute trauma to the shoulder region contribute to development of tendinitis. An inflammatory process such as rheumatoid arthritis (RA) can also cause rotator cuff tendinitis independent of impingement.

Treatment consists of rest and modalities such as hot packs, ultrasound, or cold applications, with specific ROM exercises as soon as tolerated. NSAIDs are often

beneficial; however, the most frequent treatment is injection of a depot corticosteroid into the subacromial bursa, the floor of which is contiguous with the rotator cuff (7).

Rotator Cuff Tear

An acute tear of a rotator cuff after trauma is easily recognized. The trauma may be superimposed on an already degenerative and possibly even partially torn cuff. In trauma resulting in a ruptured cuff, especially falls, fractures of the humeral head and dislocation of the joint should also be considered. However, at least one half of patients with a tear recall no trauma. In these cases, degeneration of the rotator cuff gradually occurs, resulting in a complete tear. Rotator cuff tears are classified as small (1 cm or less), medium (1–3 cm), large (3–5 cm), or massive (>5 cm) (8). Shoulder pain, weakness on abduction, and loss of motion occur in varying degrees, ranging from severe pain and mild weakness to no pain and marked weakness. A positive drop-arm sign with inability to actively maintain 90° of passive shoulder abduction may be present in large or massive tears. Surgical repair is indicated in younger patients.

Less easily diagnosed is the smaller, chronic complete (full thickness) tear of the rotator cuff or a partial (incomplete or non–full thickness) tear. Pain on abduction, night pain, weakness, loss of abduction, and tenderness on palpation can be present in both of these types of tears. A small complete tear, however, can exist despite fairly good abduction. Tears of the rotator cuff may also occur as a result of the chronic inflammation in RA, and is often present with cystic swelling around the shoulder.

Magnetic resonance imaging has become the most expeditious imaging technique to determine a tear (9). Diagnostic ultrasonography can also be used. The most definitive diagnosis of a ruptured rotator cuff is established by an abnormal arthrogram showing a communication between the glenohumeral joint and the subacromial bursa. In a partial tear, in which an intact layer of rotator cuff tissue still separates the joint space from the subacromial bursa, a small ulcerlike crater is seen on the arthrogram. Small complete tears and incomplete tears of the rotator cuff are treated conservatively with rest, physical therapy, and NSAIDs. Although their role has not yet been established by careful studies, subacromial injections of a corticosteroid may relieve pain.

Bicipital Tendinitis and Rupture of the Proximal Bicipital Tendon

This condition is manifested by pain, most often in the anterior region of the shoulder and occasionally more

tendon on both T1 and T2 weighted images (14). Alteration of activities and use of NSAIDs usually alleviate the problem, although occasionally a local corticosteroid injection is required at the medial epicondyle site.

Tendinopathy, Complete and Partial Rupture of the Distal Biceps Insertion

Tendinopathy of the distal insertion of the biceps (lacertus fibrosus) may cause dull pain throughout the antecubital fossa of the elbow (15). Palpation of the distal biceps tendon confirms the source of pain, and mild swelling may be present. Resisted elbow flexion and resisted supination may increase pain. Heat, NSAIDs, rest, and, occasionally, a local injection of corticosteroid generally are beneficial in this condition. Complete rupture of the distal biceps tendon is uncommon, and, when seen, it is in a middle-aged male who experiences a sudden forced extension against an actively contracting biceps muscle (16). A popping sensation may occur, with the onset of sudden pain and weakness of elbow flexion and supination. A bulbous deformity proximal to the insertion and ecchymosis may be seen. A palpable tendon defect is present. An MRI confirms the diagnosis and surgical repair is usually indicated. In partial rupture of the distal biceps tendon there is acute pain, some weakness of elbow flexion and forearm supination, but the tendon is still palpable and no ecchymosis or swelling is seen. Conservative treatment may be of help, but sometimes surgical repair is necessary.

Cubital Bursitis

Cubital bursitis (bicipitoradial bursitis) is manifest by a swelling of the antecubital fossa and sometimes tenderness with some restriction of pronation. It is more often seen in RA or other inflammatory arthritis conditions, but also can be secondary to trauma or overuse. It may also be seen in association with a partial tear of the distal biceps tendon. An MRI or diagnostic ultrasound may confirm the diagnosis. This condition may be treated conservatively, including an image-guided aspiration and corticosteroid injection.

Triceps Tendinitis and Triceps Tendon Rupture

In triceps tendinopathy pain is present in the posterior elbow which may be worse by extension and even more by resisted extension. Tenderness of the insertion of the tendon may be noted as well as some swelling. This syndrome occurs as a result of overuse of the upper arm

and elbow, especially in such activities as throwing and hammering and also may occur as a result of direct trauma. Treatment is conservative. Rupture of the triceps tendon at the insertion in the olecranon is rare and usually is the result of trauma, although a few cases have been in association with corticosteroid injections into the olecranon bursa, and also with heavy use of anabolic steroids. Acute pain occurs, and there is weakness of elbow extension against gravity. Swelling, tenderness, and a palpable gap in the tendon may be noted. Surgical repair is usually indicated.

Ulnar Nerve Entrapment

Entrapment of the ulnar nerve at the elbow produces numbness and paresthesia of the little finger and adjacent side of the ring finger as well as aching of the medial aspect of the elbow. Hand clumsiness can be present. Tenderness may be elicited when the ulnar nerve groove, located on the posteroinferior surface of the medial epicondyle, is compressed. The little finger may have decreased sensation and weakness on abduction and flexion. Elevating the hand by resting the forearm on the head for 1 minute may produce paresthesia. In longstanding cases, atrophy and weakness of the ulnar intrinsic muscles of the hand occur. A positive Tinel's sign, elicited by tapping the nerve at the elbow, is often present. Similar symptoms may result from subluxation of the nerve.

Ulnar nerve entrapment has many causes, including external compression from occupation, compression during anesthesia, trauma, prolonged bed rest, earlier fractures, and inflammatory arthritis. A nerve conduction test that shows slowing of ulnar motor and sensory conduction and prolonged proximal latency aids in confirming the diagnosis. Avoiding pressure on the elbow and repetitive elbow flexion may be all that is necessary for improvement, but in severe persistent cases, surgical correction is needed.

DISORDERS OF THE WRIST AND HAND

Ganglion

A ganglion is a cystic swelling arising from a joint or tendon sheath that occurs most commonly over the dorsum of the wrist. It is lined with synovium and contains thick jellylike fluid. Ganglia are generally of unknown cause but may develop secondary to trauma or prolonged wrist extension. Usually, the only symptom is swelling, but occasionally a large ganglion produces discomfort on wrist extension. Treatment, if indicated, consists of aspiration of the fluid, with or without injection of corticosteroid. Use of a splint may help prevent recurrence. In severe cases, the whole ganglion may be removed surgically.

De Quervain's Tenosynovitis

De Quervain's tenosynovitis may result from repetitive activity that involves pinching with the thumb while moving the wrist. It has been reported to occur in new mothers as a complication of pregnancy. In the past it was thought to be from repetitive diapering using safety pins, but also may be a result of injury of the wrist area from lifting of the baby (17). The symptoms are pain, tenderness, and, occasionally, swelling over the radial styloid. Pathologic findings include inflammation and narrowing of the tendon sheath around the abductor pollicis longus and extensor pollicis brevis. A positive Finkelstein test result is usually seen; pain increases when the thumb is folded across the palm and the fingers are flexed over the thumb as the examiner passively deviates the wrist toward the ulnar side. This test, however, may also be positive in osteoarthritis (OA) of the first carpometacarpal (CMC) joint and must be differentiated. Treatment involves splinting, local corticosteroid injection, and NSAIDs as indicated (13,18). Accuracy of the injection may be improved with use of guided imagery such as ultrasound. Rarely, surgical removal of the inflamed tenosynovium is needed.

Intersection Syndrome

The intersection syndrome, which is less common than de Quervain's syndrome, must be differentiated from it as both occur in the radial side of the wrist. This condition involves the site of the intersection and crossing of the extensor carpi radialis longus and brevis with the abductor pollicis longus and the extensor pollicis brevis, which is about 4 cm from the wrist. Pain is present and worse with radial or twisting motions. Swelling and tenderness of this site is present and crepitus may be palpated. It results from overuse in many types of activities, including racket sports, skiing, canoeing, and weight lifting. If a diagnosis is uncertain, MRI is very helpful (19). Conservative treatment is usually successful and includes relative rest with possibly a thumb splint, NSAIDs, ice, and a local steroid injection.

Tenosynovitis of the Wrist

Tenosynovitis occurs in other flexor and extensor tendons of the wrist in addition to those involved in de Quervain's tenosynovitis and the intersection syndrome (20). The individual tendons on the extensor side that may be vulnerable are the extensor pollicis longus, extensor indicis proprius, extensor digiti minimi, and extensor carpi ulnaris, and on the flexor side, the flexor carpi radialis, flexor carpi ulnaris, flexor digitorum superficialis, and flexor digitorum profundus.

The findings vary depending on which tendon is involved. Localized pain and tenderness are usually present, and there is sometimes swelling. Pain on resisted movement is often seen. The tenosynovitis may be misinterpreted as arthritis of the wrist.

This problem may be due to repetitive use, a traumatic episode, inflammatory arthritis, or may be idiopathic. The treatment consists of avoiding overuse, splinting, and NSAIDs. A local corticosteroid injection into the tendon sheath, avoiding direct injection into the tendon itself, is usually of benefit.

Pronator Teres Syndrome

An uncommon condition, pronator teres syndrome may be difficult to diagnose because some features are similar to carpal tunnel syndrome. In this case, however, the median nerve is compressed at the level of the pronator teres muscle. The patient may complain of aching in the volar aspect of the forearm, numbness in the thumb and index finger, weakness on gripping with the thumb, and writer's cramp. The most specific finding is tenderness of the proximal part of the pronator teres, which may be aggravated by resistive pronation of the forearm. Pronator compression often produces paresthesia after 30 seconds or less. In some patients, a positive Tinel's sign is found at the proximal edge of the pronator teres. Unlike carpal tunnel syndrome, nocturnal awakening and numbness in the morning are absent. Pronator teres syndrome is thought to result from overuse by repetitive grasping or pronation, trauma, or a space-occupying lesion.

Electrodiagnostic studies may reveal signs of denervation of the forearm muscles supplied by the median nerve but sparing the pronator teres; however, they often fail to localize the lesion. If the condition does not improve with alteration of activities and with time, exploratory surgery may be undertaken to look for fibrous or tendinous bands or a hypertrophied pronator muscle.

Anterior Interosseous Nerve Syndrome

Compression of the anterior interosseous nerve near its bifurcation from the median nerve produces weakness of the flexor pollicis longus, flexor digitorum profundus, and pronator quadratus muscles. Sensation is not affected, but a person with this syndrome cannot form an O with the thumb and index finger because motion is lost in the interphalangeal (IP) joint of the thumb and the distal interphalangeal (DIP) joint of the index finger. Electromyography may help confirm the diagnosis. Repetitive overuse, trauma, and fibrous bands are the principal causes of this syndrome. Protection from trauma usually results in improvement; if not, surgical exploration may be undertaken.

Radial Nerve Palsy

The most common type of radial nerve palsy is the spiral groove syndrome, or bridegroom palsy, in which the radial nerve is compressed against the humerus. The most prominent feature is a wrist drop with flexion of the metacarpophalangeal (MCP) joints and adduction of the thumb. Anesthesia in the web space and hypesthesia from the dorsal aspect of the forearm to the thumb, index, and middle fingers may be present. If the radial nerve is compressed more proximally through improper use of crutches or prolonged leaning of the arm over the back of a chair (Saturday night palsy), weakness of the triceps and brachioradialis muscles may also occur. Compression injuries generally heal over a period of weeks. Splinting the wrist during this recovery time prevents overstretching of the paralyzed muscles and ligaments. Electrodiagnostic studies are helpful in determining the specific point of compression.

Posterior Interosseous Nerve Syndrome

Posterior interosseous nerve entrapment in the radial tunnel produces discomfort in the proximal lateral portion of the forearm. The fingers cannot be extended at the MCP joints. The posterior interosseous nerve, a branch of the radial nerve, is primarily a motor nerve, so sensory disturbances are rare. Occupational or recreational repetitive activity with forceful supination, wrist extension, or radial deviation against resistance may be a factor. Direct trauma and such nontraumatic conditions as a ganglion also have been implicated. Interestingly, this syndrome has been seen in RA due to synovial compression of the nerve and, therefore, must be distinguished from a ruptured extensor tendon (21).

Superficial Radial Neuropathy (Cheiralgia Paresthetica)

A lesion of this sensory nerve is more common than previously thought and causes symptoms of a burning or shooting pain and sometimes numbness and tingling over the dorsoradial aspect of the wrist, thumb, and index fingers. Hyperpronation and ulnar wrist flexion may be provocative. Decreased pinprick sensation and a positive Tinel's sign may be seen. Electrodiagnostic studies are helpful in the diagnosis.

Tight wrist restraints from handcuffs or watch bands are well-known causes. Trauma to the area, repetitive wrist motion, diabetes, ganglion cyst, venipuncture, and local surgical procedures are other possible etiologies. The neuropathy may resolve with time. Treatment consists of splinting, NSAIDs, local corticosteroid injection, or surgical neurolysis in some cases.

Carpal Tunnel Syndrome

Carpal tunnel syndrome is the most common cause of paresthesias and numbness in the hands. The median nerve and flexor tendons pass through a common tunnel at the wrist, whose rigid walls are bounded dorsally and on the sides by the carpal bones, and on the volar aspect by the transverse carpal ligament (Figure 3D-2). Any process encroaching on this tunnel compresses the median nerve, which innervates the thenar muscles (for flexion, opposition, abduction); the radial lumbricales; and the skin of the radial side of the palm, thumb, second and third fingers, and the radial half of the fourth finger.

Symptoms are variable, but episodes of burning pain or tingling in the hand are common, often occurring during the night and relieved by vigorous shaking or movement of the hand. Numbness commonly affects the index and middle fingers, radial side of the ring fingers, and occasionally the thumb. Some patients experience only numbness without much pain. Numbness may also occur with activities such as driving or holding a newspaper or book. The patient may have a sensation of hand swelling when in fact no swelling is visible. Occasionally the pain spreads above the wrist into the forearm or, rarely, even above the elbow and up the arm. Bilateral disease is common.

A positive Tinel's sign or Phalen's sign may be present. Phalen's test is performed by holding the wrist flexed at 90° for 1 minute. Loss of sensation may be

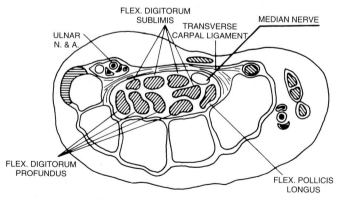

FIGURE 3D-2

Cross-section of wrist illustrating the position of the transverse carpal ligament (flexor retinaculum) and the structures occupying the osseous–fibrous carpal tunnel.

demonstrated in the index, middle finger, or radial side of the fourth finger. Weakness and atrophy of the muscles of the thenar eminence may gradually appear in chronic cases. Confirmation of the diagnosis can be obtained by demonstrating prolonged distal latency times during electrodiagnostic studies.

A variety of disorders may cause carpal tunnel syndrome, including edema from pregnancy or trauma, osteophytes, ganglia related to tenosynovial sheaths, lipomata, and anomalous muscles, tendons, and blood vessels that compress the median nerve. Carpal tunnel syndrome has been observed in various infections such as tuberculosis, histoplasmosis, sporotrichosis, coccidioidomycosis, and rubella. Rheumatoid arthritis, gout, pseudogout, and other inflammatory diseases of the wrist can cause compression of the median nerve. Amyloid deposits of the primary type or in association with multiple myeloma can occur at this site, and carpal tunnel syndrome may be the initial manifestation of the disease. The syndrome has also been reported to occur in myxedema and acromegaly. In many cases, however, no obvious cause can be found or a nonspecific tenosynovitis is evident. Many idiopathic cases may be due to occupational stress.

In milder cases, splinting the wrist in a neutral position may relieve symptoms (22). Local injections of corticosteroids into the carpal tunnel area, using a 25-gauge needle, are helpful for nonspecific or inflammatory tenosynovitis. The benefit may be only temporary, depending on the degree of compression and the reversibility of the neural injury. When conservative treatment fails, surgical decompression of the tunnel by release of the transverse carpal ligament and removal of tissue compressing the median nerve is often beneficial. Even with surgery, however, symptoms may sometimes recur.

Ulnar Nerve Entrapment at the Wrist

The ulnar nerve can become entrapped at the wrist proximal to Guyon's canal, in the canal itself, or distal to it (23). Guyon's canal is roughly bounded medially by the pisiform bone, laterally by the hook of the hamate, superiorly by the volar carpal ligament (pisohamate ligament), and inferiorly by the transverse carpal ligament. Because the ulnar nerve, on entering the canal, bifurcates into the superficial and deep branches, the clinical picture may vary, with only sensory, only motor, or both sensory and motor findings.

The complete clinical picture includes pain, numbness, and paresthesias of the hypothenar area, clumsiness, and a weak hand grip, including difficulty using the thumb in a pinching movement. Pressure over the ulnar

nerve at the hook of the hamate may cause tingling or pain. Atrophy of the hypothenar and intrinsic muscles can occur. Clawing of the ring and little fingers may be seen, resulting from weakness of the third and fourth lumbricales. Loss of sensation occurs over the hypothenar area.

If the superficial branch alone is involved, then only numbness, pain, and loss of sensation occur. Entrapment of the deep branch produces only motor weakness of the ulnar innervated muscles. The sites of motor weakness depend on the exact location of nerve compression. For example, if the compression is distal to the superficial branch but proximal to the branch of the hypothenars, then the hypothenar muscles and intrinsics may be spared, causing weakness and atrophy of only the adductor pollicis, deep head of the flexor pollicis brevis, and first dorsal interosseous muscles. The causes of ulnar neuropathy at the wrist include trauma, ganglia, bicycling, inflammatory arthritis, flexor carpi ulnaris hypertrophy, fractures, neuroma, lipomata, and diabetes.

The diagnosis is assisted by electrodiagnostic studies, indicating a prolonged distal latency of the ulnar nerve at the wrist and denervation of the ulnar innervated muscles. Treatment includes rest from offending activity, splinting, or a local corticosteroid injection; however, surgical exploration and decompression may be necessary.

Trigger Finger (Volar Flexor Tenosynovitis)

Inflammation of the tendon sheaths of the flexor digitorum superficialis and flexor digitorum profundus tendons in the palm is extremely common but often unrecognized. Pain in the palm is felt on finger flexion, but in some cases the pain may radiate to the proximal interphalangeal (PIP) and MCP joints on the dorsal side, thus misleading the examiner. The diagnosis is made by palpation and identification of localized tenderness and swelling of the volar tendon sheaths. The middle and index fingers are most commonly involved, but the ring and little fingers can also be affected. Often a nodule composed of fibrous tissue can be palpated in the palm just proximal to the MCP joint on the volar side. The nodule interferes with the normal tendon gliding and can cause a triggering or locking (trigger finger), which may be intermittent and may produce an uncomfortable sensation. Similar involvement can occur at the flexor tendon of the thumb. Volar tenosynovitis may be part of inflammatory conditions, such as RA, psoriatic arthritis, or apatite crystal deposition disease. It is seen frequently in conjunction with OA of the hands. It is important to point out that volar flexor tenosynovitis occurs in the absence of triggering. The actual trigger finger may be a late phase of the process. The most common cause of volar flexor tenosynovitis is overuse trauma of the hands from gripping with increased pull on the flexor tendons. Injection of a long-acting steroid into the tendon sheath usually relieves the problem (24,25), although surgery on the tendon sheath may be needed in unremitting cases.

Infection of the tendon sheaths in the hand requires drainage and antibiotics. People with drug addictions and diabetes may be at increased risk for such infections. Atypical mycobacterium or fungal infections also cause a chronic tenosynovitis in the hands. *Mycobacterium marinum*, which is found in infected fish, barnacles, fish tanks, and swimming pools, is a common culprit (26).

Dupuytren's Contracture

In Dupuytren's contracture, a thickening and shortening of the palmar fascia occurs. In established cases the diagnosis is obvious with typical thick, cordlike superficial fibrous tissue felt in the palm causing a contracture, usually of the ring finger. The fifth, third, and second fingers are involved in decreasing order of frequency. Initially, a mildly tender fibrous nodule in the volar fascia of the palm may be the only finding, leading to confusion with volar flexor tenosynovitis. Dimpling or puckering of the skin over the involved fascia helps identify the early Dupuytren's contracture. The initial nodules probably result from a contraction of proliferative myofibroblasts, which are the product of fibrogenic cytokines inducing fibroblasts (27). The tendon and tendon sheaths are not implicated, but the dermis is frequently involved, resulting in fixation to the fascia. Progression of the disease varies, ranging from little or no change over many years to rapid progression and complete flexion contracture of one or more digits.

The cause of this condition is unknown, but a hereditary predisposition appears to be present. Some patients also have associated plantar fasciitis, knuckle pads, and fibrosis in the shaft of the penis. The disorder is about five times more frequent in men, occurs predominantly in Caucasians, and is more common in Europe. A gradual increase in incidence of the disease occurs with age. Associations exist between Dupuytren's contracture and chronic alcoholism, epilepsy, and diabetes.

Treatment depends entirely on the severity of the findings. Heat, stretching, ultrasound, and intralesional injection of corticosteroids may be helpful in early stages. When actual contractures occur, surgical intervention may be desirable. Limited fasciectomy is effective in most instances, but more radical procedures, including digital amputation, may rarely be necessary. Palmar fasciotomy is a useful and more benign proce-

dure, but if the disease remains active, recurrence is likely.

DISORDERS OF THE HIP REGION

Trochanteric Bursitis

Although common, trochanteric bursitis frequently goes undiagnosed. It occurs predominantly in middle-aged to elderly people, and somewhat more often in women than men. The main symptom is aching over the trochanteric area and lateral thigh. Walking, various movements, and lying on the involved hip may intensify the pain. Onset may be acute, but more often is gradual, with symptoms lasting for months. In chronic cases the patient may fail to adequately locate or describe the pain, or the physician may fail to note the symptoms or interpret them correctly. Occasionally the pain may have a pseudoradiculopathic quality, radiating down the lateral aspect of the thigh. In a few cases the pain is so severe that the patient cannot walk and complains of diffuse pain of the entire thigh.

The best way to diagnose trochanteric bursitis is to palpate over the trochanteric area and elicit point tenderness. In addition to specific pain on deep pressure over the trochanter, other tender points may be noted throughout the lateral aspect of the thigh muscle. Pain may be worse with external rotation and abduction against resistance. A positive Trendelenburg sign is often present. Although bursitis is generally named as the principal problem, the condition more likely arises at the insertions of the gluteus medius and gluteus minimus tendons (28). Local trauma and degeneration play a role in the pathogenesis. In some cases calcification of the trochanteric bursa is seen. Conditions that may contribute to trochanteric bursitis, apparently by adding stress to the area, include OA of the lumbar spine or of the hip, leg length discrepancy, and scoliosis. Treatment consists of local injection of depot corticosteroid using a 22-gauge, 3½″ needle to ensure that the bursal area is reached (29). The use of fluoroscopic guidance with injection of radiopaque contrast increases the accuracy of the injections. NSAIDs, weight loss, and strengthening and stretching of the gluteus medius muscle and iliotibial band help in overall management.

Iliopsoas (Iliopectineal) Bursitis

The iliopsoas bursa lies behind the iliopsoas muscle, anterior to the hip joint and lateral to the femoral vessels. It communicates with the hip in 15% of iliopsoas bursitis cases. When the bursa is involved, groin and anterior thigh pain are present. This pain becomes worse on passive hip hyperextension and sometimes on flexion, especially with resistance. Tenderness is palpable over the involved bursa. The patient may hold the hip in flexion and external rotation to eliminate pain and may limp to prevent hyperextension. The diagnosis is more apparent if a cystic mass, which is present in about 30% of cases, is seen; however, other causes of cystic swelling in the femoral area must be excluded. A bursal mass may cause femoral venous obstruction or femoral nerve compression. As with most bursitis, acute or recurrent trauma and inflammatory conditions like RA may be a cause. The diagnosis is confirmed by plain roentgenogram and injection of a contrast medium into the bursa, or by computed tomography, ultrasonography, or MRI. Iliopsoas bursitis generally responds to conservative treatment, including corticosteroid injections under guided imagery. With recurrent involvement, excision of the bursa may be necessary.

Ischial (Ischiogluteal) Bursitis

Ischial bursitis is caused by trauma or prolonged sitting on hard surfaces as evidenced by the name, *weaver's bottom*. Pain is often exquisite when sitting or lying down. Because the ischiogluteal bursa is located superficial to the ischial tuberosity and separates the gluteus maximus from the tuberosity, the pain may radiate down the back of the thigh. Point tenderness over the ischial tuberosity is present. MRI and ultrasonography may be used to confirm the diagnosis. Use of cushions and local injection of a corticosteroid are helpful.

Piriformis Syndrome

Piriformis syndrome is not well recognized and is incompletely understood, even though it was first described in 1928 (30). The main symptom is pain over the buttocks, often radiating down the back of the leg as in sciatica. A limp may be noted on the involved side. Women are more often affected, and trauma plays a major role. Diagnosis is aided by tenderness of the piriformis muscle on rectal or vaginal examination. Pain in the involved buttock is evident on hip flexion, adduction and internal rotation (FAIR) (31). Another maneuver is performed by having the patient lie on the uninvolved side with the upper knee resting on the table. Buttock pain occurs when the knee of the involved side is lifted several inches off the table. Pain and weakness have also been noted on resisted abduction and external rotation. A carefully done local injection of lidocaine and corticosteroid, under fluoroscopic guidance, into the piriformis muscle may help.

Meralgia Paresthetica

The lateral femoral cutaneous nerve (L2–L3) innervates the anterolateral aspect of the thigh and is a sensory nerve. Compression of the nerve causes a characteristic intermittent burning pain associated with hypesthesia and sometimes with numbness of the anterolateral thigh. Extension and abduction of the thigh or prolonged standing and walking may make symptoms worse, whereas sitting may relieve the pain. Touch and pinprick sensation over the anterolateral thigh may be decreased. Pain can be elicited by pressing on the inguinal ligament just medial to the anterior superior iliac spine. This syndrome is seen more commonly in people who have diabetes, are pregnant, or are obese. Direct trauma, compression from a corset, or a leg length discrepancy may also be factors. Nerve conduction velocity studies help confirm the diagnosis. Weight loss, heel correction, and time generally alleviate the problem. Because entrapment of the nerve often occurs just medial to the anterior superior iliac spine, a local injection of a corticosteroid at that site may help.

Coccydynia

Coccydynia is manifest by pain in the coccyx area when pressure is applied to the area. This most notably occurs upon sitting. The patient squirms from buttock to buttock to relieve the pressure and consequent pain, and often chooses to sit on a cushion. The symptoms may be chronic and severe. The condition may relate to a fall on the coccyx or to dropping to a hard chair upon sitting, or to some related trauma to the coccyx. However, at times no obvious cause can be detected. Women are much more frequently affected. Perhaps this is due to the lordosis often occurring in women, which exposes the coccyx to more trauma. The diagnosis is confirmed by finding localized tenderness over the coccyx on palpation. A plain x-ray can be obtained to exclude a fracture or dislocation of the coccyx. Treatment with a local injection of a long-acting corticosteroid and 2 mL of 2% lidocaine is usually very effective (32). The exact nature of the pathology of coccydynia has not been studied but is presumed to be a bone bruise.

DISORDERS OF THE KNEE REGION

Popliteal Cysts

Popliteal cysts, also known as *Baker's cysts*, are not uncommon, and the clinician should be well aware of the possibility of dissection or rupture. A cystic swelling with mild or no discomfort may be the only initial finding. With further distention of the cyst, however, a greater awareness and discomfort is experienced, particularly on full flexion or extension. The cyst is best seen when the patient is standing and is examined from behind. Any knee disease having a synovial effusion can be complicated by a popliteal cyst. A naturally occurring communication may exist between the knee joint and the semimembranosus–gastrocnemius bursa, which is located beneath the medial head of the gastrocnemius muscle. A one-way valvelike mechanism between the joint and the bursa is activated by pressure from the knee effusion. An autopsy series has shown that about 40% of the population has a knee joint–bursa communication.

Popliteal cysts are most common secondary to RA, OA, or internal derangements of the knee. There are a few reported cases secondary to gout and reactive arthritis. A syndrome mimicking thrombophlebitis may occur, resulting from cyst dissection into the calf or actual rupture of the cyst. Findings include diffuse swelling of the calf, pain, and sometimes erythema and edema of the ankle. An arthrogram of the knee will confirm both the cyst and the possible dissection or rupture. Ultrasound is now used more often to make a diagnosis and monitor the course. History of a knee effusion is often a hint that a dissected Baker's cyst is the cause of the patient's swollen leg. A Doppler ultrasound can also exclude the possibility of concomitant thrombophlebitis. A cyst related to an inflammatory arthritis is treated by injecting a depot corticosteroid into the knee joint and possibly into the cyst itself, which usually resolves the problem. If the cyst results from OA or an internal derangement of the knee, surgical repair of the underlying joint lesion is usually necessary to prevent recurrence of the cyst.

Anserine Bursitis

Seen predominantly in overweight, middle-aged to elderly women with big legs and OA of the knees, anserine bursitis produces pain and tenderness over the medial aspect of the knee about 2″ below the joint margin. Pain is worsened by climbing stairs. The pes anserinus (Latin for "goose foot") is composed of the conjoined tendons of the sartorius, gracilis, and semitendinosus muscles. The bursa extends between the tendons and the tibial collateral ligament. The diagnosis is made by eliciting exquisite tenderness over the bursa and by relieving pain with a local lidocaine injection. The treatment is rest, stretching of the adductor and quadriceps muscles, and a corticosteroid injection into the bursa.

Anserine bursitis is often overlooked as it frequently occurs concomitantly with OA of the knee, which when present is the assumed cause of pain; however, in some cases of dual involvement, anserine bursitis is the principal source of pain.

Prepatellar Bursitis

Manifested as a swelling superficial to the kneecap, prepatellar bursitis results from trauma such as frequent kneeling, leading to the name "housemaid's knee." The prepatellar bursa lies anterior to the lower half of the patella and upper half of the patellar ligament. The pain is generally slight unless pressure is applied directly over the bursa. The infrapatellar bursa, which lies between the patellar ligament and the tibia, is also subject to trauma and swelling. Chronic prepatellar bursitis can be treated by protecting the knee from the irritating trauma.

Septic prepatellar bursitis should also be considered when swelling is noted in this area. Generally, erythema, heat, and increased tenderness and pain are present. When obtained, the history may include trauma to the knee with puncture or abrasion of the skin overlying the bursa is obtained. The bursal fluid should be aspirated and cultured, and treatment with appropriate antibiotics should be instituted if infection is demonstrated.

Medial Plica Syndrome

A plica is a synovial fold in the knee joint, and infrapatellar, suprapatellar, and medial plicae have been identified. The medial plica can sometimes cause knee symptoms (33). Patella pain may be the predominant complaint, and snapping or clicking of the knee, a sense of instability, and possible pseudolocking of the knee may be seen. The plica become symptomatic through any traumatic or inflammatory event in the knee. Diagnosis and treatment are made by arthroscopy, in which a thickened, inflamed, and occasionally fibrotic medial patella plica, leading to a bowstring process, is seen.

Popliteal Tendinitis

Pain in the posterolateral aspect of the knee may occur secondary to tendinitis of the popliteal tendons (hamstring and popliteus). With the knee flexed at 90°, tenderness on palpation may be found. Straight leg raising with or without palpation may cause pain. Running downhill increases the strain on the popliteus and can lead to tendinitis. Rest and conservative treatment are indicated; occasionally a corticosteroid injection may be beneficial.

Pellegrini–Stieda Syndrome

Pellegrini–Stieda syndrome consists of calcification of the medial collateral ligament of the knee. This syndrome generally occurs in men, is thought to result from trauma and is followed by an asymptomatic period.

Later, the symptomatic stage of medial knee pain and progressive restriction of knee movement coincides with the beginning of calcification of the medial collateral ligament, typically appearing as an elongated, amorphous shadow on roentgenogram (34). The pain is self-limited, and improvement usually occurs within several months.

Patellar Tendinitis

Patellar tendinitis, or jumper's knee, is seen predominantly in athletes engaging in repetitive running, jumping, or kicking activities. Pain and tenderness are present over the patellar tendon. Diagnostic ultrasonography adds to confirmation of diagnosis (35). Treatment consists of rest, NSAIDs, ice, knee bracing, and stretching and strengthening of the quadriceps and hamstring muscles. Corticosteroid injections are usually contraindicated due to risk of tendon rupture. In some chronic cases surgery is needed.

Rupture of Quadriceps Tendon and Patellar Tendon

When the tendons around the patella rupture, the quadriceps tendon is involved about 50% of the time; otherwise, the patellar tendon is involved. Quadriceps tendon rupture is generally caused by sudden violent contractions of the quadriceps muscle when the knee is flexed. A hemarthrosis of the knee joint may follow. Rupture of the patellar tendon has been associated with a specific episode of trauma, repetitive trauma from sporting activities, and systemic diseases. Patients with chronic renal failure, RA, hyperparathyroidism, gout, and systemic lupus erythematosus patients on steroids have been reported to have spontaneous ruptures of the quadriceps tendon. The patient experiences a sudden sharp pain and cannot extend the leg. Roentgenograms may show a high riding patella, and the diagnosis may be confirmed by MRI or ultrasonography. The tendon is generally found to be degenerated, and surgical repair is necessary.

Peroneal Nerve Palsy

In peroneal nerve palsy, a painless foot drop with a steppage gait is usually evident. Pain sensation may be slightly decreased along the lower lateral aspect of the leg and the dorsum of the foot. Direct trauma, fracture of the lower portion of the femur or upper portion of the tibia, compression of the nerve over the head of the fibula, and stretch injuries are all causes of this palsy. Generally, the common peroneal nerve is compressed, affecting the muscles innervated by the superficial peroneal nerve (which supplies the everters) and the deep peroneal nerve (which supplies the dorsiflexors of the foot and toes). An electromyogram is helpful in demonstrating slowing of nerve conduction velocities. Treatment consists of removing the source of compression, if there is one, and use of an ankle–foot orthosis if necessary. Occasionally, surgical exploration is needed.

Patellofemoral Pain Syndrome

This syndrome consists of pain and crepitus in the patellar region (36). Stiffness occurs after prolonged sitting and is alleviated by activity; overactivity involving knee flexion, particularly under loaded conditions such as stair climbing, aggravates the pain. On examination, pain occurs when the patella is compressed against the femoral condyle or when the patella is displaced laterally. Joint effusions are uncommon and usually small. The symptoms of patellofemoral pain syndrome are often bilateral and occur in a young age group. This syndrome may be caused by a variety of patellar problems, such as patella alta, abnormal quadriceps angle, and trauma. The term *chondromalacia patellae* has been used for this syndrome, but patellofemoral pain syndrome is preferred by many. Treatment consists of analgesics, NSAIDs, ice, rest, and avoidance of knee overuse. Isometric strengthening exercises for the quadriceps muscles are of benefit. In some patients, however, surgical realignment may be tried.

DISORDERS OF THE ANKLE AND FOOT REGION

Achilles Tendinitis

Usually resulting from trauma, athletic overactivity, or improperly fitting shoes with a stiff heel counter, Achilles tendinitis can also be caused by inflammatory conditions such as ankylosing spondylitis, reactive arthritis, gout, RA, and calcium pyrophosphate dihydrate crystal deposition disease (CPPD). It also has been associated with treatment with fluoroquinolones. Pain, swelling, and tenderness occur over the Achilles tendon at its attachment and in the area proximal to the attachment. Crepitus on motion and pain on dorsiflexion may be present. Ultrasonography aids in the diagnosis. Management includes NSAIDs, rest, shoe corrections, heel lift, gentle stretching, and sometimes a splint with slight plantar flexion. Because the Achilles tendon is vulnerable to rupture when involved with tendinitis, it was felt in the past that treatment by a corticosteroid injection could worsen this possibility. However, this view is being challenged and fluoroscopic guided steroid injections have been successfully performed (37).

possibly by an intermetatarsophalangeal bursa or synovial cyst may be responsible for the entrapment. Treatment usually includes a metatarsal bar or a local steroid injection into the web space. Ultimately, surgical excision of the neuroma and a portion of the nerve may be needed.

Tarsal Tunnel Syndrome

In tarsal tunnel syndrome, the posterior tibial nerve is compressed at or near the flexor retinaculum. Just distally, the nerve divides into the medial plantar, lateral plantar, and posterior calcaneal branches. The flexor retinaculum is located posterior and inferior to the medial malleolus. Numbness, burning pain, and paresthesias of the toes and sole extend proximally to the area over the medial malleolus. Nocturnal exacerbation may be reported. The patient gets some relief by leg, foot, and ankle movements. A positive Tinel's sign may be elicited on percussion posterior to the medial malleolus, and loss of pinprick and two-point discrimination may be present. Women are more often affected than men. Trauma to the foot, especially fracture, valgus foot deformity, hypermobility, and occupational factors may relate to development of tarsal tunnel syndrome. An electrodiagnostic test may show prolonged motor and sensory latencies and slowing of the nerve conduction velocities. In addition, a positive tourniquet test and pressure over the flexor retinaculum can induce symptoms. A newer test is reported to be of value in which the ankle is passively maximally everted and dorsiflexed while all of the MTP joints are maximally dorsiflexed. The position is held for 5 to 10 seconds, and in a positive test, numbness and/or pain are produced and tenderness is intensified (39). Shoe corrections and steroid injection into the tarsal tunnel may be of benefit, but often surgical decompression is needed.

DISORDERS OF THE ANTERIOR CHEST WALL

Chest wall pain of a musculoskeletal origin is fairly common. It must be differentiated from chest pain of a cardiac nature, which is the usual main concern, or from pain due to pulmonary or gastrointestinal disease. Pain can also radiate to the chest as a result of cervical or thoracic spine disease. The musculoskeletal syndromes usually associated with chest wall pain are Tietze's syndrome and costochondritis. Both conditions are characterized by tenderness of one or more costal cartilages and the terms have sometimes been used interchangeably. The two disorders, however, are generally separated by the presence of

local swelling in Tietze's syndrome but not in costochondritis (40).

Tietze's syndrome is much less common than costochondritis and is of unknown etiology. Its onset may be gradual or abrupt with swelling usually occurring in the second or third costal cartilage. Pain, which ranges from mild to severe, may radiate to the shoulder and be aggravated by coughing, sneezing, inspiration, or by various movements affecting the chest wall. Tenderness is elicited on palpation, and approximately 80% of patients have a single site.

Costochondritis is more common and is associated with pain and tenderness of the chest wall, without swelling. Tenderness is often present over more than one costochondral junction, and palpation should duplicate the described pain. In one study of 100 patients with noncardiac chest pain, 69% were found to have local tenderness on palpation and in 16% the palpation elicited the typical pain (41). Other names attached to costochondritis include anterior wall syndrome, costosternal syndrome, parasternal chondrodynia, and chest wall syndrome. Some individuals with chest wall pain are found to have fibromyalgia or localized myofascial pain. Chest wall pain can also complicate heart or lung disease, so its presence does not exclude more serious problems.

Xiphoid cartilage syndrome or xiphoidalgia, also known as hypersensitive xiphoid or *xiphodynia*, is characterized by pain over the xiphoid area and tenderness on palpation. Pain may be intermittent and brought on by overeating and various twisting movements.

These three conditions are often self-limiting. Treatment consists of reassurance, heat, stretching of chest wall muscles, or local injections of lidocaine, corticosteroid, or both.

In addition, a number of other disorders may produce chest wall pain. Sternocostoclavicular hyperostosis is manifested by a painful swelling of the clavicles, sternum, or ribs and may be relapsing. It is associated with an elevated erythrocyte sedimentation rate, pustules on the palms and soles, and progression to ossification of the chest wall lesions. Condensing osteitis of clavicles is a rare, benign condition of unknown etiology, occurring primarily in women of child-bearing age. It is characterized by sclerosis of the medial ends of the clavicles without involvement of the sternoclavicular joints. Pain and local tenderness are present.

Any condition involving the sternoclavicular joint, including spondyloarthropathy, OA, and infection, can cause chest wall pain. Stress fracture of the ribs, cough fracture, herpes zoster of the thorax, and intercostobrachial nerve entrapment are other causes of chest pain.

Thorough palpation of the chest wall must be done, including the sternoclavicular joint, costochondral junctions, sternum, and chest wall muscles. Maneuvers such as crossed-chest adduction of the arm and backward extension of the arm from 90° of abduction help in elucidating whether chest pain is of a musculoskeletal origin. Imaging studies may include plain roentgenogram of the ribs, special roentgenogram of the sternoclavicular joint, tomogram, and bone scan. A computed tomography scan or MRI provides the most detail of the sternoclavicular joint.

REFERENCES

1. Hazleman B, Riley G, Speed C. Soft tissue rheumatology. Oxford: Oxford Medical Publications; 2004.
2. Khan KM, Cook JL, Bonar F, et al. Histopathology of common tendinopathies. Update and implications for clinical management. Sports Med 1999;27:393–408.
3. Genovese, MC. Joint and soft-tissue injection. A useful adjuvant to systemic and local treatment. Postgrad Med 1998;103:125–134.
4. Kisner C, Colby LA. Therapeutic exercise: foundations and techniques, 3rd ed. Philadelphia: FA Davis; 1996.
5. 5.Biundo JJ, Hughes GM. Rheumatoid arthritis rehabilitation: practical guidelines. J Musculoskeletal Med 1991; 8:85–96.
6. Neer CR. Impingement lesions. Clin Orthop 1983;173: 70–77.
7. Goupille P, Sibilia, J. Local corticosteroid injections in the treatment of rotator cuff tendinitis (except frozen shoulder and calcific tendinitis). Clin Exp Rheumatol 1996;14: 561–566.
8. Frieman BG, Albert TJ, Fenlin JM Jr. Rotator cuff disease: a review of diagnosis, pathophysiology and current trends in treatment. Arch Phys Med Rehabil 1994;75:604–609.
9. Naredo AE, Aguado P, Padron M, et al. A comparative study of ultrasonography with magnetic resonance imaging in patients with painful shoulder. J Clin Rheumatol 1999; 5:184–192.
10. Dacre JE, Beeney N, Scott DL. Injections and physiotherapy for the painful stiff shoulder. Ann Rheum Dis 1989;48:322–325.
11. Weinstein PS, Canoso JJ, Wohlgethan JR. Long-term follow-up of corticosteroid injection for traumatic olecranon bursitis. Ann Rheum Dis 1984;43:44–46.
12. Kraushaar BS, Nirschl RP. Tendinosis of the elbow (tennis elbow). Clinical features and findings of histological, immunohistochemical, and electron microscopy studies. J Bone Joint Surg Am 1999;81:259–278.
13. Alvarez-Nemegyei J, Canoso JJ. Evidence-based soft tissue rheumatology: epicondylitis and hand stenosing tendinopathy. J Clin Rheumatol 2004;10:33–40.
14. Kijowske R, DeSmet AA. Magnetic resonance imaging findings in patients with medial epicondylitis. Skeletal Radiol 2005;34:196–202.
15. Tomaino MM, Towers MD. Clinical presentation and radiographic findings of distal biceps tendon degeneration: a potentially forgotten cause of proximal radial forearm pain. Am J Orthop 2004;33:31–34.
16. Hamilton W, Ramsey ML. Rupture of the distal tendon of the biceps brachii. U Penn Orthop J 1999;12:21–26.
17. Skoff HD. "Postpartum/newborn" deQuervain's tenosynovitis of the wrist. Am J Orthop 2001;30:428–430.
18. Anderson BC, Manthey R, Brouns MC. Treatment of de Quervain's tenosynovitis with corticosteroids. Arthritis Rheum 1991;34:793–798.
19. Costa CR, Morrison WB, Carrino JA. MRI features of intersection syndrome of the forearm. AJR Am J Roentgenol 2003;181:1245–1249.
20. Stern PJ. Tendinitis, overuse syndromes, and tendon injuries. Hand Clinics 1990;6:467–475.
21. Kishner S, Biundo JJ. Posterior interosseous neuropathy in rheumatoid arthritis. J Clin Rheumatol 1996;2:1080–1084.
22. Burke DT, Burke MM, Stewart GW, Cambré A. Splinting for carpal tunnel syndrome: in search of the optimal angle. Arch Phys Med Rehabil 1994;75:1241–1244.
23. Wu JS, Morris JD, Hogan GR. Ulnar neuropathy at the wrist: case report and review of the literature. Arch Phys Med Rehabil 1985;66:785–788.
24. Anderson B, Kaye, S. Treatment of flexor tenosynovitis of the hand ("trigger finger") with corticosteroids. Arch Intern Med 1991;151:153–156.
25. Nimigan AS, Ross DC, Gan BS. Steroid injections in the management of trigger fingers. Am J Phys Med Rehabil 2006;85:36–43.
26. Williams CS, Riordan DC. Mycobacterium marinum infections of the hand. J Bone Joint Surg Am 1973;55: 1042–1050.
27. Cordova A, Tripoli M, Corradino B, et al. Dupuytren's contracture: an update of biomolecular aspects and therapeutic perspectives. J Hand Surg 2005;30:557–562.
28. Alvarez-Nemegyei J, Canoso JJ. Evidence-based soft tissue rheumatology III: trochanteric bursitis. J Clin Rheumatol 2004;10:123–124.
29. Shbeer MI, O'Duffy D, Michet CJ Jr, et al. Evaluation of glucocorticosteroid injection for the treatment of trochanteric bursitis. J Rheumatol 1996;23:2104–2106.
30. Wyant GM. Chronic pain syndromes and their treatment. III. The piriformis syndrome. Can Anaesth Soc J 1979; 26:305–308.
31. Fishman LM, Dombi GW, Michaelsen C, et al. Piriformis syndrome: diagnosis, treatment, and outcome—a 10 year study. Arch Phys Med Rehabil 2002;83:295–301.
32. Ramsey ML, Toohey JS, Neidre A, et al. Coccygodynia: treatment. Orthopedics 2003;26:403–405.
33. Galloway MT, Jokl P. Patella plica syndrome. Ann Sports Med 1990;5:38–41.
34. Wang JC, Shapiro MS. Pellegrini–Stieda syndrome. Am J Orthop 1995;24:493–497.
35. Peers KH, Lysens RJ. Patellar tendinopathy in athletes: current diagnostic and therapeutic recommendations. Sports Med 2005;35:71–87.
36. Papageloopoulos PJ, Sim FH. Patellofemoral pain syndrome: diagnosis and management. Orthopedics 1997;20: 148–157.
37. Gill SS, Gelbke MK, Mattson SL, et al. Fluoroscopically guided low-volume peritendinous corticosteroid injection for Achilles tendinopathy. A safety study. J Bone Joint Surg Am 2004;86:802–806.

38. Churchhill RS, Sferra JJ. Posterior tibial tendon insufficiency. Its diagnosis, management, and treatment. Am J Orthop 1998;27:339–347.

39. Kinoshita M, Okuda R, Morikawa J, et al. The dorsiflexion-eversion test for diagnosis of tarsal tunnel syndrome. J Bone Joint Surg Am 2001;83:1835–1839.

40. Calabro JJ. Costochondritis. N Engl J Med 1997;296:946–947.

41. Wise CM, Semble L, Dalton CB. Musculoskeletal chest wall syndromes in patients with noncardiac chest pain: a study of 100 patients. Arch Phys Med Rehabil 1992;72:147–149.

Musculoskeletal Signs and Symptoms
E. The Fibromyalgia Syndrome

DINA DADABHOY, MD
DANIEL J. CLAUW, MD

- Fibromyalgia (FM) is a soft tissue pain syndrome that affects 4% of the population of the United States.
- American College of Rheumatology (ACR) criteria for the classification of FM include a history of chronic widespread pain involving all four quadrants of the body and the axial skeleton, plus the presence of 11 of 18 tender points on physical examination.
- A variety of nonspecific symptoms are often present in FM. These include fatigue (often worsened by physical activity), paresthesias, irritable bowel complaints, migraine headaches, and deficits of attention and memory.

- Patient education about FM is a fundamental part of the treatment process. A variety of Internet-based Web sites are available for patients.
- Exercise is a crucial element of therapy. A regular exercise program should be considered to be a full part of the pharmacological armamentarium.
- Tricyclic antidepressant (TCA) agents, such as cyclobenzaprine and amitriptyline, are usually the first-line pharmacologic treatment.

Fibromyalgia (FM) is the most common cause of chronic, widespread pain in the United States. The differential diagnosis of FM is lengthy because diffuse pain may also occur in a number of other settings (Table 3E-1). The diagnostic evaluation of an individual with diffuse pain varies depending on the duration of symptoms, as well as the findings in the history and physical examination. Diffuse pain that has been present for years is likely to be due to FM, especially if there are symptoms of fatigue, memory difficulties, and sleep disturbance, and if the physical examination reveals tenderness to palpation at soft tissue sites. In this setting, minimal workup is necessary. In contrast, an individual whose symptoms are of only a few weeks' or months' duration requires a more extensive evaluation for autoimmune, endocrine, and neurological conditions.

In performing the history, particular attention should be focused on the onset and character of the pain, accompanying symptoms, and "exposures" that could be causing the symptoms. Both prescription and over-the-counter medications are particularly important in this regard. Red flags in the history indicating the need for further investigation include a family history of myopathies, a personal history of cancer, unexplained symptoms of weight loss or associated fevers, or symptoms suggesting joint inflammation (true morning stiffness, swelling, redness, and warmth).

The examination should be detailed with a focus on the musculoskeletal and neurological exam. Signs of inflammation (e.g., synovitis) or neurological abnormalities (e.g., objective weakness) are not consistent with FM and imply other possible etiologies.

At a minimum, individuals who present with chronic, widespread pain should have a complete blood count, liver and kidney function tests, thyroid stimulating hormone level, erythrocyte sedimentation rate, and C-reactive protein measured. Careful history-taking and physical examination generally obviate the need for extensive radiological evaluations and other tests. Radiographs, cross-sectional imaging studies, nuclear medicine tests, electromyography, and nerve conduction velocities should be obtained sparingly, and only when they are designed to address specific clinical issues raised by the history or physical examination.

EPIDEMIOLOGY

Fibromyalgia affects up to 4% of the population. To fulfill the classification criteria for FM published by an American College of Rheumatology (ACR) committee

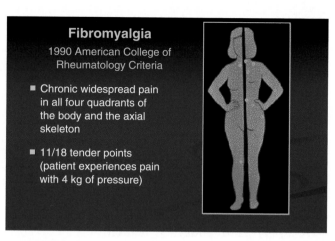

FIGURE 3E-1

1990 American College of Rheumatology classification criteria for fibromyalgia syndrome. (Reference 1).

in 1990, an individual must have both a *history* of chronic widespread pain involving all four quadrants of the body (and the axial skeleton), and the presence of 11 of 18 tender points on *physical examination* (Figure 3E-1) (1). These criteria were never intended for application as diagnostic criteria to individual patients; at least half of the individuals who have clinical diagnoses of FM do not fulfill the ACR classification criteria.

CLINICAL FEATURES

The defining features of FM are chronic, widespread pain and tenderness. The pain of FM frequently waxes and wanes, and may be migratory. In some instances patients will present with aching all over, whereas in other instances patients experience several areas of chronic regional pain. In this setting, regional musculoskeletal pain typically involves the axial skeleton and/or tender point regions, and may be diagnosed initially as a local problem (e.g., low back pain, lateral epicondylitis).

Tender points at defined anatomic sites throughout the body are considered present when an individual complains of pain when 4 kg of pressure are applied (approximately the amount of pressure required to blanch the examiner's nail). Since the publication of the ACR criteria, much has been learned about tender points. Research has shown that individuals with FM are not only tender at discrete localized areas, but have tenderness extending throughout their body (2). In addition, women with chronic widespread pain are more likely to have more tender points on examination than

TABLE 3E-1. DIFFERENTIAL DIAGNOSIS OF DIFFUSE PAIN AND/OR FATIGUE.

Mechanical overuse

Drugs
   Statins and fibrates
   Antimalarials

Endocrinopathies
   Hypothyroidism
   Hyperparathyroidism
   Cushing's syndrome
   Diabetes mellitus

Neurological
   Multiple sclerosis
   Myasthenia gravis

Malignancy

Infections
   Hepatitis C
   Human immunodeficiency virus (HIV)
   Lyme disease

Rheumatologic diseases
   Rheumatoid arthritis
   Systemic lupus erythematosus
   Sjögren's syndrome
   Ankylosing spondylitis
   Polymyalgia rheumatica
   Inflammatory myopathies

Metabolic myopathy

Osteomalacia

Tapering of steroids

Regional pain syndrome

are their male counterparts. Whereas tender points have been shown to be associated with psychological factors such as distress, tenderness (as measured through objective testing paradigms) is not. Therefore, rigidly adhering to the ACR criteria in clinical practice skews the diagnosis of FM towards identifying females with high levels of distress.

In addition to pain and tenderness, most individuals with FM also report a high lifetime and current prevalence of a variety of nonspecific symptoms that seem to defy any current organic explanation (Figure 3E-2). Fatigue, often worse with activities, is one of the most common such symptoms. Paresthesias following a nondermatomal distribution and neurological symptoms, particularly those related to attention and short-term memory, are also common.

The clustering of somatic symptoms associated with FM can give rise to a number of identifiable overlapping syndromes, including the chronic fatigue syndrome, irritable bowel syndrome, and multiple chemical sensitivity. There is also frequently overlap with other chronic pain conditions, such as tension headaches, migraines, and temporomandibular disorders.

Except for the finding of tender points, the physical examination is generally unremarkable in FM. As stated previously, the tenderness is diffuse, and not confined to tender points. The former concept of control points, previously described as areas of the body that should not be tender, has been abandoned. Laboratory testing should be highly focused on the exclusion of FM mimickers that appear to be legitimate possibilities (Table 3E-1). Fishing expeditions with laboratory tests are strongly discouraged.

Although individuals with FM may present with symptoms that can be seen early in the course of autoimmune disorders, serologic assays such as antinuclear antibodies (ANA) and rheumatoid factor should generally be avoided unless there is strong evidence for an autoimmune disorder. Such tests have very low predictive values in the setting of nonspecific symptoms.

OVERLAP WITH AUTOIMMUNE DISORDERS

The overlap between FM and autoimmune disorders deserves special mention. Symptoms that can be seen in both FM and autoimmune disorders include not only arthralgias, myalgias, and fatigue, but also morning stiffness and a history of subjective swelling of the hands and feet. In addition, symptoms suggestive of Raynaud's phenomenon (characterized, in contrast to true Raynaud's phenomenon, by paleness or erythema of the *entire hand* rather than only specific digits), malar flushing (in contrast to a fixed malar rash), and livedo reticularis are all common in FM, and can mislead the practitioner to suspect an autoimmune disorder.

Persons with established autoimmune disorders also commonly exhibit comorbid symptoms of FM. Studies have suggested that up to 25% of persons with systemic inflammatory disorders, such as systemic lupus erythematosus (SLE), rheumatoid arthritis (RA), and ankylosing spondylitis, also meet ACR criteria for FM. Because both inflammatory and non-inflammatory mechanisms cause symptoms in this setting, FM should be suspected when an individual with an autoimmune

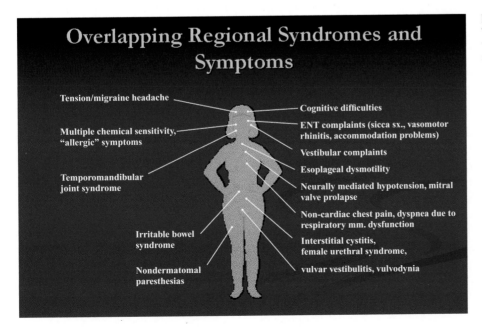

FIGURE 3E-2

Overlapping regional syndromes and symptoms.

disorder has persistent complaints despite normal inflammatory indices, or when symptoms are unresponsive to anti-inflammatory regimens. FM symptoms may become particularly prominent when individuals are being tapered from high doses of glucocorticoids (perhaps due to an effect of glucocorticoids on the sleep cycle), a phenomenon previously termed *pseudo-rheumatism*.

ETIOLOGY AND PATHOGENESIS

Genetic and Environmental Influences

Increasing evidence supports the existence of a genetic predisposition to FM. First-degree relatives of individuals with FM display an eightfold higher risk of FM than the general population (3) Although no absolute links have been ascertained, polymorphisms in the serotonin 5-HT2A receptor (T/T phenotype), the serotonin transporter, the dopamine 4 receptor, and the catecholamine *o*-methyl transferase enzyme have been detected at higher frequencies in patients with FM (4) Notably, these polymorphisms all affect the metabolism or transport of monoamines, compounds that have a critical role in both sensory processing and the human stress response.

In addition to the genetic associations, factors external to the patient can enhance symptom expression. For many patients, certain stressors have strong temporal associations with the development of either FM or chronic fatigue syndrome: physical trauma (especially involving the axial skeleton and trunk); certain infections (e.g., hepatitis C virus, Epstein–Barr virus, parvovirus, and Lyme disease); emotional stress; and other regional pain conditions or autoimmune disorders.

Abnormalities in Pain and Sensory Processing

Once a susceptible individual has symptoms of FM, the most consistently detected objective abnormalities involve the pain and sensory processing systems. Numerous experimental pain studies have demonstrated that FM patients cannot *detect* electrical, pressure, or thermal stimuli at lower levels than normal subjects, but the point at which these stimuli cause pain or unpleasantness is lower. The aberrant pain perception is likely multifactorial, but one key factor is central pain, or enhanced nociceptive sensation due to augmented central pain processing. Because peripheral pain (e.g., that caused by injury or inflammation) can lead to central pain amplification, it is possible that peripheral

input plays a role in central pain amplification in some individuals with FM. This may have some bearing on why so many patients with autoimmune disorders develop FM.

Investigators are examining the pain processing pathways to understand the neuropathology involved in augmented central pain. Just as the immune system contains pro- and anti-inflammatory cytokines, pain processing systems contain compounds and pathways that are generally pronociceptive (i.e., increase the gain on pain processing systems) or antinociceptive.

Biochemical studies performed on samples from FM patients have supported the notion that the pathology might be due to high levels of pronociceptive compounds, low levels of antinociceptive compounds, or both. Four studies have identified much higher levels of substance P in the cerebrospinal fluid (CSF) of patients with FM versus normal subjects (5). Substance P is a pronociceptive peptide stored in the secretory granules of sensory nerves and released upon axonal stimulation. Elevated substance P is not specific for FM because it occurs in other chronic pain states, and appears to be a biological marker for the presence of chronic pain.

Alternatively, there are data suggesting that FM could be related to a decrease in the activity of descending antinociceptive pathways (6). Beginning in the limbic forebrain structures or subcortical structures and passing either directly or indirectly to the spinal cord, these antinociceptive pathways exert a tonic effect, inhibiting the upward transmission of pain in normal conditions.

The two principal descending antinociceptive pathways in humans are the opioidergic and mixed serotonergic–noradrenergic pathways. Current evidence suggests that the opioidergic systems are activated to a maximum extent in groups of individuals with FM. Consequently, the deficiency may be in the other antinociceptive pathway, the serotonergic–noradrenergic pathway. Drugs that inhibit the reuptake of norepinephrine and serotonin are effective in FM. In contrast, no randomized controlled trials have confirmed efficacy for opiates in this condition.

Hypothalamic–Pituitary and Autonomic Dysfunction

Substantial data imply alterations in the hypothalamic–pituitary axes and the autonomic nervous system in subsets of persons with FM and related disorders (7). Although the findings generally indicate a hyperactivity of both the hypothalamic–pituitary adrenal axis as well as the sympathetic nervous system, there are inconsistencies in these studies' results. Recent work suggests that these abnormalities create a milieu in which the somatic symptoms may occur, rather than triggering the symptoms directly themselves.

Psychological and Behavioral Factors

There has been a longstanding debate over the role of psychiatric, psychological, and behavioral factors in FM. Population-based studies have demonstrated that distress can lead to pain, and pain to distress. In this latter instance, pain and other symptoms of FM may cause individuals to function less well in their various roles. They might have difficulties with family members and coworkers, which exacerbate symptoms and lead to maladaptive illness behaviors such as cessation of pleasurable activities and reductions in activity and exercise. In the worst cases, patients become involved with disability and compensation systems, a decision that almost ensures they will not improve. The psychosocial factors that influence the experience of pain are not, however, unique to FM, but have a prominent role in symptom expression in all rheumatic diseases.

Given the biopsychosocial nature of FM, several groups have identified positive psychological and cognitive factors might actually buffer neurobiological factors, leading to pain and distress. These psychological and cognitive factors, postulated to work by affecting the supraspinal pain modulatory pathways, include an internal locus of control (i.e., patients feel that they are empowered to do something about their pain) or low catastrophizing (a negative, pessimistic view of their pain) (8). The findings stress the value of positive coping responses and give insight into why psychological interventions such as cognitive behavioral therapy (CBT) may be efficacious in improving physical and psychological functioning in FM (9).

TREATMENT

Progress in the understanding of FM has led to improved therapeutic options for patients with this condition. Clinic-based evidence advocates a multifaceted program emphasizing education, certain medications, cognitive behavioral therapy, and exercise (Figure 3E-3).

Consider Diagnosis Label

Once an individual with the diagnosis of FM is identified, the practitioner must consider whether or not labeling the patient at that juncture is wise. For the majority of patients, having a name to apply to their disorder helps them understand their symptoms and the most appropriate treatment. On the other hand, for some individuals the diagnostic label may prove detrimental (10). The practitioner must make this decision on a case-by-case basis.

The practitioner should schedule a prolonged visit, or series of visits. This upfront time can be extremely useful for both patients and providers. It helps the physician understand precisely what is bothering the patient, and assists the patient in understanding the goals and rationale of treatment.

Education

For all patients with FM, education about the nature of this disorder is critical. Some patients who present with milder symptoms of FM want only to be told that this is a benign, nonprogressive condition. At a minimum, the physician should describe this condition in terms they feel most comfortable with, and then refer the

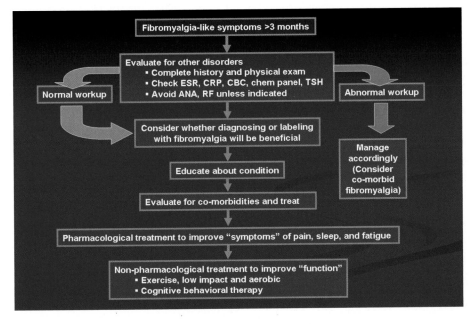

FIGURE 3E-3

Evaluation and treatment paradigm for fibromyalgia syndrome.

patient to reputable sources of information, such as the Arthritis Foundation, several national patient support organizations (e.g., the National Fibromyalgia Association, the American Fibromyalgia Syndrome Association, and the Fibromyalgia Alliance of America), or current, reputable Web sites.

Pharmacologic Therapies

Tricyclic compounds (tricyclic antidepressants; TCA), notably amitriptyline and cyclobenzaprine, have been studied most extensively; these demonstrate the strongest evidence for efficacy in the treatment of FM (9). To increase the tolerance of cyclobenzaprine and amitriptyline, these compounds should be administered several hours before bedtime, beginning at low doses (10 mg or less) and increasing slowly (10 mg every 1–2 weeks) until the patient reaches the maximally beneficial dose (up to 40 mg of cyclobenzaprine, or 50–100 mg of amitriptyline).

Because of the side effects of tricyclics, recent studies have examined the efficacy of better-tolerated compounds, specifically serotonin reuptake inhibitors (SSRIs) and dual receptor inhibitors [serotonin–norepinephrine and norepinephrine–serotonin reuptake inhibitors (SNRIs and NSRIs)]. Many experts believe that drugs targeting both the serotonin and norepinephrine pathways may be more beneficial than drugs that are purely serotonergic. The SSRI evaluated most carefully to date is fluoxetine. Aggregate data suggest that fluoxetine is most efficacious at higher doses, perhaps because it partially inhibits reuptake of norepinephrine as well as serotonin at high doses, and that the use of fluoxetine is synergistic with a TCA taken at bedtime.

The currently available SNRIs include venlafaxine and duloxetine. There is one randomized, controlled trial of venlafaxine for FM, but data from open trials indicate that higher doses than that employed in that trial (i.e., in the range of one 75 mg extended release tablet twice daily) may be necessary. Because of nausea early in the use of this class of drugs, they should be begun at a low dose (i.e., 37.5 mg/day) and escalated slowly. Duloxetine, studied in multicenter trials, is effective in improving pain, fatigue, and overall well-being with either 60 mg daily or 60 mg twice daily. The impact of duloxetine on symptoms were independent of the medication's effect on the mood of the patient, suggesting that the analgesic and other positive effects of this class of drugs in FM are not simply due to the treatment of depression.

Anticonvulsant medications are also being evaluated for the treatment of FM. Recent trials have shown the effectiveness of pregabalin (especially at doses of 450 mg/day) in improving pain, fatigue, sleep, and mood. Anecdotal evidence suggests that gabapentin, not yet tested in randomized, controlled trials, also improves these types of symptoms. Due to its sedative properties, giving a proportionally higher dose at night in the context of a three times a day schedule leads to better medication tolerance and has the additional benefit of improving sleep. Clonazepam, another anticonvulsant agent, and dopamine agonists, such as pramipexole, may also be helpful in this condition, particularly if patients suffer from the comorbid condition or restless leg syndrome.

Compounds with more prominent noradrenergic and/or dopaminergic mechanisms, such as buproprion, nefazadone, and pemoline, may have some clinical utility, especially if given during the day to patients with prominent fatigue or cognitive complaints. Other drugs may be useful for treating certain symptoms of FM, without necessarily leading to a globally beneficial effect. For example, tramadol is an effective analgesic in this disorder. For treating insomnia in persons intolerant to tricyclic compounds, bedtime doses of trazadone and zolpidem may be of benefit. In persons with symptoms suggestive of autonomic dysfunction, such as orthostatic intolerance, vasomotor instability, or palpitations, increased fluid and sodium/potassium intake, and/or low doses of beta blockers, might be of benefit.

Cognitive Behavioral Therapy

Cognitive behavioral therapy refers to a structured education program that focuses on teaching individuals skills that they can utilize to improve their illness. CBT, shown to be effective in improving patient outcomes in nearly every chronic medical illness (including FM), must be tailored to the specific condition. The skills most commonly associated with CBT for pain include relaxation training, activity pacing, pleasant activity scheduling, visual imagery techniques, distraction strategies, focal point and visual distraction, cognitive restructuring, problem solving, and goal setting.

Aerobic Exercise

Aerobic exercise improves FM outcomes, particularly those related to function. In designing aerobic exercise programs, careful planning is required to enhance tolerability and ensure long-term compliance. Especially in illnesses such as FM, patients may experience a worsening of symptoms immediately after exercise, and thus fear that any form of exercise will exacerbate their condition. To reduce the pain associated with exercise, low-impact exercises, such as aquatic exercise, walking, swimming, or stationary cycling, are recommended. Just as with medication, a "start low, go slow" approach appears to be most effective, with a gradual progression in exercise intensity and a focus on adherence to a long-term program.

Complementary Therapies

There are several different types of complementary therapies that are used to treat FM. Some of these are physical modalities, such as trigger point injections, myofascial release therapy (or other hands-on techniques), acupuncture, and chiropractic manipulation, each of which has some data supporting efficacy. Many others, however, including most nutritional supplements, diets, and devices, are to be avoided.

Because few controlled trials of these complementary therapies are available to guide the practitioner, a general approach is suggested. The practitioner should first evaluate the safety of the proposed treatment, and indicate any potential harmful effects. The physician should then consider whether this treatment is reinforcing a maladaptive belief, for example, a treatment program of prolonged bed rest, or of isolation, which in the end will be harmful to the patient. If the treatment is neither harmful nor maladaptive, then the practitioner may suggest that the patient conduct the equivalent of a clinical trial on himself or herself (as is done in "n of 1" trials). In this setting, the patient begins a single treatment (keeping all other variables constant) and determines if the treatment is beneficial. If the patient judges the treatment helpful, then the treatment should be discontinued to determine if the symptoms worsen. If the treatment withstands this test of efficacy, a placebo effect cannot be excluded, but in clinical practice, it is difficult to argue with success.

REFERENCES

1. Wolfe F, Smythe HA, Yunus MB, et al. The American College of Rheumatology 1990 Criteria for the Classification of Fibromyalgia. Report of the Multicenter Criteria Committee. Arthritis Rheum 1990;33:160–172.
2. Granges G, Littlejohn G. Pressure pain threshold in pain-free subjects, in patients with chronic regional pain syndromes, and in patients with fibromyalgia syndrome. Arthritis Rheum 1993;36:642–646.
3. Arnold LM, Hudson JI, Hess EV, et al. Family study of fibromyalgia. Arthritis Rheum 2004;50:944–952.
4. Buskila D, Neumann L. Genetics of fibromyalgia. Curr Pain Headache Rep 2005;9:313–315.
5. Russell IJ, Orr MD, Littman B, et al. Elevated cerebrospinal fluid levels of substance P in patients with the fibromyalgia syndrome. Arthritis Rheum 1994;37:1593–1601.
6. Julien N, Goffaux P, Arsenault P, Marchand S. Widespread pain in fibromyalgia is related to a deficit of endogenous pain inhibition. Pain 2005;114:295–302.
7. Crofford LJ. Neuroendocrine abnormalities in fibromyalgia and related disorders. Am J Med Sci 1998;315:359–366.
8. Gracely RH, Geisser ME, Giesecke T, et al. Pain catastrophizing and neural responses to pain among persons with fibromyalgia. Brain 2004;127:835–843.
9. Goldenberg DL, Burckhardt C, Crofford L. Management of fibromyalgia syndrome. JAMA 2004;292:2388–2395.
10. Hadler NM. Fibromyalgia, chronic fatigue, and other iatrogenic diagnostic algorithms. Do some labels escalate illness in vulnerable patients?. Postgrad Med 1997;102:161–166, 171.

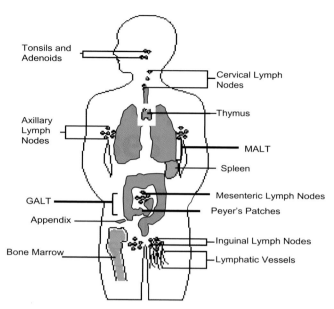

FIGURE 4-2

Immune system tissues are found throughout the body. They include large organs, such as the spleen and bone marrow, as well as aggregates of lymphatic tissue lining mucosal surfaces.

(*chemokines*) and their cognate receptors provide a flexible code for facilitating this cell trafficking. Limiting lymphocyte migration through pharmacological targeting of chemokines or their receptors is one strategy for immunosuppression. One drug that acts in this manner is *fingolimod*, a sphingosine 1-phosphate receptor agonist.

INNATE IMMUNITY

Innate immunity provides the body's initial encounter with pathogens. Phagocytic cells, that is, macrophages, dendritic cells (DCs), and neutrophils, recognize

pathogens by using pathogen-associated molecular patterns (PAMPs). PAMPs, such as viral RNA and lipopolysaccharide (LPS), are essential molecules for microbial survival, which restricts major changes in their structure. Cells recognize PAMPs using pathogen-recognition receptors (PRRs), such as Toll-like receptors (TLRs), an evolutionarily ancient mechanism that is conserved in plants and animals (1,2). Other PRRs include NLRs (NOD-like receptors), and RLRs (RIG-I-like receptors) (Table 4-1).

The engagement of PRRs leads to the activation of signaling pathways that activate inflammation. The *NF-κB signaling pathway* can be activated by most TLRs and culminates in the transcriptional activation of hundreds of pro-inflammatory genes, including many pro-inflammatory cytokines such as interleukin (IL)-1, IL-6, tumor necrosis factor (TNF), and chemokines, such as IL-8, that attract more innate immune cells. Activation of NLRs leads to the formation of a proteolytic signaling complex denoted the *inflammasome*, which processes a subset of these cytokines, leading to the secretion of IL-1 and IL-18 (3).

The importance of proinflammatory cytokines in rheumatic disease is exemplified by the effectiveness of TNF-alpha receptor antagonists like *etanercept*, *infliximab*, and *adalimumab* in the treatment of rheumatoid arthritis (RA). Conversely, dominant mutations in one of the TNF receptors (TNFR1) result in an autoinflammatory disorder termed *TRAPS* (TNFR-associated periodic syndrome). Mutations in constituents of the inflammasome give rise to diseases such as *familial Mediterranean fever* (FMF) and *neonatal onset multiorgan inflammatory disorder* (NOMID) (4). The latter disorder can be effectively treated with the IL-1 receptor antagonist *anakinra*. Mutation of proteins that recognize intracellular pathogens such as the NLR NOD2/CARD15 is associated with *Crohn's disease*.

TABLE 4-1. PATTERN RECOGNITION RECEPTORS (PRRs) IDENTIFIED IN EXPERIMENTAL ANIMALS AND HUMANS.[a]

PRR FAMILY	FAMILY MEMBERS	EXAMPLES OF PAMPs	EXAMPLES OF ASSOCIATED IMMUNE DISEASES
Toll-like receptors (TLRs)	TLR1-13	Zymosan, lipopolysaccharide, CpG oligonucleotides	Leprosy, atherosclerosis, asthma, inflammatory bowel disease
NOD-like receptors (NLRs)	NOD 1–5, NALP 1–14, CIITA, IPAF, NAIP	Low intracellular potassium, monosodium urate, peptidoglycan	Crohn's disease, Muckle–Wells syndrome, pseudogout, Familial Mediterranean fever
RIG-I-like receptors (RLRs)	RIG1, MDA5, LGP2	Double-stranded RNA	Increased susceptibility to RNA viruses

[a]Dozens of pattern recognition receptors (PRRs) have been identified in experimental animals and in humans. Although the pathogen-associated molecular pattern (PAMP) that each of these receptors recognizes has not been elucidated, mutations in PRRs have been linked to several human diseases. These include genetic mutations that lead to hyperactivation of the inflammasome (e.g. NALP3 and Muckle–Wells syndrome) and increased susceptibility to chronic inflammation (e.g., NOD2 and Crohn's disease). Chronic stimulation of the innate immune system through PRRs appears to be important in the chronic inflammation of rheumatic diseases. This is the rationale behind arthritis therapy with the drug etanercept, which blocks the action of TNF-alpha, a PRR signaling pathway target cytokine.

Innate Immune Cells

The release of pro-inflammatory cytokines activates other components of the innate and adaptive immune systems, and DCs are key to this connection (Figure 4-3) (5). Although derived from the bone marrow, DCs reside in the periphery. Most organs are thought to possess their own DC populations, where they act as sentinels for pathogens. Upon activation, they migrate to the lymph nodes and the spleen, where they present their antigens to T cells in the context of costimulatory molecules. *Adjuvants* increase the antigenicity of vaccines through their ability to activate DCs and other phagocytes. DCs produce an array of cytokines, including IL-12 and IL-23, that activate and regulate lymphocytes. Conversely, DCs and other phagocytic cells are activated by the products of lymphocytes, such as the cytokine interferon (IFN) gamma. A subset of DCs, plasmacytoid DCs, is the body's major producer of type I IFNs (6).

IFNs are critical for host defense against viruses, but overproduction of IFN is a feature of rheumatic diseases, such as systemic lupus erythematosus (SLE).

Natural killer cells are a lymphocyte subset that can be included in the innate immune system because NK cells lack rearranging antigen receptors. Among the receptors NK cells do express, some can sense stressed or damaged cells. For example, NK cells can lyse virus-infected cells and tumors that lack major histocompatibility class (MHC) I molecules. NK cells also produce significant quantities of cytokines, such as IFN-gamma, that can influence the development of T cells. NKT cells are a unique subset of T cells with properties of NK cells that recognize lipid antigens presented by the molecule CD1d via a restricted set of T-cell receptors. NK T cells appear to be vital for combating certain fungal, protozoan, bacterial, and viral infections (7).

Eosinophils, basophils, and mast cells are cellular components of the innate immune system that are often

FIGURE 4-3

Dendritic cells (DC) reside inside peripheral tissues where they survey the environment for pathogens. After contact with a pathogen, a DC migrates to the regional lymph node to activate the adaptive immune response. DCs sense pathogens in one of several ways. One method is activation of intracellular and extracellular pattern recognition receptor (PRR) signaling pathways by pathogen-associated molecular patterns (PAMPs). Dendritic cells also ingest pathogens and break them down into peptides that are then presented to T cells in the context of major histocompatibility complex (MHC) molecules. In addition, complement can bind to the surface of pathogens, and phagocytes will recognize the complement–pathogen aggregates through complement receptors. After antigen recognition, the DC activates cells of the adaptive immune response either via direct cell contact at the immune synapse or through cytokine signaling. T cells and B cells in turn secrete cytokines that offer feedback to the dendritic cells, altering the DC cytokine secretion profile and regulating DC survival. Adaptive immune cells also signal to one another as well as engage in autocrine stimulation.

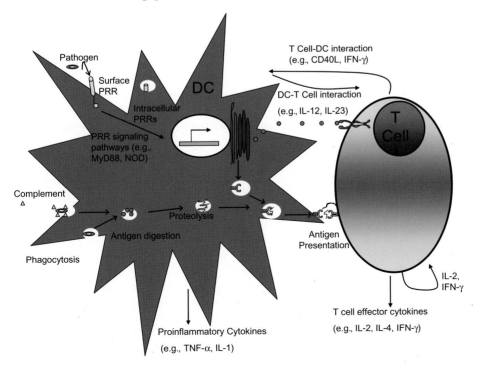

associated with allergic diseases, but these cells are also active participants in other aspects of immunity (8). Eosinophils, important for host defense against gastrointestinal parasites, secrete cytokines that regulate B cells and T cells, and exhibit strong effects on mucosal surfaces. Basophils and mast cells both express high affinity IgE receptor and release histamine. Basophils influence CD4+ T cells via the release of IL-4 and IL-13 and activate B cells via CD40 ligand. Mast cells are long-lived cells that undergo terminal differentiation and ultimately reside in well-vascularized tissues. They express TLRs, secrete pathogen-fighting toxins, respond to allergens, and secrete cytokines that influence CD4+ T-cell activity. Though mast cells are known to be involved in the pathogenesis of allergies and asthma, they also appear to be critical in the development of arthritis.

COMPLEMENT

The complement system consists of more than 30 serum and cell surface proteins that function as soluble innate immune receptors and amplifiers of antibody responses. Components of the complement system, such as C1q, C3, and mannan binding lectin (MBL), bind cellular and subcellular components of microbes as well as DNA, RNA, and membrane fragments released by endogenous cell death. The classic complement pathway begins with the activation of C1q by immunoglobulin-containing immune complexes, and the alternative complement pathway begins with the thioester activation of C3. Complement coats the surface of microorganisms. Receptors on phagocytic cells can then bind the complement, prompting ingestion of the microorganisms (*opsonization*). Complement also induces phagocytic cells to secrete cytokines through activation of the complement receptors and influences TLR signal transduction. Additionally, the inflammatory cascade initiated by complement binding recruits more phagocytes and mast cells to sites of tissue injury and promotes cytokine production that activates the adaptive immune response. Another complement function is the direct lysing of microorganisms through formation of the membrane attack complex (MAC), made up of C5-C9.

Interestingly, mutations in complement and complement regulatory protein gene deficiencies have been linked to several autoimmune and inflammatory diseases, including SLE (9). Complement H deficiency increases susceptibility to *hemolytic uremic syndrome* and *macular degeneration*. Deficiency of C1 inhibitor causes *hereditary angioedema*. C3 deficiency results in severe susceptibility to microbial pathogens, and deficiency of C5-C9 is associated with selective susceptibility to *Neisseria* species. Patients with mutations of MBL are also immunodeficient. Patients with C4 deficiency are the most susceptible to SLE and related autoimmune diseases, perhaps due to a failure to properly regulate the effects of immune complexes on adaptive immune cells.

ANTIGEN PRESENTATION AND MAJOR HISTOCOMPATIBILITY CLASS MOLECULES

An antigen can be defined as a substance that generates an immune response. What distinguishes adaptive immune cells from innate immune cells is the ability of B cells and T cells to express unique, highly antigen-specific receptors on their plasma membranes. Engagement of these receptors causes an individual B or T cell to expand into a clonal population of lymphocytes directed against the antigen-bearing pathogen. Expansion of lymphocytes that recognize host antigens rather than pathogenic antigens is one mechanism of autoimmune disease.

Although T and B cells use a similar strategy to produce their antigen-specific receptors, they recognize antigen very differently. B cells recognize soluble peptides, proteins, nucleic acids, polysaccharides, lipids, and small synthetic molecules. These antigens bind directly to the B-cell antigen receptor (BCR), a membrane-associated form of immunoglobulin. Consequently, B cells have no need for antigen-presenting cells. In contrast, T cells need antigen to be presented, that is, the T-cell antigen receptor (TCR) recognizes fragments only when they are bound to MHC molecules on the surface of other cells.

The two types of MHC molecules, class I and class II, are the most polymorphic human proteins, and expression of different MHC alleles correlates with susceptibility to autoimmune disease. In humans, the MHC [also termed *histocompatibility locus antigen (HLA)*] comprises a 3.6 Mbp DNA sequence on chromosome 6p. It is the single most gene-dense region of the human genome. HLA alleles associated with specific diseases include HLA-B27 with spondyloarthropathy and HLADRB1 with rheumatoid arthritis.

The three-dimensional structure of both classes of MHC creates a cleft, or groove, in which peptides are bound and can be recognized by T cells. Each MHC molecule binds a single peptide, but the total pool of MHC molecules can bind an array of peptides. The association of peptides with MHC molecules is determined by MHC molecule primary and secondary structures. The types of antigens that each MHC class binds are distinct: MHC class I molecules most often present endogenous peptides, while the MHC class II molecules present exogenous peptides. Class I molecules are constitutively expressed on nearly all cells except neurons and red blood cells, whereas class II molecules are limited to B cells, macrophages, DCs, activated T cells, and activated endothelial cells. Cells that present antigen to T cells in the context of MHC class II are called *antigen presenting cells* (APCs).

Although most T cells recognize peptides, gamma delta T cells, representing about 5% of peripheral blood T cells, can recognize nonpeptide antigen, such as prenyl pyrophosphate derivatives of mycobacteria. A subset of these cells, known as Vdelta2$^+$ T cells, do not need APCs to recognize antigen and may act as APCs themselves to direct other T-cell responses.

MAJOR HISTOCOMPATIBILITY CLASS CLASS I

Major histocompatibility class class I molecules are synthesized and assembled within the endoplasmic reticulum (ER). Two proteins comprise the MHC class I molecule. The alpha chain, encoded by genes within the HLA locus (HLA-A, -B, and -C), associates with a non–MHC-encoded protein, beta$_2$ microglobulin. Class I molecules bind peptides that are 9 to 11 amino acids in length. Peptides from pathogens in the cytosol, such as viruses, as well as normal cellular proteins are degraded in the proteasome and then transferred to the ER by the TAP transporter molecules, also encoded within the MHC locus. Within the ER, these endogenous peptides bind the nascent MHC class I molecules. In addition, mechanisms allow certain exogenous antigens to be cross-presented by class I, such as fusion of endosomes with the ER. This occurs most efficiently in activated DCs. The MHC I molecule–peptide complexes translocate to the plasma membrane, where they engage T cells. The T-cell accessory molecule, CD8, binds to class I molecules; thus, *CD8+ T cells are class I restricted.*

MHC CLASS II

Major histocompatibility class class II molecules bind extracellular peptides. Class II molecules are composed of two chains that are products of different MHC genes (HLA-DR, -DQ, and -DP) than MHC class I. Antigen processing by MHC class II–expressing APCs occurs in three steps: extracellular antigens are ingested, internalized, and proteolyzed (Figure 4-3). MHC class II molecules are synthesized and assembled in the ER, but they are prevented from binding endogenous antigens because the class II complex associates with a molecule called the invariant chain. After export from the Golgi complex, the invariant chain is removed by the action of proteases and HLA-DM. Endosomes containing the ingested extracellular peptides then fuse with MHC class II–containing vesicles exported from the Golgi. This action allows processed, extracellularly derived antigen to bind to class II molecules. The T-cell accessory molecule, CD4, binds to class II molecules; therefore, *CD4+ T cells are class II restricted.* The bare lymphocyte syndrome (BLS) is a primary immunodeficiency resulting from the absence of MHC class II expression.

T CELLS

The T-Cell Receptor and Antigen Recognition

Antigen-recognition and signal-transducing elements aggregate at the plasma membrane to form the T-cell receptor (TCR) complex. Four TCR genes encode the subunits responsible for antigen recognition: alpha, beta, gamma, and delta. These TCR genes are members of the immunoglobulin superfamily. Like other immunoglobulin genes, the TCR genes undergo DNA rearrangement of variable (V), diversity (D), joining (J), and constant (C) region segments. Recombination of gene segments is generated by the action of several enzymes, including the recombinase-activating genes RAG-1 and RAG-2. The rearranged genes are then transcribed and translated to produce protein subunits. Heterodimers of these subunits come together to create either the alpha beta or gamma delta receptors, which function as the T cell's antigen-recognition units. The majority of T cells in peripheral blood, lymph nodes, and spleen express alpha beta receptors.

Diversity-generating mechanisms allow humans to produce 10^{16} possible antigen-specific alpha beta T-cell receptors. V-region gene segments are highly polymorphic, and recombinant assembly of the different V, D, and J segments allows for a wide array of possible antigen receptors. The enzyme terminal deoxytransferase further expands the receptor repertoire by inserting random nucleotides at the junctions between the gene segments.

T-cell receptor genes show allelic exclusion, that is, if one chromosome undergoes rearrangement and produces a functional receptor chain, the genes on the other chromosome are prevented from rearranging. Hence, each T-cell clone expresses only one antigen receptor, and antigen-specific T cells develop in unimmunized or naive individuals independent of exposure to antigen. Subsequent antigen exposure leads to clonal selection or expansion of lymphocytes with the appropriate antigen receptors. Clonal selection improves the efficiency of the immune response and produces immunological memory.

Mutations in the genetic machinery for V(D)J recombination have been linked to a variety of *severe combined immunodeficiency* (SCID) conditions in humans (10). Deficiency in RAG-1 or RAG-2 leads to a virtual lack of all mature T and B lymphocytes, whereas impairment of RAG-1 and RAG-2 without total loss of function leads to a distinct phenotype called *Omenn syndrome*. Mutations in another recombination gene, ARTEMIS, cause *RS-SCID*, a condition with absence of mature B cells and T cells, normal NK cells, and increased radiosensitivity. Rearrangement of the TCR genes requires double-stranded breaks in the genome, and the kinase ataxia telangiectasia mutated (ATM) regulates this potentially hazardous action. ATM deficiency leads to *ataxia–telangiectasia* (A-T), an autosomal recessive genomic instability syndrome.

T-Cell Receptor Signal Transduction

T-cell receptor alpha beta or gamma delta subunits provide an elegant solution to the problem of antigen recognition, but these subunits do not transmit activation signals. The antigen-recognizing subunits associate with nonpolymorphic signaling subunits called the *invariant chains*, which include the CD3 family of molecules (gamma, delta, and epsilon) and the zeta chain (Figure 4-4). These subunits contain domains called *immune tyrosine-based activation motifs* (ITAMs), domains that are also present on B-cell and Fc receptors. The ITAMs are phosphorylated by *protein tyrosine kinases* (PTKs) and serve to recruit other signaling molecules. Some lymphocyte receptors have motifs called

FIGURE 4-4

A CD4+ T cell and an APC interact at the immune synapse. The T-cell receptor, comprised of the alpha beta subunits, CD3 invariant chains, and CD4 coreceptor, contacts the MHC–peptide complex. Costimulatory signals are transmitted through a series of molecules, including CD28 and CD40L. Engagement of peptide in the context of MHC brings the CD4-linked tyrosine kinase Lck into proximity with the beta alpha subunits and CD3, while excluding the phosphatase CD45. Lck phosphorylates immune tyrosine-based activation motifs (ITAMs) on CD3. This triggers a phosphorylation cascade that ultimately activates the transcription factors, including NFAT and NF-κB, which bind the DNA and modulate gene expression. APCs also activate T cells through cytokines, particularly via the JAK/STAT signaling pathway. Drugs that block the activation of T cells are shown in italics.

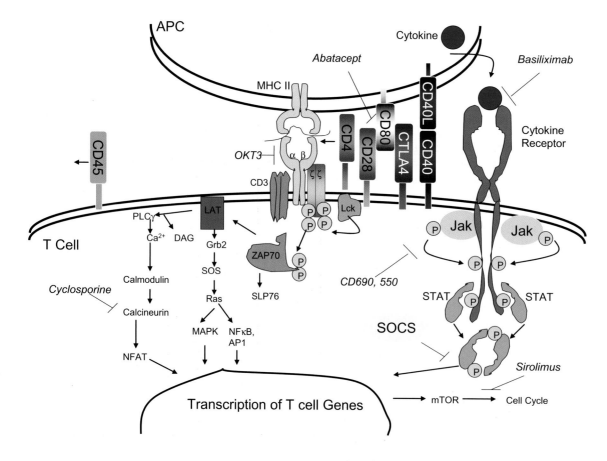

immunoreceptor tyrosine-based inhibitory motifs (ITIMs), which recruit phosphatases and attenuate signaling. In the resting T cell, a kinetic balance between PTKs and tyrosine phosphatases keeps TCR signaling through the ITAMs at a low basal level.

When the TCR engages the MHC–antigen complex of an APC, rearrangement of the plasma membrane surrounding the TCR changes the relative distribution of PTKs and tyrosine phosphatases near the cell surface; this redistribution of signaling molecules is referred to as the *immune synapse* (Figure 4-4) (11). The first step in TCR signaling is tyrosine phosphorylation of receptor subunits and adapter molecules such as LAT (linker of activated T cells) and SLP-76. This is mediated by a series of PTKs including Lck (a PTK bound to the CD4+ and CD8+ molecules), Zap-70 (zeta-associated protein of 70kDa), and members of the Tec family. This in turn leads to the elevation of intracellular calcium, which activates the phosphatase calcineurin. Calcineurin dephosphorylates NFAT (nuclear factor of activated T cells), allowing the translocation of this transcription factor to the nucleus. The immunosuppressive drugs *cyclosporine* and *tacrolimus* work by inhibiting calcineurin and NFAT activation; conversely, mutations that inhibit calcium channel function are a cause of primary immunodeficiency. TCR signaling also activates other transcription factors such as NF-κB, Fos, and Jun, which modulate the expression of genes encoding cytokines, receptors, and other proteins that carry out T-cell functions.

T cells are also activated by cytokines, some of which are made by other cells, and some of which are made by T cells themselves. Many, but not all, cytokines bind to receptors that are members of a cytokine receptor superfamily that signals via Janus kinases (JAKs). An important class of substrates for JAKs are the STATs (signal transducers and activators of transcription), a family of seven transcription factors with distinct but critical functions in host defense. Cytokine signaling is negatively regulated by inhibitors of cytokine signal transduction, including SH2-containing phosphatases (SHP), protein inhibitors of activated STATs (PIAS), and suppressors of cytokine signaling (SOCS). Absence of SHP1, SOCS1, or SOCS3 is associated with systemic autoimmune disease in mouse models. Conversely, patients with mutations of *JAK3*, or its associated receptor subunit the common gamma chain, have SCID due to failure in signaling by IL-2, IL-4, IL-7, IL-15, and IL-21. Pharmacological targeting of JAK3 is being studied as a new class of immunosuppressant drugs (12).

Costimulation

Occupancy of the T-cell receptor alone does not lead to T-cell activation; occupancy of other costimulatory molecules is necessary to provide a full activation signal (13). T cells that only receive a TCR signal can become *anergic* or unable to achieve full activation. Receptors that provide costimulation include: CD28, ICOS (inducible costimulator), PD-1, and adhesion molecules (CD11a/CD18, CD2, and others). Mutation of ICOS is one cause of common variable immunodeficiency (CVID). A number of receptors in the TNF-receptor family also function as lymphocyte costimulators. The counter-receptors for CD28 are CD80 and CD86, which are expressed on APCs. Interruption of CD28-dependent costimulation with the drug *abatacept* is efficacious in treating rheumatoid arthritis. A CD28-related molecule, CTLA-4, which also binds CD80 and CD86, downregulates immune responses; its deficiency is associated with lethal autoimmune disease in mice.

T-Cell Development

Precursor T cells originate in the bone marrow from hematopoietic stem cells and migrate to the thymus. As they mature, T cells move from the thymic cortex to the medulla. The most immature T cells, known as double-negative (DN) T cells, lack the surface markers CD4 and CD8; these cells do not express a mature TCR but do express the pre–T-cell receptor, which comprises the beta chain, an invariant protein called pre-T alpha, CD3, and zeta proteins. These cells mature into double-positive (DP) T cells, which express CD4 and CD8 and undergo alpha chain rearrangement to form TCR alpha beta heterodimers. DP thymocytes mature to become single-positive (SP) thymocytes, which express either CD4 or CD8, as well as a complete TCR. Mature SP T cells migrate out from the thymic medulla to populate the peripheral lymphoid tissues.

The development of T cells depends on signals from the thymic stroma, which direct multipotent cells towards the T-cell fate. Forkhead box N1 (FOXN1) is a transcription factor that is essential for thymic organogenesis and the attraction of hematopoietic stem cells to the thymus. Mutations of FOXN1 result in the "nude" phenotype in mice and humans, characterized by athymia and hairlessness. Another important stromal signal is Notch1 signaling; mutation of Notch1 results in developmental arrest of T cells.

The vast majority of T cell precursors generated in the thymus die there. Much of the T-cell death that occurs in the thymus is due to programmed cell death (*apoptosis*). To survive, potential T cells must first produce TCRs at the DP stage that can recognize self-MHC molecules, a process called *positive selection*. Cells lacking an appropriate receptor undergo "death by neglect," that is, they do not receive further maturation signals from the thymic stroma. Of the SP thymocytes that do develop, some recognize self-MHC molecules and self-peptides with high avidity. These potentially autoreactive T cells are also eliminated, a process called *negative selection or clonal deletion*. The removal of potentially harmful T cells in the thymus is termed *central tolerance*. Of course, not all potential self-peptides are expressed in the thymus. This problem is addressed by a transcription factor, autoimmune regulator (AIRE), which induces the ectopic transcription of organ-specific non-thymic peptides in thymic epithelium (14). Patients with mutations in *AIRE* have an autoimmune disorder called APECED (autoimmune polyendocrinopathy-candidiasis-ectodermal dystrophy) syndrome, which results from failure of negative selection of T cells responsive to tissue-specific antigens.

CD4+ T-Cell Differentiation

CD4+ T cells are also known as T-helper cells because of their role in promoting the function of other immune cells. Classically, CD4+ cells have been thought to differentiate into one of two primary effector cell types: T-helper 1 (Th1) and T-helper 2 (Th2) cells (Figure 4-1). Precisely how T-helper cell lineage differentiation occurs is the subject of intense study, but cytokines produced by DCs and macrophages are clearly important in the outcome. Macrophages and dendritic cells promote differentiation of naive CD4+ cells into Th1 cells by secreting IL-12. In addition, T-cell transcription factors, such as Stat6, GATA-3, Stat4, and T-Bet are also critical (15).

T-helper 1 cells secrete cytokines that promote cell-mediated immunity. The key Th1 cytokine is IFN-gamma, which enhances the ability of macrophages to kill ingested microorganisms, upregulates MHC class I expression on many cell types, and suppresses Th2 responses. Mutations that affect the IL-12/IFN-gamma axis cause susceptibility to intracellular microorganisms, especially atypical *Mycobacteria*. Mutation of Tyk2, the Jak kinase responsible for signaling by IL-12 and type I IFNs, is one cause of primary immunodeficiency known as *HyperIgE syndrome* (HIES).

T-helper 2 cells are essential for defense against helminth infections and the host response to allergens. IL-4 promotes the differentiation of naive CD4+ T cells into Th2 cells, which produce IL-4, IL-5, IL-10, and IL-13. These cytokines promote humoral and allergic-type responses. IL-4 inhibits macrophage activation, blocks the effects of IFN-gamma, promotes mast cell growth, and induces B cells to produce IgE. IL-5 induces eosinophilia, and IL-10 inhibits macrophage antigen presentation and decreases expression of MHC I molecules. The importance of IL-10 is underscored by the finding that IL-10 knockout mice develop severe autoimmune disease.

The simple dichotomy between Th1 and Th2 cells has recently been called into question with the discovery of other types of CD4+ cells that produce neither IFN-gamma nor IL-4, but rather produce other inflammatory cytokines. So-called Th17 cells produce IL-17, IL-6, IL-22, G-CSF (granulocyte-colony stimulating factor), and TNF-alpha (16). Th17 cell differentiation and maintenance is promoted by transforming growth factor (TGF)-beta 1, IL-6, and IL-23, and it is inhibited by both IFN-gamma and IL-4. Th17 cells are abundant in the lamina propria of the small intestine in mice and seem to be important in host defense against extracellular bacteria. IL-17 is overproduced in many autoimmune and autoinflammatory disorders, in which it appears to play a major pathogenic role. In addition, although individual mouse T cells tend to produce cytokines related to one of the above subsets, human T cells can produce a wider variety of cytokines and are not as easily classified by the above criteria.

Regulatory T Cells and Maintenance of Peripheral Tolerance

Another set of CD4+ cells, dubbed T regulatory (Treg) cells, is essential for limiting immune responses; as such, it is critical for *peripheral tolerance* (17). Tregs have the remarkable ability to suppress proliferation and cytokine production by effector T cells through mechanisms that are at present not well understood. The transcription factor FoxP3 (forkhead box P3) is both necessary and sufficient for Treg function. *Natural Treg*s (nTregs), arising in the thymus, express molecules such as CD25 and GITR that are usually restricted to activated T cells. In addition, naive T cells can be driven to differentiate into *induced* or iTregs under the influence of the cytokine TGF-beta1. Mutation of FoxP3 produces the *scurfy* phenotype in mice and *IPEX* (immune dysregulation, polyendocrinopathy, enteropathy, X-linked) syndrome in humans, both of which are manifested by T-cell attack on multiple organs and autoantibody production.

Though important, Treg cells are not the only mediators of peripheral tolerance. Another mechanism is elimination of activated T cells through repetitive stimulation. Repeatedly stimulated CD4$^+$ T cells can undergo autocrine cell death through interactions between the TNF-ligand FasL and its receptor Fas/CD95. *Autoimmune lymphoproliferative syndrome* (ALPS), characterized by lymphadenopathy, accumulation of an unusual subset of CD4$^-$CD8$^-$ double-negative peripheral T cells, and frequent autoimmune disease, is caused in most cases by dominant negative germline mutations in the gene coding for Fas. Naive T cells activated through the TCR without appropriate costimulation can also become anergic, a more temporary form of peripheral immune tolerance. Because of positive selection towards self-MHC, it is thought that most peripheral T cells are constantly receiving low levels of activation signals from self-peptide MHC complexes in the periphery, and this may modulate T-cell responses as well.

CD8+ T Cells

CD8+ T cells, also known as cytotoxic T lymphocytes (CTLs), recognize antigen in the context of MHC I molecules. Because MHC I molecules present antigens synthesized by the target cell, CTLs play a prominent role in defense against intracellular pathogens, particularly viruses, protozoa, and bacteria, as well as cancer. During primary infection, antigen-specific CTL clones expand rapidly, and at the peak of response can represent a substantial fraction of all T cells. After the infection is cleared, this initial burst is followed by a rapid depletion of these cells, probably due to the cells outgrowing their cytokine supply (Figure 4-5). A small number of CD8+ T cells then become memory T cells, allowing the host rapid, heightened responses to future infections with a specific pathogen. Although the exact events producing the memory phenotype are unknown, cytokines including IL-2, IL-7, and IL-15 are important for CD8+ memory cell generation and maintenance (15). Lack of CD4+ help or IL-2 during primary stimulation of CD8+ T cells can promote the expression of molecules like PD1, which negatively regulates proliferation, or TRAIL, which induces apoptosis and blocks effective memory cell formation. This can occur in chronic infections such as human immunodeficiency virus (HIV).

Cytotoxic T lymphocytes have several strategies for mediating cell killing. Like NK cells, CTLs kill target cells directly using perforin and granzymes. Perforin, a homologue to the complement component C9, disrupts the plasma membrane through pore formation. This allows the CTL to insert granules containing granzymes, which are proteases that rapidly activate apoptosis in

FIGURE 4-5

The immune response begins when the cells of the innate immune system and complement engage pathogens. As the pathogens are neutralized, innate immune cells secrete cytokines that increase the number of phagocytes at the site of infection. APCs also migrate to the lymphatic tissue, where they stimulate the clonal expansion of B cells and T cells. As the immune response progresses, the specificity of the reaction increases. B cells refine their immunoglobulins through isotype/class switching and somatic hypermutation. CD8+ T cells lyse infected cells, and CD4+ T cells direct the B-cell response as well as increase the ability of phagocytes to neutralize pathogens. As the infection clears, there is attenuation of the immune response accomplished by the apoptosis of clonal T cells and decreased activation of innate immune cells. Memory cells develop, allowing a rapid response to any future encounters with pathogens. Failure to resolve the initial immune response produces chronic inflammation, a state of continued innate cell activation and adaptive cell reaction.

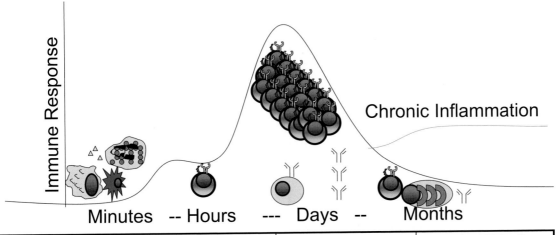

	Minutes -- Hours	--- Days --	Months
Immune Processes	Complement activation, phagocytosis, engagement of PRRs, activation of inflammasome	Migration of APCs to lymph nodes, expansion of CD8 clones, secretion of IgM then isotype switching	Apoptosis of CD8 cells, establishment of memory T cells and plasma B cells, decrease in inflammatory response
Primary Cells Involved	Macrophages, DCs, neutrophils, NK cells	B cells, T cells	B cells, T cells
Examples of Disorders	Chronic Granulomatous Disease, C3 deficiency, TRAPS, FMF	X-linked SCID, JAK3 deficiency, Hyper IgM syndrome, XLA	RA, SLE, ALPS

the target cells. CTLs also direct secretion of FasL, which binds the apoptosis-inducing receptor Fas on target cells. CTLs secrete cytokines such as TNF-alpha and IFN-gamma, which can attract phagocytes to sites of infection. Viruses can evade CD8+ T cells by down-regulating MHC class I molecules; fortunately, the loss of MHC molecules is a signal that activates NK cells. CTLs may also regulate themselves through cytotoxic activity. This is evident in patients with *familial hemophagocytic lymphohistiocytosis*, a fatal autosomal recessive disorder caused by mutations in perforin or other molecules involved in cytotoxic granule formation. These patients have uncontrolled activation of CTLs and overproduction of inflammatory cytokines.

B CELLS AND IMMUNOGLOBULINS

Another major component of the adaptive immune response is a class of lymphocytes termed *B cells*. Generated in the bone marrow, B cells produce immunoglobulins or antibodies. B cells can also function as antigen-presenting cells and share some features with innate immune cells. Immunoglobulins function as antigen receptors on B cells, but are also secreted and have major functions in host defense. Additionally, immunoglobulins are major contributors to immune-mediated disease.

Immunoglobulin molecules consist of four polypeptide chains: two identical light (L) chains and two identical heavy (H) chains, both of which have variable and constant regions. Structurally, the four chains assemble to form a Y-shaped molecule. The variable regions bind antigens, which, unlike in T cells, encompass many types of molecules, including proteins, lipids, carbohydrates, nucleic acids, or even drugs. The constant regions of the H chain form what is called the Fc region of the immunoglobulin molecule. Many of the effector functions of immunoglobulins, such as binding complement and receptors on phagocytic cells (Fc receptors), depend on the constant region of H chain.

There are two types of immunoglobulin L chains—kappa and lambda—and five types of H chains—mu, gamma, delta, epsilon, alpha. The five different classes or isotypes are designated IgM, IgG, IgD, IgE, and IgA, respectively. There are also subclasses of IgG (gamma l, gamma 2, gamma 3, and gamma 4) and IgA (alpha 1 and alpha 2). The antigen receptor on B cells is a membrane-bound form of IgM or IgD. After encounter with antigen and with the help of T cells, B cells proliferate and secrete immunoglobulins of different classes, a process known as heavy chain class or isotype switching. The secreted form of IgM molecules is a multimer of five Y-shaped immunoglobulin monomers joined by a J chain. IgA molecules form a dimer, which functions at epithelial surfaces and, when secreted, is associated with a secretory fragment.

B-Cell Development and Immunoglobulin Gene Rearrangement

Like other hematopoietic cells, B cells first develop in the fetal liver but later are produced in the bone marrow; like T cells, the cytokine milieu is important for the proliferation of stem cells and B-cell progenitors. As with T-cell development, successful B-cell development is dependent upon immunoglobulin gene rearrangement and the formation of a functional antigen receptor. As in T cells, B-cell development requires the recombination of V, D, and J genes that are separate from one another in the germline; a proper B-cell receptor repertoire is dependent upon the recombinase machinery. B-cell precursors first assemble heavy chain (chromosome 14) D and J genes, with subsequent joining of a V region to the DJ complex, forming a mu chain. H-chain rearrangements then cease. B-cell precursors that have not yet initiated immunoglobulin rearrangement are called pro-B cells, whereas precursors that express an H chain are called pre-B cells. In pre-B cells, the mu chains are mostly intracellular, but some are expressed on the cell surface in association with surrogate L chain to form the pre–B-cell receptor complex. This receptor signals the pre-B cell to proliferate and to rearrange the V and J regions of one of its L chain genes (kappa and lambda loci on chromosomes 2 and 22, respectively). Once a B-cell precursor successfully rearranges an H and L gene, the process stops, and the cell expresses surface immunoglobulin; it then is termed an immature B cell. Mature B cells express both membrane IgM and IgD.

Combinatorial rearrangement of H and L chain genes allows for 10^{11} possible antigen receptors and immunoglobulin molecules. Many precursor cells fail to make successful rearrangements or fail to express a functional pre–B-cell receptor, which results in apoptosis. In general, any mutation that impairs H-chain rearrangement or expression will block B-cell development.

B-Cell Activation and Differentiation

The B-cell receptor (BCR) signals similarly to the TCR, but unlike the TCR it has two functions. It initiates signals that activate B cells to proliferate but also binds and internalizes antigens. The antigens are processed, loaded onto class II molecules, and presented to CD4+ T cells. Structurally, the BCR consists of membrane-bound IgM associated with two transmembrane proteins: Ig-alpha and Ig-beta Similar to the TCR-associated molecules, Ig-alpha and Ig-beta have ITAMs, which are phosphorylated by PTKs such as Lyn, Blk, and Fyn. This leads to the activation of additional PTKs, including Syk and Bruton's tyrosine kinase (Btk), which activate downstream pathways. Mutations of Btk underlie the disorder *X-linked agammaglobulinemia*. The B-cell transmembrane protein CD19 enhances BCR signaling, and deficiency of this molecule is a cause of *common variable immunodeficiency* (CVID). These patients, who make inadequate amounts of immunoglobulin, can be treated with replacement intravenous immunoglobulin.

Once a B-cell precursor expresses surface immunoglobulin, it can respond to exogenous and self-antigens. However, binding of antigens to the BCR on immature B cells does not trigger cellular activation; rather, binding induces a cellular response that leads to self-tolerance. Multivalent self-antigens tend to induce programmed cell death, whereas oligovalent self-antigens render immature B cells refractory to further stimulation. Such a cell may escape anergy by rearranging another L-chain immunoglobulin gene, changing its BCR specificity, and losing its self-reactivity; this process is known as *receptor editing*.

A subset of B cells, B1 cells, is produced early in ontogeny and is present predominantly in the peritoneal cavity. They have limited diversity of their antigen receptors. Most of the circulating IgM comes from B1 cells and is specific for carbohydrate products of bacteria.

Mature B cells with non–self-reactive BCRs enter secondary lymphoid tissues, such as the spleen and lymph nodes, where they may encounter foreign antigens. B-cell antigens are divided broadly into thymus-dependent (TD) and thymus-independent (TI) antigens. TD antigens are typically soluble protein antigens that require MHC class II–mediated T-cell help for antibody production, whereas TI antigens do not require such help. TI antigens often are multivalent, for example, bacterial polysaccharides. In general, TI responses generate poor immunological memory, induce minimal germinal-center formation (see below), and trigger IgG2 secretion. B cells responding to TI antigens have a distinct phenotype and localize in the marginal zone of the spleen. Dependence on these splenic B cells for responses to TI antigens may account for the poor responses to polysaccharide antigens seen in splenectomized individuals and in infants, because marginal zone B cells do not mature until about 2 years of age. For vaccines, this deficit can be overcome by coupling polysaccharides to a carrier protein, which triggers a TD response.

In the spleen, antigen-activated B cells migrate to T cell–rich zones in the periarteriolar lymphoid sheath searching for T-cell help. Failure to find this help likely results in anergy, but successful B-cell/T-cell collaboration produces short-lived oligoclonal proliferative foci (each derived from several B cells). Many of the B cells in these foci secrete IgM and undergo isotype switching, and IgM antibodies of a given antigen specificity can be converted to IgG, IgA, or IgE. These events depend on direct costimulatory signals from T cells, such as CD40 ligand/CD40 interactions and T-cell–derived cytokines such as IL-2, IL-4, IL-6, L-10, and IL-21. Mutations of CD40 or CD40L (TNF/TNFR members on T cells and B cells, respectively) underlie *hyper-IgM syndromes*. These patients lack germinal centers and have impaired class switch recombination in B cells owing to a lack of T cell stimulation. Interference with the CD40/CD40L interaction is being studied as a means of treating autoimmune disorders.

Some B cells migrate from these proliferative foci to primary follicles and enter the germinal-center pathway. Within a primary follicle, an oligoclonal expansion of B cells forms the dark zone. Eventually, these cells migrate into a region called the light zone, where they interact with helper T cells and follicular dendritic cells that have trapped and localized antigen on their surfaces. Under these conditions, antibody affinity is further altered by the introduction of mutations in B-cell variable gene segments, a process known as *somatic hypermutation*, which does not occur in T-cell receptor variable genes. As a consequence of random hypermutation, B cells possessing high affinity BCRs are selected for survival, whereas those that do not possess this affinity die. B cells in which somatic mutations generated an autoreactive BCR also are eliminated.

Passage through the germinal center leads to the formation of plasma-cell precursors and memory B cells; few antibody-secreting cells remain within the germinal center. Plasma cells lose their membrane immunoglobulin and many of the markers that identify B cells, including CD20, the target for the drug *rituximab* (18). Instead, plasma cells uniquely express high levels of CD38. Plasma cells secrete large amounts of immunoglobulin. They are generally short-lived cells and need constant replenishment to sustain high antibody levels, although a population of long-lived plasma cells can be maintained in the bone marrow. These may account for memory immunoglobulin persistence (19). Memory B cells are long-lived cells, carry somatically mutated V genes, and are morphologically distinct from naive B cells. They can be restimulated to rapidly generate a secondary antibody response.

Together, the extrafollicular and germinal-center pathways of B-cell differentiation lead to a coordinated humoral response that provides the very rapid production of low affinity antibodies, the subsequent production of high affinity antibodies, and the potential for a rapid recall response. Cytokines such as IL-2, IL-10, IL-6, and IL-21 promote differentiation into plasma cells, whereas CD40/CD40L interactions promote memory-cell formation and inhibit plasma-cell generation. Cytokines also contribute to isotype switching. IL-4 enhances switching to IgE and IgG4; IL-10 to IgG1, IgG3, and IgA; and TGF-beta 1 to IgA. The enzyme activation-induced cytidine deaminase (AID), which participates in receptor editing, class switching, and somatic hypermutation, is key to the diverse B-cell response. AID deficiency is another cause of hyper-IgM syndromes.

AUTOIMMUNITY AND THE PATHOGENESIS OF IMMUNE-MEDIATED DISEASE

A fundamental aspect of the immune response is that pathogen-derived and MHC-disparate foreign antigens are recognized and eliminated, but the host generally does not attack its own tissues. This unresponsive state is referred to as self-tolerance, but as discussed, self/non-self recognition occurs on many levels. Innate immune cells recognize non-self through PRRs; similarly, the alternative complement pathway also recognizes microbial products. Cross-reactivity to self-antigens by PRRs could be an evolutionary hard-wired aspect of autoimmunity. For example, recognition of certain mammalian DNA or RNA sequences may be important in targeting autoantibodies to these ubiquitous molecules. Similarly, the repertoire of antigens recognized by adaptive immune cells, T and B cells, is immense and highly specific but the inherent self-reactivity of T cells and somatic mutation of B cells requires additional mechanisms, such as Tregs, to maintain peripheral immune tolerance. Fas-mediated deletion of activated T cells is another homeostatic mechanism that contributes to self-tolerance. In addition, cytokines like IL-10 and TGF-beta 1 help damp immune responses. Negative regulatory molecules also inhibit most immune activation events, for example, *pyrin* in inflammasome activation, *CTLA4* in T-cell activation, and *SOCS proteins* in cytokine signaling. Genetic ablation of many of these negative regulatory proteins in mice or mutations in humans results in autoimmune or autoinflammatory disease.

Classically, immune-mediated diseases have been characterized based on their predominant immunopathologic lesion. These categories are: immediate hypersensitivity due to production of IgE (e.g., allergies and anaphylaxis); antibodies against circulating or fixed cells (e.g., autoimmune thrombocytopenia, Goodpasture's syndrome); immune-complex disease (e.g., SLE, vasculitis); and delayed type hypersensitivity. While this classification has some utility, it is equally important to bear in mind that the components of the immune system are highly interdependent.

Some autoimmune diseases can be classified as mediated by adaptive immunity, such as diseases in which autoantibodies attack particular tissues, while others are clearly limited to the innate immune system, such as gout and the inherited periodic fevers. Most fall between these two extremes and can be thought of as resulting from pathological positive feedback between innate and adaptive immune mechanisms. For example, in rheumatoid arthritis, macrophages secrete cytokines, such as TNF and metalloproteinases, that help destroy the joint structure, but these cells depend on cytokines and cellular signals provided by T cells that are co-infiltrating the synovium. To complete the feedback loop, activated macrophages produce cytokines such as IL-12 that reinforce the production of T-cell–derived cytokines such as IFN-gamma. Rheumatoid factor–containing immune complexes present in the rheumatoid joint produced by autoreactive B cells can then amplify innate inflammatory responses through complement and Fc receptors on innate immune cells. Such an integrated model could explain why therapies directed against both the innate (e.g., anticytokine) and adaptive (e.g., anticostimulatory, anti–B cell) immune systems are effective in this disease. The extraordinary therapeutic advances that have been made recently in the treatment of rheumatologic disorders through the targeting of specific molecules with biologic agents have the added potential benefit of providing mechanistic insights that should permit even better therapies in the future.

SUMMARY

The human immune response is composed of highly antigen-specific cells that work in concert with cells involved in innate immunity. Ordinarily, this orchestrated process efficiently rids the host of pathogenic organisms, but not always. Immunological disease can occur as a consequence of dysregulation of many different parts of the immune system. Immunopathology also can occur as a byproduct of immune responses to foreign pathogens or tissue damage. Unlike rare single-gene disorders that are illustrative of the role of particular molecules in the immune system, a variety of mutations or polymorphisms in an array of separate immune system genes likely contribute to the genetic susceptibility to common rheumatologic diseases, and these loci are now being identified. The challenge for the future will be to use these insights into the immune system to design better therapies for rheumatic diseases.

REFERENCES

1. Creagh EM, O'Neill LA. TLRs, NLRs, and RLRs: a trinity of pathogen sensors that co-operate in innate immunity. Trends Immunol 2006;27:352–357.

2. Akira S, Uematsu S, Takeuchi O. Pathogen recognition and innate immunity. Cell 2006;124:783–801.

3. Ogura Y, Sutterwala FS, Flavell RA. The inflammasome: first line of the immune response to cell stress. Cell 2006;126:659–662.

4. Stojanov S, Kastner DL. Familial autoinflammatory diseases: genetics, pathogenesis and treatment. Curr Opin Rheumatol 2005;17:586–599.

5. Steinman RM, Bonifaz L, Fujii S, et al. The innate functions of dendritic cells in peripheral lymphoid tissues. Adv Exp Med Biol 2005;560:83–97.

6. Stetson DB, Medzhitov R. Type I interferons in host defense. Immunity 2006;25:373–381.

7. Brigl M, Bry L, Kent SC, Gumperz JE, Brenner MB. Mechanism of CD1d-restricted natural killer T cell activation during microbial infection. Nat Immunol 2003;4:1230–1237.

8. Prussin C, Metcalfe DD. IgE, mast cells, basophils, and eosinophils. Allergy Clin Immunol 2006;117(Suppl):S450–S456.

9. Wen L, Atkinson JP, Giclas PC. Clinical and laboratory evaluation of complement deficiency. J Allergy Clin Immunol 2004;113:585–593.

10. Kovanen PE, Leonard WJ. Cytokines and immunodeficiency diseases: critical roles of the gamma(c)-dependent cytokines interleukins 2, 4, 7, 9, 15, and 21, and their signaling pathways. Immunol Rev 2004;202:67–83.

11. Davis SJ, van der Merwe PA. The kinetic-segregation model: TCR triggering and beyond. Nat Immunol 2006;7:803–809.

12. O'Shea JJ, Husa M, Li D, et al. Jak3 and the pathogenesis of severe combined immunodeficiency. Mol Immunol 2004;41:727–737.

13. Chikuma S, Bluestone JA. CTLA-4 and tolerance: the biochemical point of view. Immunol Res 2003;28:241–253.

14. Villasenor J, Benoist C, Mathis D. AIRE and APECED: molecular insights into an autoimmune disease. Immunol Rev 2005;204:156–164.

15. Laky K, Fowlkes BJ. Receptor signals and nuclear events in CD4 and CD8 T cell lineage commitment. Curr Opin Immunol 2005;17:116–121.

16. Weaver CT, Harrington LE, Mangan PR, Gavrieli M, Murphy KM. Th17: an effector CD4 T cell lineage with regulatory T cell ties. Immunity 2006;24:677–688.

17. Kronenberg M, Rudensky A. Regulation of immunity by self-reactive T cells. Nature 2005;435:598–604.

18. Edwards JC, Cambridge G. B-cell targeting in rheumatoid arthritis and other autoimmune diseases. Nat Rev Immunol 2006;6:394–403.

19. Kalia V, Sarkar S, Gourley TS, Rouse BT, Ahmed R. Differentiation of memory B and T cells. Curr Opin Immunol 2006;18:255–264.

Suggested Reading

Abbas AK, Lichtman AH, Bell E, Bird L, eds. Cellular and molecular immunology. 5th ed. Philadelphia, PA: Saunders; Nature, 2005;435:583–627.

Janeway C. Immunobiology: the immune system in health and disease. 6th ed. New York: Garland Science; 2005.

Diamond B, Davidson A. Autoimmune diseases. N Engl J Med 2001;345:340–350.

McGonagle D, McDermott MF. A proposed classification of the immunological diseases. PLoS Med 2006;3:e297. Available at: http://medicine.plosjournals.org/perlserv/?request=get-document&doi=10.1371/journal.pmed.0030297.

Nature insight: autoimmunity 435:583–627. Available at: http://www.nature.com/nature/supplements/insights/autoimmunity/index.html.

4

CHAPTER 5

Genetics and Disease

JAMES KELLEY, PHD
ROBERT P. KIMBERLY, MD

- Most rheumatic disease are caused by a combination of genes and environment, with genetic variation predisposing or protecting and environmental factors initiating and maintaining a disease state.
- Variations in genes can occur as single nucleotide polymorphisms in coding or noncoding regions and leading to different alleles. Point mutations are rare variations occurring at less than 1% minor allele frequency. Deletion, insertion, repeated sequences of different lengths, and copy number polymorphisms are also responsible for differences in genes.
- Haplotypes, blocks of polymorphisms inherited together more often than expected by chance, can be used to identify disease-causing variants and provide information on recombination, population structure, and evolutionary pressures.
- Association of genes with disease can be performed using linkage studies or association studies. Association studies can determine the odds ratio of a particular gene variant being associated with a particular disease, but require large numbers of samples from affected and unaffected individuals.
- Linkage studies are most useful for monogenic traits with high penetrance where extended family information is available. If a particular gene has only a subtle effect, linkage studies are limited in use.

Relationships between genes and diseases have long been hypothesized. The association of a disease with a gene dates back in Western medicine as far as Hippocrates, who hypothesized epilepsy was caused by a singular hereditary unit of biological material. However, with technological advances and the completion of the human genome sequence (1), scientists can now associate specific genetic variations with clinical conditions. Genetic associations provide informative clues for developing new diagnostic and therapeutic techniques to improve patient care. Understanding the principles that underlie genetic studies will become an essential skill for clinicians if we are to appreciate the complexity of genetic contributions to disease and its treatment (Table 5-1).

THE CAUSE OF DISEASE

In most cases, diseases are not caused by either genes or the environment but by a combination of the two. Genetic variation confers a susceptible or protective effect towards an illness for a specific person when compared with a population. In this paradigm, genetic variations predispose an individual towards a particular outcome while environmental factors, such as infectious agents, chemicals, tobacco smoke, and diet, actually initiate and maintain a disease state in the presence of a set of genetic variants (2). The relative contributions of genetic and environmental factors to disease can be thought of in terms of a sliding scale (Figure 5-1). On one side of the scale, some conditions could be attributed almost entirely to the environment, for example, a car accident. On the other end of the spectrum, there are primarily genetic disorders, such as cystic fibrosis or hemoglobinopathy. Most clinical conditions, though, ranging from heart disease to rheumatoid arthritis (RA) to the common cold, involve some causal component from both an individual's genetic background and environment. For example, genes may predispose an individual to develop type II diabetes mellitus; however, diet and exercise habits ultimately lead to disease. Remembering this paradigm is important for appreciating both the advantages and limits of applying genetic research to the understanding of both health and illness. Neither genetics nor environmental factors should be evaluated alone.

When determining the genetic contribution to the cause of disease, the question arises: does one gene or many lead to illness? Mendelian, or monogenic, diseases, such as Huntington's disease or cystic fibrosis, can be associated with a single genetic variant. Most diseases, however, are complex diseases because they derive their genetic components from a combination of genetic variants, each providing subtle, additive, and personalized effects. The varying genetic components

TABLE 5.1. GLOSSARY OF SELECTED GENETIC TERMS.

TERM	DEFINITION
Admixture	Amount of genetic variation present in an individual due to descending from a particular population
Allele	One of the genetic forms possible at a specific locus, when variation at that locus occurs
Ancestry informative marker	Polymorphism occurring at varying allele frequencies between different populations
Complex (disease or trait)	Involving more than one gene
Haplotype	Group of polymorphisms that are inherited together and are observed together more often than expected by chance
Linkage disequilibrium (LD)	Likelihood that two or more polymorphisms will be inherited together as part of a haplotype
Locus (loci)	Defined position within the genome
Minor allele frequency (MAF)	The frequency of the less common allele in a population
Penetrance	Tendency for a trait to be expressed
Polymorphism	"Many bodies," genetic variation
Population structure	Background genetic variation common within and unique to a group due to a similar and isolated evolutionary history
Recombination	Rearrangement of alleles that is due to the nuclear sequence breaking and recombining during the crossing-over phase of meiosis

of complex diseases explain the different possible clinical manifestations present in one condition, such as the 11 defined possible criteria for patients with systemic lupus erythematosus (SLE), of which only four are required for diagnosis (3).

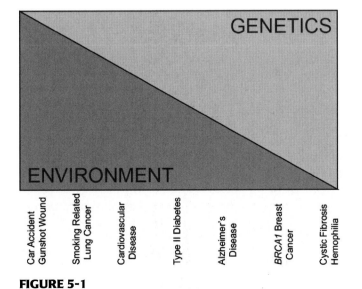

FIGURE 5-1

Relative contributions of genetic and environmental factors to disease. Each disease is caused by varying degrees of genetic and environmental factors.

TYPES OF GENETIC VARIATION

The genetic component of disease can be attributed to genetic variations present (or lacking) in affected individuals of the population. Genetic variation is found by sequencing the genomes of several individuals from a population to detect the most frequent allele and any variants at that specific locus. Single nucleotide polymorphisms (SNPs), the most common type of genetic variant, occur when more than one nucleotide is present at a single position. Nonsynonymous SNPs are those present in coding regions that change the protein's sequence. Synonymous SNPs are those present in exons that do not alter protein sequence. SNPs present in untranslated regions and introns can also affect protein function by altering splicing sites, affecting transcription factor binding, changing promoter sites, and influencing gene expression.

Point mutations are rare variants occurring at a single basepair locus with less than 1% minor allele frequency (MAF). (SNPs occur at greater than 1% MAF.) Point mutations are much more difficult to associate with disease than SNPs without larger sample sizes, which are logistically difficult to collect (2). The frequency at which a variant appears in the population is important because a disease found in a high proportion of the population should be associated with a genetic variant also occurring in a high proportion of the population.

This idea, the common disease–common variant hypothesis (4), directs researchers to which polymorphisms are more likely to influence a disease.

Deletion/insertion polymorphisms (DIPs or "indels") result from the removal or incorporation of nucleotides into the genome sequence. While most DIPs occur outside exons, they are likely to be important in complex traits and diseases, due to their potential for influencing gene expression.

Repeated sequences, or repeat elements, are another form of genetic variation. Interspersed repeat sequences, which account for almost half of the human genome sequence (1), are sections of DNA copied and distributed randomly throughout the genome. Tandemly duplicated elements, such as microsatellites (e.g., CACACACACA), are repeat sequences that, at their time of origin, were copied in a unique pattern and then translocated immediately near their original sequence. However, once present, tandemly duplicated elements are generally inherited through generations in a stable manner. These unique patterns of tandemly duplicated elements provide genetic markers that are both specific and consistent to a population or group of descendants.

Copy number polymorphisms arise when an entire gene or gene segment has been duplicated or when a gene is absent in some individuals. Entire gene duplications allow new genes with new functions to evolve while keeping a functional, backup copy of the original, ancestral gene (5). Examples of copy number polymorphisms are found in natural killer cell receptor gene families and in the major histocompatibility complex (MHC) (6), both regions important in clinical immunology.

RELATIONSHIPS BETWEEN VARIANTS: HAPLOTYPES AND LINKAGE DISEQUILIBRIUM

Haplotypes are "blocks" of polymorphisms that are inherited together more often than expected by chance. These blocks of genetic variants are often separated by regions of high recombination. Haplotypes are useful in identifying disease-causing variants in association studies and can provide information on recombination, population structure, and evolutionary pressures. Because haplotypes define groups of polymorphisms that occur together, experimentally obtaining information about one polymorphism also provides information on the other polymorphisms in the haplotype. Therefore, when attempting to associate genetic variants with disease, testing one or a selection of polymorphisms per haplotype, in a process called *haplotype tagging*, can save time and resources (7).

Assigning polymorphisms to a haplotype, when possible, requires experimental data. About half the genome contains variants that cannot be placed in haplotypes (8). Sequencing multiple samples from a population identifies the combinations and frequencies of polymorphisms possible in that population, which allows researchers to predict which polymorphisms are inherited together and belong in a common haplotype. Haplotypes are defined based on statistical predictions, not absolute certainties. Therefore, polymorphisms assigned to the same haplotype may not be inherited together in all individuals, even though it is likely that they will.

The probability that polymorphisms assigned to the same haplotype will occur together is called linkage disequilibrium (LD). In complete or strong LD, these linked alleles are inherited together within one segment of genomic information. Therefore, any evolutionary pressure or association with disease for one linked allele will inadvertently be observed as present in all polymorphisms of the same haplotype. In weak LD, variants are inherited independently, due to recombination, and a genetic event influencing one allele will not affect the other.

Linkage disequilibrium is most commonly measured with the statistics D' and r^2. The values of these measures range from 0 to 1, with 0 showing weak LD and 1 referring to strong or complete LD. Generally, polymorphisms within a defined haplotype will have a correlation coefficient or r^2 value of at least 0.8. To illustrate how LD is determined and haplotypes are defined from experimental data, an equation for calculating D' between two loci is seen below.

$$D = P_{AB} - (P_A X P_B) \qquad D_{max} = P_{AB} \qquad D' = |D/D_{max}|$$
$$D' = 1 \rightarrow \text{Complete LD}$$

The measure D is equal to the probability of both polymorphisms occurring together in an individual (P_{AB}) minus the product of the probabilities that only one of the polymorphisms will occur in an individual (i.e., P_A is the probability that only polymorphism A will occur). Please note that the probabilities mentioned above are equivalent to the appropriate allele frequencies determined from the sequencing data experimentally obtained. For example, if both polymorphisms occur together in 80% of samples and each polymorphism is observed individually in 10% of samples, then $D = 0.8 - (0.1 \times 0.1) = 0.79$. D' is equal to the absolute value of dividing D by D_{max}. D_{max} equals the probability that both polymorphisms occur in the same sample. Again, in this instance, $D' = |0.79/0.8| = 0.9875$, showing that strong LD is present between these two loci. Strong LD in the above situation is intuitive because both variants occur together in 80% of samples.

POPULATION STRUCTURE: CONSIDERING ETHNIC DIFFERENCES

Factors causing genetic variation do so in response to the development, migration, and structure of populations. Due to human history, each population has been exposed to different environments, likely creating different evolutionary pressures to preserve or delete genetic variants in their genomes (9). Cross-population studies on the genomic organization of polymorphisms have shown that Yoruban Africans (Nigeria) have shorter haplotypes and more variants than do Europeans and Asians (8). The wider range of genetic diversity in Africans occurs because humans originated there and only a subgroup of the ancestral human population (and therefore subgroup of genetic variants) migrated to other continents, leaving more genetic diversity in Africa to evolve.

Genetic variations common to a population but not to the whole species is known as *population structure*. These population-specific variants can create phenotypic alterations, including some associated with disease. Ethnic differences in allele frequencies at disease-associated loci and in disease prevalence are commonly reported, such as the increased presence of SLE in patients of African ancestry or an increase in RA in Native Americans when compared with Caucasians. Due to the presence of ethnic-specific genetic contributions, matching cases and controls by ethnicity can help prevent any false genetic associations created by population structure (10).

In addition to self-identification, samples segregated by population can be tested empirically for population admixture. Population admixture is the measurement of the number of discrepancies in allele frequencies between two populations that have been historically isolated. Therefore, admixture quantifies the proportion of an individual's genome that is unique and attributable to an ethnic background (i.e., 20% European ancestry). Population structure varies greatly among groups whose immediate ancestors no longer remained in isolation, such as Latin Americans and African Americans. Admixture can be measured by comparing evolutionarily stable microsatellites, which are exclusive to a particular population (11), or by evaluating ancestry informative markers (AIMs). AIMs are polymorphisms (or the genes containing such polymorphisms) that vary distinctly in allele frequencies between populations.

DETERMINING GENETIC COMPONENTS OF DISEASE

Two main types of studies are used to identify disease-causing genes: linkage studies and association studies. Linkage studies use standardized genetic markers, which do not necessarily produce a phenotypic effect, distributed throughout the genome to detect regions that may contain a variant influencing disease. Such studies rely on LD between these markers and a disease-associated variant. Linkage studies have proven most useful in detecting monogenic diseases, such as Huntington's disease and cystic fibrosis.

While linkage studies provided early insight into the genetic component of complex diseases, association studies are used with increasing frequency to identify variants involved in complex disorders, such as SLE, RA, and other autoimmune conditions. They compare the frequency of a variant in an appropriate number of patients with the disease to the frequency in unrelated, yet matched, controls. Matched controls have similar ages, ethnicities, and backgrounds to affected patients in an effort to reduce errors from population structure. While such studies associate the likelihood of a variant occurring simultaneously with a phenotype, they do not necessarily provide information on any functional difference leading to disease (12). During an association study, genome-wide polymorphism scans can detect specific polymorphisms that are more common in disease groups than in healthy cohorts. Using high capacity technology, this approach evaluates a panel of thousands of common polymorphisms for differences in allele frequencies between affected individuals and controls. A smaller scale technique for association studies is to select and test candidate genes for association. Candidate gene selection suggests a physiological reason for a gene's possible relationship with a particular disease, thereby focusing which genes and variants to study (13).

Statistical measures facilitate the interpretation and design of association studies. Relative risk (RR) measures the likelihood that an individual who possesses the genetic variant will (or will not) develop the associated disease (i.e., the *risk* an individual possessing the variant has of getting the disease *relative* to those without the variant). A RR of 1.5 means an individual with the associated variant is 1.5 times more likely to express the phenotype. RR can be estimated in association studies with a statistic, the odds ratio (OR). The OR can be calculated with the equation: $(A \times B)/(C \times D)$, where A equals the number of samples with the variant and the disease, B equals the number of samples without either the variant or the disease, C equals the number of samples with the variant but not the disease, and D equals the number of samples with the disease but not the variant (see Figure 5-2). Basically, the OR measures the ratio of the presence or absence of both disease and variant against the appearance of either of the two exclusively.

Statistical power, in association studies, refers to the probability of finding a genetic association when it is in fact true. Power is a function of the number of samples tested, the MAF of the variant, the presence of genetic

5

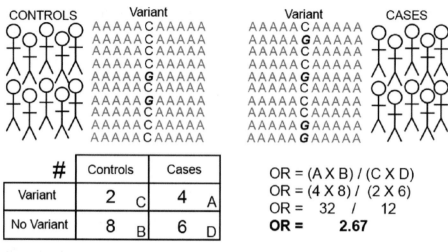

FIGURE 5-2

Associating a genetic variant with disease. Samples taken from a group of affected cases and a group of matched controls are used to determine which allele each individual in the study possesses. Note that not all individuals with disease have the studied variant and not all individuals with the variant have the disease. In this case, the variant is the G allele at position 6. By counting the number of times the variant occurs in each group, it is possible to determine the likelihood that having the variant will correlate with having the disease. This correlation is based on calculating the odds ratio (OR).

features (e.g., dominant/recessive allele), and the OR required to convince scientists the association is meaningful. This OR is arbitrarily set depending on the disease and the level of effect researchers hope to observe. A study that tests too few samples can likely lead to false-positive results, especially when testing a low frequency variant.

There are advantages and weaknesses of both linkage and association studies. Linkage studies are more useful in situations where samples are available from extended families to detect a monogenetic trait with high penetrance. When a variant only contributes a subtle phenotypic effect, linkage studies are limited in use. In this case, association studies should better detect an association; however, the large sample sizes necessary for statistical inference of association with disease can be challenging to obtain. Phenotypes tested in association studies often vary, especially in rheumatic diseases, complicating interpretation of results. For example, in SLE, patients can present a variety of symptoms; therefore, the genetic variants contributing to one individual's disease may differ from the next patient. Therefore, association studies should consider well-defined clinical subgroups during analysis to prevent missing a positive association. Replication, which is finding a positive association in another collection of samples or another population, also can confuse interpretation of association studies' results. During replication studies, positive associations can be lost when larger sample sizes are tested or when testing other populations due to the different evolutionary histories and other genetic variants

present in each group. Keeping these issues in mind is important when interpreting genetic studies because many false positives may be in the literature due to a positive publication bias; that is, studies demonstrating an association are more likely to be published than studies that fail to find an association (14).

MAJOR HISTOCOMPATIBILITY COMPLEX

While scientists have found that genetic variants from all over the genome contribute to complex disease, one region of the genome has been associated with more diseases, including rheumatic diseases, than any other: the MHC (6). A selection of genetic associations of rheumatic diseases with MHC-encoded genes is listed in Table 5-2.

The MHC is a dense cluster of over 260 genes on chromosome 6p21.3 containing a high percentage of immune-related genes, in particular the highly polymorphic human leukocyte antigen (HLA) genes involved in antigen presentation. The MHC is genomically organized into multiple regions. From the telomere to centromere, they are: extended class I region, class I region (*HLA-A, HLA-B, HLA-C*, etc.), class III region (*C4, TNF, LTA*, etc.), class II region (*HLA-DR, HLA-DQ, HLA-DP*, etc.), and the extended class II region. The class IV, or inflammatory region, is located within the class III region and contains a concentration of genes encoding inflammatory-mediating molecules (see

TABLE 5.2. SOME RHEUMATIC DISEASE ASSOCIATIONS WITH THE MAJOR HISTOCOMPATIBILITY COMPLEX.

GENE	DISEASE
HLA	Systemic sclerosis
HLA-B	Ankylosing spondylitis
HLA-B	Behcet's disease
HLA-B	Sarcoidosis
MICA	Behcet's disease
MICA	Rheumatoid arthritis
TNF	Ankylosing spondylitis
TNF	Rheumatoid arthritis
NFKBIL1	Rheumatoid arthritis
BTNL2	Sarcoidosis
HLA class II	Juvenile ankylosing spondylitis
HLA class II	Systemic lupus erythematosus[a]
HLA class II	Systemic sclerosis
HLA-DRB1	Rheumatoid arthritis
HLA-DRB1	Sarcoidosis
HLA-DRB1	Sjögren's syndrome
HLA-DRB1	Takayasu arteritis
TAP2	Rheumatoid arthritis
TAP2	Sjögren's syndrome
TAP2	Systemic lupus erythematosus

[a] Specific associations with HLA class II genes (HLA-DQ and HLA-DR) may vary with ethnicity.
Examples were taken from the Online Mendelian Inheritance in Man database (http://www.ncbi.nlm.nih.gov/sites/entrez?db=omim) and the Genetic Association Database (http://geneticassociationdb.nih.gov). Note that MHC encoded genes other than HLA have been associated with diseases.

Chapter 6B). The MHC is likely involved with so many diseases because it contains the highest density of genetic variants, areas of strong LD, and highest density of genes in the human genome (6).

Genetics will have an increased role in medicine over the coming years as genes' relationships with disease become more understood and as new genetic-based technologies are translated into the clinic. Understanding the genetic contribution to a clinical condition, both in the MHC and throughout the genome, will allow physicians and researchers the ability to find new markers for detecting and preventing an illness, to develop new diagnostic measures for evaluating potential success of drug therapies, and to predict biological malfunctions underlying a disease.

References

1. Finishing the euchromatic sequence of the human genome. Nature 2004;431:931–945.
2. Hunter DJ. Gene-environment interactions in human diseases. Nat Rev Genet 2005;6:287–298.
3. Hochberg MC. Updating the American College of Rheumatology revised criteria for the classification of systemic lupus erythematosus. Arthritis Rheum 1997;40:1725.
4. Reich DE, Lander ES. On the allelic spectrum of human disease. Trends Genet 2001;17:502–510.
5. Ohno S. Evolution by gene duplication. Berlin: Springer; 1970.
6. Kelley J, Trowsdale J. Features of MHC and NK gene clusters. Transpl Immunol 2005;14:129–134.
7. Johnson GC, Esposito L, Barratt BJ, et al. Haplotype tagging for the identification of common disease genes. Nat Genet 2001;29:233–237.
8. Gabriel SB, Schaffner SF, Nguyen H, et al. The structure of haplotype blocks in the human genome. Science 2002;296:2225–2229.
9. Bamshad M, Wooding SP. Signatures of natural selection in the human genome. Nat Rev Genet 2003;4:99–111.
10. Clayton DG, Walker NM, Smyth DJ, et al. Population structure, differential bias and genomic control in a large-scale, case-control association study. Nat Genet 2005;37:1243–1246.
11. Patterson N, Hattangadi N, Lane B, et al. Methods for high-density admixture mapping of disease genes. Am J Hum Genet 2004;74:979–1000.
12. Daly AK, Day CP. Candidate gene case-control association studies: advantages and potential pitfalls. Br J Clin Pharmacol 2001;52:489–499.
13. Risch NJ. Searching for genetic determinants in the new millennium. Nature 2000;405:847–856.
14. Ioannidis JP, Trikalinos TA, Ntzani EE, Contopoulos-Ioannidis DG. Genetic associations in large versus small studies: an empirical assessment. Lancet 2003;361:567–571.

5

Rheumatoid Arthritis
A. Clinical and Laboratory Manifestations

CHRISTOPHER V. TEHLIRIAN, MD
JOAN M. BATHON, MD

- Rheumatoid arthritis affects all ethnic groups, with females 2.5 times more likely than males to develop the disease and an overall prevalence of 1% to 2% of the population.
- Most common mode of onset is insidious fatigue, morning stiffness, and joint pain and swelling involving small distal joints [wrists, metacarpophalangeal (MCP), proximal interphalangeal (PIP), metatarsophalangeal (MTP)] in symmetrical fashion.
- In most cases, rheumatoid arthritis is a chronic progressive disease that, if left untreated, can cause joint damage and disability. Factors that predict poor outcome include severity of disease, seropositivity, low socioeconomic and educational status, and poor functional status.

- Physical findings are most notable for joint-centered swelling, deformities, and painful or reduced joint motion. Extra-articular disease occurs in seropositive patients and includes rheumatoid nodules, Sjögren's syndrome, interstitial lung disease, and vasculitis.
- Laboratory tests that support a diagnosis of rheumatoid arthritis include elevated erythrocyte sedimentation rate and C-reactive protein, positive rheumatoid factor, positive anti-cyclic citrullinated peptide (CCP) antibody. Further evidence of chronic inflammation includes anemia and hypoalbuminemia. Radiographs may reveal periarticular osteoporosis, joint space narrowing, erosions, and deformities. Magnetic resonance imaging and ultrasound may be more sensitive in early disease.

Rheumatoid arthritis (RA) is a chronic systemic autoimmune inflammatory disease that affects all ethnic groups throughout the world. Females are 2.5 times more likely to be affected than males. The onset of disease can occur at any age but peak incidence occurs within the fourth and fifth decades of life. The average annual incidence of RA in the United States is 0.5 per 1000 persons per year (1). The overall prevalence of RA is 1% to 2%, and it steadily increases to 5% in women by the age of 70 (2). However, there are differences in prevalence rates of RA in various ethnic groups, ranging from 0.1% in rural Africans to 5% in Pima or Chippewa Indians (3). Many factors contribute to the risk of developing RA and are reviewed in the following chapter (see Chapter 6B).

PATIENT HISTORY

A detailed history of the articular symptoms is of the utmost importance, with particular focus on the mode of onset (gradual vs. acute), the pattern of joints involved, and any variance in symptoms according to time of day. It is important to remember that RA is a systemic disease and individuals may therefore present with symptoms such as fever, weight loss, and fatigue; however, joint symptoms are usually the most prominent.

Most commonly, the onset of symptoms of joint pain and swelling is insidious, occurring over weeks to months (4). However, a minority of patients may present with an abrupt explosive onset polyarthritis. Still others may present with transient self-limited episodes of mono- or polyarthritis lasting days to weeks. This presentation is known as *palindromic rheumatism*. Approximately 50% of patients with palindromic rheumatism will go on to develop (i.e., fulfill criteria for) RA, and only 15% remain symptom-free after 5 years. Occasionally RA may present as a monoarthritis; however, infectious and crystalline etiologies should always be ruled out first when inflammation affects a single joint.

Rheumatoid arthritis is the most common form of inflammatory arthritis that affects diarthrodial joints. In early disease, the wrists, metacarpophalangeal (MCP) joints, proximal interphalangeal (PIP) joints of the fingers, interphalangeal joints of the thumbs, and metatarsalphalangeal (MTP) joints are most commonly affected. As the disease progresses, larger joints such as the ankles, knees, elbows, and shoulders frequently become affected. In contrast, involvement of the temporomandibular and sternoclavicular joints and cervical spine are relatively uncommon, and the distal interphalangeal (DIP) joints and thoracolumbar spine are nearly always spared.

Joint involvement is classically symmetrical in nature, and morning stiffness lasting more than an hour is a hallmark symptom of RA. Frequently patients with newly diagnosed RA arise from bed 1 to 2 hours earlier than usual to allow time in order to loosen up, and will often describe the need for a warm shower or for soaking their hands in warm water in order to enhance early morning function. Pain with turning door knobs, opening jars, and buttoning shirts is commonly reported due to pain and swelling in the wrists and small joints of the hands. Pain in the ball of the foot (metatarsalgia) upon arising from bed, and widening of the forefoot necessitating an increase in shoe size, are frequently reported and are due to inflammation of the metatarsalphalangeal joints. Neck pain and stiffness tend to occur later in disease and may signal tenosynovitis of the transverse ligament of C1, which stabilizes the odontoid process of C2. The symmetry, bilaterality, and predilection for small joints (especially early in disease) are incorpo-

rated into the Revised 1987 American Rheumatism Association (now the American College of Rheumatology) Criteria for the classification of RA (Table 6A-1).

In addition to articular symptoms, patients with early RA frequently have constitutional symptoms such as low grade fevers, fatigue, malaise, myalgias, decreased appetite, and weight loss that are due to systemic inflammation. In some individuals, constitutional symptoms may even overshadow the articular symptoms. Organ involvement other than the joints tends to occur in longstanding disease and includes firm nontender bumps (rheumatoid nodules) that occur most commonly on the elbows, Achilles tendons, and fingers; shortness of breath or chest pain due to pleuropulmonary involvement; orbital redness and pain due to scleritis; and dry eyes (keratoconjunctivitis sicca) and dry mouth (xerostomia) due to secondary Sjögren's syndrome. Extra-articular symptoms are present in approximately 40% of RA patients. Other organ systems involved will be described later in this chapter.

In most cases, RA is a chronic progressive disease that, if left untreated or inadequately treated, can cause extensive joint damage and chronic pain. A number of prognostic variables that predict a poor outcome have been identified and include female sex, strong family history, human leukocyte antigen-DR4 cluster susceptible genes (the so-called shared epitopes; see Chapter 6B), a high number of swollen/tender joints, a high score on a patient-rated instrument for measuring disability (the Health Assessment Questionnaire or HAQ),

TABLE 6A-1. THE 1987 REVISED CRITERIA FOR THE CLASSIFICATION OF RHEUMATOID ARTHRITIS (TRADITIONAL FORMAT).[a]

CRITERION	DEFINITION
1. Morning stiffness	Morning stiffness in and around the joints, lasting at least 1 hour before maximal improvement.
2. Arthritis of three or more joint areas	At least three joint areas simultaneously have had soft tissue swelling or fluid (not bony overgrowth alone) observed by a physician. The 14 possible areas are right or left PIP, MCP, wrist, elbow, knee, ankle, and MTP joints.
3. Arthritis of hand joints	At least one area swollen (as defined above) in a wrist, MCP, or PIP joint.
4. Symmetric arthritis	Simultaneous involvement of the same joint areas (as defined in item 2) on both sides of the body (bilateral involvement of PIPs, MCPs, or MTPs is acceptable without absolute symmetry).
5. Rheumatoid nodules	Subcutaneous nodules, over bony prominences, or extensor surfaces, or in juxta-articular regions, observed by a physician.
6. Serum rheumatoid factor	Demonstration of abnormal amounts of serum rheumatoid factor by any method for which the result has been positive in <5% of normal control subjects.
7. Radiographic changes	Radiographic changes typical of rheumatoid arthritis on posteroanterior hand and wrist radiographs, which must include erosions or unequivocal bony decalcification localized in or most marked adjacent to the involved joints (osteoarthritis changes alone do not qualify).

SOURCE: From *Arthritis and Rheumatism*, 1988;31:315–324, with permission.
[a] For classification purposes, a patient shall be said to have rheumatoid arthritis if he/she has satisfied at least four of these seven criteria. Criteria 1 through 4 must have been present for at least 6 weeks. Patients with two clinical diagnoses are not excluded. Designation as classic, definite, or probably rheumatoid arthritis is not to be made.

high titer of rheumatoid factor (RF), high titer of anti-cyclic citrullinated peptide (anti-CCP) antibodies, low socioeconomic status, low educational status, psychosocial problems, and the presence of erosions on joint radiographs. Several studies have demonstrated the highest predictor of disability at 5 years after diagnosis to be a high score on the HAQ at 1 year after initial diagnosis. Additional predictors of poor outcomes include elevated erythrocyte sedimentation rate (ESR) and C-reactive protein (CRP), persistently high scores on the HAQ, and persistent pain.

PHYSICAL EXAMINATION

Patients with suspected or confirmed RA should undergo a thorough initial physical exam to gauge the extent of articular and extra-articular involvement. Patients should be followed every 2 to 4 months henceforth to monitor disease activity and response to treatment, the frequency depending upon the severity of the disease and the medication regimen.

Joint Examination

Not surprisingly, the articular manifestations of RA are the most common findings on physical exam. Symmetrical swelling and tenderness of the joints is invariably observed. Careful palpation of the joint line is necessary in order to feel joint space fullness (swelling) and synovial bogginess in order to differentiate those features from joint enlargement secondary to the bony hypertrophy (osteophytes) of primary or secondary osteoarthritis. Frank synovitis can sometimes be subtle and difficult to confirm early on but, as the disease progresses,

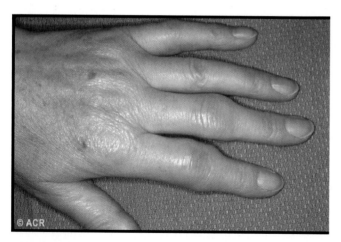

FIGURE 6A-1

Swelling of the proximal interphalangeal joints in a patient with early rheumatoid arthritis. (From the ACR slide collection on the rheumatic diseases, 3rd ed. Slide 17 (#9105020), with permission of the American College of Rheumatology.)

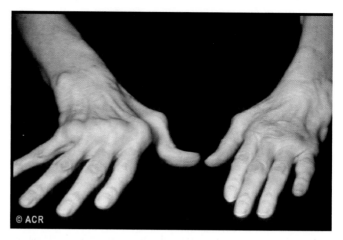

FIGURE 6A-2

Ulnar deviation and subluxation of the metacarpophalangeal joints are present in the hand on the left. Muscle atrophy is also evident in the dorsal musculature of both hands. (From the ACR slide collection on the rheumatic diseases, 3rd ed. Slide 19 (#9105030), with permission of the American College of Rheumatology.)

warmth, mild erythema, and swelling of the joints becomes more apparent. Joint swelling is usually confined within the joint capsule (in contrast to gout, e.g., which can also cause considerable periarticular edema). It is important to record the location, symmetry, and degree of swelling in each joint at the initial evaluation, and to repeat this examination at subsequent visits in order to gauge response to treatment. The examiner should also identify the joints that are painful on active and/or passive motion, the range of motion of each joint, and any deformities of the joints. The presence of joint swelling is indicative of active synovitis, whereas joint deformity, decreased range of motion, malalignment, or frank dislocation is indicative of joint damage.

Fusiform swelling of the proximal interphalangeal joints (PIP) is one of the earliest findings (Figure 6A-1), whereas deformities of the hands occur later in disease and include ulnar deviation of the fingers, dorsal subluxation of the MCP joints, and hyperextension (Swan neck) or hyperflexion (boutonniere deformity) at the proximal interphalangeal joints (Figure 6A-2). Swelling of the wrists and elbows is common and is easily palpable as both joints are superficial. Loss of extension at the elbows and wrists may result from active synovitis or from loss of cartilage; treatment should restore extension in the former, but not the latter instance. Compressive ulnar neuropathy may develop as a complication of synovitis in the elbow, whereas compressive median neuropathy (carpal tunnel syndrome) can result from synovitis in the wrist. Thus, a careful neurologic examination is important if sensory–motor symptoms are elicited during the history taking.

Synovitis in the shoulder is more difficult to assess by physical examination because the joint is deep and the joint capsule is not very distensible. If there is a complete tear in the rotator cuff, an effusion in the glenohumeral joint may extravasate into the subacromial space and become more visible. Painful synovitis in the shoulder can result rather rapidly in loss of range of motion due to contracture of the joint capsule and should be aggressively and proactively treated. Hip involvement in RA occurs in only 20% of patients. This joint, like the shoulder, is deep and therefore difficult to palpate or visualize on physical exam; thus, it is particularly important to ask about symptoms. Synovitis in the hip typically causes groin, thigh, buttock, low back, or referred ipsilateral knee pain, but early hip involvement may be asymptomatic. Knee involvement is quite common in RA and effusions are easily detected on physical exam. Large knee effusions may herniate posteriorly, creating a popliteal (Baker's) cyst that can dissect or rupture into the calf, causing calf pain, swelling, pitting edema, and bruising around the ankle (the so-called crescent sign). These symptoms may also be suggestive of a deep venous thrombosis but ultrasonography can differentiate the two entities. Synovitis in the ankle may be due to inflammation in the tibiotalar joint (which mediates flexion and extension) or in the joints of the hind foot (which mediate inversion and eversion of the ankle). Range of motion of the tibiotalar joint is usually fairly well preserved early on, while diminished inversion and eversion are more common. Synovial hypertrophy in the ankle can compress the tarsal tunnel, causing a compressive neuropathy. Tenosynovitis and frank rupture of the posterior tibialis tendon (inferomedial to the medial malleolus) is common in patients with RA, resulting in disabling heel valgus and chronic pain. Physical examination of the MTPs in early disease reveals tenderness, a widened and puffy forefoot, and frequently splaying of the toes. In more chronic disease, dorsal subluxation of the MTPs resulting in cock-up toe deformities, and hallux valgus (bunion) are commonly seen.

Early symptoms of cervical spine involvement consist primarily of neck stiffness due to tenosynovitis of the transverse ligament of C1, which stabilizes the odontoid process of C2. With persistent inflammation, erosion of the odontoid process and/or attrition and rupture of the transverse ligament may occur, leading to cervical myelopathy. The amount of neck pain does not correlate with the severity of myelopathy. Therefore, a careful neurologic exam is helpful in uncovering significant myelopathy as abnormalities of cervical spine joints are neither visible nor palpable.

Extra-Articular Examination

Because extra-articular manifestations can be seen in almost 50% of all RA patients at some point during the course of their illness (Table 6A-2) (5), an organ-specific evaluation should be done periodically and in response

TABLE 6A-2. ORGAN SYSTEMS INVOLVED IN RHEUMATOID ARTHRITIS.

Skin	Rheumatoid nodules (25%–50%)
Hematologic	Normocytic normochromic anemia (25%–30%), thrombocytosis, thrombocytopenia,[a] lymphadenopathy[a]
Felty's syndrome	Splenomegaly with neutropenia, large granular lymphocytes, thrombocytopenia[a]
Hepatic	Nonspecific transaminitis
Pulmonary	Pleural thickening, pleural effusions, pulmonary nodules, diffuse interstitial lung disease, BOOP, Caplan's syndrome, cricoarytenoid arthritis (pulmonary arteritis, PAH, shrinking lung[a])
Cardiac	Pericarditis, accelerated atherosclerotic disease, valvulitis[a]
Ophthalmologic	Keratoconjunctivits sicca (10%–15%), episcleritis, scleritis, uveitis,[a] ulcerative keratitis[a]
Neurologic	Peripheral entrapment neuropathy, cervical myelopathy due to cervical spine subluxation
Muscular	Muscle atrophy, inflammatory myositis[a]
Renal	Low grade membranous glomerular nephropathy, reactive amyloid
Vascular	Small vessel vasculitis, systemic vasculitis[a]

[a]Less than 5%.
Percentage range of rheumatoid arthritis patients reported to have this organ system involvement is presented in parentheses.

to new symptoms. The most common extra-articular manifestation of RA is Sjögren's syndrome, manifested by dry eyes (keratoconjunctivitis sicca) and dry mouth (xerostomia), and occurring in approximately 35% of patients. Rheumatoid nodules are also relatively common, with a reported frequency of approximately 25%. Rheumatoid nodules develop over pressure areas of the body such as the elbows, Achilles tendons, fingers, scalp, and ischial tuberosities (Figure 6A-3). The nodules are firm, nontender, and are frequently adherent to the underlying periosteum. Nodules are usually associated with seropositivity for rheumatoid factor. Up to 50% of RA patients will have pleural thickening on autopsy, but this is usually asymptomatic. Pleural effusions and pleurisy can be bilateral in up to 25% of the cases. The pleural fluid typically exhibits a low to modestly elevated white blood cell count, low glucose, high lactate dehydrogenase, and high protein concentration. Up to 30% of RA patients will have parenchymal lung disease including pulmonary nodules (usually asymptomatic)

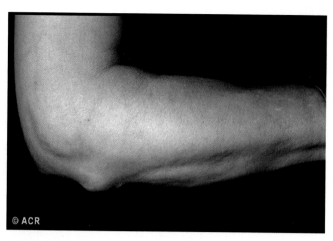

© ACR

FIGURE 6A-3

A large subcutaneous nodule is located on the extensor surface of the forearm near the elbow. (From the ACR slide collection on the rheumatic diseases, 3rd ed. Slide 37 (#9105190), with permission of the American College of Rheumatology.)

and/or diffuse interstitial lung disease that resembles idiopathic pulmonary fibrosis, obliterative bronchiolitis, bronchiectasis, or bronchiolotis obliterans organizing pneumonia (BOOP). From a cardiac standpoint, pericarditis is the most common manifestation of RA and, as with pleural disease, is generally asymptomatic and found on autopsy. Patients with RA also have a higher incidence of fatal and nonfatal cardiovascular events (myocardial infarction and stroke) than the general population, presumably due to accelerated atherosclerosis from chronic systemic and/or vascular inflammation. Hematologically, most RA patients are anemic. The most common cause is due to inflammation-induced anemia of chronic disease but iron deficiency anemia due to gastrointestinal blood loss from nonsteroidal anti-inflammatory agents also occurs (see Chapter 41). Small vessel vasculitis is relatively uncommon and is generally restricted to the digits and nailfold areas but may also cause peripheral neuropathy and/or mononeuritis multiplex presenting as wrist or foot drop.

LABORATORY FINDINGS

Routine laboratory studies at baseline are important in assessing the degree of systemic inflammation, in ruling out other potential confounding conditions, and in guiding the use of therapies that have known organ-specific toxicities. These should include a comprehensive metabolic panel, a complete blood count with differential, and inflammatory biomarkers such as the ESR and/or C-reactive protein. The serum electrolytes, liver function, and renal function are usually normal in patients with RA. Abnormal liver function tests usually signal the presence of a concomitant disease process

that may limit the use of hepatically cleared medications such as methotrexate or leflunomide. Likewise, renal insufficiency will preclude the use of nonsteroidal anti-inflammatory medications. In some individuals, high levels of systemic inflammation are associated with depressed hepatic synthesis of albumin (hypoalbuminemia) and increased gamma globulin production by B cells (hypergammaglobulinemia), leading to elevated serum levels of nonalbumin protein (so-called protein gap or gamma gap). It is important in these cases to rule out a monoclonal gammopathy. Most often in RA a broad-based polyclonal increase in gamma globulins will be observed on serum protein electrophoresis. Approximately 25% of RA patients will have a normocytic normochromic anemia as a result of chronic inflammation. If iron deficiency anemia is found, further workup is warranted to evaluate for gastrointestinal blood loss, especially if the patient chronically uses nonsteroidal anti-inflammatory medications. Rarely, RA patients may exhibit leucopenia or thrombocytopenia, which can be due to Felty's syndrome (splenomegaly and neutropenia associated with longstanding severe RA) or due to medications.

The most commonly used inflammatory biomarkers in clinical practice are the ESR and CRP. These markers are usually, but not always, elevated in RA patients with active disease and decline with treatment. Thus, the two inflammatory markers can be followed along with the patients' symptoms and joint examination to monitor disease activity over time. High ESR and CRP at the onset of disease are predictive of more aggressive disease and potentially worse prognosis.

In addition to the routine bloodwork discussed above, two autoantibodies should be assessed in patients suspected of having RA. These are the RF and anti-CCP antibodies. RFs are antibodies against the Fc portion of IgG and can be of any immunoglobulin subclass (IgA, IgG, and IgM) but are most commonly IgM. The cutoff value for a positive RF varies depending on the methodology used in the local laboratory, but a common cutoff point is greater than 45 IU/mL by enzyme-linked immunoabsorbent assay (ELISA) or laser nephelometry, or greater than a titer of 1:80 by latex fixation. Similarly, the cutoff point for a positive anti-CCP test varies according to the assay used, but greater than or equal to 80 IU/mL is commonly used.

Rheumatoid factor is detectable during the course of disease in approximately 75% to 85% of patients with RA. Approximately 50% are positive in the first 6 months of illness and 85% become positive over the first 2 years. A low level of RF can also be associated with a number of other chronic inflammatory infectious and noninfectious conditions as well (such as bacterial endocarditis, hepatitis C with cryoglobulinemia, aging, primary biliary cirrhosis), whereas a high level of RF is more likely indicative of RA. In RA patients, high levels of RF are also predictive of more aggressive erosive articular disease and poorer long-term function, and are associated with more extra-articular disease such as rheumatoid nodules and lung involvement. The sensitivity and specificity of RF for the diagnosis of RA are roughly 66% and 82%, respectively.

Anti-cyclic cirullinated peptide antibodies are also found in the sera of many patients with RA and are directed against the citrullinated residues of proteins. Citrulline is a non-naturally occurring amino acid generated by deimination of arginine residues on proteins by enzymes called *peptidylarginine deiminases*. Deiminated recombinant fillagrin protein in cyclic form is a particularly useful substrate to detect these auto antibodies. The sensitivity of the anti-CCP antibody test for RA is similiar (70%), but specificity is superior (95%) to RF. Moreover, 35% of patients with a negative RF at presentation will test positively for anti-CCP antibody (6). Thus, diagnostic yield is enhanced by measuring both RF and anti-CCP in a patient suspected of having RA. Like RF, the higher the level of anti-CCP antibody, the higher the correlation with erosive joint disease, functional disability, and extra-articular disease.

Interestingly, anti-CCP and RF have been demonstrated in sera up to 10 years *before* the onset of articular symptoms in some patients who later develop RA, and anti-CCP antibodies appear somewhat earlier than RF (Figure 6A-4) (7). This important observation has potential implications for screening individuals who are at high risk for developing RA, as well as the potential for instituting preventive therapy in the preclinical stage of disease. These types of innovative approaches are under discussion in academic centers.

A small portion of RA patients will remain seronegative throughout the course of their disease. Antinuclear antibody (ANA) can be present in 20% to 30% of patients with RA. ANA is more common in RA patients with high titer RF and extra-articular manifestations of the disease. In contrast to systemic lupus erythematosus, in which complement levels are low, complement levels in RA are usually normal or increased because complement is an acute phase reactant.

Synovial fluid analysis can also be useful in the assessment of patients suspected of having RA. Although there is no pathognomonic finding in RA, analysis of the synovial fluid is useful to rule out infectious and crystalline processes. RA patients are at an increased risk of developing septic joints (streptococcal and staphylococcal infection most commonly), which can be diagnosed based on Gram stain and culture of the synovial fluid. A total white blood cell count in the synovial fluid above 2000 cells/mm^3 is indicative of an inflammatory process. A total white blood cell count greater than 50,000 cells/mm^3 should be worrisome for an infectious process. The differential on the white blood cell count in the rheumatoid joint (whether infected or not) usually demonstrates a neutrophilic predominance. The presence of crystals or bacteria in the synovial fluid speak to an alternate diagnosis. Synovial biopsy is not routinely recommended unless a chronic infectious process such as tuberculosis is suspected.

RADIOLOGICAL FINDINGS

Radiographic abnormalities are very helpful in the diagnosis and treatment of RA. The earliest change on radiographs of the small joints of the hands and feet is periarticular osteopenia; however, this is variable, nonspecific, and nondiagnostic. More typical changes of RA are juxta-articular bony erosions and symmetrical joint space narrowing. These changes can be evident in the first 6 to 12 months of disease and accumulate over time if effective control of disease activity is not achieved.

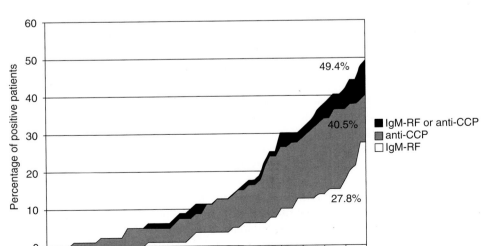

FIGURE 6A-4

Cumulative percentages of patients with one or more positive test results for IgM rheumatoid factor (IgM-RF), anti-cyclic citrullinated peptide (anti-CCP), and IgM-RF and/or anti-CCP before the onset of symptoms of rheumatoid arthritis. (From Nielen M, van Schaardenburg D, Reesink H, et al. Arthritis Rheum 2004;50:380–386, by permission of *Arthritis and Rheumatism*.)

Erosions typically appear at the margins of the joints, both medially and laterally, and on both apposing bones. Late radiographic findings include subluxation and loss of joint alignment, due not only to bone and cartilage destruction, but also due to laxity or frank rupture of the ligaments and tendons surrounding the joint. Radiographs in advanced disease may also show degenerative changes such as osteophytes. While not specific for RA, the findings of erosions, symmetric joint space narrowing, and/or subluxation indicate the presence of an inflammatory arthritis that requires urgent assessment and treatment. Radiographs of the hands, wrists, and feet should be obtained at baseline in patients with RA, and can be repeated periodically to ensure that additional damage is not occurring in the face of apparently effective treatment. Radiographs of the hands, feet, and wrists are more informative for following disease progression than radiographs of large joints because of the numerous joints available for assessment; furthermore, because the bone is thinner in these joints, erosions are identified earlier and visualized more easily than in larger joints such as the knees.

Magnetic resonance imaging (MRI) and ultrasound have proven to be more sensitive methods for detecting early joint erosions; in addition, because these methods also image soft tissues, inflammation (tenosynovitis) and integrity (rupture) of the tendons can be evaluated, and cartilage volume can be measured by MRI. In patients suspected of having early RA in whom the articular exam is particularly difficult (e.g., in the obese individual), MRI can also be very helpful in confirming the presence of synovial effusion and hypertrophy. MRI and ultrasound has largely replaced arthrography, particularly for confirmation of ruptured popliteal cysts in the knee.

DIFFERENTIAL DIAGNOSIS

A comprehensive initial evaluation of the patient, including demographic characteristics, characterization of articular and extra-articular complaints, and careful physical examination, will guide the construction of the differential diagnosis and subsequent laboratory and radiological testing. The most common causes of symmetrical inflammatory polyarthritis that may be confused with RA are the other systemic connective tissue disorders, psoriatic arthritis, and viral-induced arthritis (in particular, parvovirus B19– and hepatitis C–associated arthritis).

Other connective tissue disorders that can cause polyarthritis with a rheumatoidlike distribution include systemic lupus erythematosus, systemic sclerosis, mixed connective tissue disease, and Sjögren's syndrome. In most cases, the presence of extra-articular features such as Raynaud's phenomenon and rash, the absence of

anti-CCP reactivity, and the presence of antinuclear (and other) antibodies will help to differentiate these diseases from RA. It should be noted that RF can be present in most connective tissue diseases and occurs with particularly high frequency in Sjögren's syndrome. Patients with connective tissue diseases who have erosive arthritis should be considered to have an overlap syndrome (e.g., "rupus" as an overlap of RA and systemic lupus).

Hepatitis C–associated polyarthritis with cryoglobulinemia can present a more challenging diagnostic dilemma because cryoglobulins frequently have reactivity in the RF assay. For this reason, it is particularly important to consider hepatitis C risk factors in evaluating patients with rheumatoidlike arthritis and a positive RF. The distribution of joint involvement in patients with parvovirus B19–associated polyarthritis is generally very similar to RA but the intensity of inflammation is considerably less; furthermore, this arthritis resolves spontaneously in weeks to months in most individuals without treatment. The presence of IgM-specific parvo B19 viral antibodies will confirm the diagnosis.

Psoriatic skin involvement most commonly occurs *before* the onset of the arthritis, thus providing a clue to the diagnosis of psoriatic arthritis. Furthermore, unlike RA, psoriatic arthritis typically involves the DIP joints and is less symmetrical. Other causes of inflammatory arthritis that are less symmetrical and typically oligo- or monoarthritic in presentation include the crystalline arthropathies (gout and pseudogout), septic arthritis, and the human leukocyte antigen (HLA)-B27–associated spondyloarthropathies. In patients presenting with an inflammatory *monoarthritis*, the process should be assumed to be septic until proven otherwise. Joint aspiration should be performed and the fluid sent for Gram stain, culture, and crystal examination. Usually patients with bacterial infectious arthritis will appear septic and erosions may be present on radiographs, depending on the duration of infection within the joint. Monoarthritis that is more chronic and accompanied by radiographic damage should evoke the possibility of mycobacterial or fungal infection; in this case, a synovial biopsy for culture may be needed in order to expose the infection. Arthritis caused by disseminated *Neisseria gonorrhea* should be considered, particularly in younger female patients; skin lesions (pustules, blisters, vasculitic lesions) can provide a clue to the diagnosis along with history of vaginal discharge. If suspected, vaginal and oral cultures should be obtained along with synovial fluid cultures. In patients presenting with oligoarthritis, the spondyloarthropathies should be considered. These include ankylosing spondylitis, psoriatic arthritis (discussed above), reactive arthritis, and arthritis associated with inflammatory bowel disease. Features common to these diseases include involvement of the sacroiliac joints, asymmetric peripheral joint involvement, uveitis, and Achilles tendonitis. Lyme-associated arthritis is also, in essence, a reactive arthritis, occurring weeks to months after the acute infection. Lyme arthritis tends to occur in the knee and/or ankle as a monoarthritis or oligoarthritis. Patients should be queried about tick bites and Lyme antibody testing should be obtained if suspected. Gout and pseudogout commonly present with an intense inflammation and subcutaneous edema and can be confused with cellulitis. If inadequately treated, gout can evolve to a phase of chronic tophaceous polyarthritis that may be confused with RA.

Non-inflammatory painful conditions, such as fibromyalgia and overuse syndromes, and degenerative arthritis or osteoarthritis, should not be confused with RA as they do not exhibit prolonged morning stiffness, and swelling of the joints is relatively uncommon. In contrast to RA, the DIP joints of the hands are involved in osteoarthritis and bony enlargement (Heberden's and Bouchard's nodes) rather than soft tissue swelling is typical. Fibromyalgia presents with diffuse musculoskeletal pain and the joint examination is usually normal. Another consideration is malignancy, which can occasionally present as polyarthralgias but true synovitis is usually absent. For example, lung cancer can cause hypertrophic osteoarthropathy. In addition, if a large protein gap is present, then one should evaluate for a monoclonal gammopathy by checking a serum protein electropheresis. Certain metabolic disorders such as hypo- or hyperthyroidism can cause polyarthralgias. Also, hyperparathyroidism and other causes of hypercalcemia predispose to the development of pseudogout.

Making the diagnosis of RA early in the course of disease is imperative so that effective treatment can be initiated in a timely manner. The goals of treatment are reduction of pain and inflammation and prevention of long-term disability and extra-articular morbidity and mortality (see Chapter 6C).

REFERENCES

1. Drosos A. Epidemiology of rheumatoid arthritis. Autoimmun Rev 2004;3(Suppl 1):S20–S22.
2. Symmons D, Barrett E, Bankhead C, et al. The occurrence of rheumatoid arthritis in the United Kingdom: results from the Norfolk Arthritis Register. Br J Rheumatol 1994;33:735–739.
3. Hochberg M, Spector T. Epidemiology of rheumatoid arthritis: update. Epidemiol Rev 1990;12:247–252.
4. Jacoby R, Cosh J, Jayson M. Onset, early stages, and prognosis of rheumatoid arthritis: a clinical study with 100 patients with 11 years of follow-up. Br Med J 1973;2: 96–100.
5. Turesson C, O'Fallon W, Crowson C, et al. Extra-articular disease manifestations in rheumatoid arthritis: incidence trends and risk factors over 46 years. Ann Rheum Dis 2003;62:722–727.
6. Schellekens G, Visser H, de Jong B, et al. The diagnostic properties of rheumatoid arthritis antibodies recognizing a cyclic citrullinated peptide. Arthritis Rheum 2000;43: 155–163.
7. Nielen M, van Schaardenburg D, Reesink H, et al. Specific autoantibodies precede the symptoms of rheumatoid arthritis: a study of serial measurements in blood donors. Arthritis Rheum 2004;50:380–386.

6

Rheumatoid Arthritis
B. Epidemiology, Pathology, and Pathogenesis

JEAN-MARC WALDBURGER, MD, PHD
GARY S. FIRESTEIN, MD

- Genetic factors, including the human leukocyte antigen (HLA) shared epitope, hormonal factors, and environmental exposures such as tobacco smoke or infectious agents may predispose to the development of rheumatoid arthritis (RA).
- The primary target organ in RA is the synovial membrane. Changes include increased cellularity, increased vascularity, and infiltration with immune inflammatory cells.
- Autoantibodies in RA include rheumatoid factor and anti-cyclic citrullinated peptide (CCP) antibodies. Importance of humoral immunity is demonstrated by the efficacy of anti–B lymphocyte treatment strategies.

- T cells are involved in RA pathogenesis due to their presence in the synovium, association with HLA, presence of T-cell cytokines, and efficacy of anti–T lymphocyte treatment strategies.
- Cytokines are critical to RA pathogenesis. Proinflammatory cytokines tumor necrosis factor alpha (TNF-alpha), interleukin (IL) 1, and IL-6 have proved to be important as treatments, though many others may also play essential roles.
- Mechanisms that result in destruction of cartilage and bone lead to joint deformities and disability.

Rheumatoid arthritis (RA) is one of the most common inflammatory arthritides. Affected patients suffer from chronic articular pain, disability, and excess mortality. It primarily affects the small diarthrodial joints of the hands and feet, although larger weight-bearing and appendicular joints can also be involved. Extra-articular manifestations and systemic symptoms also occur, but in a minority of patients. RA is a heterogeneous disease of variable severity and unpredictable response to therapy. Genetic and environmental factors are clearly implicated in its etiology and pathogenesis. Translational research efforts have led to novel targeted therapies, although the treatment of RA remains a significant unmet medical need.

EPIDEMIOLOGY AND RISK FACTORS OF RHEUMATOID ARTHRITIS

The prevalence estimates for RA are between 0.5% and 1.0% in European and North American populations. The disease has a worldwide distribution but studies in Asia, including China and Japan, suggest a somewhat lower rate in those regions (0.2%–0.3%). Some Native American populations have a remarkably high prevalence (more than 5%) that is likely related to as yet poorly defined genetic factors.

Genetic Factors

Genetic background contributes disease susceptibility in RA, and the risk of developing the disease in first-degree relatives of a rheumatoid patient is 1.5-fold higher than the general population. The concordance rate is markedly higher for monozygotic twins compared with dizygotic twins (12%–15% vs. 3.5%, respectively), which supports a critical role of genes in addition to shared environmental influences between siblings. The overall heritability of RA has been estimated from twin studies to reach about 50% to 60%.

The Role of HLA-DR and the Shared Epitope Hypothesis

The most potent genetic risk for RA is conveyed by certain major histocompatibility complex alleles (MHC, or HLA for human leukocyte antigen; see Chapter 4). Early studies of MHC associations relied on serologic or cellular HLA typing, which only identified a fraction of the allelic variability. Increased prevalence of RA was reported to be associated with a subset of DR4 alleles in most Western European populations or a subset of DR1 alleles in other populations such as Spanish, Basque, and Israeli cohorts. Current HLA typing can discriminate allelic variants at the nucleotide level and reveals that a conserved amino acid sequence is over-represented in patients with RA. This sequence maps in the third hypervariable region of DR beta chains from amino acids 70 to 74. The shared epitope (SE) (1) is glutamine-leucine-arginine-alanine-alanine (QKRAA), and presence of the SE is associated with increased susceptibility to and severity of RA.

Different models have been proposed to explain the role of the shared epitope in RA. Susceptibility alleles could (1) bind efficiently to arthritogenic peptides, such as those either derived from a self-antigen or a microbial pathogen, (2) lead to the positive or negative selection of autoimmune T cells in the thymus, (3) lead to inadequate numbers of regulatory T cells, (4) become the target of T cells themselves due to molecular mimicry between QKRAA and pathogens implicated in RA, such as *Escherichia coli* DnaJ or Epstein–Barr virus (EBV) peptides.

A recent alternative hypothesis suggests that the association is not necessarily between the SE itself and the development of RA, but instead between the SE and the production of certain autoantibodies, especially anti-cyclic citrullinated peptide (CCP) antibodies. This model implies that anti-CCP antibodies rather than the SE is responsible for the genetic link. One possible explanation is that the SE confers a positive charge to the peptide binding cleft on the class II MHC that prevents the binding of peptides containing arginine. Peptidylarginine deiminases (PADIs) convert arginine to an uncharged citrulline, thereby permitting the antigen to be loaded onto the MHC and presented to autoreactive T cells. Given this functional role, it is of interest that one of the four isoforms, PADI 4, has been implicated in RA, although the association with RA appears to be mainly in Asian populations rather than Western Europeans.

Other Genetic Risk Factors

Polymorphisms in several other genes may contribute incremental risk for RA that is quantitatively lower than the MHC itself. Many genes have been implicated, although the data vary widely. Some of the putative associations relate to cytokines, chemokines, and their receptors.

The analysis of the genetic predisposition to RA has recently been expanded using genomewide scans (2). An example of a newly described susceptibility gene discovered by this approach is a functional variant (R620W) of the intracellular protein tyrosine phosphatase N22 (PTPN22). The risk of developing RA is about twofold higher in heterozygotes and fourfold higher in homozygotes who carry this polymorphism. The PTPN22 variant is also associated with other autoimmune diseases, including type I diabetes and systemic lupus erythematosus. The product of this gene is an intracellular tyrosine phosphatase that negatively regulates T-cell activity. The R620W allele results in a gain of enzymatic function that alters the threshold for T-cell receptor (TCR) signaling. Theoretically, the defect in TCR signaling caused by R620W could generate autoimmunity by modulating negative selection in the thymus. PTPN22 could also regulate other cell types because it is expressed in myeloid cells and B cells.

Nongenetic Risk Factors
Influence of Sex

Women are two to three times more likely to develop RA than men. Hormonal factors like estrogen and progesterone could potentially explain some of the gender effect. Estrogen might have detrimental effects through its ability to decrease apoptosis of B cells, potentially permitting the selection of autoreactive clones. Hormones also have a complex influence on the balance of T-cell subsets with distinct cytokine profiles. For instance, administration of estrogen in animal models can enhance or suppress T-helper (Th) 1-mediated immunity, depending on the timing and the dose used. In murine collagen–induced arthritis, exogenous administration of estrogen is protective primarily by inhibiting Th1 immunity. However, the precise explanation for the greater prevalence of RA in females and the role of hormones remains uncertain.

The situation during pregnancy exemplifies complex influence that sex has on RA. Seventy-five percent of pregnant women with RA experience spontaneous remission, although the disease typically flares within weeks after delivery. Soluble mediators released by the placenta like transforming growth factor (TGF) beta, IL-10, or alpha-fetoprotein might contribute to this effect. Alternatively, the immune system in pregnant women displays a shift towards a Th2 bias, which could suppress the characteristic Th1 profile of RA (see T-cell subsets p. 127).

The presence of fetal cells in the maternal circulation that contain potentially alloreactive, paternal HLA molecules has been implicated in immune modulation during pregnancy. Generation of alloantibodies to the MHC or competition of fetal peptides with maternal autoantigens for MHC binding could potentially modulate the disease. In one study, most pregnant women experiencing RA remission had maternal–fetal disparity in HLA class II molecules, whereas HLA mismatch was less common in pregnancies that did not show RA improvement. This association was not observed in a second study, so the immunological effects of a maternal–fetal HLA mismatch remains to be clearly established.

Tobacco

Exposure to various environmental factors increase the risk for RA, and cigarette smoke is one of the best characterized. Of interest, smoking also enhances the risk of developing anti-CCP positive RA in patients with the SE (3). The mechanism of anti-CCP antibody generation from inhaled smoke probably relates to inflammation and activation of innate immunity in the airway, which then induces peptide citrullination. In a susceptible host, such as someone carrying the SE and with genetically determined immune hyperreactivity, these repeated insults followed by chronic exposure to citrullinated peptides could lead to the production of anti-CCP antibodies and other antibodies like rheumatoid factors. While the link between autoantibody production and the onset of RA is not always exact, this situation could enhance the synovial inflammatory response when innate immunity in the joint is activated by unrelated stimuli.

Bacteria and Their Products

Infectious agents have long been considered prime candidates as initiating factors for RA, although the search for a specific etiologic agent has been unrewarding. Bacterial DNA is present in synovial tissue by sensitive polymerase chain reaction techniques, but the species are not unique and have also been identified in many other arthropathies. Other microbial components, such

as peptidoglycans, are also present in RA joints in the absence of active infection. Bacterial peptidoglycans, like prokaryotic DNA, can activate Toll-like receptors (TLR) and stimulate synovial innate immune responses. Even nonspecific bacterial products could thus play a role in synovitis by activating cytokine networks or acting enhancing adaptive autoimmune responses. Such phenomena are well described in animal models where arthritis can be induced and/or enhanced by injecting purified bacterial products, in particular lipopolysaccharide (LPS) or extracts of mycobacteria. Importantly, LPS shares a common signaling pathway with IL-1 and can substitute for this cytokine in a mouse model of antibody-mediated arthritis.

Viruses

Several viruses have been implicated as possible etiologic factors in RA. A relationship between RA and EBV was suggested by several observations. For instance, EBV is a polyclonal activator of B lymphocytes and increases the production of rheumatoid factor (RF). Rheumatoid arthritis patients have an increased EBV load, and their synovium can expresses viral RNA. The viral gp110 protein is also one of the many xeno-proteins that contains the QKRAA sequence also found in the SE. Such proteins might trigger autoimmune responses by a process known as *molecular mimicry*, leading to an inappropriate immune response directed against a similar endogenous protein. Parvovirus B19 has also been suggested as an etiologic agent in RA. B19 DNA is more often found in RA joints than in controls, although only about 5% of newly diagnosed RA patients have evidence of recent parvovirus infection. The mechanisms of B19–induced synovitis, when it does occur, could include increased invasive properties of infected fibroblastlike synoviocytes.

Based on current data, the bacterial products or viral nucleic acids detected in RA joints are not likely to be part of an active infectious process. Even so, these products could still participate indirectly to arthritis in genetically susceptible individuals by stimulating their innate immune system, which can amplify adaptive immunity.

SYNOVIAL PATHOLOGY

The synovium is the primary site of inflammation in RA. Morphological and functional studies of this target tissue have led to improved understanding of RA through systematic comparison of rheumatoid samples with other joint diseases and normal tissue. Serial biopsies are also used increasingly in clinical studies, thus providing insight into pathogenic mechanisms at the molecular level.

The Normal Synovium

The normal synovium consists of an intimal lining layer that is usually discontinuous, one to two cell layers thick, and lacks an underlying basal membrane. The sublining below the intima contains blood vessels, lymphatics, nerves, and adipocytes distributed within a less cellular, fibrous matrix. The intimal lining layer comprises roughly equal proportions of two different cell types, macrophagelike synoviocytes or type A synoviocytes, and fibroblastlike synoviocytes (FLS) or type B synoviocytes. The latter are responsible for the synthesis of extracellular matrix proteins including collagen, fibronectin, hyaluronic acid, and other molecules that facilitate the lubrication and function of cartilage surfaces. Type A cells are phagocytic and express numerous markers of the monocyte–macrophage lineage.

The Synovium in Rheumatoid Arthritis

The complex histological architecture of the synovial tissue in RA is the result of a dynamic process involving coordinated molecular signals (chemokines, adhesion molecules, cytokines, and growth factors) and cellular events (apoptosis, proliferation, cell migration, and survival). Increased numbers of both type A and B synoviocytes augment the depth of the lining layer, sometimes to 10 cell layers, and mononuclear cells infiltrate the sublining (Figure 6B-1). The lining is the primary source of inflammatory cytokines and proteases, thus participating in joint destruction in concert with activated chondrocytes and osteoclasts. Villous projections protrude into the joint cavity, invading the

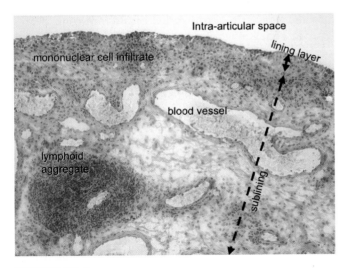

FIGURE 6B-1

Synovium in rheumatoid arthritis. Only modest synovial lining hyperplasia is present in this example, although sublining mononuclear cell infiltration, lymphoid aggregates, and vascular proliferation are prominent.

underlying cartilage and bone where the proliferating tissue is called *pannus*. In the synovial sublining region, edema, blood vessel proliferation, and increased cellularity lead to a marked increase in tissue volume.

T and B lymphocytes, plasma cells, interdigitating and follicular dendritic cells (IDC and FDC), and natural killer cells (NK cells) accumulate in rheumatoid synovium and can be distributed diffusely throughout the sublining or organized into lymphoid aggregates. The dominant cells, CD4+ T cells, are mostly of the memory CD45RO+ and display the chemokine receptors CXCR3 and CCR5 characteristic of Th1 cells. CD4+ T cells are especially enriched in aggregates, whereas CD8+ T cells are present in the periphery of the aggregates or scattered throughout the sublining. In about 15% to 20% of patients, structures typical of secondary lymphoid follicles can be found. T- and B-cell infiltrates are not specific to RA and can be found in many chronic inflammatory arthropathies.

The Synovial Fluid in Rheumatoid Arthritis

Normal joints contain a small amount of synovial fluid to lubricate articular surfaces. The volume of synovial fluid can increase dramatically in RA due to increased leakage from the synovial microvasculature. Neutrophils (polymorphonuclear leukocytes, or PMNs) are the predominant cell type, although lymphocytes, macrophages, NK cells, and fibroblasts are also present. PMNs are drawn into the articular cavity by a gradient of chemokines and other chemotactic factors, such as C5a and leukotriene B4. The dramatic influx of neutrophils into joint effusions might be due, in part, to low expression of adhesion molecules on PMNs that would retain these cells within the synovial tissues compared with mononuclear cells. The former can readily migrate out of the tissue while the latter are retained. PMNs in the synovial fluid are activated by factors such as immune complexes and cellular debris. They degranulate, generate products of oxygen metabolism, metabolize arachidonic acid, and release proteinases and cytokines. The lymphocyte population in synovial effusions differs from the synovium, with a higher number of CD8+ T cells in the fluid compared with CD4+ T-cell predominance in the tissue.

AUTOIMMUNITY AND AUTOANTIBODIES IN RHEUMATOID ARTHRITIS

The role of autoimmunity in RA was first suggested by the discovery of autoantibodies like rheumatoid factor in the sera of patients, which suggests that autoreactive

B cells are generated. Risks conveyed by the SE also serve as an argument for a pathogenic role of adaptive immunity. The advent of B- and T-cell–directed therapies provide compelling evidence that adaptive immune processes are involved in RA (see Chapter 6C).

B-Cell Autoimmunity and Autoantibodies

Antibodies directed against joint-specific and systemic autoantigens are commonly detected in the blood of RA patients. Autoantibodies are also found in immune complex deposits in rheumatoid joints and probably contribute to the local inflammation by activating complement. In mouse models of arthritis, synovitis can be induced by injecting purified antibodies directed against joint-specific proteins like type II collagen or against ubiquitous proteins that localize to joint tissue by nonspecific interactions with cartilage. Although antibodies can be arthritogenic, the arthritis generated by injection of antibodies is generally transient, whereas active production of autoantibodies and persistent disease requires T-cell help. The concept that autoantibodies and immune complexes are pathogenic fostered the development of targeted B-cell depletion in RA (see Chapter 6C) (4).

Rheumatoid Factors

Rheumatoid factors (RFs) are autoantibodies directed against the Fc portion of IgG (5). They were first detected in the sera of patients in 1940 and fostered the concept that humoral autoimmunity contributes to the pathogenesis of RA. IgG and IgM RFs are found in up to 90% of RA patients. Testing for IgM RF is about 70% sensitive and 80% specific for RA. However, these autoantibodies can also be produced during chronic infections, malignancy, and in a variety of inflammatory and autoimmune syndromes. RFs are also detectable in 1% to 4% of healthy individuals, and up to 25% of healthy individuals over the age of 60 years. They can be detected in the blood up to 10 years before the onset of RA, with an increasing incidence in the period immediately before clinical symptoms develop (see Chapter 6A). Therefore, the mere presence of RF is not sufficient to cause arthritic symptoms. The presence of RF in RA, however, has prognostic significance. Seropositive patients have more aggressive disease while seronegative patients tend to experience less severe arthritis with fewer bone erosions.

B cells isolated from RA synovium can secrete RF, indicating that the autoantibody is produced locally in the joint. The variable domains of the RF light chain from RA patients contain somatic mutations that encode high affinity antibodies, which are a hallmark of anti-

genic driven B-cell selection. In contrast, RFs produced by healthy individuals have avidity for the Fc portion of IgG several orders of magnitude lower than in RA and contain mostly germline-derived sequences.

Anti-Cyclic Citrullinated Peptide Antibodies

Anti-cyclic citrullinated peptide antibodies are another key autoantibody system in RA. Anti-CCP testing has a sensitivity of up to 80% to 90% and a specificity of 90% for RA, which increases to >95% specificity if combined with the presence of IgM RF (see Chapter 6A). Anti-CCP antibodies are occasionally produced in other inflammatory diseases, such as psoriatic arthritis, autoimmune hepatitis, and pulmonary tuberculosis (TB). Similar to RF, anti-CCP antibodies are a risk factor for more aggressive disease and are produced early in disease.

The process of citrullination involves conversion of arginine to citrulline by PADIs. Of the four isoforms, PADI 2 and PADI 4 are most abundant in the inflamed synovium. In RA, citrullination occurs in the inflamed synovium and the antibodies produced by resident B cells. A variety of citrullinated proteins are present in the rheumatoid joint, including fibrinogen, collagen, and fibronectin. The precise pathogenic role of the autoantibodies in RA is not well defined. However, anti-CP antibodies bind to intra-articular antigens in mice with collagen-induced arthritis and can enhance joint damage.

Other Autoantibodies

Many other autoantibodies can be detected in RA sera, indicating that aberrant immune responses can be directed against a broad range of autoantigens. Anti–type II collagen antibodies are especially interesting because they are pathogenic in a mouse model of arthritis. Synovial B cells in RA produce anticollagen antibodies that fix complement. However, elevated serum titers are found in only a minority of patients.

T-Cell Autoimmunity

T cells have been implicated in RA due to their presence in the synovium and the class II MHC association. Synovial T cells isolated from patients respond to some cartilage-specific proteins as well as ubiquitous antigens like heat-shock peptides. In animal models, T cells contribute at various levels to the development and progression of experimental arthritis. Several models rely on active immunization protocols against joint antigens such as type II collagen, which requires T-cell help. In one mouse model, a mutation in a signal transduction protein linked to TCR signaling causes arthritis through abnormal thymic selection of arthritogenic T cells. Despite evidence implicating T cells in RA, the results of early targeted therapies were disappointing. More recently, a biologic agent that blocks T cell costimulation (CTLA4-Ig; abatacept) demonstrated efficacy and has renewed the interest in targeting T cells to treat RA (see Chapter 6C) (6).

T-Cell Subsets

Naive CD4+ T cells can be differentiated into multiple effector types, including Th1 and Th2 phenotypes. Experimental systems have shown that precursor cells can be polarized towards one of these phenotypes depending on the nature of the antigen, characteristics of the antigen-presenting cells, and the cytokine milieu. Th1 cells are involved in the defense against intracellular pathogens and have been implicated in many autoimmune diseases. Th2 cells participate in host defense against parasitic worms but can also contribute to allergy and asthma. Each subtype is induced by cytokines present in the milieu (mainly IL-12 for Th1 cells, IL-4 for Th2 cells) and secretes characteristic effector cytokines (IFN-gamma and IL-2 by Th1 cells, IL-4 and IL-10 by Th2 cells). IL-4 and IL-10 inhibit Th1 cells, while IFN-gamma suppresses Th2 function.

Additional subsets have also been defined, including Th3 cells that produce TGF-beta and Th17 cells that produce IL-17 after precursor cells are exposed to IL-6 and TGF-beta or IL-23. Another subset, regulatory T cells (Tregs) can suppress arthritis in several experimental models of autoimmunity. Tregs co-express the surface markers CD25 and CD4 and inhibit T-cell responses by poorly defined cell-contact mechanisms. In RA, CD4+CD25+ regulatory T cells isolated from patients might be functionally compromised, and anti–TNF-alpha therapy appears to this defect.

T-Cell–Derived Cytokines

CD4+ T cells infiltrating the synovium primarily display the Th1 phenotype. Nevertheless, levels of Th1 cytokines in the rheumatoid synovium are surprisingly low. IFN-gamma can be detected in most patients, but its concentration is much less than in other Th1-mediated diseases. Another prototypic Th1 cytokine, IL-2, is also quite low in RA. However, cytokines that enhance Th1 differentiation, such as IL-12, can be readily detected in the rheumatoid joint.

Of the T-cell cytokines implicated in RA, IL-17 may be especially important. This cytokine synergizes with IL-1 and TNF-alpha in vitro to induce inflammatory cytokine production by fibroblasts and macrophages and enhance osteoclast activation. In animal models of arthritis, IL-17 deficiency or blockade markedly decrease clinical arthritis and destruction of the extracellular matrix. IL-17 has been detected in the synovium of patients with RA, although its functional role in vivo remains to be determined.

Th2 cytokines, such as IL-4 and IL-10, have also been examined in RA, in part because they tend to antagonize Th1 cells and are effective treatments when administered in animal models of arthritis. Levels of Th2 cytokines are generally very low in RA, perhaps reflecting the Th1 bias of the synovium. Of the Th2 factors present, IL-10 has been most consistently detected; however, a clinical trial of IL-10 in RA did not demonstrate significant benefit.

MACROPHAGE AND FIBROBLAST CYTOKINES IN RHEUMATOID ARTHRITIS

Cytokine Networks

Macrophages and fibroblasts are the primary sources of cytokines in the rheumatoid synovium. Synovial macrophages and fibroblasts produce a plethora of proinflammatory factors in the joint involved in the cytokine network (Figure 6B-2), including IL-1, IL-6, IL-8, IL-12, IL-15, IL-16, IL-18, IL-32, TNF-alpha, granulocyte-macrophage colony-stimulating factor (GM-CSF), and multiple chemokines (7). These cytokines can participate in paracrine and autocrine networks that enhance and perpetuate synovial inflammation. For instance, macrophages and fibroblasts in the intimal lining can activate adjacent cells that, in turn, can produce mediators that can stimulate their neighbors. The concept of cytokine networks dominated by synovial lining cells played a major role in the advent of anticytokine therapy in RA.

Although proinflammatory cytokines can be counterbalanced by the suppressive cytokines (IL-10, TGF-beta), soluble receptors (TNF-alpha), binding proteins (IL-18), and naturally occurring receptor antagonists (IL-1Ra), all of which are produced by macrophages and fibroblasts in the synovial intima, the concentrations are below those required to suppress inflammation. Although the cytokine network can be highly redundant, disease control can be achieved in many patients by inhibiting a single cytokine. TNF-alpha antagonists are the most salient example, in which one third to one half of patients have dramatic clinical responses to cytokine blockade (see Chapter 6C).

Some of the key cytokines produced by macrophages and fibroblasts in RA are discussed below. This is by no means a complete list, and the network becomes more complex with each passing year. In some cases, the contribution of more recently described proinflammatory cytokines has not been defined.

FIGURE 6B-2

Cytokine networks. Macrophages (Mφ), fibroblastlike synovioctyes (FLS), and synovial and T cells produce proinflammatory cytokines (denoted with +) that can activate either themselves (autocrine loops, *blue arrows*) or their adjacent cells within the joint (paracrine loops, *orange arrows*). They also secrete inhibitory cytokines (denoted by -) that only partially suppress the inflammation. Cytokines also stimulate osteoclasts, the main cell type responsible for bone destruction. RANKL produced by FLS and T cells (not shown in the figure) activate osteoclasts in the rheumatoid joint.

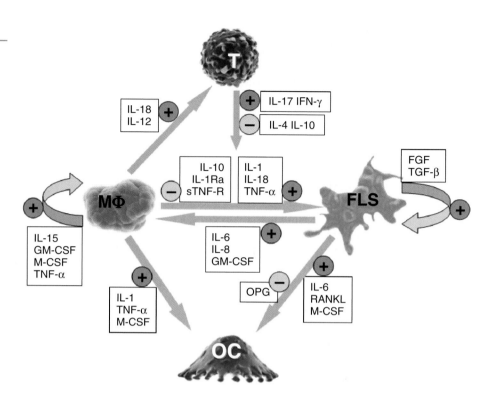

Tumor Necrosis Factor Superfamily

Tumor necrosis factor alpha is a pro-inflammataory cytokine that is synthesized as a membrane-bound protein and released after proteolytic cleavage by TNF convertase (TACE). It is the eponymous member of a larger group of related cytokines known as the TNF superfamily, many of which are also produced in the rheumatoid joint. Some members of the family regulate the subsynovial microarchitecture (lymphotoxins and LIGHT) while others participate in apoptosis (TRAIL, Fas ligand) or osteoclast activation (RANKL, receptor activator of NF-κB ligand).

In RA, TNF-alpha is mainly produced by synovial macrophages. The stimulating signals have not been defined but could involve TLRs, a family of receptors that recognize specific molecular patterns and activate the innate immune system, and other cytokines like IL-15. TNF-alpha can then bind to two ubiquitously expressed receptors (TNF-RI and TNF-RII) to induce the release of other cytokines and metalloproteases by fibroblasts, decrease the synthesis of proteoglycans by chondrocytes, and promote the differentiation of monocytes to osteoclasts in the presence of RANKL. TNF-alpha inhibitors improve signs and symptoms of RA and also decrease the progression of bone erosions due to effects on other cytokines and osteoclasts. In addition to its role in RA, TNF-alpha is an important molecule in the host response to certain infectious agents. Opportunistic infections, including reactivation of latent TB,

or defective tumor immune surveillance represent potential adverse effects of anti–TNF-alpha agents.

Interleukin 1 Family

Interleukin 1

Interleukin 1 exhibits many properties that can contribute to inflammation in RA, including increased synthesis of IL-6, chemokines, GM-CSF, prostaglandin and collagenase. It also plays a pivotal role in many animal models of inflammatory arthritis. Of the two forms of IL-1, IL-1 beta is secreted, whereas IL-1 alpha is expressed within cells and associated with cell membranes. The bioactive form of IL-1 beta is cleaved from a precursor protein by the cysteine protease caspase-1, also known as interleukin 1 converting enzyme (ICE). IL-1 acts via the type I IL-1 receptor (IL-1R1), whereas IL-1R2 is a decoy receptor that does not transduce an intracellular signal. Macrophages are the main source of IL-1 in the rheumatoid synovium. A variety of inflammatory factors induce IL-1 production in RA, including TNF-alpha, GM-CSF, immunoglobulin Fc fragments, collagen fragments and, to a lesser extent, immune complexes.

Interleukin 18

Interleukin 18 is another proinflammatory member of the IL-1 family and induces the production of IFN-gamma, IL-8, GM-CSF, and TNF-alpha by synovial macrophages. IL-18 also biases the immune responses of T cells toward the Th1 phenotype. It is expressed mainly by synovial fibroblasts and macrophages in response to TNF-alpha and IL-1 stimulation. IL-18 inhibition significantly attenuates collagen-induced arthritis in the mouse. A human IL-18 binding protein blocks IL-18 activity in vitro and is a potential therapeutic agent.

Interleukin 1 Receptor Antagonist Protein

Interleukin 1 receptor antagonist protein is a natural inhibitor of IL-1 present in the RA joint, but at concentrations too low to counteract IL-1 activity. Administration of exogenous IL-1Ra is very effective in IL-1–dependent diseases such as systemic onset juvenile idiopathic arthritis, adult Still's disease, or familial cold autoinflammatory syndrome. IL-1Ra, along with other IL-1– directed approaches like caspase-1 inhibitors and engineered IL-1 binding proteins, have modest efficacy in RA (see Chapter 6C). Taken together, these data suggest that IL-1 might not be a central cytokine regulating synovial inflammation in this disease.

Interleukin 6 Family

Interluekin 6 has pleiotropic effects and influences systemic inflammation through its actions on hematopoiesis and many cell types of the immune system. IL-6 is perhaps the major factor that induces acute phase proteins like CRP by the liver. Very high levels of IL-6 are present in the synovial fluid of RA patients and type B synoviocytes are the major source. IL-6 is also implicated in the activation of the endothelium and contributes to bone erosion by stimulating the maturation of osteoclasts. In RA, IL-6 levels decrease dramatically after treatment with TNF inhibitors. Clinical trials of IL-6 inhibitors show a degree of efficacy that is similar to TNF-alpha antagonists (see Chapter 6C).

Other Key Cytokines

The number of additional cytokines and growth factors produced by macrophages and fibroblasts in RA is extensive and a complete description is beyond the scope of this chapter. For instance, many C-C and C-X-C chemokines are produced by the synovium that recruit mononuclear cells and PMNs into the joint. IL-15 is a macrophage-derived cytokine that activates T cells and can increase endogenous TNF-alpha production. Certain macrophage products, like IL-12, can influence T-cell differentiation and bias cells towards the Th1 phenotype. Colony stimulating factors, such as

M-CSF and GM-CSF, are produced by both macrophages and fibroblasts in the intimal lining and can enhance osteoclast differentiation and macrophage activation, respectively.

MECHANISM OF JOINT DESTRUCTION

Angiogenesis and Cell Migration

The generation of new blood vessels is required to provide nutrients to the expanding synovial membrane and is an early event in the development of synovitis. The expanding tissue can ultimately outstrip angiogenesis in RA; synovial fluid oxygen tension is quite low and is associated with low pH and high lactate levels. Hypoxia is a potent stimulus for angiogenesis in the synovium, and factors that promote blood vessel growth, such as vascular endothelial growth factor (VEGF), IL-8, angiopoietin-1, and many others, are expressed in RA. Several anti-angiogenesis approaches can markedly attenuate arthritis in animal models. For instance, targeting the integrin alpha-v beta-3 expressed by proliferating blood vessels in the synovium or treating with antibodies to the type 1 VEGF receptor (VEGF-R1) suppress clinical and histologic evidence of disease.

Proinflammatory cytokines induce the expression of specialized receptors on capillaries and postcapillary venules that regulate the migration of the inflammatory cells into the synovium. E- and P-selectins, which mediate leukocyte rolling, and vascular cell adhesion molecule-1 (VCAM-1) and intercellular adhesion molecule-1 (1-IAM), which control immobilization and ingress of cells into tissue, are adhesion molecules identified on the inflamed synovial endothelium in RA. Once leukocytes have migrated into the tissue, they adhere to the matrix through surface receptors and their survival and proliferation is stimulated by the cytokine milieu.

The Role of Fibroblastlike Synoviocytes

Activated type-B synoviocytes are a major source of inflammatory mediators and metalloproteinases in RA. Synoviocytes can be grown in vitro to study signal transduction systems that relay information from the environment to the nucleus and activate gene expression. Several intracellular pathways have distinctive but overlapping functions, including NF-κB, mitogen-activated protein kinases (MAPK), and signal transducers and activators of transcription (STATs). For instance, p38 MAPK regulate production of IL-6 by

6

synoviocytes, while c-Jun N-terminal kinase (JNK) is a critical MAPK that induces collagenase expression and regulates joint destruction in experimental arthritis. These studies have contributed to the notion that targeting signaling molecules that regulate synoviocyte and macrophage activation might have therapeutic potential in RA.

Fibroblastlike cells derived from the synovium of RA patients exhibit some unique aggressive properties. Unlike synovial fibroblasts from normal or osteoarthritis donors, RA synoviocytes transferred to severe combined immunodeficient (SCID) mice invade and destroy human cartilage explants. Insufficient synoviocyte apoptosis in RA probably contributes to intimal lining hyperplasia of the synovium due to several mechanisms, including low expression of anti-apoptotic genes and abnormal function of tumor suppressor genes like p53. RA synoviocytes also express a variety of oncogenes and display some evidence of de-differentiation, as demonstrated by expression of the want family of embryonic genes.

Extracellular Matrix Damage
Cartilage Destruction

Aggressive synoviocytes at sites of pannus overgrowth, cytokine-activated chondrocytes, and PMNs are major cell types responsible for destruction of the cartilage in RA. They release destructive enzymes in response to IL-1, TNF-alpha, IL-17, and immune complexes. Once the cartilage is compromised, mechanical stress works as an accelerating factor to enhance destruction. A variety of enzymes participate in extracellular matrix degradation of the joint, such as matrix metalloproteinases (MMPs; collagenases, gelatinases, and stromelysin), serine proteases (trypsin, chymotrypsin), and cathepsins (see Chapter 11B). Reversible loss of proteoglycans occurs early, most likely due to the catabolic effect of cytokines and the production of stromelysins and aggrecanases. Cleavage of native type II collagen by collagenases is an irreversible step that permanently damages the cartilage.

Protease inhibitors are also present in the RA joint; like endogenous cytokines antagonists, they are overwhelmed by massive production of degradative enzymes. In addition to protecting the matrix, serine protease inhibitors can also prevent the activation of MMPs through limited proteolytic digestion. Tissue inhibitors of metalloproteinases (TIMPs) inhibit the active form of MMPs and are expressed by intimal lining and sublining synovial cells. The relative balance between MMPs and TIMPs is unfavorable in RA compared with osteoarthritis and

is improved in patients treated with chronic low dose methotrexate.

Bone Destruction

Focal bone erosions are a hallmark of RA that can occur early in the disease and cause significant morbidity due to subchondral and the cortical bone damage. RA is also associated with periarticular bone loss adjacent to inflamed joints and generalized osteopenia, leading to increased risk of fracture in both the appendicular and axial skeleton.

The cellular and molecular mechanisms underlying cartilage destruction and focal bone erosions are distinct. Synoviocytes, chondrocytes, and neutrophils are probably the major effectors of the former. Bone erosions are mainly caused by osteoclasts, which are derived from macrophage precursors (8). They accumulate at the pannus–bone interface and the subchondral marrow space.

Receptor activator of NF-κB (RANK) and its ligand RANKL form the most important receptor–ligand pair that modulates bone resorption in RA. RANK is expressed by osteoclasts and modulates their maturation and activation. Expression of the RANKL on T cells and fibroblastlike synoviocytes is promoted by cytokines such as TNF-alpha, IL-1, and IL-17. The RANK–RANKL system is antagonized by a soluble decoy receptor, osteoprotegerin (OPG), that binds to RANKL. Injection of OPG or deletion of the RANKL gene in animal models inhibits bone destruction but does not suppress inflammation. Of interest, anti–TNF-alpha agents can slow the progression rate of bone erosions in RA, even in patients without clinical improvement. Therefore, the inflammatory and destructive mechanisms in RA can be distinct.

CONCLUSION

The pathogenesis of RA is highly complex and involves interconnected cellular and molecular pathways ultimately causing joint inflammation and damage (9). Interaction between innate and adaptive immunity explain many aspects of RA (Figure 6B-3). Basic research and clinical studies have not clearly established a hierarchy among the different pathogenic pathways because therapies that target cytokines, T cells, or B cells exhibit a similar efficacy. The self-perpetuating mechanisms of RA are resistant to current treatments because established disease usually relapses when therapy is discontinued, even if a full remission had been achieved. A better understanding of these unre-

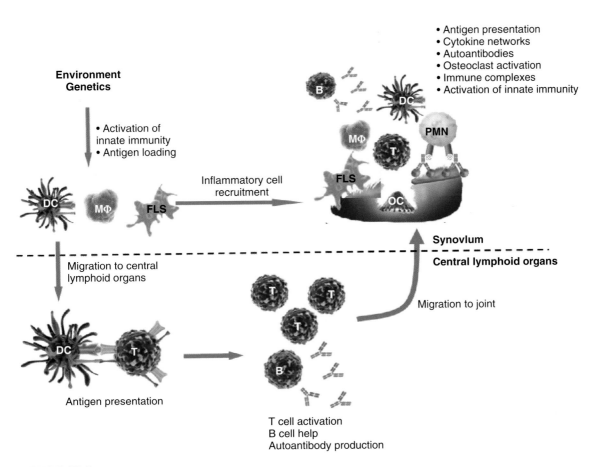

FIGURE 6B-3

Innate and adaptive immunity both contribute to the pathogenesis of RA. Genetic predisposition places individuals at risk for RA, perhaps due to abnormal T-cell selection, elevated cytokine production, or enhanced propensity to protein citrullination. Stochastic events, such as environmental exposures, might enhance immune reactivity and permit a breakdown of tolerance. Nonspecific inflammation due to environmental exposures or endogenous ligands, such as stimulation of the TLR, can also directly induce cytokine production, activate synoviocytes and macrophages that secrete chemokines, and recruit lymphocytes that can respond to local antigens. Self-antigens derived from the inflamed tissues can be processed by tissue dendritic cells, which migrate to central lymphoid organs and activate T cells. B cells and T cells activated in the central tissues can subsequently migrate back to the joint. At later stages, local cytokine networks amplify and maintain a self-sustained inflammatory loop within the joints and perhaps lead to local antigen presentation and the formation of secondary lymphoid aggregates. The activation of enzymes that degrade the matrix and osteoclasts can cause irreversible joint destruction.

solved issues will hopefully lead to improved diagnostic and prognostic tools that are needed to achieve early disease control in RA before irreversible joint damage has occurred.

REFERENCES

1. Gregersen PK, Silver J, Winchester RJ. The shared epitope hypothesis. An approach to understanding the molecular genetics of susceptibility to rheumatoid arthritis. Arthritis Rheum 1987;30:1205–1213.

2. Gregersen PK. Pathways to gene identification in rheumatoid arthritis: PTPN22 and beyond. Immunol Rev 2005; 204:74–86.

3. Klareskog L, Stolt P, Lundberg K, et al. A new model for an etiology of rheumatoid arthritis: smoking may trigger HLA-DR (shared epitope)-restricted immune reactions to autoantigens modified by citrullination. Arthritis Rheum 2006;54:38–46.

4. Cambridge G, Edwards JC. B-cell targeting in rheumatoid arthritis and other autoimmune diseases. Nat Rev Immunol 2006;6:394–403.

5. Dorner T, Egerer K, Feist E, Burmester GR. Rheumatoid factor revisited. Curr Opin Rheumatol 2004;16:246–253.

6. Kremer JM. Selective costimulation modulators: a novel approach for the treatment of rheumatoid arthritis. J Clin Rheumatol 2005;11(Suppl):S55–S62.

7. Arend WP. Physiology of cytokine pathways in rheumatoid arthritis. Arthritis Rheum 2001;45:101–106.

8. Walsh NC, Crotti TN, Goldring SR, Gravallese EM. Rheumatic diseases: the effects of inflammation on bone. Immunol Rev 2005;208:228–251.

9. Firestein GS. Evolving concepts of rheumatoid arthritis. Nature 2003;423:356–361.

Rheumatoid Arthritis
C. Treatment and Assessment

ALYCE M. OLIVER, MD, PhD
E. WILLIAM ST. CLAIR, MD

- Ongoing assessment of rheumatoid arthritis (RA) should include evaluation of tender and swollen joints, acute phase reactants [erythrocyte sedimentation rate (ESR), C-reactive protein (CRP)], subjective evaluation of pain and overall disease activity, functional limitations, and radiographs.
- The treatment goal in RA is early and effective control of synovitis to prevent joint damage, disability, and secondary consequences of chronic inflammation such as cardiovascular disease.
- Symptomatic relief of pain and swelling can be achieved using nonsteroidal anti-inflammatory drugs (NSAIDs) and glucocorticoids.

- Disease-modifying drugs, such as methotrexate, should be initiated within the first 3 to 6 months of disease and, in most cases, effective control of disease activity will require more than one medication.
- If RA cannot be controlled with one or more conventional therapies, biologic treatments such as anti–tumor necrosis factor (TNF) drugs should be used.
- Knowledge of drug toxicities and institution of appropriate monitoring is required to effectively manage RA patients.

ASSESSMENT OF RHEUMATOID ARTHRITIS

The assessment of patients with rheumatoid arthritis (RA) incorporates multiple domains, which include clinical, functional, biochemical, and imaging parameters. The history and physical examination are vital for ongoing evaluation of any patient with a diagnosis of RA. The history should document the location of the affected joints, and presence of joint pain and swelling. Morning stiffness of the joints is an important symptom that should be documented as well. While RA predominantly affects the joints, it also may lead to systemic manifestations, including fatigue, Raynaud's phenomenon, dry eyes and mouth (secondary Sjögren's syndrome), interstitial lung disease, pleuritis, pericarditis, peripheral nervous system involvement, and vasculitis, to name a few. Therefore, the history must be complete to evaluate for possible extra-articular disease. In addition, the medical history is important to assess the patient's extent of disability, including the effect of the disease on daily activities, family life, recreational pursuits, and work.

During the musculoskeletal examination, each joint is carefully palpated for tenderness, inspected for swelling, and tested for impaired range of motion. Inflamed joints are typically tender and swollen, with visible effusions. Synovitis may also be reflected by impaired or painful joint motion. Other findings, such as subcutaneous rheumatoid nodules on extensor surfaces, are associated with positive rheumatoid factor (RF) and antibodies to cyclic citrullinated peptide (CCP) and should also be documented.

Several patient-reported measures may be used in clinical practice to evaluate the activity of disease. The duration of morning stiffness often exceeds 1 hour in patients with active synovitis and tends to correlate with the amount of inflammation (e.g., more prolonged stiffness associated with more active disease). Patient self-reported pain and fatigue may be quantified using a visual analog scale. The Health Assessment Questionnaire Disability Index (HAQ-DI) measures a patient's functional ability by asking questions in different categories of functioning and can be useful in monitoring the patient's course and response to therapy.

Laboratory Studies

Once the diagnosis of RA is established and seropositivity has been determined, testing for RF and anti-CCP to follow disease activity is not useful. Acute phase reactants, such as the erythrocyte sedimentation rate (ESR) and C-reactive protein (CRP), are measures of systemic inflammation. The finding of an elevated ESR or serum CRP level is usually indicative of active disease and, if repeatedly elevated over the disease course, portends a greater risk of disease progression.

Radiographic Studies

Serial radiographs of the hands and feet may be used to monitor disease progression and the effectiveness of treatment. The accumulation of erosions or worsening of joint space narrowing implies an inadequate response to disease-modifying antirheumatic drugs (DMARDs) or biologics and may warrant a change in medical management. In fact, scoring systems (e.g., van der Heijde modification of the Sharp score) to quantify the extent of joint damage have been developed to assess radiographic progression in clinical trials of DMARDs and biologics. Magnetic resonance imaging (MRI) and ultrasonography have been increasingly utilized in patients with early RA because they are imaging modalities that can detect erosions with greater sensitivity than plain radiographs and uniquely visualize the synovium and adjacent soft tissue structures. However, they are mostly used as research tools, and are not yet validated for routine use.

Disease Activity Indices

The assessment of disease activity in RA is drawn from a composite of clinical, laboratory, and radiographic measures. In clinical practice, the number of tender and swollen joints is the dominant variable that drives the overall assessment of disease activity. However, treatment decisions are not strictly dependent on the joint count and may be influenced by other factors. For example, large joints with synovitis may assume more importance in treatment decisions because of their disproportionately greater impact on physical dysfunction. Individual patient factors, such as age and occupation, are also frequently taken into account to ensure an appropriate balance of risk and benefit. A patient's overall rating of pain, degree of functional disability, serum levels of acute phase reactants, and extent of radiographic progression of disease also influence the assessment of disease activity. A formula incorporating selected clinical and laboratory variables has been derived to produce a disease activity score (DAS28), which is calculated from the number of tender and swollen joints (28-joint count), patient self-assessment of disease activity (visual analog scale), and ESR or serum CRP level. This formula has been applied in clinical practice to monitor disease activity and guide treatment decisions and is increasingly being used as an endpoint in clinical trials.

TREATMENT OF RHEUMATOID ARTHRITIS

There has been a growing emphasis on diagnosing and treating RA early and intensively due to the recognition that disability and damage rapidly accrue during the first several years of the disease. This more intensive approach has been made possible in light of the expanding therapeutic armamentarium over the past decade. The classes of drugs used for the treatment of RA include: nonsteroidal anti-inflammatory drugs (NSAIDs) and selective cyclooxygenase-2 (COX-2) inhibitors, DMARDs, biologics, and corticosteroids. NSAIDs and COX-2 inhibitors are utilized primarily for symptomatic relief of pain and are useful cotherapies because of their anti-inflammatory and analgesic effects (see Chapter 41). DMARDs are a diverse group of therapeutic agents that reduce the signs and symptoms of RA as well as retard radiographic progression of joint damage. This class of drugs is central to the control of RA, and is part of nearly every patient's treatment regimen. The ability of a drug to slow disease progression or produce a disease-modifying effect is that property which defines it as a DMARD. The biologics are structurally engineered versions of natural molecules (e.g., monoclonal antibodies) designed to specifically target pathogenic mediators of joint inflammation and damage. In general, biologics are also considered to be DMARDs when they have been shown in large clinical trials to significantly inhibit the progression of joint damage. Corticosteroids are versatile agents with potent anti-inflammatory effects that represent yet another class of drugs (see Chapter 42). They are prescribed in a variety of clinical situations to control disease activity, but their use is limited by significant long-term toxicity. These different classes of drugs are frequently combined in a multidrug regimen to afford optimal suppression of disease activity for the individual patient.

Several overarching principles guide the treatment of RA. Most importantly, treatment decisions are based on accurate assessment of disease activity. There are no specific standards for optimal care of RA, but the outcome measures described above provide a framework for determining if patients need a change in therapy or have achieved an adequate therapeutic response. Treatment decisions are shaped by experienced clinical judgment and balanced by the possibility of improving disease control with the risks of drug toxicity. The goals of therapy are to reduce or eliminate joint pain and swelling, prevent joint damage, minimize disability, and maintain employability. Presently, treatment decisions are largely made on empiric grounds given the lack of reliable biomarkers that can tailor therapies to the individual patient. Thus, the same drugs are generally employed for the treatment of all patients with RA.

Treatment with Disease-Modifying Antirheumatic Drugs

The initiation of DMARD therapy within the first 3 to 6 months of disease onset is now the standard of care for RA. The most common DMARD of choice in this setting is methotrexate (MTX) because of its proven clinical benefits and well-understood long-term efficacy and toxicity profile. Moreover, MTX may be combined effectively with most other DMARDs, making it a highly adaptable drug. Alternatively, sulfasalazine (SSZ) and hydroxychloroquine (HCQ) may be employed for the treatment of patients with milder forms of RA. In early disease, corticosteroids may be used to provide rapid control of the signs and symptoms of RA and serve as a bridge between the initiation of DMARD therapy and its onset of action, which is often delayed by a few months.

While remission is the ultimate goal of therapy, it is usually not achievable with standard DMARD monotherapy. Thus, many different two- and three-drug combinations of DMARDs have been tested in patients with RA and found to be more effective than MTX therapy alone. For example, a popular DMARD combination is the triple therapy of MTX combined with HCQ and SSZ (1). MTX is also frequently combined with a tumor necrosis factor alpha (TNF-alpha) blocker, such as etanercept, infliximab, or adalimumab. Many other DMARD combinations with MTX as the anchor drug have proven to be more effective than MTX alone. It is also important to realize that complete remission, while desirable, is often not attainable despite treatment with an optimal, empirically derived regimen given the current available agents.

An empiric approach to the treatment of RA is the so-called step-up method in which DMARDs are added in sequential fashion until the signs and symptoms of RA are adequately controlled to reach the desired outcome (Figure 6C-1). As MTX is often the initial DMARD used for the treatment of RA, it is usually continued as other DMARDs or biologics are added to enhance clinical benefit. In some cases, MTX may be

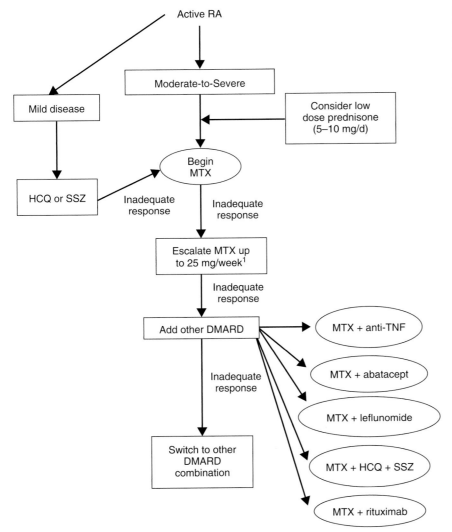

FIGURE 6C-1

Algorithm for treating active RA. In general, patients with moderate-to-severe RA are initially treated with methotrexate (MTX) therapy. Alternatively, patients with milder forms of RA may be treated initially with hydroxychloroquine (HCQ) or sulfasalazine (SSZ), and if necessary, advanced to MTX therapy depending on clinical response and disease progression. The MTX dose may be increased from 10 to 25 mg/week, as tolerated, to afford optimal control of disease activity. DMARD combinations are employed for those patients with an inadequate response to MTX therapy. If patients fail to achieve any clinical benefits from MTX therapy, or are intolerant of this drug, they are usually switched from MTX to another DMARD, such as leflunomide or an anti-TNF blocker (not shown in the figure).
[1]If inadequate response to oral weekly MTX therapy, consider switching from oral to subcutaneous route of administration to improve bioavailability.

withdrawn if the patient fails to achieve even a partial clinical response or suffers intolerable side effects. Conversely, a step-down method may be employed in which two to three DMARDs are initiated simultaneously in combination to produce a maximal clinical effect at the outset of disease. The disadvantage of this approach is that some patients with a favorable prognosis may be overtreated and exposed to unnecessary side effects. Following this paradigm, patients achieving a sustained clinical response are then weaned from some of their medications to a less intensive regimen that maintains disease control. This approach is also referred to as *induction therapy* and is based on a theory that early, intensive treatment may alter the natural history of the disease, an appealing feature of this strategy. To this point, a 52-week study investigated the use of SSZ (2 g/day), prednisolone (60 mg/day), and MTX (7.5 mg/week) in patients with early RA. Those receiving this combination regimen had significantly less joint damage at the end of 52 weeks than those receiving SSZ alone (2). Interestingly, the inhibition of disease progression was maintained in those patients receiving the combination regimen for up to 5 years (2,3). The clinical efficacy and

safety of induction regimens continues to be a focus of investigation.

Successful treatment of RA depends on a detailed knowledge of the different drugs, including their pharmacokinetics, interactions with other drugs, side effects, and monitoring (Tables 6C-1 and 6C-2). A full discussion of this information is beyond the scope of this chapter but some of the most important aspects of the individual DMARDs and biologics are described below. In clinical trials of DMARD therapy for RA, treatment responses are usually defined according to the American College of Rheumatology (ACR) criteria for improvement. These criteria are based on a composite set of disease measures, including the number of tender and swollen joints, patient self-reported assessment of pain, patient and physician assessment of overall disease severity, patient self-assessment of functional disability, and serum levels of acute phase reactants (ESR or CRP). For example, an ACR20 response is defined as a 20% improvement in the number of tender and swollen joints plus 20% improvement in at least three of the five other disease measures. The ACR20 response is a minimum amount of improvement that has

TABLE 6C-1. DISEASE-MODIFYING ANTIRHEUMATIC DRUGS (DMARDs) FOR THE TREATMENT OF RHEUMATOID ARTHRITIS: SIDE EFFECTS, MONITORING, AND OTHER CONSIDERATIONS.

DMARD	CLINICALLY IMPORTANT SIDE EFFECTS	SCREENING/MONITORING	OTHER WARNINGS AND CONSIDERATIONS
Methotrexate	Nausea, diarrhea, stomatitis, fatigue, alopecia, elevated liver enzymes, myelosuppression, pneumonitis, increased risk of infection	CBC, renal function, liver enzymes every 8–12 weeks	Viral hepatitis B and C screening; contraindicated in renal disease (creatinine ≥2 mg/dL), teratogenic
Leflunomide	Nausea, diarrhea, rash, alopecia, elevated liver enzymes	CBC, renal function, liver enzymes every 8–12 weeks	Screening for viral hepatitis B and C; teratogenic
Hydroxychloroquine	Nausea, rash, skin hyperpigmentation, retinopathy (rare)	Yearly ophthalmologic exam[a]	Adjusted dose in renal insufficiency
Sulfasalazine	Nausea, abdominal bloating, rash, granulocytopenia	CBC, liver enzymes every 8–12 weeks	Screen for G6PD deficiency; reduce dose in renal or hepatic insufficiency
Injectable gold	Stomatitis, proteinuria, myelosuppression	CBC, urinalysis prior to each dose	
Oral auranofin	GI upset, stomatitis, proteinuria, myelosuppression	CBC, urinalysis every 8–12 weeks	
Minocycline	Skin hyperpigmentation, rash, nausea, drug-induced lupus		Avoid sun exposure
Cyclosporine	Nausea, abdominal pain, nephrotoxicity, hypertension, hypertrichosis, paresthesias, tremor, gum hyperplasia, increased risk of infection	CBC, renal function	Cyclosporine levels increase with concomitant use of ketoconazole, calcium antagonists, and H2 blockers; decreased levels with use of anticonvulsants and rifampicin; contraindicated in renal insufficiency

ABBREVIATIONS: CBC, complete blood count; G6PD, glucose 6-phosphate dehydrogenase.
[a] American Academy of Ophthalmology recommends annual eye exams for individuals older than 50 years.

TABLE 6C-2. BIOLOGICS FOR THE TREATMENT OF RHEUMATOID ARTHRITIS: SIDE EFFECTS, MONITORING AND OTHER CONSIDERATIONS.

BIOLOGIC	CLINICALLY IMPORTANT SIDE EFFECTS	MONITORING	OTHER WARNINGS AND CONSIDERATIONS
TNF antagonists Etanercept Infliximab Adalimumab	Injection site reaction, infusion reaction, reactivation of latent TB, increased risk of serious bacterial and opportunistic infection, possible increased risk of lymphoma, rare occurrence of demyelinating disorders and lupuslike syndromes	Periodic CBC	Question about prior history of TB exposure and screen with tuberculin skin testing; avoid in NYHA class III–IV heart failure
Kineret	Injection site reaction, neutropenia, increased risk of serious bacterial infection		Screen with tuberculin skin testing
Abatacept	Infusion reaction, increased risk of serious bacterial infection		Screen with tuberculin skin testing; use with caution in individuals with COPD because of an increased risk of adverse events and serious infections in this group; avoid live vaccines
Rituximab	Infusion reaction, increased risk of infection	Periodic CBC	Screen for viral hepatitis B infection

ABBREVIATIONS: CBC, complete blood count; COPD, chronic obstructive pulmonary disease; NYHA, New York Heart Association; TB, tuberculosis.

been shown to distinguish between an effective drug and placebo. Compared with an ACR20 response, ACR50 and ACR70 responses correspond to 50% and 70% improvement in these same disease measures, and are viewed as more robust levels of improvement with greater clinical relevance.

METHOTREXATE

As indicated above, the mainstay of DMARD therapy for RA is methotrexate (MTX). MTX inhibits dihydrofolate reductase, an enzyme needed for DNA synthesis. Its therapeutic action was originally thought to be due to suppression of lymphocyte proliferation. However, MTX's mechanism of action is most likely due to its anti-inflammatory effects, although the specific mechanisms remain unclear. Inside cells, MTX is converted to a polyglutamated form that inhibits the enzyme 5-aminoimidazole-4-carboxamidoribonucleotide (AICAR) transformylase. This enzymatic block leads to the intracellular accumulation of AICAR and, in turn, extracellular adenosine release. Adenosine binds to specific receptors on the surface of lymphocytes, monocytes, and neutrophils, and downregulates inflammatory pathways. MTX also has been reported to inhibit neovascularization, neutrophil activity and adherence, interleukin (IL) 1 and IL-8 production by stimulated peripheral blood mononuclear cells, and TNF production by stimulated peripheral T cells.

Methotrexate can be taken orally or by subcutaneous injection. Generally, the oral form of MTX is initiated for convenience, but may be switched to the subcutaneous route to improve gastrointestinal tolerability as well as bioavailability. Initial doses of MTX range from 7.5

to 15 mg weekly and may be escalated to a maximum dose of 25 mg weekly to yield maximal disease control. Weekly MTX therapy has been shown in randomized, controlled trials to reduce the signs and symptoms of RA and slow its rate of radiologic progression (4,5). When used alone, MTX therapy is associated with an ACR20 response rate of nearly 60% (6), which compares favorably with the other most effective DMARDs. MTX also has been shown to reduce the rate of radiological progression of disease. Importantly, women of childbearing age must use appropriate contraceptive measures because of the known teratogenic effects of MTX. Because MTX is partially eliminated through the kidney, this DMARD is generally avoided in patients with a serum creatinine of greater than 2.0 mg/dL. Suppression of bone marrow occurs more commonly if renal insufficiency is present. In addition, MTX may cause an increase in serum transaminases and, rarely, liver fibrosis. Periodic laboratory monitoring of complete blood counts and liver enzymes are recommended in all patients taking MTX (see Appendix II).

LEFLUNOMIDE

Leflunomide was approved in 1997 for the treatment of RA, and represents an alternative oral agent to MTX. It inhibits an enzyme involved in pyrimidine synthesis, orotic acid dehydrogenase. Leflunomide is taken once a day orally, in doses of 10 or 20 mg. Leflunomide's active metabolite has a long half-life of 15 to 18 days, which is a notable feature of its pharmacokinetics. In a double-blind, randomized trial, leflunomide was clinically superior to placebo and showed ACR20 response rates similar to MTX or SSZ (7,8). Leflunomide also has been proven to reduce structural damage. Its use is limited to some extent by gastrointestinal side effects and potential for teratogenicity. Similar to MTX, leflunomide therapy has been associated with elevated serum transaminases and should be monitored by regular liver enzyme testing.

HYDROXYCHLOROQUINE AND SULFASALAZINE

Hydroxychloroquine and SSZ have been both shown in clinical trials to reduce the signs and symptoms of RA. They are typically used to treat milder forms of RA and in combination with other DMARDs. The mechanism of action of HCQ is not well understood but may, in part, be due to the fact that it concentrates inside cells, principally within acidic cytoplasmic vesicles. In lysosomes, accumulation of HCQ raises the intravesical pH and may thereby interfere with the processing of auto-antigenic peptides (9). The clinical efficacy of HCQ therapy has been shown in a randomized, controlled trial of patients with relatively mild disease of less than 5 years' duration (10). To date, no studies have shown that HCQ alone can decrease the rate of structural damage in RA.

Sulfasalazine was initially designed as a drug that linked an antibiotic, sulfapyridine, with an anti-inflammatory agent, 5-aminosalicyclic acid (5-ASA), which was based on a belief many decades ago that RA was an infectious disease. Approximately 30% of SSZ is absorbed from the gastrointestinal (GI) tract. The remainder is degraded in the gut to sulfapyridine and 5-ASA. Whereas the bulk of the sulfapyridine is absorbed from the gut, most 5-ASA is excreted in the feces. SSZ suppresses various lymphocyte and leukocyte functions and, like MTX, inhibits AICAR transformylase, resulting in extracellular adenosine release (11). In a randomized, double-blind, placebo-controlled trial, an ACR20 response was achieved by 56% of patients receiving SSZ after 24 weeks of treatment, compared with a 29% response rate for placebo-treated subjects (8). SSZ also has been shown to reduce the development of joint damage.

OTHER ANTIRHEUMATIC MEDICATIONS

Several well-designed controlled trials attest to the clinical efficacy of minocycline and doxycyline for the treatment of RA, but they appear to be suited primarily for mild disease. Large trials have not been performed using these agents, and they are not approved drugs for the treatment of RA. The mechanisms by which tetra-cyclines exert their ameliorating effects are unknown, but they have been shown in vitro to inhibit collagenase activity and nitric oxide production. In addition, minocycline upregulates the synthesis of IL-10, an anti-inflammatory cytokine. Minocycline and doxycycline have been shown to decrease the signs and symptoms of RA, but their effects on radiographic progression remain unclear (12).

Gold compounds are seldom used now because of their frequent toxicity and the availability of other agents with better tolerability. There are two parenteral gold formulations, gold sodium malate and myochrysine, and an oral compound, auranofin. Treatment with injectable gold and methotrexate produce similar response rates in clinical trials but gold therapy has higher rates of drug discontinuation due to toxicity (13). Auranofin has fewer side effects than gold injections, but has had limited use in clinical practice due to slow onset of action, lack of sustained clinical efficacy, and poor gastrointestinal tolerability.

In clinical trials, cyclosporine has been shown to reduce the signs and symptoms of RA, as well as slow the development of joint erosions. Cyclosporine has been shown to produce incremental clinical benefit in combination with MTX therapy (14,15). The micro-emulsion-based formulation of cyclosporine (Neoral™) has higher oral bioavailablitiy and more predictable absorption than the standard form. Cyclosporine's effectiveness may be due to its biologic activities of inhibiting IL-2 production and the proliferation of activated T cells. Its renal side effects have been a major limiting factor in long-term use.

TUMOR NECROSIS FACTOR ANTAGONISTS

Etanercept, infliximab, and adalimumab are TNF inhibitors approved for the treatment of RA. These biologic agents have revolutionized the treatment of RA because of their substantial benefits on the signs and symptoms of this disease, as well as their ability to significantly retard the radiographic progression of joint damage. These drugs were engineered to specifically inhibit TNF, which is a critical mediator of joint inflammation. TNF has been shown to be a pivotal proinflammatory cytokine that regulates the production of other proinflammatory cytokines, such as IL-1 and IL-6 (see Chapter 6B). TNF also activates endothelium, upregulates the expression of adhesion molecules, promotes the release of matrix metalloproteinases, and stimulates osteoclastogenesis. All of these pathways are believed to be important in the pathogenesis of RA.

Etanercept is a soluble receptor fusion protein that binds to soluble TNF, neutralizing its biologic activities. Infliximab is a chimeric monoclonal antibody that binds to both soluble and membrane-bound TNF, whereas adalimumab is a fully human monoclonal antibody with binding properties similar to infliximab. Etanercept and adalimumab are administered as a subcutaneous injection while infliximab is administered as an intravenous infusion. Clinical trials indicate that all of these TNF blockers, when added to MTX, produce incremental ACR20 response rates of approximately 50% to 70%. These agents have also been studied in patients with early RA and when used in combination with MTX, produce ACR50 response rates of 40% to 50%. Although etanercept and adalimumab can be used as monotherapy, the combination of MTX and a TNF blocker appears to be the most effective regimen for preventing radiographic progression of disease.

While TNF blockers have proven to be clinically efficacious in RA, their use has been associated with side effects, some of which may have serious consequences. Etanercept and adalimumab have caused injection site reactions but they are rarely severe enough to limit therapy. Infliximab has been associated with infusion reactions, which can range from rash to urticaria and fever, and rarely to anaphylaxis. Neutralizing antibodies can develop in infliximab-treated individuals that may inhibit the efficacy of the drug and predispose to infusion reactions. There is also an increased risk of serious bacterial and opportunistic infections, especially reactivation of latent tuberculosis. A long-term study of etanercept therapy for RA showed that the rate for serious infection was 4.2 per 100,000 patient years, which remained relatively stable throughout the time period (16). The German Biologics Registrar showed a relative risk of 3.0 for serious infection in patients receiving infliximab (17). Additionally, recent meta-analysis of trial data found a twofold increased risk for serious infections in RA subjects treated with anti-TNF antibodies (18). Data from the FDA in 2001 revealed 8.2 cases of tuberculosis (TB) in the United States for every 100,000 patient years of etanercept or infliximab therapy, although more cases of reactivated TB have been reported with infliximab therapy. There have also been cases of TB reported with the use of adalimumab. Because of the increased risk for reactivation of latent TB, it is now standard practice to screen individuals for prior TB exposure and with skin testing before starting a TNF antagonist. The rate of TB infection while using TNF antagonists appears to be declining due in large part to this routine screening.

Use of anti-TNF agents may also confer an increased risk for lymphoproliferative disorders, namely lymphoma. The strength of this link remains unclear because of the fact that RA itself is associated with an increased risk of lymphoma and that the magnitude of this risk appears to rise with increasing disease severity. Patients with RA have an increased risk of lymphoma, corresponding to a standardized incidence ratio (SIR) of 1.9.

In trials, the SIR increases to 2.6 and 3.8 with the use of infliximab and etanercept, respectively (19). Based on trial data, a meta-analysis has shown that infliximab and adalimumab therapy has a pooled odds ratio of 3.3 for malignancies, including nonmelanoma skin cancers, suggesting a possible relationship between TNF blockers and an increased risk for solid tumors (19).

Other rare side effects of note include demyelinating disorders and drug-induced lupus reactions. The anti-TNF agents should not be used in patients with New York Heart Association (NYHA) class III to V heart failure because these drugs may exacerbate heart failure.

ANAKINRA

Anakinra is a human recombinant anti–IL-1 receptor antagonist that has been approved for the treatment of RA. It is administered as a daily 100 mg subcutaneous injection and has been shown to improve the signs and symptoms of RA. However, in a randomized, controlled trial the ACR20 response rates using this drug were only 38% (20). Modest reductions in radiographic progression of joint disease were also seen using this drug compared to controls (21). Overall, the clinical benefits of anakinra are less than those of the TNF blockers. For this reason, the use of anakinra in RA has been limited to selective patients with refractory disease.

ABATACEPT AND RITUXIMAB

Abatacept and rituximab are among the recent additions to the biologics available for the treatment of moderate-to-severe RA. They are currently approved for patients with active RA who have had an inadequate response to other DMARDs or have failed treatment with an anti-TNF agent. Abatacept (CTLA-4Ig) is a recombinant fusion protein consisting of the extracellular domain of human CTLA-4 and the Fc domain of human IgG1. Abatacept binds to CD80/CD86 on the surface of antigen-presenting cells, thus preventing their binding to CD28 on T cells. Blockade of CD28 binding prevents the so-called second signal of T-cell activation. A randomized, double-controlled trial has shown that abatacept therapy produces an ACR20 response of 50% in patients with active RA who had previously failed an anti-TNF drug, compared to placebo rate of 19% (22). Abatacept has also been shown to be effective in patients with an inadequate response to MTX therapy. Moreover, in those taking a combination of both abatacept and methotrexate, radiographic progression was reduced in comparison to controls (22).

Initially approved in 1997 for non-Hodgkin's lymphoma, rituximab is a chimeric anti-CD20 monoclonal antibody now approved for the treatment of moderate-to-severe RA. Rituximab depletes B cells that have CD20 on their surface. Its mechanism of action is incompletely understood but may involve inhibition of T-cell activation through reduction of antigen presentation by B cells or reduction of B-cell cytokines. Despite the depletion of peripheral B cells by more than 97%, immunoglobulin levels usually remain within the normal range. RF may decline; however, clinical improvement often starts before the RF titers decline. Rituximab is infused at a dose of 1000 mg and repeated 2 weeks later.

Initial studies of rituximab therapy were performed in patients who had failed MTX therapy. In one study, they were treated for 24 weeks with MTX alone, rituximab alone, MTX and rituximab, and rituximab and cyclophosphamide. An ACR20 was achieved by 38%, 65%, 73%, and 76%, respectively (23). To reduce the likelihood of infusion reactions, intravenous methylprednisolone was given with the infusion followed by tapering doses of oral prednisone. A subsequent study has found that such corticosteroid therapy has no effect on efficacy, but that methylprednisolone given at the time of the infusion does decrease the severity and rate of infusion reactions (24). In rituximab-treated individuals, B cells remain depleted for greater than 3 months. Repopulation of B cells occurs at a mean of 8 months and repopulation occurs preferentially with naive B cells (25). Repeated rituximab dosing appears to be effective in restoring disease control. Remarkably, rituximab therapy has been generally well tolerated except for infusion reactions of mild-to-moderate severity, although little is known about the long-term risks of repeated rituximab dosing.

COMORBIDITIES

Osteoporosis is a major comorbidity in RA and can result from both the disease itself and the use of corticosteroids. Most patients are routinely advised to take calcium and vitamin D to prevent osteoporosis. Bone densitometry should be performed in patients with risk factors for osteoporosis to address the need for a bisphosphonate or a selective estrogen receptor blocker.

Cardiovascular (CV) disease is the number one cause of death in RA patients. Indeed, RA itself is a CV risk factor. It is unclear if intensive treatment of RA influences this risk, though available data suggest that MTX and anti-TNF treatment reduces the rate of CV events. Low dose aspirin should be considered in patients over the age of 50 years as primary prevention for CV disease. Cholesterol levels should be regularly monitored and cholesterol-lowering medications prescribed as needed. Other CV risk factors, such as hypertension, diabetes, and obesity, should be treated according to usual recommendations.

SUMMARY

The assessment of RA demands a careful history and examination, with a detailed joint count to determine disease activity. The level of clinical disease activity largely determines the need for therapy. DMARDs are central to the control of disease activity and resulting joint damage. The availability of an expanding array of DMARDs and biologics has created new opportunities to effectively intervene in this condition. The standard of care for RA continues to evolve with increasing evidence that persistent joint inflammation leads to irreversible damage and disability. As a result, combination DMARD regimens are being employed to afford optimal disease control in order to avert permanent joint injury.

REFERENCES

1. O'Dell J, Haire CE, Erikson N, et al. Treatment of rheumatoid arhtritis with methotrexate alone, sulfasalazine and hydroxychloroquinne, or a combination of all three medications. N Engl J Med 1996;334:1287–1291.
2. Boers M, Verhoeven AC, Markusse HM, et al. Randomised comparison of combined step-down prednisolone, methotrexate and sulphasalazine with sulfasalzine alone in early rheumatoid arthritis. Lancet 1997;350:309–338.
3. Landewé RB, Boers M, Verhoeven AC, et al. COBA combination therapy in patients with early rheumatoid arthritis: long-term structural benefits of a brief intervention. Arthritis Rheum 2002;46:347–356.
4. Andersen PA, West SG, O'Dell JR, et al. Weekly pulse methotrexate in rheumatoid arthritis. Clinical and immunologic effects in a randomized, double-blind study. Ann Intern Med 1985;103:489–496.
5. Weinblatt ME, Polisson R, Blotner SD, et al. The effects of drug therapy on radiographic progression of rheumatoid arthritis. Results of a 36-week randomized trial comparing methotrexate and auranofin. Arthritis Rheum 1993;36:613–619.
6. Bathon JM, Martin RW, Fleischmann RM, et al. A comparison of etanercpt and methotrexate in patients with early rheumatoid arthritis. N Engl J Med 2000;343:1586–1593.
7. Strand V, Cohen S, Schiff M, et al. Treatment of active rheumatoid arthritis with luflunomide compared with placebo and methotrexate. Arch Intern Med 1999;159:2542–2550.
8. Smolen JS, Kalden JR, Scott DL, et al. Efficacy and safety of leflunomide compared with placebo and sulphasalazine in active rheumatoid arthritis: a double-blind, randomised, multicentre trial. Lancet 1999;353:259–266.

9. Fox RI. Mechanism of action of hydroxychloroquine as an antirheumatic drug. Semin Arthritis Rheum 1993;23:82–91.

10. Clark P, Casas E, Tugwell P, et al. Hydroxychloroquinne compared with placebo in rheumatoid arhtritis. A randomized controlled trial. Ann Intern Med 1993;119:1067–1071.

11. Gadangi P, Langaker M, Naime D, et al. The anti-inflammatory mechanism of sulfasalazine is related to adenosine release at inflamed sites. J Immunol 1996;156:1937–1941.

12. Alarcon GS. Minocycline for the treatment of rheumatoid arthritis. Rheum Dis Clin North Am 1998;24:489–499.

13. Lehman AJ, Esdaile JM, Klinkhoff AV, et al. A 48-week, randomized, double-blind, double-observer, placebo-controlled multicenter trial of combination methotrexate and intramuscular gold therapy in rheumatoid arthritis: results of the METGO study. Arthritis Rheum 2005;53:1360–1370.

14. Marchesoni A, Battafarano N, Arreghini M, et al. Radiographic progression in early rheumatoid arthritis: a 12-month randomized controlled study comparing the combination of cyclosporin and methotrexate with methotrexate alone. Rheumatology 2003;42:1545–1549.

15. Gerards AH, Landewe RB, Prins AP, et al. Cyclosporin A monotherapy versus cyclosporin A and methotrexate combination therapy in patients with early rheumatoid arthritis: a double blind randomised placebo controlled trial. Ann Rheum Dis 2003;62:291–296.

16. Moreland LW, Weinblatt ME, Keystone EC, et al. Etanercept treatment in adults with established rheumatoid arthritis: 7 years of clinical experience. J Rheumatol 2006;33:854–861.

17. Listing J, Strangfeld A, Kary S, et al. Infections in patients with rheumatoid arhtritis treated with biologic agents. Arthritis Rheum 2005;52:3403–3412.

18. Bongartz T, Sutton AJ, Sweeting MJ, et al. Anti-TNF antibody therapy in rheumatoid arthritis and the risk of serious infections and malignancies. JAMA 2005;295:2275–2285.

19. Wolf F, Michaud K. Lymphoma in rheumatoid arthritis: the effect of methotrexate and anti-tumor necrosis factor therapy in 18,572 patients. Arthritis Rheum 2004;50:1740–1751.

20. Cohen SB, Moreland LW, Cush JJ, et al. A multicentre, double blind, randomised, placebo controlled trial of anakinra (Kineret), a recombinant interleukin 1 receptor antagonist, in patients with rheumatoid arthritis treated with background methotrexate. Ann Rheum Dis 2004;63:1062–1068.

21. Bresnihan B, Newmark R, Robbins S, et al. Effects of anakinra monotherapy on joint damage in patients with rheumatoid arthritis. Extension of a 24-week randomized, placebo-controlled trial. J Rheumatol 2004;31:1103–1111.

22. Genovese MC, Becker JC, Schiff M, et al. Abatacept for rheumatoid arthritis refractory to tumor necrosis factor alpha inhibition. N Engl J Med 2005;353:1114–1123.

23. Edwards JC, Szczepanski L, Szechinski J, et al. Efficacy of B-cell targeted therapy with rituximab in patients with rheumatoid arthritis. N Engl J Med 2004;350:2572–2581.

24. Emery P, Fleischmann R, Filipowicz-Sosnowska A, et al. The efficacy and safety of rituximab in patients with active rheumatoid arthritis despite methotrexate treatment: results of a phase IIb randomized, double-blind, placebo-controlled, dose-ranging trial. Arthritis Rheum 2006;54:1390–1400.

25. Leandro MJ, Cambridge G, Ehrenstein MR, et al. Reconstitution of peripheral blood B cells after depletion with rituximab in patients with rheumatoid arthritis. Arthritis Rheum 2006;54:613–620.

Juvenile Idiopathic Arthritis
A. Clinical Features

DANIEL J. LOVELL, MD, MPH

- Juvenile idiopathic arthritis (JIA) is the most common form of childhood arthritis and one of the more common chronic childhood illnesses.
- JIA is an umbrella term that refers to a group of disorders that have in common chronic arthritis.

- Diagnosis requires a combination of data from history, physical examination, and laboratory testing.
- For the vast majority of patients with JIA, the immunogenetic associations, clinical course, and functional outcome are quite different from adult-onset rheumatoid arthritis.

Juvenile idiopathic arthritis (JIA) is the most common form of childhood arthritis and one of the more common chronic childhood illnesses. As the term indicates, the cause is unknown. In fact, JIA is an umbrella term that refers to a group of disorders that have in common chronic arthritis. Diagnosis requires a combination of data from history, physical examination, and laboratory testing. For the vast majority of patients with JIA, the immunogenetic associations, clinical course, and functional outcome are quite different from adult-onset rheumatoid arthritis (RA). However, approximately 5% to 10% of those with JIA (those classified as polyarthritis rheumatoid factor positive) have a disease that resembles adult-onset RA much more than other types of JIA. The JIA nomenclature has in most instances replaced the older classification for chronic idiopathic arthritis in childhood—juvenile rheumatoid arthritis (JRA). The differences and similarities in the two classifications will be discussed below. In fact, this is the first edition in which the term *juvenile idiopathic arthritis* is being used in the *Primer on the Rheumatic Diseases*.

EPIDEMIOLOGY

The prevalence of JIA has been estimated to be between 57 and 220 per 100,000 children younger than 16 years in population-based studies (1–8). In a meta-analysis including both practitioner- and clinic-based studies, a prevalence of 132 per 100,000 [95% confidence interval (95% CI), 119,145] was reported (9). In a population-based study from Sweden, Andersson-Gäre and Fasth

reported that 50% of JIA patients have active disease that persists into adulthood (5). Many of the published prevalence studies have not included adult-age JIA patients, resulting in an underestimation. The incidence ranges between 7 to 21 per 100,000 people in studies of US- and Northern European–based populations (1,9,10). All the incidence and prevalence estimates have wide confidence intervals because of the relative rarity of JIA and the small number of actual cases detected in even the largest studies. This leads to enormous differences between the lower and upper estimates of actual JIA cases. The most commonly cited figure is 70,000 to 100,000 cases (active and inactive) of JIA in the US population under age 16 (1). Using Andersson-Gäre and Fasth's report on disease persisting into adulthood, an estimated 35,000 to 50,000 people over age 16 have active JIA in the United States (5).

Juvenile idiopathic arthritis affects a much smaller portion of the US population than adult-onset RA. However, compared to other pediatric-onset chronic illnesses, JIA is relatively common, affecting approximately the same number of children as juvenile diabetes, at least four times as many children as sickle cell anemia or cystic fibrosis, and at least 10 times as many as hemophilia, acute lymphocytic leukemia, chronic renal failure, or muscular dystrophy (6).

CLINICAL FEATURES

The criteria for JIA require disease onset before the 16th birthday, persistent objective arthritis in one or more joints for at least 6 weeks, and exclusion of other causes of childhood arthritis (7,11,12). Misdiagnosis often results when one or more of the following four key points are missed: (1) objective arthritis must be present and is defined as swelling, effusion, or the presence of two or more of the following—limitation of motion, tenderness, pain on motion, or joint warmth (i.e., arthralgia alone is not sufficient); (2) the arthritis must be consistently present for at least 6 weeks; (3) more than 100 other causes of chronic arthritis in children must be excluded; and (4) no specific laboratory or other test can establish the diagnosis of JIA, that is, it is a diagnosis of exclusion.

Juvenile idiopathic arthritis is subdivided into seven categories: systemic, polyarthritis rheumatoid factor positive, polyarthritis rheumatoid factor negative, oligoarthritis (subcategories of persistent and extended), psoriatic arthritis, enthesitis-related arthritis and undifferentiated arthritis (11,12; Table 7A-1). These subtypes demonstrate unique clinical presentations, immunogenetic associations, and clinical courses (Table 7A-2). The categories of JIA are meant to be mutually exclusive so that the inclusion criteria for one classification are also used as exclusion criteria for the other categories. For those patients who fit into more than one

TABLE 7A-1. CLASSIFICATION CRITERIA FOR JUVENILE IDIOPATHIC ARTHRITIS, SECOND REVISION, EDMONTON, 2001.

CLASSIFICATION	DESCRIPTION	PERCENTAGE OF JIA POPULATION
Systemic	Arthritis with or preceded by daily fever of at least 2 weeks duration, documented to be quotidian for at least 3 days, and accompanied by at least one of the following: rheumatoid rash, generalized lymphadenopathy, hepato- or splenomegaly and serositis Exclusions: a,b,c,d	2%–17%
Oligoarthritis, subcategory persistent	Arthritis in ≤four joints at any time during the onset or course of the disease Exclusions: a,b,c,d,e	12%–29%
Oligoarthritis, subcategory extended	Arthritis in ≤four joints in first 6 months of disease but affecting a cumulative total of ≥five joints after the first 6 months Exclusions: a,b,c,d,e	12%–29%
Polyarthritis rheumatoid factor negative	Arthritis affecting ≥five joints during first 6 months with negative tests for rheumatoid factor Exclusions: a,b,c,d,e	10%–28%
Polyarthritis rheumatoid factor positive	Arthritis affecting ≥five joints during first 6 months and positive test for rheumatoid factor at least twice at least 3 months apart Exclusions: a,b,c,e	2%–10%
Enthesitis-related arthritis	Arthritis and enthesitis or arthritis or enthesitis plus any two of the following: Sacroiliac joint tenderness and/or inflammatory lumbosacral pain Positive HLA-B27 Physician-diagnosed HLA-B27–associated disease in first- or second-degree relative Symptomatic anterior uveitis Male > 6 years old at onset of arthritis or enthesitis Exclusions: a,d,e	3%–11%
Psoriatic arthritis	Arthritis and psoriasis or arthritis and at least two of the following: Physician-diagnosed psoriasis in first-degree relatives Dactylitis Nail abnormalities (pitting or onycholysis) Exclusions: b,c,d,e	2%–11%
Undifferentiated	Arthritis but does not fulfill any of the above categories or fits into more than one category Exclusions: Not applicable	2%–23%

Source: Data from Petty RE, Southwood TR, Manners P, et al. J Rheumatol 2004;31:390–392, *Journal of Rheumatology.*
Exclusion criteria:
(a) Psoriasis or a history of psoriasis in the patient or a first-degree relative.
(b) Arthritis in an HLA-B27–positive male beginning after the 6th birthday.
(c) Ankylosing spondylitis, enthesitis-related arthritis, sacroiliitis with inflammatory bowel disease, Reiter's syndrome, or acute anterior uveitis, or a history of one of these disorders in a first-degree relative.
(d) The presence of IgM rheumatoid factor on at least two occasions at least 3 months apart.
(e) The presence of systemic JIA in the patient.

TABLE 7A-2. JUVENILE IDIOPATHIC ARTHRITIS CATEGORY CHARACTERISTICS.

CHARACTERISTIC	sJIA	poJIA RF+	poJIA RF−	oJIA, PERSISTENT	oJIA, EXTENDED	pJIA	eJIA	uJIA
Number of joints with arthritis at onset	Variable	≥5	≥5	≥4	≥5	Variable	Variable	Variable
Sex ratio (F:M)	1:1	3:1	3:1	4:1	4:1	1:1	1:7	1:1
Frequency of uveitis (% of patients in that JIA category)	0%–2%	3%–10%	3%–10%	30%–50%	15%–20%	5%–20%	≤25% (acute)	••
Frequency of +RF on at least two occasions in first 6 months of disease (% of patients in the JIA category)	0%	100%	0%	0%	0%	0%	0%	3%–5%
Frequency of ≥5 joints involved during course of disease (% of patients in the JIA category)	50%	100%	100%	0%	100%	6–55%	50%	••
Percentage in clinical remission at last F/U[a]	33%–80%	0%–15%	23%–46%	43%–73%	12%–35%	–	–	–
Percentage in Steinbrocker functional class III or IV at last F/U[a]	0%–65%	5%–38%	3%–41%	0%–7%	36%–43%	–	–	–
Percentage with radiographic evidence of joint damage at last F/U[a]	14%–75%	75%–77%	40%–43%	5%–27%	25%–33%	–	–	–

ABBREVIATIONS: eJIA, enthesis-related JIA; F/U, last follow-up visit in published studies; JIA, juvenile idiopathic arthritis; oJIA, oligoarticular JIA; pJIA, psoriatic JIA; poJIA, polyarthritis JIA; RF, rheumatoid factor; sJIA, systemic JIA; uJIA, undifferentiated JIA.
[a]Data taken from meta-analysis of outcome studies in JIA and JRA populations.[17]

category or who do not satisfy all the inclusion criteria for one of the other categories, the undifferentiated arthritis category is to be used. In both the older JRA criteria, and even more so with the JIA criteria, the concept is that these systems are classifying within a single umbrella term different forms of chronic arthritis (11,12). The JIA classification was intended to have ongoing validation by both clinical and immunogenetic methods to assess the homogeneity and stability of the diagnostic categories and, if necessary, change the categories on the basis of published data (12).

In addition to the inclusion criteria, for each of the JIA categories the relevant *exclusion criteria* for that category will be indicated using the letter of the criteria in this listing:

(a) psoriasis in the patient or a first-degree relative;
(b) arthritis in a human leukocyte antigen (HLA)-B27–positive male with arthritis onset after 6 years of age;
(c) anklyosing spondylitis, enthesitis-related arthritis, sacroiliitis with inflammatory bowel disease, reactive arthritis, or acute anterior uveitis in a first-degree relative;
(d) presence of IgM rheumatoid factor on at least two occasions more than 3 months apart;
(e) presence of systemic JIA in the patient.

JUVENILE IDIOPATHIC ARTHRITIS, SYSTEMIC CATEGORY

Approximately 2% to 17% of children with JIA have systemic juvenile idiopathic arthritis (sJIA) (12). Classification as systemic JIA requires that the child demonstrate daily fever of at least 2 weeks duration that for at least three of those days is documented to be quotidian (defined as a daily recurrent fever that rises to ≥39°C once a day and returns to 37°C or below between fever spikes) and at least *one* of the following: (a) an evanescent, nonfixed, erythematous rash; (b) generalized lymph node enlargement; (c) hepatomegaly and/or splenomegaly; (d) serositis (pericardial, pleural or peritoneal). Systemic JIA is excluded if criteria a, b, c, or d from the list of exclusion criteria are present.

The characteristic rash is pale pink, blanching, transient (lasting minutes to a few hours), nonpuritic in 95% of cases, and characterized by small macules or maculopapules. Children with sJIA often have growth delay, osteopenia, diffuse lymphadenopathy, hepatosplenomegaly, pericarditis, pleuritis, anemia, leukocytosis, thrombocytosis, and elevated acute-phase reactants. Positive rheumatoid factor (RF) and uveitis are rare. The extra-articular features are usually mild to moderate in severity and almost always self-limited. Most systemic features will resolve when the fevers resolve; however, sJIA patients can develop pericardial tamponade, severe vasculitis with secondary consumptive coagulopathy, and macrophage activation syndrome, all of which require intense steroid therapy.

The long-term prognosis for sJIA is determined by the severity of the arthritis, which usually develops concurrently with the fever and systemic features, but in some patients does not develop for weeks or months after the onset of the fever. sJIA may develop at any age <16 years, but the peak age of onset is 1 to 6 years old. Boys and girls are equally affected.

JUVENILE IDIOPATHIC ARTHRITIS, POLYARTHRITIS RHEUMATOID FACTOR POSITIVE AND RHEUMATOID FACTOR NEGATIVE CATEGORIES

To be characterized as having polyarthritis juvenile idiopathic arthritis (poJIA), a child must have arthritis in five or more joints during the first 6 months of the disease. To be classified as poJIA, exclusion criteria a, b, c, and e must be absent. To be considered RF+, the patient must have at least two positive results for RF at least 3 months apart during the first 6 months of disease.

Approximately 2% to 10% of all children with JIA have polyarthritis juvenile idiopathic arthritis rheumatoid factor positive (poJIA RF+) and 10% to 28% have polyarthritis juvenile idiopathic arthritis rheumatoid factor negative (poJIA RF–) (12). poJIA RF+ patients are almost always girls with later disease onset (at least 8 years old) who are usually HLA-DR4 positive, have symmetric small joint arthritis, and are at greater risk for developing erosions, nodules, and poor functional outcome compared with RF– patients. poJIA RF+ resembles adult-onset RA more than any other JIA subset. Clinical manifestations and outcome of both poJIA categories are highly variable, and include fatigue, anorexia, protein–caloric malnutrition, anemia, growth retardation, delay in sexual maturation, and osteopenia. poJIA may develop at any age less than 16 years, and girls with poJIA outnumber boys with this form 3 to 1.

JUVENILE IDIOPATHIC ARTHRITIS, OLIGOARTHRITIS

To be characterized as having oligoarthritis juvenile idiopathic arthritis (oJIA), a child must have arthritis in four or more joints during the first 6 months of the disease. Relevant exclusion criteria are a, b, c, d, and e. oJIA patients are divided into two subcategories: persistent and extended. Persistent oJIA patients never have a cumulative total of more than four joints with arthritis during the course of the disease and extended oJIA patients demonstrate a cumulative total during the course of the disease of arthritis in five or more joints after the first 6 months of the disease. oJIA is the most frequent of the JIA categories (24%–58% of all JIA patients) (12). Persistent oJIA has the best overall articular outcome of all JIA categories. Up to half of the persistent oJIA patients will demonstrate monoarticular involvement in a knee joint (13). The severity of joint symptoms in these patients is usually very mild and it is not uncommon for these children to present with normal or near normal overall physical function, joint swelling, and loss of motion in the knee. Up to 50% of oJIA cases will evolve to the extended subcategory and 30% will do so in the 2 years after disease onset. Risk factors in the first 6 months of disease onset for developing oJIA, extended subcategory (i.e., more extensive and severe articular involvement), are arthritis in the wrist, hand or ankle; symmetric arthritis, arthritis in more than one joint; elevated erythrocyte sedimentation rate (ESR) and positive antinuclear antibodies (ANA) (13). Patients with oJIA are commonly younger (1–5 years old at onset), are more likely to be girls (girls outnumber boys 4 to 1), are often ANA positive, and have the greatest risk for developing chronic eye inflammation (7). Eye involvement occurs in 30% to 50% of oJIA patients (7,13). The inflammatory process primarily involves the

7

TABLE 7A-3. AMERICAN ACADEMY OF PEDIATRICS GUIDELINES FOR SCREENING EYE EXAMINATIONS ADAPTED FOR JUVENILE IDIOPATHIC ARTHRITIS.

DISEASE SUBGROUP	FREQUENCY OF SCREENING
Any JIA category except sJIA, ≤6 years old at JIA onset, ANA+	Every 3–4 months for 4 years, then every 6 months for 3 years, then annually
Any JIA category except sJIA, ≤6 years old at JIA onset, ANA–	Every 6 months for 4 years, then annually
Any JIA category except sJIA, ≥7 years old at JIA onset, ANA+/–	Every 6 months for 4 years, then annually
sJIA	Annually

SOURCE: Adapted from Cassidy J, Kivlin J, Lindsley C, Nocton J, Pediatrics 2006;117:1843–1845, by permission of *Pediatrics*.
ABBREVIATIONS: JIA, juvenile idiopathic arthritis; sJIA, systemic JIA.

anterior chamber of the eye and is associated with minimal, if any, symptoms in more than 80% of affected children. Because severe, irreversible eye changes, including corneal clouding, cataracts, glaucoma, and partial or total visual loss, can occur, patients should be screened at regular intervals and treated by experienced eye specialists (Table 7A-3).

The risk for persistent articular disease is very different for the oJIA subtypes. In one study, 75% of the patients with persistent oJIA achieved remission by adulthood compared to only 12% of those with extended oligoarticular JIA (13).

JUVENILE IDIOPATHIC ARTHRITIS, PSORIATIC ARTHRITIS

In contrast to the JRA criteria, patients demonstrating arthritis in association with psoriasis are included in the JIA classification. Patients manifesting chronic arthritis in association with psoriasis with an onset at or before the age of 16 are said to have psoriatic juvenile idiopathic arthritis (pJIA). However, the classic psoriatic rash may not appear for many years after the onset of the arthritis. In published studies, 33% to 62% of the patients will not, in the past or at the time the arthritis develops, demonstrate any of the dermatologic manifestations. Only about 10% of children have the onset of the rash and the arthritis at the same time. In the rest of the patients (33%–67%), the rash comes first (7). Accordingly, the JIA criteria allow for children to be classified as having psoriatic arthritis if they have arthritis and at least two of the following three criteria: dactylitis, nail pitting or onycholysis, and psoriasis in a first-degree relative. The psoriasis has to be diagnosed by a physician. The relevant

exclusion criteria are b, c, d, and e. In the JIA criteria, *dactylitis* is defined as swelling of one or more digits, usually in an asymmetric distribution, that extends beyond the joint margin and *nail pitting* is defined as a minimum of two pits on one or more nails at any time. *Onycholysis* is not specifically defined in the JIA criteria but refers to the partial loosening or complete detachment of the nail from the nail bed. pJIA accounts for 2% to 11% of all JIA cases (12).

In the vast majority of cases of pJIA, the arthritis is peripheral, asymmetric, and often involves the knees, ankles, and small joints of the hands and feet. The dactylitis ("sausage digit") involves inflammation of not only the small joints of the toes or fingers but also the tendon sheath. The dactylitis is often surprisingly asymptomatic despite obvious swelling and loss of motion in the digit. At onset, about 70% of the pJIA patients have arthritis in four or more joints. In longitudinal studies, during the course of the disease, about 40% (range, 11%–100%) of pJIA patients demonstrated involvement of the sacroiliac joint (7).

Asymptomatic chronic anterior chamber uveitis clinically indistinguishable from that seen in oJIA develops in up to 20% of these patients (7,13). Accordingly, following the usual recommendations for routine slit lamp of the eyes, as described in Table 7A-3, is required in pJIA.

JUVENILE IDIOPATHIC ARTHRITIS, ENTHESITIS RELATED

This category addresses the fact that in children the axial manifestations of spondyloarthropathy may not become evident for many years. Children are classified as enthesitis juvenile idiopathic arthritis (eJIA) if they have both arthritis and enthesitis or have either arthritis or enthesitis with any two of the five following manifestations: (1) sacroiliac tenderness and/or inflammatory lumbosacral pain; (2) positive HLA-B27; (3) onset of arthritis in a male ≥6 years old; (4) acute (symptomatic) anterior uveitis; and (5) presence in a first-degree relative of ankylosing spondylitis, enthesitis-related arthritis, inflammatory bowel disease with sacroiliitis, reactive arthritis or acute anterior uveitis. The relevant exclusion criteria are a, d, and e. About 10% of all JIA patients are classified as eJIA (12).

Enthesitis refers to inflammation at the insertion of the tendon, ligament, joint capsule, or fascia into the bone. The most frequent manifestations are pain and tenderness at the enthesis but swelling is also seen at the site. Enthesitis is not specific for pJIA and is sometimes seen in other JIA categories, systemic lupus erythematosus (SLE), and healthy active children (7). The most common sites for enthesitis include the superior curve of the patella, infrapatellar at the tibial tuberosity, attachment of the Achilles tendon, back of the foot (attachment of plantar fascia to the calcaneous), and sole of the foot at the metatarsal heads (7).

In contrast to the JRA criteria, patients with arthritis in association with inflammatory bowel disease can be classified as eJIA if the inclusion and exclusion criteria are satisfied. In patients with inflammatory bowel disease, the articular involvement may precede the gastrointestinal (GI) inflammation by months to years. Clues to the presence of GI involvement include fatigue, weight loss, growth failure, nocturnal bowel movement, mouth ulcers, erythema nodosum, pyoderma gangrenosum, and anemia (more severe than normally seen in association with the extent of the arthritis).

Patients with eJIA may also demonstrate involvement in other areas. Acute uveitis characterized by intermittent episodes of red, photophobic, painful ocular inflammation (usually unilateral) may occur in up to 25% of eJIA patients. Aortic involvement with aortic valve insufficiency has been rarely reported in children with eJIA (7).

At disease onset, the articular involvement includes peripheral arthritis in approximately 80% of eJIA patients and only 25% will have symptoms or physical findings involving the sacroiliac or lumbar spine areas. In about 85% of the patients, the arthritis will involve four or more joints. Because the eJIA criteria are relatively new and the axial manifestations can evolve very slowly, no publications provide longitudinal data specific to eJIA. Data from older related diagnostic categories can be used to give some insight as to the risk for axial involvement over time. In children diagnosed as having seronegative enthesitis and arthritis syndrome (SEA syndrome), after 11 years of follow-up, 65% had evolved to have clinically important axial involvement. In those diagnosed with juvenile ankylosing spondylitis, over 90% eventually manifest clinically important lumbar spine and/or sacroiliac (SI) joint involvement (7).

In eJIA, tests for ANA and RF are negative, and plain radiographs often do not show the characteristic changes in the SI or lumbosacral spine for many years. Bone scans are seldom helpful because radioisotope uptake is typically increased in the SI joints and the lumbar spine in all children as a consequence of skeletal growth. Computed tomography (CT) and magnetic resonance imaging (MRI) scans can be useful studies if interpreted by a radiologist familiar with axial imaging of children. There are no pathognomonic laboratory tests.

JUVENILE IDIOPATHIC ARTHRITIS, UNDIFFERENTIATED

Patients are placed in the undifferentiated juvenile idiopathic arthritis (uJIA) category if the manifestations do not fulfill the inclusion criteria for any category or the patient fulfills criteria for more than one category. In the published series, 2% to 23% of all JIA patients were classified as uJIA. In those classified as uJIA, 60% failed to demonstrate characteristics that fulfilled the eligibility criteria for one of the other JIA categories and 40% demonstrated criteria from more than one JIA category (12). In those fitting more than one category, the overlap was most commonly between the poJIA RF– category and either the eJIA or the pJIA categories. Some children overlapped the oJIA category with either the eJIA or pJIA categories (12). Longitudinal studies need to be performed to determine the eventual diagnoses in the patients placed in the uJIA category to see how many will remain as uJIA and how many will evolve to fulfill the criteria for one of the other JIA categories or diseases other than JIA.

OCULAR INVOLVEMENT IN JUVENILE IDIOPATHIC ARTHRITIS

A unique manifestation of JIA is chronic uveitis. A meta-analysis of 21 published studies on uveitis in children with JIA with a combined 4598 JIA patients (13). The data demonstrated that there are obvious differences in the incidence of uveitis in JIA patients based on geographic distribution. In Scandinavian studies, 18.5% of patients demonstrated uveitis, in studies from the United States 14.5% of patients demonstrated uveitis, and in studies from East Asia only 4.5% of patients demonstrated uveitis. The frequency of uveitis varies by JIA subtype—12% of children with oJIA, 4.3% of poJIA, and 1.8% of sJIA patients developed chronic uveitis. Other studies have documented that up to 20% of children with pJIA will develop chronic uveitis identical to the chronic uveitis associated with oJIA in terms of manifestations, chronicity, and ocular outcomes (7).

Uniform adoption of early and routine screening guidelines have been developed and recently updated (2006) by the American Academy of Pediatrics Sections of Ophthalmology and Rheumatology for children with JRA (Table 7A-3) (14). The recommendations were based on factors known to be associated with an increased frequency of developing uveitis in children with JRA: articular features, age at onset of the arthritis, duration of disease, and presence of ANA. These same factors relate to the uveitis risk for JIA categories and should be applied as shown in Table 7A-3. Despite general adoption of routine screening for uveitis and rapid institution of treatment, the outcome for chronic uveitis in children with JIA is still associated with an unacceptably high frequency of serious complications. In this meta-analysis, in the JIA patients with uveitis, 20% developed cataracts, 19% developed glaucoma,

7

and 16% developed band keratopathy (13). The identi-fication of effective treatments for JIA-associated uveitis that are able to avoid or minimize the eye damage associated with chronic steroid treatment and chronic inflammation of the eyes is an important and unsolved problem at this time.

OUTCOME

In a recent meta-analysis of outcome studies in children with chronic idiopathic arthritis, only 2 of the 21 studies reviewed used the JIA classification criteria (15). In a summary of published outcome studies, more than 30% of people with childhood-onset idiopathic chronic arthritis (most frequently classified as having one of the JRA subtypes) had significant functional limitations after 10 or more years of follow-up (16). Twelve percent were in Steinbrocker classes III (limited self-care) or IV (bed or wheelchair bound) 3 to 7 years after disease onset, but 48% were classified in class III or IV 16 or more years after disease onset (7). Active synovitis can be detected in 30% to 55% of the patients 10 years after disease onset (16). In a longitudinal study of JRA patients referred to a pediatric rheumatologist within the first 6 months of disease onset, 28% of the pJRA, 54% of the poJRA, and 45% of the sJRA patients demonstrated either erosions or joint-space narrowing on standard radiographs during follow-up (16). In an analysis of outcome studies published after 1994 that are thought to reflect the positive impact of at least some of the recent therapeutic advances, only 40% to 60% of the JIA patients demonstrated either inactive disease or remission, and on average 10% demonstrated severe functional limitation (Steinbrocker functional class III or IV) (17).

Mortality estimates have ranged from 0.29 to 1.10 per 100 patients. These estimates represent a mortality rate 3 to 14 times greater than the standardized mortality rate for a similarly aged US population (16).

The outcome for JRA patients with uveitis has significantly improved over the past several decades, but is still associated with an unacceptably high rate of ocular complications. In the most recent study of ocular outcomes, at a mean follow-up of 9.4 years since onset of eye disease, 85% of patients had normal visual acuity but 15% had significant visual loss, including 10% who were blind in at least one eye (7).

SUMMARY

Juvenile idiopathic arthritis is the most common chronic arthritis in children, the most common inflammatory rheumatic disease in children, and still a cause of significant morbidity and increased mortality. Each of the JIA categories has characteristic manifestations, complications, and outcomes. Familiarity with the different types of JIA will facilitate earlier diagnosis, awareness of potential problems, and, initiation of proper treatment.

REFERENCES

1. Singsen BH. Rheumatic diseases of childhood. Rheum Dis Clin North Am 1990;16:581–599.
2. Towner SR, Michet CJJ, O'Fallen WM, Nelson AM. The epidemiology of juvenile arthritis in Rochester, Minnesota. Arthritis Rheum 1983;26:1208–1213.
3. Hochberg MC, Linet MS, Sills EM. The prevalence and incidence of juvenile rheumatoid arthritis in an urban black population. Am J Public Health 1983;73:1202–1203.
4. Andersson-Gäre BA, Fasth A. Epidemiology of juvenile chronic arthritis in Southwestern Sweden—5-year prospective population study. Pediatrics 1992;90:950–958.
5. Andersson-Gäre BA, Fasth A. The natural history of juvenile chronic arthritis: a population based cohort study. II. Outcome. J Rheumatol 1995;22:308–319.
6. Gortmaker S. Chronic childhood disorders. Prevalence and impact. Pediatr Clin North Am 1984;31:3–18.
7. Cassidy JT, Petty RE, Laxer RM, Lindsley CB. Textbook of pediatric rheumatology, 5th ed. Philadelphia: Elsevier Saunders; 2005.
8. Borchers AT, Seemi C, Chema G, Keen CL, Sheonfeld Y, Gershwin ME. Juvenile idiopathic arthritis. Autoimmune Rev 2006;5:279–298.
9. Oen KG, Cheang M. Epidemiology of chronic arthritis in childhood. Semin Arthritis Rheum 1996;26:575–591.
10. Berntson L, Andersson-Gäre B, Fasth A, et al. Incidence of juvenile idiopathic arthritis in Nordic countries. A population based study with special reference to the validity of ILAR and EULAR criteria. J Rheumatol 2003;30:2275–2282.
11. Petty RE, Southwood TR, Manners P, et al. International League of Associations for Rheumatology classification of juvenile idiopathic arthritis: second revision, Edmonton, 2001. J Rheumatol 2004;31:390–392.
12. Hofer M, Southwood TR. Classification of childhood arthritis. Best Pract Res Clin Rheumatol 2002;16:379–396.
13. Weiss JE, Ilowite NT. Juvenile idiopathic arthritis. Pediatr Clin N Am 2005;52:413–442.
14. Cassidy J, Kivlin J, Lindsley C, Nocton J. Ophthalmologic examination in children with juvenile rheumatoid arthritis. Pediatrics 2006;117:1843–1845.
15. Adib N, Silman A, Thomson W. Outcome following onset of juvenile idiopathic inflammatory arthritis: I. Frequency of different outcomes. Rheumatology 2005;44:995–1001.
16. Levinson JE, Wallace CA. Dismantling the pyramid. J Rheumatol 1992;19:6–10.
17. Ravelli A. Toward an understanding of the long-term outcome of juvenile idiopathic arthritis. Clin Exp Rheum 2004;22:271–275.

Juvenile Idiopathic Arthritis
B. Pathology and Pathogenesis

PATRICIA WOO, BSC, MBBS, PHD, MRCP, FRCP, CBE

- Juvenile idiopathic arthritis (JIA) is an umbrella term for a heterogeneous group of childhood onset, inflammatory forms of arthritis.
- T-cell and cytokine profiles vary according to the JIA subtype.

- Gene variations in the human leukocyte antigen (HLA) region of chromosome 6 are associated with different types of subtypes of JIA except systemic-onset JIA.

Juvenile idiopathic arthritis (JIA) is the umbrella term for a heterogeneous group of childhood onset arthritides lasting more than 6 weeks. The current international classification system proposed by International League of Associations for Rheumatology (ILAR) (1) defines clinical differences between the groups. However, within each group there is also a clinical spectrum of disease duration and severity. Some of this may be defined by genetic markers/susceptibility genes. This chapter aims to describe common and discriminative features between the groups from the pathological and genetic points of view.

OLIGOARTICULAR JUVENILE IDIOPATHIC ARTHRITIS

Children with oligoarticular JIA have four or fewer joints affected at the onset of disease. There are two recognizable clinical subtypes with different disease courses: persistent oligoarthritis (PO) and extended oligoarthritis (EO). Oligoarthritis patients have milder disease and many have spontaneous remission. In addition, all patients in this group can have anterior uveitis.

The Synovium and Synovial Fluid

There is no distinction in the histology of the synovial tissues in inflamed joints, whether adult onset or childhood onset; that is, there is infiltration of lymphocytic and monocytic cells as well as abundant neutrophils. However, there are differences in the types of T

cells and the cytokines produced between the JIA subtypes.

The immunohistochemistry of the synovial membranes of a mixed group of JIA patients were examined for cytokine production by T cells and a type 1 immune response was found (2). Furthermore, the analysis of synovial fluid (SF) T-cell markers has shown that the difference between T cells in PO and EO is the presence of regulatory T cells in the milder PO, consistent with the current hypothesis that there is a better balance of the immune system in the milder disease (3).

Laboratory Findings

In monoarthritis and mild PO patients, there is often no sign of acute phase response in the serum, such as a raised erythrocyte sedimentation rate (ESR) or C-reactive protein (CRP). In the more severe cases and in EO patients, the ESR and CRP are raised. Rheumatoid factor is not present, but low titer antinuclear antibodies (ANA) are frequently seen. There are no other autoantibodies.

Uveitis

The anterior uveitis that is found in JIA patients is particularly indolent and predominantly affects the anterior uveal tract, with cells visible in the anterior chamber of the eye on slit lamp examination. The pathogenesis is not clear and there are differences between the clinical nature of the inflammation in this and the other types of uveitis, such as sarcoid, Behçets, and infection-related types. Studies reported that a positive ANA was a risk factor/associated marker, but when using more sensitive tests for ANA, such as the use of Hep2 cells in the test, the correlation is less strong.

Inflammatory Cytokines and Joint Damage

There have been many studies that measure various inflammatory and anti-inflammatory cytokines in the serum and synovial fluid of oligoarticular JIA, and these studies have often been limited by the technical problems of sample collections and the assays themselves. For example, interleukin 1 (IL-1) and tumor necrosis factor (TNF) are easily degraded ex vivo and levels of IL-6 and TNF are often increased during the blood clotting procedure. There are some consistent findings, however. TNF and its natural inhibitor, soluble TNF receptors (TNFR), are usually found in synovial fluid, along with IL-6 and IL-18 and a number of chemotactic factors, such as macrophage inhibitory protein-1 alpha (MIP-1 alpha), all of which will attract lymphocytes, monocytes, and neutrophils to the synovium. Joint damage is less in the PO versus polyarticular JIA and one current hypothesis is that insufficient inhibition of proinflammatory cytokines can prolong disease, thus leading to more damage. Consistent with this hypothesis is the observation in the study of Rooney and colleagues (4), where the authors showed a higher sTNFR/TNF ratio (sTNFR is a natural inhibitor of TNF) in the SF of the PO patients versus polyarticular JIA patients.

Damage to cartilage and bone erosion are both seen in JIA, but the rate and degree of damage, as seen on radiological imaging, is less in PO. There is often uneven local acceleration of growth of epiphyses in the inflamed area, leading to growth deformities.

Genetic Predisposition

There is good evidence that there is a strong genetic component to oligoarticular JIA. In the biggest collection of affected siblings with JIA, known as affected sibling pairs (ASP), a high proportion of the ASP show concordance of disease onset type (53% of the ASPs were concordant for the oligoarticular onset type). In addition, there is a strong autoimmune disease background in the family history of the ASP. These observations suggest a strong genetic background to this group of diseases (5). Approximately 17% of the risk of a sibling developing JIA has been estimated to be due to the influence of a region on chromosome 6 (6p), where the HLA are found (5). There was significant sharing of HLA-DR alleles (6) in the ASPs with respect to onset type and disease course in the oligoarticular group. The HLA genes are classically found significantly associated with autoimmune diseases, and the replication of disease association in different populations shows that the associated genes mentioned above are likely to contribute to pathology by modifying adaptive immunity responses. These consist of the presentation of protein fragments to the effector arm of the immune system (T and B lymphocytes) via these HLA molecules, causing the lymphocytes to become activated, divide and multiply, and differentiate into further subtypes. Further linkage analyses of the ASP have confirmed the contribution of genes in this region of the chromosome, as well as many other possible regions (7).

Nonhuman leukocyte antigen genetic polymorphisms associated with oligoarticular JIA include protein tyrosine phosphatase N22 (PTPN22) (8), a TNF haplotype (9), SLC11A1 (10), and a genetic variant of macrophage inhibitory factor (MIF) that may determine levels of MIF production (11). IL-10 is a cytokine that suppresses the expression of proinflammatory cytokines and its production is genetically determined by a particular genetic variant of IL-10. Crawley and colleagues showed the association of this genetic variant of IL-10 with the more severe EO subtype (12) and also showed that low IL-10 production is inherited from the parents in the EO patients (13). Thus, a complex inheritance pattern is emerging of genes that confer different levels of risk to the child and which may lead to differing disease course and severity.

Cause of the Disease

The prevailing hypothesis is that given a specific autoimmune genetic background, diverse stimuli can trigger the disease. Indeed, many JIA patients will have a history of upper respiratory infections or, sometimes, vaccinations preceding the onset of arthritis. The composite genetic background in the individual will determine the severity of the arthritis. The true extent of the contribution of different areas of the genome is still being characterized. There is no single microorganism that has been implicated to be the cause of oligoarticular JIA.

SYSTEMIC JUVENILE IDIOPATHIC ARTHRITIS

This group of patients represents approximately 10% of all JIA in Caucasian series. Its proportion is reported to be greater in other ethnic groups, such as the Japanese and Chinese. There is a wide spectrum of disease severity.

Laboratory Findings

There are no specific laboratory tests for systemic JIA (sJIA), but there are characteristic patterns of laboratory abnormalities. There is typically a very high level of CRP, high ESR, neutrophilia, thrombocytosis, and a hypochromic, microcytic anemia. Liver enzymes and coagulation screen might be abnormal in the more severe cases and in the complication often seen in severe sJIA, macrophage activation syndrome (MAS). The factors that have the most specificity in the diagnosis of MAS, as distinct from a flare of sJIA, have been identified to be decreased platelet count, fibrinogen, high ferritin, raised liver enzymes, and decreased white blood cell count (14). Confirmation of MAS with a bone marrow aspirate, or trephine biopsy makes the diagnosis. There are no autoantibodies or rheumatoid factor (RF) detectable in JIA serum and complement levels are normal or high. Immunological abnormalities include the presence of polyclonal hypergammaglobulinemia, raised proinflammatory cytokines, such as IL-1, IL-6, IL-18, and TNF, as well as chemokines, such as IL-8 (CXCL8) in the serum or plasma (15–17). Occasionally a fulminant presentation of sJIA can take the form of MAS and polyarthritis with aneurysms in medium-sized arteries, demonstrable by angiography.

Apart from severe joint destructions in patients at the more severe end of the spectrum, secondary complications include MAS, generalized osteoporosis, growth retardation/failure, and amyloidosis. All of these features suggest generalized and systemic inflammation affecting all parts of the body, not just the joints.

Pathogenesis

Infectious agents have often been reported as having triggered the onset of the disease, but there is no single agent that can be identified as the culprit in microbiological and virological examinations. In fact, by definition, sJIA is not an infectious disease because a negative septic screen is necessary for diagnosis. The frequent association of the complication MAS with severe sJIA is unusual and research, so far, shows reversible defects in natural killer (NK) cell activity, as well as reversible expression of the perforin gene on NK cells (18,19). These defects may be part of the pathology of sJIA and triggering of disease flares by infectious agents would suggest that the mechanisms for ridding the child of these agents are defective, NK cell function being one of them.

There is some evidence that genetic predisposition to sJIA comprises at least part of the etiology of sJIA. There are very few sibling pairs with this type of JIA in a large sibling pair cohort from North America (5). Despite earlier reports of associations with different HLA alleles in small cohorts, these results were not replicated in other case control studies. Furthermore, there is no association between HLA and sJIA in a larger cohort of UK Caucasians, in sharp contrast with other types of JIA, where there are multiple reports of disease association with HLA (20).

On the other hand, non-HLA genes, such as the gene encoding macrophage migration inhibitory factor (MIF), have been shown to be associated with JIA as a whole (10), but in particular, a MIF single nucleotide variant that correlated with higher MIF levels in serum and synovial fluids has been found to be associated with sJIA (21). Another non-HLA genetic variant, the 174G-allele of IL-6, found to correlate with significantly higher serum IL-6 levels, has been confirmed as a susceptibility gene for sJIA by family studies (22,23). These genes code for proteins that can be grouped broadly as proinflammatory according to their effects and many hypothesize that such genetic variants predispose the patient to a more than usually vigorous inflammatory response to stimuli, such as infectious agents. Secretion of IL-1 beta, another major proinflammatory cytokine, has also been found to be high in patients with sJIA (24). Open-label pilot trials of biologic agents blocking the signaling of IL-1 and IL-6 have shown highly encouraging results (24–26). Such putative genetic imbalances echo the more recent discovery of genetic defects in innate immunity and anti-inflammatory pathways in the autoinflammatory syndromes. Examples of these autoinflammatory syndromes are familial Mediterranean fevers (FMF), hyperIgD or familial Dutch fevers, Muckle-Wells syndrome (MWS), chronic infantile neurological cutaneous arthropathy syndrome (CINCA, also known as NOMID), and familial Hibernian fever or tumor necrosis receptor–associated periodic fever syndromes (TRAPS). sJIA can also be regarded as an autoinflammatory syndrome from the clinical picture of generalized inflammation, as well as its association with certain pro- and anti-inflammatory gene variants.

POLYARTICULAR JUVENILE IDIOPATHIC ARTHRITIS

These are usually chronic and severe conditions that require disease-modifying therapies. There are two subgroups as defined by ILAR: RF negative and RF positive.

Rheumatoid factor positive polyarticular JIA is similar to adult-onset rheumatoid arthritis (RA) with severe widespread erosive joint disease. The similarities between juvenile- and adult-onset RA include the presence of rheumatoid factor, as well as other more specialized antibodies, such as anti-cyclic citrullinated peptides (anti-CCP) and anti-Bip, and association with certain HLA genes. Caution has to be made in the diagnosis of this in children, because RF can be transiently raised due to infection. The ILAR definition clearly stipulates that the classification is made only if there are two positive results found at least 3 months apart.

7

Rheumatoid factor negative polyarticular JIA is by far the most common and is heterogeneous in terms of age of onset as well as disease course. Many of the younger patients also have anterior uveitis, similar to oligoarticular JIA patients and, similarly, it is often associated with a positive ANA. The histology of the synovium is similar to oligoarthritis, but there may be subtle differences in the proportion of T-cell subsets (3) and cytokine production (4).

Infections can trigger its onset, but there often appears to be no external trigger. Thus, genetic predisposition also contributes to the pathogenesis of this group. The HLA-DRB1*0801 gene variant, found to be associated with oligoarthritis, is also associated with polyarticular JIA, but there are other different genetic associations, as seen in a genomewide linkage study performed in the North American ASP cohort (20). These are preliminary data that will need to be refined and worldwide collaboration among groups working on JIA genetics are being proposed to resolve these questions.

ENTHESITIS-RELATED ARTHRITIS AND PSORIATIC ARTHRITIS

These arthritides are classified using clinical criteria and, as yet, not much is known in terms of pathogenesis. In the enthesitis-related arthritis (ERA) subtype, some of the patients will develop sacroiliitis and spondylitis in late teenage or adult years. Many of these will have a positive HLA-B27, which is significantly associated with adult ankylosing spondylitis. Current hypothesis for the pathogenesis for ERA is defective presentation of microorganisms from the gut by the HLA-B27 molecule to the immune system (27). Other non-HLA genes may modify the clinical presentation of the disease, including the IL-1 gene cluster (28,29).

The pathogenesis of psoriatic arthritis is unknown. The genetic component has, so far, been shown to be that of psoriasis itself, that is, HLA-Cw6 (30), but why a minority of psoriasis patients have arthritis and what determines the age of onset is currently unclear.

SUMMARY

Gene variants in the HLA region of chromosome 6 are associated with JIA, except for sJIA, similar to other autoimmune diseases. The gene variants appear to be different in each clinical subtype and this may constitute the reason for the differences in the clinical spectrum. Modifying influences from non-HLA genes also contribute to the clinical spectrum. sJIA is a systemic inflammatory disease and pathological and genetic studies, so far, suggest that this may be better classified as an autoinflammatory syndrome, with genetic variations in genes within the inflammation networks that predispose the patient to a proinflammatory state.

REFERENCES

1. Petty RE. Growing pains: the ILAR classification of juvenile idiopathic arthritis. J Rheumatol 2001;28:927–928.
2. Murray KJ, Grom AA, Thompson SD, Lieuwen D, Passo MH, Glass DN. Contrasting cytokine profiles in the synovium of different forms of juvenile rheumatoid arthritis and juvenile spondyloarthropathy: prominence of interleukin 4 in restricted disease. J Rheumatol 1998;25:1388–1398.
3. de Kleer IM, Wedderburn LR, Taams LS, et al. CD4(+)CD25(bright) regulatory T cells actively regulate inflammation in the joints of patients with the remitting form of juvenile idiopathic arthritis. J Immunol 2004;172:6435–6443.
4. Rooney M, Varsani H, Martin K, et al. Tumour necrosis factor alpha and its soluble receptors in juvenile chronic arthritis. Rheumatology (Oxford) 2000;39:432–438.
5. Glass DN, Giannini EH. Juvenile rheumatoid arthritis as a complex genetic trait. Arthritis Rheum 1999;42:2261–2268.
6. Prahalad S, Ryan MH, Shear ES, Thompson SD, Giannini EH, Glass DN. Juvenile rheumatoid arthritis: linkage to HLA demonstrated by allele sharing in affected sibpairs. Arthritis Rheum 2000;43:2335–2338.
7. Thompson SD, Moroldo MB, Guyer L, et al. A genome-wide scan for juvenile rheumatoid arthritis in affected sibpair families provides evidence of linkage. Arthritis Rheum 2004;50:2920–2930.
8. Hinks A, Barton A, John S, et al. Association between the PTPN22 gene and rheumatoid arthritis and juvenile idiopathic arthritis in a UK population: further support that PTPN22 is an autoimmunity gene. Arthritis Rheum 2005;52:1694–1699.
9. Zeggini E, Thomson W, Kwiatkowski D, Richardson A, Ollier W, Donn R. Linkage and association studies of single-nucleotide polymorphism-tagged tumor necrosis factor haplotypes in juvenile oligoarthritis. Arthritis Rheum 2002;46:3304–3311.
10. Runstadler JA, Saila H, Savolainen A, et al. Association of SLC11A1 (NRAMP1) with persistent oligoarticular and polyarticular rheumatoid factor-negative juvenile idiopathic arthritis in Finnish patients: haplotype analysis in Finnish families. Arthritis Rheum 2005;52:247–256.
11. Donn R, Alourfi Z, Zeggini E, et al. A functional promoter haplotype of macrophage migration inhibitory factor is linked and associated with juvenile idiopathic arthritis. Arthritis Rheum 2004;50:1604–1610.
12. Crawley E, Kay R, Sillibourne J, Patel P, Hutchinson I, Woo P. Polymorphic haplotypes of the interleukin-10 5' flanking region determine variable interleukin-10 transcription and are associated with particular phenotypes of

juvenile rheumatoid arthritis. Arthritis Rheum. 1999;42: 1101–1108.

13. Crawley E, Kon S, Woo P. Hereditary predisposition to low interleukin-10 production in children with extended oligoarticular juvenile idiopathic arthritis. Rheumatology (Oxford) 2001;40:574–578.

14. Ravelli A, Magni-Manzoni S, Pistorio A, et al. Preliminary diagnostic guidelines for macrophage activation syndrome complicating systemic juvenile idiopathic arthritis. J Pediatr 2005;146:598–604.

15. de Jager W, Wedderburn LR, Rijkers GT, Kuis W, Prakken BJ. Simultaneous detection of 30 soluble mediators in plasma and synovial fluid of patients with JIA. Clin Exp Rheumatol 2004;22:538.

16. Mangge H, Gallistl S, Schauenstein K. Long-term follow-up of cytokines and soluble cytokine receptors in peripheral blood of patients with juvenile rheumatoid arthritis. J Interferon Cytokine Res 1999;19:1005–1010.

17. Woo P. Cytokines and juvenile idiopathic arthritis. Curr Rheumatol Rep 2002;4:452–457.

18. Wulffraat NM, Rijkers GT, Elst E, Brooimans R, Kuis W. Reduced perforin expression in systemic juvenile idiopathic arthritis is restored by autologous stem-cell transplantation. Rheumatology (Oxford) 2003;42:375–379.

19. Grom AA, Villanueva J, Lee S, Goldmuntz EA, Passo MH, Filipovich A. Natural killer cell dysfunction in patients with systemic-onset juvenile rheumatoid arthritis and macrophage activation syndrome. J Pediatr 2003;142: 292–296.

20. Thomson W, Barrett JH, Donn R, et al. Juvenile idiopathic arthritis classified by the ILAR criteria: HLA associations in UK patients. Rheumatology (Oxford) 2002;41: 1183–1189.

21. De Benedetti F, Meazza C, Vivarelli M, et al. Functional and prognostic relevance of the -173 polymorphism of the macrophage migration inhibitory factor gene in systemic-onset juvenile idiopathic arthritis. Arthritis Rheum 2003; 48:1398–1407.

22. Fishman D, Faulds G, Jeffery R, et al. The effect of novel polymorphisms in the interleukin-6 (IL-6) gene on IL-6 transcription and plasma IL-6 levels, and an association with systemic-onset juvenile chronic arthritis. J Clin Invest 1998;102:1369–1376.

23. Ogilvie EM, Fife MS, Thompson SD, et al. The -174G allele of the interleukin-6 gene confers susceptibility to systemic arthritis in children: a multicenter study using simplex and multiplex juvenile idiopathic arthritis families. Arthritis Rheum 2003;48:3202–3206.

24. Pascual V, Allantaz F, Arce E, Punaro M, Banchereau J. Role of interleukin-1 (IL-1) in the pathogenesis of systemic onset juvenile idiopathic arthritis and clinical response to IL-1 blockade. J Exp Med 2005;201:1479–1486.

25. Woo P, Wilkinson N, Prieur AM, et al. Open label phase II trial of single, ascending doses of MRA in Caucasian children with severe systemic juvenile idiopathic arthritis: proof of principle of the efficacy of IL-6 receptor blockade in this type of arthritis and demonstration of prolonged clinical improvement. Arthritis Res Ther 2005;7:R1281–R1288.

26. Yokota S, Miyamae T, Imagawa T, et al. Therapeutic efficacy of humanized recombinant anti-interleukin-6 receptor antibody in children with systemic-onset juvenile idiopathic arthritis. Arthritis Rheum 2005;52:818–825.

27. Colbert RA. The immunobiology of HLA-B27: variations on a theme. Curr Mol Med 2004;4:21–30.

28. Brown MA, Brophy S, Bradbury L, et al. Identification of major loci controlling clinical manifestations of ankylosing spondylitis. Arthritis Rheum 2003;48:2234–2239.

29. Timms AE, Crane AM, Sims AM, et al. The interleukin 1 gene cluster contains a major susceptibility locus for ankylosing spondylitis. Am J Hum Genet 2004;75:587–595.

30. Korendowych E, McHugh N. Genetic factors in psoriatic arthritis. Curr Rheumatol Rep 2005;7:306–312.

7

Juvenile Idiopathic Arthritis
C. Treatment and Assessment

PHILIP J. HASHKES, MD, MSc
RONALD M. LAXER, MD, FRCPC

- Most patients with juvenile idiopathic arthritis (JIA) do not achieve a remission and require long-term treatment.
- Discovery and use of new therapies such as methotrexate and biologics have improved the outcome of JIA.

- Evidence-based guidelines are available for the treatment of some subtypes of JIA.
- Assessment tools have improved the documentation of individual and clinical trial outcome.

RATIONALE OF CURRENT TREATMENT APPROACH

The medical treatment of juvenile idiopathic arthritis (JIA) has changed dramatically over the past 15 years. This change has been related to data showing that most children never achieve a long-term remission, and thus the burden of disease to the patient, family, and, ultimately, society is enormous. Until 1990, treatment was based on the pyramid approach beginning with various nonsteroidal anti-inflammatory drugs (NSAIDs) and corticosteroids and gradually advancing to other medications. Studies in the late 1980s indicated that previous assumptions on the course and outcome of JIA were incorrect. Radiologic joint damage, previously thought to develop late in the disease course, occurs in most patients with systemic and polyarthritis within 2 years and in oligoarthritis within 5 years (1). Early cartilage damage, often in the first year of disease, was demonstrated using magnetic resonance imaging (MRI).

The assumption that JIA will usually resolve by adulthood also was found to be incorrect. Studies have shown that between 50% to 70% of patients with poly- or systemic arthritis and 40% to 50% of patients with oligoarthritis will continue to have active disease in adulthood. Only a few patients seem to achieve long-term, medication-free remission (1–3). Between 30% to

40% of patients have significant long-term functional disabilities including unemployment, and between 25% to 50% need major surgery, including joint replacement (2).

Juvenile idiopathic arthritis is associated with a mortality rate of 0.4% to 2%, about three times the standardized mortality rate for the US population. Most deaths are in patients with systemic arthritis, with amyloidosis (almost exclusively in Europe) and the macrophage activation syndrome being the main causes (1).

The outcome of uveitis has improved significantly in recent years, but there is still a high prevalence of ocular complication and vision loss. Five to 16% of patients have significant visual deficits, and even blindness, and 16% to 26% develop cataracts, 14% to 24% develop glaucoma, and 11% to 22% develop band keratopathy (4).

Several predictors of a poor outcome can help determine patients requiring early aggressive therapy. Patients with polyarthritis and positive rheumatoid factor (RF), antibodies to cyclic citrullinated peptides anti-CCP), the presence of human leukocyte (HLA)-DR4, nodules, and early-onset symmetric small joint involvement have a worse prognosis. Patients with systemic arthritis who are corticosteroid dependent for control of systemic symptoms and have a platelet count >600,000 after 6 months of disease have a worse outcome.

MEDICAL TREATMENT OF JUVENILE IDIOPATHIC ARTHRITIS

Nonsteroidal Anti-Inflammatory Drugs

Only about 25% to 33% of JIA patients, mainly those with oligoarthritis, respond well to NSAIDs (5). A 4- to 6-week trial of an individual NSAID is necessary to assess its efficacy. Because NSAIDs do not alter the disease course or prevent joint damage, they are used more to treat pain, stiffness, and the fever associated with systemic arthritis. No individual NSAID has been shown to have a clear advantage over others in treating arthritis. Some patients not responsive to one NSAID may respond to another (Tables 7C-1 and 7C-2).

Nonsteroidal anti-inflammatory drugs approved by the Food and Drug Administration (FDA) for JIA and currently available on the market in the United States include naproxen, ibuprofen, meloxicam, and tolmetin sodium. Liquid preparations are available for the former three. For reasons of compliance it is preferable to use an NSAID which is administered only once or twice per day. Thus, the need to administer aspirin three times per day, to monitor serum levels, and the association of aspirin with the Reye syndrome have largely resulted in other NSAIDs replacing aspirin in treating JIA.

Serious gastrointestinal (GI) adverse effects are rare, although many children develop GI symptoms. In order to prevent these symptoms, NSAIDs should be administered with food. GI symptoms can be treated by changing NSAIDs or by using H2 blockers or proton pump inhibitors. Mild elevations of liver enzymes are common. Other adverse effects include pseudoporphyria, most often associated with the use of naproxen in fair-hair Caucasians, and central nervous system effects, including headaches and disorientation, especially from indomethacin. Renal adverse effects are uncommon in children, but are more frequent during concurrent use of more than one NSAID. The issue of cardiovascular adverse effects has not been formally studied but there are no case reports of these events in children with JIA treated with NSAIDs.

Corticosteroids

Due to many deleterious effects, especially the effect on bone and growth, the use of systemic corticosteroids for JIA should be minimized. There is no evidence that systemic corticosteroids are disease modifying. The main indications for systemic use of corticosteroids are uncontrolled fever, serositis, and the macrophage activation syndrome in systemic arthritis. Another indication

TABLE 7C-1. MAJOR MEDICATIONS AND INDICATIONS FOR TREATMENT OF JUVENILE IDIOPATHIC ARTHRITIS.

MEDICATION	ARTHRITIS SUBTYPE	INDICATION
NSAIDs	All types	Symptomatic: pain, stiffness
Intra-articular corticosteroids	All types, mainly oligoarthritis	Injection of few swollen joints
Systemic corticosteroids	Systemic, polyarthritis	Fever, serositis, bridging medication, macrophage activation syndrome
Methotrexate	All types, less effective in systemic	Disease modifying
Sulfasalazine	Oligoarthritis, polyarthritis, enthesitis-related	Disease modifying
Leflunomide	Polyarthritis	Disease modifying
Cyclosporine A	Systemic	Macrophage activation syndrome, steroid sparing
Thalidomide	Systemic	Possibly anti-TNF
Anti-TNF (etanercept infliximab, adalimumab)	Polyarthritis, enthesitis-related (less effective in systemic)	Biologic modifying
Anti–IL-1 (anakinra)	Systemic	Biologic modifying
Anti–IL-6 (tocilizumab)	Systemic	Biologic modifying (currently not available outside studies)
IVIg	Systemic	Steroid sparing

ABBREVIATIONS: IL, interleukin; IVIg, intravenous immunoglobulin; NSAIDs, nonsteroidal anti-inflammatory drugs; TNF, tumor necrosis factor.
Hydroxychloroquine, gold, and penicillamine not effective in JIA. Abatacept, rituximab, and minocycline not studied in JIA.

7

TABLE 7C-2. DOSES AND ADVERSE REACTIONS OF MAJOR MEDICATIONS USED TO TREAT JUVENILE IDIOPATHIC ARTHRITIS.

MEDICATION	DOSE	MAIN ADVERSE REACTIONS
NSAIDs		GI, liver enzymes, headaches, interstitial nephritis
Naproxen	7.5–10 mg/kg (max 500 mg) twice daily	As above, pseudoporphyria
Ibuprofen	10–15 mg/kg (max 800 mg) 3–4 times daily	As above
Meloxicam	0.25–0.375 mg/kg (max 15 mg) once daily	As above
Methotrexate	10–15 mg/m^2/week (parenteral if >12.5 mg/m^2)	GI, mouth sores, liver enzymes, cytopenia
Sulfasalazine	15–25 mg/kg (max 1500 mg) twice daily	GI, rashes, cytopenia
Leflunomide	<20 kg: 10 mg every other day 20–40 kg: 10 mg/day >40 kg: 20 mg/day	GI, liver enzymes
Etanercept	0.4 mg/kg (max 25 mg) SC injection twice weekly	Injection site reaction, UR symptoms, infections
Adalimumab	24 mg/m^2 (max 40 mg) SC injection every other week	Injection site reaction, UR symptoms, infections
Infliximab	3–6 mg/kg, intravenously at weeks 0, 2, and 6, then every 6–8 weeks	Infusion reactions (allergic), infections
Anakinra	1–2 mg/kg/day (max 100 mg) SC injection	Injection site reaction, UR symptoms, infections
Triamcinolone hexacetonide	For large joints 1 mg/kg (max 40 mg) IA injection	Subcutaneous atrophy

ABBREVIATIONS: GI, gastrointestinal; IA, intra-articular; NSAIDs, nonsteroidal anti-inflammatory drugs; SC, subcutaneous; UR, upper respiratory.

is use as a bridging medication until other medications become effective. In some patients, periodic intravenous pulses of corticosteroids (30 mg/kg/dose, maximal 1 g) are used instead of high dose daily oral corticosteroids, although there are no controlled studies showing fewer adverse effects of this modality in children.

There is excellent evidence for the efficacy of intra-articular injections of corticosteroids, mainly in patients with oligoarthritis. Several studies have shown that as many as 70% of patients with oligoarthritis do not have reactivation of disease in the injected joint for at least 1 year and in 40% for more than 2 years (6). MRI studies have shown a marked decrease in synovial volume after injection without a deleterious effect on the cartilage. One study reported significantly fewer patients with leg length discrepancies when intra-articular corticosteroid injections are used early (7). The efficacy is less in other JIA subtypes, especially systemic arthritis.

There are few adverse effects associated with these injections. One that can be seen is the development of periarticular subcutaneous atrophy. This may be preventable by injecting small amounts of saline while withdrawing the needle following the injection and by applying pressure to the injection site. Repeated injections over time to an individual joint have not been found to be associated with joint or cartilage damage.

Several controlled studies, including a study of simultaneous injections of bilateral inflamed joints in individual patients, have found that the long-acting triamcinolone hexacetonide was more effective and had a longer effect than other forms of injectable corticosteroids (8). Younger children and children needing multiple joint injections usually require sedation during the procedure.

Methotrexate

The use of methotrexate (MTX) is the cornerstone of the medical management plan for most patients with JIA and polyarthritis (9). The initial dose is 10 mg/m^2/week given orally or parenterally. If not effective the MTX dose should be increased to 15 mg/m^2/week and given parenterally (10). There is no additional advantage in giving higher doses.

The efficacy of MTX differs by the subtype of JIA, with the greatest efficacy seen in patients with extended oligoarthritis, while less effective in systemic arthritis (11). MTX may slow the radiologic damage progression rate as demonstrated in two small series.

Because food decreases the bioavailability of MTX, it is advised to give MTX on an empty stomach. MTX at doses ≥12 mg/m^2 should be given parenterally, because oral MTX is not absorbed well at those doses.

In order to decrease adverse effects of nausea, oral ulcerations, and perhaps liver enzyme abnormalities, MTX should be administered with folic acid (1 mg/day) or folinic acid, 25% to 50% of the MTX dose, given 24 hours after MTX administration.

Nausea and other GI symptoms are frequent. Strategies to decrease the severity of these phenomena include taking MTX before bed, switching the mode of administration (oral to parenteral) and using anti-emetics. Some children develop a psychologic aversion to MTX that can be alleviated by teaching relaxation or self-hypnosis techniques.

The collective long-term experience of MTX use for JIA remains one of remarkable safety. Tests to monitor for MTX toxicity, complete blood counts, liver enzymes, and renal function are recommended at least every 3 months (12). While mild elevations of liver enzymes occur frequently through the course of treatment, no cases of severe, irreversible liver fibrosis have been reported in JIA. Thus, routine liver biopsies are not recommended (13). Pulmonary toxicity and severe infections are extremely rare in children. Children should avoid live vaccinations while using MTX but other vaccinations can be given and seasonal influenza vaccine is recommended. If possible, children should receive varicella vaccine prior to starting MTX. MTX should be skipped during an acute infection, especially Epstein–Barr virus (EBV; see below). While rare case reports of lymphoma have been reported, current data do not suggest that the rate of malignancies is greater than in the general child population. Some of the lymphomas developed in association with EBV infection.

Other Disease-Modifying Antirheumatic Drugs and Immunosuppressive Medications

Sulfasalazine and leflunomide may be alternatives to methotrexate. A controlled study showed that sulfasalazine is effective in the treatment of oligo- and polyarthritis; the effect may persist for years after sulfasalazine is discontinued (14). Sulfasalazine may also slow the progression of radiologic damage (15). Sulfasalazine seems to be most effective in older males with oligoarthritis, representing, perhaps, children with enthesitis-related arthritis. Adverse reactions were frequently reported, especially rashes, GI symptoms, and leukopenia, frequently necessitating discontinuation of sulfasalazine. Adverse effects may be especially severe in patients with systemic arthritis. Leflunomide was shown to be effective in polyarthritis, although in a controlled study significantly more responders were found in patients receiving MTX (16).

Cyclosporine A may be more beneficial for fever control and corticosteroid dose reduction than for the treatment of arthritis in patients with systemic arthritis and may be especially effective in patients with the macrophage activation syndrome. Thalidomide may be effective in the treatment of refractory systemic arthritis, both for systemic features and arthritis. In addition to the teratogenic effect, careful observation for the development of peripheral neuropathy is necessary (17).

Most controlled studies in children did not find hydroxychloroquine, oral gold, D-penicillamine, or azathioprine to be effective in the treatment of JIA (5). There are no controlled studies of minocycline use or of combination disease-modifying antirheumatic drugs (DMARD) therapy with or without MTX in JIA.

Biologic-Modifying Medications
Anti-Tumor Necrosis Factor Medications

Recent studies have shown these medications to be highly effective in patients with polyarthritis, including patients who failed MTX. There are three anti-tumor necrosis factor (TNF) medications: etanercept, a soluble TNF receptor, and two anti-TNF antibodies, infliximab, based on a mouse protein, and adalimumab, a humanized protein. Trials of all three medications have shown similar efficacy, but currently etanercept is the only drug approved by the FDA (18). More than 50% of patients have a response greater than the American College of Rheumatology (ACR) Pediatric 70 level for all three medications. Anti-TNF medications also appear to be highly effective in enthesitis-related arthritis (juvenile spondyloarthropathy) but are significantly less effective in systemic arthritis (19). Infliximab is more effective than etanercept for JIA-related uveitis (20,21). It is still not clear whether the combination of anti-TNF and MTX is more effective than either alone but initial data support the use of combination therapy. Anti-TNF medications may slow radiologic damage progression and may increase bone density.

Adverse effects of etanercept are generally mild, mainly injection site inflammation for etanercept and adalimumab and infusion-related allergic reactions for infliximab. To prevent or minimize infliximab allergic reactions, premedication with acetaminophen, diphenhydramine, and, occasionally, hydrocortisone are sometimes needed. Other common mild adverse effects include upper respiratory infections and headaches. However, some patients develop severe adverse effects including neurologic (demyelinating diseases), psychiatric, severe infectious (especially related to varicella), cutaneous vasculitis, pancytopenia, and development of other autoimmune diseases (18,19). One case of each of tuberculosis and histoplasmosis have been reported in the use of anti-TNF medications for JIA.

No cases of malignancy have been reported in children. Adult screening guidelines for tuberculosis, at a minimum using purified protein derivative (PPD) skin testing prior to anti-TNF therapy, are adopted in pediatric practice.

Other Biologic-Modifying Drugs

Interleukin (IL)-1 Receptor Antagonists

Initial very promising results using anakinra, an IL-1 receptor antagonist, for systemic arthritis have been reported for both the systemic and articular components, including patients not responsive to anti-TNF medications. IL-1 appears to be a major mediator of inflammation in systemic arthritis (22). Anakinra is less effective for polyarthritis than anti-TNF medications.

Anti-Interleukin-6 Receptor Antibody

Interleukin 6 is also an important cytokine in the pathogenesis of systemic arthritis. Two open series of 29 patients with systemic arthritis given intravenous tocilizumab, an anti-IL6 receptor antibody, reported significant improvements in the majority of the patients as soon as after the second dose (23). Tocilizumab is still under study.

Intravenous Immunoglobulin

Two controlled studies did not find intravenous immunoglobulin (IVIg) to be effective in the treatment of the arthritis component of systemic and polyarthritis JIA. There may be more benefit for IVIg for the treatment of the systemic features of systemic arthritis.

Other Medications

There are no reports or studies in JIA of new medications found to be effective in rheumatoid arthritis, including rituximab (anti-CD20 mature B-cell antibodies) or abatacept (anti-CD28, T-cell co-stimulator antibodies).

Autologous Stem-Cell Transplantation

In patients with longstanding and unresponsive systemic and polyarthritis JIA there may be a role for autologous stem-cell transplantation (ASCT) (24). However, there is a significant mortality rate associated with ASCT (15%), thus ASCT must still be regarded as an experimental procedure in JIA.

EVIDENCE-BASED GUIDELINES FOR THE TREATMENT OF JUVENILE IDIOPATHIC ARTHRITIS SUBTYPES

Suggested treatment guidelines were published based on a systematic review of the controlled studies done in JIA (25). Thirty-six controlled trials were identified, 30 of them were double blind. This brief summary of the recommendations emphasizes that the treatment plan needs to be individualized based on the arthritis subtype.

Oligoarthritis

Only a minority of patients respond completely to NSAIDs. In those not responsive or patients presenting with flexion contractures, intra-articular corticosteroid injections, especially triamcinolone hexacetonide, are effective for most patients. Patients not responsive to corticosteroid injections or with extended oligoarthritis or small joint involvement should be treated as patients with polyarthritis.

Polyarthritis

Nonsteroidal anti-inflammatory drugs are mostly not effective as disease-modifying medications and are used mostly as symptomatic treatment. MTX should be started early, initially at $10\,mg/m^2$/week, and if not effective increased to $15\,mg/m^2$/week, given parenterally. Alternatives include sulfasalazine and leflunomide. If not effective, anti-TNF medications should be used.

Systemic Arthritis

There is a particular lack of evidence for systemic arthritis. NSAIDs and systemic corticosteroids are often needed for symptomatic (fever, serositis) relief. Intra-articular corticosteroid injections, MTX, and anti-TNF medications appear to be less beneficial than in other JIA subtypes, both for the systemic and arthritis components. Among the medications currently available there may be an advantage to using anakinra as a first-line corticosteroid-sparing medication. IVIg may have some benefit as a corticosteroid-sparing effect on the systemic component. Treatment for the macrophage activation syndrome includes high dose intravenous corticosteroids pulses and if not rapidly effective cyclosporine should be added. Tocilizumab, still available only in research trials, shows initial promise.

Enthesitis-Related Arthritis

Sulfasalazine may be beneficial, particularly for older males with peripheral arthritis. Anti-TNF medications are highly effective.

Psoriatic Arthritis

There are no studies of the treatment of psoriatic arthritis in children. The presentation of psoriatic arthritis can be as oligo-, poly-, and enthesitis-related arthritis and until other evidence is reported should be treated as the parallel JIA subset.

Uveitis

The treatment of uveitis should be directed by ophthalmologists with experience in treating this disorder with the guidance of pediatric rheumatologists experienced in managing immunosuppressive and biologic-modifying medications. Usually, initial treatment consists of topical corticosteroid drops. Subtenon corticosteroid injections may also be beneficial. Immunosuppresive therapy should be started early in patients with severe uveitis or in those who become corticosteroid dependent. MTX is the most common medication used (21,26). For patients not responsive to MTX, infliximab, but not etanercept, appears to be effective (19,20).

OTHER FACETS OF TREATING JUVENILE IDIOPATHIC ARTHRITIS

The medical treatment of JIA, while most important, is only one facet of JIA therapy. A multidisciplinary team incorporating pediatric rheumatologists, ophthalmologists, orthopedic surgeons, dentists, physical and occupational therapists, dietitians, social workers, psychologists, and educational and vocational counselors are involved in treating patients with JIA.

Many patients continue to have pain despite adequate disease control with modern medications and often pain is not adequately treated. Patients should receive adequate pain medications, including narcotics if necessary. Other pain modalities should be considered, including physical therapy, physical measures like heat or cold, splints, orthotics, acupuncture and massage, and various behavioral and stress-reducing techniques.

A critical part of the treatment regimen is physical therapy. The main purposes of physical therapy are to maintain range of motion of the affected joints, improve muscle strength, prevent deformities, and to correct or minimize damage and loss of function. Methods used include guided and home exercise programs for range of motion and muscle strengthening exercises, splints, orthotics, and various modalities to decrease pain. Aquatic exercise is often tolerated more than land exercises, especially in patients with significant lower extremity arthritis. Splints are used for knee flexion contractures. Some patients with persistent knee contractures may benefit from serial casting. Orthotics are often used for ankle or subtalar arthritis or for foot deformities in order to decrease pain when walking, improve gait, as an arch support for flatfoot, and to minimize pressure on metatarsal heads, thus preventing the formation of callus or subluxations of the toes. Patients with leg length discrepancy occasionally need shoe lifts in the shorter leg.

The role of occupational therapy is to maintain and improve the normal life function. Techniques used include hand exercises; wrist, hand and finger splints; teaching joint protection techniques; and fitting various aids for daily activities. These depend on the extent of the disease and include aids for writing, dressing (also shoes), eating utensils, adapting bathrooms and other household equipment for patients with arthritis, and mobility aids, if needed (canes, walkers, wheelchairs). Heat pads or bottles, bathing, and paraffin baths may help decrease morning stiffness.

Dietary consultation may be needed because some patients with significant arthritis have anorexia and lack adequate growth from several factors, including active disease, arthritis of the temporomandibular joint, and various medications (NSAIDs, methotrexate). Dietary consultation is also important for patients treated with corticosteroids in preventing excessive weight gain, hypertension, and bone loss, and includes advice on adequate calcium and vitamin D intake.

Physical activity is encouraged but should be tailored by the degree of arthritis and the joints involved. Children are encouraged to set their own limits but should not persist in an activity that causes pain in an arthritic joint. In general, activities that are less weight bearing, such as swimming and cycling, are preferred, but most sports that do not involve significant contact (football, hockey, wrestling, boxing) are tolerated. Patients with neck arthritis need to limit activities that can result in cervical spine damage (diving, certain types of jumping).

It is important to discuss school issues with the patients, family, and, if needed, school officials. In general, patients with JIA attain similar school achievements as healthy students. However, JIA patients are often absent due to flares, infections, and visits to physicians and other therapists. Patients may arrive late to school due to morning stiffness. Gym performance, moving from class to class, and writing may be affected. Children with uveitis may need adjustments due to visual difficulties. Common school adjustments include allowing elevator use, more time to get from class to class, stretching in class, more time to write tests, computer

7

use, having a second set of books, and gym modifications. In the United States, the Americans with Disability Act (504 plan) mandates allowing for every child to receive education in the least restrictive environment. In more severe cases a formal individualized educational plan (IEP) can be employed (see Chapter 7D).

As in any chronic disease, especially one with chronic medication use, psychological support is often needed. Patients and families should be encouraged to seek support early before a crisis occurs. This support is often needed to deal with medication issues such as body image changes from corticosteroids, nausea from methotrexate, or to increase compliance with the medication regimen (see Chapter 7D for a discussion of adherence). Social workers can assist with the financial burden caused by the disease and the cost of medications.

An important issue is the transition to adulthood, including transition of medical care to adult rheumatologists, education, and vocational planning. These issues should start to be discussed and planned well in advance of the youth's 18th birthday. Data show that transition to adult health care results in improved outcomes if the transition is planned and the disease is well controlled at the time of the transfer to the adult rheumatologist (27). A transition policy has been adopted by the major primary care physician groups (American Academy of Pediatrics, American Academy of Family Physicians, and the American College of Physicians) (28) and there are special medical issues for the young adult who has grown up with JIA.

Patient advocacy groups, such as the Juvenile Arthritis Alliance, sponsored by the Arthritis Foundation, can also give support. The Arthritis Foundation supports regional and national meetings, arthritis camps, educational materials, newsletters, and discussion forums on JIA (http://www.arthritis.org). Other important sources of educational material on JIA include the American College of Rheumatology (http://www.rheumatology.org) and the Pediatric Rheumatology International Trials Organization (PRINTO; http://www.printo.it). The latter site has information on JIA in more than 30 languages.

TOOLS TO ASSESS JUVENILE IDIOPATHIC ARTHRITIS OUTCOMES

Several assessment tools have been developed for the purposes of following individual patients as well as for clinical trials and outcome studies (Table 7C-3). These tools assess various domains of JIA. A validated comprehensive global disease activity scale has not been developed yet. Disease activity tools commonly used include active joint count (joints with swelling or tender/pain on motion), joints with limitation of motion, and

TABLE 7C-3. ASSESSMENT AND OUTCOME MEASURE TOOLS FOR JUVENILE IDIOPATHIC ARTHRITIS.

DOMAIN	ASSESSMENT TOOLS
Disease activity	Active joint count, acute phase reactants
Global assessment	Physician, patient visual analog scale
Functional assessment	Childhood Health Assessment Questionnaire (CHAQ), Juvenile Arthritis Functional Assessment Report (JAFAR), Juvenile Arthritis Functional Status Index (JASI)
Quality-of-life assessment	Childhood Health Questionnaire (CHQ), Peds-Quality of Life (QOL)–rheumatology subset, pain visual analog scale
Radiologic damage	Poznanski, Dijkstra scores
Disease-related irreversible damage	Juvenile Arthritis Damage Index (JADI)
Clinical trial outcome measures	American College of Rheumatology (ACR) Pediatric 30, criteria for inactive disease or clinical remission

acute phase reactants, for example, the erythrocyte sedimentation rate (ESR) and C-reactive protein (CRP). It is important to note, however, that many patients with active arthritis have normal acute phase reactants. Subjective, but well-validated global assessment tools include visual analog scales used by physicians and parents.

Several functional assessments tools have been developed (29). These include the Childhood Health Assessment Questionnaire (CHAQ), Juvenile Arthritis Functional Assessment Report (JAFAR), and Juvenile Arthritis Self-Report Index (JASI). These tools have all been validated, and are reliable, sensitive to change, include items applicable to all children with JIA at all ages, and are easy to use and score (except the JASI, which is limited to children >8 years old and is very lengthy). Most are completed by parents and/or patients. These tools provide an overall functional assessment by a composite score and also enable determination of particular functional deficits. The CHAQ, translated and validated in more than 30 languages, is the most commonly used. Various studies did not find significant differences between the measures, thus all appear valid for use in clinical practice and trials. There are several problems with the functional assessment tools, especially a ceiling effect in patients with mild oligoarthritis and minimal functional problems.

Most functional tools do not address issues of overall quality of life (QOL), especially general health and psychosocial issues related to JIA (29). These are most commonly assessed in JIA by use of the Juvenile Arthritis Quality of Life Questionnaire (JAQQ) and the Childhood Health Questionnaire (CHQ). The CHQ also allows comparisons between diseases for research studies. It has been translated and validated in more than 30 languages and is the most used tool. In the United States, there is also widespread use of the Pediatric Quality of Life generic questionnaire and the rheumatology module (PedsQL-RM).

Until recently the only radiologic assessment tool was the Poznanski scale that looked at wrist damage by comparing the ratio of the length of the carpus bones to the length of the second metacarpal bone. A more comprehensive scale was recently developed and validated by the Dutch JIA Study Group (15). The Dijkstra composite score is based on inflammation (swelling, osteopenia), damage (joint space narrowing, cysts, erosions), and growth abnormality subscores for 19 joints or joint groups.

Most recent clinical trials for JIA have used the well-validated ACR Pediatric 30 scale as the primary outcome measure of responsiveness (30). This scale, developed in 1997, defines patients as responders or nonresponders. This scale was modified for defining disease flares necessary for some clinical trials of rapidly acting biologic-modifying medications utilizing a withdrawal design, that is, patients defined as responders in the open phase of the trial were randomized to continue the medication or to receive placebo. Due to the advent of potent biologic-modifying medications, rheumatologists no longer aim only for improvement, but aspire to induce remission. Preliminary criteria defining clinical remission of all JIA subtypes on and off medications were defined and validated in a large series of patients (3,31).

A global damage assessment tool, the Juvenile Arthritis Damage Index (JADI), was recently developed and validated (32). The JADI includes two components. The JADI-A assesses articular damage based on persistent findings of joint contractures, deformities, or major surgery in 36 joints or joint groups lasting at least 6 months and not related to active arthritis. The JADI-E assesses extra-articular damage to the eyes, skin, nonarticular musculoskeletal system, endocrine system, and secondary amyloidosis.

SUMMARY AND FUTURE RESEARCH

The development of new therapies has markedly increased our ability to effectively treat children with JIA. Indeed, there are indications that patients treated aggressively early in the disease course with MTX and/or biologic-modifying medications appear to improve significantly faster than patients treated later in the disease course. However, recent sobering studies have shown our inability to induce long-term, medication-free remission in most patients. There also is a lack of evidence-based medicine in the treatment of some JIA subtypes. Controlled studies for new medications for systemic arthritis, including anti–IL-6 receptor antibodies, new anti–IL-1 medications, and thalidomide or other combinations are necessary. Studies of new medications shown to be effective in rheumatoid arthritis, such as abetacept and rituximab, need to be studied in polyarthritis.

A high priority for investigation should be the early effect of aggressive therapy on the disease course, including the potential use of remission induction therapy that could include combining various methods of administering corticosteroids with MTX and a biologic-modifying medication to be followed with step-down maintenance therapy in both poly- and systemic arthritis. While intuitively logical in the short term, these protocols need to be validated for long-term effects as well as for potential increases in adverse reactions. The results of these studies should fill gaps in evidence-based guidelines in order to assure quality care of children with arthritis. New outcome tools will enable us to study the long-term disease-modifying effects of MTX and biologic-modifying medications on remission rates, radiologic changes, functional capabilities, and the prevention of irreversible articular and extra-articular damage.

REFERENCES

1. Wallace CA, Levinson JE. Juvenile rheumatoid arthritis: outcome and treatment for the 1990s. Rheum Dis Clin North Am 1991;17:891–905.
2. Oen K, Malleson PN, Cabral DA, et al. Disease course and outcome of juvenile rheumatoid arthritis in a multicenter cohort. J Rheumatol 2002;29:1989–1999.
3. Wallace CA, Huang B, Bandeira M, et al. Patterns of clinical remission in select categories of juvenile idiopathic arthritis. Arthritis Rheum 2005;52:3554–3562.
4. Carvounis PE, Herman DC, Cha S, et al. Incidence and outcomes of uveitis in juvenile rheumatoid arthritis, a synthesis of the literature. Graefes Arch Clin Exp Ophthalmol 2006;244:281–290.
5. Giannini EH, Cawkwell GD. Drug treatment in children with juvenile rheumatoid arthritis. Pediatr Clin North Am 1995;42:1099–1125.
6. Padeh S, Passwell JH. Intraarticular corticosteroid injections in the management of children with chronic arthritis. Arthritis Rheum 1998;41:1210–1214.
7. Sherry DD, Stein LD, Reed AM, et al. Prevention of leg length discrepancy in young children with pauciarticular juvenile rheumatoid arthritis by treatment with intraarticular steroids. Arthritis Rheum 1999;42:2330–2334.
8. Zulian F, Martini G, Gobber D, et al. Triamcinolone acetonide and hexacetonide intra-articular treatment of

symmetrical joints in juvenile idiopathic arthritis: a double-blind trial. Rheumatology 2004;43:1288–1291.

9. Giannini EA, Brewer EJ, Kuzmina N, et al. Methotrexate in resistant juvenile rheumatoid arthritis: results of the U.S.A.-U.S.S.R. double-blind, placebo-controlled trial. N Engl J Med 1992;326:1043–1049.

10. Ruperto N, Murray KJ, Gerloni V, et al. A randomized trial of parenteral methotrexate comparing an intermediate dose with a higher dose in children with juvenile idiopathic arthritis who failed to respond to standard doses of methotrexate. Arthritis Rheum 2004;50:2191–2201.

11. Woo P, Southwood TR, Prieur AM, et al. Randomized, placebo-controlled, crossover trial of low-dose oral methotrexate in children with extended oligoarticular or systemic arthritis. Arthritis Rheum 2000;43:1849–1857.

12. Passo MH, Hashkes PJ. Use of methotrexate in children. Bull Rheum Dis 1998;47:1–5.

13. Ortiz-Alvarez O, Morishita K, Avery G, et al. Guidelines for blood test monitoring of methotrexate toxicity in juvenile idiopathic arthritis. J Rheumatol 2004;31:2501–2506.

14. van Rossum MA, Fiselier TJ, Franssen MJ, et al. Sulfasalazine in the treatment of juvenile chronic arthritis: a randomized double-blind placebo-controlled, multicenter study. Arthritis Rheum 1998;41:808–816.

15. van Rossum MA, Boers M, Zwinderman AH, et al. Development of a standardized method of assessment of radiographs and radiographic changes in juvenile idiopathic arthritis: introduction of the Dijkstra composite score. Arthritis Rheum 2005;52:2865–2872.

16. Silverman E, Mouy R, Spiegel L, et al. Leflunomide or methotrexate for juvenile rheumatoid arthritis. N Engl J Med 2005;352:1655–1666.

17. Lehman TJ, Schechter SJ, Sundel RP, et al. Thalidomide for severe systemic onset juvenile rheumatoid arthritis. J Pediatr 2004;145:856–857.

18. Lovell DJ, Giannini EH, Reiff A, et al. Etanercept in children with polyarticular juvenile rheumatoid arthritis. N Engl J Med 2000;342:763–769.

19. Quartier P, Taupin P, Bourdeaut F, et al. Efficacy of etanercept for the treatment of juvenile idiopathic arthritis according to the onset type. Arthritis Rheum 2003;48:1093–1101.

20. Smith JA, Thompson DJ, Whitcup SM, et al. A randomized, placebo-controlled double-masked clinical trial of etanercept for the treatment of uveitis associated with juvenile idiopathic arthritis. Arthritis Rheum 2005;53:18–23.

21. Saurenmann RK, Levin AN, Rose JB, et al. Tumor necrosis factor inhibitors in the treatment of childhood uveitis. Rheumatology 2006;45:982–989.

22. Pascual V, Allantaz F, Arce E, et al. Role of interleukin-1 in the pathogenesis of systemic onset juvenile idiopathic arthritis and clinical response to IL-1 blockade. J Exp Med 2005;201:1479–1486.

23. Woo P, Wilkinson N, Prieur AM, et al. Open label phase II trial of single, ascending doses of MRA in Caucasian children with severe systemic juvenile idiopathic arthritis: proof of principle of the efficacy of IL-6 receptor blockade in this type of arthritis and demonstration of prolonged clinical improvement. Arthritis Res Ther 2005;7:R1281–R1288.

24. De Kleer IM, Brinkman DM, Ferster A, et al. Autologous stem cell transplantation for refractory juvenile idiopathic arthritis: analysis of clinical effects, mortality, and transplant related morbidity. Ann Rheum Dis 2004;63:1318–1326.

25. Hashkes PJ, Laxer RM. Medical treatment of juvenile idiopathic arthritis. JAMA 2005;294:1671–1684.

26. Foeldvari I, Wierk A. Methotrexate is an effective treatment for chronic uveitis associated with juvenile idiopathic arthritis. J Rheumatol 2005;32:362–365.

27. McDonough JE, Southwood TR, Shaw KL. The impact of a coordinated transitional care programme on adolescents with juvenile idiopathic arthritis. Rheumatology 2006;46:161–168.

28. American Academy of Pediatrics, American Academy of Family Physicians, American College of Physicians-American Society of Internal Medicine. A consensus statement on health care transitions for young adults with special health care needs. Pediatrics 2002;110:1304–1306.

29. Duffy CM. Measurement of health status, functional status, and quality of life in children with juvenile idiopathic arthritis: clinical science for the pediatrician. Pediatr Clin North Am 2005;52:359–372.

30. Giannini EH, Ruperto N, Ravelli A, et al. Preliminary definition of improvement in juvenile arthritis. Arthritis Rheum 1997;40:1202–1209.

31. Wallace CA, Ruperto N, Giannini E, et al. Preliminary criteria for clinical remission for select categories of juvenile idiopathic arthritis. J Rheumatol 2004;31:2290–2294.

32. Viola S, Felici E, Magni-Manzoni S, et al. Development and validation of a clinical index for assessment of long-term damage in juvenile idiopathic arthritis. Arthritis Rheum 2005;52:2092–2102.

Juvenile Idiopathic Arthritis
D. Special Considerations

Carol B. Lindsley, MD

- Youth with juvenile idiopathic arthritis (JIA) require special attention to managing growth abnormalities, both local and general, as well as osteopenia.
- Adherence to medical regimens is often suboptimal and can be improved by paying attention to

- educational, organizational, and behavioral approaches
- Management of youth with JIA should take in account the psychological, educational, and transition to adulthood issues to maximize their outcome.

Many rheumatic diseases that occur in adults also affect children, albeit less frequently. Additionally, some diseases such as systemic-onset or pauciarticular pattern of juvenile rheumatoid arthritis occur predominantly in children. In all of these diseases, the clinical manifestations are often impacted by the child's growth and development.

EXAMINATION

Performing a valid and complete examination on a child who is ill or in pain can be difficult. Yet an accurate exam is necessary if the correct diagnosis is to be made. Children at different ages and developmental levels respond differently to examination. Rheumatic disease manifestations can also vary with age. It may be helpful to keep certain guidelines in mind. Height and weight should be obtained at each visit and these growth parameters plotted on an appropriate growth chart. Inadequately controlled disease or medication side effects can impair normal growth.

In infants and toddlers, observation skills are particularly important. By looking for movements that cause pain or irritability as well as lack of movement of any joint, one can ascertain much before the patient is ever examined. Using toys, talking, and keeping eye contact with the child may help alleviate the child's fear. Having the child sit on the parent's lap and even having the parent assist with the examination may make a more thorough examination possible. Swelling can be subtle in a chubby child and careful attention to range of

motion is critical. A single swollen digit may be the only sign of arthritis.

Most school-aged children like to actively participate in the examination, particularly if they are in comfortable clothing such as T-shirt and shorts. It is generally best to examine any painful area last, after completing the general and remainder of the musculoskeletal examination. In addition to joint examination, careful attention should be paid to gait, leg length, and muscle strength. Having a child perform a sit-up or climb a few stairs can be a helpful screen for muscle weakness.

In adolescents, the examination itself is not difficult but relating to the patient can be. It is again important that the patient is as comfortable as possible and that rapport is established with the adolescent, not just the parent. In situations where the parent continues to dominate the interactions, it may be helpful to ask to speak to the adolescent alone. The examination should include a scoliosis screen as part of the musculoskeletal examination.

GROWTH

Juvenile rheumatoid arthritis (JRA) is a chronic disease and has long been known to affect growth of the child. Historically, this clinical effect was noted by Still in 1897 and later described by Kuhns in 1932. Its cause is multifactorial, including not only the disease itself but medication side effects, nutrition, and mechanical problems. The roles of growth hormone and insulin-like growth factors are gradually being elucidated, as described below.

General

It is clear that the onset subtype of JRA is important, with little or no general adverse effect on growth seen in the pauciarticular group. However, this group may have severe local growth disturbances at the sites of inflammation, particularly leg length discrepancy and mandibular asymmetries.

Patients with polyarticular and systemic disease who have never received corticosteroid therapy may have general growth retardation, generally related to the severity and duration of disease. In one study, one fourth of both disease groups lost greater than 1 height Z score over the 14-year follow-up period (1). [Z score $= (X_1 - X_2)/\text{SD}$, where X_1 = subject's measurement, X_2 = mean of the reference population for age and gender, and SD = standard deviation of the mean for the reference population.] Growth impairment was generally not severe except in a small number of systemic patients. Height velocity during puberty was especially vulnerable. The degree of catch-up growth was unpredictable.

In another study with 64 prepubertal children with primarily mild pauciarticular and polyarticular JRA, growth velocity decreased in the first year of disease postdiagnosis and then increased to normal range with treatment and 4-year follow-up. The greatest effect on velocity was seen in children with more severe polyarticular disease. There were only two systemic patients in the study (2). A long-term follow-up study of adults who had JRA and had received corticosteroids showed reduced final height and arm-span (3).

Local

Local growth disturbances occur as a result of inflammation and the accompanying increase in vascularity, which may result in either over- or undergrowth of the affected bone. Examples of local growth abnormalities are the following: (1) The hip is a frequently involved joint in JRA and occasionally this leads to a small femoral head within a larger acetabulum. This was noted in five patients undergoing hip arthroplasty. The small size was thought to be secondary to destruction of the articular cartilage (4). Of note, all patients had disease onset prior to age 3. (2) The knee is the most frequently involved joint in JRA and persistent synovitis, particularly in an asymmetric fashion, can lead to significant leg length discrepancy. The distal femoral epiphysis accounts for approximately 70% of femoral growth, so persistent inflammation leads to overgrowth on the involved side in a child whose epiphyses have not yet closed. Often the medial side predominates, leading to additional knee valgus. Increased use of intra-articular steroids may reduce this risk and appears to

have a low level of adverse effects (5). (3) Micrognathia and malocclusion are known as common sequelae of JRA. Unilateral disease may lead to chin deviation. Sixty-nine percent of youth with polyarticular and systemic disease had orthodontic abnormalities (6). Polyarticular patients often have small, short facies with underdeveloped mandibles. These consequences of temporomandibular joint (TMJ) arthritis are difficult to treat. Magnetic resonance imaging (MRI) may detect early changes. Orthodontic consultation is recommended. Corticosteroid injection may be helpful in selected patients and costochondral grafts have been used in severely affected patients. (4) Other sites frequently involved include the wrist, with undergrowth of the ulnar head, and the vertebrae, with undergrowth of the cervical spine.

Osteopenia and Osteoporosis

Osteopenia is low bone mass for age and the child with JRA is at great risk for failure to achieve adequate postpubertal bone mass. The introduction of dual-energy x-ray absorptiometry (DXA) has enabled assessment of osteopenia and has led to realization of the magnitude of the problem. Both the cortical appendicular skeleton and the axial trabecular bone are affected, but the cortical to a greater degree (7). Osteopenia appears to correlate with disease activity and severity (7). Other factors, including decreased physical activity, immobility, decreased sun exposure, and decreased dietary intake of calcium and vitamin D, are additional contributing factors. Peak bone mass is normally reached during adolescence and this achievement is important to minimize future risk for osteoporosis and fractures. Often in JRA the bone density fails to undergo expected pubertal increase. Significant axial osteopenia of lumbar spine and femoral neck was found in patients with polyarticular disease (8). In a 2-year prospective, controlled study in early juvenile idiopathic arthritis (JIA; includes JRA, psoriatic arthritis, and ankylosing spondylitis), moderate reduction of bone mass gain, bone turnover, and total lean body mass was observed (9).

Therapy includes weight-bearing exercise, appropriate nutrition, calcium and vitamin D supplementation, and, most importantly, adequate disease control with suppression of inflammation. Early study of bisphosphonate therapy in children with rheumatic disease has been encouraging but not without adverse effects (10). Behavioral intervention may also be helpful in increasing calcium intake (11).

In addition to generalized osteopenia, involved joints often show local juxta-articular demineralization even on early radiographs. Patients may benefit from DXA monitoring at selected intervals.

Endocrine Factors

Osteocalcin

Low levels of osteocalcin, along with decreased bone mineral content, were found in children with active inflammation but both parameters were normal in children with inactive disease (12). Osteocalcin levels in patients with heights less than the third percentile were below normal, suggesting decreased osteoblast activity (13). In this study, osteocalcin levels correlated with decreased insulin-like growth factor 1 (IGF-l) levels. However, these patients were also on corticosteroid therapy, which can decrease osteocalcin levels.

Insulin-like Growth Factor 1

Insulin-like growth factor 1 is a peptide produced in the liver and is the main periperal mediator of growth hormone. It promotes collagen formation. Serum levels of this peptide have been reduced in most JRA studies, especially in systemic disease (14). Levels appear to correlate with the degree of inflammation as measured by acute phase reactants. Levels returned to normal with recombinant growth hormone (rGH) therapy in one study (13).

Interleukin 6 (IL-6)

This cytokine is markedly elevated in systemic disease and appears to correlate with the degree of inflammation. Studies in transgenic mice show that IL-6 mediates a decrease in IGF-1 production, which might represent a mechanism by which chronic inflammation affects growth (15).

Vascular Endothelial Growth Factor

This factor is a mitogen for vascular endothelial cells and a mediator of vascular permeability. Serum levels correlate with disease activity in polyarticular JRA and may play a role in inflammation that could affect growth (16).

Growth Hormone

Children with JRA and short stature have low human growth hormone (hGH) secretion and some had inadequate or no response to exogenous hGH administration, suggesting an additional defect in the response pathway or growth hormone insensitivity (17). Other studies have shown levels not significantly different from controls (13).

Growth Hormone Therapy

In one study, 14 children with JRA on corticosteroid therapy received 1.4 IU rGH/kg/week with a partial response. The mean height velocity increased from 1.9 to 5.4 cm/year with an accompanying 12% increase in lean body mass. However, at the end of 1 year the height velocity decreased to pretreatment levels (18).

In another study, rGH increased height velocity during the year of therapy (mean, 3.1 cm/year) but the long-term effect was unknown. There was no correlation between growth hormone secretion and rGH therapy response, raising the question of a target cell defect or peripheral defect regarding growth hormone mediation. Fifty percent of the children in this study had borderline or poor caloric intake (13). Growth hormone therapy may be beneficial in some patients but the response is unpredictable. In a 4-year study of growth hormone therapy in children with polyarticular or systemic disease receiving corticosteroids, improvement of 1 SD was seen in bone mineral content compared to controls (19).

Thyroid Disease

Other endocrine disease may affect both symptoms and growth. Stagi and colleagues found an increased prevalence of autoimmune thyroiditis, subclinical hypothyroidism, and celiac disease in children with JIA (20). In a separate study, antithyroid antibodies were found in a higher frequency in children with arthritis, especially pauciarticular disease, than in the general population (21). These findings suggest that careful monitoring of thyroid function in children with arthritis is indicated.

Nutrition

Adequate nutrition, both caloric and protein, are critical to optimize growth in children with JRA. Up to 30% of children with JRA have some growth abnormality (22). Using anthropometric measurements, up to 40% have poor nutritional status and muscle mass is frequently low. Protein stores as well as specific nutrients such as iron, selenium, vitamin C, and zinc have been reported as low (23). In a recent study, undernutrition was present in 16% of the children with arthritis, including those with pauciarticular disease (24). Inflammatory cytokines, such as IL-1, IL-6, and tumor necrosis factor (TNF) likely modulate some of the nutritional abnormalities. In addition, some patients have mechanical feeding problems related to jaw or upper extremity disease. Aggressive early therapy and use of newer biologic agents, such as anti-TNF agents, can dramatically improve individual patient's nutritional status and growth. However, long-term studies are not yet available.

7

Monitoring of serial weights during clinic visits should be routine. Dietary logs, nutrient analysis, and consultation with a dietitian is needed for a child with continued poor weight gain. Nutritional supplementation may be beneficial, as may behavioral therapy.

EYE DISEASE

Inflammatory eye disease, especially uveitis, occurs with increased frequency in children with arthritis. Reported incidence varies from 5% to as high as 50%, but recent studies show an incidence of 12% to 25% (25,26). The known risk factors include age <6 years at disease onset, pauciarticular pattern of disease, and antinuclear antibody (ANA) positivity. Current guidelines for frequency of ophthalmologic examination are available (27). As uveitis can develop after the onset of arthritis, ongoing monitoring is important. Long-term outcome for adult patients with childhood-onset uveitis is still poor, with visual acuity impaired in 40%, poor in 20%, and lost in 10% (28). Current arthritis therapeutic regimens, especially methotrexate and anti-TNF agents, appear effective in uveitis. Therefore, the outcome of uveitis with onset in the past 5 to 10 years will likely be much better than the existing reports (see Chapter 7A for more information) (29).

ADHERENCE

Optimal treatment of pediatric rheumatic disease often requires complex therapeutic strategies that can be both confusing and time consuming to patients and their families. Strategies often involve a coordinated list of activities, including taking regular medication, complex exercise regimens, dietary modifications, regular clinic visits and laboratory tests for monitoring the patient, and, in some children, wearing of therapeutic splints. This is complicated by the fact that there is often delayed benefit for good compliance. It is easy to understand why adherence to these regimens is often compromised. In fact, estimates are that only 50% to 54% of patients with chronic pediatric disease adhere adequately with their recommended therapy (30). In JRA, the medication adherence was found to be of similar frequency, ranging from 38% to 59% (31). In a study of prednisone therapy in children with systemic lupus erythematosus (SLE) or dermatomyositis, compliance ranged from 33% to 78%, which is similar to that reported in pediatric cancer patients (32). Surprisingly in the prednisone study, two thirds of patients overmedicated themselves, possibly when they felt poorly. Adherence with exercise regimens are likely to be lower than with medication, ranging from 47% to 67% by parent report (33). One must also

differentiate between complete nonadherence and periodic nonadherence.

The consequences of nonadherence are multiple, not only for the patient but also for the health care system. The patients' risk for disease complications and long-term sequelae are generally increased with noncompliance. Poor or dishonest communication between patient and physician or health care provider also stresses the relationship and may lead to needless changes of medication or unnecessary testing. All of these are inefficient and lead to increased health care costs.

Factors Affecting Adherence

Many factors may impede adherence. These can generally be grouped into three categories: (1) factors relating to the disease; (2) factors related to the patient and family; and (3) those related to the regimen itself. There is no typical noncompliant patient and no consistent correlations with obvious demographic factors. However, certain states that lead to noncompliance have been reported (33) and are included in Tables 7D-1 and 7D-2.

Factors Related to Treatment Regimen

The health care provider can increase the likelihood of good adherence by making the treatment regimen as simple as possible and by anticipating some of the

---

TABLE 7D-1. ADHERENCE: FACTORS RELATING TO PATIENT/FAMILY.

1. Negative reactions from the child, including complaints, refusal, discomfort, or embarrassment, or more general oppositional behavior.

2. Lack of understanding of the disease and treatment, especially in younger children.

3. Misunderstanding of the disease and treatment.

4. Lack of patient autonomy and low self-esteem.

5. Dissatisfaction with the provider or the therapeutic intervention.

6. Inadequate family resources.

7. Language barriers.

8. Family instability or disagreement.

9. Other family demands, for example, parental illness.

10. Parental resentment or anger over the illness.

11. Family's coping abilities and strategies.

TABLE 7D-2. ADHERENCE: FACTORS RELATED TO DISEASE.

1. Duration, often prolonged with unpredictable exacerbations—compliance tends to decrease over time.

2. Age of onset—younger patients are less compliant.

3. Asymptomatic periods. When a patient is asymptomatic or in remission, there is often a temptation to discontinue medication because the patient feels well. This is enhanced by a commonly seen delay in therapeutic response of days to weeks and also by the delay in occurrence of negative effects (recurrence of symptoms) with missed medication.

4. Severity of disease—no clear correlation with compliance.

known negative factors, including bad-tasting medication, dosing frequency, forgetting (exercise vs. medication), high cost, complexity, delay in therapeutic response, and transportation concerns. Exercise regimens may be especially problematic because the child may experience discomfort and express anger or resentment toward the parent.

Children with chronic disease may be asked to alter their lifestyle in a way that restricts their sports interests or peer-related social activity or reduces their leisure time. Such changes are especially difficult for active children and adolescents. Parental supervision and appropriate involvement are critical in providing the children with needed support. Delay in receiving or lack of subspecialty care and implementation of appropriate therapeutic regimens may also contribute to poor functional outcomes.

Assessment of Adherence

Assessment of adherence can be direct or indirect. Indirect means include parental observation, self-report, medication diary, prescription renewals, and presence of predictable side effects. Direct means include pill count, measurement of laboratory parameters such as drug levels, and electronic devices that record and store the time and date a pill container is opened (34).

Improving Adherence

Strategies used to improve compliance can be categorized into three types: educational, organizational, and behavioral. These can be used singly or in combination (33).

Educational strategies include providing information, helping prioritize, re-education, written handouts, reminder systems, community and national resources, positive feedback, and appropriate discipline techniques. Information should be age, culture, and language appropriate and take into account the child's

cognitive abilities. It is important not to overwhelm the family early in the process.

Organizational strategies include counseling, increasing supervision, decreasing complexity, decreasing costs, and increasing palatability of medication. The regimens should fit into the family daily routine as much as possible. Therapeutic exercise and play can often be combined.

Behavioral strategies can include self-management training to increase self-esteem, training for parents to deal with oppositional behavior, and monitoring adherence and using reinforcement or a reward system for good adherence. Reinforcement programs are time consuming and require parental training but can improve adherence (33). Reward systems where tokens are exchanged for privileges can be successful. The child's responsibilities for the treatment regimen should increase as the child gets older but parents should not completely withdraw their supervision.

Regular clinic visits are important to re-educate and reinforce adherence strategies and adapt treatment. They also help build and maintain a cooperative and trusting relationship between clinician and patient. Visits should allow enough time for adherence discussion and reinforcement. Good documentation is also important to facilitate monitoring of adherence. The clinician must relate to the child, who needs to be an active partner in his or her treatment program. Judgmental attitudes are not helpful. A multidisciplinary team approach is optimal. Further studies are needed to identify children and families at high risk for nonadherence, further define successful family coping mechanisms that can be taught and reinforced, and to evaluate strategies for improving compliance.

PSYCHOSOCIAL AND EDUCATIONAL ISSUES

Chronic disease has a major impact on the development and daily functioning of a child as well as on the family. Unfortunately, there are few and often contradictory studies on the nature of the impact and the contributing factors. Different assessment methods, varying population size, and a mixture of disease subtypes, particularly with JRA, contribute to the different conclusions. Some epidemiological studies concluded that there is more risk for psychosocial problems in JRA patients (35), others less (36). A controlled study used self-report questionnaires combined with personal interviews to study children (age 7–11) and adolescents (age 12–16) with arthritis (37). Self-esteem, perceived competence, and body image were similar to healthy controls. The arthritis patients did have less energy to participate in social activities and adolescents received more emotional support from family, peers, and professionals.

The amount of support received correlated positively with disease severity. Other studies showed that children with chronic illness do not have a higher incidence of psychiatric disease nor is there any correlation between psychological test scores and disease functional measurements (38).

Family Impact

Long-term psychosocial outcome appears to be favorable overall. Chronic family difficulties predicted psychosocial functioning in patients with JRA in a 9-year follow-up study, without correlation with disease activity (39). The most frequent psychiatric disturbance on follow-up was anxiety disorder. No children had depressive disorder and 15% had mild-to-moderate impairment in psychosocial functioning (39).

Positive family factors may play an important role in the child's ability to cope with chronic illness. In one study a highly cohesive family structure correlated with a high level of social adjustment in children with JRA (37). An environment with flexibility, individual freedom, and an emphasis on self-mastery appears optimal. Family coping skills can be enhanced by educational programs such as those sponsored by the Arthritis Foundation, and by retreats or workshops directed by professionals (40). These also can reduce family stress and improve parent–child relationships.

Pain

Inadequate attention is often given to pain in children with arthritis. Young children usually do not verbalize discomfort or pain and even the older child may have become accustomed or tolerant to a certain level of pain. Tools are available to help the clinician ascertain the child's perception of pain and can be used as serial measurements. The Pain Coping Questionnaire has been validated in children and adolescents and is good at assessing the child's pain coping strategies. It is simple and applicable over a wide age range (41). Less coping effectiveness has been related to higher levels of pain. Use of the Visual Analogue Scale of Pediatric Pain Questionnaire is also a simple tool that can be used during clinic visits to monitor pain levels in patients at risk. Higher patient perceived pain intensity correlates with higher incidence of depressive and anxiety symptoms (42).

School and Educational Achievement

Many factors affect school attendance but it is generally high except for more severely affected patients. In one study, school absence was associated with decreased adherence with physical therapy and the presence of psychological problems but not with age or duration of illness (43). School problems for children with arthritis include handwriting, opening doors, lateness to class, physical education participation, carrying books, fatigue, absences, and inadequate understanding by teachers and peers. School success is critical to the normal development of the child and school status and educational progress should be assessed regularly at clinic visits. In a controlled study of 44 adults with JRA surveyed 25 years after disease onset, there were equivalent levels of educational achievement, income, and insurance coverage but lower rates of employment, daily energy levels, and exercise tolerance (44).

During the past decade, the overall prognosis for children with rheumatic disease has steadily improved. However, for optimal treatment and outcome attention must be given to their special needs.

REFERENCES

1. Polito C, Strano CG, Olivieri AN, et al. Growth retardation in non-steroid treated juvenile rheumatoid arthritis. Scand J Rheumatol 1997;26:99–103.
2. Saha MT, Verronen P, Liappala P, Lenko HL. Growth of prepubertal children with juvenile chronic arthritis. Acta Paediatr 1999;88:724–728.
3. Zak M, Muller J, Karup-Pedersen F. Final height, armspan, subischial leg length and body proportions in juvenile chronic arthritis. A long-term follow-up study. Horm Res 1999;52:80–85.
4. Hastings DE, Orsini E, Myers P, Sullivan J. An unusual pattern of growth disturbance of the hip in juvenile rheumatoid arthritis. J Rheumatol 1994;21:744–747.
5. Sherry DD, Stein LD, Reed AM, Schanberg LE, Kredich, DW. Prevention of leg length discrepancy in young children with pauciarticular juvenile rheumatoid arthritis by treatment with intraarticular steroids. Arthritis Rheum 1999;42:2330–2334.
6. Ronchezel MV, Hilario MO, Goldenberg J, et al. Temporomandibular joint and mandibular growth alterations in patients with juvenile rheumatoid arthritis. J Rheumatol 1995;22:1956–1961.
7. Cassidy JT. Osteopenia and osteoporosis in children. Clin Exp Rheumatol 1999;17:245–250.
8. Kotaniemi A. Growth retardation and bone loss as determinants of axial osteopenia in juvenile chronic arthritis. Scand J Rheumatol 1997;26:14–18.
9. Lien G, Selvaag AM, Flato B, et al. A two-year prospective controlled study of bone mass and bone turnover in children with early juvenile idiopathic arthritis. Arthritis Rheum 2005;52:833–840.
10. Cimaz R. Osteoporosis in childhood rheumatic diseases: prevention and therapy. Best Pract Res Clin Rheumatol 2005;16:397–340.
11. Stark LJ, Janicke DM, McGrath AM, Mackner LM, Hommel KA, Lovell D. Prevention of osteoporosis: a randomized clinical trial to increase calcium intake in

children with juvenile rheumatoid arthritis. J Pediatr Psychol 2005;30:377–386.

12. Reed A, Haugen M, Pachman LM. Abnormalities in serum osteocalcin values in children with chronic rheumatic diseases. J Pediatr 1990;116:574–580.

13. Davies UM, Jones J, Reeve J, et al. Juvenile rheumatoid arthritis. Effects of disease activity and recombinant human growth hormone on insulin-like growth factor 1, insulin-like growth factor binding proteins 1 and 3, and osteocalcin. Arthritis Rheum 1997;40:332–340.

14. Cimaz R, Rusconi R, Cesana B, et al. A multicenter study on insulin-like growth factor-I serum levels in children with chronic inflammatory diseases. Clin Exp Rheum 1997;15:691–696.

15. DeBenedetti F, Alonzi T, Moretta A, et al. Interleukin 6 causes growth impairment in transgenic mice through a decrease in insulin-like growth factor-I. A model for stunted growth in children with chronic inflammation. J Clin Invest 1997;99:643–650.

16. Maeno N, Takei S, Imanaka H, et al. Increased circulating vascular endothelial growth factor is correlated with disease activity in polyarticular juvenile rheumatoid arthritis. J Rheumatol 1999;26:2244–2248.

17. Hopp RJ, Degan J, Corley K, Lindsley CB, Cassidy, JT. Evaluation of growth hormone secretion in children with juvenile rheumatoid arthritis and short stature. Nebr Med J 1995;80:52–57.

18. Simon D, Touati G, Prieur AM, Ruiz JC, Czernichow P. Growth hormone treatment of short stature and metabolic dysfunction in juvenile chronic arthritis. Acta Paediatr Suppl 1999;88:100–105.

19. Bechtold S, Ripperger P, Hafner R, Said E, Schwarz HP. Growth hormone improves height in patients with juvenile idiopathic arthritis: 4-year data of a controlled study. J Pediatr 2003;143:512–519.

20. Stagi S, Giani T, Simonini G, Falcini F. Thyroid function, autoimmune thyroiditis and celiac disease in juvenile idiopathic arthritis. Rheumatology (Oxford) 2005;44: 517–520.

21. Apigiani MG, Cerboni M, Bertini I, et al. Endocrine auto-immunity in young patients with juvenile chronic arthritis. Clin Exp Rheumatol 2002;20:565–568.

22. Henderson CT, Lovell DJ. Assessment of protein energy malnutrition in children and adolescents with JRA. Arthritis Care Res 1989;2:108–113.

23. Bacon MC, White PH, Raith DJ, et al. Nutritional status and growth in JRA. Semin Arthritis Rheum 1990;20: 97–106.

24. Cleary AG, Lancaster GA, Annan F, Sills JA, Davidson JE. Nutritional impairment in juvenile idiopathic arthritis. Rheumatology (Oxford) 2004;43:1569–1573.

25. Berk AT, Kocak N, Unsal E. Uveitis in juvenile arthritis. Ocul Immunol Inflamm 2001;9:243–251.

26. Kodsi SR, Rubin SE, Milojevic D, Ilowite N, Gottlieb B. Time of onset of uveitis in children with juvenile rheumatoid arthritis. J AAPOS 2002;6:373–376.

27. Cassidy J, Kivlin J, Lindsley C, Nocton J, Section of Rheumatology, Section of Opthalmology. Opthalmologic examinations in children with juvenile rheumatoid arthritis. Pediatrics 2006;117:1843–1845.

28. Ozdal PC, Vianna RN, Deschenes J. Visual outcome of juvenile rheumatoid arthritis-associated uveitis in adults. Ocul Immunol Inflamm 2005;13:33–38.

29. Paroli MP, Speranza S, Marino M, Pirraglia MP, Pivetti-Pezzi P. Prognosis of juvenile rheumatoid arthritis-associated uveitis. Eur J Ophthalmol 2003;13:616–621.

30. Rapoff MA, Belmont J, Lindsley C, Olson N, Morris J, Padur J. Prevention of nonadherence to nonsteroidal anti-inflammatory medications for newly diagnosed patients with juvenile rheumatoid arthritis. Health Psychol 2002; 21:620–623.

31. Rapoff MA. Compliance with treatment regimens for pediatric rheumatic diseases. Arthritis Care Res 1989; 2(Suppl):40–47.

32. Pieper KB, Rapoff MA, Purviance MR, Lindsley CB. Improving compliance with prednisone therapy in pediatric patients with rheumatic disease. Arthritis Care Res 1989;2:132–135.

33. Rapoff MA. Adherence to pediatric medical regimens. New York: Kluwer Academic/Plenum Publishers; 1999.

34. Rapoff MA, Belmont JM, Lindsley CB, Olson NY. Electronically monitored adherence to medications by newly diagnosed patients with juvenile rheumatoid arthritis. Arthritis Rheum 2005;53:905–910.

35. Gortmaker SL, Walker DK, Weitzman M, Sobol AM. Chronic conditions, socio-economic risks and behavioral problems in children and adolescents. Pediatrics 1990;85: 267–276.

36. Vandvik IH. Mental health and psychosocial functioning in children with recent onset of rheumatic disease. J Child Psychol Psychiatry 1990;31:961–971.

37. Huygen ACJ, Kuis W, Sinnema G. Psychological, behavioural, and social adjustment in children and adolescents with juvenile chronic arthritis. Ann Rheum Dis 2000;59: 276–282.

38. Frank RG, Hagglund KJ, Schopp LH, et al. Disease and family contributors to adaptation in juvenile rheumatoid arthritis and juvenile diabetes. Arthritis Care Res 1998; 11:166–176.

39. Aasland A, Flato B, Vandvik IH. Psychosocial outcome in juvenile chronic arthritis: a nine-year follow-up. Clin Exp Rheumatol 1997;15:561–568.

40. Hagglund KJ, Doyle NM, Clay DL, Frank RG, Johnson JC, Pressly TA. A family retreat as a comprehensive intervention for children with arthritis and their families. Arthritis Care Res 1996;9:35–41.

41. Reid GJ, Gilbert CA, McGrath PJ. The pain coping questionnaire: preliminary validation. Pain 1998;76:83–96.

42. Varni JW, Rapoff MA, Waldron SA, Gragg RA, Bernstein BH, Lindsley CB. Chronic pain and emotional distress in children and adolescents. J Dev Behav Pediatr 1996;17:154–161.

43. Sturge C, Garralda ME, Boissin M, Doré CJ, Woo P. School attendance and juvenile chronic arthritis. Br J Rheumatol 1997;36:1218–1223.

44. Peterson LS, Mason T, Nelson AM, O'Fallon WM, Gabriel SE. Psychosocial outcomes and health status of adults who have had juvenile rheumatoid arthritis: a controlled, population-based study. Arthritis Rheum 1997; 40:2235–2240.

Psoriatic Arthritis
A. Clinical Features

DAFNA D. GLADMAN, MD, FRCPC

- Psoriatic arthritis (PsA) occurs in approximately 26% of patients with psoriasis, leading to prevalence in the population of 0.3% to 1%.
- There are multiple clinical subsets of PsA reflecting variable clinical patterns including: distal joint disease, arthritis mutilans, oligoarthritis (less than or equal to four joints), rheumatoid arthritis (RA)-like polyarthritis, and spondylitis.

- Other musculoskeletal features include dactylitis (sausage digit), tenosynovitis, and enthesitis.
- Patients with PsA may also have iritis, urethritis, nonspecific colitis, and cardiovascular manifestations.
- Diagnosis is made on clinical grounds in patients with psoriasis having skin, scalp, or nail changes. Rheumatoid factor should be negative.

Psoriatic arthritis (PsA) is an inflammatory arthritis associated with psoriasis (1). Psoriasis is an inflammatory skin condition that presents with a red scaly rash often on the extensor surfaces but may also affect the scalp and flexural areas as well as palms and soles (2). It commonly affects the nails with either pits or onycholysis. Up to one third of patients with psoriasis may develop an inflammatory arthritis presenting with pain and stiffness in the affected joints. Both psoriasis and PsA affect men and women equally. PsA was distinguished from rheumatoid arthritis (RA), the prototype inflammatory arthritis, in the middle of the past century with the discovery of rheumatoid factor (RF). Whereas 85% of patients with RA are RF positive, patients with psoriatic arthritis are usually seronegative for RF. Earlier studies using the latex fixation test suggested that up to 15% of patients with PsA were seropositive (3), but more recent studies using either nephelometry or enzyme-linked immunosorbent assay (ELISA) tests reveal a prevalence of only 4% to 5% (4).

Several other features distinguish PsA from RA, including the equal gender frequency, the pattern of joint involvement, the presence of spinal involvement, and specific radiologic features. Because of the seronegative RF, the spinal involvement, and other extra-articular features seen among patients with PsA, as well as the association with human leukocyte antigen (HLA)-B27, PsA has been classified among the seronegative spondyloarthropathies.

EPIDMEMIOLOGY OF PSORIATIC ARTHRITIS

Prevalence of Psoriatic Arthritis

The exact prevalence of PsA is unknown. Estimates have varied from 0.1% to over 1% of the population (5,6). This variation may be related to the fact that there are no valid diagnostic criteria for the disease and various studies have used different case definitions. Moreover, some studies used administrative databases, some used population surveys, and others used clinical observations within hospital admissions or clinic attendees. The incidence of PsA has also varied and its true value remains unknown.

The prevalence of PsA among patients with psoriasis has varied from 6% in the Mayo Clinic (7) study to 30% in the European survey (Table 8A-1) (8). It should be noted that the Mayo Clinic study was based on an administrative database and accepted the database diagnosis of psoriasis, whereas the European survey was administered to members of a psoriasis association. A recent survey performed through the National Psoriasis Foundation in the United States identified an overall prevalence of PsA among patients with psoriasis at 11%, but this value increased to 56% when the extent of psoriasis exceeded 10 palms (9). An Italian study that was based at a clinic where dermatologists and rheuma-

TABLE 8A-1. FREQUENCY OF PSORIATIC ARTHRITIS AMONG PATIENTS WITH PSORIASIS.

AUTHOR (YEAR; REFERENCE)	CENTER	NUMBER OF PATIENTS STUDIED	PERCENTAGE PSA
Leczinsky (1948) (64)	Sweden	534	7
Vilanova (1951) (65)	Barcelona	214	25
Little (1975) (66)	Toronto	100	32
Leonard (1978) (67)	Rochester	77	39
Green (1981) (68)	Cape Town	61	42
Scarpa (1984) (10)	Naples	180	34
Stern (1985) (69)	Boston	1285	20
Zanelli (1992) (70)	Winston-Salem	459	17
Falk (1993) (71)	Kautokeino	35	17
Barisic-Drusko (1994) (72)	Osijek region	553	10
Salvarani (1995) (73)	Reggio-Emilia	205	36
Shbeeb (2000) (7)	Mayo Clinic	1056	6.25
Brockbank (2001) (74)	Toronto	126	31
Alenius (2002) (75)	Sweden	276	48
Zachariae (2003) (8)	Denmark	5795	30
Gelfand (2005) (9)	United States	601	11

tologists see patients together, identified 33% of the patients as having psoriasis (10). As can be seen in Table 8A-1, the frequency estimates for PsA among patients with psoriasis average 26%. If the prevalence of psoriasis is 1% to 3% of the population, then the true prevalence of PsA is more likely between 0.3% and 1%. A definite prevalence figure awaits valid diagnostic criteria for this disease.

Classification Criteria

Several sets of classification criteria for PsA have been proposed, although only one was derived from clinical data (11). Taylor and colleagues (12) compared several classification criteria sets for PsA. Most criteria sets were highly sensitive and specific, but the Fournie criteria (11) require HLA typing and therefore 24% of patients could not be classified. The CASPAR (Classification of Psoriatic Arthritis) group, an international group gathered to develop classification criteria for PsA, recently completed its study of the classification of PsA (4). It proposed a new set of criteria for classification of PsA which were 99% specific and 92% sensitive for PsA (Table 8A-2).

CLINICAL FEATURES OF PSORIATIC ARTHRITIS

Clinical Subsets of Psoriatic Arthritis

Psoriatic arthritis affects both peripheral joints and the axial skeleton. Wright and Moll described the clinical patterns of PsA (1). These include (1) a predominantly distal joint disease, which they identified in about 5% of their patients, and which have been variably recognized by other groups (3,10,13–21); (2) arthritis mutilans, a very destructive form of arthritis, which they identified in 5% of the patients, but which may be more frequent; (3) oligoarthritis, affecting four or fewer joints, often in an asymmetric distribution which they observed in 70% of the patients; (4) polyarthritis, indistinguishable from RA, which they detected in 15% of the patients; (5) spondyloarthritis, which occurs alone in about 5% of the patients, but may be associated with one of the other forms in about 40% of the patients. It has now been recognized that while these patterns may be helpful at disease onset, they do not stay stable over time (17,22,23). Moreover, it has been recognized that

8

TABLE 8A-2. CASPAR CRITERIA.

INFLAMMATORY ARTICULAR DISEASE (JOINT, SPINE, OR ENTHESEAL)

With 3 or more points from the following:

1. Evidence of psoriasis (one of a, b, c)	(a) Current psoriasis[a]	Psoriatic skin or scalp disease present today as judged by a rheumatologist or dermatologist
	(b) Personal history of psoriasis	A history of psoriasis that may be obtained from patient, family doctor, dermatologist, rheumatologist, or other qualified health care provider
	(c) Family history of psoriasis	A history of psoriasis in a first- or second-degree relative according to patient report
2. Psoriatic nail dystrophy		Typical psoriatic nail dystrophy including onycholysis, pitting, and hyperkeratosis observed on current physical examination
3. A negative test for rheumatoid factor		By any method except latex but preferably by ELISA or nephelometry, according to the local laboratory reference range
4. Dactylitis (one of a, b)	(a) Current	Swelling of an entire digit
	(b) History	A history of dactylitis recorded by a rheumatologist
5. Radiological evidence of juxta-articular new bone formation		Ill-defined ossification near joint margins (but excluding osteophyte formation) on plain x-rays of hand or foot

SOURCE: The CASPAR Study Group, Arthritis Rheum 2006;54:2665–2673, with permission of *Arthritis and Rheumatism*.
Specificity, 98.7%; sensitivity, 91.4%.
[a] Current psoriasis scores 2, whereas all other items score 1.

the symmetry is a function of the number of joints involved (24). Indeed, with established disease most patients with PsA present with polyarthritis (3,6).

We have recorded the patterns according to distal, oligoarthritis, polyarthritis alone or in combination with spinal disease, as well as isolated spinal disease (3,19). Because arthritis mutilans could occur within any of these groups it has not been identified as an isolated group. This classification was found to be 97% sensitive and 99% specific for PsA (12). A review of 705 patients followed prospectively at the University of Toronto PsA Clinic reveals that at presentation, 3.7% have predominantly distal joint disease but over 50% of the patients have distal joint involvement in association with another pattern. Arthritis mutilans, defined as at least one totally destroyed joint, was detected in 19.5%, whereas five or more totally destroyed joints were detected in 8.2% of the patients (Table 8A-3).

Peripheral Arthritis in Psoriatic Arthritis

The arthritis of PsA is inflammatory in nature, presenting with pain, swelling, and stiffness in the affected joints. Any joint may be affected. Early in the disease course the arthritis tends to be oligoarticular, but may become polyarticular as more joints are accrued over time. There are several clinical characteristics of the peripheral arthritis in PsA regardless of the clinical pattern. Patients with PsA are not as tender as patients

with RA (25). This has practical implications both in terms of recognizing the presence of arthritis by the patients and physicians, and therefore the ability to diagnose the condition, and in terms of recognizing the need for therapy. Many patients present with deformity and joint damage, not having perceived any pain during the inflammatory phase of their disease. The presence of a bluish/purplish discoloration over the inflamed joint is typical for seronegative disease, including PsA, and may help differentiate PsA from RA even in the absence of obvious psoriasis (26). The distribution of the affected joints is another typical feature of PsA. Whereas RA tends to involve joints along the same level (all metacarpophalangeal joints, all proximal interphalangeal joints) in a symmetric distribution, PsA affects all the joints of one digit, in a ray pattern, giving the asymmetric distribution typical for the disease. Thus, the presence of distal joint inflammation as well as the ray pattern are key features in PsA (Figure 8A-1).

Psoriatic Spondyloarthritis

Spinal involvement in PsA includes inflammation in both the sacroiliac joints and the apophyseal joints of the spine. The distribution in PsA tends to be asymmetric, with only one sacroiliac joint involved and the other being spared, or with a different degree of involvement noted on sacroiliac radiographs. Likewise, the spinal involvement tends to be asymmetric, and with skip lesions (Figure 8A-2). Nonetheless, all levels of the spine may be involved (27–30). The prevalence of spinal

TABLE 8A-3. PATTERNS OF PSORIATIC ARTHRITIS.[a]

Number of patients	705
Age at onset skin (mean [SD])	28.8 (14.4)
Age at onset joints	36.1 (13.2)
Gender	57% male, 43% female
Age at presentation	43.7 (13.3)
Number of inflamed joints	10.2 (9.6)
Number of damaged joints Clinical Radiological	 3.2 (7.5) 4.8 (8.1)

PATTERN	AT PRESENTATION (%)	LAST VISIT (%)
Distal	3.7	1.6
Oligoarthritis	14.7	8.5
Polyarthritis	39.3	30.6
Back alone	2.4	1.4
Back plus distal	2.6	1.1
Back plus oligoarthritis	7.4	10.1
Back plus polyarthritis	29.9	45.7
Remission	0	1.1
Arthritis mutilans ≥1 joint with stage 4 radiological damage ≥5 joints with stage 4 radiological damage	 19.5 8.2	 36.4 18.2

[a] Data from the University of Toronto Clinic, Toronto, Ontario, Canada.

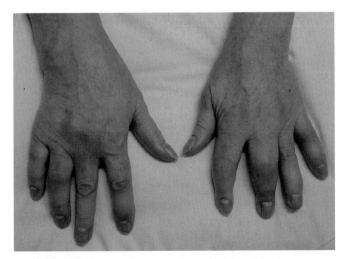

FIGURE 8A-1

Ray distribution peripheral arthritis. Note the involvement of the second, third, and fifth digits on the left hand, while the third right digit is totally spared.

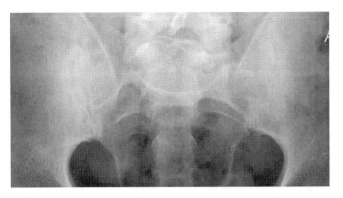

FIGURE 8A-2

Asymmetric sacroiliitis, skip syndesmophytes.

involvement in PsA has been variable, partly due to the definition used by the investigators. If radiographs are performed on each patient, then sacroiliitis may be detected quite frequently. In one study it was reported in 78% of the patients (30). After 10 years of observation, some 50% of the patients in the University of Toronto PsA Clinic have demonstrated evidence of spinal involvement defined by the presence of sacroiliitis and/or syndesmophytes. However, only a portion of these patients have clinical complaints of either pain or morning stiffness. Indeed, patients with psoriatic spondylitis do not complain of as much pain, and do not exhibit as much spinal limitation as patients with idiopathic ankylosing spondylitis (31). This may be the result of the generalized lower pain threshold noted among these patients, as well as from the fact that the disease itself may not be as severe, because fewer patients with psoriatic spondyloarthritis present with grade 4 sacroiliitis and they have fewer syndesmophytes than patients with ankylosing spondylitis (31).

OTHER ARTICULAR MANIFESTATIONS IN PSORIATIC ARTHRITIS

Dactylitis

Dactylitis, or sausage digit, is a typical feature of PsA. It refers to inflammation of the whole digit. It likely results from both synovitis in the joints of the digit, as well as tenosynovitis, particularly in the flexor tendons (32,33). Dactylitis most commonly affects the toes, but fingers are affected as well (34). Joints within digits that demonstrated acute dactylitis were more likely to develop erosions than those in digits without dactylitis, suggesting that the presence of dactylitis is prognostic for disease progression (34). It should be noted that dactylitis may become chronic, such that it is no longer painful or red, but remains as a chronically swollen digit, which may not respond to therapeutic intervention. Helliwell and colleagues (35) proposed a method for assessing dactylitis that may be useful in clinical trials and in clinical observational cohort studies. Recently, swelling of the extremity has been recognized as a feature of PsA (36). The exact mechanism of this peripheral edema is unclear but both lymphedema and tenosynovitis may play a role (37).

Tenosynovitis

Tendonitis or tenosynovitis occurs frequently among patients with PsA. Inflammation may affect the flexor tendons of the fingers, as well as the extensor carpi ulnaris, sites that are commonly affected in RA. Achilles tendonitis is commonly seen, as is plantar fasciitis. These may interfere with function and may lead to disability. In PsA, tendonitis may be associated with tendon nodules and significant functional limitation.

Enthesitis

Inflammation of the enthesis, site of insertion of tendon into bone, is another typical feature of PsA. Enthesitis may occur at any tendon insertion site, but most commonly affects the plantar fascia, Achilles tendon insertion, insertion of tendons at the knee and shoulder, as well as the pelvic bones. It has been suggested that enthesitis alone in the presence of psoriasis may be sufficient for the diagnosis of PsA (38). Indeed, the CASPAR criteria require the presence of any inflammatory musculoskeletal features, including enthesitis, together with three other features to classify a patient as having PsA (4).

EXTRA-ARTICULAR FEATURES OF PSORIATIC ARTHRITIS

Skin Disease

Skin psoriasis is a prerequisite for the diagnosis of psoriatic arthritis. There are several clinical presentations of psoriasis (2). Psoriasis vulgaris is the most common type and the most commonly associated with psoriatic arthritis. If affects the extensor surfaces, particularly elbows and knees. Psoriasis vulgaris may also affect the scalp, the gluteal folds, as well the anal cleft. Psoriasis may affect flexural areas primarily, in which case it would be hidden unless the patients are asked about it, or are totally undressed for the physical examination. Guttate psoriasis may also be associated with psoriatic arthritis, but is less common than psoriasis vulgaris (6). The most severe form of psoriasis is the erythrodermic type.

The relationship between skin and joint disease is variable (39,40). There may be a stronger association in patients whose skin and joint manifestations began simultaneously (40). It has been noted that in clinical trials for PsA the degree of skin disease is not as high as it is in clinical trials in psoriasis patients. Nail lesions have been observed in a higher frequency among patients with PsA compared to uncomplicated psoriasis (41). These may be associated with distal interphalangeal joint disease.

Other Extra-Articular Manifestations

Iritis is an extra-articular feature common to all spondyloarthropathies and is also seen among patients with PsA. Some 7% of patients with PsA present with iritis, and it can also be seen among patients with psoriasis without arthritis (3,41).

Urethritis is also a feature of seronegative disease. It is less common in PsA than in the other members of the spondyloarthritis group.

Bowel involvement may occur in patients with PsA and is usually nonspecific colitis (42,43).

Cardiac abnormalities have been reported among patients with PsA, including dilatation of the base of the aortic arch which occurs in ankylosing spondylitis. More recently it has been recognized that patients with PsA are at risk for cardiovascular disease (44). This may be related to the metabolic abnormalities associated with PsA, including hyperlipidemia, hyperuricemia, as well as lifestyle factors such as obesity and smoking (44,45).

DIAGNOSING PSORIATIC ARTHRITIS

The diagnosis of PsA should be considered in any patient who presents with an inflammatory arthritis in the presence of psoriasis. However, not all patients with psoriasis presenting with arthritis have PsA. PsA must be distinguished from RA. Because psoriasis occurs in 1% to 3% of the population and RA occurs in about 1%, the chance of a patient having both RA and psoriasis is 1:10,000. If a patient with psoriasis and inflammatory arthritis has rheumatoid nodules, they are more likely to have coexistence of RA with psoriasis. On the other hand, if they are RF negative, have distal interphalangeal joint disease, and have nail lesions, they are much more likely to have PsA even if they present with a symmetric polyarthritis. The presence of spinal disease also tips the balance towards PsA. Because of the involvement of distal joint disease, PsA must be distinguished from osteoarthritis. Osteoarthritis is primarily not an inflammatory disease. Therefore, if the distal interphalangeal joints are inflamed with redness and swelling, especially in the context of nail lesions, the patient is much more likely to have PsA. In patients with mono- or oligoarticular presentation, PsA must be differentiated from gout. Because patients with PsA may have an elevated serum uric acid, it is important to obtain synovial fluid for crystal analysis to determine the underlying pathophysiology.

Patients with PsA who present with inflammatory spinal disease must be differentiated from other spondyloarthropathies. Because psoriasis may be associated with Crohn's disease, with the latter being associated with spondylitis, it may be difficult to differentiate. However, as noted above, the spinal involvement in PsA tends to be asymmetric, whereas in ankylosing spondylitis and inflammatory bowel disease the spinal disease tends to be symmetric. The presence of nail lesions suggests the diagnosis of PsA (46).

COURSE AND OUTCOME IN PSORIATIC ARTHRITIS

In the past, patients with PsA were thought to have a milder disease than patients with rheumatoid arthritis (47). However, over the past 20 years it has become clear that the disease is more severe than previously thought. A study of 220 patients with PsA demonstrated that 67% of the patients had erosive disease at presentation to clinic, and 20% of the patients had a very severe form of arthritis, similar to what had been reported for RA (3). More recently, 47% of the patients with PsA seen in clinic within 5 months of onset were found to have erosive disease by 2 years (48). Patients with PsA demonstrate disease progression over time, with more patients developing polyarthritis and an increase in joint damage both clinically and radiologically (23,49). While progression of damage may be determined first by radiographs, clinical damage may be observed at each clinic visit and should be recorded (50).

Predictors for Disease Progression

Predictors for the progression of clinical damage include polyarticular presentation and a high medication level at presentation to clinic (51,52). The number of actively inflamed joints present at each visit predict progression of clinical damage in subsequent visits (53). HLA markers may influence outcome in both positive and negative ways (see Chapter 8B). However, 17.6% of the patients with PsA sustained a remission, defined as no actively inflamed joints for at least 1 year (11,54). The remission lasted 2.6 years on average, and was associated with male gender and less active and severe disease at presentation to clinic.

Quality of Life in Psoriatic Arthritis

Patients with PsA demonstrate reduced quality of life and function compared to the general population (55,56). Indeed, quality of life among patients with PsA was similar to that of patients with RA (57). Patients with PsA exhibited more vitality, but also more bodily pain than patients with RA (58). While 28% of the patients did not demonstrate disability over a 10-year period, female sex and older age were associated with more disability, while longer disease duration was associated with no change in disability (59).

Mortality in Psoriatic Arthritis

Patients with PsA are at an increased risk of death compared to the general population (60). While the causes of death are similar to those seen in the general population, disease activity and severity at presentation are predictive of early mortality in patients with PsA (61). Survival in PsA seems to have improved in the past 30 years, with the most recent standardized mortality ratio reducing from 1.62 to 1.36 (62). It is possible that more aggressive therapeutic approaches have helped improve survival (63). A recent study demonstrated that there is no increased malignancy risk among patients with PsA followed over 25 years.

SUMMARY

Psoriatic arthritis is an inflammatory arthritis associated with psoriasis, usually seronegative for RF. It presents in a number of clinical patterns. PsA may be severely disabling and is associated with an increased mortality risk. Patients with PsA should be diagnosed early and treated promptly and aggressively in order to prevent these untoward outcomes.

REFERENCES

1. Wright V, Moll JMH. Psoriatic arthritis. In: Seronegative polyarthritis. Amsterdam: North Holland Publishing; 1976:169–223.
2. Langley RGB, Krueger GG, Griffiths CEM. Psoriasis: epidemiology, clinical features and quality of life. Ann Rheum Dis 2005;64:18–23.
3. Gladman DD, Shuckett R, Russell ML, et al. Psoriatic arthritis (PSA)—an analysis of 220 patients. Q J Med 1987;62:127–141.

8

Psoriatic Arthritis
B. Pathology and Pathogenesis

Christopher Ritchlin, MD

- Psoriatic arthritis (PsA) histopathology differs from rheumatoid arthritis (RA), with the most striking difference in the characteristic of the synovial vasculature.
- Psoriatic arthritis is triggered by interaction between genetic and environmental factors with initiating events occurring in the skin and/or gut.

- Cellular immunity and cytokines, including tumor necrosis factor alpha (TNF-alpha), are important mediators of PsA.
- Osteoclasts are important mediators of dysregulated bone remodeling in PsA.

Psoriatic arthritis (PsA) is an inflammatory arthritis associated with psoriasis that is usually negative for rheumatoid factor (RF). Inflammation can target a range of musculoskeletal structures, including the axial skeleton, peripheral joints, attachment sites of ligaments, tendons or joint capsules onto bone (entheses), and tendon sheaths. Joint manifestations may be highly localized and mild in some patients, while others may experience widespread inflammation and damage that results in significant functional decline. Moreover, as discussed in the previous chapter, several clinical subsets of PsA have been described (symmetric polyarthritis, asymmetric oligoarticular arthritis, spondylitis, arthritis mutilans, and predominant distal interphalangeal disease) and it is not known whether these distinct clinical entities are orchestrated by the same disease mechanisms. Joint dysfunction can arise not only as a result of bone resorption and cartilage degradation, but also from diffuse soft tissue inflammation (dactylitis) and new bone formation in the form of ankylosis or periostitis.

PATHOLOGY

The histologic changes in the peripheral joints are similar to those observed in rheumatoid arthritis (RA) but important distinctions have been noted. One of the most prominent features is a striking increase in synovial vascularity, characterized at the macroscopic level by dilated and tortuous blood vessels that contrast sharply with the linear pattern observed in RA (1). At the histologic and ultrastructural level, psoriatic syno-

vial vasculature displayed endothelial cell swelling, inflammatory cell infiltration, and marked thickening of the vessel wall (2). Monocytoid cells infiltrate the sub-synovium but in PsA the numbers are less than in RA. Immunopathologic features observed more commonly in PsA compared to RA were increased vascularity, prominent neutrophil infiltration, and increased expression of the mature monocyte marker CD163 by subsynovial monocytes (3). Infiltrating CD4+ lymphocytes predominate in the synovial tissue, whereas CD8+ T cells are present in the synovial fluid (4,5). Ectopic lymphoid aggregates have been noted in psoriatic synovium. No significant pathologic differences were found between oligo- or polyarticular PsA and the psoriatic synovial histology was more similar to other forms of spondyloarthropathies (SpA) than to RA (6).

The inflamed synovial membrane or pannus, comprised of fibroblastoid cells and activated macrophages, is invasively destructive. Fibroblastoid cells release metalloproteinases (MMP)-1, 2, and 3, which degrade cartilage, while MMP-9 is localized to vessel walls (7). Osteoclasts are present in deep resorption pits at the bone–pannus junction. Biopsies of entheseal inflammation sites revealed CD8+ T cells in the underlying subchondral bone and macrophages infiltrating the tendon (8,9). Studies of bone and synovium from patients with axial PsA have not been performed, but imaging studies suggest an entheseal-based pathology with prominent osteitis in the underlying bone (Figure 8B-1) (10). Dactylitis is most likely a form of flexor tenosynovitis, although pathologic studies of involved digits have not been published.

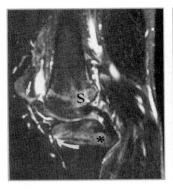
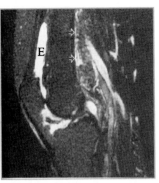

FIGURE 8B-1

Fat-suppressed T2 weighted magnetic resonance imaging (MRI) scans in PsA and RA. In the left panel, a psoriatic knee demonstrates extensive bone marrow edema in three areas: the anterior patella (*straight arrow*), superior insertion of the posterior cruciate ligament (S), and marked subchondral bone marrow edema in the tibial plateau, especially at the patellar tendon insertion (*curved arrow*) and the inferior insertion of posterior cruciate ligament (*). In the right panel, a rheumatoid knee shows a joint effusion (E) and focal increased signal limited to vessels behind the femur. (Modified from McGonagle D et al., *Arthritis Rheum* 1998;41:694–700, with permission of *Arthritis and Rheumatism* and Wiley Periodicals, Inc.)

PATHOGENESIS

In the current paradigm, PsA is triggered by a complex interaction between genetic and environmental factors. Given the temporal relationship with psoriasis, it is likely that the initiating events involve both innate and acquired immune responses that arise in the skin and spread to the joint in susceptible individuals. Recent studies have underscored the central role of inflammatory cytokines in joint inflammation and destruction. Treatment interventions directed at these molecules have provided effective treatment options and uncovered novel disease mechanisms.

Genetic Basis of Psoriatic Arthritis

Moll and Wright found that 5.5% of first-degree relatives of PsA probands developed inflammatory arthritis—an inheritability risk that is greater than observed in psoriasis (11). Several genetic loci have been implicated in the predisposition to psoriasis and PsA, but the strongest effect has been linked to alleles in the major histocompatibility complex (MHC). Earlier association studies in PsA focused attention on HLA-Cw6, in addition to HLA-B13 and -B17 (B57). These associations reflect the strong linkage disequilibrium between HLA-Cw6 and HLA-B57, and HLA-Cw6 and HLA-B13, which extends into the MHC class II region. In individuals with PsA, the association with HLA-Cw6

is slightly weaker than in psoriasis. A smaller proportion of cases have an association with HLA-B27, chiefly in patients with predominant spinal disease. HLA-B27 in the presence of HLA-DR7 and HLA-DQw3 in the absence of HLA-DR7 predict progression, while HLA-B22 is protective. Other reports noted an association with HLA-B38 and -B39, as well as with other alleles in linkage disequilibrium. The presence of HLA-DR*04 shared epitope is associated with worse radiological damage (12,13).

Major histocompatibility complex class I molecules could promote PsA by presenting arthritogenic peptides to CD8+ lymphocytes or by selection of a T-cell repertoire that is autoreactive in skin and joints. Another mechanism recently described indicates that natural killer (NK) cell activity is controlled through interactions between killer immmunoglobulinlike receptors (KIR) and MHC class I genes, particularly Cw6. PsA patients have a genetic profile of KIR alleles that lower the threshold for NK activations (14). Two recent reports have also found associations of PsA with interleukin 1 (IL-1) and tumor necrosis factor (TNF) alleles (15,16).

It should be emphasized that the great majority of these studies have been performed in cases or families ascertained by the presence of psoriasis. Thus, to dissect disease associations specific to arthritis, two separate cohorts of psoriasis patients (with and without arthritis) must be characterized and genotyped. Furthermore, the finding that relevant HLA class I MHC alleles occur in less than 50% of PsA patients may reflect involvement of non-HLA genes in the causal pathway.

Environmental Factors

Compelling evidence suggests that trauma and infection play a role in the etiologic pathway of PsA. Koebner phenomenon, described as psoriatic lesions arising at sites of trauma, occurs in 24% to 52% of psoriasis patients (17). The development of PsA following trauma to a joint, with the suggested name of the *deep Koebner phenomenon*, has also been reported in the Toronto longitudinal observational cohort, where 50 of 203 (24.6%) patients reported a traumatic event prior to the diagnosis of PsA (18). Subclinical trauma may also contribute to the distal interphalangeal (DIP) joint arthritis, dactylitis, and enthesitis, although this relationship has not been formally studied. It is also important to note that a history of trauma has been reported in only a minority of PsA patients.

Some studies suggest involvement of bacterial agents in psoriasis and possibly PsA. A strikingly high association between guttate psoriasis and preceding streptococcal pharyngitis and tonsillitis exists in children (19). The link between Gram-positive infection and PsA was suggested by high levels of circulating antibodies to

8

microbial peptidoglycans and elevated levels of group A streptococcus 16S RNA in the peripheral blood of PsA patients (20). Both streptococcal and staphylococcal superantigens promote inflammation and upregulation of keratinocyte TNF in noninvolved psoriatic skin, but not other inflammatory dermatoses, elucidating the potential importance of this novel immune pathway in psoriasis (21).

Cellular Activation and Cytokine Pathways in Psoriatic Arthritis

Recent evidence indicates that cells of the innate immune system may direct the early events in psoriatic joint inflammation. The effector cells of the innate response are keratinocytes, dendritic cells, neutrophils, monocytes/macrophages, and NK cells. In a mouse model of PsA, targeted keratinocyte deletion of JunB and c-Jun, components of the AP-1 transcription factor that is involved in cellular differentiation and proliferation, resulted in psoriasiform skin lesions and subsequent arthritis with features of joint destruction and new bone formation (22). This model demonstrated that disruption of keratinocye function could promote an inflammatory response in the skin that spreads to the joint via mechanisms that involve T cells and TNF signaling pathways. Activated plasmacytoid and monocytoid dendritic cells (DC) have been detected in the dermis of psoriasis plaques and both of these DC subsets were isolated from PsA joint fluid (23). As previously mentioned, prominent neutrophil and monocyte infiltrates are present in psoriatic skin and synovium. The role of NK cells in PsA has not been elucidated, but the finding that specific alleles associated with NK cell receptor are associated with susceptibility to psoriasis and PsA suggests that they may contribute to the pathogenesis (14). Moreover, cytokines involved in the innate immune response have been detected in psoriatic synovium, including IL-1, IL-8, IL-15, and TNF-alpha (24).

Several lines of evidence demonstrate that TNF-alpha is a pivotal cytokine in psoriatic joint inflammation. First, elevated levels of TNF-alpha have been detected in joint fluid and in psoriatic synovial supernatants (24). Second, immunohistochemical studies demonstrated upregulation of TNF-alpha in the psoriatic synovial membrane and skin (25,26). Third, histopathologic analysis of synovial specimens from PsA patients treated with anti-TNF agents revealed decreased vascularity, synovial lining thickness, and mononuclear cell infiltration following treatment (Figure 8B-2) (27,28). Fourth, clinical trials revealed that anti-TNF agents significantly lessen inflammation in the psoriatic plaque, entheses, flexor tendons, and the axial skeleton (see Chapter 8C) (29).

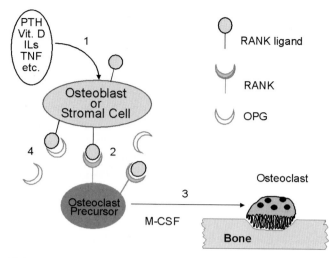

FIGURE 8B-2

Representative images of CD3+ and CD68+ immunohistochemical staining and TUNEL assay in psoriatic synovial tissues at baseline and 48 hours after initiation of infliximab therapy. A significant decline in infiltrating CD3+ T cells and CD68+ macrophages was noted. Therapy was not associated with increased apoptosis as measured by the TUNEL assay. (From Goedkoop AY et al., Ann Rheum Dis 2004;63:769–773, with permission of *Annals of the Rheumatic Diseases*.)

The role of the acquired immune response in psoriatic joint disease is not well understood but the strong association of psoriatic arthritis with MHC class I molecules suggests that CD8+ T lymphocytes may be pivotal in pathogenesis. Immunohistologic studies on psoriatic synovial membranes, however, revealed a predominance of CD45RO+ memory T cells in the synovial lining mononuclear cell infiltrate (30). In contrast, CD8+ T cells are the principal lymphocytes in synovial fluid, some of which demonstrate oligoclonal expansion of T-cell receptor (TCR) B chains, suggesting the presence of an antigen-driven response (5). Additional support for T-lymphocyte involvement came from studies on psoriatic synovial explant tissues which produced higher levels of the helper-T-lymphocyte (Th1) cytokines IL-2 and interferon gamma (INF-gamma) protein than explants similarly cultured from osteoarthritis and rheumatoid patients (24). In contrast, IL-4 and IL-5 were not identified in psoriatic explants. This Th1 profile has been observed in both psoriasis and RA. A similar pattern of cytokine production in psoriatic synovium was shown using immunohistochemical techniques (25).

Dysregulated Bone Remodeling in Psoriatic Arthritis

In regard to bone, psoriatic joint biopsies demonstrate large multinucleated osteoclasts in deep resorption pits at the bone–pannus junction (31). Osteoclastogenesis (differentiation of osteoclasts) is a contact-dependent process directed by osteoblasts and stromal cells in the bone marrow (Figure 8B-3) (32). These cells release two different signals necessary for differentiation of an osteoclast precursor (OCP), derived from the CD14+ monocyte population, into an osteoclast. The first, macrophage-colony stimulating factor (M-CSF) and the second, receptor activator of NF-κB ligand (RANKL), a member of the TNF superfamily, bind to RANK on the surface of OCP and osteoclasts. This ligand–receptor interaction stimulates proliferation and differentiation of OCP and activation of osteoclasts. Because permissive quantities of M-CSF are constitutively expressed in the bone microenvironment, it has been proposed that the relative expression of RANKL and its natural antagonist osteoprotegerin (OPG) ultimately control osteoclastogenesis. Interestingly, RANKL is also expressed by infiltrating T cells and synovial fibroblastoid cells in the synovial lining of inflamed joints.

In psoriatic synovial tissues, marked upregulation of RANKL protein and low expression of OPG was detected in the adjacent synovial lining Osteoclasts were also noted in cutting cones traversing the subchondral bone supporting a bidirectional attack on the bone

in psoriatic joints (31). In addition, OCP, derived from circulating CD14+ monocytes, were markedly elevated in the peripheral blood of PsA patients compared to healthy controls. Treatment of PsA patients with anti-TNF agents significantly decreased the level of circulating OCP, thus supporting a central role for TNF-alpha in the generation of this precursor population.

The mechanisms responsible for new bone formation in the psoriatic joint are poorly understood. Transforming growth factor (TGF) beta and vascular endothelial growth factor (VEGF) may be pivotal in this process given that TGF-alpha is strongly expressed in synovial tissues isolated from ankylosing spondylitis patients and synergizes with VEGF to induce bone formation in animal models (33,34). Male DBA/1 mice caged together develop an ankylosing enthesitis remarkably similar to lesions in PsA and bone morphogenetic proteins (BMP) 2 and 7 are upregulated in regions of pathologic new bone formation (35). In addition, expression of phosphorylated Smad 1 and Smad 5, important signaling molecules in the downstream BMP signaling pathway, was markedly increased in regions of new bone formation taken from the calcaneous in a patient with Achilles tendonitis and periostitis.

Before After

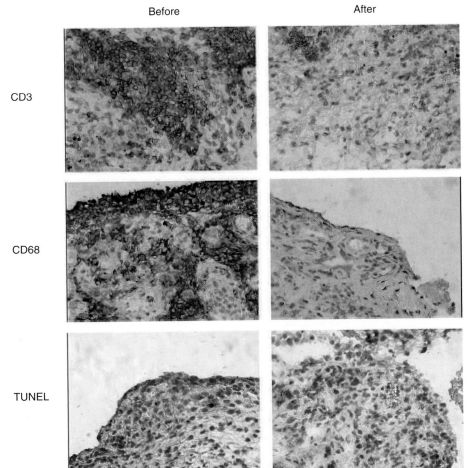

CD3

CD68

TUNEL

FIGURE 8B-3

Osteoclast differentiation. RANKL is expressed by osteoblasts and stromal cells in response to a variety of stimuli. In the inflamed joint, RANKL is expressed by fibroblastoid lining cells and infiltrating T lymphocytes. RANKL binds to the RANK receptor expressed on OCP and OC. In the presence of M-CSF and RANKL, OCP mature into OC capable of resorbing bone. OPG, a physiologic decoy molecule, can bind to RANKL and inhibit OC differentiation and activation. Abbreviations: RANKL, receptor activator of NF-κB ligand; OCP, osteoclast precursor; M-CSF, monocyte colony stimulating factor; OPG, osteoprotegerin.

8

Pathogenesis of Extra-Articular Psoriatic Arthritis

Gut and eye involvement are present in a subset of PsA patients. Subclinical gut inflammation was noted in 16% of 64 PsA patients on ileocolonoscopy, and this finding was limited to patients with oligoarthritis or spinal disease but not those with polyarthritis (36). Furthermore, PsA patients have an increased risk of inflammatory bowel disease compared to controls. Uveitis, both unilateral and bilateral, can occur in PsA patients, particularly in the subset with axial disease. Furthermore, both uveitis and bowel inflammation often respond to anti-TNF therapy. These clinical observations suggest a link between bowel inflammation, spondylitis, and eye disease in a subset of PsA patients that may be mediated in part by TNF. An alternative view has been proposed based on the concept of psoriatic disease in which psoriasis is viewed as a systemic disease that involves different anatomical sites in the same patient (37).

Taken together, the evidence suggests that trauma or infection in a genetically susceptible individual triggers PsA and that the initial inciting event probably occurs in the skin, resulting in activation of monocytes and T cells (Figure 8B-4). In the subset with spondylitis, the early events may arise in the gut. In some patients with psoriasis, local events in the joint promote angiogenesis followed by mononuclear cell activation accompanied by increased expression of TNF-alpha and RANKL. Circulating OCP enter the joint after binding to activated endothelial cells and undergo osteoclastogenesis and resorb bone. Elevated production of BMP and VEGF contribute to new bone formation, while MMPs released by synovial lining cells degrade cartilage and engage in blood vessel remodeling. Presumably, perpetual release of proinflammatory cytokines,

FIGURE 8B-4

PsA pathogenesis model. The major events in PsA begin in the skin (step 1) and spread to the joint (step 2). The genetic factors associated with skin or joint disease may not be identical. In step 1, DC are triggered by trauma, infection, or other signals to activate T cells. Activated T cells promote entry of monocytes into the dermis and release of TNF and other cytokines that lead to keratinocyte hyperplasia and PMNs infiltration. In step 2, activated monocytes and T cells leave the skin and enter the joint that has been subjected to trauma or infection, after binding to primed ECs. Vascular remodeling is directed by VEGF, MMP-9, and ang-2. TNF and other cytokines released by these infiltrating cells drive synovial cell hyperplasia. The lining cells promote osteoclastogenesis and subsequent bone resorption via RANKL expression and they release MMPs which mediate cartilage degradation. Inflammatory events in the subchondral bone foster enthesitis and osteitis. Activation of BMPs leads to new bone formation. Abbreviations: EC, endothelial cell; MΦ, monocyte/macrophage; MHC, major histocompatibility complex; MMP: metalloproteinase; ang-2, angiopoietin 2; VEGF, vascular endothelial growth factor; PMN, neutrophils; BMP, bone morphogenetic protein; KIR, killer immunoglobulin receptor.

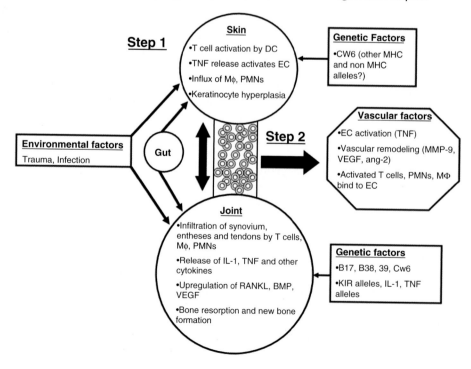

particularly TNF, leads to persistent synovitis, enthesitis, and progressive matrix degradation. The events that drive the chronic influx of mononuclear cells into the joint and sustained release of proinflammatory cytokines have not been elucidated.

REFERENCES

1. Reece RJ, Canete JD, Parsons WJ, Emery P, Veale DJ. Distinct vascular patterns of early synovitis in psoriatic, reactive, and rheumatoid arthritis. Arthritis Rheum 1999;42:1481–1484.
2. Espinoza LR, Vasey FB, Espinoza CG, Bocanegra TS, Germain BF. Vascular changes in psoriatic synovium. A light and electron microscopic study. Arthritis Rheum 1982;25:677–684.
3. Baeten D, Kruithof E, De Rycke L, et al. Infiltration of the synovial membrane with macrophage subsets and polymorphonuclear cells reflects global disease activity in spondyloarthropathy. Arthritis Res Ther 2005;7:R359–R369.
4. Smith MD, O'Donnell J, Highton J, Palmer DG, Rozenbilds M, Roberts-Thomson PJ. Immunohistochemical analysis of synovial membranes from inflammatory and non-inflammatory arthritides: scarcity of CD5 positive B cells and IL2 receptor bearing T cells. Pathology 1992;24:19–26.
5. Costello PJ, Winchester RJ, Curran SA, et al. Psoriatic arthritis joint fluids are characterized by CD8 and CD4 T cell clonal expansions appear antigen driven. J Immunol 2001;166:2878–2886.
6. Kruithof E, Baeten D, De Rycke L, et al. Synovial histopathology of psoriatic arthritis, both oligo- and polyarticular, resembles spondyloarthropathy more than it does rheumatoid arthritis [see comment]. Arthritis Res Ther 2005;7:R569–R580.
7. Kane D, Jensen LE, Grehan S, Whitehead AS, Bresnihan B, Fitzgerald O. Quantitation of metalloproteinase gene expression in rheumatoid and psoriatic arthritis synovial tissue distal and proximal to the cartilage-pannus junction. J Rheumatol 1274;31:1274–1280.
8. Laloux L, Voisin MC, Allain J, et al. Immunohistological study of entheses in spondyloarthropathies: comparison in rheumatoid arthritis and osteoarthritis. Ann Rheum Dis 2001;60:316–321.
9. McGonagle D, Marzo-Ortega H, O'Connor P, et al. Histological assessment of the early enthesitis lesion in spondyloarthropathy. Ann Rheum Dis 2002;61:534–537.
10. McGonagle D, Gibbon W, O'Connor P, Green M, Pease C, Emery P. Characteristic magnetic resonance imaging entheseal changes of knee synovitis in spondyloarthropathy. Arthritis Rheum 1998;41:694–700.
11. Moll JM. Psoriatic spondylitis: clinical radiological and familial aspects. Proc Roy Soc Med 1974;67:46–50.
12. Gladman DD, Farewell VT, Kopciuk K, et al. HLA markers and progression in psoriatic arthritis. J Rheumatol 1998;25:730–733.
13. Korendowych E, Dixey J, Cox B, Jones S, McHugh N. The Influence of the HLA-DRB1 rheumatoid arthritis shared epitope on the clinical characteristics and radiological outcome of psoriatic arthritis. J Rheumatol 2003;30:96–101.
14. Martin MP, Nelson G, Lee JH, et al. Cutting edge: susceptibility to psoriatic arthritis: influence of activating killer Ig-like receptor genes in the absence of specific HLA-C alleles. J Immunol 2002;169:2818–2822.
15. Rahman P, Sun S, Peddle L, et al. Association between the interleukin-1 family gene cluster and psoriatic arthritis. Arthritis Rheum 2006;54:2321–2325.
16. Rahman P, Siannis F, Butt C, et al. TNFalpha polymorphisms and risk of psoriatic arthritis. Ann Rheum Dis 2006;65:919–923.
17. Stankler L. An experimental investigation on the site of skin damage inducing the Koebner reaction in psoriasis. Br J Dermatol 1969;81:534–535.
18. Langevitz P, Buskila D, Gladman DD. Psoriatic arthritis precipitated by physical trauma. J Rheumatol 1990;17:695–697.
19. Rasmussen JE. The relationship between infection with group A beta hemolytic streptococci and the development of psoriasis. Pediatr Infect Dis J 2000;19:153–154.
20. Wang Q, Vasey FB, Mahfood JP, et al. V2 regions of 16S ribosomal RNA used as a molecular marker for the species identification of streptococci in peripheral blood and synovial fluid from patients with psoriatic arthritis. Arthritis Rheum 1999;42:2055–2059.
21. Travers JB, Hamid QA, Norris DA, et al. Epidermal HLA-DR and the enhancement of cutaneous reactivity to superantigenic toxins in psoriasis [comment]. J Clin Invest 1999;104:1181–1189.
22. Zenz R, Eferl R, Kenner L, et al. Psoriasis-like skin disease and arthritis caused by inducible epidermal deletion of Jun proteins. Nature 2005;437:369–375.
23. Jongbloed S, Lebre M, Fraser A, et al. Enumeration and phenotypical analysis of distinct dendritic cell subsets in psoriatic arthritis and rheumatoid arthritis. Ann Rheum Dis 2005;8:R14.
24. Ritchlin C, Haas-Smith SA, Hicks D, Cappuccio J, Osterland CK, Looney RJ. Patterns of cytokine production in psoriatic synovium. J Rheumatol 1998;25:1544–1552.
25. Danning CL, Illei GG, Hitchon C, Greer MR, Boumpas DT, McInnes IB. Macrophage-derived cytokine and nuclear factor kappaB p65 expression in synovial membrane and skin of patients with psoriatic arthritis. Arthritis Rheum 2000;43:1244–1256.
26. Austin LM, Ozawa M, Kikuchi T, Walters IB, Krueger JG. The majority of epidermal T cells in psoriasis vulgaris lesions can produce type 1 cytokines, interferon-gamma, interleukin-2, and tumor necrosis factor-alpha, defining TC1 (cytotoxic T lymphocyte) and TH1 effector populations: a type 1 differentiation bias is also measured in circulating blood T cells in psoriatic patients. J Invest Dermatol 1999;113:752–759.
27. Canete JD, Pablos J, Sanmarti R, et al. Antiangiogenic effects of anti-tumor necrosis factor therapy with infliximab in psoriatic arthritis. Arthritis Rheum 2004;50:1636–1641.
28. Goedkoop AY, Kraan MC, Teunissen MB, et al. Early effects of tumour necrosis factor alpha blockade on skin

8

and synovial tissue in patients with active psoriasis and psoriatic arthritis. Ann Rheum Dis 2004;63:769–773.

29. Mease PJ, Antoni CE. Psoriatic arthritis treatment: biological response modifiers. Ann Rheum Dis 2005; 64(Suppl 2):ii78–ii82.

30. Costello P, Bresnihan B, O'Farrelly C, Fitzgerald O. Predominance of CD8+ T lymphocytes in psoriatic arthritis. J Rheumatol 1999;26:1117–1124.

31. Ritchlin CT, Haas-Smith SA, Li P, Hicks DG, Schwarz EM. Mechanisms of TNF-alpha- and RANKL-mediated osteoclastogenesis and bone resorption in psoriatic arthritis. J Clin Invest 2003;111:821–831.

32. Gravallese EM. Bone destruction in arthritis. Ann Rheum Dis 2002;61(Suppl 2):ii84–ii86.

33. Braun J, Bollow M, Neure L, et al. Use of immunohistologic and in situ hybridization techniques in the examination of sacroiliac joint biopsy specimens from patients with ankylosing spondylitis. Arthritis Rheum 1995;38:499–505.

34. Peng H, Wright V, Usas A, et al. Synergistic enhancement of bone formation and healing by stem cell-expressed VEGF and bone morphogenetic protein-4. J Clin Invest 2002;110:751–759.

35. Lories RJ, Derese I, Luyten FP. Modulation of bone morphogenetic protein signaling inhibits the onset and progression of ankylosing enthesitis. J Clin Invest 2005;115: 1571–1579.

36. Schatteman L, Mielants H, Veys EM, et al. Gut inflammation in psoriatic arthritis: a prospective ileocolonoscopic study. J Rheumatol 1995;22:680–683.

37. Scarpa R, Ayala F, Caporaso N, Olivieri I. Psoriasis, psoriatic arthritis, or psoriatic disease? J Rheumatology 2006; 33:210–212.

Psoriatic Arthritis
C. Treatment and Assessment

Philip J. Mease, MD

- Multiple instruments are available for assessment of skin, joints, and quality of life in psoriasis and psoriatic arthritis (PsA).
- Management of skin and arthritis can often be accomplished with similar agents.

- Destructive arthritis should be managed by traditional disease-modifying drugs or biologic therapies.
- Tumor necrosis factor (TNF) inhibitors have shown the greatest efficacy to date in PsA.

The framework for the treatment of psoriatic arthritis (PsA) is constituted by proper diagnosis and assessment of severity of the domains of disease activity involved in PsA: peripheral arthritis, enthesitis, dactylitis, spine inflammation, and skin and nail lesions, which may be differentially active. The degree of disease activity in these domains, along with background contextual factors for the individual (age, gender, psychological and socioeconomic factors, comorbidities, etc.) determine the impact of disease on quality of life, function, and life expectancy.

Typically, a patient will be aware of having the skin condition psoriasis long before the associated arthritis occurs. In just 15% to 25% of patients will the arthritis manifest simultaneously or subsequently (1,2). Thus, many patients will be under the care of a dermatologist or primary care physician (PCP) for management of skin lesions and, as such, are in an ideal position to be queried about symptoms of musculoskeletal pain and stiffness. PsA can occur in up to 30% of patients with psoriasis, depending on method of ascertainment and severity of psoriasis (see Chapter 8A). Because other forms of arthritis may occur in a patient with psoriasis, such as osteoarthritis, rheumatoid arthritis (RA), other spondyloarthritides, and gout (see Chapter 8A), it may be prudent for the dermatologist or PCP to obtain a rheumatology consult to help clarify what type of arthritis condition is present, supplement education for the patient and family, and strategize about treatment approaches based on the diagnosis and severity (3).

Although this review will focus on pharmacotherapy of PsA, it must be recognized that optimal therapy also comprises nonpharmacotherapy approaches, including patient and family education about the disease process and therapy, exercise, nutrition, psychological counseling, physical and occupational therapy, and orthopedic surgery. There have been few studies of these modalities in PsA per se, although there has been extensive research on their value and utility in the management of arthritis in general and RA specifically, from which we can extrapolate regarding their value and utility in PsA. A key role for the rheumatologist and rheumatology office staff is to serve as a central triage point for such adjunct therapy.

ASSESSMENT OF DISEASE ACTIVITY AND THERAPY OUTCOME

Determination of disease severity and effectiveness of therapies in clinical trials and in practice requires assessment tools that have generally been adapted from similar measures used in assessment of RA and psoriasis (Table 8C-1) (4–9). These have been used in clinical trials and clinical registries of PsA patients. These measures have been shown to effectively assess peripheral joint and skin symptoms and signs, function, quality of life, and fatigue, as well as distinguish treatment from placebo. Approaches to assessment of enthesitis, dactylitis, and spine involvement are still in development. Adaptation of RA methodologies to assess change of radiographs in PsA has occurred in a number of recent clinical trials (7,8), suggesting that such approaches are appropriate in PsA despite its differences from RA. Several studies have documented the effectiveness of ultrasound and magnetic resonance imaging (MRI) in detecting

TABLE 8C-1. PSORIATIC ARTHRITIS OUTCOME MEASURES USED IN CLINICAL TRIALS.

Arthritis response
  American College of Rheumatology Response Criteria
    (including DIP and CMC joints)
  Psoriatic Arthritis Response Criteria (PsARC)
  Disease Activity Score (DAS, DAS 44, DAS 28)

Radiographic assessment
  Modified (for PsA) Sharp
  Modified (for PsA) van der Heijde/Sharp

Skin response
  Psoriasis Area and Severity Index (PASI)
  Target Lesion score
  Physician Global Assessment (PGA) of Psoriasis

Quality of life/function improvement
  Short-Form 36 Health Survey (SF-36)
  Health Assessment Questionnaire (HAQ) Disability Index
  Dermatology Life Quality Index (DLQI)
  Functional Assessment of Chronic Illness Therapy (FACIT)

SOURCE: Data from references 4 through 9.
ABBREVIATIONS: CMC, carpometacarpal; DIP, distal interphalangeal.

inflammation in the joints and enthesium of SpA patients, as well as the extent of structural damage (8).

PSORIASIS MANAGEMENT

The patient's individual experience with psoriasis therapies, prior to development of PsA, will have depended on the severity of skin disease. Milder disease, for example, involving less than 5% body surface area (BSA), showing less severe induration and scale, and not involving important functional or cosmetic areas such as the hands, scalp, or other visible areas, may be treated with topical corticosteroid and/or vitamin D or A analogues, as well as ultraviolet (UV) light therapy (10–12). Patients with moderate-to-severe skin disease may have been treated with systemic therapies, such as methotrexate, cyclosporine, and acitretin, as well as UV light therapy, often in a cyclic fashion to maximize therapeutic effect while minimizing treatment side effects (10–17). When psoriasis clears it does not leave residual damage, so dermatologists typically treat till clear and then withdraw therapy until lesions return. A number of strategies have been developed for intermittent as well as combination therapy, based on assessment of skin lesion severity, to achieve optimal results (17). It is important to take into account previous tolerability and effectiveness of systemic medicines used for psoriasis when considering therapeutic options for inflammatory arthritis when it develops.

In recent years, there has been extensive uptake of the biologic response modifier medications in psoriasis,

all administered parenterally, based on successful clinical trials of the anti–tumor necrosis factor (anti-TNF) agents etanercept, infliximab, and adalimumab (18–20) and the T-cell modulating agents, alefacept and efalizumab (21,22). Etanercept, infliximab, and efalizumab have been approved in the United States and Europe for psoriasis and alefacept has been approved for use in the United States. Clinical studies and clinical experience, including safety and tolerability issues, with these agents in psoriasis have been extensively reviewed elsewhere (9,10,13,17,23–25). The first biologic agents approved in the United States were the T-cell modulatory agents alefacept and efalizumab, based on the key role played by T lymphocytes in psoriasis pathogenesis (26). Both block T-cell stimulation; alefacept promotes apoptosis of memory T cells and efalizumab inhibits migration of lymphocytes to the site inflammation. Both show clinically meaningful reductions in skin lesional activity and improved quality of life. A typically greater and more rapid improvement of psoriasis has been seen with the anti-TNF agents, along with correlated improvements of fatigue and quality of life and return to normal work and social life. These drugs offer an alternative to other systemic therapies or time-consuming UV light or topical therapies.

PSORIATIC ARTHRITIS MANAGEMENT

Nonsteroidal Anti-Inflammatory Drugs in Psoriatic Arthritis

Nonsteroidal anti-inflammatory drugs (NSAIDs) are a cornerstone of therapy for most PsA patients with musculoskeletal pain symptoms, either used alone in mild disease or in combination with other therapies. Typically a patient may have already tried an over-the-counter formulation, such as ibuprofen and naprosyn, so will have a sense of their relative effectiveness and tolerability. Switching among choices of NSAIDs may be indicated to try to achieve maximum convenience, effectiveness, and tolerability. There is scant trial experience with NSAIDs in PsA documenting efficacy (27), so support for their use is primarily derived from trials in rheumatoid arthritis (RA) and osteoarthritis (OA) as well as clinical experience. There are isolated case reports of psoriasis exacerbation related to NSAID use, but this has not been felt to be of significant consequence (27).

Nonsteroidal anti-inflammatory drugs have been found to be efficacious for the treatment of spinal pain in ankylosing spondylitis, on which evidence it is reasonable to extrapolate efficacy in management of PsA spondylitis (28).

Glucocorticoids in Psoriatic Arthritis

Episodic intra-articular steroid injections can be symptomatically helpful, especially for patients with monoarticular PsA, oligoarticular disease, or a situation wherein a polyarticular patient has one or a few joints inadequately controlled by systemic therapy. Enthesitis and tendonitis may also be helped by selective steroid injection. Results tend to be short lived, thus of limited long-term use if inflammation is recurrent in that site. However, if the inflammation is transient in that site, then local injection therapy can be quite helpful. Systemic glucocorticoids should be used more judiciously than in other inflammatory arthritides because of the chance that psoriasis skin lesions will severely flare upon withdrawal of therapy (27).

Traditional Disease-Modifying Antirheumatic Drugs in Psoriatic Arthritis

Utilization of systemic disease-modifying drugs in PsA has generally been modeled after their use in psoriasis and RA. Those that are considered traditional include the oral agents methotrexate, sulfasalazine, and cyclosporine. Injectable and oral gold and azathioprine would also be considered in this group, but have been infrequently used and, in the case of injectable gold therapy, have generally fallen out of favor.

Leflunomide, a pyrimidine antagonist approved for the treatment of RA, is typically considered along with this group of agents.

Methotrexate

Methotrexate (MTX) is one of the most commonly used systemic medications in PsA, yet controlled trial evidence for its effectiveness is scant. In 1984, Willkens published a small controlled trial using dosages of the drug that were then considered potentially appropriate in the treatment of inflammatory arthritis, 7.5 mg and 15 mg per week (29). In this trial, only the physician global assessment of arthritis showed statistically significant improvement, and not the tender and swollen joint count. Skin improvements were modest. However, clinical experience with standard doses in the 15 to 20 mg per week range would suggest that the drug can be efficacious in many patients and it remains one of the most commonly used disease-modifying antirheumatic drugs (DMARDs).

Increasingly it has been recognized that MTX only partially inhibits the progression of structural damage in RA (30). This has not been prospectively assessed in PsA, but a 2-year retrospective analysis of matched PsA patients who were either on or off MTX therapy did not

show any difference in radiologic progression scores in the two groups (31). Patients on chronic MTX therapy must have regular blood monitoring (blood counts, liver function tests, and creatinine). Significant elevation of liver tests or drop in blood counts should lead to adjustment of dose or cessation of therapy. A further consideration is that based on older liver biopsy studies, the suggestion has been made that there is greater proclivity to MTX hepatotoxicity in a psoriasis population than in patients with RA (32). Thus, there is often a preference by the dermatologist to limit overall use of MTX, or, if continued, to assess for liver toxicity by periodic liver biopsy (33). This is in contrast to the rheumatology experience wherein liver function tests are periodically assessed, but not liver biopsies, and MTX is used continuously and often in combination with other medications (34). Nevertheless, the practice of routine liver biopsies based on MTX dose has been questioned in the literature as more data are acquired (33–35).

Although the combination of MTX and TNF inhibitors has in RA been shown to be superior in all clinical parameters of efficacy, including inhibition of structural damage (30), this has not been assessed in PsA. Thus, in the treatment of PsA in clinical practice, MTX may sometimes be discontinued after initiation of biologic therapy and only reinitiated if the patient experiences inadequate control of disease with biologic monotherapy. Response of spinal joints has not been assessed in PsA. In ankylosing spondylitis, MTX has not been shown to benefit spinal measures of disease activity (28,36).

Sulfasalazine

The largest number of controlled trials of traditional DMARD therapy has been conducted with sulfasalazine (27). In the largest of these, 221 PsA patients were treated with sulfasalazine, 2 g/day, for 36 weeks (37). Although a composite arthritis score showed statistically significant improvement in the treatment group, the only individual measure within the responder index to do so was the patient global assessment, indicating that the effect was not strong. Further, there was no benefit to the skin and gastrointestinal intolerability was an issue. As with MTX, spine response was not assessed and controlled trials with this agent in ankylosing spondylitis have not shown efficacy in the spine domain (28).

Cyclosporine

Although cyclosporine can achieve rapid improvement of the skin lesions of psoriasis, its effectiveness in PsA has been minimally studied other than showing some effectiveness in open trials (27). Its utility is limited by concerns regarding the adverse effects of hypertension

8

and renal insufficiency. Regarding the combination of cyclosporine with MTX, 72 patients with incomplete response to MTX were randomized to placebo or addition of cyclosporine (38). At 48 weeks, significant improvements in tender and swollen joint count, C-reactive protein (CRP), psoriasis area and severity index (PASI), and synovial ultrasound score occurred in the combination group, but statistical differentiation between the combination and MTX-alone group occurred just in PASI and ultrasound score.

Leflunomide

Leflunomide, a pyrimidine antagonist approved in RA at a dose of 20 mg/day, was assessed in 188 PsA patients. The Psoriatic Arthritis Response Criteria (PsARC) response, the primary endpoint, was met by 59% of leflunomide-treated patients compared with 29.7% of placebo-treated patients ($p < 0.0001$). American College of Rheumatology (ACR) 20 response was achieved by 36.3% and 20%, respectively ($p = 0.0138$), and PASI 75 response by 17.4% and 7.8%, respectively ($p = 0.048$) (39). As with MTX, liver function test abnormalities may be noted and need to be monitored. Leflunomide did not benefit the spine in AS (28,36).

Tumor Necrosis Factor Alpha Inhibitors in Psoriatic Arthritis

The anti–tumor necrosis factor alpha (TNF-alpha) compounds, etanercept (Enbrel®) (40), infliximab (Remicade®) (41), and adalimumab (Humira®) (42) are approved for use in PsA as well as psoriasis skin disease.

Etanercept

Etanercept is a soluble receptor for TNF, administered subcutaneously in a dose of 25 mg twice a week or 50 mg once a week for PsA, now approved in RA, PsA, psoriasis, and ankylosing spondylitis. In the placebo-controlled portion of the phase III etanercept trial in PsA ($n = 205$), utilizing 25 mg administered subcutaneously twice a week, ACR20 response was achieved by 59% of etanercept treated patients versus 15% in the placebo group (42% and 41% on background MTX, respectively; $p < 0.0001$; 43). Skin response, as measured by the PASI score in patients with BSA involvement ≥ 3%, showed a 75% improvement in 23% and 3%, respectively, at 24 weeks ($p = 0.001$). A change of 0.51 units of the Health Assessment Questionnaire (HAQ), a measure of physical function, was noted in the etanercept group, both statistically significant and clinically meaningful (44). Improvement in quality of life, as measured by the Short Form 36 (SF-36) questionnaire, was also demonstrated in the treatment group. Inhibition of

progression of joint space narrowing and erosions was shown, with 1 unit of modified total Sharp score (mTSS) progression in the placebo group and none (−0.03 units) in the etanercept group ($p = 0.001$). In the open label extension of this study, at 2 years, effectiveness was maintained in joint response, and skin response further improved to a PASI 75 response in 38%. Originally placebo patients achieved a similar degree of effectiveness in joints and skin as well as inhibition of further structural damage (45). The drug was well tolerated and no safety issues emerged apart from those seen in clinical trial and general clinical experience with etanercept in RA.

Infliximab

Infliximab is a chimeric monoclonal anti-TNF antibody now approved in RA, Crohn's, PsA, psoriasis, and ankylosing spondylitis. A phase III study of infliximab in 200 PsA patients (IMPACT II) showed significant benefit (46). Baseline demographic and disease activity characteristics were similar to those of the etanercept phase III trial. At week 14, 58% of infliximab patients and 11% of placebo patients achieved an ACR20 response ($p < 0.001$). Presence of dactylitis and enthesitis, assessed by palpation of the Achilles tendon and plantar fascia insertions, decreased significantly in the infliximab group (46). In skin evaluation, at 24 weeks, PASI 75 was achieved by 64% of the evaluable treatment group and 2% of the placebo group ($p < 0.001$). Utilizing the van der Heijde-Sharp scoring method (hands and feet), modified for PsA, infliximab-treated patients showed inhibition of radiographic disease progression at 24 weeks, although PsA-specific radiographic features, including pencil-in-cup deformities and gross osteolysis, did not differ between the treatment groups, as has been observed in other anti–TNF-alpha trials, presumably due to the more fixed nature of theses changes (47). HAQ score improved for 59% of infliximab patients, compared with 19% of placebo patients, while both the physical and mental components of SF-36 scores improved for patients receiving infliximab. Improvement was sustained at 1 year (46).

Adalimumab

Adalimumab is a fully human anti–TNF-alpha monoclonal antibody administered subcutaneously, 40 mg, every other week or weekly and is approved for RA and PsA. It was studied in a phase III study ($n = 313$), the Adalimumab Effectiveness in Psoriatic Arthritis Trial (ADEPT) (48). At 12 weeks, 58% of patients receiving adalimumab 40 mg every other week achieved ACR20 response compared with 14% of patients receiving placebo ($p < 0.001$). This response rate did not differ between patients taking adalimumab in combination with MTX (50% of patients) and those taking adalimumab alone, similar to observations made in the etanercept and infliximab trials. Mean improvement in enthesitis and dactylitis was greater for patients receiving adalimumab, but this result did not achieve statistical significance. PASI 75 was achieved by 59% in the adalimumab-treated group and 1% in the placebo group ($p < 0.001$) in those evaluable for PASI scoring. Radiographic progression of disease was significantly inhibited by adalimumab, as evaluated by x-rays of hands and feet, using a modified Sharp score (48). Mean change in TSS was −0.2 for patients receiving adalimumab and 1.0 for patients receiving placebo ($p < 0.001$). Mean change in HAQ was −0.4 for adalimumab patients and −0.1 for placebo patients ($p < 0.001$). Mean change in the physical component of the SF-36 was 9.3 for the treatment group and 1.4 for the placebo group ($p < 0.001$).

Spine disease was not assessed in these trials, due to variability of expression of this domain in this patient group. However, significant efficacy of anti-TNF treatment of axial symptoms and signs has been demonstrated in a closely related disease, ankylosing spondylitis (28,36,49). Relative inefficacy of methotrexate, sulfasalazine, and leflunomide has been noted in ankylosing spondylitis, suggesting preference for use of the anti-TNF agents in this domain. It is unknown if the same holds true in PsA, although extrapolation of this experience to PsA seems reasonable.

In summary, the anti–TNF-alpha medications have shown the greatest efficacy of any treatment to date in the various clinical aspects of PsA. Their efficacy in joint disease activity, inhibition of structural damage, function, and quality of life are similar. There may be some differentiation in efficacy in the skin and enthesium, but all have excellent effects in these domains. These agents tend to be well tolerated and patients generally acclimate to their parenteral administration, especially when they experience significant efficacy. Safety concerns are present, such as risk for infection, but no new concerns have arisen in the PsA population compared to the more extensively studied RA patient experience (see Chapter 6C). Recent studies have also demonstrated the cost-effectiveness of anti–TNF-alpha therapy in PsA (50–52). New anti–TNF-alpha agents are being developed for use in PsA, including cimzia and golimumab, each with advantages of infrequent subcutaneous administration. Experience in management of RA with currently available anti-TNF agents suggests that when a clinician switches from one of these agents to another, if the first has not had or has lost efficacy, or caused side effects, that a substantial percentage of patients will respond to another medication in this class. Anecdotally, a similar experience has been noted in the management of PsA patients.

Other Biologic Agents

Alefacept

Alefacept is a fully human fusion protein that blocks interaction between LFA-3 on the antigen-presenting cell and CD2 on the T cell, or by attracting natural killer lymphocytes to interact with CD2 to yield apoptosis of particular T-cell clones (53). It is approved for treatment of psoriasis (21,54) and is administered weekly as a 15 mg intramuscular injection, in an alternating 12 weeks on, 12 weeks off regimen in order to allow return of depleted CD4 cells in the off period. A phase II controlled trial of alefacept in PsA ($n = 185$) showed that 54% of patients given a combination of alefacept and MTX had an ACR20 response as compared to 23% in the MTX alone group ($p < 0.001$) at week 24. PASI 75 results were 28% and 24%, respectively (55).

Efalizumab

Efalizumab is a humanized monoclonal antibody to the CD11 subunit of LFA-1 on T cells, which inteferes with its coupling with ICAM-1 on antigen-presenting and endothelial cells. It interferes with activation of T lymphocytes and migration of cells to the site of inflammation. It is administered subcutaneously, once per week and is approved for use in psoriasis (22). In a 12-week trial of efalizumab in patients with PsA, 28% of patients achieved an ACR20 response versus 19% in the placebo group ($p = 0.2717$). Because this response was not statistically significant, it is not recommended for treatment of arthritis (56).

Abatacept

Abatacept (CTLA4-Ig) is a recombinant human fusion protein that binds to the CD80/86 receptor on an antigen-presenting cell, thus blocking the second signal activation of the CD28 receptor on the T cell. It is administered intravenously once per month and has been approved for use in RA (57). A phase II trial for use in psoriasis has been conducted (58). It is anticipated that this drug will be evaluated in PsA.

Other Potential Treatments

A pilot trial of anti-interleukin (IL) 15 compound has shown efficacy in PsA (59). An IL-1 antagonist, anakinra, has not shown significant efficacy (60). A monoclonal antibody to the IL-6 receptor (MRA) is in phase III development for the treatment of RA, and will likely be tested in PsA (61). Several inhibitors of IL-12 are being evaluated in psoriasis, with good success (62), and will likely be assessed in PsA.

8

CONCLUSION

A number of systemic treatments for PsA, such as inhibitors of TNF-alpha, have demonstrated significant benefit for all disease domains, including inflammation in the joints, enthesium, and skin, inhibition of joint damage as assessed by radiographic progression, and improved quality of life and functional status. Traditional immune-modulating drugs can beneficially affect many of these domains as well. Agents that block the cell–cell interactions required to activate T cells are effective in the skin and may benefit the joints. Observation of the effectiveness of these agents has helped elucidate the pathogenesis of PsA and psoriasis which, in turn, may lead to more novel and effective interventions. Mild disease in the joints and skin can be treated with anti-inflammatories and topical treatments.

Development of targeted therapies has also increased interest in the accurate diagnosis and assessment of PsA, which facilitates the institution of appropriate therapy in a timely fashion. Because in the great majority of patients, the skin manifestations of psoriasis develop long before arthritis symptoms develop, the dermatologist or PCP is in an ideal position to educate about and screen for arthritis in order to make an early diagnosis and through appropriate treatment and coordinated care with rheumatologists, help prevent progressive structural damage in those that are likely to progress. Significant efforts are under way to further develop and validate outcome measures that accurately map the natural history of PsA and demonstrate the impact of increasingly effective emerging therapies on patients' function and quality of life.

REFERENCES

1. Gladman D, Antoni C, Mease P, Clegg DO, Nash P. Psoriatic arthritis: epidemiology, clinical features, course, and outcome. Ann Rheum Dis 2005;64(Suppl 2):ii14–ii17.
2. Mease PJ, Goffe BS. Diagnosis and treatment of psoriatic arthritis. J Am Acad Dermatol 2005;52:1–19.
3. Gordon KB, Ruderman EM. The treatment of psoriasis and psoriatic arthritis: an interdisciplinary approach. J Am Acad Dermatol 2006;54(Suppl 2):S85–S91.
4. Gladman DD, Helliwell P, Mease PJ, Nash P, Ritchlin C, Taylor W. Assessment of patients with psoriatic arthritis: a review of currently available measures. Arthritis Rheum 2004;50:24–35.
5. Mease P, Antoni C, Gladman DD, Taylor W. Psoriatic arthritis assessment tools in clinical trials. Ann Rheum Dis 2005;64(Suppl 2):ii49–ii54.
6. Feldman SR, Krueger G. Psoriasis assessment tools in clinical trials. Ann Rheum Dis 2005;64(Suppl 2):ii65–ii68.
7. van der Heijde D, Sharp J, Wassenberg S, et al. Psoriatic arthritis imaging: a review of scoring methods. Ann Rheum Dis 2005;64(Suppl 2):ii61–ii64.
8. Mease P, van der Heidje D. Joint damage in psoriatic arthritis: how is it assessed and can it be prevented? Int J Adv Rheumatol 2006;4:38–48.
9. Mease PJ, Menter MA. Quality-of-life issues in psoriasis and psoriatic arthritis: outcome measures and therapies from a dermatological perspective. J Am Acad Dermatol 2006;54:685–704.
10. Lebwohl M. A clinician's paradigm in the treatment of psoriasis. J Am Acad Dermatol 2005;53(Suppl 1):S59–S69.
11. Lebwohl M, Ting P, Koo J. Psoriasis treatment: traditional therapy. Ann Rheum Dis 2005;64(Suppl 64):ii83–ii86.
12. Koo JY. New developments in topical sequential therapy for psoriasis. Skin Therapy Lett 2005;10:1–4.
13. Fairhurst DA, Ashcroft DM, Griffiths CE. Optimal management of severe plaque form of psoriasis. Am J Clin Dermatol 2005;6:283–294.
14. Naldi L, Griffiths CE. Traditional therapies in the management of moderate to severe chronic plaque psoriasis: an assessment of the benefits and risks. Br J Dermatol 2005;152:597–615.
15. Norris DA. Mechanisms of action of topical therapies and the rationale for combination therapy. J Am Acad Dermatol 2005;53(Suppl 1):S17–S25.
16. Krueger G, Ellis CN. Psoriasis–recent advances in understanding its pathogenesis and treatment. J Am Acad Dermatol 2005;53(Suppl 1):S94–S100.
17. Feldman SR, Koo JY, Menter A, Bagel J. Decision points for the initiation of systemic treatment for psoriasis. J Am Acad Dermatol 2005;53:101–107.
18. Leonardi CL, Powers JL, Matheson RT, et al. Etanercept as monotherapy in patients with psoriasis. N Engl J Med 2003;349:2014–2022.
19. Reich K, Nestle FO, Papp K, et al. Infliximab induction and maintenance therapy for moderate-to-severe psoriasis: a phase III, multicentre, double-blind trial. Lancet 2005;366:1367–1374.
20. Langley R, Leonardi CL, Hoffman R. Long-term safety and efficacy of Adalimumab in the treatment of moderate to severe chronic plaque psoriasis. Paper presented at: American Academy of Dermatology Annual Meeting; February 18–20, 2005; New Orleans, LA.
21. Krueger GG, Papp KA, Sough DB, et al. A randomized, double-blind, placebo-controlled phase III study evaluating efficacy and tolerability of 2 courses of alefacept in patients with chronic plaque psoriasis. J Am Acad Dermatol 2002;47:821–833.
22. Lebwohl M, Tyring SK, Hamilton TK, et al. A novel targeted T-cell modulator, efalizumab, for plaque psoriasis. N Engl J Med 2003;349:2004–2013.
23. Fiorentino D, Mease P. The skin in psoriatic arthritis. Int J Adv Rheumatol 2005;3:110–117.
24. Winterfield L, Menter A, Gordon KB, Gottlieb A. Psoriasis treatment: current and emerging directed therapies. Ann Rheum Dis 2005;64(Suppl 64):ii87–ii90.

25. Krueger G, Ellis CN. Psoriasis–recent advances in understanding its pathogenesis and treatment. J Am Acad Dermatol 2005;53(Suppl 1):S94–S100.

26. Krueger JG. The immunologic basis for the treatment of psoriasis with new biologic agents. J Am Acad Dermatol 2002;46:1–23; quiz 6.

27. Nash P, Clegg DO. Psoriatic arthritis therapy: NSAIDs and traditional DMARDs. Ann Rheum Dis 2005;64(Suppl 2):ii74–ii77.

28. Braun J, Baraliakos X, Godolias G, Bohm H. Therapy of ankylosing spondylitis–a review. Part I: Conventional medical treatment and surgical therapy. Scand J Rheumatol 2005;34:97–108.

29. Willkens RF, Williams HJ, Ward JR, et al. Randomized, double-blind, placebo controlled trial of low-dose pulse methotrexate in psoriatic arthritis. Arthritis Rheum 1984;27:376–381.

30. van der Heijde D, Klareskog L, Rodriguez-Valverde V, et al. Comparison of etanercept and methotrexate, alone and combined, in the treatment of rheumatoid arthritis: two-year clinical and radiographic results from the TEMPO study, a double-blind, randomized trial. Arthritis Rheum 2006;54:1063–1074.

31. Abu-Shakra M, Gladman DD, Thorne JC, Long JA, Gough J, Farewell VT. Long-term methotrexate therapy in psoriatic arthritis: clinical and radiological outcome. J Rheumatol 1995;22:241–245.

32. Whiting-O'Keefe QE, Fye KH, Sack KD. Methotrexate and histologic hepatic abnormalities: a meta-analysis. Am J Med 1991;90:711–716.

33. Roenigk HH Jr, Auerbach R, Maibach H, Weinstein G, Lebwohl M. Methotrexate in psoriasis: consensus conference. J Am Acad Dermatol 1998;38:478–485.

34. Kremer JM, Alarcon GS, Lightfoot RW Jr., et al. Methotrexate for rheumatoid arthritis. Suggested guidelines for monitoring liver toxicity. American College of Rheumatology. Arthritis Rheum 1994;37:316–328.

35. Thomas JA, Aithal GP. Monitoring liver function during methotrexate therapy for psoriasis: are routine biopsies really necessary? Am J Clin Dermatol 2005;6:357–363.

36. Braun J, Baraliakos X, Brandt J, Sieper J. Therapy of ankylosing spondylitis. Part II: biological therapies in the spondyloarthritides. Scand J Rheumatol 2005;34:178–190.

37. Clegg DO, Reda DJ, Mejias E, et al. Comparison of sulfasalazine and placebo in the treatment of psoriatic arthritis. A Department of Veterans Affairs Cooperative Study. Arthritis Rheum 1996;39:2013–2020.

38. Fraser AD, van Kuijk AW, Westhovens R, et al. A randomised, double blind, placebo controlled, multicentre trial of combination therapy with methotrexate plus cyclosporin in patients with active psoriatic arthritis. Ann Rheum Dis 2005;64:859–864.

39. Kaltwasser JP, Nash P, Gladman D, et al. Efficacy and safety of leflunomide in the treatment of psoriatic arthritis and psoriasis. Arthritis Rheum 2004;50:1939–1950.

40. Enbrel® (etanercept) prescribing information. Thousand Oaks, CA: Immunex Corporation; 2003.

41. Remicade (infliximab) prescribing information. Malvern, PA: Centocor Inc; 2003.

42. Humira™ (adalimumab) prescribing information. North Chicago, IL: Abbott Laboratories; 2003.

43. Mease P, Kivitz A, Burch F, et al. Etanercept treatment of psoriatic arthritis: safety, efficacy, and effect on disease progression. Arthritis Rheum 2004;50:2264–2272.

44. Mease P, Ganguly L, Wanke E, Yu E, Singh A. How much improvement in functional status is considered important by patients with active psoriatic arthritis: applying the outcome measures in rheumatoid arthritis clinical trials (OMERACT) group guidelines. Ann Rheum Dis 2004;63(Suppl 1):391.

45. Mease PJ, Kivitz AJ, Burch FX, et al. Continued inhibition of radiographic progression in patients with psoriatic arthritis following 2 years of treatment with etanercept. J Rheumatol 2006;33:712–721.

46. Antoni C, Krueger GG, de Vlam K, et al. Infliximab improves signs and symptoms of psoriatic arthritis: results of the IMPACT 2 trial. Ann Rheum Dis 2005;64:1150–1157.

47. van der Heijde D, Kavanaugh A, Beutler A, et al. Infliximab inhibits progression of radiographic damage in patients with active psoriatic damage in patients with arthritis: results from IMPACT 2 trial. Ann Rheum Dis 2005;64(Suppl 3):109.

48. Mease P, Gladman D, Ritchlin C. Adalimumab in the treatment of patients with moderately to severely active psoriatic arthritis: results of ADEPT. Arthritis Rheum 2005;58:3279–3289.

49. Zochling J, van der Heijde D, Dougados M, Braun J. Current evidence for the management of ankylosing spondylitis: a systematic literature review for the asas/eular management recommendations in ankylosing spondylitis. Ann Rheum Dis 2006;65:423–432.

50. Bansback N, Barkham N, Ara R, et al. The economic implications of TNF-inhibitors in the treatment of psoriatic arthritis. Arthritis Rheum 2004;50(Suppl 9):S509.

51. Guh D, Bansback N, Nosyk B, Melilli L, Anis A. Improvement in health utility in patients with psoriatic arthritis treated with adalimumab (Humira). Ann Rheum Dis 2005;64(Suppl 3):401.

52. Marra CA. Valuing health states and preferences of patients. Ann Rheum Dis 2005;64(Suppl 3):36.

53. Kraan MC, van Kuijk AW, Dinant HJ, et al. Alefacept treatment in psoriatic arthritis: reduction of the effector T cell population in peripheral blood and synovial tissue is associated with improvement of clinical signs of arthritis. Arthritis Rheum 2002;46:2776–2784.

54. Lebwohl M, Christophers E, Langley R, Ortonne JP, Roberts J, Griffiths CE. An international, randomized, double-blind, placebo-controlled phase 3 trial of intramuscular alefacept in patients with chronic plaque psoriasis. Arch Dermatol 2003;139:719–727.

55. Mease PJ, Gladman DD, Keystone EC. Alefacept in combination with methotrexate for the treatment of psoriatic arthritis: results of a randomized, double-blind, placebo-controlled study. Arthritis Rheum 2006;54:1638–1645.

8

56. Papp KA, Caro I, Leung HM, Garovoy M, Mease PJ. Efalizumab for the treatment of psoriatic arthritis. J Cutan Med Surg 2007;11:57–66.

57. Kremer JM, Westhovens R, Leon M, et al. Treatment of rheumatoid arthritis by selective inhibition of T-cell activation with fusion protein CTLA4Ig. N Engl J Med 2003; 349:1907–1915.

58. Abrams JR, Lebwohl M, Guzzo C. CTLA4Ig-mediated blockade of T cell co-stimulation in patients with psoriasis vulgaris. J Clin Invest 1999;103:1243–1252.

59. McInnes IB, Gracie JA. Interleukin-15: a new cytokine target for the treatment of inflammatory diseases. Curr Opin Pharmacol 2004;4:392–397.

60. Gibbs A, Gogarty M, Veale D, Bresnihan B, Fitzgerald O. Efficacy of anakinara (Kineret) in psoriatic arthritis, a clinical and immunohistological study. Ann Rheum Dis 2006;65(Suppl 2):216.

61. Nishimoto N, Yoshizaki K, Miyasaka N, et al. Treatment of rheumatoid arthritis with humanized anti-interleukin-6 receptor antibody: a multicenter, double-blind, placebo-controlled trial. Arthritis Rheum 2004;50:1761–1769.

62. Krueger C, Langley R, Leonardi C, Lebwohl M. Results of a phase II study of CNTO 1275 in the treatment of psoriasis. J Am Acad Dermatol 2006;54: AB10.

Ankylosing Spondylitis
A. Clinical Features

DÉSIRÉE VAN DER HEIJDE, MD, PHD

- Ankylosing spondylitis (AS) is the prototypical form of seronegative spondyloarthropathies, a group of disorders that involves chronic inflammation of the sacroiliac joints and spine as well as extraspinal lesions involving the eye, bowel, and heart.
- The prevalence of AS ranges from 0.1% to 6.0% across different populations, with figures for most populations near the lower end of that range.
- Human leukocyte antigen (HLA)-B27 is a strong genetic risk factor for AS. However, this gene is neither necessary nor sufficient to cause the disease.
- The principal musculoskeletal lesions associated with AS are sacroiliitis, synovitis, and enthesitis (inflammation at the site of tendinous insertions into bone).

- Sacroiliitis, the most common initial feature, causes pain in the buttocks, typically alternating in severity between the left and right sides.
- When synovitis is present, the hips, knees, ankles, and metatarsophalangeal joints are affected most commonly.
- Acute anterior uveitis, characteristically unilateral, is the typical ocular lesion. Patients present with a red, painful, photophobic eye.
- A sizable minority (10%–15%) of patients with AS have full-blown inflammatory bowel disease.
- Conventional radiographs of the sacroiliac joints are usually the most helpful diagnostic test. In earlier cases, findings on magnetic resonance imaging may also be diagnostic.

Ankylosing spondylitis (AS) is a chronic inflammatory disease of the sacroiliac joints and spine that may be associated with a variety of extraspinal lesions involving the eye, bowel, and heart. AS usually begins in young adulthood. The natural history of AS involves progressive stiffening of the spine, with ankylosis (fusion of some or all spinal joints) occurring after some years of disease in about two thirds of the patients. Patients with long-standing severe disease are at increased risk of premature death, but overall the life span of individuals with AS appears to be normal. AS shares many features with the arthritides associated with psoriasis, inflammatory bowel disease, and reactive arthritis. Together, these conditions comprise the spondyloarthritis family and are sometimes termed the *seronegative spondyloarthropathies* ("seronegative" because they are not associated with rheumatoid factor) (1). Typical spondylitis may be present in each of the other spondyloarthritides.

EPIDEMIOLOGY

The prevalence of AS in different populations varies from 0.1% in some African and Eskimo populations, through 0.5% to 1.0% among white populations in the United Kingdom and United States, to around 6% in the Haida Native Americans in Northern Canada. The prevalence generally, but not exclusively, reflects the prevalence of human leukocyte antigen (HLA)-B27 in the different populations. Because few population surveys have been undertaken, much of the available data have been drawn from selective hospital-based surveys and from information on other related spondyloarthritides.

Ankylosing spondylitis is more common in men, with a male:female ratio of approximately 2:1. Expression of disease may vary slightly between men and women, but earlier reports exaggerated this disparity to the under-estimation of women with AS, many of whom experienced unnecessary delays in diagnosis (2). Some investigators have suggested that the true sex ratio is closer to unity if based on population data.

ETIOLOGY

In spite of dramatic advances in recent years, the etiology of AS remains unclear. A strong multigenic inherited component is evident, although HLA-B27 remains the strongest association in almost all populations (3).

Animal and laboratory studies suggest that the HLA-B27 molecule itself plays a key role, and that involvement of class I major histocompatibility complex (MHC) antigens in the presentation of microbial peptides is central to the pathogenic mechanism (4).

Infective mechanisms also have been proposed. However, aside from the occurrence of spondylitis in some patients with another form of spondyloarthropathy—reactive arthritis—no clear evidence implicates infection in the etiology of AS. *Klebsiella aeruginosa* has been implicated on the basis of molecular mimicry with HLA-B27 and clinical studies, although its true significance remains unclear. Subclinical mucosal inflammation in the large and small bowel undoubtedly is present in many individuals with AS; this finding could provide the basis for an immune or infective mechanism for the spinal disease.

CLINICAL FEATURES

The principal musculoskeletal lesions associated with AS are enthesitis and synovitis, with sacroiliitis also involving adjacent bone. Inflammatory eye lesions, myocardial changes, gut mucosal lesions, and skin lesions are inconsistent but characteristic features of AS.

PRESENTING FEATURES

Spinal features of AS seldom appear before the age of 16 to 18 years. Before this age, children and teenagers may develop oligoarthritis—typically a swollen knee or metatarsophalangeal (MTP) joint—sometimes associated with iritis and/or enthesitis (5). Juvenile AS is remarkable because it does not involve the spine. For many, symptoms begin early in the third decade of life; the average age at onset is 26 years. Although the disease rarely begins after the age of 40 years, it is not uncommon for the diagnosis to be made only years later, well after that age. Earlier symptoms often are mild, ignored, or not recognized as being part of AS.

The usual presenting symptom is inflammatory back pain that is insidious in onset, persistent for more than 3 months, worsened by rest and improved by exercise. Night pain is a frequent symptom. Sacroiliitis, the most common initial feature, causes pain in the buttocks, typically alternating between right and left in severity. This pain sometimes radiates down the thighs but never below the knee. Although clinical examination is unreliable as a means of diagnosing sacroiliitis, pain in the buttocks may be elicited in some patients by pushing firmly with both hands on the sacrum when the patient is prone. A minority of patients present with oligoarthritis or enthesitis that particularly affects the heel, or hip pain due to aggressive synovitis. Fatigue, a common and troublesome symptom, may be caused in large part by impaired sleep caused by pain and stiffness. Other constitutional features may include fever and weight loss. Overt or subclinical depression, accompanied by a loss of libido and reduced capacity for work, also may contribute to lack of well-being.

Spinal discomfort and stiffness typically ascend the spine over a period of years, producing progressive spinal pain and restriction. One of the first clinical signs is the disappearance of the lumbar lordosis. This progression affects the costovertebral joints, reducing respiratory excursion, and the cervical spine, limiting neck movement. Thoracic spine involvement may be associated with anterior chest pain and sternal/costal cartilage tenderness, which can be particularly distressing for patients. Osteoporosis (which may be prevented by appropriate therapy) may lead to vertebral and other fractures later in life (6). Spinal fractures are more common in patients who have severe involvement with rigidity. Aseptic spondylodiscitis may occur in patients with AS, especially in the thoracic spine.

Enthesitis

The central feature of AS is inflammation at entheses, the sites where tendons and ligaments attach to bone. These inflammatory lesions initially lead to radiographic appearances of osteopenia or lytic lesions, but subsequently reactive bone forms a new, more superficial enthesis, which develops into a radiologically detectable bony overgrowth or spur (7). In the spine, enthesitis occurs at capsular and ligamentous attachments and discovertebral, costovertebral, and costotransverse joints, with involvement also at bony attachments of interspinous and paravertebral ligaments.

Enthesitis accounts for much of the pain, stiffness, and restriction at sacroiliac and other spinal joints. The phenomenon also occurs at extraspinal sites, producing potentially troublesome symptoms. Such lesions most commonly affect the plantar fascia and Achilles tendon insertions to the calcaneus, leading to disabling heel pain. Plantar fasciitis typically leads to the formation of fluffy calcaneal spurs visible on heel radiographs after 6 to 12 months. Similar lesions may occur around the pelvis, costochondral junctions, tibial tubercles, and elsewhere, causing marked local tenderness. More widespread diffuse lesions lead to insidious stiffness and generalized discomfort. Sternal and costochondral pain also reflect a combination of local enthesitis and referred pain from the thoracic spine. This development frequently produces chest pain that must be distinguished from myocardial ischemia.

Sacroiliitis

Inflammation of the sacroiliac joints develops most frequently in the late teens or in the third decade of life, producing bilateral or occasionally, unilateral buttock pain, usually worse after inactivity and sometimes aggravated by weight bearing. Changes principally affect the lower anterior (synovial) portion of the sacroiliac joints and are associated with juxta-articular osteopenia and osteitis. This condition leads to radiographic appearances of widening of the sacroiliac joint. Endochondral ossification as a consequence of the osteitis gives the radiographic appearance of erosion along the lower part of the sacroiliac joints. Osteitis appears as increased water content of adjacent bone, as seen on magnetic resonance imaging (MRI). MRI is a valuable imaging modality for assessment of inflammation in both the sacroiliac joints and the spine. This can frequently be an important aid in establishing an early diagnosis. Capsular enthesopathy also occurs over the anterior and posterior aspect of the joint throughout its length, leading to sheets of ossification that ultimately obscure the joint completely on standard radiographs, depicted as ankylosis of the sacroiliac joint.

Synovitis

Peripheral synovitis in AS is distinctive because of by the distribution of joints affected rather than because of distinct histological changes. Synovitis is indistinguishable histologically and immunohistochemically from typical rheumatoid disease. Peripheral joint synovitis may precede, accompany, or follow the onset of spinal symptoms. Hips, knees, ankles, and MTP joints are affected most commonly. With the exception of the shoulders, upper limb joints are almost never involved in AS, particularly in the absence of psoriasis. In further contrast to rheumatoid arthritis, peripheral joint synovitis usually is oligoarticular, often asymmetrical, and frequently episodic rather than persistent. Joint erosions, especially at the MTP joints, may lead to subluxation and deformity. Peripheral joint involvement is indistinguishable from that seen in the other spondyloarthritides. Temporomandibular joints may be affected, leading to reduced mouth opening and discomfort on chewing. Dactylitis may lead to pain in one or more toes that lasts many months.

Eye Lesions

Acute anterior uveitis (iritis) develops at some time during the course of the disease in approximately one third of patients with AS, and may be recurrent (Figure 9A-1). The typical pattern is alternating, unilateral eye inflammation associated with pain, redness, lacrimation, photophobia, and blurred vision. The occurrence of uveitis typically does not coincide with flares of arthritis. Untreated or inadequately treated iritis may lead rapidly

Acute Anterior Uveitis

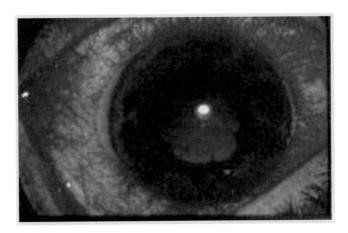

FIGURE 9A-1

Acute anterior uveitis in AS, typically unilateral and associated with redness, pain, and photophobia.

to considerable scarring, irregularity of the pupil, and visual impairment. Red, sore, gritty eyes or blurring of vision in a patient with AS require urgent ophthalmologic examination.

Inflammatory Bowel Disease

Sacroiliitis occurs in 6% to 25% of people with Crohn's disease or ulcerative colitis. Patients with Crohn's disease or ulcerative colitis frequently have unilateral sacroiliitis, and may also suffer from peripheral arthritis and enthesitis. Similarly, inflammatory bowel disease may be present or develop in people with preexisting AS. Indeed, approximately 60% of people with AS have subclinical changes in the small or large bowel (8). There is speculation that these changes may relate to the pathogenesis of AS, but their true significance is unknown. Even though some AS lesions closely resemble those of Crohn's disease, the great majority of such lesions never become symptomatic. Only about 10% to 15% of the patients with AS have overt ulcerative colitis or Crohn's disease. The link between AS and inflammatory bowel disease appears to be indirect, as variations in inflammatory activity of each disease appear to occur independently. However, in a patient with AS altered bowel habits with diarrhea and abdominal discomfort, with or without passage of blood or mucus, requires investigation.

In a minority of people with colitis and peripheral arthritis, peripheral joint disease may diminish substantially after total colectomy. Conversely, however, many

9

patients complain of a disorder resembling fibromyalgia that produces mild but widespread discomfort after colectomy. Active inflammatory bowel disease increases the risk and severity of osteoporosis. Crohn's disease with extensive small bowel involvement also may lead to impaired vitamin D absorption and osteomalacia, producing ill-defined musculoskeletal pain and difficulty with walking.

Cardiovascular Involvement

Cardiac conduction abnormalities and myocardial dysfunction have been recorded in a significant minority of people with AS (9). Aortitis with dilatation of the aortic valve ring and aortic regurgitation has been demonstrated in approximately 1% of patients. The risk of occurrence of aortic insufficiency and cardiac conduction abnormalities increase with age, disease duration, presence of HLA-B27, and peripheral joint involvement.

Pulmonary Involvement

Approximately 1% of patients develop progressive upper lobe fibrosis of the lungs (10). Rigidity of the chest wall results in the inability to extend the chest fully and to mild restrictive lung function impairment, but rarely leads to ventilation insufficiency due to the compensation by increased diaphragmatic contribution.

Neurologic Lesions

Neurologic deficits are associated most often with cord or root lesions following spinal fracture. Nerve root pain may arise from the cervical spine, especially when there is marked flexion deformity. Long-tract signs, including quadriplegia, may follow spinal fracture dislocation after relatively minor trauma and complicate spontaneous atlantoaxial subluxation. Subluxation also may lead to severe occipital headache. Weakness of the legs occasionally occurs in association with a cauda equina syndrome. This syndrome is particularly associated with the development of dural ectasia demonstrable on MRI.

Skin Involvement

In various series, between 10% and 25% of the patients with typical AS have concomitant psoriasis lesions.

Renal Consequences

Although rarely seen today, secondary amyloidosis caused by longstanding AS is well described.

IMAGING

Radiographic damage of the spine and axial joints is a key characteristic of patients with AS. By definition, all patients fulfilling the modified New York criteria show signs of sacroiliitis on radiographs. However, about 30% of the patients do not develop damage of the spine visible on radiographs. If patients show no spinal damage after a certain disease duration (about 10 years), it is unlikely that the patient will develop radiographic abnormalities of the spine at all. On the other hand, patients who have spinal damage are prone to develop more damage.

The most widely used imaging technique is conventional radiography. However, MRI and ultrasound are being used more frequently. Characteristic features on radiographs of the sacroiliac joints are pseudowidening of the joint space, sclerosis, erosions, and ankylosis (Figure 9A-2). At late stages, there is complete ankylosis of the joint. The sacroiliac joint has a complicated, irregular anatomy; computed tomography (CT), which provides views through slices of the joint space, can be helpful when the presence of sacroiliitis is in question. Many AS-related changes can be seen in the spine; squaring of the vertebrae, sclerosis, erosions, syndesmophytes, bony bridging, and spondylodiscitis are the most relevant (Figures 9A-3 and 9A-4).

Syndesmophytes are characterized by axial growth that may lead to bridging phenomena. For making a diagnosis, conventional radiography is still the preferred option. However, if the radiographs are persistently normal in the setting of high disease suspicion, MRI of the sacroiliac joints and spine can add information. In contrast to conventional radiographs, MRI has the potential to demonstrate inflammation, not merely the end results of inflammation on bone. Among MRI

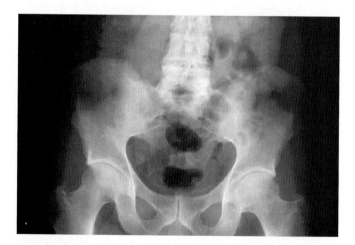

FIGURE 9A-2

Anteroposterior radiographs of the pelvis showing complete ankylosis of both sacroiliac joints and syndesmophyte formation in the lower lumbar vertebrae.

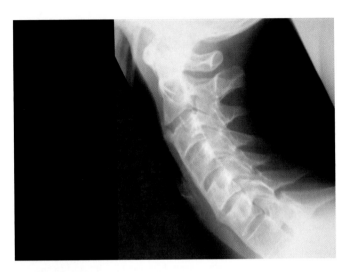

FIGURE 9A-3

Radiograph of the lateral cervical spine, demonstrating the formation of extensive bridging syndesmophytes that involve almost the entire cervical spine.

techniques for delineating inflammation, the short tau inversion recovery (STIR) technique is preferred (Figure 9A-5). MRI is also useful in visualizing enthesitis, for example, of the heel or Achilles tendon insertion.

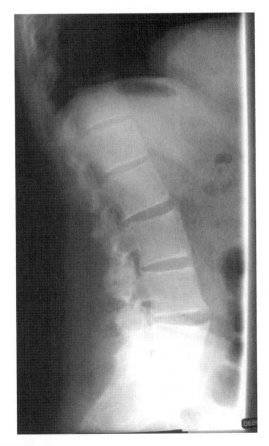

FIGURE 9A-4

Radiograph of the lateral lumbar spine with squaring of L1 and syndesmophyte formation from L3 to L5.

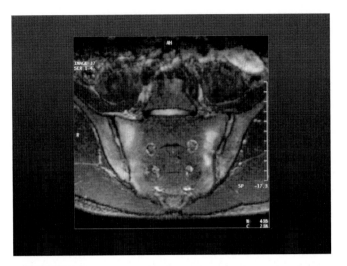

FIGURE 9A-5

Short tau inversion recovery (STIR) image of the sacroiliac joints revealing extensive inflammation (*white*) involving both the sacral and iliac sides of the joints bilaterally.

MAKING THE DIAGNOSIS

As in many other diseases in which the etiology is not clearly defined (e.g., by the isolation of a specific causative pathogen), the diagnosis of AS must rest on the combination of clinical features, radiological findings, and laboratory results. There are no established diagnostic criteria for AS. On the other hand, classification criteria, used for the purpose of categorizing patients in research studies, are available. The most widely used classification criteria for AS are the modified New York criteria (Table 9A-1) (11). Although the New York criteria are useful in established disease, their heavy reliance on the demonstration of radiographic sacroiliitis diminishes their applicability in patients with early disease.

9

TABLE 9A-1. MODIFIED NEW YORK CRITERIA FOR ANKYLOSING SPONDYLITIS.

Criteria

1. Low back pain for at least 3 months' duration improved by exercise and not relieved by rest.
2. Limitation of lumbar spine motion in sagittal and frontal planes.
3. Chest expansion decreased relative to normal values for age and sex.
4a. Unilateral sacroiliitis grade 3–4.
4b. Bilateral sacroiliitis grade 2–4.

Definite ankylosing spondylitis if (4a OR 4b) AND any clinical criterion (1–3)

SOURCE: From Van der Linden et al., Arthritis Rheum 1984;27:361–368, with permission of *Arthritis and Rheumatism*.

Classification criteria for spondyloarthritis, although clearly not intended for diagnostic purposes, are used frequently in clinical practice aids to the identification of atypical or undifferentiated cases. Amor's criteria (Table 9A-2) (12) and the European Spondyloarthropathy Study Group criteria (Table 9A-3) (13) are often employed in this manner. Ongoing studies are designed to evaluate the use of classification criteria for the purpose of diagnosis when applied to patients at early stages of disease.

The optimal role of HLA-B27 in establishing the diagnosis of AS remains under investigation. For many years, HLA-B27 was not recommended for use as a diagnostic test. In certain clinical situations,

TABLE 9A-2. AMOR'S CLASSIFICATION CRITERIA FOR SPONDYLOARTHRITIS.

A	CLINICAL SYMPTOMS OR HISTORY OF	SCORING
1	Lumbar or dorsal pain at night or morning stiffness of lumbar or dorsal pain	1
2	Asymmetrical oligoarthritis	2
3	Buttock pain	1
	If alternate buttock pain	2
4	Sausagelike toe or digit	2
5	Heel pain or other well-defined enthesopathy	2
6	Iritis	1
7	Nongonococcal urethritis or cervicitis within 1 month before the onset of arthritis	1
8	Acute diarrhea within 1 month before the onset of arthritis	1
9	Psoriasis, balanitis, or inflammatory bowel disease (ulcerative colitis or Crohn's disease)	2
B	RADIOLOGICAL FINDINGS	
10	Sacroiliitis (bilateral grade 2 or unilateral grade 3)	3
C	GENETIC BACKGROUND	
11	Presence of HLA-B27 and/or family history of ankylosing spondylitis, reactive arthritis, uveitis, psoriasis, or inflammatory bowel disease	2
D	RESPONSE TO TREATMENT	
12	Clear-cut improvement within 48 hours after NSAIDs intake or rapid relapse of the pain after their discontinuation	2

Source: From Amor B et al., Rev Rheum Mal Ostéoart 1990;57:85–89, by permission of *Revue du rheumatisme et des maladies ostéo-articulaires*.
Abbreviations: NSAIDs, nonsteroidal anti-inflammatory drugs.
A patient is considered as suffering from a spondylarthropathy if the sum is ≥6.

TABLE 9A-3. THE EUROPEAN SPONDYLARTHROPATHY STUDY GROUP CRITERIA.

Inflammatory spinal pain

OR

Synovitis (asymmetric, predominantly in lower extremities)

AND one or more of the following:
- Family history: first- or second-degree relatives with ankylosing spondylitis, psoriasis, acute iritis, reactive arthritis, or inflammatory bowel disease
- Past or present psoriasis, diagnosed by a physician
- Past or present ulcerative colitis or Crohn's disease, diagnosed by a physician and confirmed by radiography or endoscopy
- Past or present pain alternating between the two buttocks
- Past or present spontaneous pain or tenderness at examination of the site of the insertion—the Achilles tendon or plantar fascia (enthesitis)
- Episode of diarrhea occurring within 1 month before onset of arthritis
- Nongonococcal urethritis or cervicitis occurring within 1 month before onset of arthritis
- Bilateral grade 2–4 sacroiliitis or unilateral grade 3 or 4 sacroiliitis [grades are 0, normal, 1, possible, 2, minimal, 3, moderate, 4, completely fused (ankylosed)]

Source: From Dougados M et al., Arthritis Rheum 1991;34:1218–1230, by permission of *Arthritis and Rheumatism* and Wiley Periodicals, Inc.

however, when moderate to high suspicion of spondyloarthritis exists, HLA-B27 testing may play an important role (14). At present, only radiographic sacroiliitis is included in the various criteria sets. However, MRI studies confirming the presence of inflammation even before the occurrence of radiographically evident joint damage may contribute to earlier diagnosis.

REFERENCES

1. Khan MA. An overview of clinical spectrum and heterogeneity of spondyloarthropathies. Rheum Dis Clin N Am 1992;18:1–10.
2. Kidd B, Mullee M, Frank A, et al. Disease expression of ankylosing spondylitis in males and females. J Rheumatol 1988;15:1407–1409.
3. Wordsworth P. Genes in the spondyloarthropathies. Rheum Dis Clin North Am 1998;24:845–863.
4. Gonzalez S, Martina-Barra J, Lopez-Larrea C. Immunogenetics. HLA-B27 and spondyloarthropathies. Curr Opin Rheumatol 1999;11:257–264.
5. Burgos-Vargas R, Vasquez-Mellado J. The early recognition of juvenile onset ankylosing spondylitis and its differentiation from juvenile rheumatoid arthritis. Arthritis Rheum 1995;38:835–844.
6. Will R, Palmer R, Bhalla A, et al. Osteoporosis in early ankylosing spondylitis: a primary pathological event? Lancet 1989;2:1483–1485.

7. Vernon-Roberts B. Ankylosing spondylitis; pathology. In: Klippel JH, Dieppe PA, eds. Rheumatology. 2nd ed. London: Mosby; 1998:6.18.1–6.18.6.

8. Leirisalo-Repo M, Repo H. Gut and spondyloarthropathies. Rheum Dis Clin North Am 1992;18:23–35.

9. O'Neill TW, Bresnihan B. The heart in ankylosing spondylitis. Ann Rheum Dis 1992;51:705–706.

10. Rosenow E, Strimlan CV, Muhm JR, et al. Pleuropulmonary manifestations of ankylosing spondylitis. Mayo Clin Proc 1977;52:641–649.

11. Van der Linden SM, Valkenburg HA, Cats A. Evaluation of diagnostic criteria for ankylosing spondylitis: a proposal for modification of the New York criteria. Arthritis Rheum 1984;27:361–368.

12. Amor B, Dougados M, Mijiyawa M. Critères de classification des spondylarthropathies. Rev Rhum Mal Ostéoart 1990;57:85–89.

13. Dougados M, Van der Linden S, Juhlin R, et al. The European Spondylarthropathy Study Group preliminary criteria for the classification of spondyloarthropathy. Arthritis Rheum 1991;34:1218–1230.

14. Rudwaleit M, van der Heijde D, Kahn A, et al. How to diagnose axial spondyloarthritis early? Ann Rheum Dis 2004;63:535–543.

9

Ankylosing Spondylitis
B. Pathology and Pathogenesis

JUERGEN BRAUN, MD

- Human leukocyte antigen (HLA)-B27 is the major genetic risk factor for ankylosing spondylitis (AS), reactive arthritis, psoriatic arthritis, spondyloarthropathy associated with inflammatory bowel disease, and isolated acute anterior uveitis.
- These diseases are linked by the frequency of inflammation involving the entheses (the sites where tendons and ligaments join to bones) and the axial skeleton, and the common finding of micro- or macroscopic gut inflammation, even in patients without overt gastrointestinal symptoms.
- HLA-B27 transgenic rats develop a spondyloarthropathy.
- HLA-B27 is present in >90% of patients with AS, as well as 50% to 75% of patients with other forms of spondyloarthritides. In contrast, only 5% to 15% of the general population is HLA-B27 positive.
- The contribution of HLA-B27 to AS susceptibility is estimated to be 30%.
- Fewer than 5% of HLA-B27–positive individuals develop SpA.
- Among the HLA class B molecules that determine the antigen binding cleft, HLA-B27 has a unique B pocket that likely influences the peptide repertoire.
- The subtypes of HLA-B27, of which there are more than 30, differ in part only by single amino acids. Only a few HLA-B27 subtypes are associated with AS.
- Intracellular misfolding of HLA-B27 may lead to aberrant expression of B27 homodimers on the cell surface, with possible influences on antigen presentation.

Ankylosing spondylitis (AS) and other spondyloarthritides (SpA) are characterized by inflammation and new bone formation in the axial skeleton and entheses. Peripheral joints and other organs, such as the eye, skin, heart, and gut, may also be involved. Details of the pathogenesis of AS and other SpA remain unresolved, but much has been learned in the three decades since the discovery of HLA-B27, a major histocompatibility complex (MHC) class I allele that is the major genetic factor in these interrelated diseases. HLA-B27 is present not only in most patients with AS, but also in many with other forms of SpA: reactive arthritis (ReA), psoriatic SpA, inflammatory bowel disease (IBD)–associated SpA, and isolated acute anterior uveitis.

Some important considerations related to the origin of AS and related diseases stem from clinical observations. First, the entheses and the axial skeleton are affected much more strongly in patients with SpA than in other rheumatic diseases. Second, microscopic and macroscopic gut inflammation are more frequent in patients with SpA than in other rheumatic diseases (1). The gastrointestinal immune response to pathogens and even normal flora may play a role in causing these disorders.

Several interesting features of the HLA-B27 molecule itself may contribute to disease pathogenesis in the SpA. The following points are explored in further detail in this chapter:

1. Among the HLA class B molecules that determine the antigen binding cleft, HLA-B27 has a unique B pocket that likely influences the peptide repertoire.
2. There are more than 30 subtypes of HLA-B27, which differ in part only by single amino acids. Only a few HLA-B27 subtypes are associated with AS.
3. Intracellular misfolding of HLA-B27 may lead to aberrant expression of B27 homodimers on the cell surface, with possible influences on antigen presentation.
4. HLA-B27 itself can be presented by HLA class II as an autoantigen, and could be recognized by CD4+ T cells.
5. HLA-B27 transgenic rats develop an SpA-like disease.
6. Data suggest that intracellular handling of microbes by HLA-B27 transfected cell lines is altered.

Both genetic and nongenetic factors contribute to AS. In addition to HLA-B27 and other MHC-related genetic factors, current hypotheses implicate both innate and adaptive immune responses. *Chlamydia, Yersinia,*

Salmonella, and other species contribute directly to the etiology of ReA, for example, and autoantigens such as the G1 domain of aggrecan have been linked to AS.

Human Leukocyte Antigen-B27

The discovery of the link between HLA-B27 and AS was a major contribution to understanding the pathogenesis of this disease (2). HLA-B27 is present in >90%

of patients with AS, as well as 50% to 75% of patients with other forms of SpA. In contrast, only 5% to 15% of the general population is HLA-B27 positive, with variations based on ancestry. The overall contribution of HLA-B27 to AS susceptibility is estimated to be 30%, but the gene is neither necessary nor sufficient to cause the disease. Fewer than 5% of HLA-B27–positive individuals develop SpA, but the individual risk is higher in the setting of a positive family history of SpA (Figure 9B-1) (3). The dominant effect of HLA-B27 in AS

FIGURE 9B-1

Unique intracellular and extracellular functions of HLA-B27 that may affect susceptibility to spondyloarthritis. (a) The HLA-B27 heavy chain is transcribed off ribosomes in macrophages, and retained in the endoplasmic reticulum (ER) by the molecular chaperone calnexin and ERp57. The latter is a protein disulfide isomerase that reduces and oxidizes disulfide bonds. HLA-B27 is then folded into its tertiary structure and bound to beta-2-microglobulin. Calnexin releases the complex, which becomes associated with calreticulum, which in turn chaperones the formation of the peptide loading onto the complex of heavy chain, beta-2-microglobulin and antigenic peptide, via the TAP proteins and tapasin. Thence the trimolecular peptide complex (HLA-B27 heavy chain, beta-2-microglobulin, and peptide) travels to the cell surface, where the antigenic peptide is presented either to CD8+ T lymphocytes or to natural killer (NK) cells. (b) The HLA-B27 heavy chain misfolds in the endoplasmic reticulum, forming B27 homodimers and other misfoldings, where they either (b1) accumulate causing an proinflammatory ER stress response; or (b2) migrate to the cell surface, where they become antigenic themselves or present peptide to receptors on other inflammatory cells. (c) Intracellular impairment of peptide processing or loading into HLA-B27 by viruses or intracellular bacteria causes a selective impairment of the immune response. (d) Either the trimolecular complex presents processed peptide to CD4+ T lymphocytes, or free HLA-B27 heavy chains or HLA-B27 homodimers are recognized as antigenic by the T-cell receptor thence, or processed antigenic fragments of HLA-B27 are presented to the T-cell receptor of CD4–positive T lymphocytes.

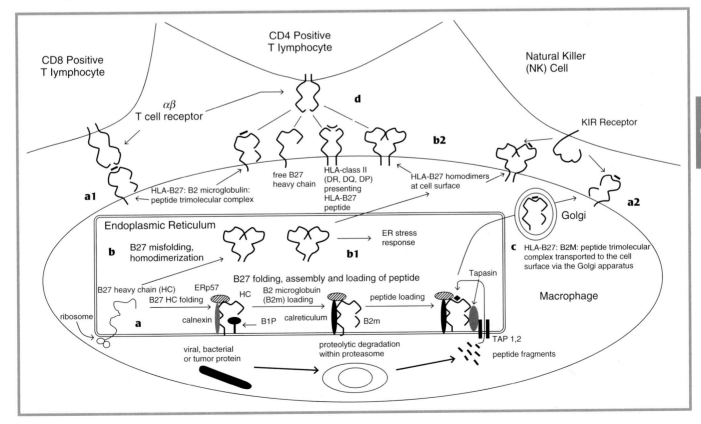

makes this disease rather unique among rheumatic conditions. It is clear, however, that other genes also contribute to the risk of AS.

Human leukocyte antigen-B27 is an MHC class I molecule and, as such, participates in antigen presentation. HLA-B27 binds an accessory molecule—beta-2 microglobulin—that helps the heavy chain maintain its proper conformation. Genetic evidence from humans and data from animal models suggest that HLA-B27 has one or more unique characteristics that can promote inflammation. Among individuals with HLA-B27, the protein is expressed ubiquitously but most abundantly on antigen-presenting cells such as macrophages and dendritic cells (DC). HLA-B27 expression is upregulated by proinflammatory stimuli. The peptides displayed by HLA-B27 and related MHC class I molecules are normally derived from self-proteins, but when cells are infected with microbes such as viruses or other intracellular pathogens, foreign peptides are presented.

Peptide-loaded MHC class I molecules are recognized by receptors on several different types of immune cells. T-cell receptors (TCRs) on cytotoxic CD8+ T cells recognize MHC class I complexes. The ability of TCRs on CD8+ T cells to recognize MHC class I molecules and distinguish different alleles or different peptides displayed by the same allele (e.g., viral vs. self-peptide) plays a critical role in the adaptive immune response to viruses.

Hypotheses about the role of HLA-B27 in AS can be considered in terms of two distinct paradigms: one invokes immunological recognition of HLA-B27 expressed on the cell surface, either as classic trimolecular complexes of heavy chain/peptide/beta-2 microglobulin, or beta-2-microglobulin free forms of the heavy chain that exist as dimers or perhaps monomers. The other paradigm posits that intracellular effects of HLA-B27 are responsible for influences on bacterial killing, either due to HLA-B27 misfolding (4) or some other as yet unrecognized consequence of its expression (Table 9B-1). Potential links to pathogenesis from misfolding include endoplasmic reticulum (ER) stress and activation of the unfolded protein response, while enhanced bacterial survival may lead to persistent infection. These concepts also differ in terms of whether the fundamental abnormality is one of adaptive (arthritogenic peptides) or innate immunity (immune receptor recognition, misfolding, altered bacterial survival).

Arthritogenic Peptides

The basis for this concept is essentially that of molecular mimicry; that is, self-peptides displayed by folded HLA-B27 heavy chain/beta-2 microglobulin complexes are targeted by autoreactive CD8+ T cells because they resemble microbial peptides (5). In this model, the cytotoxic T cells and the unique peptide binding specificity

TABLE 9B-1. OVERVIEW OF THE FOUR MAIN THEORIES ON THE PATHOGENESIS OF SPONDYLOARTHRITIDES RELATED TO HLA-B27.

The Arthritogenic Peptide Hypothesis
HLA-B27 binds a unique set of antigenic peptides, bacterial or self, which gives rise to an HLA-B27–restricted cytotoxic T-cell response to such peptides which are presented by disease-associated HLA-B27 subtypes but not by other HLA class I molecules.

Self-Association of the HLA-B27 Molecule
A unique property of HLA-B27 is that its heavy chains can form homodimers in vitro that are dependent on disulfide binding through their cysteine-67 residues in the alpha-1 domain. These homodimers occur as a result of B27 misfolding within the endoplasmic reticulum. The accumulation of misfolded protein may result in a proinflammatory intracellular stress response. Alternatively, B27 homodimers can migrate to the cell surface where they either become antigenic themselves or present peptide to other inflammatory cells.

Alteration of Intracellular Handling of Microbes Due to HLA-B27
HLA-B27 leads to a less effective elimination of microbes, such as salmonella, in conjunction with an upregulated production of cytokines.

Recognition of HLA-B27 as an Autoantigen
HLA-B27 itself can be recognized by CD4+ T cells, when presented by HLA class II (DR, DQ, and DP) heterodimers as an autoantigen. This was also part of the classic molecular mimicry hypothesis, wherein homology of peptides from the HLA-B27 molecule shared striking sequence homology with those from bacterial sources.

of HLA-B27 are the main causes of the chronic inflammation. HLA-B27-restricted CD8+ T-cell clones with specificity for bacteria or possibly self-peptides have been detected in both the synovial fluid and peripheral blood of patients with ReA and AS. With regard to ReA, several HLA-B27–binding *Yersinia*- and *Chlamydia*-derived peptides have been identified in synovial fluid that may account for the CD8+ T-cell response. Whether these immune responses are beneficial or detrimental to the patient remains unclear. Autoreactive self-peptides that might be targeted by these T cells have not been defined.

Indirect evidence that antigens might be driving the inflammation comes from analyses of the TCR beta chain (TCRB) repertoire using TCRB CDR3 size spectratyping: HLA-B27+ twin pairs who were concordant for AS exhibited increased T-cell oligoclonality in both CD8+ and CD4+ T-cell subsets, suggesting a role for conventional T-cell antigens in AS pathogenesis.

Although triggering bacterial infections have as yet not been identified in AS, several HLA-B27–binding candidate peptides have been studied. The peptide LRRYLENGK, for example, known to be part of both the HLA-B27 heavy chain and proteins from enterobacteriae, was recognized more often by HLA-B27–restricted CD8+ T cells from AS patients compared to controls.

Aberrant Cell Surface Heavy Chains

Human leukocyte antigen-B27 heavy chains exist in aberrant forms on the cell surface. Purified HLA-B27 molecules can refold in vitro without beta-2 microglobulin, for which the formation of disulfide-linked dimers through the unpaired Cys 67 residue (Cys^{67}) is functional. Such dimers form when cell surface heavy chains lose beta-2 microglobulin and undergo endosomal recycling. Furthermore, relatively stable monomeric HLA-B27 heavy chains exist on the cell surface (6). Thus, MHC class I receptors on leukocytes might recognize aberrant forms of HLA-B27 in a specific manner, leading to modification of leukocyte function. The extent to which other alleles form cell surface dimers is less clear.

Enhanced Bacterial Survival

The strong relationship between HLA-B27 and ReA leads to the question of whether HLA-B27 might influence the invasion and the handling of intracellular bacteria. Enhanced survival of intracellular *Salmonella* has been reported in monocytic cells and fibroblasts that express HLA-B27 after DNA transfection. The effect of HLA-B27 seems to depend on the Glu^{45} residue, which may be a major determinant of HLA-B27 misfolding. Data on this point are not conclusive, however, as other experiments have failed to demonstrate an effect of HLA-B27 expression on synoviocytes on the clearance of *Salmonella*.

Protein Misfolding and Endoplasmic Reticulum Stress

Evidence of abnormalities in HLA-B27 folding was first reported a few years ago. HLA-B27 heavy chains, even those expressed under normal physiologic conditions, were described as undergoing ER-associated degradation (ERAD) shortly after synthesis. ERAD is a quality control pathway that cells use to dispose of proteins that do not fold efficiently. Abnormally folded HLA-B27 complexes have been found in the ER, with abnormalities relating to aberrant inter- and intrachain disulfide bonds.

In normal cells, the dimers that form in the ER do not contribute to the cell surface population. About 25% of newly synthesized HLA-B27 heavy chains form disulfide-linked complexes in the ER, whereas only about 6% become disulfide-linked on the cell surface. Another critical feature of misfolding is prolonged

binding of the heavy chain to the ER chaperone BiP. Misfolding has not been seen in other MHC class I alleles. HLA-B27 misfolding and cell surface dimerization are distinct processes.

The tendency of HLA-B27 to misfold is a consequence of residues that comprise the B pocket of the peptide-binding groove. The B pocket renders HLA-B27 inefficient at loading peptides because of resistance to the peptide-induced conformational change that promotes folding. Prolonged retention of the HLA-B27 heavy chain in the ER in an unfolded conformation results in aberrant disulfide bond formation, with possible involvement of the unpaired Cys at position 67 (Cys^{67}). Aberrant disulfide bond formation may contribute to the accumulation of heavy chains bound to BiP. The amino acid residue in HLA-B27 most detrimental to efficient folding, not surprisingly, is Glu^{45} in the B pocket. Some proteins that misfold are not eliminated efficiently and may lead to stress in the ER by activating a process known as the unfolded protein response.

Human Leukocyte Antigen-B27: A Causative Factor for Disease in Animal Models

The immunologic function of HLA-B27 is to bind peptides derived from proteins degraded in the cytosol and display them on the cell surface, where they can be recognized by CD8+ T cells. In transgenic animal models, HLA-B27 and human beta-2-microglobulin were expressed in mice without producing inflammatory joint disease. In other HLA-B27 transgenic mice models, a higher frequency of ankylosing enthesopathy was reported, but this phenotype occurs also in wild-type mice.

The strongest experimental evidence that HLA-B27 plays a direct role in disease pathophysiology comes from transgenic rats, where overexpression of HLA-B27 and human beta-2-microglobulin results in spontaneous inflammation in the gastrointestinal tract and joints (7). The skin and nail lesions in this transgenic rat model resemble those seen in psoriasis HLA-B27/human beta-2-microglobulin transgenic (B27-Tg) rats, which develop colitis initially and subsequently manifest inflammation in other locations. Expression of the disease phenotype depends on the specific genetic background of the rat. When raised under entirely germ-free conditions, B27-Tg rats do not develop disease. Colonization of the gastrointestinal tract with normal gut flora, however (e.g., *Bacteroides* sp.), is sufficient to trigger inflammation. B27-Tg rats do not provide a precise phenocopy of human AS because they do not develop ankylosis of the axial skeleton. Further, the colitis observed in the B27-Tg rats is more prominent than that which occurs in human AS patients.

THE ROLE OF MICROBES AND THE GUT

Several gastrointestinal or genitourinary pathogens have been implicated as triggers of HLA-B27–associated ReA in humans, including *Campylobacter*, *Chlamydia*, *Salmonella*, and *Shigella*. DNA from these organisms can be detected by polymerase chain reaction (PCR) in synovial samples, and the lipopolysaccharide (LPS) of *Salmonella*, *Yersinia*, and *Shigella* has also been found. The presence of bacterial products in joints provides a potential link between gut infection and joint inflammation in ReA (1). More than two thirds of patients with SpA have microscopic lesions of the gut: polymorphonuclear infiltration of ileal villi and crypts, and granulocytes, lymphocytes, and plasma cells in the lamina propria. Patients who develop overt inflammatory bowel disease are more likely to have symptoms of active AS, and SpA patients with gut inflammation have a higher risk of developing AS.

In juvenile AS patients without gastrointestinal symptoms, radionuclide labeling of lymphocytes indicate homing to the gut in almost half of the patients. Positive scans are in patients with active joint disease and correlate with nonspecific mucosal inflammatory changes on biopsy. Thus, subclinical gut inflammation may be important in disease pathogenesis. In this regard, CD163+ macrophages are overrepresented in the gut mucosa of patients with SpA and Crohn's disease, but not ulcerative colitis. These findings have underscored the close relationship between gut inflammation and arthritis in the SpA.

Human Leukocyte Antigen-B27 SUBTYPES

Human leukocyte antigen-B27 constitutes the greatest known risk factor for AS. However, HLA-B27 is not just one molecule: more than 30 different subtypes have now been described (http://www.ebi.ac.uk/imgt/hla/). Most of these subtypes only differ by a few amino acids, but these differences may be sufficient to alter the peptide binding properties of the molecule.

Human leukocyte antigen-B*2705, found in all populations, appears to be the original or parent HLA-B27 molecule. Most of the other subtypes have probably evolved from three pathways, defined by the pattern of amino acid substitutions in the first (alpha-1) and second (alpha-2) domains (Figures 9B-2 and 9B-3). The finding of particular HLA-B27 subtypes in populations tends to have strong geographic patterns. The most common subtypes—*HLA-B*2705, -B*2702, -B*2704, -B*2707*—are clearly associated with SpA.

The HLA-B27 subtypes are distributed unevenly around the world. Whereas HLA-B*2709 is found pri-

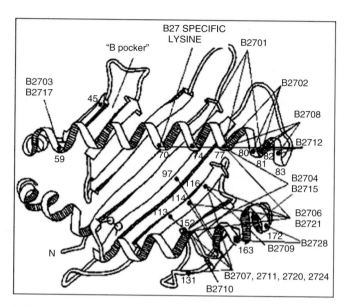

FIGURE 9B-2

The crystallized HLA-B27 molecule, indicating positions of amino acid substitutions in selected HLA-B27 subtypes.

marily in Sardinia and regions of mainland Italy, -B*2706 is common in native Indonesians. Although neither -B*2709 nor -B*2706 appears to be associated with AS, B*2709 has been reported in patients with undifferentiated forms of SpA (uSpA).

Variations in the clinical phenotype associated with HLA-B27 subtypes likely relate to amino acid differences in the B pocket of the antigen binding cleft, which could alter the nature of the peptides presented by these HLA-B27 subtypes. The only xdifference between these subtypes and the major AS-associated subtypes is the exchange at position 116 of an aspartate for a histidine residue. Position 116, located within the peptide binding groove at the floor of the F pocket, plays a pivotal role in anchoring the C-terminal peptide residue. Other subtypes of HLA-B27 are too rare to have had their clinical associations established, but cases of AS have occurred in carriers of -*B*2701, *2703, *2704, *2707, *2708, *2710, *2714, *2715,* and **2719*.

Until recently, the only known differences between these subtypes was their peptide binding specificity, which has been used to support the concept that disease pathogenesis is a consequence of peptide display differences. For the VIP1R$_{400-408}$ peptide, this is clearly not the case because it is presented by both -B*2705 and -B*2709. However, there are interesting differences between -B*2706 and other disease-associated alleles. Comparing -B*2704, -B*2705, -B*2706, and -B*2709, -B*2706 is the only subtype that does not interact appreciably with the peptide loading complex (8). The -B*2706 heavy chain also folds faster than other subtypes. This raises the possibility that the -B*2706 heavy chain might show a diminished capacity to misfold and cause ER stress because mutations that enhance the

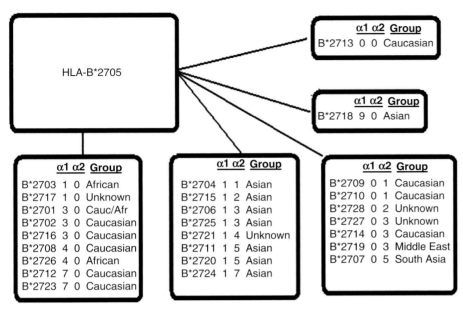

FIGURE 9B-3

Possible evolutionary pathway of HLA-B27 subtypes from the parent *HLA-B*2705*. The three major families of HLA-B27 subtypes are denoted in relationship to the parent subtype *HLA-B*2705* (*HLA-B*2713* and *B*2718* are assumed to have evolved separately). The numbers of amino acid substitutions from B*2705 in the first (alpha-1) and second (alpha-2) domains are indicated, as well as the predominant ethnic group in which the subtype was described. For example, *HLA-B*2704* differs from HLA-B27 by one amino acid substitution in the alpha-1 and one amino acid substitution in the alpha-2 domain. Of note, at the time of this writing, we are unable to find the sequences of four HLA-B27 subtypes that have been described only in the past few months (*B*2729–B*2732*).

rate of -B*2705 folding reduce misfolding. If this is responsible for the lack of association with disease, then another explanation would be necessary for -B*2709.

OTHER MAJOR HISTOCOMPATIBILITY COMPLEX GENES AND ANKYLOSING SPONDYLITIS SUSCEPTIBILITY

Human leukocyte antigen-B27 constitutes only part of the overall risk for SpA. Fewer than 5% of HLA-B27–positive individuals in the general population develop an SpA. In contrast, up to 20% of HLA-B27–positive relatives of AS patients will develop an SpA in time. Family studies have shown that HLA-B27 contributes less than 40% of the overall genetic risk for SpA. The entire effect of the MHC, on the other hand, is about 50%.

Identifying other MHC genes that may be involved in AS susceptibility is generally complicated because of the tight linkage disequilibrium found within the MHC. However, there is some evidence from studies of individual MHC genes that other non-B27 MHC genetic effects are present in patients with AS. These genes are listed in Table 9B-2.

NON–MAJOR HISTOCOMPATIBILITY COMPLEX GENES AND ANKYLOSING SPONDYLITIS SUSCEPTIBILITY

The strength of the association of B27 and of the linkage of the MHC with AS has obscured the role of other genetic factors for decades. The concordance rate for B27-positive dizygotic (DZ) twin pairs (23%), considerably lower than that of monozygotic (MZ) twin pairs (63%), points clearly to the presence of non-B27 susceptibility factors (9).

The total number of genes involved in susceptibility to AS is unknown, but family recurrence risk modeling suggests that the number is limited. The reduction of disease concordance with distant relatives of patients is determined by the number and the interactions of the involved genes. In AS, an oligogenic model appears to be operative, with multiplicative interactions between loci.

Non-major histocompatibility complex genetic effects appear to also have significant influence on disease severity, as demonstrated by a complex segregation study (10). A high degree of familiality was observed

9

7. Hammer RE, Maika SD, Richardson JA, et al. Spontaneous inflammatory disease in transgenic rats expressing HLA-B27 and human b_2-m: an animal model of HLA-B27-associated human disorders. Cell 1990;63:1099–1112.

8. Brown MA, Wordsworth BP, Reveille JD. Genetics of ankylosing spondylitis. Clin Exp Rheumatol 2002;20(Suppl 28):S43–S49.

9. Brown MA, Kennedy LG, MacGregor AJ, et al. Susceptibility to ankylosing spondylitis in twins: the role of genes, HLA, and the environment. Arthritis Rheum 1997;40:1823–1828.

10. Hamersma J, Cardon LR, Bradbury L, et al. Is disease severity in ankylosing spondylitis genetically determined? Arthritis Rheum 2001;44:1396–1400.

11. Brown MA. Non-major-histocompatibility-complex genetics of ankylosing spondylitis. Best Pract Res Clin Rheumatol 2006;20:611–621.

12. Brown MA, Brophy S, Bradbury L, et al. Identification of major loci controlling clinical manifestations of ankylosing spondylitis. Arthritis Rheum 2003;48:2234–2239.

13. Zou J, Rudwaleit M, Brandt J, et al. Upregulation of the production of tumour necrosis factor alpha and interferon gamma by T cells in ankylosing spondylitis during treatment with etanercept. Ann Rheum Dis 2003;62:561–564.

14. Lories RJ, Derese I, Luyten FP. Modulation of bone morphogenetic protein signaling inhibits the onset and progression of ankylosing enthesitis. J Clin Invest 2005;115:1571–1579.

CHAPTER 9

Ankylosing Spondylitis
C. Treatment and Assessment

JOHN C. DAVIS, JR., MD, MPH

- Multiple modalities for the therapy of ankylosing spondylitis (AS) are available, including physical therapy and patient education, nonsteroidal anti-inflammatory drugs (NSAIDs), glucocorticoids, disease-modifying antirheumatic drugs (DMARDs), and anti–tumor necrosis factor (TNF) agents.
- Combination approaches to therapy are often required to relieve symptoms, improve function, and potentially modify disease progression.
- In assessing patient outcomes in clinical trials, disease activity is measured by the Bath Ankylosing Disease Activity Index (BASDAI), which includes six patient-oriented questions based on fatigue, overall back and hip pain, peripheral arthritis, entheses, and the duration and intensity of morning stiffness.

- Physical therapy and stretching exercises are cornerstones of AS treatment, regardless of which other therapies are employed.
- Indomethacin is the most commonly prescribed NSAID for AS treatment, but other NSAIDs are comparable to indomethacin in efficacy and safety.
- Tumor necrosis factor inhibitors (etanercept, infliximab, and adalimumab) demonstrate striking efficacy in the majority of patients with AS.
- For patients with AS and concomitant inflammatory bowel disease, a monoclonal antibody approach to the inhibition of TNF (i.e., either infliximab or adalimumab) is preferred.

Ankylosing spondylitis (AS) is the prototype of chronic inflammatory diseases of the spine known as the spondyloarthropathies (SpA). Patients present with significant inflammatory back pain and may progress, in severe forms, to fusion of the entire spine. AS may also involve peripheral joints, entheses, and non-articular structures (such as the gut and anterior chamber of the eye). Accordingly, these manifestations should be taken into account when assessing and treating the patient. Recently, the treatment goal in AS has evolved from providing only symptomatic relief to inducing major clinical responses and potentially disease-modifying benefits. Multiple modalities are available, including physical therapy and patient education, nonsteroidal anti-inflammatory drugs (NSAIDs), glucocorticoids, disease-modifying antirheumatic drugs (DMARDs), and anti–tumor necrosis factor (TNF) agents (Table 9C-1). No single modality treats all manifestations of a patient with AS. Combination approaches to therapy are often required to relieve symptoms, improve function, and potentially modify disease progression.

DISEASE ACTIVITY AND CLINICAL ASSESSMENT

Other than a complete medical history and physical examination, a core set of domains and instruments has been recommended by the Assessments in Ankylosing Spondylitis Working group (ASAS) for monitoring patients in the clinical setting (Table 9C-2) (1). These include measures of physical function, pain, spinal mobility, patient's global assessment, duration of morning stiffness, involvement of peripheral joints and entheses, acute phase reactants, and fatigue. Overall disease activity should be measured by the Bath Anky-losing Spondylitis Disease Activity Index (BASDAI), which includes six patient-oriented questions based on fatigue, overall back and hip pain, peripheral arthritis, entheses, and the duration and intensity of morning stiffness (Table 9C-2). In addition, a physician global assessment, taking into account available clinical, laboratory, and imaging data, should be performed using either a visual analog scale or a numeric ranking scale.

may represent differences in dosing regimens. Commonly reported side effects include drowsiness, constipation, dizziness, headache, nausea/vomiting, and paresthesias. Peripheral neuropathy (often irreversible) is an important long-term concern with thalidomide.

Sulfasalazine

Sulfasalazine (SSZ), a salicyclic acid derivative created by covalent linkage of 5-amino-salicyclic acid (5-ASA) to sulfapyridine, is cleaved by bacteria in the colon. The 5-ASA absorption is limited to the colonic wall, where the drug is effective in inflammatory bowel disease. The sulfapyridine moiety, absorbed through the gastrointestinal wall, acts as systemic effects in several autoimmune diseases (21). A meta-analysis of five randomized, controlled trials involving a total of 272 patients was published in 1990 (22). Doses ranged from 2 to 3 g/day for 3 to 11 months. Benefit was demonstrated in clinical and laboratory parameters, including the severity and duration of morning stiffness and the severity of pain. General well-being, acute phase reactants, and spinal mobility measurements showed nonsignificant trends in favor of SSZ. Only one of the five trials in this meta-analysis evaluated response rates in axial versus peripheral symptoms, with a nonstatistically significant trend favoring response of peripheral symptoms (23).

METHOTREXATE

The limited studies of methotrexate (MTX) available have shown little benefit in the treatment of AS, in contrast to the proven long-term efficacy and tolerability in rheumatoid arthritis and psoriatic arthritis. In an open-label study of MTX (7.5–15 mg once a week), 9 of 11 patients who had previously demonstrated inadequate response to either NSAIDs or sulfasalazine were evaluated at 24 weeks. The small study reported a reduction in the number of swollen joints in patients with a predominance of peripheral arthritis (24). Two patients with significant extra-articular disease (both with enthesitis and iridocyclitis) discontinued MTX due to continued disease activity. A randomized, placebo-controlled trial of MTX in AS failed to demonstrate significant benefit in either axial or peripheral arthritis, but there was a trend toward a reduction in peripheral symptoms (25). A more recent small study evaluated MTX in a dose of only 7.5 mg/week in patients with AS treated for 24 weeks (26). This study reported a composite response rate of over 50% ($n = 17$) in those receiving MTX, compared with 17% in the placebo group (despite the relatively low dose of MTX used in the study). Long-term data in MTX-treated patients are not available.

BIOLOGIC AGENTS

There is no evidence that the conventional therapies discussed so far actually modify disease progression. In contrast, there is a growing body of evidence that demonstrates the clinical efficacy of TNF blockade. Multiple studies have demonstrated that TNF-alpha appears to play a key role in promoting inflammation in AS. Increased TNF-alpha expression is found in the sacroiliac joints, peripheral synovial tissue, and serum of patients with AS (27–31). Following a series of randomized, controlled clinical trials, three TNF inhibitors are either approved for the treatment of AS or the subject of ongoing study—etanercept, infliximab, and adalimumab.

Etanercept

Etanercept is a soluble fusion protein containing an Fc fragment of human IgG_1 fused to two extracellular domains of the p75 TNF receptor. The medication's mechanism of action is to bind soluble forms of TNF-alpha, thereby preventing attachment of the cytokine to cell surface receptors. Etanercept is given in doses of 50 mg subcutaneously per week (alternatively 25 mg twice weekly). The efficacy of etanercept in AS was demonstrated in a double-blind, placebo-controlled trial of 40 patients with active spondylitis (32). Patients had moderate-to-severe disease despite stable doses of NSAIDs, DMARDs, or glucocorticoids. Patients randomized to the etanercept group demonstrated a rapid and sustained response in four primary outcome measures: duration of morning stiffness, nocturnal pain, patient's global assessment, and functional index. A number of secondary outcomes also improved, including spinal and chest range of motion, enthesitis, and acute phase reactants. The most frequent side effects were injection-site reactions and minor infections, which did not differ statistically between the two groups. These results were confirmed in a larger randomized, placebo-controlled trial in patients with moderate to severe disease (33). A significant percentage of patients achieved the primary outcome, defined by the ASAS Working Group 20% improvement criteria (ASAS20) compared to placebo at both 12 and 24 weeks. These results were sustained through 2 years (34).

Early evidence of the benefit of etanercept by MRI was published in an uncontrolled study of 10 patients with active spondylitis (35). Repeated MRIs demonstrated a 86% reduction or resolution in acute inflammatory bone lesions over 24 weeks. Moreover, no new bone lesions were identified over this period. These results were confirmed by a larger MRI substudy of the large randomized study that demonstrated significant reduction in inflammatory lesions (36).

Infliximab

Infliximab is a chimeric monoclonal IgG$_1$ antibody that binds both soluble and cell bound forms of TNF-alpha. In AS, infliximab is usually given at a slightly higher dose than in rheumatoid arthritis patients. Dosing for AS is 5 mg/kg intravenously at baseline, week 2, week 6, and then every 6 weeks thereafter. In an early study, a 3-month randomized study compared infliximab in doses of 5 mg/kg intravenously to placebo in AS patients with active disease (37). A larger proportion of patients experienced a response in terms of the BASDAI than placebo. This has been shown to be sustained to 3 years (38). These results have been confirmed by a larger randomized placebo-controlled trial over 24 weeks (39). A significantly larger proportion of patients achieved an ASAS20 compared to placebo over the 24 weeks. MRI results also demonstrated a significant decrease in inflammatory lesions.

Adalimumab

Adalimumab is a fully humanized IgG$_1$ monoclonal antibody that inhibits. The usual dose is 40 mg, administered subcutaneously every other week. Results from a small open-label trial in which AS patients were treated with adalimumab showed significant improvement in disease activity, acute phase reactants, pain, and morning stiffness (40). Results from a large, randomized, placebo-controlled study demonstrated a significant clinical response in the ASAS20 as well as many secondary outcome measures when adalimumab was administered over a 24-week period (41).

TREATMENT RECOMMENDATIONS AND BEST PRACTICE GUIDELINES

A systematic literature review and Delphi exercise was performed on all treatment modalities for AS and recently published (Table 9C-3) (42). In addition, treatment recommendations for the use of anti-TNF agents have been published by the ASAS and modified for use in the United States by the Spondyloarthritis Research and Treatment Network (SPARTAN) (Table 9C-4) (43–45). Patients who are symptomatic, regardless of their predominant manifestation (peripheral arthritis, axial arthritis, enthesitis) should be given a trial of at least two NSAIDs. Patients with moderate disease activity or greater [BASDAI score of 4 or above and a physician global score of at least 2 (range, 0–4)], should be given additional therapy. For patients with pronounced peripheral symptoms, a trial of SSZ or MTX should be considered. For patients with purely axial manifestations, no trial of SSZ or MTX is required and an anti-TNF agent should be prescribed. For those with concomitant inflammatory bowel disease, a monoclonal antibody is preferred. Strict adherence to screening and treatment of latent tuberculosis infection is required prior to the initiation of anti-TNF therapy. In

TABLE 9C-3. SUMMARY OF APPROVED ANTI–TUMOR NECROSIS FACTOR AGENTS USED IN THE TREATMENT OF PATIENTS WITH ANKYLOSING SPONDYLITIS.

AGENT	DESCRIPTION	DOSING	CLINICAL RESPONSE	DISEASE-MODIFYING PROPERTIES
Etanercept	Dimeric fusion protein of the TNF-alpha receptor linked to the Fc portion of human IgG1	Subcutaneous injection of 50 mg once a week or 25 mg twice weekly	ASAS 20/50/70 BASDAI 50 ASAS 5/6 Partial remission	DXA improvement in lumbar spine Reduction in acute MRI changes Limited plain radiographic data
Infliximab	Monoclonal IgG1 anti-TNF antibody with a mouse variable region	Intravenous infusion of 5 mg/kg at 0, 2, and 6 weeks and then every 6 weeks	ASAS 20/50/70 BASDAI 50 ASAS 5/6 Partial remission	DXA improvement in lumbar spine and hip Improvement in cartilage and bone metabolism measures Reduction in acute MRI changes Limited radiographic data Effective in patients with IBD
Adalimumab	Fully humanized monoclonal antibody directed against TNF-alpha	Subcutaneous injection of 40 mg every other week	ASAS 20/50/70 BASDAI 50 ASAS 5/6 Partial remission	Reduction in acute MRI changes Limited data on efficacy in patients with IBD

ABBREVIATIONS: ASAS, Assessments in Ankylosing Spondylitis Working Group; BASDAI, Bath Ankylosing Spondylitis Disease Activity Index; DXA, dual-energy x-ray absorptiometry; IBD, inflammatory bowel disease; MRI, magnetic resonance imaging; TNF, tumor necrosis factor.
Data from References 33 and 39.

TABLE 9C–4. BEST CLINICAL PRACTICE GUIDELINES FOR THE USE OF ANTI–TUMOR NECROSIS FACTOR AGENTS IN ANKYLOSING SPONDYLITIS.

Patient acceptance including and understanding of risk and benefits of long-term or potentially lifelong anti-TNF therapy and unknown effects on pregnancy/lactation.

Diagnosis and/or associated features

Modified NY Criteria or other evidence of SpA, including inflammatory back pain, persistently elevated acute phase reactants, baseline radiographic damage and/or rapid radiographic progression, spinal inflammation on imaging modality including MRI and ultrasound.

Suggested disease activity

BASDAI Score of ≥4 (0–10).

Physician global assessment of at least moderate disease activity based upon either a score of ≥2 on a Lickert scale (0–4) or VAS score of ≥4 (0–10).

Clinical presentation and extra-articular features

Three clinical presentations: axial, peripheral arthritis (excluding hip), and entheseal. Predominant feature guides the previous treatment requirements.

For axial, peripheral, and entheseal presentations–failure of at least two NSAIDs either due to inefficacy or toxicity.

For peripheral features–arthritis or ethesitis: NSAID failure and failure of methotrexate or sulfasalazine at maximally tolerated doses for 3 months.

For axial predominance: NSAID failure and no DMARD failure required.

Intra-articular or entheseal injections of glucocorticoids as clinically indicated.

Response

Reduction in BASDAI score and physician global score of at least 50%.

Timing of response

Response expected within 12 weeks of initiation of treatment.

Agents

Etanercept 50 mg/wk sq

Infliximab 5 mg/kg at 0, 2, and 6 weeks, then every 6 weeks intravenously.

Adalimumab 40 mg every other week sq

Precautions/contraindications

Active or recurrent infection including untreated evidence of latent TB or recent TB exposure.

SLE or MS symptom/history.

Other per package insert.

ABBREVIATIONS: BASDAI, Bath Ankylosing Spondylitis Disease Activity Index; DMARD, disease-modifying antirheumatic drug; MRI, magnetic resonance imaging; MS, multiple sclerosis; NSAIDs, nonsteroidal anti-inflammatory drugs; SLE, systemic lupus erythematosus; SpA, spondyloarthropathies; TB, tuberculosis; TNF, tumor necrosis factor; VAS, visual analog scale.
Data from References 43 through 45.

addition, if during treatment there are signs/symptoms of infection or recent contact, screening and evaluation should be pursued.

SURGICAL INTERVENTION

Advances in orthopedic surgery have also proven to be highly effective in patients with disabling manifestations (in particular, severe pain) of AS. The disease commonly involves the hip joint, a finding that portends more severe disease and a worse prognosis. Additionally, kyphosis can lead to significant loss of function and disability. Surgical intervention—total hip arthroplasty and osteotomy and fixation—may greatly improve a patient's level of mobility and quality of life. Appropriate referrals should be made to an orthopedist.

Acknowledgment. This work supported by the Rosalind Russell Medical Center for Arthritis Research, The University of California San Francisco.

REFERENCES

1. van der Heijde D, Calin A, Dougados M, et al. Selection of instruments in the core set for DC-ART, SMARD, physical therapy, and clinical record keeping in ankylosing spondylitis. Progress report of the ASAS Working Group. Assessments in Ankylosing Spondylitis. J Rheumatol 1999;26:951–954.
2. Dougados M, Dijkmans B, Khan M, et al. Conventional treatments for ankylosing spondylitis. Ann Rheum Dis 2002;61(Suppl 3):iii40–iii50.
3. Dagfinrud H, Kvien TK, Hagen KB. Physiotherapy interventions for ankylosing spondylitis. Cochrane Database Syst Rev 2004;CD002822.

4. van Tubergen A, Hidding A. Spa and exercise treatment in ankylosing spondylitis: fact or fancy? Best Pract Res Clin Rheumatol 2002;16:653–666.

5. Van Tubergen A, Boonen A, Landewe R, et al. Cost effectiveness of combined spa-exercise therapy in anky-losing spondylitis: a randomized controlled trial. Arthritis Rheum 2002;47:459–467.

6. Koh WH, Pande I, Samuels A, et al. Low dose amitripty-line in ankylosing spondylitis: a short term, double blind, placebo controlled study. J Rheumatol 1997;24:2158–2161.

7. Dougados M, Behier J, Jolchine I, et al. Efficacy of cele-coxib, a cyclooxygenase 2-specific inhibitor, in the treat-ment of ankylosing spondylitis: a six-week controlled study with comparison against placebo and against a con-ventional nonsteroidal antiinflammatory drug. Arthritis Rheum 2001;44:180–185.

8. Wanders A, van der Heijde D, Landewe R, et al. Non-steroidal antiinflammatory drugs reduce radiographic progression in patients with ankylosing spondylitis: a ran-domized clinical trial. Arthritis Rheum 2005;52:1756–1765.

9. Peters ND, Ejstrup L. Intravenous methylprednisolone pulse therapy in ankylosing spondylitis. Scand J Rheuma-tol 1992;21:134–138.

10. Mintz G, Enriquez R, Mercado U, et al. Intravenous methylprednisolone pulse therapy in severe ankylosing spondylitis. Arthritis Rheum 1981;24:734–736.

11. Maugars Y, Mathis C, Berthelot J, et al. Assessment of the efficacy of sacroiliac corticosteroid injections in spon-dyloarthropathies: a double-blind study. Br J Rheumatol 1996;35:767–770.

12. Luckman SP, Hughes DE, Coxon F, et al. Nitrogen-con-taining bisphosphonates inhibit the mevalonate pathway and prevent post-translational prenylation of GTP-binding proteins, including Ras. J Bone Miner Res 1998;13:581–589.

13. Sansoni P, Passeri G, Fagnonoi F, et al. Inhibition of antigen-presenting cell function by alendronate in vitro. J Bone Miner Res 1995;10:1719–1725.

14. Pennanen N, Lapinjoki S, Urtti A, et al. Effect of liposo-mal and free bisphosphonates on the IL-1 beta, IL-6 and TNF alpha secretion from RAW 264 cells in vitro. Pharm Res 1995;12:916–922.

15. Maksymowych WP, Jhangri G, Fitzgerald A, et al. A six-month randomized, controlled, double-blind, dose-response comparison of intravenous pamidronate (60 mg versus 10 mg) in the treatment of nonsteroidal antiinflam-matory drug-refractory ankylosing spondylitis. Arthritis Rheum 2002;46:766–773.

16. Maksymowych WP, Jhangri G, Leclercq S, et al. An open study of pamidronate in the treatment of refractory anky-losing spondylitis. J Rheumatol 1998;25:714–717.

17. Calabrese L, Fleischer AB. Thalidomide: current and potential clinical applications. Am J Med 2000;108:487–495.

18. Breban M, Gombert B, Amor B, et al. Efficacy of thalido-mide in the treatment of refractory ankylosing spondylitis. Arthritis Rheum 1999;42:580–581.

19. Wei JC, Chan T, Lin H, et al. Thalidomide for severe refractory ankylosing spondylitis: a 6-month open-label trial. J Rheumatol 2003;30:2627–2631.

20. Huang F, Gu J, Zhao W, et al. One-year open-label trial of thalidomide in ankylosing spondylitis. Arthritis Rheum 2002;47:249–254.

21. Taggart A, Gardiner P, McEvoy F, et al. Which is the active moiety of sulfasalazine in ankylosing spondylitis? A randomized, controlled study. Arthritis Rheum 1996;39:1400–1405.

22. Ferraz MB, Tugwell P, Goldsmith C, et al. Meta-analysis of sulfasalazine in ankylosing spondylitis. J Rheumatol 1990;17:1482–1486.

23. Nissila M, Lehtinen K, Leirisalo-Repo M, et al. Sulfasala-zine in the treatment of ankylosing spondylitis. A twenty-six-week, placebo-controlled clinical trial. Arthritis Rheum 1988;31:1111–1116.

24. Creemers MC, Franssen MJ, van de Putte LB, et al. Meth-otrexate in severe ankylosing spondylitis: an open study. J Rheumatol 1995;22:1104–1107.

25. Roychowdhury B. Is methotrexate effective in ankylosing spondylitis? Rheumatology (Oxford) 2002;41:1330–1332.

26. Gonzalez-Lopez L, Garcia-Gonzalez A, Vazquez-Del Mercado M, et al. Efficacy of methotrexate in ankylosing spondylitis: a randomized, double blind, placebo con-trolled trial. J Rheumatol 2004;31:1568–1574.

27. Braun J, Bollow M, Neure L, et al. Use of immunohisto-logic and in situ hybridization techniques in the examina-tion of sacroiliac joint biopsy specimens from patients with ankylosing spondylitis. Arthritis Rheum 1995;38:499–505.

28. Canete JD, Llena J, Collado A, et al. Comparative cyto-kine gene expression in synovial tissue of early rheuma-toid arthritis and seronegative spondyloarthropathies. Br J Rheumatol 1997;36:38–42.

29. Grom AA, Murray KJ, Luyrink L, et al. Patterns of expression of tumor necrosis factor alpha, tumor necrosis factor beta, and their receptors in synovia of patients with juvenile rheumatoid arthritis and juvenile spondyloar-thropathy. Arthritis Rheum 1996;39:1703–1710.

30. Toussirot E, Lafforge B, Boucraut J, et al. Serum levels of interleukin 1-beta, tumor necrosis factor-alpha, soluble interleukin 2 receptor and soluble CD8 in seronegative spondyloarthropathies. Rheumatol Int 1994;13:175–180.

31. Gratacos J, Collado A, Filella X, et al. Serum cytokines (IL-6, TNF-alpha, IL-1 beta and IFN-gamma) in ankylos-ing spondylitis: a close correlation between serum IL-6 and disease activity and severity. Br J Rheumatol 1994;33:927–931.

32. Gorman JD, Sack KE, Davis JC Jr. Treatment of ankylos-ing spondylitis by inhibition of tumor necrosis factor alpha. N Engl J Med 2002;346:1349–1356.

33. Davis JC Jr, van der Heijde D, Braun J, et al. Recombi-nant human tumor necrosis factor receptor (etanercept) for treating ankylosing spondylitis: a randomized, con-trolled trial. Arthritis Rheum 2003;48:3230–3236.

34. Davis JC, van der Heijde D, Braun J, et al. Sustained durability and tolerability of etanercept in ankylosing spondylitis for 96 weeks. Ann Rheum Dis 2005;64:1557–1562.

35. Marzo-Ortega H, McGonagle D, O'Connor P, et al. Effi-cacy of etanercept in the treatment of the entheseal pathology in resistant spondyloarthropathy: a clinical and magnetic resonance imaging study. Arthritis Rheum 2001;44:2112–2117.

9

36. Baraliakos X, Davis J, Tsuji W, et al. Magnetic resonance imaging examinations of the spine in patients with ankylosing spondylitis before and after therapy with the tumor necrosis factor alpha receptor fusion protein etanercept. Arthritis Rheum 2005;52:1216–1223.

37. Braun J, Brandt J, Listing J, et al. Treatment of active ankylosing spondylitis with infliximab: a randomised controlled multicentre trial. Lancet 2002;359:1187–1193.

38. Braun J, Brandt J, Listing J, et al. Persistent clinical response to the anti-TNF-alpha antibody infliximab in patients with ankylosing spondylitis over 3 years. Rheumatology (Oxford) 2005;44:670–676.

39. van der Heijde D, Dijkmans B, Geusens P, et al. Efficacy and safety of infliximab in patients with ankylosing spondylitis: results of a randomized, placebo-controlled trial (ASSERT). Arthritis Rheum 2005;52:582–591.

40. Haibel H, Rudlaweit M, Brandt HC, et al. Adalimumab reduces spinal symptoms in active ankylosing spondylitis: clinical and magnetic resonance imaging results of a fifty-two-week open-label trial. Arthritis Rheum 2006;54:678–681.

41. Van der Heijde D, Kivitz A, Schiff MH, et al. Efficacy and safety of adalimumab in patients with ankylosing spondylitis: results of a multicenter, randomized, double-blind, placebo-controlled trial. Arthritis Rheum 2006;54:2136–2146.

42. Zochling J, van der Heijde D, Burgos-Vargas R, et al. ASAS/EULAR recommendations for the management of ankylosing spondylitis. Ann Rheum Dis 2006;65:442–452.

43. Braun J, Davis J, Dougados M, et al. First update of the International ASAS Consensus Statement for the use of anti-TNF agents in patients with ankylosing spondylitis. Ann Rheum Dis 2005.

44. Braun J, Pham T, Sieper J, et al. International ASAS consensus statement for the use of anti-tumour necrosis factor agents in patients with ankylosing spondylitis. Ann Rheum Dis 2003;62:817–824.

45. Ward M, Bruckel J, Colbert R. Summary of the 2005 annual research and education meeting of the Spondyloarthritis Research and Therapy Network (SPARTAN). J Rheumatol 2006;33:978–982.

CHAPTER 10

Reactive and Enteropathic Arthritis

ROBERT D. INMAN, MD

- In reactive arthritis (ReA), exposure of the host to infectious agents leads to the development of an inflammatory arthritis and other manifestations of systemic disease in the absence of an ongoing infectious process.
- Approximately 50% of ReA and undifferentiated oligoarthritis cases can be attributed to a specific pathogen by a combination of culture and serology. The predominant organisms are *Chlamydia, Salmonella, Shigella, Yersinia,* and *Campylobacter* species.
- The annual incidence of ReA, found to be 28/100,000 individuals in one study, may exceed that of rheumatoid arthritis.
- In a study of 91 individuals exposed to food-borne *Salmonella enteritidis,* 17 (19%) individuals developed ReA. Other studies have estimated the frequency of ReA following exposure to potential etiologic agents to be on the order of 10%.
- Reactive arthritis characteristically involves the joints of the lower extremities in an asymmetric, oligoarticular pattern.
- A dactylitis ('sausage digit') pattern in the feet is typical of ReA.

- Enthesopathy (inflammation at the sites of insertion of tendons and ligaments into bone) and anterior uveitis are often found in ReA, as in other seronegative spondyloarthropathies.
- Cutaneous manifestations of ReA include: keratoderma blenorrhagicum, a papulosquamous rash affecting the palms and soles; nail dystrophy; circinate balanitis, characterized by shallow ulcers on the glans or the shaft of the penis; and oral ulcers, typically painless.
- Enteropathic spondyloarthritis is the inflammatory arthritis that often accompanies ulcerative colitis or Crohn's disease.
- The peripheral arthritis of enteropathic spondyloarthritis is typically pauciarticular, asymmetric, and migratory. It has a predilection for joints of the lower extremities.
- The axial disease of enteropathic spondyloarthritis is indistinguishable clinically from that of primary ankylosing spondylitis.

REACTIVE ARTHRITIS

The role of infection as a triggering factor in the pathogenesis of the various forms of spondyloarthritis (SpA) is implicated with varying degrees of certainty among the SpA subcategories. The very definition of reactive arthritis (ReA)—a sterile synovitis following an extra-articular infection—clearly implicates infection in its defining features, and ReA occupies the conceptual ground somewhere between septic arthritis and the classic autoimmune rheumatic diseases, such as rheumatoid arthritis (RA). An etiologic classification has fueled the search for definitive links between particular pathogens and ReA. Many of these studies are based on guilt by association, in that the demonstration of a particular immune response profile by serology or cellular responses leads to identification of the causative pathogen even when there is no direct demonstration of the organism or its antigens in synovial tissues or fluid. The predictive power of a diagnostic microbiology test, however, critically depends on the prevalence of positives in the healthy population at large (1), and this is an important consideration in the case for causality in ReA.

Epidemiology

Studies on the epidemiology of ReA have provided insight into the frequency of this complication of enteric infections. Data indicate that approximately 50% of ReA and undifferentiated oligoarthritis cases can be attributed to a specific pathogen by a combination of culture and serology. The predominant organisms are *Chlamydia, Salmonella, Shigella, Yersinia,* and *Campylobacter* species (2). Species-specific analysis of serological responses to pathogens might increase this detection rate further (3). A prospective study of the annual incidence of inflammatory joint disease in Sweden found that the annual incidence of ReA (28/100,000) exceeded that of RA (24/100,000), emphasizing the importance of ReA in the overall burden of rheumatic diseases (4). Studies on both sporadic (5) and outbreak-related (6) *Salmonella typhimurium* infections have provided further support for the role of *Salmonella* spp in triggering ReA. The frequency of ReA in this context has generally been in the range of 10% (6), but in a study of 91 individuals exposed to food-borne *Salmonella enteritidis*, 17 individuals developed ReA, indicating that this might be more frequent than previously thought (7). In a population-based study, it was determined that ReA is common after campylobacter infections, with an annual incidence of 4.3/100,000 (8). These incidence figures are no doubt strongly influenced by the unique aspects of a particular population under study: ReA appears to be more prevalent in Alaskan Eskimo populations (9), for example, and the incidence of ReA after a salmonella outbreak appears to be lower in children than adults (10).

Clinical Features of Reactive Arthritis

Reactive arthritis is characteristically a lower extremity, asymmetric oligoarthritis. The pattern may be additive. Hip disease is uncommon and exclusively upper extremity involvement is extremely rare. The joints are typically warm, swollen, and tender, and can mimic a septic arthritis, reminding that aspiration of synovial fluid and cultures are mandatory when assessing such patients. A dactylitis pattern in the feet is not uncommon.

Enthesitis (inflammation at sites of ligamentous attachment to bone) is a characteristic feature of ReA. Achilles tendonitis and plantar fasciitis are the most common sites, but pain in the iliac crests, ischial tuberosities, and back can be seen. This aspect of the disease can be disabling, with marked restriction in weight bearing and ambulation.

Low back pain and buttock pain, reflecting sacroiliac joint inflammation, occurs in up to 50% of cases, but progression to ankylosing spondylitis (AS) is uncommon. The latter event is strongly associated with human leukocyte antigen (HLA)-B27.

The extra-articular features of ReA can often be helpful in diagnosis, particularly in circumstances when it is difficult to identify a triggering infection. Keratoderma blenorrhagicum is a papulosquamous rash most commonly affecting palms and soles. The lesions can be indistinguishable clinically and histopathologically from pustular psoriasis. Nail dystrophy can occur with ReA, further highlighting the clinical overlap of some features with psoriatic arthritis. Circinate balanitis presents as shallow ulcers on the glans or the shaft of the penis, and is plaquelike and hyperkeratotic. Dysuria and pyuria present an interesting clinical feature because urethritis can be the clue to the inciting infection (as in

chlamydial urethritis) or can be an extra-articular feature of postdysenteric ReA. The distinction is important because there may be great concern on the part of the patient about a possible sexually transmitted disease when genital symptoms occur, and a discussion with the patient (and often the spouse) becomes a key element in care. Oral ulcers on the hard palate or tongue are typically painless, so the patient may be unaware of their presence in the mouth. Acute anterior uveitis occurs in 20% of patients at some point during the course of ReA. As in the case of evolution into AS, whether the uveitis is triggered by the antecedent infection or is a feature of a common genetic predisposition has not been resolved.

Pathogenesis of Reactive Arthritis

With respect to ReA, the most common triggering urogenital agents are urogenital (*Chlamydia* spp) and enteric (*Shigella*, *Salmonella*, *Yersinia*, and *Campylobacter* spp) pathogens (11). Substantial regional differences are evident, however, particularly with regard to the enteric pathogens (12). *Chlamydia* spp are regarded as the most common causative agents in ReA. *Chlamydia* DNA, mRNA, rRNA, and intact *Chlamydia*-like cells have been found in synovial tissues and peripheral blood of ReA patients (13,14). The mechanisms accounting for the persistence of *Chlamydia* and the thwarting of host immune defenses have been studied from several perspectives. In chronic disease, altered regulation of specific *Chlamydia* genes is apparent, with reduced expression of the major outer membrane protein and increased expression of heat shock protein (HSP) and lipopolysaccharide (LPS). *Chlamydia* spp can also downregulate the expression of major histocompatibility complex (MHC) antigens on the surface of infected cells. *Chlamydia* spp may induce T-cell apoptosis by stimulating the local production of tumor necrosis factor (TNF) (15). There is also evidence that *Chlamydia* spp can alter host response to the organisms by inhibition of host cell apoptosis, by reducing the release of cytochrome C, and by sequestering protein kinase C delta in the membrane of the organisms' vacuoles (16). Newer analytic techniques are being used to probe synovial fluids and tissues for evidence of prior or current microbes (17,18).

Serological studies have previously provided suggestive evidence that certain Gram-negative bacteria, notably *Klebsiella pneumoniae*, contribute to the pathophysiology of AS. The implication of such studies is that AS may be a form of ReA. One recent analysis, however, which addressed both humoral and cellular host immune responses, found no evidence to support the notion that *K. pneumoniae* has a pathogenic role in AS (19). LPS in synovial tissue is a potent macrophage stimulator and this could set the stage for persistence of activated macrophages within the synovium and for ensuing chronic inflammation. One unresolved issue is the mechanism by which antecedent infection can induce inflammation and erosions in a joint in the absence of viable organisms. Synovial fibroblasts might have an intermediary role in this sequence of events. In laboratory models, synovial fibroblasts infected with *S. typhimurium* mediate osteoclast differentiation and activation (20).

Human Leukocyte Antigen-B27 and Direct Host–Pathogen Interactions

The conventional role ascribed to class I HLA molecules such as HLA-B27 is the presentation of processed peptides to CD8+, cytotoxic T lymphocytes (CTL). It has been difficult to demonstrate that such CTL mediate the chronic inflammation that is the hallmark of SpA, however. Two points related to HLA-B27 may be relevant. First, HLA-B27–positive cells kill *Salmonella* less efficiently than do control cells (21). Second, LPS stimulation results in a more pronounced increase in nuclear factor κB activation and TNF secretion in HLA-B27–positive cells (22).

This phenomenon of more permissive intracellular replication of *Salmonella* might depend on the unique characteristics of the HLA-B27 B pocket, in particular the glutamic acid residue at position 45 (23). In contrast, some investigators have found that HLA-B27 expression alters neither the rates of infection nor the rate of replication of *C. trachomatis* in cell lines (24). Using synoviocytes harvested from HLA-B27–positive patients, it was observed that HLA-B27 had no direct role in either the internalization of *S. typhimurium* or in the kinetics of intracellular killing (25). A biochemical approach has been used to examine endogenously labeled HLA-B27–bound peptides by mass spectrometry (26). This technique allows investigators to radiolabel peptides that are specifically bound to the HLA-B27 molecule, and thereafter to isolate these peptides for characterization. Using this approach, there was no evidence of significant changes in the range of peptides that were bound by the HLA-B27 molecule after infection of the target cells with *S. typhimurium*. Although this does not exclude a role for altered CTL recognition of infected HLA-B27–positive target cells, harvesting arthritogenic peptides using such a biochemical approach will be an extremely challenging undertaking using current methods.

Human Leukocyte Antigen-B27 and Host Immune Responses

The strong association between HLA-B27 and SpA has indirectly implicated microbial antigen-specific, MHC class I–restricted CD8+ CTLs as having a role in the pathogenesis of these diseases. CD8+ T cells in synovial fluid can express a heterogeneous array of natural killer (NK) cell receptors (27), which might modulate their cytotoxicity and contribute to disease pathogenesis. An analysis of the specificity of T-cell clones demonstrated that target cells pulsed with *Yersinia* HSP60, but not with other *Yersinia* proteins, were successfully lysed by CTLs, and that this killing was controlled by B27 (28). A single nonamer derived from *Yersinia* HSP60 was the dominant epitope in this recognition event. Using a computer-generated algorithm that incorporated HLA-B27 binding motifs and proteosome-generated motifs, an approach has been undertaken to identify immunodominant peptides from *C. trachomatis* (29). Nine peptides identified using this method proved to be stimulatory for CD8+ T cells, and many of these same peptides were recognized by CD8+ T cells derived from patients with ReA. A recent study successfully used HLA-B27 tetramers to identify low frequency antigen-specific T cells in *Chlamydia*-induced reactive arthritis (30). Such cells could be expanded ex vivo, suggesting a functional capability that might contribute to the arthritis.

Molecular Mimicry

Whether microbial peptides share functional homology with self-proteins such as HLA-B27 itself remains unknown. There is some supportive evidence for this notion of molecular mimicry in SpA (31). This theory postulates that an autoimmune process can ensue after an infection if there is some degree of cross-reactivity in host and microbial antigens. But several important questions need to be addressed. For example, the target organ specificity of seronegative spondyloarthropathies remains unexplained, as does the apparent frequency of homologous sequences, even among bacteria not commonly thought to be arthritogenic on clinical grounds.

An immunodominant epitope from the *S. typhimurium* GroEL chaperonin molecule (a member of the HSP60 protein family) was recognized by CTLs after natural infection in mice (32). These CTLs cross-reacted with peptides derived from mouse HSP60. A dodecamer derived from the intracytoplasmic tail of HLA-B27 was found to be a natural ligand for disease-associated HLA-B27 subtypes, but not for non–disease-associated subtypes. This peptide showed striking homology to a region of the DNA primase from *C. trachomatis*, indicating that some molecular mimicry exists between HLA-B27–derived and chlamydial peptides (33). In a study investigating CTL recognition in B27-transgenic animals (34), it was observed that these animals are tolerant to immunization with B27 DNA, but if splenocytes from these animals are exposed to *Chlamydia* spp in vitro, then autoreactive B27-specific CTLs are

10

generated. This indicates a dynamic interrelationship between the pathogen and host B27 that might have important implications for the pathogenesis of ReA. These interactions might result in a break in self-tolerance, or perhaps an impaired clearance of the organism on the basis of impaired recognition of the organism as non-self.

Therapy for Reactive Arthritis

First-line treatment of ReA includes nonsteroidal anti-inflammatory drugs (NSAIDs), which in most cases prove adequate for control of the acute synovitis and enthesitis. Intra-articular corticosteroid injections can be useful for a monoarthritis. Second-line agents for persistent synovitis have included sulfasalazine and methotrexate, but there are few controlled trials to objectively evaluate efficacy. Because the triggering event in ReA is infection, there has been particular interest in the role of antibiotics in the treatment of ReA. Some studies to date indicate that only *Chlamydia*-induced ReA is responsive to antibiotic treatment, raising the question of fundamental differences between ReA induced by this pathogen and disease triggered by enteric pathogens. The cellular basis for such differences, if genuine, are not clear.

A 3-month, double-blind, randomized, placebo-controlled study found no benefit of ciprofloxacin treatment in patients with ReA and undifferentiated oligoarthritis (35). In subgroup analysis, however, ciprofloxacin was better than placebo in *Chlamydia*-induced ReA, but not in *Salmonella*- or *Yersinia*-induced ReA. A subsequent report showed that lymecycline therapy decreased the duration of acute arthritis in *Chlamydia*-induced ReA, but not in patients with ReA induced by other pathogens (36). Of 17 patients followed for 10 years in this study, 1 patient had AS, 3 had radiographic sacroiliitis, and 3 had radiographic changes in peripheral joints, but long-term lymecycline treatment did not change the natural history of the disease.

A 3-month trial of doxycycline for chronic SpA showed this drug to be no better than placebo for reducing pain or improving functional status, but the causative organism was only identified in a few patients (37). In a group of patients with undifferentiated SpA, it was reported that a combination of doxycycline and rifampin was superior to doxycline alone, although no placebo was included in the design (38). In a 4- to 7-year follow-up of an earlier ReA trial, it was noted that chronic arthritis developed in 41% of patients initially treated with placebo, in contrast to 8% of patients initially treated with ciprofloxacin, suggesting that long-term prognosis might be favorably influenced by antibiotic treatment (39). Recently the results of a 3-month, placebo-controlled trial of azithromycin in ReA were reported (40). Azithromycin, given orally for 13 weeks, was ineffective in ReA, based on the data from 152 patients who were analyzed for a response.

ENTEROPATHIC SPONDYLOARTHRITIS

The arthritis accompanying the inflammatory bowel diseases (IBDs)—Crohn's disease (CD) and ulcerative colitis (UC)—is included in the family of spondyloarthritis because so many clinical features of this arthritis are shared with other members of this family of disorders. In contrast, the arthritis associated with Whipple's disease and celiac disease, albeit enteropathic by definition, are generally not considered part of the spondyloarthritis spectrum. Arthritis occurs in 10% to 22% of patients with IBD, with a higher prevalence in CD than in UC. Arthritis may precede the gastrointestinal (GI) symptoms by lengthy periods of time, and the patients may be regarded as undifferentiated SpA until the IBD declares itself. The studies of Mielants and Veys have provided evidence that patients with undifferentiated spondyloarthropathies (uSpA) and even AS may have subclinical bowel inflammation that plays an important role in triggering and perpetuating joint inflammation (41). One 20-year follow-up study of patients with IBD reported musculoskeletal features in 30% (42). Another study, employing computed tomography scans, detected sacroiliitis in 45% of patients with CD complaining of back pain (43). Magnetic resonance imaging (MRI) is the most sensitive means of detecting sacroiliitis in IBD patients. Asymptomatic sacroiliitis may occur in 14% of patients with IBD (44). HLA-B27–positive patients with CD have a high likelihood of progressing to frank AS. Enteropathic arthritis can occur in a peripheral, axial, or mixed pattern.

Peripheral Arthritis

The arthritis is typically pauciarticular and asymmetric, and may occur in a migratory pattern in some patients. In one study, 6% of uSpA patients developed CD 2 to 9 years after the onset of arthritis (45). The arthritis is typically nonerosive, occurring in intermittent attacks lasting up to 6 weeks (46). There is a predilection for lower extremity joints. Dactylitis and enthesitis reiterate the close relationship to the SpA family. The activity of the peripheral arthritis generally correlates well with the degree of active bowel inflammation, particularly in UC. Indeed, colectomy performed for control of UC can be associated with a complete arthritis remission. The same is not true of surgical interventions for CD.

Axial Arthritis

The axial pattern of enteropathic arthritis is indistinguishable clinically and radiographically from primary AS, although some studies have observed that severity, defined by spinal mobility impairment, is enhanced in IBD-related spondylitis in comparison with primary AS (47). Unlike the peripheral arthritis, axial disease in IBD does not parallel the activity of the bowel disease, and may precede it. Similarly, surgical therapy of UC or CD has no impact on the associated spondylitis. An association with HLA-B27 is seen in axial but not in the peripheral form of enteropathic arthritis.

Nonarticular Complications of Inflammatory Bowel Disease

Skin lesions can be seen in up to 25% of patients. Erythema nodosum tends to mirror the activity of the bowel disease and can often parallel the activity of the peripheral arthritis. Pyoderma gangrenosum, with painful deep skin ulcerations, is a more serious skin manifestation but is less common. Acute anterior uveitis can be seen in up to 11% of patients and is usually the unilateral, transient pattern of eye inflammation characteristic of SpA patients. CD may also be associated with a granulomatous uveitis that is more chronic. Recurrent oral ulcerations may reflect the activity of underlying CD.

Diagnostic Studies

Anemia is common in enteropathic SpA, reflecting both the anemia of chronic disease and GI blood loss. C-reactive protein and erythrocyte sedimentation rate are usually elevated when the disease is active. Rheumatoid factors and antinuclear antibodies are absent in most patients. Radiographic studies of peripheral joints generally do not reveal erosive changes, but a destructive process in the hip can occur. Imaging of the sacroiliac joints and spine are usually similar to primary AS, although a higher frequency of asymmetric sacroiliitis and zygapophyseal joint ankylosis has been reported (48).

Genetics

The peripheral arthritis of IBD is not associated with HLA-B27, whereas the axial form of arthritis is, although to a lesser extent than primary AS (33% B27-positive for the former vs. 85% for the latter). CD has been associated with mutation in the *NOD2* (*CARD15*) gene on chromosome 16. This is of interest in the pathogenesis of CD because *NOD2* plays an important role in innate immunity to pathogens and indirectly implicates microbial triggers in IBD. But studies to date have found no significant relationship between CARD15 and SpA and indicate no enhanced risk for primary AS associated with this gene. However, CARD15 mutations may be found more commonly among patients with CD complicated by sacroiliitis (49).

Treatment

Therapies for enteropathic arthritis follow the same principles as those guiding treatment of SpA in general. NSAIDs are first-line treatment for joint inflammation in both axial and peripheral disease. The cautionary note in these patients, however, is that NSAIDs may exacerbate underlying IBD, particularly UC. NSAID-related adverse events may also mimic a flare of IBD and complicate management. Decisions on NSAID use should be undertaken jointly by the rheumatologist and the gastroenterologist.

Sulfasalazine, which has a role in the treatment of colonic inflammation in IBD, has been effective in treating peripheral, but not axial, arthritis in these patients. Studies that address the efficacy of methotrexate in the peripheral form of enteropathic arthritis are lacking. Intra-articular glucocorticoid injections can be used for flares of the peripheral arthritis. Budesonide, a glucocorticoid with first-pass hepatic metabolism and fewer systemic side effects as a result, has been used increasingly for CD flares, but there are no studies to date addressing the effect of this steroid on enteropathic arthritis. In RA, budesonide has not found to be superior to prednisone therapy (50).

Anti-tumor necrosis factor therapies have had a major impact on the therapeutic approach to IBD and to the associated joint diseases. Striking differences in IBD are apparent between different modes of TNF inhibition, however, with infliximab (a monoclonal antibody) showing efficacy for many patients with IBD—particularly CD—but etanercept (a soluble fusion protein) being ineffective. Etanercept can control the arthritis associated with CD while having no effect on the bowel disease itself (51). Infliximab mediates the healing of fistulas in CD and also helps maintain disease control. Recent studies have demonstrated that infliximab is as effective for both axial and peripheral arthritis associated with CD as it is for primary AS (52).

REFERENCES

1. Sieper J, Rudwaleit M, Braun J, et al. Diagnosing reactive arthritis. Arthritis Rheum 2002;46:319–327.
2. Fendler C, Laitko S, Sorensen H, et al. Frequency of triggering bacteria in patients with reactive arthritis and undifferentiated oligoarthritis and the relative importance of the tests used for diagnosis. Ann Rheum Dis 2001;60:337–343.

10

3. Nikkari S, Puolakkainen M, Narvanen A, et al. Use of a peptide based enzyme immunoassay in diagnosis of *Chlamydia trachomatis* triggered reactive arthritis. J Rheumatol 2001;28:2487–2493.

4. Soderlin MK, Borjesson O, Kautiainen H, et al. Annual incidence of inflammatory joint diseases in a population-based study in southern Sweden. Ann Rheum Dis 2002;61:911–915.

5. Buxton JA, Fyfe M, Berger S, et al. Reactive arthritis and other sequelae following sporadic *Salmonella typhimurium* infection in British Columbia, Canada - a case control study. J Rheumatol 2002;29:2154–2158.

6. Hannu T, Mattila L, Siitonen A, Leirisalo-Repo M. Reactive arthritis following an outbreak of *Salmonella typhimurium* phage type 193 infection. Ann Rheum Dis 2002;61:264–266.

7. Locht H, Molbak K, Krogfelt KA. High frequency of reactive arthritis symptoms after an outbreak of *Salmonella enteritidis*. J Rheumatol 2002;29:767–771.

8. Hannu T, Mattila L, Rautelin H, et al. Campylobacter-triggered reactive arthritis: a population-based study. Rheumatol 2002;41:312–318.

9. Boyer GS, Templin DW, Bowler A, et al. Spondyloarthropathy in the community: clinical syndromes and disease manifestations in Alaskan Eskimo populations. J Rheumatol 1999;26:1537–1544.

10. Rudwaleit M, Richter S, Braun J, Sieper J. Low incidence of reactive arthritis in children following a salmonella outbreak. Ann Rheum Dis 2001;60:1055–1057.

11. Colmegna I, Cuchacovich R, Espinoza LR. HLA-B27-associated reactive arthritis: pathogenetic and clinical considerations. Clin Microbiol Rev 2004;17:348–369.

12. Soderlin MK, Kautiainen H, Puolakkainen M, et al. Infections preceding early arthritis in southern Sweden: a prospective population-based study. J Rheumatol 2003;30: 425–429.

13. Gerard HC, Branigan PJ, Schumacher HR Jr, et al. Synovial *Chlamydia trachomatis* in patients with reactive arthritis/Reiter's syndrome are viable but show aberrant gene expression. J Rheumatol 1998;25:734–742.

14. Kuipers JG, Jurgens-Saathoff B, Bialowons A, et al. Detection of *Chlamydia trachomatis* in peripheral blood leukocytes of reactive arthritis patients by polymerase chain reaction. Arthritis Rheum 1998;41:1894–1895

15. Jendro MC, Fingerle F, Deutsch T, et al. *Chlamydia trachomatis*-infected macrophages induce apoptosis of activated T cells by secretion of tumor necrosis factor-alpha in vitro. Med Microbiol Immunol 2004;193:45–52.

16. Tse SML, Mason D, Botelho RJ, et al. Accumulation of diacylglycerol in the Chlamydia inclusion vacuole. Possible role in the inhibition of host cell apoptosis. J Biol Chem 2005;280:25210–25215.

17. Chen T, Rimpilainen M, Luukkainen R, et al. Bacterial components in the synovial tissue of patients with advanced RA or OA; analysis with gas chromatography-mass spectrometry and pan-bacterial polymerase chain reaction. Arthritis Rheum 2003;49: 328–334.

18. Zhang X, Pacheco-Tena C, Inman RD. Microbe hunting in the joints. Arthritis Rheum 2003;49:479–482.

19. Stone MA, Payne U, Schentag C, Rahman R, Pacheco-Tena C, Inman RD. Comparative immune responses to candidate arthritogenic bacteria do not confirm a role for *Klebsiella pneumoniae* in the pathogenesis of familial ankylosing spondylitis. Rheumatology 2004;43:148–155.

20. Zhang X, Aubin J, Kim TH, et al. Synovial fibroblasts infected with Salmonella enterica serovar typhimurium mediate osteoclast differentiation and activation. Infect Immun 2004;72:7183–7189.

21. Ekman P, Saarinen M, He Q, et al. HLA-B27-transfected and HLA-A2-transfected human monocytic U937 cells differ in their production of cytokines. Infect Immun 2002;70:1609–1614.

22. Pentinnen MA, Holmberg CI, Sistonen LM, Granfors K. HLA-B27 modulates NFkB activation in human monocytic cells exposed to lipopol/saccharide. Arthritis Rheum 2002;46:2172–2180.

23. Pentinnen MA, Heiskanen KM, Mohaptra R, et al. Enhanced intracellular replication of Salmonella enteritidis in HLA B27-expressing human monocytic cells. Arthritis Rheum 2004;50:2225–2263.

24. Young JL, Smith L, Matyszak MK, Gaston JS. HLA-B27 expression does not modulate intracellular *Chlamydia trachomatis* infection of cell lines. Infect Immun 2001;69: 6670–6675.

25. Payne U, Inman RD. Determinants of synovocyte clearance of arthritogenic bacteria. J Rheumatol 2003;30:1291–1297.

26. Ringrose JH, Meiring HD, Spiejer D, et al. Major histocompatibility complex class I peptide presentation and *Salmonella enterica* serovar typhimurium infection assessed via a stable isotope tagging of the B27-presented peptide repertoire. Infect Immun 2004;72:5097–5105.

27. Dulphy N, Rabian C, Douay C, et al. Functional modulation of expanded CD8+ synovial fluid T cells-NK cell receptor expression in HLA-B27-associated reactive arthritis Int Immunol 2002;14:471–479.

28. Ugrinovic S, Mertz A, Wu P, et al. A single nonamer from the *Yersinia* 60-kDa heat shock protein is the target of HLA-B27-restricted CTL response in *Yersinia*-induced arthritis. J Immunol 1997;159:5715–5723.

29. Kuon W, Holzhutter HG, Appel H, et al. Identification of HLA-B27-restricted peptides from the *Chlamydia trachomatis* proteome with possible relevance to HLA-B27-associated diseases. J Immunol 2001;167:4738–4746.

30. Appel H, Kuon W, Wu P, et al. Use of HLA-B27 tetramers to identify low-frequency antigen-specifiv T cells in Chlamydia-triggered reactive arthritis. Arthritis Res Ther 2004;6:521–534.

31. Lopez-Larrea C, Gonzalez S, Martinez-Borra J. The role of HLA-B27 polymorphism and molecular mimicry in spondyloarthropathy. Mol Med Today 1998;4:540–549.

32. Lo WF, Woods AS, DeCloux A, et al. Molecular mimicry mediated by MHC class Ib molecules after infection with gram-negative pathogens. Nat Med 2000;6:215–218.

33. Ramos M, Alvarez I, Sesma L, et al. Molecular mimicry of HLA-B27-derived peptide ligand of arthritis-linked subtypes with chlamydial proteins. J Biol Chem 2002;277: 37573–37581.

34. Popov I, Dela Cruz CS, Barber BH, Chiu B, Inman RD. Breakdown of CTL D, tolerance to self HLA-B*2705

induced by exposure to *Chlamydia trachomatis*. J Immunol 2002;169:4033–4038.

35. Sieper J, Fendler C, Laitko S, et al. No benefit of long-term ciprofloxacin treatment in patients with reactive arthritis and undifferentiated oligoarthritis: a three-month, multicenter, double-blind, randomized, placebo-controlled study. Arthritis Rheum 1999;42:1386–1396.

36. Laasila K, Lassonen L, Leirisalo-Repo M. Antibiotic treatment and long term prognosis of reactive arthritis. Ann Rheum Dis 2003;62:655–658

37. Smieja M, MacPherson DW, Kean W, et al. Randomised, blinded, placebo-controlled trial of doxycycline in chronic seronegative arthritis. Ann Rheum Dis 2001;60:1088–1094.

38. Carter JD, Valeriano J, Vasey FB. Doxcycline versus doxycycline and rifampin in undifferentiated spondyloarthropathy, with special reference to Chlamydia-induced arthritis. A prospective, randomized 9-month comparison. J Rheumatol 2004;31:1973–1980.

39. Yli-Kerttula T, Luukkainen R, Yli-Kerttula U, et al. Effect of a three-month course of ciprofloxacin on the late prognosis of reactive arthritis. Ann Rheum Dis 2003;62:880–884.

40. Kvien TK, Gaston JSH, Bardin T, et al. Three month treatment of reactive arthritis with azithromycin: a EULAR double-blind, placebo-controlled study. Ann Rheum Dis 2004;63:1113–1119.

41. Mielants H, Veys EM, Cuvelier C, De Vos M, Botelberghe L. HLA-related arthritis and bowel inflammation. Ileocolonoscopy and bowel histology in patients with HLA-B27 related arthritis. J Rheumatol 1985;12:294–298.

42. Veloso FT, Carvalho J, Magro F. Immune-related manifestations of inflammatory bowel disease—a prospective study of 792. J Clin Gastroenterol 1988;83:703–709.

43. Steer S, Jones H, Hibbert J, et al. Low back pain, sacroiliitis and the relationship with HLA-B27 in Crohn's disease. J Rheumatol 2003;30:518–522.

44. Turkcapar N, Toruner M, Soykan I, et al. The prevalence of extraintestinal manifestations and HLA association in patients with inflammatory bowel disease. Rheum Int 2005;34:387–391.

45. Mielants H, Veys EM, Cuvelier C, et al. The evolution of spondyloarthropathies in relation to gut histology. Relation between gut and joint. J Rheumatol 1995;22:2279–2284.

46. Palm O, Moum B, Jahnsen J, Gran JT. The prevalence and incidence of peripheral arthritis in patients with inflammatory bowel disease: a prospective population study. Rheumatology 2001;40:1256–1261.

47. Brophy S, Pavy S, Lewis P, et al. Inflammatory eye, skin and bowel disease in spondyloarthritis: genetic, phenotypic and environmental factors. J Rheumatol 2001;28:2667–2673.

48. Helliwell PS, Hickling P, Wright V. Do the radiologic changes of classic ankylosing spondylitis differ from the changes found in spondylitis associated with inflammatory bowel disease, psoriasis and reactive arthritis. Ann Rheum Dis 1998;57:135–140.

49. Peeters H, Van der Cruyssen B, Laukens D, et al. Radiologic sacroiliitis, a hallmark of spondylitis is linked with CARD15 gene polymorphisms in patients with Crohn's disease. Ann Rheum Dis 2004;63:1131–1134.

50. Kirwan JR, Hallgren R, Mielants H, et al. A randomized, placebo-controlled 12-week trial of budesonide and prednisolone in rheumatoid arthritis. Ann Rheum Dis 2004;63:688–695.

51. Marzo-Ortega H, McGonagle D, O'Connor P, Emery P. Efficacy of etanercept for treatment of Crohn's-related spondyloarthroarthritis but not colitis. Ann Rheum Dis 2003;62:74–76.

52. Rispo A, Scarpa R, Di Girolamo E, et al. Infliximab in the treatment of extra-intestinal manifestations of Crohn's disease. Scand J Rheumatol 2005;34:387–391.

10

Osteoarthritis
A. Clinical Features

PAUL DIEPPE, MD

- Osteoarthritis (OA) is the most common form of joint disease in humans.
- The most commonly affected are apophyseal joints of the cervical and lumbar spine, interphalangeal joints of the hand, the thumb base, the first metatarsophalangeal joint, the hips, and the knees.
- Osteoarthritis is strongly age related. Additional risks include family history, female sex, obesity, and trauma.

- The symptoms of OA are pain, short-lasting stiffness, cracking of joints, joint swelling, fatigue, and functional limitation.
- Osteoarthritis is characterized on physical exam by firm swelling around the joint line, crepitus, and restricted range of motion.
- Diagnosis of OA can usually be made by history and physical exam, but radiographs demonstrating joint space loss, osteophytes, and changes in the subchondral bone are diagnostic.

Osteoarthritis (OA) is the most common form of joint disease in humans. Our ancestors' skeletons show that it has been with us for many centuries. However, it was only differentiated from other forms of arthritis about 100 years ago (1), when a combination of pathological and radiographic studies made it clear that there were two quite distinct types of synovial joint damage: atrophic arthritis, in which there is periarticular osteoporosis and erosive changes, in addition to cartilage loss; and hypertrophic arthritis, in which the cartilage loss is accompanied by an increase in bone density and bone formation around the joint.

The atrophic subset was subsequently differentiated into a variety of infectious and inflammatory conditions, including rheumatoid arthritis (RA). Hypertrophic arthritis is what we now know as OA. It is clear that this too includes a variety of different conditions, but we have made less progress in our understanding of this group, and the differentiation of distinct entities has proved elusive. *Osteoarthritis*, then, is a term that describes a heterogeneous group of common conditions, with similar pathological and radiographic features.

EPIDEMIOLOGY

Osteoarthritis is a strongly age-related disorder. It is uncommon before the age of 40, but its prevalence rises rapidly with age thereafter, such that most people over the age of 70 have the pathological changes of OA in some of their joints (although they may remain asymptomatic).

The most important risk factors for OA are shown in Table 11A-1. But, as indicated, some risk factors are more important for OA of a particular joint than others. For example, OA of the knee is strongly associated with women and obesity, and is more common in blacks than whites, whereas hip OA has a more equal sex incidence, a less strong association with obesity, and is rare in Chinese people.

CLINICAL FEATURES

Osteoarthritis is, by definition, a disorder of synovial joints. It can affect any one of the 200 or so synovial joints in the body, but whereas it is common in some, it rarely affects others. The most frequently affected sites are the apophyseal joints of the cervical and lumbar spine, the interphalangeal joints of the hand, the thumb base, the first metatarsophalangeal joint, the knee and the hip. Shoulders, ankles, and metacarpophalangeal joints are amongst the less common sites of OA.

Osteoarthritis is also a focal disease of joints. Unlike inflammatory arthropathies, it does not always affect the whole joint. For example, in the knee the most common parts to be affected are the medial tibiofemoral and lateral patellofemoral compartments, and the superior pole of the hip is the most likely area of that joint to be damaged.

TABLE 11A-1. RISK FACTORS FOR OSTEOARTHRITIS.

Increasing age (all sites)

Female sex or gender (some sites, particularly knee and hand)

Race or ethnicity (variable at different joint sites)

Genetic predisposition (all sites)

Obesity (most sites, but more marked for the knee than other joints)

Trauma, and some occupations involving repetitive activities (specific sites)

How can we explain this? If the OA process is driven by mechanical factors, one plausible hypothesis is that it is an age-related disorder of evolution (2). Our musculoskeletal system evolved to suit our ancestors, who walked around on four legs and did not have a prehensile grip. In evolutionary terms, we stood up and started to grip things between fingers and thumbs a relatively short time ago, so that the skeleton has not had time to adapt to these changes in posture and joint use. One result of this is that the shape of certain parts of our joints, such as the superior pole of the hip, are not well suited to the mechanical stresses that our everyday activities submit them to.

HISTORY

Despite the fact that OA is described as a heterogeneous group of disorders, shared clinical features bind the group together. The two cardinal symptoms of OA are use-related pain, and relatively short-lasting stiffness or gelling of the joints after inactivity.

We know surprisingly little about OA pain—either about the patient experiences of pain or about its pathogenesis. Most people describe pain that is exacerbated by use of the joint, but the discomfort often continues for some time after activity ceases, wearing off slowly. Some people experience particularly severe but short-lasting bouts of pain on a particular movement or activity, and some experience such bouts spontaneously. In others pain can occur at night, disrupting sleep. A wide variety of adjectives are used to describe the pain or discomfort. The amount of pain experienced obviously depends on what people do, and to what extent they avoid particular activities or movements that are most likely to exacerbate it, making the assessment of pain in OA problematic.

Similarly, gelling of joints is a somewhat mysterious symptom. The most common phenomenon seems to be difficulty initiating joint movement after inactivity, epitomized by the problems older people with OA have in

"getting started" after sitting down for a while. It is not known what causes this. People may present with a variety of other symptoms, including cracking of joints (audible crepitus), joint locking, swelling, fatigue, and, of course, difficulty with daily activities.

PHYSICAL EXAMINATION

The osteoarthritic joint generally has evidence of mild-to-moderate firm swelling around the joint line, palpable creaking on movement (crepitus), and restricted range of motion with pain at the end of the range. The swelling is usually due to the formation of chondrophytes or osteophytes at the joint margin, and these may be tender. There may also be tenderness over the joint line itself. In some cases there is evidence of mild inflammation, with some warmth over the joint line and an effusion. Other common signs include weakness and wasting of the muscles acting on the joint, and areas of periarticular tenderness. In advanced cases, deformities and instability of the joints are seen.

INVESTIGATIONS

In the majority of cases, OA can and should be diagnosed from the history and clinical signs alone, without recourse to any investigations. It is a localized disorder, without any systemic features, so blood tests are all normal [with the caveat that small increases in serum C-reactive protein (CRP) can occur]. Joint images, including x-rays and magnetic resonance imaging (MRI), are abnormal, reflecting the joint pathology. The plain radiograph is the investigation most frequently used to confirm the clinical diagnosis, and for the definition of the condition for research studies. The main radiographic features of OA are narrowing of the joint space (due to loss of articular cartilage), osteophytes, and a variety of changes in the subchondral bone, including cysts, sclerosis, shape changes, and loss of bone volume (Figure 11A-1) (3).

If synovial fluid is aspirated from a joint with OA, it is generally relatively viscous and translucent in comparison with that from a patient with RA, which tends to be thinner and more opaque due to the higher number of cells related to a greater degree of intra-articular inflammation.

There is a great deal of current interest in another type of laboratory investigation in OA—the search for so-called biochemical markers of the disease process, products of abnormal breakdown or synthesis of connective tissue components in the joint, but such investigations have proved to be of limited value as yet, even as a research tool, and they have no clinical relevance.

11

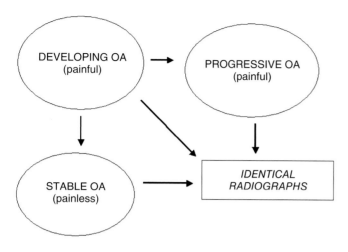

FIGURE 11A-3

Diagram summarizing an hypothesis about OA x-rays and disease progression. This hypothesis, outlined in the text, considers OA to be a phasic disease process that is a response to abnormal joint biomechanics and an attempt at joint repair. While the disease is active, changing joint anatomy, it can cause direct nocioceptive pain. Pain sensitization may also occur, in which case pain may persist when the disease process has ceased to be active. The plain radiograph, the most frequently used investigation in OA, will look the same whether the disease is evolving, inactive, or progressing, and whether the pain is due to direct nocioception, to periarticular problems, or results from peripheral or central pain sensitization.

need a joint replacement. It follows that either the joint damage and/or the symptoms cannot progress in the majority. Most cases stabilize after a period of change in joint anatomy, some progress, and a small minority improve spontaneously (especially hip OA) (8).

It seems likely that OA is a pathological process characterized by phases of activity within the joint, interspersed with periods in which the process is quiescent (9). Perhaps relatively minor degrees of change in biomechanics trigger the process. The process itself can be seen as an attempt of the joint to repair damage; thus, the formation of osteophytes and thickening of the capsule can be seen as the attempt of the joint to splint itself, and the changes in the subchondral bone, which alter joint shape, can be seen as an attempt to normalize load bearing. These processes, which are accompanied by cartilage loss (within this hypothesis cartilage is the innocent bystander) inevitably lead to x-ray changes, but not to symptoms. However, it is also probable that

as the joint anatomy is changing pain is generated, along with a change in pain sensitization both in the periphery and centrally, in which case normal movements may become painful, and this activity-related pain (due to sensitization of the pain system) may persist even when the process has become quiescent. If this is the case, it may help us explain the discordance between x-rays and symptoms, as outlined in Figure 11A-3.

Osteoarthritis, then, is not necessarily a progressive disorder, and the prognosis is not inevitably a bad one. However, OA is a disease affecting older people, in whom a combination of advancing years and comorbidities are taking their toll on health. For these reasons, many—perhaps most—people with OA do get worsening of disability over the years, making it appear that their OA has deteriorated. But the comorbidities may be much more important than the OA. For example, in people with OA, walking speed may be as dependent on the presence of a cataract as it is on the joint disease.

REFERENCES

1. Nichols E, Richardson F. Arthritis deformans. J Med Res 1909;21:149–221.
2. Lim K, Rogers J, Shepstone L, Dieppe P. The evolutionary origins of osteoarthritis: a comparative study of hand disease in two primates. J Rheumatol 1995;22:2132–2134.
3. Watt I, Doherty M. Plain radiographic features of osteoarthritis. In: Brandt K, Doherty M, Lohmander S, eds. Osteoarthritis. 2nd ed. Oxford, England: Oxford University Press; 2003.
4. Englund M, Lohmander S. Risk factors for symptomatic knee osteoarthritis fifteen to twenty-two years after menisectomy Arthritis Rheum 2004;50:2811–2819.
5. Nakashima E, Kitoh H, Maeda K, et al. Novel COL9A3 mutation in a family with multiple epiphyseal dysplasia. Am J Med Genet A 2005;132:181–184.
6. Sarzi-Puttini P, Atzeni F. New developments in our understanding of DISH (diffuse idiopathic skeletal hyperostosis). Curr Opin Rheumatol 2004;16:287–292.
7. Steultjens M, Dekker J, Bijlsma J. Coping, pain and disability in osteoarthritis. J Rheumatol 2001;28:1068–1072.
8. Perry G, Smith M, Whiteside C. Spontaneous recovery of the joint space in degenerative hip disease. Ann Rheum Dis 1979;31:440–448.
9. Kirwan J, Elson C. Is the progression of osteoarthritis phasic? Evidence and implications. J Rheumatol 2000; 27:834–836.

Osteoarthritis
B. Pathology and Pathogenesis

FRANCIS BERENBAUM, MD, PhD

- Changes in articular cartilage and subchondral bone are the characteristic histopathological changes of osteoarthritis (OA).
- Osteoarthritis results from a failure of chondrocytes to maintain the balance between degradation and synthesis of extracellular matrix.
- Increased breakdown of cartilage involves proteinases such as matrix metalloproteinase.
- Proinflammatory cytokines synthesized by chondrocytes and synoviocytes may drive production of cartilage-degrading enzymes. Other mediators of inflammation including prostaglandins and reactive oxygen species also contribute to OA pathogenesis.
- Mechanical factors are essential for maintaining normal cartilage homeostasis and mechanical stress contributes significantly to disease initiation and progression.

PATHOLOGY

Osteoarthritis (OA) can be defined as a gradual loss of articular cartilage, combined with thickening of the subchondral bone, bony outgrowths (osteophytes) at joint margins, and mild, chronic nonspecific synovial inflammation. The difference between physiologic aging of the cartilage and OA cartilage is not sharp. However, three cartilage stages can be identified: stage I, normal cartilage; stage II, aging cartilage; and stage III, OA cartilage.

Normal Cartilage

Normal cartilage has two main components. One is the extracellular matrix, which is rich in collagens (mainly types II, IX, and XI) and proteoglycans (mainly aggrecan). Aggrecan is a central core protein bearing numerous glycosaminoglycan chains of chondroitin sulfate and keratan sulfate, all capable of retaining molecules of water. The second component consists of isolated chondrocytes, which lie in the matrix. The matrix components are responsible for the tensile strength and resistance to mechanical loading of the articular cartilage.

Passage of Normal Cartilage to Aging Cartilage

Fissures that develop in cartilage during aging are due mainly to stress fractures of the collagen network. Several structural and biochemical changes involving the noncollagenous component of the matrix occur during aging. These changes alter biomechanical properties of the cartilage that are essential for the distribution of forces in the weight-bearing zone. Glycosaminoglycans are modified qualitatively; they become shorter as the cartilage ages. The concentration of type 6 keratan sulfate (KS) increases during aging, to the detriment of type 4 KS. Also, an age-related reduction in total proteoglycan synthesis after skeletal maturation has been reported. This reduction could be due, at least in part, to a reduction in chondrocyte numbers with advancing age. These quantitative and qualitative changes in proteoglycan reduce the capacity of the molecules to retain water. A prominent feature of aging is the modification of proteins by nonenzymatic glycation leading to the accumulation of advanced glycation end products (AGEs). Once they are formed, AGEs cannot be removed from the collagens, and, therefore, they accumulate in articular cartilage. The accumulation of

AGEs in cartilage leads to inferior mechanical properties. Moreover, chondrocytes can express receptors that are capable of binding AGEs and can modulate cell function. The best characterized AGE receptor is called the receptor for advanced glycation end products (RAGE). Thus, AGEs trigger RAGE on chondrocytes, leading to increased catabolic activity and therefore to cartilage degradation (1). In conclusion, aging cartilage contains less water, which alters the biochemical properties of the cartilage, less chondrocytes, which decreases the capacity of cartilage to synthesize matrix, and altered collagens.

Osteoarthritic Joints

Osteoarthritic joints have abnormal cartilage and bone, with synovial and capsular lesions (2). Macroscopically, the most characteristic elements are reduced joint space, formation of ostephytes (protrusions of bone and cartilage) mostly at the margins of joints, and sclerosis of the subchondral bone. These changes are the result of several histologic phases.

Phase 1: Edema and Microcracks

The first recognizable change in OA is edema of the extracellular matrix, principally in the intermediate layer. The cartilage loses its smooth aspect, and microcracks appear. There is a focal loss of chondrocytes, alternating with areas of chondrocyte proliferation.

Phase 2: Fissuring and Pitting

The microcracks deepen perpendicularly in the direction of the forces of tangential cutting and along fibrils of collagen. Vertical clefts form in the subchondral bone cartilage. Clusters of chondrocytes appear around these clefts and at the surface.

Phase 3: Erosion

Fissures cause fragments of cartilage to detach and "fall" into the articular cavity, creating osteocartilaginous loose bodies and uncovering the subchondral bone, where microcysts develop. The loose bodies cause the mild synovial inflammation of OA. The resulting synovial inflammation often is more focal, though often just as intense, than inflammation that occurs in rheumatoid synovitis. Histologically, OA synovitis is characterized by nonspecific lymphoplasmocytic and histiocytic infiltration.

There is sclerosis of the subchondral bone, due to the apposition of small strips of new bone. Osteophytes form around this zone, their surface covered with fibrilar cartilage. Subchondral sclerosis increases with disease progression. Specific changes in the architecture of the subchondral trabecular bone are due to accelerated bone turnover.

PATHOGENESIS

The physiologic homeostasis of the articular cartilage is driven by chondrocytes, which synthesize collagens, proteoglycans, and proteinases. Osteoarthritis result from a failure of chondrocytes within the joint to synthesize a good quality matrix, in terms of resistance and elasticity, and to maintain the balance between synthesis and degradation of the extracellular matrix.

The change in the quality of the matrix synthesized is due to alterations in the differentiation process of chondrocytes (3). Chondrocyte hypertrophy can contribute to the progression of OA via effects including dysregulation of matrix repair through reduced expression of collagen II and aggrecan, increased expression of type X collagen, upregulation of matrix metalloproteinase 13 (MMP-13), and promotion of pathologic calcification. OA cartilage typically develops foci of maturation of cells to hypertrophic differentiation (4). A recapitulation of embryonic skeletal development also occurs in the deep and calcified zones where the hypertrophic chondrocyte-specific type X collagen is expressed, and in the upper middle zone where type III collagen expression is detected. Chondrocyte dedifferentiation has also been described. The main evidence of chondrocyte dedifferentiation in OA is the presence of types I and III collagens, and the chondroprogenitor splice variant type IIA collagen—none of which usually are present in adult articular cartilage—and the production of greater than normal amounts of type VI collagen.

The imbalance between synthesis and degradation of the extracellular matrix is caused by increasing synthesis of proteinases that breakdown collagens and aggrecans, and decreased synthesis of natural inhibitors of these proteinases, the tissue inhibitor of metalloproteinases (TIMPs). This abnormal chondrocyte synthesis is the result of tissue activation by cytokines, lipid mediators (mainly prostaglandins), free radicals (NO, H_2O_2), and constituents of the matrix itself, such as fibronectin fragments. Activated chondrocytes become capable of synthesizing certain proteinases and proinflammatory mediators. Although the role of the chondrocyte seems to be fundamental, the synovial tissue helps perpetuate chondrocyte activation. Synovial cells phagocytize the fragments of cartilage released into the joint, which causes synovial inflammation. Then, OA synovial cells become capable of producing a range of mediators that are released in the cavity, such as MMPs and cytokines, which in turn can alter the cartilage matrix and activate chondrocytes. Finally, the subchondral bone may contribute to the degradation of cartilage. Osteoblasts isolated from subchondral OA bone demonstrate an altered phenotype. In comparison to normal osteoblasts, they produce more alkaline phosphatase, osteocalcin, insulinlike growth factor (IGF)-1, and urokinase. OA osteoblast phenotype contributes to cartilage degradation by inhibiting cartilage matrix component synthesis and by increasing MMP synthesis by articular chondrocytes (5).

Enzymes Involved in Cartilage Degradation

The main proteinases involved in the destruction of cartilage in OA are the MMPs (6). There are at least 18 members of this gene family of neutral Zn^{2+} metalloproteinases. Because they are active at neutral pH, the MMPs can act on the cartilaginous matrix at some distance from the chondrocytes. They can be synthesized by chondrocytes and synoviocytes under the influence of cytokines.

Aggrecanase, the enzyme that cleaves the Glu^{373}-Ala^{374} bond of the interspherical domain of aggrecan, also plays a major role in the degradation of the matrix. Two aggrecanases have been cloned. They belong to the MMP family, specifically the ADAMTS (disintegrin and metalloproteinases with thrombospondin motifs) family. They are called aggrecanase 1 (or ADAMTS-4) and aggrecanase 2 (or ADAMTS-11).

The activities of MMPs are strictly controlled by stoichiometric inhibition with specific inhibitors, TIMP1-4. Therefore, the balance between the amounts of MMPs and TIMPs in cartilage determines if cartilage is degraded (7). MMPs produced by the chondrocyte and released into the extracellular matrix are activated by an enzyme cascade involving serine proteinases (plasminogen activator, plasminogen, plasmin), free radicals, cathepsins, and some membrane-type MMPs. This enzymatic cascade is regulated by natural inhibitors, including the TIMPs and the inhibitors of the plasminogen activator. MMP-13 is elevated in OA joint tissues, particularly in articular cartilage, and colocalizes with type II collagen cleavage epitopes in regions of matrix depletion in OA cartilage. The other enzymes that can degrade type II collagen and proteoglycans are the cathepsins. They are active only at low pH and include the aspartate proteinases (cathepsin D) and cysteine proteinases (cathepsins B, H, K, L, and S) that are stored in chondrocyte lysosomes and released into the pericellular microenvironment. Glycosidases also may be important, because proteoglycans are very rich in carbohydrate chains. Although hyaluronidases are not present in cartilage, other glycosidases may contribute to the degradation of proteoglycans.

CYTOKINES

Although OA is often classified as a non-inflammatory disease, numerous studies have shown that inflammatory cytokines provide essential biomechanical signals that stimulate chondrocytes to release cartilage-degrading enzymes. Proinflammatory cytokines synthesized by chondrocytes and synoviocytes bind to specific receptors on chondrocytes. These bound cytokines cause transcription of the MMP genes, and the genes' products are exported from the cell in an inactive form. It is generally accepted that interleukin (IL) 1 is the pivotal cytokine released during inflammation of the osteoarthritic joint (8). Other cytokines are released, including chemokines (IL-8, GRO alpha, MIP-1 alpha and MIP-1 beta). Some of these cytokines and chemokines may be regulatory [e.g., IL-6, IL-8, lymphocyte inhibitory factor (LIF)], or inhibitory (e.g., IL-4, IL-10, IL-13, interferon gamma). IL-1 receptor antagonist, IL-4, IL10, and IL-13 prevent the secretion of some MMPs and may increase the synthesis of TIMPs. In a more general way, IL-4 and IL-13 counteract the catabolic effects of IL-1. Finally, IL-1 alters the quality of the cartilage matrix by causing synthesis of type II and IX collagens to decrease, while increasing the synthesis of type I and type III collagens.

A new family of cytokines, called adipokines (for cytokines produced by adipose tissue), has been recently implicated in the pathophysiology of OA. Adipokines such as leptin, adiponectin, and resistin are detected both in the plasma and in the synovial fluid obtained from OA patients. Various tissues obtained from human OA-affected joints, including synovium, infrapatellar fat pad, meniscus, cartilage, and bone, release leptin and adiponectin. The roles of adopokines in OA pathophysiology remain largely unknown.

Lipid Mediators

The eicosanoids also can take part in chondrocyte activation (9). Prostaglandins, produced after activation of phospholipases A2, cyclooxygenases (mainly the cyclooxygenase-2 isoform) and prostaglandin synthases (mainly the microsomal prostaglandin E synthase-1) by proinflammatory cytokines can favor the synthesis of MMPs by activating the cell via specific cellular or/and nuclear prostaglandin receptors. Among eicosanoids, prostaglandin E2 seems to be the main lipid mediator produced by synovial cells, chondrocytes, and subchondral osteoblasts and involved in cartilage degradation in OA.

Reactive Oxygen Species

Reactive oxygen species (ROS) play a crucial role in the regulation of a number of basic chondrocyte activities,

11

such as cell activation, proliferation, and matrix remodeling. However, when ROS production exceeds the antioxidant capacities of the cell, an oxidative stress occurs, leading to structural and functional cartilage damages like cell death and matrix degradation (10).

Nitric oxide (NO) is a gas synthesized by way of the oxidation of L-arginine by the NO synthases (NOS). Chondrocytes produce large amounts of NO after upregulation of the iNOS gene by cytokines. Most in vitro studies indicate that NO is partly responsible for the blocking of glycosaminoglycan and collagen synthesis by IL-1, and may contribute to the activation of the latent forms of MMPs. NO also may mediate the IL-1–stimulated synthesis of MMP mRNA and protein, and may contribute to chondrocyte cell death by interfering with survival signals from the extracellular matrix. However, NO may have anabolic and anticatabolic effects in cartilage under certain conditions. Therefore, the actual role of NO in the degradative process of OA is not clear (11).

Matrix Degradation Products

The products of matrix degradation, such as fibronectin fragments, can activate chondrocytes through intergrin-type receptors, causing the synthesis of MMPs. These products can stimulate or activate other factors, such as catabolic cytokines, that amplify the damage. The damage, in turn, enhances the concentrations of the degradation products themselves, as in a positive feedback loop.

Mechanical Stress

Along with chemical mediators, biophysical mediators could also be directly involved in chondrocyte activation in OA. Compressive, but also shear and stretch, stresses occur on cartilage. Interestingly, there is considerable evidence that interactions between biomechanical factors and proinflammatory mediators are involved in the initiation and the progression of OA (12). In vivo studies have shown increased concentrations of inflammatory cytokines and mediators in the joint in mechanically induced models of osteoarthritis. In vitro explant studies confirm that mechanical load is a potent regulator of matrix metabolism, cell viability, and the production of proinflammatory mediators such as NO and prostaglandin E2. Chondrocytes have receptors for responding to mechanical stress and can respond to direct biomechanical perturbation by upregulating synthetic activity or inflammatory cytokines, which are also produced by other joint tissues. Chondrocytes express several members of the integrin family, and these can serve as receptors for fibronectin (alpha 5 beta 1), types II and VI collage (alpha 1 beta 1, alpha

5 beta 1, alpha 10 beta 1), laminin (alpha 6 beta 1), and vitronectin and osteopontin (alpha V beta 3). Some of these receptors are sensitive to prolonged changes in pressure (mechanoreceptors). Injurious static or dynamic compression stimulates depletion of proteoglycans and damage to the collagen network and decreases the synthesis of cartilage matrix proteins, whereas low intensity dynamic compression increases matrix synthetic activity. Certain types of mechanical stress and cartilage matrix degradation products are capable of stimulating the same signaling pathways as those induced by IL-1 and tumor necrosis factor alpha (TNF-alpha). These pathways involve cascades of kinases, including the stress-activated protein kinases (SAPKs), also termed c-Jun N-terminal kinases (JNKs) and p38 MAP kinase, IκB kinases, and phosphatidylinositol-3′-kinase (PI-3K) and NF-κB. Because these pathways may also induce the expression of the genes encoding these cytokines, it remains controversial whether inflammatory cytokines are primary or secondary regulators of the progressive cartilage destruction in OA.

Attempts to Repair Cartilage

There is evidence of attempted repair of the OA-damaged joint, particularly of the cartilage and subchondral bone, at least in the early stages of OA (13). Growth factors involved in the physiological matrix synthesis, such as platelet-derived growth factor, IGF-1, and transforming growth factor beta (TGF-beta), are produced in excess by OA chondrocytes, subchondral bone, and synovial tissues. TGF-beta, IGF-I, and basic fibroblast growth factor have anabolic effects in matrix synthesis, can inhibit the effects of the proinflammatory cytokines, and possess mitogenic properties for the chondrocyte. These growth factors also have a high affinity for matrix. When they are synthesized they become trapped in the cartilage, which acts as a reservoir for these factors. The factors are released when the matrix is broken down, and tend to repair lesions.

There is considerable interest in the role of subchondral bone in this attempted repair. The metabolism of subchondral bone is increased during OA, which leads to the production of growth factors, such as the bone morphogenic protein 2 (BMP-2). Experiments have shown that this protein can repair a cartilaginous defect. However, attempted repair of cartilage defects is in vain for the following reasons: (1) Alterations in the differentiation process of the chondrocytes results in the synthesis of a matrix with poor biomechanical properties. (2) Not enough growth factors and TIMPs are produced to counteract the effect of cytokines and proteinases. (3) The bioavailability of certain growth factors is decreased (e.g., IGF-I activity is reduced because of excess IGF-binding proteins and receptor desensitization).

Initiation of Osteoarthritis

The initiation of OA is not well understood. It involves local, systemic, genetic, and environmental factors. Numerous mechanical factors can directly or indirectly increase cartilage vulnerability. Experimentally, increased pressure on cartilage alters the matrix architecture, which probably explains the high incidence of knee OA in obese people. The ligaments around the joints become more lax with age, leading to instability and injury. With age, strength gradually decreases and peripheral neurologic responses that protect the joints slow. All these factors contribute to an abnormal distribution of pressure on the cartilage, resulting in shear stress.

Osteoarthritis also may be triggered by changes in the structure of the subchondral bone. This hypothesis is based on the observation that sclerosis of subchondral bone precedes cartilaginous defects in some patients. Repeated microtraumas affecting the joint could provoke microfractures of the subchondral bone that, in turn, may modify the biomechanical qualities of the cartilage in the environment of these microfractures. These changes would cause the bone to synthesize growth factors that can result in the production of osteophytes and osteosclerosis.

Epidemiological studies on the prevalence of OA in women after menopause suggest that one or more hormonal factors are involved in the initiation of OA. Chondrocytes bear estrogen receptors, and stimulation of these receptors triggers the synthesis of growth factors. The plasma concentration of estrogens decreases after menopause, which could result in decreased synthesis of growth factors by chondrocytes. This theory is being examined, particularly in OA of the hand and knee, two sites more frequently affected in this population.

CONCLUSION

The simple hypothesis that a passive deterioration of cartilage is the main cause of OA has given way to a more exciting view (Figures 11B-1, 11B-2). It is clear that the pathogenesis of OA is due to altered chondrocyte phenotype mediated by different autocrine and paracrine signals, leading to the synthesis of many mediators of inflammation and degradation that alter the matrix. Moreover, recent experimental studies emphasize the predominant role of mechanical stresses on chondrocyte activation. It is quite likely that research carried out over the next decade will result in increased understanding of the interaction between biomechanics and molecular biology of chondrocytes, and of the interaction between bone and cartilage in the pathogenesis of OA.

FIGURE 11B-1

Modulation of chondrocyte activation by catabolic pathways. Signaling pathways are activated by the binding of catabolic mediators on specific receptors. Activation of these signaling cascades lead to transcription and post-transcriptional modifications of a set of genes [MMPs, aggrecanases (ADAMTS), cytokines, NO, and prostaglandins]. Some of them may feedback/regulate or amplify these responses. These catabolic factors include biochemical [proinflammatory cytokines, reactive oxygen species (ROS), prostaglandins, ligands for the receptor of advanced glycation end products (RAGE), extracellular matrix (ECM) components] and biophysical factors (mechanical stresses).

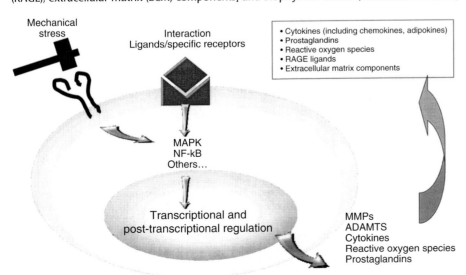

11

FIGURE 11B-2

Hypothetical model for initiation and perpetuation of osteoarthritis. Accumulation of risk factors on aging cartilage triggers the initiation of the osteoarthritic process. For didactic reasons, two phases are described, early OA and late OA, but the passage from one to the other is progressive and generally lasts many years. Structural treatment of OA should be more efficient at the early stage when chondrocytes keep a high metabolic activity rather than at the late stage when chondrocytes lose their ability to synthesize matrix. Abbreviations: KS, keratan sulfate; AGE, advanced glycation end products.

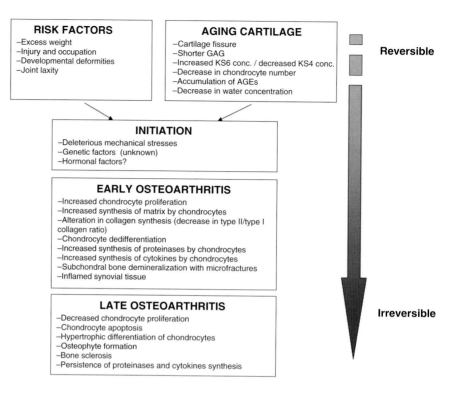

REFERENCES

1. Loeser RF, Yammani RR, Carlson CS, et al. Articular chondrocytes express the receptor for advanced glycation end products: potential role in osteoarthritis. Arthritis Rheum 2005;52:2376–2385.
2. Pritzker KPH. Pathology of osteoarthritis. In: Brandt KD, Doherty M, Lohmander S, eds. Osteoarthritis. New York: Oxford University Press; 1998;50–61.
3. Goldring MB. The role of the chondrocyte in osteoarthritis. Arthritis Rheum 2000;43:1916–1926.
4. Cecil DL, Johnson K, Rediske J, Lotz M, Schmidt AM, Terkeltaub R. Inflammation-induced chondrocyte hypertrophy is driven by receptor for advanced glycation end products. J Immunol 2005;175:8296–8302.
5. Lajeunesse D, Hilal G, Pelletier JP, Martel-Pelletier J. Subchondral bone morphological and biochemical alterations in osteoarthritis. Osteoarthritis Cartilage 1999;7:321–322.
6. Cawston T. Matrix metalloproteinases and TIMPs: properties and implications for the rheumatic diseases. Mol Med Today 1998;4:130–137.
7. Dean DD, Martel-Pelletier J, Pelletier JP, Howell DS, Woessner JF Jr. Evidence for metalloproteinase and metalloproteinase inhibitor imbalance in human osteoarthritic cartilage. J Clin Invest 1989;84:678–685.
8. Jacques C, Gosset M, Berenbaum F, Gabay C. The Role of IL-1 and IL-1Ra in joint inflammation and cartilage degradation. Vitam Horm 2006;74:371–403.
9. Goldring MB, Berenbaum F. The regulation of chondrocyte function by proinflammatory mediators: prostaglandins and nitric oxide. Clin Orthop 2004;(Suppl):S37–S46.
10. Henrotin Y, Kurz B, Aigner T. Oxygen and reactive oxygen species in cartilage degradation: friends or foes? Osteoarthritis Cartilage 2005;13:643–654.
11. Abramson SB, Attur M, Amin AR, Clancy R. Nitric oxide and inflammatory mediators in the perpetuation of osteoarthritis. Curr Rheumatol Rep 2001;3:535–541.
12. Guilak F, Fermor B, Keefe FJ, et al. The role of biomechanics and inflammation in cartilage injury and repair. Clin Orthop 2004;17–26.
13. van der Kraan PM, van den Berg WB. Anabolic and destructive mediators in osteoarthritis. Curr Opin Clin Nutr Metab Care 2000;3:205–211.

Osteoarthritis
C. Treatment

LEENA SHARMA, MD

- Nonpharmacologic treatments of osteoarthritis (OA) include education, weight management, and appropriate exercise, which may delay disease progression, reduce symptoms, and improve function.
- Nutritional supplements such as glucosamine and chondroitin sulfate have been studied in OA, may benefit some patients, and have low toxicity.

- Pharmacologic approaches to treatment include non-narcotic analgesics such as acetaminophen and nonsteroidal anti-inflammatory drugs (NSAIDs).
- Intra-articular injection of glucocorticoids or hyaluronan may be useful for isolated joint involvement.
- Surgical joint replacement, especially at the hip and knee, can reduce pain and improve function in appropriate candidates.

It is estimated that 12% of Americans between ages 25 and 75 years have clinical signs and symptoms of osteoarthritis (OA). The increase in the prevalence of symptomatic OA with age, the inadequacy of current symptom-relieving treatments, and the lack of disease-modifying treatment each contribute to the overall burden of OA. Given the frequency of periarticular syndromes that mimic OA symptoms, it is important to establish, as much as is possible, that the given symptoms are a result of the OA itself (see Chapter 11A). The variation in responsiveness to standard treatments may be explained by the heterogeneity of OA as a clinical syndrome and the several other potential sources of pain.

Four sources of guidelines for the management of lower-limb OA include recommendations for nonpharmacological therapy and pharmacological therapy: the American College of Rheumatology (ACR; Table 11C-1) (1); the task force of the European League Against Rheumatism Standing Committee for International Clinical Studies Including Therapeutics (EULAR; Table 11C-2) (2,3); Algorithms for the Diagnosis and Management of Musculoskeletal Complaints (4); and the Institute for Clinical Systems Improvement (5). Pencharz and colleagues provide a critical appraisal of some of these sets of guidelines (6).

NONPHARMACOLOGIC THERAPY

An array of nonpharmacologic interventions for OA has been described, each in various stages of development, investigation, and application. Interventions from this burgeoning field take advantage of gains in understanding of causes of symptoms, disease progression, function loss, and disability in persons with OA. The category of nonpharmacologic therapy in OA encompasses physical activity, exercise, weight loss, education, inserts, footwear, bracing, therapeutic ultrasound, and pulsed electromagnetic field therapy. For many of these interventions, further investigation is necessary to better define their place in OA management.

For knee OA in particular, results from ongoing studies suggest that interventions targeting knee laxity, symptoms of knee instability, proprioceptive acuity, muscle function, agility, self-efficacy, and specific combinations of nonpharmacologic therapies may be especially effective and should be further developed and tested.

Some nonpharmacologic interventions for OA may ultimately be shown to contribute to secondary prevention, that is, prevention of disease progression. At present, these approaches are applied predominantly to

TABLE 11C-1. RECOMMENDATIONS (2000) FOR THE MANAGEMENT OF KNEE OSTEOARTHRITIS FROM THE AMERICAN COLLEGE OF RHEUMATOLOGY.

Nonpharmacologic therapy for patients with osteoarthritis
  Patient education
  Self-management programs (e.g., Arthritis Foundation Self-
    Management Program)
  Personalized social support through telephone contact
  Weight loss (if overweight)
  Aerobic exercise programs
  Physical therapy
  Range-of-motion exercises
  Muscle-strengthening exercises
  Assistive devices for ambulation
  Patellar taping
  Appropriate footwear
  Lateral-wedged insoles (for genu varum)
  Bracing
  Occupational therapy
  Joint protection and energy conservation
  Assistive devices for activities of daily living (ADL)

Pharmacologic therapy for patients with osteoarthritis
  Oral
    Acetaminophen
    COX-2-specific inhibitor
    Nonselective NSAID plus misoprostol or a proton pump
      inhibitor
    Nonacetylated salicylate
    Other pure analgesics (tramadol, opioids)
  Intra-articular
    Glucocorticoids
    Hyaluronan
  Topical
    Capsaicin
    Methylsalicylate

SOURCE: From Altman RD, et al. Arthritis Rheum 2000;43:1905–1915, by permission of *Arthritis and Rheumatism*.

treat symptoms and maintain or improve functioning. Many nonpharmacologic interventions are low cost, incorporate self-management approaches, and are home based, and, as such, may ultimately have substantial public health impact. Some specific suggestions are offered in Table 11C-3.

It is well documented that regular physical activity and exercise benefit symptoms, function, and quality of life, and they are crucial components of OA management. Exercise for OA should address range of motion, flexibility, aerobic conditioning, and muscle function. Muscle performance can be enhanced not only by strengthening exercise but also by functional exercise to improve muscle endurance and motor control. The daily exercise regimen—particularly exercises targeting muscle strength—should take into consideration the local joint pathology and impairments such as malalignment and laxity. In theory, exercise and activity benefits on pain and function in OA may be mediated through a variety of routes, including improvement in strength,

endurance, cardiovascular fitness, and self-efficacy and reduction in excess body weight, depression, and anxiety. The reviews of Van Baar and colleagues (7) and of Baker and McAlindon (8) suggest that the effectiveness of isolated strengthening exercise is less than more comprehensive interventions that include aerobic exercise, pain modalities, and education. A small number of studies suggest that proprioceptive acuity may be improved by exercise or by orthoses as simple as a neoprene sleeve.

There is abundant epidemiologic evidence to suggest that excess body weight increases the risk of incident knee OA. Less is known about the impact of body weight on OA progression and there is a paucity of trial data concerning the discrete effects of weight reduction on OA outcomes. Nevertheless, there is a strong

TABLE 11C-2. RECOMMENDATIONS (2003) FOR THE MANAGEMENT OF KNEE OSTEOARTHRITIS FROM A TASK FORCE OF THE EULAR STANDING COMMITTEE FOR INTERNATIONAL CLINICAL STUDIES INCLUDING THERAPEUTICS (ESCISIT).

The optimal management of knee OA requires a combination of nonpharmacological and pharmacological treatment modalities.

The treatment of knee OA should be tailored according to:
  Knee risk factors (obesity, adverse mechanical factors, physical activity)
  General risk factors (age, comorbidity, polypharmacy)
  Level of pain intensity and disability
  Sign of inflammation, e.g., effusion
  Location and degree of structural damage

Nonpharmacological treatment of knee OA should include regular education, exercise, appliances (sticks, insoles, knee bracing), and weight reduction.

Paracetamol is the oral analgesic to try first and, if successful, the preferred long-term oral analgesic.

Topical applications (NSAID, capsaicin) have clinical efficacy and are safe.

NSAIDs should be considered in patients unresponsive to paracetamol. In patients with an increased gastrointestinal risk, nonselective NSAIDs and effective gastroprotective agents, or selective COX-2 inhibitors should be used.

SYSADOA (glucosamine sulphate, chondroitin sulphate, ASU, diacerein, hyaluronic acid) have symptomatic effects and may modify structure.

Intra-articular injection of long-acting corticosteroid is indicated for flare of knee pain, especially if accompanied by effusion.

Joint replacement has to be considered in patients with radiographic evidence of knee OA who have refractory pain and disability.

SOURCE: From Jordan KM, et al. Ann Rheum Dis 2003;62:1145–1155, with permission from *Annals of the Rheumatic Diseases*.

TABLE 11C-3. SPECIFIC SUGGESTIONS FOR NONPHARMACOLOGIC INTERVENTION IN OSTEOARTHRITIS.

Address psychosocial factors
    Enhance self-efficacy, using individualized approaches +
        arthritis self-management courses
    Educate about OA
    Improve coping skills
    Prevent/treat anxiety and depression
    Improve social support

Improve/maintain aerobic capacity, conditioning, strength, and
    ADL performance
    Increase physical activity
    Promote home exercise (aerobic + resistance)
    Refer for physical and occupational therapy
    Provide assistive devices

Address local factors
    Adjust footwear
    Refer for inserts/insoles
    Promote resistance exercise cognizant of individual pathologic
        anatomy (i.e., physical therapy referral to learn optimal
        exercises for malaligned or unstable knee)
    Refer for agility training

Provide weight loss program for those who are overweight

rationale that weight reduction in persons with knee OA who are overweight may delay disease progression, reduce symptoms, improve function, and lower the impact of comorbidities.

Several nutritional products are available and touted as beneficial for OA, but few have undergone rigorous testing. Among these, glucosamine and chondroitin sulfate have been evaluated in clinical trials, most of which received some manufacturer support. A meta-analysis suggested efficacy for symptoms, but also described evidence of publication bias, suggesting that the magnitude of the beneficial effect may be less than what has been reported (9). Studies of glucosamine published since the meta-analysis have had mixed results, with some trials suggesting no or very modest difference between treatment and placebo. A recent report from an National Institutes of Health–funded multicenter trial suggests that glucosamine and chondroitin (alone or in combination) were not better than placebo in reducing pain in the overall group of patients with knee OA, but that the combination may be effective in persons with moderate-to-severe knee pain (10).

There is some epidemiologic evidence that dietary intake of vitamin C and vitamin D may be associated with a reduced risk of knee OA progression and a trial of vitamin D in knee OA is ongoing. Data are insufficient at present to support a therapeutic dose of vitamins C or D for prevention or treatment of OA.

Patient education is highly recommended in the management of OA. OA patient education may have a specific focus, for example, relaxation, cognitive pain management, or exercise, or may be a multicomponent program. The Arthritis Self-Management Program (ASMP), taught by trained lay leaders at weekly sessions, includes patient education regarding disease processes, medication side effects, exercise, as well as cognitive–behavioral techniques, and a communication exercise in which participants learn to elicit support from family and friends (11). A body of literature suggests that the ASMP leads to improvement in symptoms, psychological well-being, perceived helplessness, levels of physical activity, use of cognitive pain management techniques, use of self-management behaviors such as exercise, communication with physicians, with long-term retention of initial gains. ASMP sessions are sponsored and/or organized by the national Arthritis Foundation in the United States and other organizations in Canada and the United Kingdom. A major mechanism of the beneficial effect of the ASMP is enhanced self-efficacy, a key determinant of physical functioning over time in epidemiologic studies.

Varus alignment substantially increases the likelihood of progression of subsequent medial tibiofemoral OA. For years, wedge osteotomy has been undertaken with the goal of reducing forces in the medial compartment in varus knees. Conservative approaches have also emerged. The use of a lateral wedge insole orthosis is believed to lower medial compartment load and reduce lateral tensile forces by enhancing valgus correction of the calcaneus, whether or not varus deformity at the knee is lessened. A small number of controlled trials have been reported, most of which suggest a beneficial effect on knee symptoms. Larger trials of longer duration are ongoing.

Kerrigan and colleagues found that wearing high-heeled shoes leads to a striking increase in forces across the medial and patellofemoral compartments (12). Although long-term effects of this footwear have not been elucidated, it seems prudent to minimize the wearing of high-heeled shoes.

The goal of the valgus unloading brace in medial knee OA is to produce an abduction moment to shift the joint contact force away from the stressed medial compartment. Most studies suggesting a beneficial effect on symptoms were uncontrolled or inadequately controlled. Systematic reviews suggest that there is insufficient evidence as yet to advocate either therapeutic ultrasound or pulsed electromagnetic field therapy in the management of OA.

SYSTEMIC PHARMACOLOGIC THERAPY

Pharmacologic treatment categories for OA are typically set up to designate whether drugs are symptom relieving or disease modifying. However, there is insufficient evidence as yet that any drug has a disease-modifying effect in OA.

11

Non-Narcotic Analgesic Medication

The most recent ACR guidelines for the medical management of OA suggest acetaminophen as an effective initial approach for mild-to-moderate pain. In keeping with this, the most recent EULAR guidelines suggest paracetamol as the initial approach as well as the best long-term choice. While some studies have shown that the effect of acetaminophen and nonsteroidal anti-inflammatory drugs (NSAIDs) is comparable, others have revealed that NSAIDs may be more efficacious and preferred by patients. The ACR guidelines suggest NSAIDs as an alternative approach in those with moderate-to-severe pain and signs of inflammation. However, given the superior safety profile for acetaminophen, its over-the-counter availability and low cost, and concerns about the potential cardiovascular and gastrointestinal effects of NSAIDs, it seems reasonable to initiate therapy with regularly dosed acetaminophen.

Doses of acetaminophen should not exceed 4000 mg/day and the minimally effective dose should be used. As acetaminophen may increase the half-life of warfarin sodium, warfarin dosage may need to be adjusted in persons who start high dose acetaminophen. Acetaminophen-associated hepatic toxicity is rare in persons on doses used in the setting of OA but may be more likely in those with liver disease or who abuse alcohol.

Narcotic Analgesic Medication

Narcotic analgesic medication should be reserved for persons with severe OA and pain that is refractory to regularly dosed non-narcotic analgesia coupled with nonpharmacologic measures. A central goal of pain management is to provide a sufficient level of symptom improvement to allow healthy levels of physical activity and exercise that, in turn, may help to prevent function loss and disability. Given the potential negative consequences of undertreating or overtreating OA pain, the involvement of a multidisciplinary pain service should be considered, especially in the management of persons with severe OA who are ineligible for or who have opted against total joint replacement.

Nonsteroidal Anti-Inflammatory Drugs

If treatment with a non-narcotic analgesic is not effective, therapy with a nonselective NSAID or a cyclooxygenase-2 (COX-2)–selective NSAID may be initiated (see Chapter 41). NSAIDs inhibit the enzymatic activity of cyclooxygenase (COX), which is essential for the production of prostaglandins. Two isoforms of this enzyme exists, with the COX-2 isoform being most important for synthesis of prostaglandins that cause pain and inflammation. All NSAIDs inhibit COX-2, while the nonselective NSAIDs inhibit both COX-1 and COX-2. The effect of both nonselective and selective NSAIDs on symptoms may relate to their analgesic as well as their anti-inflammatory effects.

For both nonselective and COX-2–selective NSAIDs, it is recommended that a patient be started on the lowest therapeutic dose and that the dose be gradually increased until the response is satisfactory, the maximal recommended dose is reached, or the patient experiences an adverse effect. If the response is inadequate at the full dose of a given NSAID, it may be beneficial to try other NSAIDs. Efficacy does not differ substantially between nonselective and COX-2–selective NSAIDs in clinical trials. However, different NSAIDs may be more or less effective in individual patients. The use of two or more NSAIDs simultaneously does not improve efficacy but does increase the risk of toxicity. NSAIDs and acetaminophen may be used concurrently, and this combination may be more effective than using either medication alone.

Monitoring for possible occult side effects during the regular use of any NSAIDs is recommended. This should include the following: at 2 weeks or so after the institution of therapy, an examination of blood pressure, a complete blood cell count, and laboratory tests of hepatic and renal function; every 4 to 6 months, blood pressure, a complete blood cell count, hepatic and renal function tests, urinalysis, and a stool occult blood test. With routine use of NSAIDs in patients with OA, there is an increased risk of upper gastrointestinal toxicity (e.g., gastric and duodenal ulcers) and gastrointestinal bleeding, though this risk may be reduced with COX-2–selective NSAIDs. The 2000 ACR guidelines for the medical management of OA recommend either misoprostol or a proton-pump inhibitor with a nonselective NSAID in a patient at increased risk for an adverse gastrointestinal effect. Gastroprotective therapy is not felt to be necessary in those with a low risk for adverse gastrointestinal effects.

Renal toxicity (e.g., renal insufficiency, fluid retention, hyperkalemia) also occurs with all NSAIDs. Only nonselective NSAIDs are associated with disrupted platelet function, a function of COX-1 inhibition. Certain COX-2–selective NSAIDs have been associated with an increased risk for serious cardiovascular events. However, new labeling requirements are in place regarding cardiovascular effects for all NSAIDs to emphasize the possibility that all these drugs may be associated with risk. Given the toxicity issues associated with nonselective and COX-2–selective NSAIDs, it seems most prudent to individualize this aspect of pharmacological management of OA depending upon comorbidities and individual risks.

LOCALIZED PHARMACOLOGIC THERAPY

Intra-articular administration of corticosteroids may result in pain reduction in OA joints, an effect that may be more likely in joints that show signs of inflammation. The duration of a beneficial effect may be only a few days but may last for a few months. Such therapy should not be repeated more than three times into the same joint in 1 year. A greater frequency is discouraged based predominantly on animal model data suggesting that intra-articular therapy may accelerate cartilage loss. Intra-articular steroid did not accelerate radiographic knee OA progression in one study. The effect of instilled steroid on OA progression by magnetic resonance imaging (MRI) has not been reported. Corticosteroid injection therapy should not be considered as a primary or scheduled form of therapy, but rather as an adjunct to other pharmacologic and nonpharmacologic treatment.

Intra-articular hyaluronan may result in a modest improvement in symptoms. The response appears to be slightly better in knees at earlier stages of OA. Available preparations are instilled weekly for 3 to 5 weeks. A potential adverse effect is the development of synovitis and effusion after the injection.

Topical capsaicin has some pain-relieving effect in osteoarthritic knees and hands. The best effect is associated with adherence to the recommended schedule, that is, application three to four times per day to the painful joint. Burning at the applied site diminishes with regular use. Capsaicin may be highly irritating to mucous membranes; careful hand washing after application helps to prevent mucous membrane contact.

SURGERY

Surgical options should be considered for patients with symptoms and functional loss refractory to nonsurgical pharmacologic and nonpharmacologic therapies. In patients with advanced OA coupled with severe pain and reduced function, total joint replacement is a highly effective intervention in the vast majority of patients, especially when the involved joint is the hip or the knee. Total joint replacement at other joint sites is at present less predictable than at the hip or the knee. Successful outcome hinges not only on operative factors and prevention of medical complications but on the quality of physical therapy before and after surgery.

With advances in prosthetic design and fixation, the typical number of years during which loosening is very rare has increased. However, given the probable life span of most prostheses and implantation techniques, and the fact of a greater likelihood of complications with revision surgery, total joint replacement is avoided in younger individuals.

In theory, osteotomy could help to unload a stressed compartment in a malaligned knee without severe OA, and thereby prevent disease progression. However, specific indications for osteotomy in the joint with mild-to-moderate OA are not clear, and this is made more complex by the concept that removal of periarticular bone stock may make future joint replacement for that knee more complex. Recent findings suggest that arthroscopic meniscal debridement may not improve outcome in OA knees (13). Whether there are categories of meniscal pathology in OA knees that should be debrided remains to be elucidated.

REFERENCES

1. Altman RD, Hochberg MC, Moskowitz RW, Schnitzer TJ. Recommendations for the medical management of osteoarthritis of the hip and knee: 2000 update. Arthritis Rheum 2000;43:1905–1915.
2. Jordan KM, Arden NK, Doherty M, et al. EULAR recommendations 2003: an evidence-based approach to the management of knee osteoarthritis: report of a task force of the Standing Committee for International Clinical Studies Including Therapeutic Trials (ESCISIT). Ann Rheum Dis 2003;62:1145–1155.
3. Zhang W, Doherty M, Arden N, et al. EULAR evidence-based recommendations for the management of hip osteoarthritis: report of a task force of the EULAR Standing Committee for International Clinical Studies Including Therapeutics (ESCISIT). Ann Rheum Dis 2005;64:669–681.
4. Algorithms for the diagnosis and management of musculoskeletal complaints. Am J Med 1997;103:3S–6S.
5. Lee JA. Adult degenerative joint disease of the knee: maximizing function and promoting joint health: Institute for Clinical System Integration. Postgrad Med 1999;105:183–197.
6. Pencharz JN, Grigoriadis E, Jansz GF, Bombardier C. A critical appraisal of clinical practice guidelines for the treatment of lower-limb osteoarthritis. Arthritis Res 2002;4:36–44.
7. van Baar ME, Assendelft WJJ, Dekker J, Oostendorp RAB, Bijlsma WJ. The effectiveness of exercise therapy in patients with osteoarthritis of the hip or knee. Arthritis Rheum 1999;42:1361–1369.
8. Baker K, McAlindon T. Exercise for knee osteoarthritis. Curr Opin Rheumatol 2000;12:456–463.
9. McAlindon TE, LaValley MP, Gulin JP, Felson DT. Glucosamine and chondroitin for treatment of osteoarthritis; a systematic quality assessment and meta-analysis. JAMA 2000;283:1469–1475.

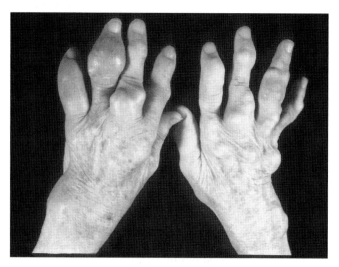

FIGURE 12A-1

The hands of a patient with advanced gout reveal large tophi over all digits as well as the right fifth metacarpophalangeal joint and both wrists.

The incidence of gout increases with age as well as with the degree of hyperuricemia. In the Normative Aging Study, the cumulative incidence of gouty arthritis among subjects with uric acid levels between 7.0 and 8.0 mg/dL was 3%, and subjects with urate levels of 9.0 mg/dL or more had a 5-year cumulative incidence of 22% (1). However, the vast majority of people with hyperuricemia never develop symptoms associated with uric acid excess, such as gouty arthritis, tophi, or kidney stones.

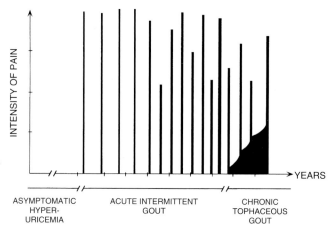

FIGURE 12A-2

The three stages of disease progression in classic gout. The period of asymptomatic hyperuricemia lasts decades, followed by acute intermittent gout with painless intercritical segments, leading to advanced gout with progressive background pain and joint destruction in untreated patients.

Acute Intermittent Gout

The initial episode of acute gout usually follows decades of asymptomatic hyperuricemia. Thomas Sydenham, the famous 17th-century physician who wrote of his personal experiences with gout, eloquently described the initial hours of an acute attack:

> He goes to bed and sleeps well, but about Two a Clock in the Morning, is waked by the Pain, seizing either his great Toe, the Heel, the Calf of the Leg, or the Ankle; this Pain is like that of dislocated Bones, with the Sense as it were of Water almost cold, poured upon the Membranes of the part affected; presently shivering and shaking follow with a feverish Disposition; the Pain is first gentle, but increased by degrees-till dash towards Night it comes to its height, accompanying itself neatly according to the Variety of the bones of the Tarsus and Metatarsus, whose Ligaments it seizes, sometimes resembling a violent stretching or tearing of those ligaments, sometimes gnawing of a dog, and sometimes a weight; more over, the Part affected has such a quick and exquisite Pain, that it is not able to bear the weight of the cloths upon it, nor hard walking in the Chamber (2).

This classic description captures the intense pain frequently associated with acute gouty arthritis, and it is this clinical picture most commonly evoked by the term *gout*.

In men, the first attacks usually occur between the fourth and sixth decades of life. In women, the age of onset is older and varies with several factors, including the age of menopause and the use of thiazide diuretics. The onset of a gouty attack usually is heralded by the rapid development of warmth, swelling, erythema, and pain in the affected joint. Pain escalates from the faintest twinges to its most intense level over an 8- to 12-hour period. The initial attack usually is monarticular and, in one half of patients, involves the first metatarsophalangeal (MTP) joint. Involvement of the first MTP joint, which occurs eventually in 90% of individuals with gout, is known as *podagra* (from the Greek for "foot-trap"; Figure 12A-3). Other joints that frequently are involved in this early stage are the midfoot, ankles, heels, and knees, and less commonly, the wrists, fingers, and elbows. The intensity of pain characteristically is very severe, but may vary among subjects. As Sydenham observed, patients find walking difficult or impossible when lower extremity joints are involved.

Systemic symptoms, such as fever, chills, and malaise may accompany acute gout. Fevers of higher than 38°C are seen in approximately 30% of gout patients during the early phases of acute attacks (3). The cutaneous erythema associated with the gouty attack may extend beyond the involved joint and resemble bacterial cellulitis (Figure 12A-3). The natural course of untreated

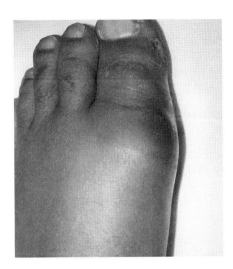

FIGURE 12A-3

Acute gouty arthritis involving the first metatarsophalangeal joint.

acute gout varies from episodes of mild pain that resolve in several hours ("petit attacks") to severe attacks that last 1 to 2 weeks. Early in the acute intermittent stage, episodes of acute arthritis are infrequent, and intervals between attacks sometimes last for years. Over time, the attacks typically become more frequent, longer in duration, and involve more joints.

Intercritical periods of acute intermittent gout are just as characteristic of this stage as are the acute attacks. Previously involved joints are virtually free of symptoms. Despite this, MSU crystals often can be identified in the synovial fluid. In one study, these crystals were found in the synovial fluids of 36 of 37 knees that previously had been inflamed. Synovial fluids containing crystals also had a higher mean cell count than those with no crystals, 449 cells/mm^3 versus 64 cells/mm^3 (4). These subtle differences may reflect ongoing subclinical inflammation.

Advanced Gout

Advanced gout (sometimes referred to as *chronic tophaceous gout*) usually develops after 10 or more years of acute intermittent gout, although patients have been reported with tophi as their initial clinical manifestation (5). The transition from acute intermittent gout to chronic tophaceous gout occurs when the intercritical periods no longer are free of pain. The involved joints become persistently uncomfortable and swollen, although the intensity of these symptoms is much less than during acute flares. Gouty attacks continue to occur against this painful background, and without therapy, they may recur as often as every few weeks. The amount of background pain also steadily increases with time if appropriate intervention is not started

(see Figure 12A-2). Clinically evident tophi may or may not be detected on physical examination during the first few years of this stage of gout. However, periarticular tophi detected by magnetic resonance imaging (MRI) (6) and synovial "microtophi" discovered through the arthroscope certainly are present early in this stage of gout and may in fact be present during the earlier acute intermittent phase of gout. Polyarticular involvement becomes much more frequent during this time. With diffuse and symmetric involvement of small joints in the hands and feet, chronic tophaceous gout can occasionally be confused with the symmetrical polyarthritis of rheumatoid arthritis.

The development of tophaceous deposits of MSU is a function of the duration and severity of hyperuricemia (7). Hench found that untreated patients developed tophi 11.7 years after the onset of acute gout, on average (8). In a study of 1165 people with primary gout, those without tophi had serum uric acid levels of 10.3 ± 1.3 mg/dL and those with extensive deposits had levels of 11.0 ± 2.0 mg/dL. Other factors associated with the development of tophi include early age of gout onset, long periods of active but untreated gout, an average of four attacks per year, and a greater tendency toward upper extremity and polyarticular episodes (9). In untreated patients, the interval from the first gouty attack to the beginning of advanced arthritis or the development of visible tophi is highly variable, ranging from 3 to 42 years, with an average of 11.6 years (10).

The subcutaneous tophus is the most characteristic lesion of advanced gout (Figure 12A-3). Tophi may be found anywhere over the body, but occur most commonly in the fingers, wrists, ears, knees, olecranon bursa, and such pressure points as the ulnar aspect of the forearm and the Achilles tendon. In people with nodal osteoarthritis, tophi have a propensity for forming in Heberden's nodes. Tophi also may occur in connective tissues at other sites, such as renal pyramids, heart valves, and sclerae. Similar appearing nodules are observed in other rheumatic conditions, such as rheumatoid arthritis and multicentric reticulohistiocytosis (11,12). Before antihyperuricemic agents were available, as many as 50% of patients with gout eventually developed clinical or radiographic evidence of tophi. Since the introduction of allopurinol and the uricosuric agents, the incidence of tophaceous gout has declined.

Much of the knowledge about sequential development of the mature, multilobulated gouty tophus comes from the classic histopathologic descriptions of Sokoloff (13) and Schumacher (14), and the more recent immunohistochemical studies of Palmer and colleagues (15). Figure 12A-4 represents a theoretical sequence of how a noncrystalline, cellular locus (macrophage acinus) progresses through stages of crystal precipitation, coronal hypertrophy, and finally, crystal coalescence and cellular atrophy, to eventually form the clinically

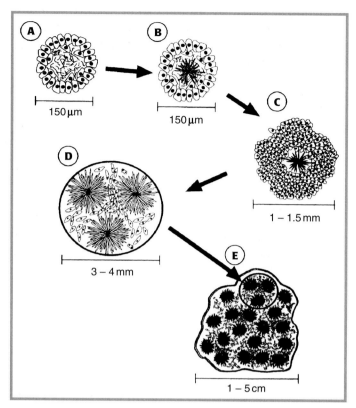

FIGURE 12A-4

The stages of development of a gouty tophus. (A) The crystal-free macrophage acinus is the earliest organized phase of a gouty tophus. (B) The amorphous center of the acinus fosters urate crystal formation. (C) As the crystalline mass expands, the surrounding corona of macrophages likewise undergoes hypertrophy. (D) Further crystallization results in a thinning of the corona until only fibrous septae separate one nidus of crystal formation from another. (E) A fully mature tophus.

observable subcutaneous tophus (7). The macrophage acinus (Figure 12A-4A) is the earliest structure observed by light microscopy in tophus development. The acinus has a core of noncrystalline, amorphous material surrounded by a rosette of mononuclear phagocytes. The

central amorphous material is believed to be detritus from a collection of monocytes that conjugates at the locus in response to some inciting event.

Some time after the acinus is formed, a small, eccentric collection of radially arranged MSU crystals form in the amorphous core of monocyte-derived material [Figure 12A-4(B)]. The macrophages do not phagocytize the MSU crystal, but as the crystalline mass expands and contacts the surrounding cells, this shell that is 1- to 2-cells thick proliferates to form a tightly packed, 8- to 10-cell-thick corona [Figure 12A-4(C)]. As the tophus matures, this corona is lost and replaced by fibrous septae [Figure 12A-4(D)] that contain some fibroblastic cells and occasional multinucleated giant cells. Adjacent crystalline deposits coalesce to form multilobulated tophi [Figure 12A-4(E)] measuring 1 to 10cm in diameter, interlaced with fibrous strands containing few cells and encapsulated by a sometimes tenuous and sometimes thick fibrous tissue. The cellular and crystalline components of a gouty tophus are easily demonstrated by magnetic resonance imaging (Figure 12A-5).

UNUSUAL PRESENTATIONS

Early-Onset Gout

Between 3% and 6% of patients with gout have symptom onset before age 25. Early-onset gout represents a special subset of cases that generally have a genetic component, show a more accelerated clinical course, and require more aggressive antihyperuricemic therapy. In large epidemiologic studies of classic gout, a family history of gout and/or nephrolithiasis is present in 25% to 30% of cases. In early-onset gout, the incidence of family history is approximately 80%. In this younger group, detailed questioning about the kindred over several generations may yield enough information to suggest a mode of inheritance (X-linked or autosomal dominant or recessive).

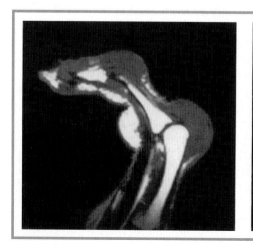
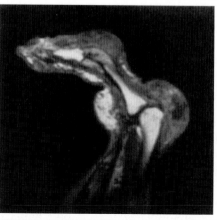

FIGURE 12A-5

(Left) Midline sagittal section magnetic resonance image of a finger with advanced tophaceous deformities. (Right) T1 weighted, spin echo technique with gadolinium contrast reveals the deep soft tissue anatomy. The heterogeneous composition of the tophus dorsal to the proximal interphalageal joint and distal phalanx is clearly revealed. The central crystalline deposit remains low intensity, but surrounding tissue enhances.

Like classic gout, early-onset gout may be caused by overproduction of urate or reduced renal clearance of uric acid. Diseases associated with overproduction of urate in children and young adults include enzymatic defects in the purine pathway, glycogen storage diseases, and hematologic disorders, such as hemoglobinopathies and leukemias. The complete deficiency of hypoxanthine-guanine phosphoribosyltransferase (HGPRT) is an X-linked inherited inborn error of purine metabolism with a characteristic clinical presentation known as the Lesch–Nyhan syndrome. These boys, who have severe neurologic abnormalities, develop gout and kidney stones in the first decade of life if not treated early with allopurinol. The partial deficiency of HGPRT (the Kelley–Seegmiller syndrome) results in early-onset gout or uric acid nephrolithiasis and also is also an X-linked trait. People with this syndrome have minor or no neurologic problems.

Glycogen storage disease types I, III, V, and VII, inherited as autosomal recessive diseases, are associated with early-onset gout. Sickle cell disease, beta-thalassemia, and nonlymphocytic leukemias may be complicated by gouty arthritis in the young adult years.

Conditions associated with uric acid underexcretion in young patients include a specific renal tubular disorder known as familial juvenile hyperuricemic nephropathy (16). This autosomal dominant disorder causes hyperuricemia from a very young age, before any evidence of renal insufficiency. The condition may lead to progressive renal failure and end-stage kidney disease by age 40. Other nephropathies associated with early-onset gout include polycystic kidney disease, chronic lead intoxication, medullary cystic disease, and focal tubulointerstitial disease.

Gout in Organ Transplantation Patients

Hyperuricemia develops in 75% to 80% of heart transplant recipients who routinely take cyclosporine to prevent allograft rejection (17). A slightly lower frequency (approximately 50%) of kidney and liver transplant recipients develop hyperuricemia, presumably because lower doses of cyclosporine are used in these individuals. Whereas asymptomatic hyperuricemia progresses to clinical gout in only 1 in 30 subjects in the general population, cyclosporine-induced hyperuricemia leads to gout in 1 in every 6 patients (18). Other differences between primary and cyclosporine-induced gout include the marked shortening of the asymptomatic hyperuricemia and acute intermittent gout stages, with the rapid appearance of tophi. The stage of asymptomatic hyperuricemia lasts for 20 to 30 years in classic gout, but is present for only 6 months to 4 years in cyclosporine-induced disease. Similarly, the duration of the acute intermittent stage is only 1 to 4 years in transplant recipients, but it may last 8 to 15 years in classic gout. Because organ transplant recipients use other medications, such as systemic corticosteroids and azathioprine, their gouty symptoms frequently are more atypical and less dramatic than those of patients with classic gout.

Gout in Women

Unlike most other rheumatic conditions, gout is less common in women than in men. In most large reviews, women account for no more than 5% of all people with gout (19). Ninety percent of women are postmenopausal at the time of their initial attack. Postmenopausal gout is similar clinically in presentation and course to classic gout, except that the age of onset is later in women than in men. Conditions that are much more commonly associated with gout in postmenopausal women than with gout in men include diuretic use (95%), hypertension (73%), renal insufficiency (50%), and preexisting joint disease, such as osteoarthritis (20).

Premenopausal gout has a strong hereditary component. Most women who develop gout before menopause have hypertension and renal insufficiency. The rare woman with premenopausal gout and normal renal function should be evaluated for the autosomally inherited familial juvenile hyperuricemic nephropathy (16) or the even more rare non–X-linked inborn errors of purine metabolism (20).

Normouricemic Gout

The most frequent explanations for apparent gout with normal levels of uric acid are that (1) gout is not the correct diagnosis or (2) the patient actually is chronically hyperuricemic but the serum urate is normal at the time it is measured (for a potential explanation of this phenomenon, see below).

Several articular conditions can mimic gout closely, including crystalline arthropathies of calcium pyrophosphate dehydrate (pseudogout), basic calcium (apatite), and liquid lipid (21). Other causes of acute monoarthropathies, such as infection, sarcoidosis, and trauma, also should be considered (22). The clinical suspicions of gout should be confirmed by crystal analysis of synovial fluid. Without this confirmation, the diagnosis remains in question.

Misunderstanding the definition of hyperuricemia also can contribute to misdiagnosis of normouricemic gout. A sustained serum urate level above 7.0 mg/dL provides a permissive environment for MSU crystal formation, but people with acute and chronic gout may have urate values below this biochemical definition of hyperuricemia. In fact, as many as one third of people presenting with acute gout to have a serum urate below

12

7.0 mg/dL during the episode of severe pain (23). This condition probably results from uricosuric effects of ACTH release and adrenal stimulation, which are caused by the stress of the painful process. Normalization of serum urate values during acute gouty flares may be more common in alcoholics than in nondrinkers. Aside from such standard urate-lowering agents as allopurinol, probenecid, and sulfinpyrazone, high dose salicylates, angiotensin II receptor blockers, fenofibrate, glucocorticoids, warfarin, glycerol guaiacholate, and x-ray contrast agents also may lower serum urate values in people with gout and lead to the false impression of normouricemic gout.

Yu reported that 1.6% of 2145 gout patients had sustained normouricemia months after discontinuing use of allopurinol or uricosuric agents (24). In most of these cases, hyperuricemia eventually returned, although several patients with very mild gouty symptoms remained normouricemic over a prolonged period.

PROVOCATIVE FACTORS OF ACUTE ATTACKS

Why crystals form in some hyperuricemic fluids and not in others is unclear. When synovial fluids are balanced for urate concentrations, the fluids from gouty patients have a far greater propensity for promoting crystal formation than similar fluids from people with osteoarthritis or rheumatoid arthritis. A number of synovial fluid proteins have been reported to function as promoters or inhibitors of crystal nucleation. The current list of physiologically important nucleators is short, with the leading contenders being type I collagen and a gamma globulin subfraction (10).

The degree of hyperuricemia correlates positively with the overall risk of acquiring gout. However, rapid increases or decreases in the concentration of synovial fluid urate are related more closely to actual precipitation of the acute gouty attack. A rapid flux in urate level is a triggering mechanism in gout induced by trauma, alcohol ingestion, and drugs.

Trauma frequently is reported to be an inciting event for acute gouty episodes. The trauma may be as minor as a long walk and may not have caused pain during the activity, but it caused intra-articular swelling. When the joint is allowed to rest, there is a relatively rapid efflux of free water from the joint fluid. This results in a sudden increase in synovial fluid urate concentration, which may allow precipitation of urate crystals and a gout attack. This mechanism may explain why gouty attacks commonly occur at night.

Alcohol ingestion may predispose to gout through several mechanisms. The consumption of lead-tainted moonshine results in chronic renal tubular damage that leads to secondary hyperuricemia and saturnine gout (the word *saturnine*, meaning of or relating to lead, is derived from the belief of the ancients that this metal comprised the planet Saturn). The ingestion of any form of ethanol can raise uric acid production acutely by accelerating the breakdown of intracellular adenosine triphosphate (25). Beer consumption has an added impact on gout because it contains large quantities of guanosine, which is catabolized to uric acid (26).

Drugs may precipitate gout by rapidly raising or lowering urate levels. Thiazide diuretics selectively interfere with urate excretion at the proximal convoluted tubule. Low dose aspirin (less than 2 g/day) also can raise serum urate levels, but higher doses have a uricosuric effect and may lower the serum urate concentration. A rapid increase or reduction in the serum urate level can provoke gouty attacks; allopurinol is the drug most often responsible for this effect. The mechanism for this paradoxic response appears to be the destabilizing of microtophi in the gouty synovium when the urate concentration of the synovial fluid is changed rapidly. As the microtophi break apart, crystals are shed into the synovial fluid and the gouty episode is initiated (27).

CLINICAL ASSOCIATIONS

Renal Disease

The only consistent visceral damage caused by hyperuricemia is its effect on the kidneys. Three forms of hyperuricemia-induced renal disease are recognized, including (1) chronic urate nephropathy, (2) acute uric acid nephropathy, and (3) uric acid nephrolithiasis.

Chronic urate nephropathy is a distinct entity caused by deposition of MSU crystals in the real medulla and pyramids and is associated with mild albuminuria. Although chronic hyperuricemia is thought to be the cause of urate nephropathy, this form of kidney involvement is essentially never seen in the absence of gouty arthritis. Progressive renal failure is common in people with gout, but the attribution of renal failure to chronic urate nephropathy itself is often difficult owing to the frequent confluence of multiple comorbid conditions in patients with gout. As described in further detail below, the hypertension, diabetes, obesity, and ischemic heart disease that often accompany gout are also risk factors for renal dysfunction. To a large extent, the role of hyperuricemia as a single factor in chronic parenchymal disease of the kidney remains controversial. Other chronic effects of hyperuricemia on the kidney may not be caused by crystal deposition but rather by the direct action of the soluble uric acid molecule on the afferent arteriolar vessels of glomeruli (28).

Acute renal failure can be caused by hyperuricemia in the acute tumor lysis syndrome, which occurs in patients given chemotherapy for rapidly proliferating lymphomas and leukemias. With massive liberation of purines during cell lysis, uric acid precipitates in the distal tubules and collecting ducts of the kidney. Acute uric acid nephropathy can result in oliguria or anuria. This form of acute renal failure can be distinguished from other forms by a ratio of uric acid to creatinine greater than 1.0 in a random or 24-hour urine collection.

Uric acid renal stones occur in 10% to 25% of all people with gout. The incidence correlates strongly with the serum urate level, and the likelihood of developing stones reaches 50% when the serum urate is above 13 mg/dL. Symptoms of renal stones precede the development of gout in 40% of patients. Calcium-containing renal stones occur 10 times more frequently in gouty subjects than in the general population.

Hypertension

Hypertension is present in 25% to 50% of people with gout, and 2% to 14% of people with hypertension have gout. Because serum urate concentration correlates directly with peripheral and renal vascular resistance, reduced renal blood flow may account for the association between hypertension and hyperuricemia. Factors such as obesity and male gender also link hypertension and hyperuricemia (29,30).

Obesity

Hyperuricemia and gout correlate highly with body weight for both men and women, and individuals with gout commonly are overweight, compared with the general population. Obesity may be a factor linking hyperuricemia, hypertension, hyperlipidemia, and atherosclerosis.

Hyperlipidemia

Serum triglycerides are elevated in 80% of people with gout. The association between hyperuricemia and serum cholesterol is controversial, although serum levels of high density lipoprotein generally are decreased in patients with gout. These abnormalities of serum lipids likely reflect overindulgence rather than a genetic link.

RADIOGRAPHIC FEATURES

The radiographic findings of gout often are unremarkable early in the disease course. In acute gouty arthritis, the only finding may be soft tissue swelling around the affected joint. In most instances, bone and joint abnormalities develop only after many years of disease and are indicative of the deposition of urate crystals. Most frequently, the abnormalities are asymmetric and seen in the feet, hands, wrists, elbows, and knees.

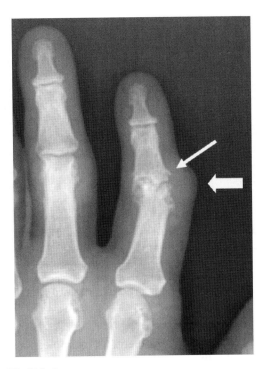

FIGURE 12A-6

Radiographic changes of advanced gout include the typical gouty erosions with overhanging edge (*white arrows*) and soft tissue swellings of gouty tophi.

The bony erosions of gout are radiographically distinct from the erosive changes of other inflammatory arthritides. Gouty erosions usually are slightly removed from the joint, but rheumatoid erosions typically are in the immediate proximity of the articular surface (Figure 12A-6). The characteristic gouty erosion has features that are both atrophic and hypertrophic, leading to erosions with an overhanging edge. The joint space is preserved in gout until very late in the disease process. Juxta-articular osteopenia, a common and early finding in rheumatoid arthritis, is absent or minimal in gout.

LABORATORY FEATURES AND DIAGNOSIS

An elevated serum urate level has long been considered a cornerstone in the diagnosis of gout. In reality, this laboratory finding is of limited value in establishing the diagnosis. The vast majority of hyperuricemic subjects will not develop gout, and serum urate levels may be normal during gouty attacks (31). Far too many patients are diagnosed with gout based on the clinical triad of an acute monoarthritis, hyperuricemia, and a dramatic improvement of articular symptoms in response to treatment. A diagnosis by these parameters is presumptive only, and the physician should remain alert to other possibilities.

Gout
B. Epidemiology, Pathology, and Pathogenesis

Hyon K. Choi, MD, MPH, DrPH, FRCPC

- The prevalence of gout, which occurs predominantly among men and postmenopausal women, is approximately 2.7%.
- The incidence of primary gout has doubled over the past 20 years in both sexes.
- Gout prevalence rises with advancing age, reaching a level of 9% in men older than 80 years of age, and 6% in women.
- There appears to be a higher prevalence of gout among individuals of lower family income levels, likely reflecting a greater number of risk factors for gout—for example, obesity, hypertension, and a Western dietary pattern with a greater red meat component.
- Two major genetic mutations are known to result in gout, urolithiasis, and other disturbances: Mutations in the 5′-phosphoribosyl 1-pyrophosphate (PRPP)

synthetase genes can result in overactivity of the pathway, leading to increased rate of PRPP, purine nucleotide, and urate production. Mutations in the gene encoding hypoxanthine-guanine phosphoribosyl transferase (HPRT) are associated with a spectrum of disease in children that ranges from hyperuricemia alone to hyperuricemia with profound neurological and behavioral dysfunction (Lesch–Nyhan syndrome).

- Ethanol administration increases uric acid production by net adenosine triphosphate (ATP) degradation to adenosine monophosphate (AMP), which is rapidly degraded to uric acid, leading to hyperuricemia. Alcohol consumption, uric acid levels, and risk of gout have a strong dose–effect relationship.

Gout is a form of inflammatory arthritis triggered by the crystallization of uric acid within the joints (1). Acute gout, characteristically intermittent, is one of the most painful conditions experienced by humans. Chronic tophaceous gout develops usually after years of acute intermittent gout. Beyond the morbidity associated with gout itself, the disease is associated with important medical conditions including the insulin resistance syndrome, hypertension, nephropathy, alcohol abuse, and disorders associated with increased cell turnover. Gout is often associated with hyperuricemia.

EPIDEMIOLOGY

Gout occurs predominantly among men and postmenopausal women. The disease rarely occurs in men before adolescence or in women before menopause. According to the Third National Health and Nutrition Examination Survey (1988–1994), the prevalence of self-reported, physician-diagnosed gout among US adults is approxi-

mately 2.7%. The prevalence rises with advancing age, reaching a level of 9% in men older than 80 years of age, and 6% in women.

Serum urate concentrations in men are about 1 mg/dL higher on average than in women (2), but after menopause the serum levels of uric acid in women tend to approach those in men. The sex differences in uric acid levels may stem from the effects of estrogen on the renal tubular handling of uric acid; premenopausal levels of estrogens in women may promote more efficient renal clearance of urate (2). The prevalence appears to be higher among African Americans than among Caucasians, possibly reflecting the increased prevalence of hypertension among African Americans (3). Once termed *the patrician malady*, gout has been considered a disease of the affluent, primarily observed in middle-aged men of wealthy status. Recent epidemiologic data, however, suggest a higher prevalence of gout among individuals of lower family income levels, likely reflecting a greater number of risk factors for gout—for example, obesity, hypertension, and a Western dietary pattern with a greater red meat component—in lower socioeconomic classes.

The incidence of primary gout, defined as the occurrence of this disease in the absence of a clear cause (e.g., the Lesch–Nyhan syndrome or diuretic use) has doubled over the past 20 years in both sexes (4). Diet and lifestyle trends, increasing frequencies of obesity, metabolic syndrome, hypertension, organ transplantation, and increasing use of certain medications (e.g., low dose salicylate and diuretics) may explain the increasing incidence of gout.

PATHOGENESIS OF HYPERURICEMIA AND GOUT

Humans are the only mammals who are known to develop gout spontaneously, probably because hyperuricemia only commonly develops in humans (1). In most fish, amphibians, and nonprimate mammals, uric acid generated from purine metabolism undergoes oxidative degradation via the uricase enzyme, producing the more soluble compound allantoin. In humans, the uricase gene is crippled by two mutations that introduce premature stop codons (1). The absence of uricase, combined with extensive reabsorption of filtered urate, results in urate levels in human plasma that are approximately 10 times than those of most other mammals (0.5–1.0 mg/dL). Urate's role as the primary antioxidant in human blood may account for its evolutionary advantage (1).

Solubility of Urate

Uric acid is a weak acid (pKa = 5.8) that exists largely as urate, the ionized form, at physiological pH. In general, the risk of supersaturation and crystal formation rises in parallel with the concentration of urate in physiologic fluids. Population studies indicate a direct correlation between serum urate levels and risk of future gout (5). Conversely, lowering uric acid levels is associated with a substantially lower risk of recurrent gout, confirming the causal relation between uric acid levels and risk of gouty arthritis (6). The solubility of urate in joint fluids is influenced by other factors as well, however, including temperature, pH, cation concentration, articular hydration state, and the presence of nucleating agents around which urate crystals may coalesce (e.g., nonaggregated proteoglycans, insoluble collagens, and chondroitin sulfate).

Variation in these factors may account for some of the difference in the risk for gout associated with a given elevation in urate level. Moreover, these risk factors may explain several of the interesting clinical features of gout: (1) predilection for the first metatarsophalangeal joint, that is, podagra (caused by the lower temperature at this peripheral body site); (2) tendency

to occur in osteoarthritic joints (because such joints contain nucleating debris); and (3) the frequency of nocturnal onset (the result of intra-articular dehydration that may occur at night) (1).

Urate Metabolism

The amount of urate in the body depends on the balance between dietary intake, synthesis, and excretion of this molecule. Hyperuricemia results from the overproduction of urate (10%), underexcretion of urate (90%), or often a combination of the two. The purine precursors come from exogenous (dietary) sources or endogenous metabolism (synthesis and cell turnover).

The dietary intake of purines makes a substantial contribution to the blood uric acid. For example, substitution of an entirely purine-free formula diet over a period of days can reduce blood uric acid of healthy men from an average of 5.0 mg/dL to 3.0 mg/dL (1). The bioavailable purine content of particular foods depends on their relative cellularity as well as the transcriptional and metabolic activity of their cellular content. Little is known, however, about the precise identity and quantity of individual purines in most foods, especially when cooked or processed (1,7). Ingested purine precursors go though steps in digestion, including (1) the breakdown of nucleic acids into nucleotides by pancreatic nucleases; (2) breakdown of oligonucleotides into simple nucleotides by phosphodiesterases; and (3) removal of phosphate and sugar groups from nucleotides by pancreatic and mucosal enzymes. The addition of dietary purines to purine-free dietary protocols has revealed a variable increase in blood uric acid, depending on the formulation and dose of purines administered (1,7). For example, RNA has a greater effect than an equivalent amount of DNA; ribomononucleotides a greater effect than nucleic acid; and adenine a greater effect than guanine.

A large prospective study showed that men in the highest quintile of meat intake had a 41% higher risk of gout compared with those in the lowest quintile, and that men in the highest quintile of seafood intake had a 51% higher risk compared with those in the lowest quintile (7). In a representative sample of US men and women, higher levels of meat and seafood consumption were associated with higher serum uric acid levels. The variation in the risk of gout associated with different purine-rich foods may be explained by varying amounts and type of purine content and their bioavailability for purine to uric acid metabolism. At the practical level, these data suggest that dietary purine restriction in patients with gout or hyperuricemia (8) may be applicable to purines of animal origin but not to purine-rich vegetables, which are excellent sources of protein, fiber, vitamins, and minerals. Similarly, implications of these findings for dietary recommendation for patients with

FIGURE 12B-1

Dietary influences on the risk for gout and their implications within a Healthy Eating Pyramid. Data on the relationship between diet and the risk for gout are primarily derived from the recent Health Professionals Follow-Up Study. Upward solid arrows denote an increased risk for gout, downward solid arrows denote a decreased risk, and horizontal arrows denote no influence on risk. Broken arrows denote potential effect but without prospective evidence for the outcome of gout. (Adapted from Choi HK, et al. Ann Intern Med 2005;143:499–516, with permission from *Annals of Internal Medicine*.)

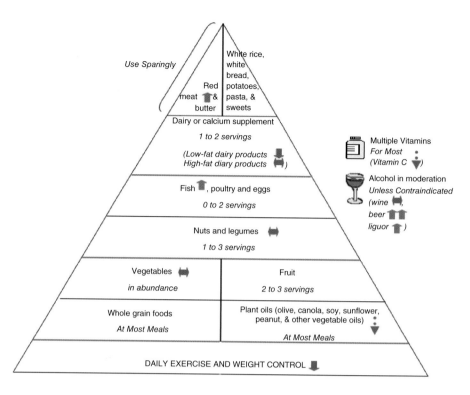

hyperuricemia or gout are generally consistent with a new Healthy Eating Pyramid, except for fish intake (Figure 12B-1) (1). The use of plant-derived omega-3 fatty acids or supplements of eicosapentaenoic acid and docosahexaenoic acid in place of fish consumption could be considered to provide the benefit of these fatty acids without increasing the risk of gout.

Urate Production Pathways and Inborn Errors of Metabolism

The steps in the urate production pathways implicated in the pathogenesis of hyperuricemia and gout are displayed in Figure 12B-2. The vast majority of patients with endogenous overproduction of urate have the condition as a result of *salvaged* purines arising from increased cell turnover in proliferative and inflammatory disorders (e.g., hematologic malignancies and psoriasis); pharmacologic intervention resulting in increased urate production (e.g., chemotherapy); or tissue hypoxia. Only a small fraction of those with urate overproduction (10%) have an inborn error of metabolism such as superactivity of 5′-phosphoribosyl 1-pyrophosphate (PRPP) synthetase or deficiency of hypoxanthine-guanine phosphoribosyl transferase (HPRT; Figure 12B-2) (2,7,9).

Mutations in the PRPP synthetase genes can result in overactivity of the pathway. Superactivity of PRPP synthetase leads to increased rate of PRPP, purine nucleotide, and urate production, in association with gout and urate urolithiasis. Mutations in the gene encod-

ing HPRT are associated with a spectrum of disease that ranges from hyperuricemia alone to hyperuricemia with profound neurological and behavioral dysfunction (Lesch–Nyhan syndrome) (2,7,9) Hypoxanthine cannot be reutilized without HPRT, and can only be degraded to urate. Both the underutilization of PRPP and decrease in inosine monophosphate and guanosine monophosphate levels in the salvage pathway contribute to hyperuricemia by feedback inhibition on de novo purine synthesis (Figure 12B-2) (2,7,9). Because both of these enzyme defects are X-linked traits, homozygous males are affected. In addition, postmenopausal gout and urinary tract stones can occur in carrier females. Hyperuricemia in prepubertal boys always suggests one of these enzymatic defects (2).

Alcohol and Gout

Conditions associated with net adenosine triphosphate (ATP) degradation lead to accumulation of adenosine diphosphate (ADP) and adenosine monophosphate (AMP), which can be rapidly degraded to uric acid, leading to hyperuricemia (Figure 12B-2, Table 12B-1). Examples of this include acute, severe illnesses such as the adult respiratory distress syndrome, myocardial infarction, or status epilepticus, in which tissue hypoxia impairs the mitochondrial synthesis of ATP from ADP. Another example relates to alcohol consumption. Ethanol administration increases uric acid production by net ATP degradation to AMP. Decreased urinary excretion associated with dehydration and metabolic

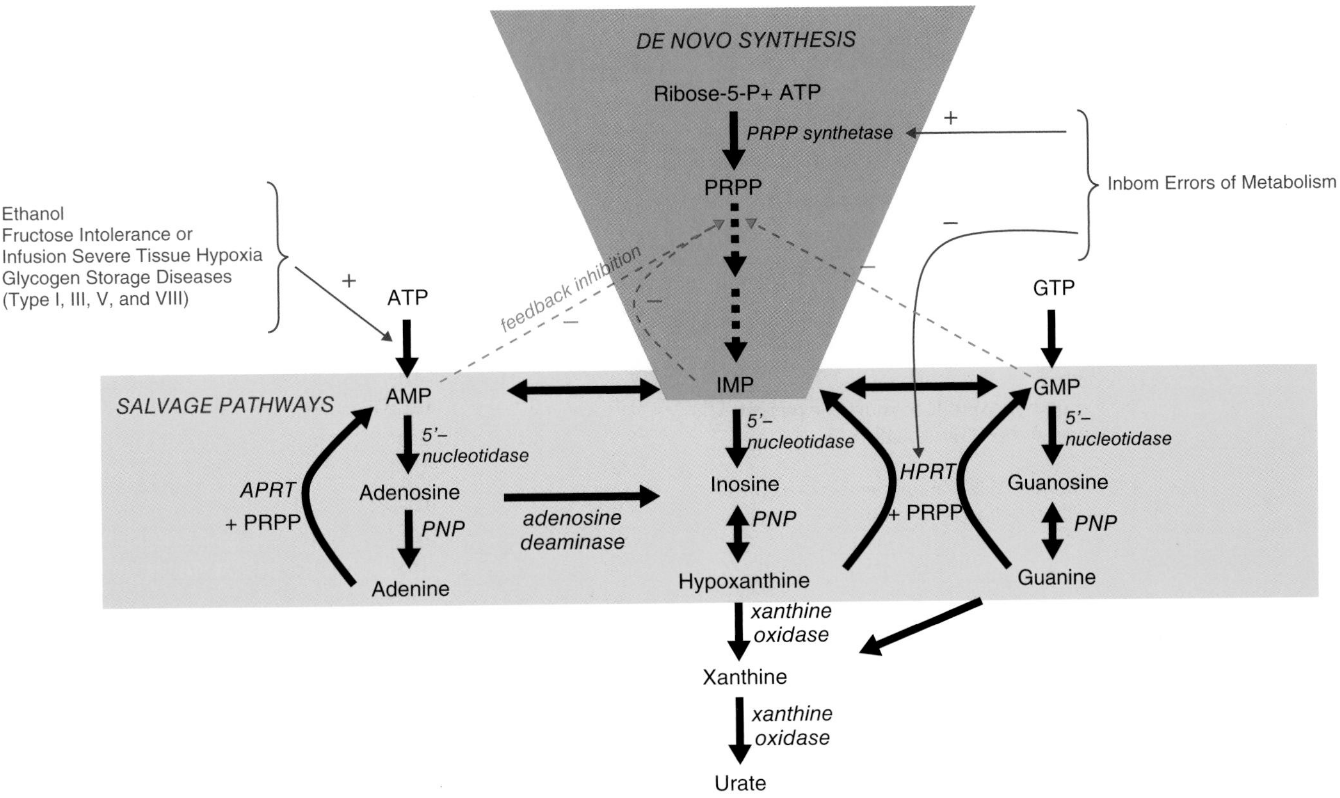

FIGURE 12B-2

Urate production pathways implicated in the pathogenesis of hyperuricemia and gout. The de novo synthesis starts with 5′-phosphoribosyl 1-pyrophosphate (PRPP), which is produced by addition of a further phosphate group from adenosine triphosphate (ATP) to the modified sugar ribose-5-phosphate. This step is performed by the family of PRPP synthetase (PRS) enzymes. In addition, purine bases derived from tissue nucleic acids are reutilized through the salvage pathway. The enzyme hypoxanthine-guanine phosphoribosyl transferase (HPRT) salvages hypoxanthine to inosine monophosphate (IMP) and guanine to guanosine monophosphate (GMP). Only a small proportion of patients with urate overproduction have the well-characterized inborn errors of metabolism, such as superactivity of PRS and deficiency of HPRT. Furthermore, conditions associated with net ATP degradation lead to the accumulation of adenosine diphosphate (ADP) and adenosine monophosphate (AMP), which can be rapidly degraded to uric acid. These conditions are displayed in left upper corner. Plus sign denotes stimulation, and minus sign denotes inhibition. Abbreviations: APRT, adenine phosphoribosyl transferase; PNP, purine nucleotide phosphorylase. (Adapted from Choi HK, et al. Ann Intern Med 2005;143:499–516, with permission from *Annals of Internal Medicine*.)

acidosis also may contribute to the hyperuricemia associated with ethanol ingestion. A prospective study confirmed the dose–response relationships between ethanol consumption, uric acid levels, and risk of gout (9).

The same study found that the risk of gout varies according to type of alcoholic beverage: beer confers a larger risk than liquor, whereas moderate wine drinking did not increase the risk (9). These findings suggest that certain nonalcoholic components within alcoholic beverages play an important role in urate metabolism. The effect of purines ingested from beer on blood uric acid may be sufficient to augment the hyperuricemic effect of alcohol itself, producing a greater risk of gout than liquor or wine (9).

Adiposity, Insulin Resistance, and Hyperuricemia

An increased adiposity and the insulin resistance syndrome are both closely associated with hyperuricemia (10). Whereas body mass index, waist-to-hip ratio, and weight gain are all associated with gout in men (11), weight reduction is associated with a decline in urate levels and risk of gout. Weight reduction leads to lower de novo purine synthesis and lower serum urate levels. Exogenous insulin can reduce the renal excretion of urate in both healthy and hypertensive subjects, thus providing an additional link between adiposity, insulin resistance, type II diabetes, and gout. Insulin may

12

TABLE 12B-1. CAUSES OF HYPERURICEMIA AND URATE-LOWERING AGENTS.

Causes of hyperuricemia

Uric acid overproduction
  Inherited enzyme defects
    HGRT deficiency, PRPP synthetase overactivity
  Increased cell turnover
Myeloproliferative and lymphoproliferative disorders,
    polycythemia vera, malignant diseases, hemolytic diseases,
    psoriasis
  Purine-rich foods
  Obesity
  Accelerated ATP degradation
Ethanol, fructose, severe tissue hypoxemia or muscle exertion,
    glycogen storage diseases (types I, III, V, and VII)
  Urate Increasing Agents
Cytotoxic drugs, warfarin, vitamin B12 (patients with pernicious
    anemia), ethylamino-1,3,4-thiadiazole, 4-amino-5-imidazole
    carboxamide riboside

Uric acid underexcretion
  Clinical disorders associated with uric acid underexcretion
Renal failure, hypertension, metabolic syndrome, obesity
  Certain nephropathy
Lead nephropathy, polycystic kidney disease, medullary cystic
    kidney disease, familial juvenile hyperuricemic nephropathy
  Agents increasing urate reabsorption through trans-stimulation
    of URAT1
Pyrazinamide, salicylate (low dose), nicotinate, lactate, beta-
    hydroxybutyrate, acetoacetate
  Agents decreasing renal urate excretion, maybe through
    URAT1 or other mechanisms
Diuretics, ethambutol, insulin, beta-blockers

Urate Lowering Agents
  Inhibition of xanthine oxidase
Allopurinol, febuxostat
  Uricase
  Agents decreasing urate reabsorption through direct inhibition
    of URAT1
Probenecid, sulfinpyrazone, benzbromarone, losartan, salicylate
    (high dose)
  Uricosuric agents, maybe through inhibition of URAT1 or other
    mechanisms
Amlodipine, fenofibrate, vitamin C, estrogen, angiotensin II,
    parathyroid hormone

ABBREVIATIONS: ATP, adenosine triphosphate; HGRT, hypoxanthine-guanine phosphoribosyl transferase; PRPP, 5′-phosphoribosyl 1-pyrophosphate; URAT1, urate transporter-1.

enhance renal urate reabsorption via stimulation of urate–anion exchanger URAT1 (12) and/or the Na$^+$-dependent anion cotransporter in brush border membranes of the renal proximal tubule. Some investigators have suggested that leptin and increased adenosine levels may contribute to hyperuricemia. The epidemic of obesity and the insulin resistance syndrome thus presents a substantial challenge in the prevention and management of gout.

RENAL TRANSPORT OF URATE

Renal urate transport follows a four-component model: (1) glomerular filtration, (2) nearly complete reabsorption of the filtered urate, (3) subsequent secretion, and (4) postsecretory reabsorption in the remaining proximal tubule (1). The molecular target for uricosuric agents, an anion exchanger responsible for the reabsorption of filtered urate by the renal proximal tubule, was identified recently (1,11). The authors searched the human genome database for novel gene sequences within the organic anion transporter (OAT) gene family and identified URAT1 (SLC22A12), a novel transporter expressed at the apical brush border of the proximal nephron (11). Urate–anion exchange activity similar to that of URAT1, initially described in brush border membrane vesicles (BBMV) from urate-reabsorbing species such as rats and dogs, was subsequently confirmed in human kidneys (1). *Xenopus* oocytes injected with URAT1-encoding RNA transport urate and exhibit pharmacological properties consistent with data from human BBMV (11). These and other experiments indicate that uricosuric compounds (e.g., probenecid, benzbromarone, sulfinpyrazone, and losartan) directly inhibit URAT1 from the apical side of tubular cells (cis-inhibition). In contrast, anti-uricosuric substances (e.g., pyrazinoate, nicotinate, lactate, pyruvate, beta-hydroxybutyrate, and acetoacetate) serve as the exchanging anion from inside cells, thereby stimulating anion exchange and urate reabsorption (trans-stimulation) (Table 12B-1).

Urate transporter-1 is crucial for urate homeostasis: a handful of patients with renal hypouricemia were shown to carry loss-of-function mutations in the human *SLC22A12* gene encoding URAT1, indicating that this exchanger is essential for the proximal tubular reabsorption (12). Furthermore, pyrazinamide, benzbromarone, and probenecid failed to affect urate clearance in subjects with homozygous loss-of-function mutations in *SLC22A12*, indicating that URAT1 is essential for the effect of both anti-uricosuric and uricosuric agents.

Anti-uricosuric agents exert their effect by stimulating renal reabsorption rather than inhibiting tubular secretion (1). The mechanism appears to involve a priming of renal urate reabsorption, via the Na$^+$-dependent loading of proximal tubular epithelial cells with anions capable of a trans-stimulation of urate reabsorption. A transporter in the proximal tubule brush border mediates Na$^+$-dependent reabsorption of pyrazinoate, nicotinate, lactate, pyruvate, beta-hydroxybutyrate, and acetoacetate, all of which are monovalent anions that are also substrates for URAT1 (1). Increased plasma concentrations of these antiuricosuric anions result in their increased glomerular filtration and greater reabsorption by the proximal tubule. The augmented intra-epithelial concentrations, in turn, induce the reabsorption of urate by promoting the URAT1-dependent anion exchange of filtered urate (trans-stimulation).

Urate reabsorption by the proximal tubule thus exhibits a form of *secondary* Na^+ dependency, in that Na^+-dependent loading of proximal tubular cells stimulates brush border urate exchange. Urate itself is not a substrate for the Na^+–anion transporter. The molecular identity of the relevant Na^+-dependent anion cotransporter(s) remains unclear. However, a leading candidate gene is *SLC5A8*, which encodes a Na^+-dependent lactate and butyrate cotransporter (1). The SLC5A8 protein may also transport both pyrazinoate and nicotinate, potentiating urate transport in *Xenopus* oocytes that co-express URAT1 (1).

The anti-uricosuric mechanism explains the long-standing clinical observations that hyperuricemia is induced by increases in beta-hydroxybutyrate and acetoacetate in diabetic ketoacidosis, lactic acid in alcohol intoxication, or nicotinate and pyrazinoate in niacin and pyrazinamide therapy, respectively (Table 12B-1). Urate retention is provoked also by a reduction in extracellular fluid volume and by excesses of angiotensin II, insulin, and parathyroid hormone. URAT1 and the Na^+-dependent anion cotransporter(s) may be targets for these stimuli (Table 12B-1).

Certain anions that interact with URAT1 have the dual potential to either increase or decrease renal urate excretion, through either trans-stimulation or cis-inhibition of apical urate exchange in the proximal tubule (1). For example, a low concentration of pyrazinoate stimulates urate reabsorption through trans-stimulation. A higher concentration, in contrast, reduces urate reabsorption via extracellular cis-inhibition of URAT1. Biphasic effects on urate excretion, that is, anti-uricosuria at low dose and uricosuria at high dose, are also well described for salicylate (1). Salicylate cis-inhibits URAT1, explaining the high dose uricosuric effect; low anti-uricosuria reflects a trans-stimulation of URAT1 by intracellular salicylate, which is evidently a substrate for the Na^+–pyrazinoate transporter.

PATHOLOGY OF GOUT

Neutrophilic synovitis is the hallmark of acute gouty attack. Acute gouty synovitis shows diffuse superficial and perivascular infiltration with polymorphonuclear leukocytes in the synovium, as well as exudate containing polymorphonuclear neutrophilic leukocytes and fibrin adhering to the synovial surface (13). Some proliferation of synovial cells and infiltration of lymphocytes, macrophages, and occasional plasma cells have also been observed during the acute gouty synovitis.

The tophus represents the most characteristic lesion of gout and can be found in the synovium as well as elsewhere (13). Crystals in the tophi in synovium and elsewhere are needle shaped and often are arranged radially in small clusters. The histopathology of tophi shows foreign body granulomas surrounding a core of amorphous mass or monosodium urate (MSU) crystals by mono- and multinucleated macrophages, fibroblasts, and lymphocytes. Other components of tophi include lipids, mucopolysaccharides, and plasma proteins. At least in some cases, tophi in the synovium have been observed at the time of first gouty attack (13). These synovial tophi often lie near the joint surface and are weakly encapsulated so that minor trauma or changes in the crystal equilibrium within the tophus would likely allow release of crystals into the joint to precipitate attacks (13).

URATE CRYSTAL–INDUCED INFLAMMATION

Urate crystals in joint fluid at the time of the acute attack may derive from rupture of preformed synovial deposits or precipitate de novo (2). However, the finding of crystals in synovial fluids of asymptomatic joints illustrates that factors other than the presence of crystals are important in modulating the inflammatory reaction (14).

Urate crystals initiate, amplify, and sustain intense inflammatory attacks by stimulating the synthesis and release of humoral and cellular mediators (1,2). Urate crystals interact with the phagocyte through two broad mechanisms. First, they activate the cells through opsonized and phagocytosed particles, eliciting a stereotypical phagocyte response of lysosomal fusion, respiratory burst, and release of inflammatory mediators. The other mechanism involves the particular properties of the urate crystal to interact directly with lipid membrane and proteins via cell membrane perturbation and cross-linking of membrane glycoproteins in the phagocyte. This interaction leads to the activation of several signal transduction pathways including G proteins, phospholipase C and D, Src tyrosine kinases, the mitogen-activated protein kinases ERK1/ERK2, 9c-Jun N-terminal kinase, and p38 mitogen-activated protein kinase (1,2). These steps are critical for crystal-induced interleukin (IL) 8 expression in monocytic cells, which plays a key role in the neutrophil accumulation (1,2). Recently, innate immune responses involving Toll-like receptors (TLR) 2 and 4 have been implicated in the chondrocyte and macrophage signaling (14). Furthermore, induction of triggering receptor expressed on myeloid cells 1 (TREM-1) has been implicated as another potential mechanism for the early, induced innate immune response to amplification of acute gouty inflammation (15).

12

Gout
C. Treatment

Robert A. Terkeltaub, MD

- The three major considerations on comprehensive gout therapy include: (1) the treatment of acute flares; (2) management of the complications of chronic tophaceous gout; and (3) prophylaxis through urate-lowering agents designed to prevent disease flares and long-term sequelae.
- In the absence of contraindications, nonsteroidal anti-inflammatory drugs (NSAIDs) are considered first-line therapy for acute gout.
- Systemic glucocorticoids, also effective therapy for acute gout, are very useful for patients in whom NSAIDs are contraindicated.
- Intra-articular glucocorticoid injections may be effective if only one or two joints are affected by acute gout.

- Colchicine (generally 0.6 mg once or twice daily) is an appropriate therapy for prophylaxis against recurrent gout flares.
- The two standard urate-lowering therapies are allopurinol (most popular) and the uricosuric agents, for example, probenecid.
- Asymptomatic hyperuricemia does not require treatment.
- The dose of allopurinol must be decreased in the setting of renal insufficiency.
- Febuxostat, a relative newcomer to gout therapy, also achieves its effects through the inhibition of xanthine oxidase, albeit through a different mechanism than allopurinol.

Gout management involves two primary components: (1) treatment and prophylaxis of acute joint and bursal inflammation and (2) lowering of serum urate levels with the objectives of avoiding recurrent, painful inflammatory flares, suppressing progression of joint damage, and preventing the occurrence of urolithiasis. All too often, current strategies for treating gouty arthritis and lowering urate levels are based more on practitioner preferences than on evidence-based medicine (1).

MANAGEMENT OF ACUTE GOUTY ARTHRITIS

Choices for both anti-inflammatory and antihyperuricemic therapy in gout are reviewed below.

Nonsteroidal Anti-Inflammatory Drugs and Other Analgesic Agents

The primary goal in treatment of acute gout is rapid, safe resolution of pain and functional incapacity. Because acute gout attacks are self-limited, results of clinical trials for this condition warrant careful consideration. Nonsteroidal anti-inflammatory drugs (NSAIDs) typically produce major symptom reduction within 24 hours. In the absence of contraindications, NSAIDs are considered first-line therapy for acute gout. No specific NSAID has clear superiority over others in the treatment of gout. Ibuprofen in full doses (e.g., 800 mg q.i.d.), for example, is as likely to be effective as indomethacin (50 mg t.i.d.). Unfortunately, NSAID gastrointestinal and renal toxicity are major concerns in many patients. The comparable efficacy of etoricoxib and indomethacin in a head-to-head comparison in acute gout (2) suggests that selective cyclooxygenase-2 (COX-2) inhibition provides an alternative approach when nonselective COX inhibitors are contraindicated in the acute setting. However, cardiac safety of selective COX-2 inhibitors remains controversial. Opiates are useful adjuncts for analgesia early in acute gout treatment, though this has not been evaluated in controlled clinical trials (1).

Glucocorticosteroids and Adrenocorticotrophic Hormone

Glucocorticosteroids (systemic or local) and adrenocorticotrophic hormone (ACTH) are reliably effective second-line treatments for acute gout. These drugs also are limited by the potential for toxicity, particularly the exacerbation of hyperglycemia. Relatively large doses of systemic glucocorticosteroids often are required to treat acute gout effectively, particularly when the arthritis is polyarticular or when it affects a large joint such as the knee. A typical regimen in such a scenario would be prednisone, initiated at 30 to 60 mg/day (perhaps in divided doses), with a steady taper to discontinuation over 10 to 14 days. The use of a tapering oral methylprednisolone dose package regimen has not yet been systematically evaluated for acute gout. The effectiveness of intra-articular injection of a depot glucocorticosteroid ester for gout affecting one or two large joints has been supported by small, open-label studies (1).

Synthetic ACTH appears to be effective within hours for acute oligoarticular and polyarticular gout and was superior to indomethacin in acute gout treatment in one controlled clinical trial (1). A controlled study of patients with acute gout suggested that systemic anti-inflammatory doses of glucocorticosteroids and ACTH have comparable effectiveness (1). Peripheral anti-inflammatory effects of ACTH mediated by melanocortin receptor 3 activation, preceding induction of adrenal glucocorticosteroid release, could be responsible for the rapidity of ACTH efficacy in acute gout. ACTH is relatively expensive, however, and is not universally available. Primary treatment of acute gout with systemic glucocorticosteroids or ACTH also can be associated with rebound arthritis flares. Therefore, initiation of low dose prophylactic colchicine simultaneously with systemic glucocorticosteroids or ACTH is often useful as an adjunctive treatment.

Colchicine

Colchicine, administered either orally or intravenously, was once a standard approach to the treatment of acute gout attacks. Colchicine is no longer recommended for the treatment of acute gout flares, however, because of the length of time required for oral colchicine to sup-

press an attack and the narrow therapeutic window and high potential for serious toxicities associated with intravenous colchicine. In nearly all patients, NSAIDs, glucocorticoids, or ACTH provide better options for the treatment of acute gout. As discussed below, colchicine continues to play a major role in the prophylaxis against gout attacks.

Prophylactic Therapy for Acute Gouty Arthritis

Low dose colchicine (i.e., 0.5 or 0.6 mg p.o. once or twice daily) is a highly appropriate choice for prophylaxis of recurrent acute gout (1). Although colchicine is not a potent anti-inflammatory agent, the medication is particularly effective for prophylaxis against gout and calcium pyrophosphate dehydrate deposition disease (CPPD) crystal-induced inflammation. Even low concentrations of colchicine modulate neutrophil adhesion to the endothelium (3). High concentrations of colchicine suppress urate crystal-induced activation of the NALP3 inflammasome (4). It is less clear that low dose NSAIDs work reliably for gout prophylaxis.

Gouty arthritis is a particularly common event in the first few months after initiation of uric acid–lowering treatment. Standard clinical practice is to prescribe daily oral colchicine (0.6 mg p.o. bid in patients with intact renal function) for the first 6 months of antihyperuricemic therapy. The dosage of low dose prophylactic colchicine should be lowered in the presence of renal dysfunction and with age over 70 (1). Even so, caution is needed, as low dose daily colchicine may be associated with severe toxicities, including neuromyopathy and bone marrow suppression. Concurrent treatment with erythromycin, statin drugs, gemfibrozil, and cyclosporine predispose to colchicine toxicity by altering colchicine elimination (1). Because colchicine is not dialyzable, it should not be employed in dialysis-dependent renal failure (1).

Uric Acid Lowering Approaches

The decision to initiate antihyperuricemic therapy in gout requires thoughtful consideration, as antihyperuricemic agents have multiple potential drug interactions and toxicities. Gout does not always progress in the absence of urate-lowering therapy, and in some patients serum urate levels can be normalized through lifestyle changes, without antihyperuricemic drugs. Lifestyle alterations that may affect urate levels include cessation of alcohol abuse, weight reduction, and the replacement of thiazide diuretics with another class of antihypertensive agent. Conventional purine-restricted diets are unpalatable and only modestly effective in lowering serum urate. A palatable, calorie-restricted, low carbohydrate diet tailored to improve insulin sensitivity appears to diminish hyperuricemia by 15% to 20% (5). Other dietary measures, such as specifically limiting beer consumption and increasing low fat dairy product consumption, merit further direct investigation.

Pharmacologic Antihyperuricemic Treatments

The two major indications for chronic uric acid–lowering therapy in gout are macroscopic subcutaneous tophi and unacceptably frequent attacks of gouty arthritis (e.g., three or more per year). Standard practice is to delay initiating uric acid–lowering treatment until resolution of the inflammatory phase of acute gout. This practice is due to concern that antihyperuricemic therapy could worsen acute gout by mobilizing urate crystals from remodeling microscopic and macroscopic tophi. Precipitation of acute gout through this mechanism is a common side effect in the first few months after initiation of antihyperuricemic therapy (1,6).

The currently available pharmacotherapies for serum urate lowering are: (1) allopurinol, a xanthine oxidase inhibitor, which reduces uric acid production; or (2) uricosuric agents (exemplified by probenecid), which increase renal uric acid excretion. Probenecid and other uricosurics act through inhibition of the organic anion exchanger URAT1 in the proximal renal tubule, thereby inhibiting urate reabsorption.

In traditional evaluations of gout, patients were divided into two groups on the basis of 24-hour urine uric acid exretion results: uric acid overproducers and underexcreters. Overproducers—the great majority of gout patients—have been defined as those gout patients whose daily urinary uric acid excretion exceeds 800 mg. Unfortunately, such urine collections are inconvenient to patients, prone to inaccuracy, and may fail to identify combined uric acid overproduction and underexcretion. Moreover, 24-hour urine collections fail to identify uric acid overproduction reliably in subjects with creatinine clearances <60 mL/min. Measurement of uric acid in spot urine samples does not distinguish reliably between uric acid overproduction from underexcretion (1). Thus, in practice, the usual approach to therapy once the need for urate-lowering therapy is determined is allopurinol, regardless of the 24-hour uric acid excretion measurement. Twenty-four–hour urine uric acid collections may be used to screen for uric acid overproduction in the absence of an obvious cause of hyperuricemia such as renal failure, diuretic use, or myeloproliferative disease. This test is particularly useful in subjects presenting with gout before the age of 30 or with gout and a history of urolithiasis. The optimal target level for serum urate reduction is held to be below 6.0 mg/dL, given that this is approximately 1 mg/dL lower than the

level of urate solubility in physiologic solutions in vitro. Standard clinical practice is to achieve this level of serum urate lowering via gradual escalation of antihyperuricemic drug dosages over the first few months of therapy (1). However, lowering serum urate to levels above 6.0 mg/dL is associated with at least partial clinical efficacy in many patients. Allopurinol and uricosuric therapy promote shrinkage of tophi at similar rates when serum urate is also diminished to a similar level.

Allopurinol is the most frequently used antihyperuricemic agent among practitioners, due to the convenient single daily dosing and the generally predictable efficacy of allourinol irrespective of etiology of the hyperuricemia in gout (1). The usual starting dose of allopurinol for most patients should be on the order of 100 mg/day (lower for patients with renal insufficiency, possibly higher for young patients with normal renal function). This dose is titrated upward over a period of several weeks according to the serum uric acid level. Doses of up to 300 mg/day and even higher may be used. A broad issue limiting effective allopurinol use appears to be poor patient compliance, which challenges practitioners to educate patients better regarding the long-term objectives of antihyperuricemic therapy.

Side effects of allopurinol include minor hypersensitivity reactions such as pruritus and dermatitis, which occur in approximately 2% of patients (1). Approximately half of the patients with such minor reactions have been reported to be desensitized successfully in small, open-label studies (1). However, allopurinol toxicity, including hepatic damage and major hypersensitivity reactions, can become severe. A mortality rate of ~20% is seen with the allopurinol major hypersensitivity syndrome, which is dose dependant and typically manifests as severe dermatitis, accompanied by features including vasculitis, fever, eosinophilia, hepatic and renal dysfunction (1). Renal insufficiency and possibly concomitant thiazide therapy are predisposing factors for the severe allopurinol hypersensitivity syndrome. In Han Chinese, human leukocyte antigen (HLA)-B5801 is strongly linked to severe allopurinol cutaneous hypersensitivity (7). Fortunately, major allopurinol hypersensitivity syndrome is uncommon and it is believed that adjusting the initial daily dose of allopurinol in direct proportion to creatinine clearance may reduce the risk of developing this drug toxicity (1). Overly aggressive attempts to bring serum urate below 6.0 mg/dL with allopurinol may be hazardous in subjects with advanced renal insufficiency because of dose-dependent toxicities of allopurinol.

When a uricosuric agent is required (e.g., in the setting of allopurinol hypersensitivity), probenecid is usually the agent of choice. Probenecid increases renal uric acid clearance and can be employed effectively for patients with substantially decreased renal uric acid excretion but creatinine clearance ≥60 mL/min (1). Uricosuric agents require good renal function in order to be effective. Probenecid is started at a dosage of 500 mg twice daily and titrated upward to a maximum dosage of 1 g twice daily (or until the target serum uric acid level is achieved). Subjects taking probenecid are at increased risk for uric acid urolithiasis and should be compliant and able to consume at least 2 L of fluid orally on a daily basis to reduce urolithiasis risk. Low dose acetylsalicylic acid, which reduces renal uric acid excretion, does not appear to significantly block the antihyperuricemic activity of probenecid. Other potent uricosuric agents include sulfinpyrazone and benzbromarone, but these drugs are limited by toxicity and are not universally available (1). Less potent uricosuric agents include the angiotensin 1 (AT1) receptor antagonist losartan, and the lipid-lowering agents atorvastatin and fenofibrate. Among these three agents, fenofibrate has the greatest capacity to decrease serum urate levels. The uricosuric effect of losartan appears to have limited sustainability. Use of losartan, atorvastatin, and fenofibrate as a serum urate-lowering primary or adjunctive approach may have potential for selected patients with moderate hyperuricemia associated with gout and comorbid conditions such as hypertension, metabolic syndrome, and hyperlipidemia. However, the place in management of these agents is not yet established and uric acid urolithiasis is a risk as with other uricosuric modalities.

Considerations Regarding Comorbidities in Patients with Gout and Asymptomatic Hyperuricemia

Implicit in the medical management of gout patients is recognition and appropriate therapy of medical conditions commonly associated with gout that may affect both urate levels and longevity. These conditions include the metabolic syndrome, hyperlipidemia, hypertension, alcohol abuse, renal disorders, and myeloproliferative diseases. Asymptomatic hyperuricemia alone does not appear to cause clinically significant renal disease. However, hyperuricemia is both an independent risk factor for atherosclerosis and a powerful predictor of adverse outcomes of ischemic cardiovascular diseases (8). Serum urate positively correlates with blood pressure in children, and extensive studies in rodents have suggested that hyperuricemia exerts direct, deleterious and pro-atherogenic effects on arterial endothelial and smooth muscle cells, as well as toxic effects on the glomerular microvasculature, renal function, and systemic blood pressure (8). There is no evidence basis to support treatment of asymptomatic hyperuricemia at this time.

Gout in the Patient with Organ Transplantation

A striking example of refractory gout is provided by patients with major organ transplantation. In such patients, cyclopsporine or tacrolimus are critical to the success of the allograft (1). In this condition, nephropathic and renal urate transport–altering effects of cyclosporine or tacrolimus drive the potential for marked hyperuricemia and remarkably accelerated tophi development. Consequently, the diagnosis of transplantation-associated gout nearly always calls for the institution of antihyperuricemic therapy. Low dose cyclosporine microemulsion regimens and ongoing development of cyclosporine-free immunosuppression regimens for major organ transplant recipients should diminish the scope and extent of this iatrogenic condition.

Treatment of Refractory Gout Patients: Current Options and Drugs in Advanced Development

Limitations in antihyperuricemic therapy often become a major clinical problem in subjects. The most common issues are intolerance to allopurinol, renal insufficiency or urolithiasis (rendering uricosuric agents ineffective or contraindicated), and extensive tophi. Several potential new agents for the treatment of gout—oxypurinol, febuxostat, and uricase—are discussed below.

Limitations of allopurinol are not confined to hypersensitivity and other forms of drug intolerance. The major active metabolite of allopurinol, oxypurinol, binds to the reduced form of xanthine oxidase with very high affinity but does not efficiently bind and inhibit the oxidized form of xanthine oxidase. This may contribute to lack of efficacy of allopurinol seen in some patients at doses as high as 300 mg daily (6). Oxypurinol is tolerated in some allopurinol-hypersensitive patients, but the oral absorption of oxypurinol is poor relative to that of allopurinol, and oxypurinol doses may need extended titration to achieve satisfactory reduction of serum urate. Cross-reactivity with allopurinol and dependence on intact renal function for efficient elimination of oxypurinol may further limit the utility of oxypurinol in the treatment of refractory gout in allopurinol-intolerant patients.

Febuxostat, which inhibits xanthine oxidase through a different mechanism than allopurinol and oxypurinol, blocks substrate access to xanthine oxidase by occupying a channel in the enzyme leading to the active site (9). This leads to the potent inhibition of both the oxidized and reduced forms of xanthine oxidase, but has minimal effects on other enzymes involved in purine and pyrimidine metabolism. Furthermore, unlike the

12

currently available xanthine oxidase inhibitors, febuxostat is metabolized primarily by hepatic glucuronide formation and oxidation and is excreted in approximately equal amounts in stool and urine. The efficacy of febuxostat (80 and 120 mg daily) in serum urate–lowering in gout patients with starting serum urate levels of ≥8.0 mg/dL was superior to that of allopurinol 300 mg daily in a phase III study in which the primary endpoint was the percentage of patients with serum urate level <6.0 mg/dL (6). Nevertheless, after 1 year of treatment, reductions in the incidence of gout flares and in the size of tophi were seen in similar fractions of subjects in all treatment groups (6).

The hepatic enzyme uricase, the expression of which is lacking in human beings, oxidizes relatively insoluble uric acid in a reaction that generates highly soluble allantoin, and also generates the oxidant hydrogen peroxide as well as reactive intermediates of uric acid oxidation. Uricase has the capacity to lower serum urate levels profoundly and to promote accelerated tophus dissolution (debulking). Recombinant unmodified *Aspergillus flavus* uricase (Rasburicase) is US Food and Drug Administration–approved for prevention of the hyperuricemia-mediated tumor lysis syndrome. However, this form of uricase is highly immunogenic and can trigger severe and potentially lethal side effects including anaphylaxis. Administration of unmodified uricase beyond a single, short-term course is limited by hypersensitivity reactions and development of uricase-neutralizing antibodies. Reduced antigenicity and prolonged half-life of uricase activity are being optimized via mutation of specific amino acids in uricase and by polyethyleneglycol (PEG) modification of the recombinant enzyme (10). PEGylated uricase has appeared promising in studies of gout patients, though intravenous infusion may be superior to subcutaneous injection with respect to immunogenicty (10). However, uricase-induced injection or infusion reactions are a concern, as is redox stress. In this context, uricase can induce hemolysis and methemoglobinemia, most predictably so in patients with glucose-6-phosphate dehydrogenase (G6PD) deficiency. Therefore, the therapeutic niche for modified uricases in the treatment of gout will most likely be for the short-term induction of tophus de-bulking in carefully selected patients intolerant or unresponsive to other forms of antihyperuricemic therapy.

REFERENCES

1. Terkeltaub RA. Clinical practice. Gout. N Engl J Med 2003;349:1647–1655.
2. Rubin BR, Burton R, Navarra S, et al. Efficacy and safety profile of treatment with etoricoxib 120 mg once daily compared with indomethacin 50 mg three times daily in acute gout: a randomized controlled trial. Arthritis Rheum 2004;50:598–606.
3. Cronstein BN, Terkeltaub R. The inflammatory process of gout and its treatment. Arthritis Res Ther 2006;8(suppl 1):S3.
4. Martinon F, Petrilli V, Mayor A, Tardivel A, Tschopp J. Gout-associated uric acid crystals activate the NALP3 inflammasome. Nature 2006;440:237–241.
5. Dessein PH, Shipton EA, Stanwix AE, Joffe BI, Ramokgadi J. Beneficial effects of weight loss associated with moderate calorie/carbohydrate restriction, and increased proportional intake of protein and unsaturated fat on serum urate and lipoprotein levels in gout: a pilot study. Ann Rheum Dis 2000;59:539–543.
6. Becker MA, Schumacher HR Jr, Wortmann RL, et al. Febuxostat compared with allopurinol in patients with hyperuricemia and gout. N Engl J Med 2005;353:2450–2461.
7. Hung SI, Chung WH, Liou LB, et al. HLA-B*5801 allele as a genetic marker for severe cutaneous adverse reactions caused by allopurinol. Proc Natl Acad Sci U S A. 2005;102:4134–4139.
8. Kanellis J, Feig DI, Johnson RJ. Does asymptomatic hyperuricaemia contribute to the development of renal and cardiovascular disease? An old controversy renewed. Nephrology 2004;9:394–399.
9. Okamoto K, Eger BT, Nishino T, Kondo S, Pai EF, Nishino T. An extremely potent inhibitor of xanthine oxidoreductase. Crystal structure of the enzyme-inhibitor complex and mechanism of inhibition. J Biol Chem 2003;278:1848–1855.
10. Ganson NJ, Kelly SJ, Scarlett E, Sundy JS, Hershfield MS. Control of hyperuricemia in subjects with refractory gout, and induction of antibody against poly(ethylene) glycol (PEG), in a phase I trial of subcutaneous PEGylated urate oxidase. Arthritis Res Ther 2005;8:R12.

CHAPTER 13

Calcium Pyrophosphate Dihydrate, Hydroxyapatite, and Miscellaneous Crystals

GERALDINE MCCARTHY, MD, FRCPI

- The incidence and prevalence of calcium pyrophosphate dihydrate (CPPD) are unknown, though there is an increasing prevalence of radiographic chondrocalcinosis with age, and trauma may predispose to the disease. Several metabolic diseases are associated with CPPD.
- Overproduction of extracellular pyrophosphate in abnormal cartilage matrix contributes to CPPD.
- Acute pseudogout is the inflammatory host response to CPPD crystals shed from cartilaginous tissues. Because of the common occurrence of these crystals in osteoarthritic cartilage, there is a strong association of pseudogout with osteoarthritis (OA).
- There are multiple clinical manifestations of CPPD, including pseudogout, pseudo-osteoarthritis, pseudo–rheumatoid arthritis, pseudo–neuropathic arthropathy, and asymptomatic chondrocalcinosis (lanthanic CPPD).
- Diagnosis is made by identifying CPPD crystals in synovial fluid of affected joints.
- There is no practical way to remove calcium pyrophosphate crystals from the joints and symptomatic treatment is with nonsteroidal anti-inflammatory drugs (NSAIDs), colchicines, and local or systemic glucocorticoids.
- Basic calcium phosphate crystals (BCP) frequently deposit in articular tissues and may involve dysregulation of extracellular pyrophosphate homeostasis. BCP crystals can cause diverse clinical conditions including destructive arthritis (Milwaukee shoulder) and calcific periarthritis/tendonitis.

Calcium pyrophosphate dihydrate (CPPD) and hydroxyapatite crystals are the most common calcium-containing crystals associated with joint and periarticular disorders. Deposition of these crystals is frequently asymptomatic or can be intermittently symptomatic. However, common clinical manifestations of calcium crystal deposition include acute or chronic inflammatory and degenerative arthritides, and certain forms of periarthritis. In addition to these, a number of other crystalline materials have been identified less commonly in synovial or bursal fluid. These include calcium oxalate, cholesterol, lipids, and synthetic corticosteroid crystals.

CALCIUM PYROPHOSPHATE DIHYDRATE DEPOSITION DISEASE

Specific identification of calcium pyrophosphate dihydrate (CPPD) crystals ($Ca_2P_2O_7.H_2O$) in synovial fluid (SF) or articular tissue allows the clinician to differentiate between CPPD crystal deposition disease and other inflammatory and degenerative arthritides. The term *chondrocalcinosis* generally refers to the characteristic radiographic features of CPPD deposition in articular cartilage. Calcium-containing crystals other than CPPD may also deposit in articular cartilage, producing radiographically detectable densities in cartilage as well as joint inflammation or degeneration. Deposition of CPPD crystals is not limited to articular cartilage. Less frequently, CPPD crystals are deposited in synovial lining, ligaments, tendons, and, on rare occasions, periarticular soft tissue, much like gouty tophi.

Calcium pyrophosphate dihydrate crystal deposition disease may be asymptomatic or may manifest in a variety of ways. The term *pseudogout* refers to the acute, goutlike attacks of inflammation that occur in some individuals with CPPD deposition disease. CPPD deposition may also cause symptoms similar to septic arthritis, polyarticular inflammatory arthritis (which can be mistaken for rheumatoid arthritis), or osteoarthritis (OA). The incidence and prevalence of clinically important CPPD deposition disease are unknown.

Radiographic surveys show a steadily increasing prevalence of chondrocalcinosis with age. Data from the Framingham study showed an overall prevalence of radiographic chondrocalcinosis of 8.1% in the population over the age of 63, showed prevalence rates of 20% in knee joints of patients over the age of 60, and rates as high as 50% in patients over the age of 90 (1).

Classification

Categorization based on etiology results in four patient groups: hereditary, sporadic/idiopathic, associated with a metabolic abnormality, or post-traumatic. Although most cases of CPPD deposition disease are nonfamilial, many multicase families with CPPD deposition disease have been reported in the literature. Most familial cases appear to be inherited in an autosomal dominant manner, with early onset and varying severity (2). Susceptibility to familial CPPD deposition disease has been most commonly localized to the short arm of chromosome 5. Of particular interest is the gene located at the CCAL2 locus on chromosome 5p, the ANKH gene. The ANKH gene codes for the multipass transmembrane protein AHKH, which transports inorganic pyrophosphate (PPi) from the cell. Gain-of-function mutations in ANKH causes familial autosomal dominant CPPD deposition, of which several variants have been reported. Other genetic conditions are associated with chondrocalcinosis. Gitelman's and Bartter's diseases are both associated with CPPD deposition, possibly due to their association with chronic hypomagnesemia. Magnesium is a cofactor of alkaline phosphatase, and it is postulated that these conditions lead to mild functional hypophosphatasia. Iron and copper overload, associated with haemochromatosis and Wilson's disease, respectively, are thought to favor calcium crystal nucleation as well as inhibiting alkaline phosphatase activity. Genetic factors could also participate in so-called sporadic cases, as a familial pattern has been identified in some case series of apparently sporadic CPPD deposition disease. However, the late onset of the arthritis phenotype makes family studies of CPPD deposition disease difficult.

A number of metabolic disease and physiologic stresses, such as aging and trauma, have been associated with CPPD crystal deposition (Table 13-1). Only aging and previous joint surgery have been proven to be associated. Nonetheless, circumstantial evidence suggests that many of these other associations are valid. Therefore, the routine study of a patient newly diagnosed with CPPD crystal deposition should include evaluation of serum calcium, ferritin, magnesium, phosphorus, alkaline phosphatase, and thyroid-stimulating hormone. Further studies should be obtained if abnormal values are found.

TABLE 13-1. CONDITIONS ASSOCIATED WITH CALCIUM PYROPHOSPHATE DIHYDRATE CRYSTAL DEPOSITION DISEASE.

Strongly associated
  Age
  Previous joint surgery
  Osteoarthritis
  Trauma
  Gout
  Hyperparathyroidism
  Hemochromatosis
  Hypophosphatasia
  Hypomagnesemia

Weakly associated
  Hypothyroidism

Potentially associated
  Wilson's disease
  Acromegaly
  Hyaluronidase deficiency
  X-linked hypophosphatemic rickets
  Familial hypocalciuric hypercalcemia
  Ochronosis

Pathogenesis of Inflammation and Cartilage Degeneration

Acute pseudogout is believed to represent a dose-related inflammatory host response to CPPD crystals shed from cartilaginous tissues contiguous to the synovial cavity. Phagocytosis of crystals by neutrophils, as invariably demonstrated by compensated polarized light microscopy in fluids removed from acutely inflamed joints of patients with pseudogout, results in the release of lysosomal enzymes and cell-derived chemotactic factors. Phagocytosis by synovial-lining cells leads to cell proliferation and release of prostaglandins, cytokines, and matrix metalloproteases capable of matrix degradation, such as collagenase and stromelysin.

The relationship between OA and CPPD deposition is complex. A study of SF sampled at the time of knee replacement demonstrated that 60% of 53 unselected patients with a preoperative diagnosis of OA contained either CPPD or hydroxyapatite or both (3). It has been suggested that most SF from patients with OA may contain CPPD or hydroxyapatite too small or too infrequent to detect by routine microscopy. The frequency of association of CPPD crystal deposits may result from the biological effects of CPPD crystals as they interact with fibroblasts or mononuclear synovial lining cells. These include a well-documented mitogenic response, resulting in tissue hypertrophy. Stimulated lining cells secrete proteolytic enzymes and cytokine release. Proteolytic enzymes may damage cartilage and other articular structures and cytokine release can enhance further protease production by synovial lining cells or chondrocytes. Such effects have been demonstrated for CPPD crystals in vitro.

Pathogenesis of Crystal Deposition

Overproduction of extracellular PPi, the anionic component of the crystal, contributes to CPPD crystal deposition (4). Synovial fluid PPi concentration is elevated in most joints with CPPD deposition, in contrast to plasma and urinary excretion levels. Furthermore, chondrocytes from CPPD-containing cartilage produce more extracellular PPi than normal and OA control cartilages. Articular chondrocytes likely contribute to SF PPi because they liberate PPi, an effect which can be enhanced by transforming growth factor beta (TGF-beta), ascorbate, retinoic acid, and thyroid hormones. PPi may be made de novo by chondrocyte ectoenzymes, which hydrolyze nucleoside triphosphates. In addition, intracellular PPi may be transported across cell membranes by the multipass transmembrane protein ANK or other proteins. Calcium is also necessary for CPPD crystal formation and calcium concentrations are increased in cartilages from patients with CPPD.

Changes in the pericellular matrix and matrix vesicles (MV) of articular cartilage have been implicated in CPPD crystal formation. MV are small membrane-bound extracellular organelles that bud off chondrocytes which, when isolated from articular cartilage, can produce CPPD crystals in vitro. CPPD crystals are formed in areas of abnormal pericellular matrix, but not in normal matrix. Affected cartilage matrix contains damaged collagen type II fibers and increased calcium-binding matricellular proteins. Type I collagen, not usually present in normal cartilage, is found in increased quantities in CPPD-containing cartilage and fewer large proteoglycans are present. Current data also supports a role for transglutaminases, which post-translationally modify extracellular matrix proteins in CPPD crystal formation.

Clinical Features and Diagnosis

At least five clinical presentations have been associated with articular CPPD (5).

Pseudogout

Acute pseudogout is an inflammatory process manifest by joint effusions and symptoms and signs of articular inflammation in one or more joints. These self-limited attacks can be as abrupt in onset and as severe as acute gout. Patients typically experience pain, stiffness, and swelling in the affected joint. Signs include swelling with variable erythema and warmth. Systemic manifestations during an attack may include a fever of 99°F to 103°F, leukocytosis of 12,000 to 15,000 cells/mm^3 and elevated erythrocyte sedimentation rate (ESR) and serum acute phase reactants. Compared to true gout, pseudogout attacks may take longer to reach peak intensity, and are often considerably longer lasting than gout attacks, as symptoms can last 3 to 120 days despite therapy (6). Pseudogout is more common in large than in small joints. The knee is the most commonly involved joint, followed by the wrist, ankle, elbow, toe, shoulder, and hip. As with gout, pseudogout attacks can occur spontaneously or can be provoked by trauma, surgery, or post–parathyroidectomy or severe illness, such as stroke or myocardial infarction. Patients are usually asymptomatic between episodes. Differentiation from gout or septic joint may be difficult and requires arthrocentesis followed by culture and examination of the SF for crystals. About 25% of people with CPPD deposition exhibit the pseudogout pattern of disease.

Pseudo-Osteoarthritis

Most patients with clinically apparent CPPD crystal deposition have an unusually severe, oddly distributed, degenerative arthritis resembling OA. They present with the gradual onset of joint pain and stiffness, typically involving knees, wrists, metacarpophalangeal (MCP) joints, hips, shoulders, spine, elbows, and ankles. Half of these patients will have acute attacks superimposed on their chronic symptoms. Flexion contractures of the affected joints and deformities of the knees are common. Valgus knee deformities are especially suggestive of underlying CPPD crystal deposition. This type of presentation can be difficult to differentiate from OA and consequently may be significantly underrecognized. In one series, 30% of patients diagnosed with OA had CPPD crystals in their affected joints at the time of total knee replacement (3).

Pseudo–Rheumatoid Arthritis

About 5% of patients with CPPD deposition manifest multiple joint involvement with symmetric distribution and low grade inflammation. Accompanying morning stiffness, fatigue, synovial thickening, flexion contractures, and elevated ESR often lead to a misdiagnosis of rheumatoid arthritis. In addition, 10% of individuals with CPPD crystal deposits have low titers of rheumatoid factor, which provide further diagnostic confusion. The presence of high titer rheumatoid factor, anti-cyclic citrullinated peptide (anti-CCP) antibodies, and radiographic evidence of typical rheumatoid bony erosions favor the diagnosis of true rheumatoid arthritis.

Pseudo–Neuropathic Arthropathy

Some patients with CPPD deposition disease have a severe destructive monoarthritis similar to that seen in neuropathic joints. These patients have no neurologic abnormalities and yet present with a painful monoarthritis, associated with dramatic destructive radiographic changes. The natural history of patients with this type of CPPD deposition disease is not well described.

Lanthanic

Some individuals with radiographic or pathologic evidence of articular chondrocalcinosis have no clinically apparent arthritis. This finding has been termed *lanthanic CPPD deposition* and is of uncertain significance. These patients have not been rigorously studied to see if they develop signs and symptoms of clinical arthritis with a greater frequency than the unaffected population.

Calcium pyrophosphate dihydrate crystals are not commonly found in tissue other than cartilage. Even in synovium, CPPD crystals typically form in areas of chondometaplasia. Tophaceous CPPD crystal deposits are well described and can cause nerve compression syndromes. Neurologic manifestations of CPPD deposition in the axial skeleton can occur. Spinal ligaments seem particularly prone to CPPD crystal deposition. Affected patients may present with myelopathy. Almost 25% of patients undergoing decompressive laminectomy for lumbar spinal stenosis had CPPD crystal deposits in their ligamenta flava. Clinically, patients with CPPD crystals had more acute onset of symptoms than those without CPPD crystals.

Diagnosis of CPPD-associated disease is most commonly and accurately made by identifying CPPD crystals by polarizing light microscopy in the SF of affected joints (Figure 13-1). The weak birefringence of CPPD

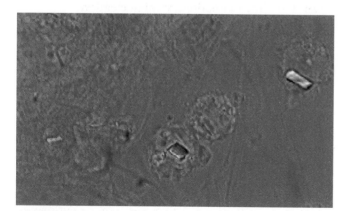

FIGURE 13-1

Rod-shaped calcium pyrophosphate dihydrate (CPPD) crystals in synovial fluid analyzed by compensated polarized light microscopy.

TABLE 13-2. REVISED DIAGNOSTIC CRITERIA FOR CALCIUM PYROPHOSPHATE DIHYDRATE CRYSTAL DEPOSITION DISEASE.

Criteria

I. Demonstration of CPPD crystals in tissue or synovial fluid by definitive means (e.g., characteristic x-ray diffraction or chemical analysis)

II. (a) Identification of monoclinic or triclinic crystals showing weakly positive or no birefringence by compensated polarized light microscopy
   (b) Presence of typical radiographic calcification

III. (a) Acute arthritis, especially of knees or other large joints.
   (b) Chronic arthritis, especially of knee, hip, wrist, carpus, elbow, shoulder, or metacarpophalangeal joint, especially if accompanied by acute exacerbations. The following features help differentiate chronic arthritis from osteoarthritis:
      1. Uncommon site—wrist, metacarpophalangeal, elbow, and shoulder
      2. Radiographic appearance—radiocarpal or patellofemoral joint space narrowing, especially if isolated (patella "wrapped around" the femur)
      3. Subchondral cyst formation
      4. Severity of degeneration—progressive, with subchondral bony collapse and fragmentation with formation of intra-articular radiodense bodies
      5. Osteophyte formation—variable and inconstant.
      6. Tendon calcifications, especially triceps, Achilles, obturators

Categories

A. Definite disease: Criteria I or II(a) plus II (b) must be fulfilled
B. Probable disease: Criteria II (a) or II (b) must be fulfilled
C. Possible disease: Criteria III (a) or III (b) should alert the clinician to the possibility of underlying CPPD crystal deposition

crystals render them more difficult to discern than monosodium urate (MSU) crystals. They can be quite sparse in number. SF characteristics can vary from inflammatory to non-inflammatory in CPPD deposition disease. In pseudogout, SF may be turbid, watery, or hemorrhagic. Average white cell counts are in the region of 12,000 cells/mm^3 in pseudogout. Histologic examination of cartilage or synovial biopsies can be helpful as long as tissue preparation methods preserve crystals. Diagnostic criteria for CPPD deposition disease have been established (Table 13-2).

Radiographic Features

The typical appearance of punctate and linear densities in hyaline or fibrocartilagenous tissues is helpful diagnostically (Figure 13-2). The most characteristic sites of crystal deposition include knee articular cartilage and menisci, acetabular labrum of hip joint, fibrocartilagenous symphysis pubis, triangular cartilage of the wrist, and the annulus fibrosis of intervertebral discs. When the deposits are typical and unequivocal, the radio-

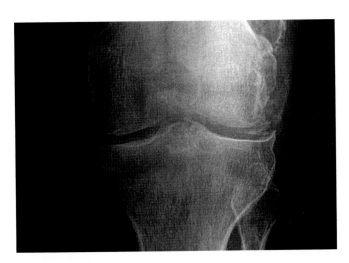

FIGURE 13-2

Chondrocalcinosis involving lateral meniscus of left knee.

graphic appearance is reasonably specific, but interpretation of atypical or faint deposits often is difficult. Calcific deposits also may appear in the articular capsule, ligaments, and tendons. Although the earliest calcific deposits occur in radiographically normal cartilage, degenerative changes often supervene. An individual can be screened for CPPD deposits with four radiographs: an anterposterior (AP) view of both knees (preferably not standing), an AP view of the pelvis for visualization of the symphysis pubis and hips, and a posteroanterior (PA) view of each hand to include the wrists. If these views show no evidence of crystal deposits, it is most unlikely that further study will prove fruitful.

Changes in the metacarpophalangeal joints, such as squaring of the bone ends, subchondral cysts, and hooklike osteophytes, are characteristic features of the arthritis associated with hemochromatosis (see Chapter 28), but are also found in patients with CPPD deposition alone. These changes occur more frequently in patients with CPPD crystal deposits and hemochromatosis than in those with only crystal deposits. In addition to the difference in pattern of affected joints, the finding of isolated patellofemoral joint space narrowing or isolated wrist degeneration differentiates CPPD from OA. Such differences may provide helpful clinical clues and are incorporated into the proposed diagnostic criteria given in Table 13-2 (7).

Treatment

In contrast to monosodium urate crystals in gout, there is no practical way to remove CPPD crystals from joints. Treatment of associated diseases, such as hyperparathyroidism, hemochromatosis, or myxedema, does not

result in resorption of CPPD crystal deposits. Acute attacks in large joints can be treated through aspiration alone or aspiration combined with injection of corticosteroids. Nonsteroidal anti-inflammatory drugs (NSAIDs) are recommended for most patients. The effectiveness of oral colchicine is less predictable in pseudogout than in gout, but the number and duration of acute attacks are reduced significantly by colchicine taken on a daily basis for prophylaxis. Corticotropin or systemic corticosteroid therapy has been used successfully in patients with gout or pseudogout. Phosphocitrate is a promising agent that inhibits CPPD crystal formation and cellular responses to CPPD, but it is not currently clinically available.

Apatite/Basic Calcium Phosphates

Basic calcium phosphate crystals (BCP), consisting of carbonate-substituted hydroxyapatite, octacalcium phosphate, and, rarely, tricalcium phosphate, frequently deposit in articular tissues, but may also be found in skin, arteries, breast, and other tissues. In the musculoskeletal system, crystals may be found in tendons, intervertebral discs, joint capsule, synovium, and cartilage. Studies have suggested that dystrophic tendon calcification occurs as a consequence of local trauma, ischemia, and necrosis of tendons. Some evidence suggests that calcifying tendonitis is an active, cell-mediated process in which local vascular and mechanical changes result in focal transformation of tendinous tissues into fibrocartilagenous material containing chondrocytes. This is followed by local deposition of hydroxyapatite crystals within extracellular matrix vesiclelike structures derived from these chondrocytes. The mechanism of intraarticular BCP crystal deposition is incompletely understood but likely involves matrix vesicles and local dysregulation of extracellular PPi homeostasis. PPi is a potent inhibitor of apatite crystal nucleation.

Basic Calcium Phosphate Crystal Identification

Although BCP crystals are common, particularly in OA, their presence in SF is recognized infrequently because of the lack of a simple, reliable test for detection. Polarized light microscopy, which effectively identifies MSU and CPPD crystals, is unable to detect BCP crystals, which are too small to be resolved by light microscopy (20–100nm). Despite the small size of individual crystals, they tend to aggregate into larger masses that occasionally may be observed by light microscopy as refractile "shiny coins" up to 5mm in diameter. The larger BCP aggregates have been detected by Alizarin red S staining, but this method lacks sensitivity and

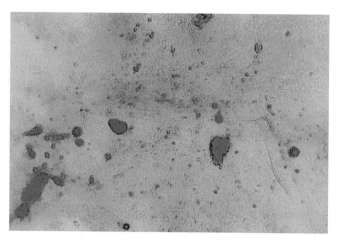

FIGURE 13-3

Alizarin red–stained clumps of apatite in joint fluid.

specificity (Figure 13-3). Techniques that are more specific for BCP crystal identification include x-ray diffraction, scanning or transmission electron microscopy with energy dispersive analysis, electron microprobe, Raman spectroscopy, atomic force microscopy, and a binding assay utilizing [^{14}C]ethane-1-hydroxy-1,1-diphosphonate. Unfortunately, these methods typically are unavailable or too costly for the handling of routine clinical specimens (8).

Clinical Features

Osteoarthritis

Concurrence of BCP crystals and OA is well established (9). The incidence of BCP crystals in SF from patients with knee OA is at least 30% to 60%. Indeed, it has recently been suggested that many OA fluids contain clusters of BCP crystals that are too small or too few in number to be identified by conventional techniques. Ample data supports the role of BCP crystals in cartilage degeneration as their presence correlates strongly with severity of radiographic OA, and larger joint effusions are seen in affected knee joints when compared with joint fluid from OA knees without crystals. Furthermore, in vitro studies of BCP crystal-induced cell activation support the active role of BCP in OA pathogenesis as they have numerous biologic effects, including the ability to induce mitogenesis in and matrix metalloproteases and prostaglandin synthesis by synovial fibroblasts and chondrocytes. Although the basis of cartilage damage by crystals has been the subject of numerous investigations, there are ongoing controversies concerning the relationship between calcium-containing crystals and OA and whether the crystals cause damage or are present as a result of joint damage.

There is no known therapy for prevention or removal of BCP crystals from joints or for interfering specifically with the biological effects of BCP crystals.

Large Joint Destructive Arthritis/Milwaukee Shoulder Syndrome

A distinctive type of destructive arthropathy of the shoulder has been described in elderly individuals (10). Typically, these patients are elderly women and manifest large, non-inflammatory synovial effusions, severe radiographic damage, and large rotator cuff tears. Patients typically have pain on shoulder use and also pain at night. There is reduced active and passive range of motion, sometimes associated with pronounced joint instability. Marked bone-on-bone crepitus is typical. The rotator cuff is generally completely destroyed. Joint effusion may be massive and typically yields 5 to 130 mL of SF that is frequently blood tinged and has a low, predominantly mononuclear cell count. BCP crystals are identified in most fluids. Some contain CPPD crystals in addition. Radiographs typically show upward subluxation and deformity of the humeral head and calcification of the tendinous rotator cuff (Figure 13-4). Treatment is generally unsatisfactory. A conservative approach, including analgesics and NSAIDs and repeated shoulder aspirations with or without steroid injections, has sometimes controlled symptoms satisfactorily. Surgical intervention is sometimes successful. Pain may subside with time alone.

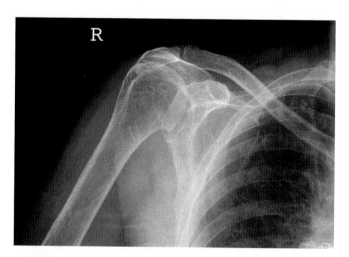

FIGURE 13-4

Anteroposterior radiograph of the shoulder joint affected by hydroxyapatite-associated destructive arthritis (Milwaukee shoulder). The extensive destruction of the periarticular tissues, including the rotator cuff, has led to instability of the shoulder with upward subluxation of the humerus. Note the associated glenohumeral degeneration and soft tissue evidence of joint effusion. Periarticular calcific deposition is noted at the acromioclavicular joint.

Calcific Periarthritis

Periarticular calcifications are occasionally observed on shoulder or other radiographs (Figure 13-4). The most common site of calcification is the rotator cuff. Most calcifications remain asymptomatic. If a patient has chronic shoulder pain, the radiographic finding of a calcification in the supraspinatus tendon or another tendon in the rotator cuff supports a diagnosis of chronic calcific tendinitis. In a few cases, particularly those with large calcific deposits, a severe attack of joint pain is precipitated by dispersal of crystals into surrounding tissues, the subdeltoid bursa, or the shoulder joint. These crystals elicit a major local inflammatory response. Patients present with severe pain and joint swelling, with warmth and erythema. The diagnosis is suspected upon radiographic observation of a rotator cuff calcification. Other diagnoses are likely to be considered, including sepsis, trauma, fracture, gout, or pseudogout. The radiographic features may evolve over time, with the calcific deposit becoming smaller, fragmenting, or disappearing. Needle aspirate of the calcific deposit may yield chalky material, and, in the case of the shoulder, may shorten the attack. Improvement also occurs following administration of NSAIDs or local corticosteroid injection. Ultrasound has been suggested as a method of breaking up calcific deposits. Untreated, the involved area may remain symptomatic for a few days or for several weeks. Smaller joints, such as the first metatarsal of the foot (hydroxyapatite pseudopodagra) and small joints of the hand, may undergo similar inflammatory attacks, particularly in younger women.

Acute Arthritis

In rare situations, BCP crystal may cause acute inflammation in joints. BCP crystal have been found in finger joints that exhibit inflammation and erosive changes. BCP crystal may have a role in inflammatory OA, a subgroup of OA associated with erythema, synovial thickening, and severe radiographic damage in proximal and distal interphalangeal joints of the hands.

Calcinosis/Idiopathic Tumoral Calcinosis

Calcinosis is the soft tissue deposition of BCP crystals. A wide variety of diseases has been associated with dystrophic calcification. Some of these conditions include the connective tissue diseases (limited scleroderma, myositis, systemic lupus erythematosus), calcification following following severe neurologic injury, and calcification following triamcinolone hexacetonide injection of joints. Idiopathic tumoral calcinosis is a rare syndrome characterized by the presence of irregular calcifying masses in periarticular soft tissue. These masses can be observed around the shoulders, hips, and elbows. They may be uni-or multifocal. Complications include skin ulceration with secondary infection, draining sinus, cachexia, and amyloidosis.

MISCELLANEOUS CRYSTALS

Oxalate Crystals

To date, oxalates have been described in joints of patients with overt renal failure only. Acute or chronic arthritis resulting from oxalate deposition can occur in a variety of joints, with the most frequently involved being the knees and hands. There are also reports of involvement of wrists, ankles, feet, tendon sheaths, and bursae. Joint fluid leukocyte counts are generally less than 2000/mm³. Definitive diagnosis is by crystal identification in joint fluid or biopsy of joints, bones, or other tissues. SF crystals can be pleomorphic but characteristically include at least some with bipyramidal or envelopelike shapes. Sizes range from 5 to 30 μm. Most crystals are brightly birefringent although some of the smaller rod-shaped crystals could be confused with CPPD. Oxalate accumulation in hemodialysis patients may be slowed by avoiding use of vitamin C, which is metabolized to oxalate.

Depot Corticosteroid-Induced Iatrogenic Inflammation

Iatrogenic inflammation typically occurs during the first 8 hours following steroid injection. It appears more common following triamcinolone hexacetonide injection than with other preparations. Diagnosis can be supported by aspiration and identification of pleomorphic crystals that include irregular shaped rods and squares with intense positive or negative birefringence. Relief can be expedited by use of local ice packs.

Other Crystals with Possible Pathogenic Potential

These include liquid lipid crystals, cholesterol, other lipids, and foreign bodies. Management of inflammatory episodes related to these less common crystals generally involves NSAIDs when the clinical situation permits. Foreign bodies are best managed by removal.

REFERENCES

1. Felson DT, Anderson JJ, Naimark A, Kannel W, Meenan RF. The prevalence of chondrocalcinosis in the elderly and its association with knee osteoarthritis: the Framingham Study. J Rheumatol 1989;16:1241–1245.

2. Zaka R, Williams CJ. Genetics of chondrocalcinosis. Osteoarthritis Cartilage 2005;13:745–750.
3. Derfus BA, Kurian JB, Butler JJ, et al. The high prevalence of pathologic crystals in pre-operative knees. J Rheumatol 2002;29:570–574.
4. Kirsch T. Determinants of pathological mineralization. Curr Opin Rheumatol 2006;18:174–180.
5. McCarty DJ. Calcium pyrophosphate dihydrate crystal deposition disease—1975. Arthritis Rheum 1976;19:275–286.
6. Masuda I, Ishikawa K. Clinical features of pseudogout attack. a survey of 50 cases. Clin Orthop 1988;173–181.
7. Ryan LM, McCarty DJ. Calcium pyrophosphate crystal deposition disease; pseudogout; articular chondrocalcinosis. In: McCarty D, ed. Arthritis and allied conditions. Philadelphia: Lea and Febiger; 1985:1515–1546.
8. Rosenthal AK, Mandel N. Identification of crystals in synovial fluids and joint tissues. Curr Rheumatol Rep 2001;3:11–16.
9. O'Shea FD, McCarthy GM. Basic calcium phosphate crystal deposition in the joint—a potential therapeutic target in osteoarthritis. Curr Opin Rheumatol 2004;16:273–278.
10. McCarty DJ, Halverson PB, Carrera GF, Brewer BJ, Kozin FK. Milwaukee shoulder: association of microspheroids containing hydroxyapatite crystals, active collagenase, and neutral protease with rotator cuff defects, I: clinical aspects. Arthritis Rheum 1981;24:464–473.

Infectious Disorders
A. Septic Arthritis

George Ho, Jr., MD

- Septic joints signal the presence of a potentially life-threatening infection. For nongonococcal joint infections, the mortality rate among adults ranges from 10% to greater than 50%.
- The most common pathway to a septic joint is through hematogenous seeding from an extra-articular site of infection, for example, pneumonia, pyelonephritis, or skin infection.
- The causes of adult nongonococcal septic arthritis are Gram-positive cocci (75%–80%) and Gram-negative bacilli (15%–20%). *Staphylococcus aureus* is most common organism in both native and prosthetic joint infections.
- Arthrocentesis and synovial fluid analysis are the cornerstones for the diagnosis of septic arthritis. If the synovial fluid white blood cell (WBC) count is extremely high (e.g., >100,000/mm^3), treatment for presumed septic arthritis should be initiated pending culture result of the fluid.
- Cell count, differential, Gram stain, culture, and examination for crystals are the crucial tests to be performed on synovial fluid. This boils down to the 3 Cs: cell count, culture, and crystals.
- In the setting of nongonococcal septic arthritis, Gram stains of infected synovial fluid are positive only 60% to 80% of the time. Blood cultures are positive in approximately 50% of patients.
- In cases of suspected septic arthritis, antibiotic treatment should begin immediately once proper samples for microbiologic studies have been collected.
- Selection of the initial antibiotic approach is guided by the result of the synovial fluid Gram stain and the organisms most likely to be responsible for the infection, based upon the clinical scenario.

Nongonococcal bacterial infections are the most serious infections affecting the joints. Normal joints, diseased joints, and prosthetic joints are all vulnerable to bacterial infection. The fact that septic joints signal the presence of a potentially life-threatening infection cannot be overemphasized, nor can the importance of early diagnosis and prompt, effective therapy. Mortality rates among adults range from 10% to greater than 50%. Full recovery is possible, but poor outcomes are common among those with preexisting arthritis, especially rheumatoid arthritis (RA). This chapter discusses acute nongonococcal bacterial arthritis in adults. Septic arthritis in children, gonococcal joint infection, and septic bursitis are also briefly discussed.

RISK FACTORS

Independent risk factors for acute nongonococcal septic arthritis are age greater than 80 years, diabetes mellitus, preexisting RA, the presence of a prosthetic joint in the knee or the hip, recent joint surgery, and skin infection (1). Compared to diseased or prosthetic joints, normal joints are very resistant to infection. An important predisposing factor to septic arthritis is an impaired immune system. RA, liver cirrhosis, chronic renal failure, and malignancies are often present among patients with septic arthritis. Hemodialysis patients and intravenous drug abusers are predisposed to bacterial joint infections at axial skeleton sites such as the sternoclavicular joint and the sacroiliac joint. Other susceptible hosts are patients with acquired immunodeficiency syndrome, hemophilia, organ transplantation, or hypogammaglobulinemia (2).

PATHOGENESIS

The most common pathway to a septic joint is bacteremic seeding of the affected joint from an extra-articular site of infection such as pneumonia, pyelonephritis, or skin infection. Direct inoculation of the pathogen into a joint is much less common. A cat bite can introduce

achieved rapidly. Tidal lavage to wash out the joint and arthroscopic procedures are intermediate steps that may benefit some patients and avoid the morbidity of arthrotomy. Under a variety of circumstances, however, surgical drainage may be necessary. Such circumstances include: (1) if when needle aspiration is technically difficult or does not provide thorough drainage of the joint; (2) if sterilization of the joint fluid is delayed; (3) if the infected joint has is already been damaged by preexisting arthritis; or (4) if infected synovial tissue or bone needs debridement (7). Involving the orthopedic surgeon and the physical therapist early in the course of treatment will facilitate the best choice of drainage procedure and result in the best functional outcome.

The optimal duration of antibiotic treatment has not been studied prospectively. For uncomplicated native joint infections, antibiotic treatment can be as brief as 2 weeks (but more often 4 weeks) if the organism is highly susceptible to the antibiotic selected. This treatment duration is typically more prolonged, between 4 and 6 weeks, for more serious infections in the compromised host. For prosthetic joint infections, the antibiotic course is usually quite protracted. For most cases of infected joint replacement, the prosthesis is removed and antibiotic treatment is continued until the site is sterile before reimplantation is considered. Antibiotic-impregnated cement or beads are sometimes employed in the reimplantation, either during multistaged procedures or during an exchange arthroplasty. On rare occasions, antibiotic treatment is continued indefinitely in the patient in whom the risk of removing the infected prosthesis is deemed too great and the microorganism responsible for the infection can be reasonably suppressed by the use of an oral antibiotic agent.

OUTCOME

Retrospective observations indicate that factors portending a poor outcome include young age, old age, virulent microorganisms, delay in the diagnosis and/or initiation of treatment, presence of underlying joint disease, and infection of particular joints (e.g., the shoulder or hip). But a prospective study confirmed that only old age, preexisting joint diseases such as RA, and the presence of a prosthetic joint constituted poor prognostic factors (8).

Avoiding delays in diagnosis, ensuring adequate decompression to prevent avascular necrosis willingness to consider alternative drainage methods when progress is not evident, and being proactive with rehabilitation are within the control of the clinician.

Although evidence-based data are lacking, intuition tells us that these considerations may improve the outcome of those with unfavorable prognostic factors.

PREVENTION

Opportunities to prevent septic arthritis are limited but should be kept in mind in patients with underlying arthritis, especially RA, and or patients with total joint replacements. For most patients who have undergone total joint replacements, antibiotic prophylaxis is not indicated routinely before dental procedures. However, in 2003 the American Dental Association and American Academy of Orthopedic Surgeons modified an earlier advisory statement regarding the use of antibiotic prophylaxis before invasive dental procedures (9). It states that antibiotic prophylaxis is not routinely indicated for most dental patients with total joint replacements. However, all patients with a total joint replacement within 2 years of the implant procedure and some immunocompromised patients with total joint replacements are at high risk for hematogenous infections should be considered for antibiotic prophylaxis before invasive dental procedures. The recommended antibiotic agents are based on an empiric regimen directed against the most common microorganisms responsible for late prosthetic joint infections (S. epidermidis).

The issue of the cost effectiveness of antibiotic prophylaxis to prevent late infections in prosthetic joints remains extremely controversial due to the lack of reliable data. No long-term observational studies or prospective trials have been done.

The incidence of late infection of a prosthetic joint as a result of procedure-related bacteremia appears to be extremely low, perhaps between 10 to 100 cases per 100,000 patients with total joint replacement per year. Until future studies provide definitive data on cost effectiveness, the decision regarding the use of antibiotic prophylaxis must be based on the physician's estimation of the potential risks, the possible benefits for individual patients, and discussions between patient and doctor.

Any local or systemic bacterial infections must be treated promptly to minimize the possible spread of the infection to the artificial joint. When confronted with an elective procedure that is likely to lead to transient bacteremia (any degree of bleeding at a site that is not normally sterile), the opportunity for antibiotic prophylaxis should be discussed and the final decision is made in consultation with the patient (Table 14A-3).

TABLE 14A-3. COUNSELING PATIENTS WITH A TOTAL JOINT REPLACEMENT REGARDING ANTIBIOTIC PROPHYLAXIS BEFORE AN INVASIVE PROCEDURE THAT LEADS TO TRANSIENT BACTEREMIA.

(1) You have (this condition, these conditions, or no condition) that may make you more susceptible to infections.

(2) The procedure that you are about to undergo may cause these kinds of bacteria to enter your bloodstream briefly. This normally results in no problems. (Brushing your teeth or moving your bowels may result in a small number of bacteria entering your bloodstream briefly in a similar manner.)

(3) Taking this antibiotic drug beforehand may reduce the likelihood of the bacteria causing problems in the replaced joint. But there is no proof or guarantee that this preventive step is 100% effective.

(4) The antibiotic medication is not very expensive. But taking it is associated with a slight risk of unpredictable side effects, similar to ones that what you may encounter with taking other medications (skin rash, nausea, vomiting, joint pain).

(5) The risk of total joint replacement infection as the result of the procedure is very small (estimated to be between 1 in 10,000 and 1 in 10,000), and taking an antibiotic beforehand may reduce the risk even further, but it will not reduce the chance to zero.

(6) If the artificial joint becomes infected, it usually means that it has to be removed and the infection has to be treated until it is cured, and then another total joint replacement procedure can be considered.

(7) In my opinion (recommend one of the three choices): a, b, or c
  (a) You most likely do not need to take an antibiotic before this procedure.
  (b) Even though taking an antibiotic before your procedure is associated with a small risk, I believe that assuming this small risk would be worthwhile in your case because of the significant implications of a joint infection and the possibility (however small) that such an infection might occur.
  (c) I believe that taking the antibiotic beforehand is worthwhile in your case.

I would be happy to review any of these points with you again before you make your decision.

SEPTIC ARTHRITIS IN CHILDREN

Septic arthritis in children is monoarticular more than 90% of the time. Knee and hip joints account for about two thirds of all cases. Children less than 2 years old are more susceptible to septic arthritis than older children. Signs of joint disease in the neonate and infant may be minimal or absent. After *S. aureus*, group B streptococcus and Gram-negative microorgan-

isms are important pathogens in the neonate and young infant. *Candida* and Gram-negative bacilli are usually acquired in the hospital or in another health care setting.

With the decline in *H. influenzae* septic arthritis in children less than 5 years old, microorganisms such as *Kingella kingae* account for a greater percentage of patients. Gonococcal infection must always be considered in the sexually active adolescent with migratory arthritis and pustular skin lesions.

Septic arthritis and osteomyelitis can coexist or complicate each other in the very young child because the metaphyseal and epiphyseal blood vessels communicate and the metaphyses of some long bones are within the joint capsule. Avascular necrosis of the femoral head is unique to septic arthritis of the hip in children. Early surgical decompression to reduce the high intra-articular pressure will restore blood flow to the femoral head. The outcome of treatment of septic arthritis in children is more favorable than in adults. Leg length discrepancy, limitation of joint mobility, and secondary degenerative joint disease are late sequelae in 25% of cases.

GONOCOCCAL JOINT DISEASE

Migratory arthritis and tenosynovitis with or without skin lesions in a sexually active adult should raise the suspicion of disseminated gonococcal infection (DGI). Joint infections caused by *Neisseria gonorrhoeae* differ from nongonococcal disease. In contrast to patients with nongonococcal arthritis, who are often elderly or have serious underlying illnesses, individuals with gonococcal (GC) arthritis are typically young, healthy adults. Women are more susceptible to DGI than men. Positive GC cultures at extra-articular sites, for example, genitourinary tract, rectum, and throat, can help confirm the diagnosis because the synovial fluid Gram stain and culture are typically negative.

Prompt response to antibiotic therapy is the rule and residual problems in the affected joint are uncommon. Resistance to penicillin is on the rise and it is wise to use a third-generation cephalosporin as the initial treatment for DGI.

SEPTIC BURSITIS

The bursae throughout the body facilitate joint mobility and many are located in close proximity to the synovial joints. The superficial bursae are more susceptible to bacterial infection than the deep bursae (10). The most common sites of septic bursitis are the olecranon and the prepatellar bursa. The pathogenesis of septic bursitis is the direct extension of a superficial skin infection into the adjacent bursa. Some of the activities that cause trauma to the superficial bursae are carpet laying, mining, plumbing, roofing, gardening, wrestling, gymnastics, and hemodialysis. *S. aureus* is the most common pathogen, responsible for greater than 80% of all cases.

Extensive cellulitis surrounding the bursa and distal edema on the affected limb are common. A careful search for skin lesions as the portal of bacteria invasion is often rewarding. A bursal effusion or fluctuance of the bursal sac on physical examination should lead to aspiration of the content.

The bursal fluid is usually inflammatory and the Gram stain is positive for Gram-positive cocci. A bactericidal antistaphylococcal agent is the initial drug of choice. In mild infections, an oral agent will suffice with outpatient follow-up and adequate drainage. If the infection is severe and the patient appears toxic, admission to the hospital for parenteral antibiotic treatment is advisable. In draining the bursa, a large bore needle is necessary when the content is thick or contains particulate matter. Surgical drainage or bursectomy is rarely necessary. The outcome of treatment of septic bursitis of the superficial bursae is usually excellent.

REFERENCES

1. Kaandorp CJE, Van Schaardenburg D, Krijnen P, et al. Risk factors for septic arthritis in patients with joint disease: a prospective study. Arthritis Rheum 1995;38: 1819–1825.
2. Franz A, Webster AD, Furr PM, et al. Mycoplasmal arthritis in patients with primary immunoglobulin deficiency: clinical features and outcome in 18 patients. Br J Rheumatol 1997;36:661–668.
3. Ho G Jr. Pseudoseptic arthritis. R I Med 1994;77:7–9.
4. Dubost J, Fis I, Denis P, et al. Polyarticular septic arthritis. Medicine 1993;72:296–310.
5. Epstein JH, Zimmermann B, Ho G Jr. Polyarticular septic arthritis. J Rheumatol 1986;13:1105–1107.
6. Post JC, Ehrlich GD. The impact of the polymerase chain reaction in clinical medicine. JAMA 2000;283: 1544–1546.
7. Ho G Jr. How best to drain an infected joint: will we ever know for certain? J Rheumatol 1993;20:2001–2003.
8. Kaandorp CJE, Krijnen P, Moens HJB, et al. The outcome of bacterial arthritis: a prospective community-based study. Arthritis Rheum 1997;40:884–892.
9. American Dental Association/American Academy of Orthopaedic Surgeons. Advisory statement: antibiotic prophylaxis for dental patients with total joint replacements. J Am Dent Assoc 2003;134:895–899.
10. Zimmermann B III, Mikolich DJ, Ho G Jr. Septic bursitis. Semin Arthritis Rheum 1995;24:391–410.

Infectious Disorders
B. Viral Arthritis

Leonard H. Calabrese, DO

- Three general patterns of virus-associated illness are observed in rheumatic disease: acute, self-limited illness; chronic infection; and latent infection, with potential for reactivation.
- Parvovirus B19 can cause a polyarticular, small-joint arthritis that mimics rheumatoid arthritis (RA).
- The "slapped cheek" rash characteristic of parvovirus B19 infections in children is seen rarely in adults.
- In contrast to RA, the duration of joint symptoms in B19 infections almost never persists beyond 1 month, and the joint disease is never erosive.
- Rubella infections are associated with fever, constitutional symptoms, cervical and posterior occipital lymphadenopathy, and a characteristic maculopapular rash.
- Hepatitis C can be associated with a variety of rheumatic complaints, none of which are associated ultimately with joint erosions: A nonerosive, nonprogressive arthritis associated with tenosynovitis and

joint symptoms out of proportion to physical findings; intermittent mono- and oligoarticular arthritis; and symmetrical polyarthritis involving small joints and resembling RA.
- The majority of patients with hepatitis C virus infections are rheumatoid factor positive, often in high titer. This frequently leads to diagnostic confusion.
- Acute hepatitis B infections are associated with the sudden onset of an inflammatory polyarthritis and often with an urticarial or maculopapular rash.
- The arthritis of hepatitis B generally precedes the onset of jaundice by days to weeks, then subsides once jaundice begins.
- Human immunodeficiency virus (HIV) infection should be considered in individuals who present with features of reactive arthritis, psoriatic arthritis, or unusual inflammatory joint complaints.

The potential relationships between many viral infections and rheumatic syndromes are confounded by the ubiquity of viral agents, and by the fact that all individuals are afflicted intermittently by viral infections of some kind. Three patterns of viral illness are useful when considering the possibility of a virus-associated rheumatic disease:

- **Acute but self-limited illness.** The pathogen produces a short-lived infection and survives by moving on to the next host. Many respiratory viruses, e.g., parvovirus B19 and rubella, fit this pattern.
- **Chronic infection**. The viral agents establish ongoing infections following the primary stage in all or only some of the patients whom they infect. Examples of viruses known to lead to chronic infections include hepatitis B (HBV), hepatitis C (HCV), and the human immunodeficiency virus (HIV).
- **Latent infection, with potential for re-activation**. In this pattern, typified by herpesviruses such as *Varicella zoster*, the primary infection may be either apparent or subclinical.

This chapter focuses on viral pathogens associated with the first two of these clinical disease patterns, as the acute (but self-limited) and chronic infection patterns are most likely to cause articular complaints. Table 14B-1 provides a full list of viral infections known to produce clinically significant forms of arthritis (1).

PARVOVIRUS B19

Parvovirus B19, a small DNA virus, is the cause of fifth disease, also known as erythema infectiosum, which is principally a disease of childhood. In addition, B19 can cause a polyarticular, small-joint arthritis that mimics rheumatoid arthritis (RA). B19 occurs in outbreaks and is spread by respiratory secretions. The secondary transmission rate to adults is about 50%. Up to 50% of healthy adults are positive for anti-B19 IgG antibodies but negative for IgM directed against this virus, indicating previous exposure to this agent and (in most cases) asymptomatic infection at some point in the past. Seronegative individuals in contact with school-aged

TABLE 14B-1. COMMON VIRAL INFECTIONS WITH PROMINENT JOINT INVOLVEMENT.

PATHOGEN	MOST CHARACTERISTIC ARTICULAR MANIFESTATIONS
Parvovirus B19	Rheumatoid arthritis–like illness lasting days to weeks after infection
Rubella virus	Morbilliform rash and self-limited polyarthritis following natural infection or vaccination
Hepatitis C virus	Chronic polyarthralgias or polyarthritis; mimic of rheumatoid arthritis
Hepatitis B virus	Acute polyarthritis in prodromal phase of hepatitis; chronic polyarthritis with systemic vasculitis
Human immunodeficiency virus (HIV)	Changing patterns of rheumatic morbidity in modern era of HIV therapy

children or with an actively infected individual are at highest risk. Eliciting a history of such contacts is essential in the evaluation of patients with an acute polyarthritis (2).

Articular symptoms in adult B19 infection generally include the acute onset of polyarthralgias or, less commonly, polyarthritis. Although the ultimate pattern of joint involvement is similar to classic RA, the arthritis of B19 infection may start in one or a few joints and spread with an additive pattern. For the purposes of diagnosis in adults, unfortunately, the striking "slapped cheek" rash so often evident in children is seen rarely. The median duration of joint symptoms is about 10 days, but pain and stiffness may persist for longer and may recur (3). In contrast to RA, however, the duration of joint symptoms almost never persists beyond 1 month in B19 infections, and the joint disease is never erosive.

Most patients with parvovirus B19 arthropathy lack rheumatoid factor, although occasional patients have been noted to have positive rheumatoid factors, antinuclear antibodies (ANAs), anti-DNA, and other autoantibodies. Other rheumatic syndromes have also been described including a lupus-like syndrome, vasculitis, and cytopenias.

The diagnosis of B19-associated arthritis depends on a high degree of clinical suspicion, often driven by the critical medical history of exposure to sick children, the appropriate clinical picture, and the detection of anti-B19 IgM antibodies. The presence of anti-B19 IgG is insufficient, as this merely indicates past infection. The detection of B19 DNA in serum by polymerase chain reaction (PCR) can also secure the diagnosis, but this is

rarely necessary. The essential elements of treatment are recognizing the self-limited nature of the condition and not confusing it with RA. Treatment is generally symptomatic, though in rare cases of chronic arthritis following acute B19 infection the administration of intravenous immunoglobulin has been reported to efficacious (3).

RUBELLA

Rubella, a small RNA virus, is spread by airborne droplets. Two or three weeks after the infection, rubella produces an exanthemous illness characterized by fever, constitutional symptoms, cervical and posterior occipital lymphadenopathy, and a characteristic maculopapular rash. Before the widespread application of vaccines, rubella occurred in epidemic patterns every 6 to 9 years. Since the introduction of aggressive immunization programs, the rates of new infections have become a mere fraction of those previously seen. Thus, many clinicians overlook rubella in the differential diagnosis of acute arthritis (1).

In the course of natural infection with rubella, symmetrical arthralgias or arthritis associated with morning stiffness may mimic RA. A more migratory pattern of joint involvement may occur, as well. Periarthritis, tenosynovitis, and carpal tunnel syndrome have also been reported. The articular phase of the illness is self-limited and generally lasts less than 2 weeks (4). Antirubella IgM antibodies appear within a few weeks of infection and persist for 4 to 6 months; thus their detection in the appropriate clinical setting is diagnostic.

Rubella can be prevented by vaccination. Postvaccination rheumatic symptomatology, however, including arthralgias, arthritis, myalgias, and paresthesias, have lessened overall enthusiasm for universal vaccination. The vaccine is a live attenuated virus that has undergone modification in recent years in the interest of diminishing arthritogenicity. Despite these modifications, adult immunization is associated with arthropathy in about 15% of individuals. These generally occur 2 weeks after immunization and last less than a week. Children undergoing immunization may develop a peculiar lumbar radiculoneuropathy that produces popliteal pain, dubbed "catcher's crouch," upon arising in the morning. This may occur 1 to 2 months following immunization and generally resolves without therapy. Rubella arthritis is managed conservatively with analgesics and nonsteroidal anti-inflammatory agents.

HEPATITIS C VIRUS

Hepatitis C virus is the major cause of post-transfusion and community acquired non-A, non-B chronic hepatitis. The natural history of HCV is generally one of a subclinical infection followed by chronicity in 70% to 80% of individuals. The incidence of HCV is 150,000 new cases each year in the United States, resulting in 93,000 cases of chronic hepatitis C. Hepatitis C, currently estimated to infect 3.5 million people nationwide, is transmitted predominantly by parenteral routes. Most patients never develop progressive liver disease, but in about 20% of cases cirrhosis or hepatocellular carcinoma ensues over two to three decades. HCV is associated with a wide variety of extrahepatic manifestations, many of which are rheumatic and immunologically driven (Table 14B-2) (5).

Articular disease manifested by painful joints is common in the setting of HCV infection. Remarkably little is known or agreed upon with regard to the articular manifestations of HCV: their clinical features, pathogenesis, natural history, or optimal therapy. Data on the prevalence of articular symptoms in HCV infection vary markedly among studies, probably due to major differences in design (e.g., reliance upon questionnaires as opposed to detailed physical examinations). Whereas studies utilizing physical examination suggest arthritis as a complication of HCV in less than 5% of patients, those employing questionnaire methodology describe joint complaints in up to 30% of infected individuals (1).

Whether HCV is associated with a distinct form of inflammatory joint disease is still unsettled, though a growing number of observational reports suggest it is. One syndrome recently described depicts a nonerosive, nonprogressive arthritis associated with tenosynovitis and joint symptoms out of proportion to physical findings. Others have found an RA-like picture, as well as an intermittent mono- and oligoarticular arthritis, all without erosive changes. On physical examination, joint tenderness is common but frank synovitis less so. Joint effusions are distinctly rare.

One of the most frequent challenges in the HCV-infected population is differentiating true RA from the polyarthritis of HCV infection. The differential diagnosis is complicated by the fact that HCV-infected individuals have a high prevalence of rheumatoid factor (RF; 50%–60%) activity as well as other laboratory

TABLE 14B-3. ESTIMATED PREVALENCE OF SEROLOGIC ABNORMALITIES IN PATIENTS WITH HEPATITIS C VIRUS INFECTION.

SEROLOGIC FINDING	PREVALENCE
Rheumatoid factor	50%–60%
Cryoglobulins	30%–40%
Antinuclear antibody	10%–40%
Monoclonal gammopathy	10%–15%
Antithyroid antibodies	5%–10%
Antiphospholipid antibodies	20%
Antismooth muscle antibody	7%–20%
Antineutrophil cytoplasmic antibody (ANCA)*	10%

SOURCE: Adapted from Vassilopoulos D, Calabrese LH. Curr Rheumatol Rep 2003;5:200–204, with permission of *Current Rheumatology Reports*.
*ANCA is hepatitis C virus infection is not directed against proteinase or myeloperoxidase.

manifestations of autoimmunity (Table 14B-3). The high proportion of HCV-infected patients who are positive for RF is explained in part by the high prevalence of cryoglobulins among HCV-infected individuals. (The IgM component of mixed cryoglobulinemia has RF activity; i.e., reacts with the Fc portion of the IgG component; see Chapter 21E.)

Although the presence of RF does not correlate with articular symptoms, it has led to much confusion in differentiating articular syndromes in HCV infection from true RA. Antibodies to CCP are of higher diagnostic sensitivity than is RF for the diagnosis of RA (6). RA patients also tend to have much more in the way of objective joint changes (i.e., frank synovitis) than patients with HCV infection, in whom arthralgias are more common. Finally, HCV-associated joint disease is not associated with erosive changes. Evidence of joint destruction or bone erosions invoke other diagnoses.

The management of HCV-associated articular manifestations remains problematic. A recent uncontrolled study of interferon-based therapy suggested that HCV-related articular manifestations may respond to aggressive antiviral therapy, but controlled trials and better clinical definitions of disease and response are needed (7). Given the potential for exacerbation of the underlying hepatic disease, all therapies must be administered with caution.

HEPATITIS B INFECTION

Hepatitis B virus (HBV) is an enveloped, partially double-stranded DNA virus. HBV is transmitted by both parenteral and sexual routes. With an estimated

TABLE 14B-2. AUTOIMMUNE CONDITIONS ASSOCIATED WITH HEPATITIS C VIRUS INFECTION.

Cryoglobulinemic vasculitis

Autoantibody production

Autoimmune cytopenias

Membranoproliferative glomerulonephritis

Sicca-like syndrome

Arthralgias and arthritis

Infectious Disorders
C. Lyme Disease

Linda K. Bockenstedt, MD

- Lyme disease is a tick-borne zoonosis caused by spirochetes of the genus *Borrelia burgdorferi sensu lato*.
- The majority of Lyme disease cases are localized to endemic foci in the United States, Europe, and Asia.
- In the United States, more than 90% of cases occur in only nine states: New York, Connecticut, New Jersey, Pennsylvania, Massachusetts, Maryland, Rhode Island, Wisconsin, and Minnesota.
- *B. burgdorferi* species are transmitted by hard-shelled ticks of the *Ixodes* complex, for example, *Ixodes scapularis* in the northeastern and north central United States.
- Upon infecting humans, *B. burgdorferi* replicates in the skin and then disseminates via the bloodstream to other organs, leading to extracutaneous disease manifestations.
- Seventy to eighty percent of Lyme disease patients develop a characteristic skin rash, erythema migrans (EM), at the site of tick feeding. The rash usually appears within days to weeks of the tick bite (range, 3–30 days).

- The hallmark of disseminated Lyme disease is the appearance of multiple EM lesions. These arise in about 50% of untreated patients with early localized disease. Secondary lesions are similar to the primary lesion, although are generally smaller in size and can appear anywhere on the body.
- Fever, malaise, myalgias, and arthralgias generally accompany dissemination of the *Borrelia* infection.
- Cardiac involvement in Lyme disease occurs in 4% to 10% of untreated patients, usually as varying degrees of atrioventricular heart block.
- Acute peripheral nervous system disease may take several forms in Lyme disease: cranial nerve palsies (unilateral or bilateral seventh nerve palsy is the most common neurological manifestation), sensorimotor radiculopathies, and mononeuritis multiplex.
- Late manifestations of Lyme disease may occur in the joints, nervous system, and skin. At this stage, joint involvement usually presents as an intermittent, oligoarticular arthritis. The knee is most commonly affected.

Lyme disease is a tick-borne zoonosis caused by spirochetes of the genus *Borrelia burgdorferi sensu lato* (1). The disease was first recognized in 1976 with evaluation of a clustering of children with presumed juvenile rheumatoid arthritis in the area around Lyme, Connecticut. The onset of arthritis was often heralded by a characteristic skin rash, erythema migrans (EM), which had been linked previously to the bite of *Ixodes ricinus* ticks in Europe and the subsequent appearance of neurologic abnormalities (Bannworth's syndrome). With time, it became apparent that arthritis was one manifestation of a multisystem disorder that involved the skin, heart, joints, and nervous system. In 1981, Willy Burgdorfer isolated the causative agent that bears his name, *Borrelia burgdorferi*, from *Ixodes scapularis* ticks collected on Long Island. The subsequent demonstration of antibodies to *B. burgdorferi* in the sera of patients with Lyme disease along with the eventual culture of the organism from tissues and body fluids confirmed the spirochetal etiology of the disorder.

EPIDEMIOLOGY

Lyme disease is widespread, with the majority of cases localized to specific endemic foci in the United States, Europe, and Asia (2). In each of these locations, *B. burgdorferi* species are transmitted by hard-shelled ticks of the *Ixodes* complex: *Ixodes scapularis* in the northeastern and north central United States, *I. pacificus* along the United States west coast, *I. ricinus* in Europe, and *I. persulcatus* in Asia. The *B. burgdorferi* species transmitted by *Ixodes* ticks differs among continents, with exclusively *B. burgdorferi sensu stricto* in North America, and *B. burgdorferi sensu stricto*, *B. afzelii*, and *B. garinii* in Europe and Asia. Although similar in genetic make-up, these Borrelia species are not identical and disease manifestations resulting from infection can vary across species. Arthritis is more common after *B. burgdorferi sensu stricto* infection. Neurologic disease is associated more strongly with *B. garinii*, and chronic skin disease with *B. afzelii* (see below).

Lyme disease is the most common vector-borne disease in the United States, with 19,804 cases reported in 2004 to the Centers for Disease Control (CDC) (3). The incidence of Lyme disease parallels the prevalence of infected ticks, with more than 90% of cases originating from just nine states: New York, Connecticut, New Jersey, Pennsylvania, Massachusetts, Maryland, Rhode Island, Wisconsin, and Minnesota. The seasonal variation of Lyme disease relates to the 2-year life cycle and feeding patterns of *Ixodes* ticks. In the northeast, larval ticks first acquire *B. burgdorferi* by feeding on small rodent reservoir hosts (especially the white-footed mouse), then molt into nymphs, the predominant vector for human disease. The peak incidence of Lyme disease occurs during the late spring and summer, when nymphal ticks feed, as adult ticks prefer to feed on white-tailed deer. Transovarial transmission of *B. burgdorferi* from infected adult female tick to egg does not occur, so a competent reservoir host, such as the white-footed mouse, is required to maintain *B. burgdorferi* in nature. This may explain the paucity of cases of Lyme disease in warmer climates, where larvae preferentially feed on noncompetent reservoirs such as lizards. Although the primary reservoir for *B. burgdorferi* is mammals, the organism can also survive in birds.

CLINICAL MANIFESTATIONS

The clinical manifestations of Lyme disease largely reflect the biology of *B. burgdorferi* as it replicates in the skin and then disseminates via the bloodstream to other internal sites where disease can be seen. Typically signs and symptoms appear in overlapping stages as early localized disease, early disseminated infection, or late disease (1,4).

Early Localized Disease

Within days to weeks of the tick bite (range, 3–30 days), 70% to 80% of infected individuals develop a characteristic skin rash, erythema migrans (EM), at the site of tick feeding [Figure 14C-1(A)]. As ticks preferentially feed in skin folds or where clothing grips the skin, common sites are the axilla, popliteal fossa, groin, and abdomen. EM typically begins as a single painless erythematous macule or papule that expands rapidly (2–3 cm/day), with some lesions more than 70 cm in diameter (most, however, are on the order of 5 cm). These features distinguish EM from reactions to the tick bite itself, which usually begins within hours and is associated with significant pruritis.

Although classically reported as a bull's eye rash, EM more commonly appears as an expanding macular lesion, occasionally with a vesicular or necrotic center. It is unusual for EM to produce local symptoms other than tingling and burning or occasionally mild pruritis.

FIGURE 14C-1

(A) Erythema migrans rash with central clearing on the shoulder of a patient. Note the central hyperpigmentation at prior tick bite site (punctum). *Borrelia burgdorferi* was isolated from a biopsy culture performed at the periphery of the lesion. (B) Multiple erythema migrans lesions on the back of a patient whose primary lesion is depicted in (A). Note absence of central papule or postinflammatory skin change. (From Nadelman RE, Wormser GP, Am J Med 1995;98:16S, with permission from Excerpta Medica, Inc.)

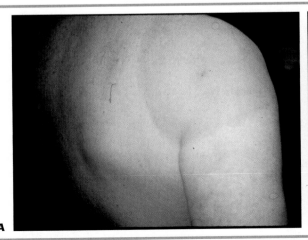
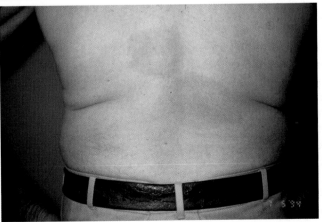

EM can be associated with systemic viral-like symptoms including malaise, fever, headache, stiff neck, myalgia, and arthralgia. These latter symptoms without EM can be the presenting manifestation in up to 18% of patients, and can be distinguished from other viral syndromes by the absence of upper respiratory or gastrointestinal involvement. Histopathology of EM lesions reveals mononuclear and lymphoplasmacytic infiltrates.

Erythema migrans must be distinguished from another EM-like rash associated with the bite of the lone star tick, *Amblyomma americanum*, found in the southeastern and south-central states. Patients with Southern tick-associated rash illness (STARI) develop a bull's eye rash but are seronegative for Lyme disease (5). A noncultivable spirochete, *Borrelia lonestari*, has been identified in *A. americanum* ticks, and one patient has been described in whom *B. lonestari* DNA was detected in a skin biopsy of the rash and in the biting tick.

Another recognized but rare skin manifestation seen in European Lyme disease is borrelial lymphocytoma, which typically presents on the earlobe or nipple as a solitary bluish-red nodule. It arises with EM or somewhat later, but may persist for months or more than a year, in contrast with EM, which usually disappears without specific therapy within weeks.

Early Disseminated Infection

Weeks to months after the onset of infection, spirochetes can disseminate to internal organs, with disease primarily seen in the skin, joints, heart, and nervous system. The hallmark of disseminated Lyme disease is the appearance of multiple EM lesions [Figure 14C-1(B)], which arise in about 50% of untreated patients with early localized disease. Secondary lesions are similar to the primary lesion, although are generally smaller in size and can appear anywhere on the body. Patients generally are ill during this phase, with fever, malaise, myalgias, and arthralgias.

Musculoskeletal involvement in Lyme disease is common at all stages of infection, but inflammatory arthritis appears in <10% of infected individuals and is considered a manifestation of late disease (see below). Fleeting migratory pains in muscles, joints, and periarticular structures, lasting only hours to days, can be seen in both early localized infection as well as in acute disseminated disease. Although myalgia is a common symptom, true myositis with elevation in muscle enzymes and abnormalities on muscle biopsy is rare.

Cardiac involvement in Lyme disease occurs in 4% to 10% of untreated patients, and typically manifests as varying degrees of atrioventricular heart block. Electrophysiology studies have demonstrated that conduction system disease occurs most commonly above the bundle of His and involves the atrioventricular node, but can involve multiple levels. Although myopericarditis can rarely occur, acute valvular disease and congestive heart failure are not found in Lyme carditis, distinguishing *B. burgdorferi* infection from acute rheumatic fever or viral myopericarditis. Lyme carditis resolves without specific therapy, but in some cases temporary pacemakers are required.

Lyme disease can affect both the peripheral and the central nervous systems. Neurologic involvement, once seen in 10% to 15% of untreated patients, has declined with earlier recognition and treatment of Lyme disease. Acute peripheral nervous system disease results in cranial nerve palsies, sensorimotor radiculopathies, and mononeuritis multiplex. Unilateral or bilateral seventh nerve palsy is the most common neurological manifestation in the United States. Even in endemic areas, however, Lyme disease accounts for only about 25% of cases of seventh nerve palsies arising during the periods of nymphal tick feeding (spring/summer). Acute central nervous system involvement presents as a lymphocytic meningitis and rarely encephalomyelitis, the latter more commonly seen in Europe. Cerebrospinal fluid examination of patients with isolated seventh nerve palsy can reveal an asymptomatic lymphocytic pleocytosis, but given the favorable outcome with oral antibiotic regimens that penetrate the central nervous system (CNS), performance of lumbar puncture is not generally recommended in the absence of suggestive signs and symptoms of meningitis or encephalomyelitis.

Disseminated *B. burgdorferi* infection can result in abnormalities in other organ systems, including the eye (keratitis), the liver (hepatitis), the spleen (necrosis), and subcutaneous tissue (panniculitis). Disease in these organ systems is rare and generally associated with more classic manifestations of Lyme disease. Routine screening for Lyme disease in the absence of other suggestive signs of *B. burgdorferi* infection in this setting is unwarranted.

Late Disease

A minority of patients develops late manifestations of Lyme disease, principally confined to the joints, nervous system, and the skin. At this stage, joint involvement may present as an intermittent, oligoarticular arthritis. The knee is most commonly affected, followed by the shoulder, the elbow, the temporomandibular joint, and the wrist. Joint effusions can be quite large (50–100 cc in the knee) but not particularly painful. Synovial fluid is inflammatory; cell counts average $25,000/mm^3$, with a neutrophil predominance. Periarticular symptoms such as bursitis and tendonitis can also be seen. Patients with Lyme arthritis can experience recurrent attacks of joint inflammation with the frequency and duration of attacks diminishing with time. Lyme arthritis can mimic other causes of mono- or pauciarticular arthritis, including the seronegative spondyloarthropathies and juvenile rheumatoid arthritis. Low back pain and spinal involvement is rare in Lyme disease, however. Less than 10% of patients with recurrent Lyme arthritis evolve a pattern of chronic unremitting synovitis involving a single joint, especially the knee. In these individuals, the spirochete DNA can no longer be detected by polymerase chain reaction (PCR) of joint fluid and synovial specimens, and further treatment with antibiotics does not alter the time to resolution, which generally occurs within 5 years.

Late neurologic manifestations of Lyme disease include encephalomyelitis, peripheral neuropathy, and encephalopathy. Encephalomyelitis is primarily seen in Europe and presents as a slowly progressive, unifocal or multifocal disease involving the white matter. A lymphocytic pleocytosis, elevated protein, and normal glucose are characteristic cerebrospinal fluid (CSF) features. Magnetic resonance imaging of the brain reveals contrast-enhancing areas of inflammation with increased signal on T2 imaging. The peripheral neuropathy of late Lyme disease presents with intermittent paresthesias in a stocking-glove distribution, occasionally associated with radicular pain. Reduced vibratory sensation can be found on physical examination, and electrophysiology studies are consistent with mononeuritis multiplex. Late encephalopathy presents with mild impairment in cognitive function and memory testing that is demonstrable on neuropsychology testing. CSF examination in this rare manifestation of Lyme disease is generally normal. Brain imaging is either normal or reveals minor, nonspecific abnormalities.

In Europe, *B. afzelii* infection can result in a chronic skin lesion, *acrodermatitis chronica atrophicans*. This skin lesion first appears as an erythematous hyperpigmented lesion that evolves to a chronic stage of hypopigmentation and atrophic, cellophane-like skin. *Acrodermatitis chronica atrophicans* responds to antibiotics if treated during the inflammatory phase. Because *B. afzelii* is not found in North America, *acrodermatitis chronic atrophicans* is not a manifestation of Lyme disease acquired on that continent.

PATHOGENESIS

Lyme disease begins when spirochetes are transmitted to humans serving as incidental bloodmeal hosts for infected ticks. *B. burgdorferi* resides in the midgut of unfed ticks and migrates to the salivary glands during the first 24 hours of tick feeding. During this period, spirochetes bind host plasminogen to disseminate within the tick, downregulate outer surface protein (Osp) A, a midgut adhesin, and upregulate Osp C, a protein required for mammalian infection. The immunomodulatory properties of *Ixodes* tick saliva promote the initial survival of spirochetes within the mammal. As an extracellular pathogen, spirochetes evade host defense mechanisms through several features, including (1) inhibition of complement through *erp* and *CRASP* gene products that bind factor H and factor H-like protein I and (2) by defeating antibody-mediated clearance through antigenic variation, especially of the *vlsE* gene. *B. burgdorferi* also expresses proteins that promote establishment of infection in the extracellular matrix and dissemination through the vasculature. These include the fibronectin-binding protein BBK32, decorin-binding proteins A and B, the integrin-binding protein p66, and the glycosaminoglycan-binding protein Bgp.

A characteristic feature of Lyme disease is that symptoms can be severe despite a paucity of organisms in tissues; much of the pathology is believed to be due to the host immune response to spirochete components. Highly inflammatory *B. burgdorferi* lipoproteins activate innate immune cells through the Toll-like receptor (TLR) family of pattern recognition receptors, principally TLR2/1 and TLR2/6 heterodimers. TLR stimulation results in a cascade of immune events, including production of inflammatory cytokines and chemokines, upregulation of adhesion molecules on endothelial cells, and priming of the adaptive T- and B-cell response. Macrophages expressing TLRs readily ingest and kill *B. burgdorferi*, but human polymorphonuclear leukocytes (PMNs) require opsonization of spirochetes for efficient phagocytosis. PMNs produce the zinc-binding protein calprotectin, which inhibits *B. burgdorferi* growth in vitro at concentrations of calprotectin found within inflamed joints.

Humoral immunity is a key host defense against *B. burgdorferi* infection. Antibodies that arise in the absence of T-cell help are sufficient to resolve inflammation and prevent challenge infection in the mouse model of Lyme borreliosis. Sera from patients with late Lyme disease contain protective antibodies. Immune complexes, found in the serum of patients with Lyme disease, are concentrated in the joints of those with Lyme arthritis. Analysis of plasma cells derived from the synovium of patients with treatment-resistant Lyme arthritis reveals evidence of expansion of the antibody a response, but the driving antigens have not been identified.

B. burgdorferi infection primes both CD4+ and CD8+ T cells and the predominance of T-helper 1–type responses correlates with more severe arthritis. The synovium of Lyme arthritis patients resembles rheumatoid synovium, with mononuclear cell infiltration and pseudolymphoid follicles formed by T cells, B cells, and plasma cells. There is an association between T- and B-cell responses to Osp A and the development of chronic antibiotic-resistant Lyme arthritis (6).

HLADRB1*0401, 0101 and related alleles are more commonly found in patients with this form of arthritis, and it has been proposed that in these individuals, Osp A immune responses are perpetuated through molecular mimicry with host proteins after *B. burgdorferi* has been cleared. Although an Osp A T-cell epitope reactive with a human LFA-1 peptide has been identified, available evidence points away from this self-peptide as a driving force for persistent inflammation. Because even treatment-resistant Lyme arthritis subsides with time (within 5 years), the immune responses detected may be appropriate and directed toward eliminating persisting antigens rather than viable organisms. Prolonged arthritis may also be due to the persistence of an abnormal immune regulatory state after the pathogen and its inflammatory products have been eliminated.

The pathogenesis of neurologic disease is more enigmatic. Peripheral neuropathy has been associated with a vasculopathy resembling endarteritis obliterans, which may secondarily lead to nerve ischemia, mononeuritis multiplex, and other manifestations of nerve dysfunction. Patients with Lyme disease rarely develop persistent neurologic abnormalities, most notably subtle cognitive changes with radicular pain or distal paresthesias. These symptoms are not responsive to antibiotics and may represent sequelae from irreversible tissue injury.

DIAGNOSIS

The diagnosis of Lyme disease should be suspected in individuals who have an appropriate clinical history and a reasonable risk of exposure to *B. burgdorferi*–infected ticks (7). The hallmark skin lesion EM is a diagnostic criterion for early Lyme disease and is sufficiently distinctive to warrant treatment without further testing. In contrast, other manifestations require supporting laboratory evidence to secure the diagnosis. Although culture is a gold standard for many bacterial infections, *B. burgdorferi* is only rarely detected by this method from diseased sites, the exception being the leading margin of EM lesions. Routine laboratory tests are nonspecific, with occasional elevation in the white blood cell count, erythrocyte sedimentation rate, and mild abnormalities of liver function tests. As noted above, analysis of synovial fluid from patients with Lyme arthritis reveals an inflammatory infiltrate (cell counts ranging from 3,000–100,000/mm³; mean, ~25,000/mm³) and the synovial histopathology is indistinguishable from that of rheumatoid arthritis or reactive arthritis. CSF examination in patients with CNS disease reveals lymphocytic pleocytosis, but oligoclonal bands are not present.

Serologic tests are the mainstay of diagnosis because they provide evidence of *B. burgdorferi* exposure. A two-tiered approach is recommended, using an enzyme-linked immunosorbent assay (ELISA) to measure serum IgM and IgG reactivity to *B. burgdorferi* as a screening tool, followed by immunoblot (Western blot) to confirm specificity (Table 14C-1). IgM reactivity usually appears within 2 to 3 weeks of infection and should be used to support a diagnosis of Lyme disease in patients with signs and symptoms present for less than 4 weeks. IgG responses are detectable after 1 month of illness and should be positive in patients with a clinical history of longer duration; IgG reactivity alone should not be used for diagnosis in these individuals. A persistently positive IgM response without IgG seroconversion is consistent with a false-positive test. Both rheumatoid factor and antinuclear antibodies can give rise to positive Lyme serology by ELISA. An IgM and IgG immunoblot of *B. burgdorferi* antigens separated by molecular weight should be used to confirm antibody specificities for all positive or equivocal ELISA samples, but should not be routinely performed on negative ELISA samples. Patients with Lyme disease may test negative within the first 1 to 2 weeks of infection. A synthetic C6 peptide ELISA, which measures antibodies to a constant region of the VlsE protein, may be useful in the early diagnosis of Lyme disease. The high specificity (99%) and sensitivity (74% in acute Lyme disease to 100% in late Lyme disease) of this assay are particularly helpful when patients present with only viral-like symptoms in the absence of EM. In the case of Lyme meningitis, intrathecal antibodies to *B. burgdorferi* can be detected. Evidence of an elevated CSF to serum IgG ratio is supportive of CNS infection. Positive serologic tests must be interpreted in the clinical setting; the rate of seropositivity in asymptomatic individuals may be as high as 4% in endemic areas. The vast majority of patients with disseminated infection are seropositive; in those with initially negative or equivocal tests, a follow-up convalescent titer 2 weeks after the first sample will often be positive, even with antibiotic therapy. Once positive, IgM and

TABLE 14C-1. CRITERIA FOR WESTERN BLOT INTERPRETATION IN THE SEROLOGIC CONFIRMATION OF LYME DISEASE.

ISOTYPE TESTED	CRITERIA FOR POSITIVE TEST
IgM	Two of the following three bands are present: 23 kDa (OspC), 39 kDa (BmpA), and 41 kDa (Fla)
IgG	Five out of 10 bands are present: 18 kDA, 21 kDa, 28 kDa, 39 kDa, 41 kDa, 45 kDa, 58 kDa (not GroEL), 66 kDa, and 93 kDa

SOURCE: Adapted from Centers for Disease Control and Prevention, Recommendations for test performance and interpretation from the Second National Conference on Serologic Diagnosis of Lyme Disease, MMWR 1995; 44:590–591.

IgG antibody titers may remain elevated for months to years after treatment and should not be used to monitor response to therapy.

Other methods for detecting *B. burgdorferi* infection include PCR amplification of spirochete DNA targets from tissues and body fluids. This technique has been used with variable success to detect *B. burgdorferi* DNA in synovial fluid and CSF specimens from patients with Lyme disease. Up to 85% of synovial fluid specimens may test positive, whereas *B. burgdorferi* DNA could be detected in less than 40% of CSF specimens from patients with Lyme meningitis. Other tests, such as a urine antigen test and blood microscopy for borrelia have not been validated.

Imaging modalities for CNS disease can provide supporting evidence of neurologic abnormalities, but no imaging findings are diagnostic of CNS Lyme disease. Magnetic resonance imaging of the brain is generally normal, but 25% of patients with encephalopathy may have white matter lesions. Absence of oligoclonal bands in the CSF helps distinguish patients with CNS Lyme disease from those with multiple sclerosis, in whom oligoclonal bands are typically present and serologic tests for Lyme disease are negative.

TREATMENT AND PROGNOSIS

Recommendations for treatment of Lyme disease, recently revised, are summarized in Table 14C-2 (8). Doxycycline, amoxicillin, and cefuroxime axetil are effective therapies for early localized or early disseminated Lyme disease in the absence of neurologic manifestations or high degree atrioventricular block. Doxycycline is the preferred antibiotic because it is also effective against another tick-borne pathogen, *Anaplasma phagocytophilum*, which causes human granulocytic anaplasmosis. Macrolides are not as effective as the other antimicrobials and should not be used as first-line therapy. First generation cephalosporins are ineffective. Most manifestations of Lyme disease can be managed with oral therapy, the exceptions being any neurologic involvement other than isolated cranial nerve palsy, cardiac disease with advance atrioventricular block, and recurrent arthritis after oral therapy.

In general, the response to therapy correlates with duration of signs and symptoms, with late manifestations requiring weeks to months for improvement or resolution. Antibiotic therapy may not hasten the resolution of cranial nerve palsies or carditis, which resolve without therapy, but patients should be treated to avoid other complications from Lyme disease. Individuals with early Lyme disease who present with more severe viral-like symptoms or who have persistent fever after 48 hours of antibiotic therapy should be evaluated for evidence of co-infection with *A. phagocytophilum* or *Babesia microti*, particularly if there is associated unexplained leucopenia, thrombocytopenia, or anemia. Patients with Lyme arthritis who fail to respond completely to oral therapy should receive a second course of either oral or intravenous therapy. If arthritis persists and PCR analysis of synovial tissue or fluid is negative for *B. burgdorferi* DNA, then treatment with nonsteroidal anti-inflammatory drugs, intra-articular corticosteroid injections, or disease-modifying antirheumatic drug (DMARD) therapy with plaquenil may be considered. Synovectomy for chronic Lyme arthritis can be curative. Individuals with late neurologic abnormalities may not respond completely to antibiotic therapy because of irreversible tissue injury. Re-treatment of this subgroup of patients is not generally recommended unless there is objective evidence of relapse or progression of disease. Serologies and intrathecal antibody production are not useful to assess response to therapy as successfully treated patients may have positive tests that persist for years.

Treatment of Lyme disease in pregnancy follows the same recommendations as for the nonpregnant state except that doxycycline should be avoided. While maternal–fetal transmission of *B. burgdorferi* can occur, there is no evidence that *B. burgdorferi* infection results in fetal abnormalities or demise in cases where the mother has received recommended antibiotic therapy. *B. burgdorferi* infection cannot be transmitted by ingestion of breast milk.

About 10% of patients may experience a Jarisch–Herxheimer reaction within 24 to 48 hours of initiation of antibiotic therapy. This condition is self-limited; supportive care with reassurance and nonsteroidal anti-inflammatory agents may help relieve symptoms. Most patients with Lyme disease respond to the recommended courses of antibiotics without significant objective sequelae, but a minority may complain of persistent fatigue, musculoskeletal pain, and cognitive dysfunction. Objective findings are generally lacking. In a study of these individuals with a previously well-documented history of Lyme disease, an extended course of antibiotics (30 days of intravenous ceftriaxone followed by 60 days of oral doxycycline) had no effect on symptoms when compared to a placebo group (9). The conclusion regarding these subjective complaints is that Lyme disease may result in a post-Lyme syndrome similar to fibromyalgia or chronic fatigue syndrome. There are, however, numerous reports of patients with chronic subjective complaints in whom serologic tests are negative yet who receive extended courses of antibiotics for Lyme disease (10). Many of these individuals report a partial response rate to therapy, which may be a placebo effect or due to anti-inflammatory properties of the antibiotics themselves that are unrelated to antimicrobial actions. When evaluated at academic medical

TABLE 14C-2. RECOMMENDED TREATMENT OF LYME DISEASE.[a,b]

MANIFESTATION	DRUG	ADULT DOSAGE	PEDIATRIC DOSAGE	DURATION (RANGE)
Erythema migrans (Recommended)	Doxycycline[c]	100 mg po b.i.d.	<8 years, not recommended ≥8 years, 4 mg/kg/day in two divided doses (max 100 mg/dose)	14 days (10–21 days)
	Amoxicillin	500 mg po t.i.d.	50 mg/kg/day in three divided doses	14 days (10–21 days)
	Cefuroxime axetil	500 mg po b.i.d.	30 mg/kg/day in two divided doses	14 days (10–21 days)
Erythema migrans (Alternative)[d]	Azithromycin	500 mg po q.i.d.	10 mg/kg q.i.d. (max 500 mg/day)	7–10 days
	Clarithromycin	500 mg po b.i.d	7.5 mg/kg b.i.d.	14–21 days
	Erythromycin	500 mg po q.i.d.	12.5 mg/kg q.i.d. (max 500 mg/dose)	14–21 days
Acute neurologic disease Cranial nerve palsy[e] Meningitis or radiculopathy[f] (Alternative IV)	Same as oral regimens for erythema migrans			14 days (10–21 days)
	Ceftriaxone	2 g IV q.i.d.	50–75 mg/kg IV q.i.d. in single dose (max 2 g/day)	14 days (10–28 days)
	Cefotaxime	2 g IV q8h	150–20 mg/kg/d IV in three to four divided doses (max 6 g/day)	
	Penicillin G	18–24 million units	200,000–400,000 U/kg/day divided q4h (max 18–24 million U/day)	
Cardiac disease[g]	Same as for erythema migrans *or*			14 days (10–21 days)
	IV regimen as for neurologic disease			14 days (10–21 days)
Late disease Arthritis without neurologic	Same as for erythema migrans			28 days (28 days)
Recurrent arthritis after oral regimen	Repeat oral regimen *or*			
	IV regimen as for neurologic disease			14 days (14–28 days)
Central or peripheral nervous system disease	IV regimen as for acute neurologic disease			14 days (14–28 days)

SOURCE: Adapted from Wormser GP, et al., Clin Infect Dis 2006;43:1089–1134, by permission of *Clinical Infectious Diseases*.

[a,b] Complete response to treatment may be delayed beyond the treatment period, regardless of the clinical manifestation, and relapse may recur. Patients with objective signs of relapse may need a second course of treatment.

[c] Tetracyclines are relatively contraindicated in pregnant or lactating women and in children <8 years of age.

[d] Due to their lower efficacy, macrolides are reserved for patients who are unable to take or who are intolerant of tetracyclines, penicillins, and cephalosporins.

[e] Patients without clinical evidence of meningitis may be treated with an oral regimen. The recommendation is based on experience with seventh cranial nerve palsy. Whether oral therapy would be as effective for patients with other cranial neuropathies is unknown; the decision between oral and parenteral therapy should be individualized.

[f] For nonpregnant adult patients intolerant of beta-lactam agents, doxycycline 200–400 mg/day orally (or IV if unable to take oral medications) in two divded doses may be adequate. For children ≥8 years of age, the dosage of doxycycline for this indication is 4–8 mg/kg/day in two divided doses (maximum daily dosage of 200–400 mg).

[g] A parenteral antibiotic regimen is recommended at the start of therapy for patients who have been hospitalized for cardiac monitoring; an oral regiment may be substituted to complete a course of therapy or to treat outpatients. A temporary pacemaker may be required for patients with advanced heart block.

centers, the majority of such patients do not have objective evidence of *B. burgdorferi* exposure or infection. Some have other treatable diseases.

PREVENTION

The most effective strategy to prevent Lyme disease is to limit potential exposure to infected ticks through environmental and personal protective measures. Eliminating brushy areas and spraying properties with insecticides can reduce the local tick population. For individuals in endemic areas, wearing protective cloth-

ing, topical application of DEET-containing insect repellents, and daily personal surveillance to remove ticks can reduce the risk of infection. For individuals bitten by *Ixodes* ticks that have been attached for ≥36 hours, a single 200 mg dose of doxycycline (or 4 mg/kg for children ≥8 years of age) is effective at preventing Lyme disease, but no data are available regarding other tick-borne diseases. This therapy is not recommended unless the tick was acquired in an area where the tick infection rate is ≥20%. A recombinant Osp A–based Lyme disease vaccine received US Food and Drug Administration approval and was briefly available for prevention of Lyme disease. Although phase I to III studies demonstrated that the vaccine was safe and 80% effective at preventing Lyme disease after three doses, it was withdrawn in part because of public concern for potential vaccine-related side effects, especially Osp A–associated arthritis.

REFERENCES

1. Steere AC, Coburn J, Glickstein L. The emergence of Lyme disease. J Clin Invest 2004;113:1093–1101.
2. Dennis DT, Hayes EB. Epidemiology of Lyme borreliosis. In: Kahl O, Gray JS, Lane RS, Stanek G, eds. Lyme borreliosis: biology, epidemiology and control. Oxford: CABI Publishing; 2002:251–280.
3. Lyme disease statistics. Centers for Disease Control Web site. Available at: http://www.cdc.gov/ncidod/dvbid/lyme/ld_statistics.htm.
4. Bockenstedt LK. Lyme disease. In: Imboden JB, Hellmann DB, Stone JH, eds. Current diagnosis and treatment in rheumatology. 2nd ed. New York: McGraw-Hill. 2007:372–382.
5. James AM, Liveris D, Wormser GP, et al. *Borrelia lonestari* infection after a bite by an *Amblyomma americanum* tick. J Infect Dis 2001;183:1810–1814.
6. Steere AC, Falk B, Drouin EE, et al. Binding of outer surface protein A and human lymphocyte function-associated antigen 1 peptides to HLA-DR molecules associated with antibiotic treatment-resistant Lyme arthritis. Arthritis Rheum 2003;48:534–550.
7. Aquero-Rosenfeld ME, Wang G, Schwartz I, et al. Diagnosis of Lyme borreliosis. Clin Microbiol Rev 2005; 18:484–509.
8. Wormser GP, Dattwyler RJ, Shapiro ED, et al. The clinical assessment, treatment, and prevention of lyme disease, human granulocytic anaplasmosis, and babesiosis: clinical practice guidelines by the Infectious Diseases Society of America. Clin Infect Dis 2006;43:1089–1134.
9. Klempner MS, Hu LT, Evans J, et al. Two controlled trials of antibiotic treatment in patients with persistent symptoms and a history of Lyme disease. N Engl J Med 2001;345:85–92.
10. Cairns V, Godwin J. Post-Lyme borreliosis syndrome: a meta-analysis of reported symptoms. Int J Epidemiol 2005;34:1340–1345.

Infectious Disorders
D. Mycobacterial, Fungal, and Parasitic Arthritis

STEVEN R. YTTERBERG, MD

- Osteoarticular involvement occurs in about 5% of patients with tuberculosis (TB), with estimated percentage ranging from about 2% of all TB cases in the United States to more than 6% in developing countries.
- Pott's disease (spinal tuberculosis) is the most common form of osteoarticular infection with *Mycobacterium tuberculosis*.
- Articular TB is usually due to reactivation of a hematogenously seeded focus and need not be associated with active disease elsewhere; it can also spread from adjacent osteomyelitis.
- Lengthy delays in diagnosis—on the order of 3 to 4 years—are reported.
- Poncet's disease is a form of reactive arthritis occurring during active TB.
- *Mycobacterium marinum* infection is often associated with such aquatic exposures as fish tank water, fish hook lacerations, skin punctures by fish spines, and cuts from boat motor propellers.

- The syndrome of erythema nodosum leprosum, manifested as crops of subcutaneous nodules, fever, and arthralgia or arthritis, occurs in patients with lepromatous leprosy.
- *Valley fever* (or *desert rheumatism*) are terms used for an immune complex–mediated syndrome associated with cocciodiomycosis infection. This syndrome, which is self-limited, is characterized by joint complaints, fever, rash, erythema nodosum, erythema multiforme, eosinophilia, and hilar adenopathy.
- Sporotrichosis, which usually presents as a painful erythematous nodule at the site of a skin wound. Inoculation of the organism *Sporothrix schenckii* into the skin through gardening or landscape exposures to soil or plant material is the mode of pathogenesis (the classic exposure is to a rose thorn).

Mycobacteria, fungi, and parasites are unusual causes of musculoskeletal infections. Infections with these organisms are seen with growing frequency in the United States, however, for two major reasons: (1) increasing numbers of persons who are immunosuppressed because of the presence of debilitating diseases, medical therapy, advanced age, or human immunodeficiency virus (HIV) infection; and (2) greater immigration from developing countries endemic for these infections. These agents should be considered in patients with chronic monoarticular arthritis, but they may present with other manifestations, including osteomyelitis, spondylitis, tendonitis, and erythema nodosum (Table 14D-1). Definitive diagnosis usually depends on identification of the responsible organism in pus, synovial fluid, or tissue. Some agents, however, may cause inflammatory disease without direct infection, resembling reactive arthritis.

MYCOBACTERIA

Mycobacterium Tuberculosis

Infection with *M. tuberculosis*, usually acquired by inhalation, begins as nonspecific pneumonitis, followed by lymphatic and hematogenous spread to upper lobes of the lung and other organs. In immunocompetent hosts, infection is limited by cellular immunity. Reactivation may occur during a period of diminished host immunity, with multiplication of bacilli in dormant foci, and spread via lymphatics or blood. Osteoarticular involvement occurs in about 5% of patients with tuberculosis (TB), with estimated percentages ranging from about 2% of all TB cases in the United States to more than 6% in developing countries (1). In children, bone infection typically occurs via hematogenous seeding during primary pulmonary infection. In contrast, in adults,

TABLE 14D-1. TYPICAL PRESENTATIONS OF OSTEOARTICULAR INFECTIONS CAUSED BY MYCOBACTERIA AND FUNGI.

Mycobacteria

Tuberculosis	Spondylitis (Pott's disease)
	Monarticular arthritis of large weight-bearing joints
	Osteomyelitis and dactylitis
	Bursitis and tenosynovitis
	Reactive arthritis (Poncet's disease)
BCG treatment	Migratory arthritis or arthralgia
Atypical mycobacteria	Arthritis or tendonitis of hand or wrist
	Multifocal bone, joint, or tendon infection
Leprosy	Polyarthritis with erythema nodosum leprosum
	Destructive arthritis of small bones and joints of hands and feet
	Neuropathic arthritis of wrists or ankles

Fungi

Candidiasis	Polyarthritis with osteomyelitis in seriously ill infants
	Monarticular arthritis of knee in seriously ill patients past infancy
Coccidioidomycosis	Polyarthritis with erythema nodosum
	Monarticular arthritis of knee
	Osteomyelitis
Sporotrichosis	Monarticular arthritis of knee, wrist, or hand
	Polyarthritis with disseminated cutaneous lesions
Blastomycosis	Osteomyelitis
	Spondylitis
	Monarticular arthritis of weight-bearing joints with lung and cutaneous lesions
Cryptococcosis	Osseous infection
	Spondylitis
	Rare monarticular arthritis
Histoplasmosis	Polyarthritis with erythema nodosum

ABBREVIATION: BCG, Bacillus Calmette-Guerin.

bone infection usually occurs from either a quiescent pulmonary focus or an extrapulmonary site. Tuberculin skin tests are positive in most patients with osteoarticular TB, but chest radiographs are often normal. The definitive diagnosis is made by the demonstration of *M. tuberculosis* in tissue or synovial fluid.

The classic presentation of osteoarticular infection is spinal TB, or Pott's disease. Infections at peripheral sites, especially weight-bearing joints, tendons, bursae, or bones, also occur. Reactive arthritis (Poncet's disease) has been reported (see below).

Spinal Tuberculosis

Pott's disease is the most common form of osteoarticular infection with *M. tuberculosis* (2). Thoracic vertebrae are involved most frequently, followed by lumbar, and, less commonly, cervical and sacral vertebrae. In regions endemic for TB, spinal TB is primarily a disease of children and young adults. In the United States and Europe, most cases are in adults, occurring by reactivation of dormant foci (3).

Infection characteristically begins in the anterior portion of the vertebral bodies, with subsequent disc involvement, disc space narrowing, destruction of vertebral end plates, and collapse of the anterior portion of the vertebral body, causing the characteristic gibbus deformity (Figure 14D-1) (1,4). Infection often extends to adjoining discs or vertebrae, or to distant sites. Localized soft tissue inflammation, for example, paravertebral or psoas abscesses or sinus tracts may ensue, accompanied by neurologic injury.

Spinal TB can mimic vertebral osteomyelitis (spondylodiskitis) caused by pyogenic bacteria, but usually has a longer duration of symptoms. Fever is less common in Pott's disease (5). Back pain and tenderness are present in most patients. Neurologic manifestations from compression of spinal cord or roots occur in 12% to 50% of patients. Active pulmonary TB may be absent, but there is often evidence of past disease.

Radiographs typically show disc space narrowing with vertebral collapse and paraspinous abscess (4). Computerized tomography (CT) can define the bony anatomy and paraspinal masses. Magnetic resonance imaging (MRI) can reveal the extent of inflammation and impingement of neural structures. The differential diagnosis is broad, including other infections, neoplasm, and sarcoidosis; bacteriologic confirmation is required. Diagnosis is best made by CT-guided or open biopsy.

Therapy is complicated by the increase in drug-resistant TB. Six to nine months of combination chemotherapy including rifampin is recommended (6). The role of surgery is not clearly defined. Indications for surgery have included the presence of motor deficits, spinal deformity, a nondiagnostic needle biopsy, and noncompliance with or lack of response to medical therapy. However myelopathy and functional impairment can resolve with chemotherapy alone (6). Although adjunctive glucocorticoids are recommended for some extrapulmonary manifestations of TB, such treatment is not recommended for musculoskeletal involvement (6).

Tuberculous Arthritis

Tuberculous arthritis occurs mainly as monoarticular arthritis affecting a hip or knee, but may involve other joints (1,7,8). Most patients are middle-aged or older, often with underlying medical disorders. The onset is

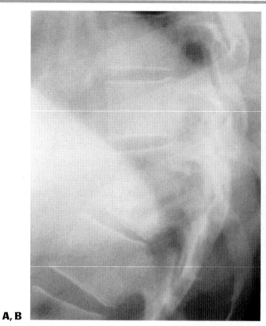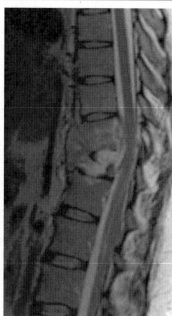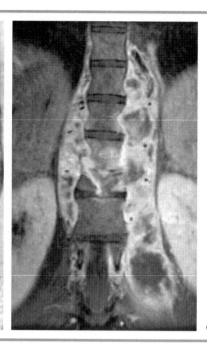

FIGURE 14D-1

Tuberculous spondylitis (Pott's disease). (A) A lateral radiograph of the thoracic spine shows destruction of adjacent vertebral endplates of the T10 and T11 vertebrae with disc space narrowing and vertebral collapse, resulting in a gibbus deformity. (B) A lateral T2 weighted magnetic resonance imgaing (MRI) scan of the thoracic spine in the same patient demonstrates inflammation in the area of collapse and extension anteriorly. (C) An anterioposterior T2 weighted MRI image of the thoracic spine of the same patient demonstrates a multilocular soft tissue mass extending above and below the area of vertebral collapse. (Courtesy of Dr. Timothy Maus, Mayo Clinic, Rochester, MN.)

typically insidious. Joint pain and swelling are usually present, but signs of inflammation may be limited. Lengthy delays in diagnosis—on the order of 3 to 4 years—are reported. Articular TB is usually due to reactivation of a hematogenously seeded focus and need not be associated with active disease elsewhere; it can also spread from adjacent osteomyelitis. Tuberculous osteomyelitis can occur without joint involvement. In adults, a single lesion is most common, usually involving the metaphysis of a long bone. In children, the hands and feet may be involved, causing tuberculous dactylitis.

Characteristic radiographic findings of tuberculous arthritis are juxta-articular osteoporosis, marginal erosions, and gradual joint space narrowing (Phemister's triad). Similar changes can occur in other forms of infection or rheumatoid arthritis. Compared with pyogenic joint infections, however, joint space is preserved early in TB arthritis. Additional radiographic findings that may be present include soft tissue swelling, subchondral cysts, bony sclerosis, periostitis, and calcifications.

The synovial fluid white blood cell count is generally elevated, usually with a predominance of neutrophils but occasionally of lymphocytes (9). The glucose in the synovial fluid is usually low. Synovial fluid acid-fast

smears are positive in about 20% of cases, and culture is positive in up to 80%. The diagnosis of tuberculous arthritis is best made by histologic and microbiologic examination of synovium. Synovial cultures are positive in over 90% of cases. Histology may demonstrate caseating or noncaseating granulomas.

Tuberculous arthritis usually responds to combination chemotherapy (1,6,8). Surgery may be needed for synovectomy, debridement, joint stabilization, or removal of infected prostheses.

Poncet's Disease

Poncet's disease is a form of reactive arthritis occurring during active TB (10). Polyarticular arthritis typically involves the hands and feet. Joint fluid and tissue samples are sterile. Symptoms abate with antituberculous treatment.

Mycobacterium Bovis and Bacillus Calmette-Guerin

Mycobacterium bovis infection is now rare, but musculoskeletal symptoms have been related to attenuated *M. bovis* as a component of Bacillus Calmette-Guerin

(BCG) (11). Intravesicular BCG instillation for bladder cancer has been associated with fever, malaise, and migratory polyarticular arthralgia or arthritis in a minority of patients. Symptoms worsen with repeated treatments and can be prevented by isoniazid. Considerable debate exists within the literature about whether the inflammation is an immune-mediated response, or whether it represents a manifestation of active BCG infection. Some musculoskeletal complications of this therapy, for example, monoarticular arthritis accompanied by the isolation of *M. bovis* from joints, are clearly related to active infection. Reactive arthritis and Sjögren's syndrome have also been reported.

Atypical Mycobacteria

Musculoskeletal involvement with atypical (nontuberculous) mycobacteria can mimic TB and include bone, joint, tendon, and bursal infection. Infections are indolent, with insidious onset. The peak age incidence is 40 to 69 years, with a male-to-female ratio of 3:1 (12). The majority of infections are caused by *M. marinum, M. kansasii,* and *M. avium* complex. Various other mycobacterial species are identified in the remaining cases. A history of prior trauma, surgery, or intra-articular injection is usual, but occasionally hematogenous seeding occurs. Glucocorticoid use and underlying arthritis are additional risk factors. *M. marinum* infection is often associated with such aquatic exposures as fish tank water, fish hook lacerations, skin punctures by fish spines, and cuts from boat motor propellers.

Any joint, bursa, or tendon sheath may be infected, but the hands are most frequently involved, followed by the wrists and knees. Polyarticular involvement occurs in less than one fourth of patients. The most common presentation is joint swelling, followed by joint pain and limited motion. Carpal tunnel syndrome may arise from synovitis involving the flexor tendons of the wrist. A slowly healing cutaneous wound may be present. Constitutional symptoms, such as fever, chills, weight loss, and malaise are infrequent.

Radiographs of affected joints are often normal. If abnormalities are present, they are usually soft tissue swelling, effusion, bony erosion, or joint destruction. A pattern of preservation of the central joint space with marginal erosion containing sclerotic borders of adjacent bone has been described.

Synovial fluid may be noninflammatory or markedly inflammatory. Pathology typically demonstrates noncaseating granulomas, but the absence of granulomas does not exclude the diagnosis. Diagnosis is made by demonstration of mycobacteria in synovial fluid or tissue. Negative cultures do not rule out infection, as these organisms can be difficult to cultivate.

Treatment of atypical mycobacterial joint infections involves a combination of antituberculous therapy and surgery. Most strains of nontuberculous mycobacteria are resistant to antituberculous drugs to some degree. Combination chemotherapy is required for most.

Mycobacterium Leprae

Leprosy can cause several forms of arthritis (13,14). Erythema nodosum leprosum occurs in patients with lepromatous leprosy. Manifestations include crops of subcutaneous nodules, fever, and arthralgias or arthritis. The joint symptoms usually are mediated by an immunologic mechanism, but septic arthritis with *M. leprae* in synovial fluid occurs infrequently. Chronic erosive arthritis of large and small joints resembling rheumatoid arthritis, which improves with treatment of the leprosy, is also described. In late stages of leprosy, Charcot joints may develop due to sensory neuropathy and repeated trauma.

FUNGI

Most fungal musculoskeletal infections have an insidious onset, an indolent course, and generally mild inflammation. Other than positive cultures, laboratory findings are nonspecific.

Candida

Candida species are commensal organisms in humans. They are the most common cause of opportunistic infection among fungi, but rarely cause joint infection (15). Fungi, most commonly *Candida albicans*, cause only 1% of infected prosthetic joints (16). Arthritis can arise from direct inoculation or hematogenous spread of organisms (16,17). Intra-articular inoculation may occur during joint surgery or arthrocentesis. Infection is typically indolent, monarticular, and chronic. Symptoms may not develop until 2 years after surgery. Loosening of prosthetic components is seen radiographically. When related to arthrocentesis, infection is usually caused by species other than *C. albicans*.

Hematogenous spread of *C. albicans* to joints can occur during disseminated candidiasis. Disseminated candidiasis is associated with drug abuse; among non–drug abusers, it is seen in seriously ill patients receiving intensive medical care, notably hospitalized infants. In infants, *Candida* arthritis is usually polyarticular and associated with local osteomyelitis. Older patients with disseminated candidiasis typically have a serious illness treated with antibiotics, chemotherapy, and/or immunosuppressive agents. The clinical course may be acute, with marked synovitis, or milder and more indolent. Arthritis is monarticular in about 75% of cases. Septic bursitis may occur.

The diagnosis is made by culture of synovial fluid or tissue. Treatment with systemic or intra-articular amphotericin B has been successful. 5-Fluorocytosine may be helpful as an adjunct to amphotericin B, but should not be used alone because of resistance. Ketoconazole and fluconazole have been successful in treating candidal infection, but the *Candida* species causing infection must be identified, as some nonalbicans species are resistant (18). Treatment of infected prosthetic joints usually requires removal of the prosthesis and debridement.

Coccidioidomycosis

Coccidioidomycosis is caused by *Coccidioides immitis*, a soil fungus endemic in semi-arid areas of the southwestern United States, Central America, and South America. Osteoarticular involvement can occur during primary or disseminated infection.

Primary infection is often asymptomatic, but about 40% of patients develop self-limited symptoms that range from flulike complaints to pneumonia. *Valley fever* or *desert rheumatism* are terms used for a self-limited, immune complex–mediated syndrome of arthralgias or arthritis that can occur during primary infection. Fever, rash, erythema nodosum, erythema multiforme, eosinophilia, and hilar adenopathy may occur. The arthritis, usually polyarticular and migratory, resolves within 4 weeks without treatment (15).

Chronic pulmonary infection occurs in about 2% of patients and disseminated disease is seen in about 0.2%. Arthritis and osteomyelitis can occur during disseminated infection. The most frequent articular manifestation is chronic arthritis of one knee. Nodular cutaneous lesions and draining sinuses may be present (19). Radiographs show lytic lesions and bony erosions. Delay in diagnosis averages over 4 years. Osteomyelitis occurs in 10% to 20% of patients with disseminated disease, most often involving ends of long bones, the skull, vertebrae, and ribs.

Synovial fluid samples rarely yield *C. immitis*. The diagnosis is best made by demonstration of organisms in tissue. Treatment involves surgical drainage of pus, debridement, or synovectomy, and chemotherapy with amphotericin B. Early infections have been treated with azole antifungal agents, but infection may recur after stopping therapy (15,18). Intra-articular amphotericin B has been reported to be useful.

Sporotrichosis

Sporotrichosis, caused by *Sporothrix schenckii*, is usually limited to cutaneous disease, presenting as a painful erythematous nodule at the site of a skin wound. Inoculation of the organism into the skin through gardening or landscape exposures to soil or plant material is the mode of pathogenesis (the classic exposure is to a rose thorn). Infection is spread by lymphatic drainage or local extension.

Extracutaneous disease primarily affects musculoskeletal structures, causing arthritis, tenosynovitis, oste-

itis, or granulomatous myositis (19). Cutaneous findings are present in most patients with musculoskeletal disease. The arthritis, usually chronic, may be monoarticular or polyarticular, involving the knees, wrists, small joints of the hands, ankles, and elbows. Disseminated sporotrichosis is rare, usually occurring in immunosuppressed or systemically ill patients. Most patients with disseminated sporotrichosis have bone or joint involvement or both. Radiographs show lytic lesions with minimal periostitis.

Synovial pathology demonstrates chronic, noncaseating granulomatous inflammation. Diagnosis is based on culture of organisms from joint fluid or tissue. Amphotericin B with or without surgical debridement is often curative, but prolonged treatment may be necessary (15,18). Azole antifungal agents and intra-articular amphotericin B have been reported to be effective.

Blastomycosis

Blastomyces dermatitidis is endemic in the Ohio and Mississippi River valleys and in the mid-Atlantic portion of the United States. Primary pulmonary infection occurs after inhalation of infectious spores; other sites are seeded by hematogenous or lymphatic spread. Skeletal infection occurs in up to 60% of patients (19). Osteomyelitis is most common, involving vertebrae, ribs, tibiae, and skull. Vertebral infection mimics TB. Arthritis is typically monoarticular but can be polyarticular (15). Patients with blastomycosis usually have constitutional symptoms and their arthritis tends to be acute in onset, characteristics that lead generally to quicker diagnoses compared with other fungal causes of arthritis. A knee is most frequently involved, followed by an ankle or elbow. Articular disease may arise from hematogenous spread or from extension from nearby osteomyelitis.

Stains of synovial fluid may reveal organisms, but definitive diagnosis requires culture. Blastomycosis can be treated with amphotericin B, ketoconazole, or itraconazole. Surgery may be required for patients who fail treatment with these drugs.

Cryptococcosis

Inhalation of *Cryptococcus neoformans* can cause clinically silent or overt pulmonary infection. Hematogenous spread may seed other organs, notably the central nervous system. Most clinically apparent disseminated cases occur in immunosuppressed patients. Osseous infection occurs in 5% to 10% with dissemination, involving the long bones, vertebrae, ribs, tarsals, and carpals with a subacute or chronic course (19). Vertebral infection may mimic TB. Radiographs show lytic lesions with little periosteal reaction. Cryptococcal arthritis is infrequent, usually due to direct extension of adjacent osteomyelitis (15,19). The diagnosis is made by demonstration of organisms in synovial fluid or tissue. Treatment is usually with amphotericin B, with or without 5-fluorocytosine. Fluconazole may be sufficient for immunocompetent hosts.

Histoplasmosis

Histoplasmosis, caused by *Histoplasma capsulatum,* is endemic in the Mississippi and Ohio River valleys of the United States. Most infections are subclinical and self-limited. During primary infection, acute self-limited migratory polyarthritis or arthralgias may occur, with or without erythema nodosum or erythema multiforme. Arthritis in these cases is immunologically mediated (15,19). Dissemination occurs in less than 0.1%, usually in elderly or immunosuppressed patients (19). Arthritis, osteomyelitis, tenosynovitis, and carpal tunnel syndrome are rarely described in disseminated histoplasmosis. Diagnosis is based on the culture of *H. capsulatum* from tissue or histologic demonstration of organisms. Successful treatment has been accomplished with amphotericin B, itraconazole, and fluconazole, but surgical debridement may be required.

Other Fungal and Related Organisms

A variety of other fungi have been reported rarely as causes of infectious arthritis (19). Invasive *Aspergillus* infection can involve a variety of organs, most often the lungs and sinuses. Direct extension of infection can result in osteomyelitis of vertebrae, ribs, or skull. Vertebral involvement can mimic Pott's disease. Articular involvement is rare (15,19). Paracoccidioidomycosis is caused by *Paracoccidioides brasiliensis*, endemic to South America. The organism may disseminate and cause osteomyelitis with extension to joints (14).

Maduromycosis, or mycetoma, is a chronic infection of skin, subcutaneous tissue, and bone, most often involving the foot (14). Maduromycosis is caused by a variety of organisms, including true fungi and actinomyces (which are actually bacteria). Infection begins with subcutaneous inoculation of organisms and local extension, with eventual development of granule-draining sinus tracts.

PARASITES

Parasites are organisms that live on or in a host organism and derive their nourishment from the host. Some parasites may persist in the host for extended periods. Parasites can be grouped as protozoa, helminths, and arthropods. Immune responses induced by parasitic infections can cause tissue injury and musculoskeletal manifestations, including hypersensitivity reactions and immune complex deposition. Such manifestations are usually benign and often resolve with treatment of the underlying infestation. Arthralgia is more common than arthritis, but the frequency of joint involvement is not clearly known (20).

Among protozoa, *Giardia lamblia* has been reported as a cause of acute-onset, mild, recurrent seronegative arthritis, similar to reactive arthritis. Other protozoa associated with arthralgia and arthritis include *Entamoeba histolytica, Trichomonas vaginalis,* and *Toxoplasma gondii.*

Several helminths have been associated with joint symptoms (20). Dracunculosis can produce arthralgia, as well as acute or chronic monarticular arthritis due to joint invasion or death of the worm in situ near a joint. Among patients with filariasis, monoarticular arthritis, often involving knee or ankle may occur. Reactive arthritis and sacroiliitis have been described with *Strongyloides stercoralis* and schistosomiasis. *Echinococcus granulosus,* which causes hydatid cysts, can lead to cystic infection of bone and pathologic fractures.

REFERENCES

1. Leonard MKJ, Blumberg HM. Musculoskeletal tuberculosis. In: Schlossberg D, ed. Tuberculosis & nontuberculous mycobacterial infections. 5th ed. New York: McGraw-Hill; 2006:242–263.
2. Martini M, Ouahes M. Bone and joint tuberculosis: a review of 652 cases. Orthopedics 1988;11:861–866.
3. Cormican L, Hammal R, Messenger J, Milburn HJ. Current difficulties in the diagnosis and management of spinal tuberculosis. Postgrad Med J 2006;82:46–51.
4. Ridley N, Shaikh MI, Remedios D, Mitchell R. Radiology of skeletal tuberculosis. Orthopedics 1998;21:1213–1220.
5. Perronne C, Saba J, Behloul Z, et al. Pyogenic and tuberculous spondylodiskitis (vertebral osteomyelitis) in 80 adult patients. Clin Infect Dis 1994;19:746–750.
6. Blumberg HM, Burman WJ, Chaisson RE, et al. American Thoracic Society/Centers for Disease Control and Prevention/Infectious Diseases Society of America: treatment of tuberculosis. Am J Respir Crit Care Med 2003;167:603–662.
7. Garrido G, Gomez-Reino JJ, Fernandez-Dapica P, Palenque E, Prieto S. A review of peripheral tuberculous arthritis. Semin Arthritis Rheum 1988;18:142–149.
8. Malaviya AN, Kotwal PP. Arthritis associated with tuberculosis. Best Pract Res Clin Rheumatol 2003;17:319–343.
9. Allali F, Mahfoud-Filali S, Hajjaj-Hassouni N. Lymphocytic joint fluid in tuberculous arthritis. A review of 30 cases. Joint Bone Spine 2005;72:319–21.
10. Dall L, Long L, Stanford J. Poncet's disease: tuberculous rheumatism. Rev Infect Dis 1989;11:105–107.
11. Tinazzi E, Ficarra V, Simeoni S, Artibani W, Lunardi C. Reactive arthritis following BCG immunotherapy for urinary bladder carcinoma: a systematic review. Rheumatol Int 2006;26:481–488.
12. Yangco BC, Espinoza CG, Germain BF. Nontuberculous mycobacterial joint infections. In: Espinosa L, Goldenberg

TABLE 14E-1. MODIFIED JONES' CRITERIA FOR DIAGNOSIS OF ACUTE RHEUMATIC FEVER.[a]

Major criteria
  Carditis
  Polyarthritis
  Chorea
  Erythema marginatum
  Subcutaneous nodules

Minor criteria
  Fever
  Arthralgia
  Elevated acute phase reactant (C-reactive protein or
    erythrocyte sedimentation rate)
  Prolonged PR interval on electrocardiogram

Supporting evidence of antecedent Group A streptococcal
  infection
  Positive throat culture or rapid antigen test
  Elevated or rising streptococcal antibody titer

[a]Diagnosis requires two major criteria or one major and two minor criteria, plus supporting evidence of antecedent group A streptococcal infection.

regurgitation without a murmur do not fulfill this criterion. Myocarditis manifests as tachycardia that is disproportionate to the degree of fever and is best assessed during sleep. Pericarditis is the least common finding in rheumatic carditis. It usually manifests as a pericardial effusion and/or friction rub. Myocarditis and/or pericarditis in the absence of valvular involvement is very unlikely to be due to ARF, and in this circumstance, other diagnoses should be explored.

Sydenham chorea (St. Vitus dance) is the manifestation of central nervous system involvement in ARF and occurs in 10% to 15% of patients. It is usually a later manifestation of ARF, occurring several months after the inciting streptococcal infection. Cross-reactive immune responses that affect the basal ganglia neurons are thought to be the etiology. The characteristic features of chorea are purposeless involuntary movements (but not stereotyped like a tic), incoordination, difficulty with handwriting, facial grimacing, and emotional lability. In one recent pediatric series, hemichorea was seen in 29% of patients (3). Chorea is a self-limited illness, and full recovery takes several months. Rarely, symptoms can occur over years and are exacerbated by stress, pregnancy, oral contraceptives, and intercurrent illnesses.

Erythema marginatum occurs in fewer than 2% of patients. It is characteristically an erythematous, serpiginous macular rash with pale central clearing. The rash usually occurs on the trunk and extremities and characteristically spares the face. The rash waxes and wanes, may be transient and is exacerbated by warmth.

Subcutaneous nodules occur in fewer than 1% of cases of ARF, most often in those with severe carditis. The nodules are firm, nontender, and are usually less than 2cm in diameter. They are typically located over bony prominences or tendon sheaths. Nodules usually resolve spontaneously without permanent sequelae.

Minor Clinical Criteria

The fever in ARF is usually greater than 39.0°C. It is usually present at the onset of illness and resolves over several weeks, even without treatment. Arthralgia may fulfill a minor criterion in the revised Jones' criteria, but only in the absence of polyarthritis. Arthralgia may be migratory, and pain may be severe, even without objective signs of arthritis.

DIAGNOSTIC TESTS

Approximately one third of patients presenting with ARF have no history of a recent symptomatic pharyngeal infection, and, therefore, it is necessary to find laboratory evidence of a recent streptococcal infection. This can be done either by (a) obtaining history of a throat culture or a GAS rapid antigen test positive for GAS from a throat swab, or by (b) documenting an elevated or rising serum antistreptococcal antibody titer. It is important for the clinician to recognize that normal values of antistreptococcal antibodies in the general population vary by patient age, geographic location, and season of the year, with highest values observed in 10 to 12 year olds and at the end of the streptococcal season (late spring) (4). The use of normal ranges established for adults for interpretation of pediatric values is misleading.

The antistreptolysin O (ASO) titer is the most commonly used streptococcal antibody test to establish a recent streptococcal infection. An ASO titer of 240 Todd units or higher in adults or in excess of 320 Todd units in children is considered modestly elevated. ASO titers above 500 Todd units are uncommon in healthy individuals and therefore more reliably serve as evidence of a recent streptococcal infection (4).

Because ASO titers can be normal in approximately 20% of ARF patients, other streptococcal antibody tests are useful to help establish a recent GAS infection; these include antideoxyribonuclease B (anti-DNase B), antistreptokinase, and antihyaluronidase. If all antistreptococcal antibody titers are normal on initial presentation and ARF remains a clinical concern, it is highly advisable to repeat these tests a few weeks later to see if the antibody titers have risen because a single low antistreptococcal antibody titer does not exclude the diagnosis of ARF.

SPECIAL TESTS

Synovial fluid analysis of the arthritis of ARF reveals a sterile inflammatory fluid typically with 10,000 to 100,000 white blood cells/mm^3 (with a predominance of neutrophils), normal glucose level, and a protein concentration of approximately 4g/dL.

The nonclinical (laboratory) minor criteria of the revised Jones' criteria include an increased PR interval on electrocardiogram (which does not per se indicate carditis) and elevated acute phase reactants (C-reactive protein and/or erythrocyte sedimentation rate). Acute phase reactants are almost always greatly elevated in ARF patients presenting with polyarthritis or acute carditis, but are often normal in patients presenting with chorea alone.

DIFFERENTIAL DIAGNOSIS

Other than ARF, the most frequently encountered diseases in the differential for acute polyarticular arthritis include juvenile rheumatoid arthritis, systemic lupus erythematosus (SLE), serum sickness, and gonococcal arthritis. Choreiform movements can occur in SLE, neoplasms involving the basal ganglia, Wilson's disease, and Huntington's disease. Chorea can occasionally be encountered in pregnancy (chorea gravidarum).

PATHOGENESIS

The pathogenesis of ARF is not completely understood, but it appears to involve immune responses to GAS antigens that then cross-react with human tissue through molecular mimicry (Figure 14E-1). Only a small percentage of individuals with untreated GAS pharyngitis go on to develop ARF. ARF is not considered a sequela of cutaneous GAS infection (5). Recent evidence supports the conclusion that ARF has declined markedly in the United States over the past four decades because of a decline in rheumatogenic types of GAS causing pharyngitis (6).

Host genetic factors appear to influence the susceptibility to ARF. Observational studies in the 19th century recognized familial tendencies to develop ARF, and in the early 1940s, studies showed familial clustering of the disease, with greatest risk occurring in children if both parents had rheumatic heart disease (7). Genetic susceptibility to develop ARF has been characterized as autosomal recessive or autosomal dominant with variable penetrance and has been linked with human leukocyte antigen (HLA) types. Significant increases in the frequency of DRB1*0701, DR6, and DQB1*0201 confer susceptibility to ARF in several international studies (8). However, monozygotic twins usually do not both develop ARF, clearly indicating that there are also important environmental factors involved in the pathogenesis of the disease (9).

TREATMENT

Treatment of ARF requires anti-inflammatory treatment, prevention of future streptococcal infections, and symptomatic care (Table 14E-2). Upon diagnosis, a dose of intramuscular benzathine penicillin or 10 days of oral penicillin or erythromycin (for penicillin-allergic patients) is recommended regardless of streptococcal

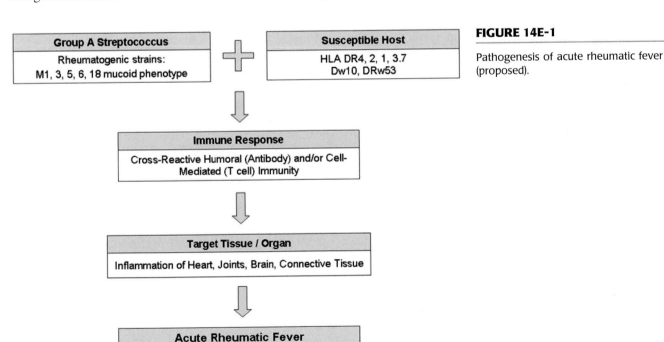

FIGURE 14E-1

Pathogenesis of acute rheumatic fever (proposed).

TABLE 14E-2. TREATMENT OF ACUTE RHEUMATIC FEVER.

CONDITION	ANTI-INFLAMMATORY TREATMENT
Mild or no carditis	Aspirin 50–100 mg/kg/day in four divided doses for 2–4 weeks, then taper over 4–6 weeks
Moderate or severe carditis	Prednisone 2 mg/kg/day in two doses for 2–4 weeks, then taper over about 4 weeks, with addition of aspirin when prednisone is ≤ 0.5 mg/kg/day.
Primary antistreptococcal therapy	1.2 million units of benzathine penicillin G IM or oral penicillin or erythromycin for 10 days
Prophylaxis of GAS infection	1.2 million units benzathine penicillin G IM q.i.d. 4 weeks or sulfadiazine 500 mg po q.i.d. (≤ 27 kg) or 1.0 g po q.i.d. (≥ 27 kg) or penicillin V 250 mg po b.i.d
Medications to control cardiac symptoms (if needed)	Diuretic, angiotension-converting enzyme inhibitor, and/or cautious use of digoxin
Medications to control chorea (if needed)	Haloperidol or phenobarbitol
Infective endocarditis prophylaxis	As recommended by the American Heart Association

throat culture results. Anti-inflammatory treatment includes oral salicylates (50–100 mg/kg/day) in four daily doses. This is continued for 2 to 4 weeks, then is gradually tapered over 4 to 6 weeks. Corticosteroid treatment should be reserved for those patients with congestive heart failure or at least moderate cardiomegaly on chest radiograph. Corticosteroids are tapered slowly over about 6 weeks; during the taper of corticosteroids, salicylates are added. Supportive care for cardiac dysfunction includes diuretics, antihypertensives, or digoxin. For patients with Sydenham chorea, haloperidol or phenobarbital may be of some benefit.

Prevention of GAS infection is of utmost importance to prevent recurrent attacks of ARF that can be associated with increased severity of cardiac disease or with development of cardiac disease not previously present. All patients with ARF should receive antimicrobial prophylaxis with intramuscular benzathine penicillin G every 4 weeks or twice daily oral penicillin, or once daily sulfadiazine if penicillin allergic, or erythromycin if

penicillin and sulfa allergic. The recommendations for the duration of secondary prophylaxis of streptococcal infection are based upon likelihood of recurrence and years since last ARF episode. The current American Heart Association recommendations for duration of antimicrobial prophylaxis of ARF are listed in Table 14E-3 (10). In addition, patients with rheumatic heart disease should receive infective endocarditis prophylaxis as recommended by the American Heart Association.

PROGNOSIS

The only long-term manifestation of ARF is that of rheumatic heart disease, and the prognosis of patients with ARF is generally attributable to the degree of cardiac involvement, to consequences of infective endocarditis, and to the risk of recurrent ARF secondary to recurrence of GAS pharyngitis. Patients presenting only with chorea or polyarthritis may develop rheumatic heart disease if they develop recurrent ARF, thus emphasizing the importance of prophylactic antibiotics.

TABLE 14E-3. RECOMMENDATIONS OF DURATION OF ANTIMICROBIAL PROPHYLAXIS IN PATIENTS WITH ACUTE RHEUMATIC FEVER.

CONDITION	TREATMENT DURATION
Patients with rheumatic fever with carditis and residual heart disease	At least 10 years since last episode and at least until age 40, sometimes lifelong prophylaxis
Rheumatic fever with carditis but no residual heart disease (no valvar disease)	10 years or well into adulthood, whichever is longer
Rheumatic fever without carditis	5 years or until age 21 years, whichever is longer

POSTSTREPTOCOCCAL REACTIVE ARTHRITIS

General Considerations

Those patients who do not fulfill the diagnostic criteria for ARF but who develop arthritis after a streptococcal infection are deemed to have poststreptococcal reactive arthritis (PSRA). This arthritis is predominantly associated with GAS infections but has also been reported after infection with group C and G streptococci. There appears to be a bimodal age distribution of PSRA, with peak incidence at ages 8 to 14 years and 21 to 37 years. In Caucasians, PSRA is associated with the class II HLA antigen DRB1*01 (11,12).

Clinical Findings

The arthritis of PSRA is generally acute and nonmigratory and predominantly affects the large joints of the lower limbs, occasionally causing tenosynovitis. It may be mono- or polyarticular, and symmetrical or asymmetrical. The axial skeleton is affected in about 20% of patients. During the antecedent GAS infection, fever with or without a scarlatiniform rash may be present, but they are not usually when arthritis has manifested. The interval between the inciting streptococcal infection and the onset of arthritis (onset usually 3–14 days after infection) is generally shorter than that of ARF. The symptoms of PSRA resolve slowly over a few weeks to several months (mean of 2 months). Characteristically, PSRA patients have a gradual response to nonsteriodal anti-inflammatory drug (NSAID) therapy in contrast to ARF patients, who typically have a dramatic and prompt response to NSAIDs (11,13,14). Recurrences have been reported after subsequent streptococcal pharyngitis episodes. The most concerning possible sequela is that of late-onset carditis; in the original description of PSRA, this occurred in 4 of 13 (31%) patients with PSRA who did not meet the criteria for and did not have a clinical history of ARF; these patients developed evidence of cardiac disease 1 to 18 years after their original diagnosis. Substantially lower rates of development of late carditis have been observed in more recent series. Other possible extra-articular manifestations of PSRA include glomerulonephritis (which is very rare with ARF) and uveitis in the minority of patients.

Diagnostic Criteria

The diagnostic criteria for PSRA are not clearly defined, but the criteria proposed by Ayoub and colleagues (15) are detailed in Table 14E-4.

Treatment

Patients with PSRA generally respond much less dramatically to aspirin or other NSAIDs than do those with classic ARF, but these agents can be used to treat this form of arthritis. Some experts recommend both a baseline echocardiogram and a follow-up echocardiogram 1 to 2 years later because of the concern of occult carditis. The American Heart Association (AHA) currently recommends that patients with PSRA should be followed while receiving antistreptococcal prophylaxis for 1 to 2 years to assess for evidence of cardiac involvement, and

TABLE 14E-4. PROPOSED DIAGNOSTIC CRITERIA FOR DIAGNOSIS OF POSTSTREPTOCOCCAL REACTIVE ARTHRITIS.

A. Characteristics of arthritis
1. Acute in onset, symmetric or asymmetric, usually nonmigratory
2. Persistent or recurrent symptoms
3. Lack of a dramatic response to nonsteroidal anti-inflammatory drugs

B. Evidence of an antecedent group A streptococcal infection (previous positive throat culture or rapid antigen test positive for GAS, or elevated or rising antistreptolysin O and/or anti-DNase B titers)

C. Does not fill the modified Jones criteria for acute rheumatic fever

that prophylaxis should be discontinued after 1 to 2 years if no evidence of carditis is found. Penicillin is recommended as first-line therapy, and erythromycin is appropriate for penicillin-allergic patients. Some experts suggest that the same prophylaxis recommendations for ARF patients also should apply to those with PSRA because the time of onset of documented carditis can be widely variable, but this recommendation has not been endorsed by the AHA or other organizations.

REFERENCES

1. Carapetis JR, Steer AC, Mulholland EK, Weber M. The global burden of group A streptococcal diseases. Lancet Infect Dis 2005;5:685–694.
2. Guidelines for the diagnosis of rheumatic fever. Jones Criteria, 1992 update. Special Writing Group of the Committee on Rheumatic Fever, Endocarditis, and Kawasaki Disease of the Council on Cardiovascular Disease in the Young of the American Heart Association. JAMA 1992;268:2069–2073.
3. Zomorrodi A, Wald ER. Sydenham's chorea in western Pennsylvania. Pediatrics 2006;117:e675–e679.
4. Kaplan EL, Rothermel CD, Johnson DR. Antistreptolysin O and anti-deoxyribonuclease B titers: normal values for children ages 2 to 12 in the United States. Pediatrics 1998;101:86–88.
5. Stollerman GH. Rheumatic fever in the 21st century. Clin Infect Dis 2001;33:806–814.
6. Shulman ST, Stollerman G, Beall B, Dale JB, Tanz RR. Temporal changes in streptococcal M protein types and the near-disappearance of acute rheumatic fever in the United States. Clin Infect Dis 2006;42:441–447.
7. Wilson M, Schweitzer, MG, Lubschez R. The familial epidemiology of rheumatic fever. J Pediatr 1943;22:461–491.
8. Guedez Y, Kotby A, El-Demellawy M, et al. HLA class II associations with rheumatic heart disease are more evident and consistent among clinically homogeneous patients. Circulation 1999;99:2784–2790.

9. Taranta A TS, Metrakos JD. Rheumatic fever in mono-zyogotic and dizygotic twins. Circulation 1959;20:778–792.

10. Dajani A, Taubert K, Ferrieri P, Peter G, Shulman S. Treatment of acute streptococcal pharyngitis and prevention of rheumatic fever: a statement for health professionals. Committee on Rheumatic Fever, Endocarditis, and Kawasaki Disease of the Council on Cardiovascular Disease in the Young, the American Heart Association. Pediatrics 1995;96:758–764.

11. Mackie SL, Keat A. Poststreptococcal reactive arthritis: what is it and how do we know? Rheumatology (Oxford) 2004;43:949–954.

12. Ahmed S, Ayoub EM, Scornik JC, Wang CY, She JX. Poststreptococcal reactive arthritis: clinical characteristics and association with HLA-DR alleles. Arthritis Rheum 1998;41:1096–1102.

13. Herold BC, Shulman ST. Poststreptococcal arthritis. Pediatr Infect Dis J 1988;7:681–682.

14. Shulman ST, Ayoub EM. Poststreptococcal reactive arthritis. Curr Opin Rheumatol 2002;14:562–565.

15. Ayoub EM, Ahmed S. Update on complications of group A streptococcal infections. Curr Probl Pediatr 1997;27:90–101.

Systemic Lupus Erythematosus
A. Clinical and Laboratory Features

JILL P. BUYON, MD

- Systemic lupus erythematosus (SLE) is a common autoimmune disorder occurring predominantly in women during reproductive years and having strong minority representation.
- The hallmark of SLE is its diversity of presentation with accumulation of manifestations over time and undulating disease course.
- Essentially any organ system can be affected by SLE with constitutional symptoms, mucocutaneous, musculoskeletal, renal, and central nervous system (CNS) being most common.
- Presence of autoantibodies, the unifying manifestation of SLE, is useful for diagnosis and the pattern

- of autoantibodies may help to predict clinical manifestations. Anti–double-stranded DNA antibodies are useful, along with changes in complement levels, for predicting disease flares in some patients.
- Special attention during pregnancy may help to avoid disease flares and adverse fetal outcome.
- Many drugs can trigger a lupuslike illness associated with autoantibodies, but typically with fewer disease manifestations and temporal association with the offending agent.

In sharp distinction to organ-specific autoimmune diseases such as thyroiditis, diabetes, or myasthenia gravis, systemic lupus erythematosus (SLE) is a constellation of signs and symptoms classified as one nosologic entity. Indeed, it is the diversity of presentation, accumulation of manifestations over time, and undulating disease course that challenge the most astute of clinicians. With rare exception, the unifying laboratory abnormality is the presence of circulating antinuclear antibodies (ANA). Acknowledging the complexity of this disease, its broad differential diagnosis, and the need to develop better and more specific therapies, the American College of Rheumatology (ACR) has designated 11 diagnostic criteria (presented in Table 15A-1) (1,2). These criteria reflect the major clinical features of the disease (mucocutaneous, articular, serosal, renal, neurologic) and incorporate the associated laboratory findings (hematologic and immunologic). The presence of four or more criteria is required for diagnosis. They need not necessarily present simultaneously: a single criterion such as arthritis or thrombocytopenia may recur over months or years before the diagnosis can be confirmed by the appearance of additional features. While there is incomplete agreement among rheumatologists as to whether these criteria need to be strictly

applied in a practice setting, or reserved only for formal academic studies, they do facilitate a methodologic approach to evaluate a patient.

As one reviews the clinical descriptions, it will become apparent that not only is just about every bodily part potentially targeted by lupus, but in each organ different structural components can be involved with varying frequencies, as exemplified in evaluating a large Canadian cohort (Figure 15A-1) (3). In addition, nonspecific constitutional features of SLE, some of which dominate the clinical picture, are fatigue, fever, and weight loss. Demographic characteristics, such as overwhelming female predominance (approximately 9:1), typical onset during the reproductive years, and strong minority representation, are helpful clues to diagnosis. Factors to consider that might precipitate the onset or exacerbation of systemic disease or isolated organ involvement include recent sun exposure, emotional stress, infection, certain drugs, such as sulfonamides, and surgery.

Happily, over 90% of SLE patients survive at least 2 years after diagnosis compared to about 50% three decades ago (4). Recent data support an 80% to 90% survival at 10 years (5). A bimodal mortality curve is prevalent in SLE (6,7). Patients who die within 5 years of diagnosis usually have active disease requiring high

TABLE 15A-1. THE REVISED CRITERIA FOR THE DIAGNOSIS OF SYSTEMIC LUPUS ERYTHEMATOSUS[a]

CRITERION	DEFINITION
1. Malar rash	Fixed erythema, flat or raised, over the malar eminence, tending to spare the nasolabial folds
2. Discoid rash	Erythematous raised patches with adherent keratotic scaling and follicular plugging; atrophic scarring may occur in older lesions
3. Photosensitivity	Skin rash as a result of unusual reaction to sunlight, by patient history or physician observation
4. Oral ulcers	Oral or nasopharyngeal ulceration, usually painless, observed by a physician
5. Arthritis	Nonerosive arthritis involving two or more peripheral joints, characterized by tenderness, swelling or effusion
6. Serositis	(a) Pleuritis; convincing history of pleuritic pain or rub heard by physician or evidence of pleural effusion OR (b) Pericarditis; documented by electrocardiogram or rub or evidence of pericardial effusion
7. Renal disorder	(a) Persistent proteinuria > 500 mg per day or > 3+ if quantitation not performed OR (b) Cellular casts: may be red cell, hemoglobin, granular, tubular or mixed
8. Neurologic disorder	(a) Seizures: in the absence of offending drugs or known metabolic derangement; e.g., uremia, ketoacidosis, or electrolyte imbalance OR (b) Psychosis: in the absence of offending drugs or known metabolic derangement; e.g., uremia, ketoacidosis, or electrolyte imbalance
9. Hematologic disorder	(a) Hemolytic anemia: with reticulocytosis OR (b) Leukopenia: < 4000/mm³ total OR (c) Lymphopenia: < 1500/mm³ on two or more occasions OR (d) Thrombocytopenia: < 100,000/mm³ in the absence of offending drugs
10. Immunologic disorder[b]	(a) Anti-DNA: antibody to native DNA in abnormal titer OR (b) Anti-SM: presence of antibody to SM nuclear antigen OR (c) Positive finding of antiphospholipid antibodies based on (1) an abnormal serum level of IgG or IgM anticardiolipin antibodies, (2) a positive test result for lupus anticoagulant using a standard method, or (3) a false-positive serologic test for syphilis known to be positive for at least 6 months and confirmed by Treponema pallidum immobilization or fluorescent treponemal antibody absorption test
11. ANA	Abnormal titer of ANA by immunofluorescence or equivalent assay at any point in time, in the absence of drugs known to be associated with drug-induced lupus syndrome

Source: From Tan EM, Cohen AS, Fries JF, et al. (1), by permission of Arthritis Rheum.
[a]This classification is based on 11 criteria. For the purpose of identifying patients in clinical studies, a person must have SLE if any 4 or more of the 11 criteria are present, serially or simultaneously, during any interval of observation (1).
[b]The modifications to criterion number 10 were made in 1997 (2).

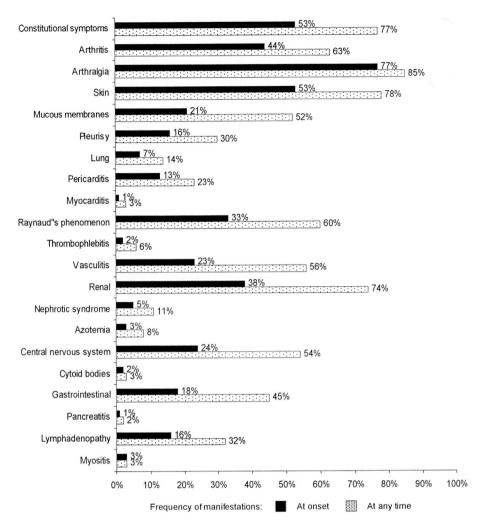

FIGURE 15A-1

Frequency of manifestations at onset and at any time during the course of systemic lupus erythematosus, in a large Canadian cohort (3). The frequency at onset is based on 376 patients diagnosed at Lupus Clinic (University of Toronto), and frequency at point is for 750 patients registered prior to July 1995. Estimates of the frequency of each manifestation differ in some studies; therefore, in the body of the text of this chapter, frequencies are reported that may be at variance with the above cohort. The reader is referred to two major books on systemic lupus erythematosus (50,51).

15

doses of corticosteroids, intense immunosuppression, and concomitant infections. In contrast, late deaths are often the result of cardiovascular disease. This latter point has received major attention at both the bench and bedside. While SLE is not considered curable, patients can enjoy periods of extended remission with virtually no clinical activity and even the disappearance of antinuclear antibodies.

MORE COMMONLY INVOLVED ORGAN SYSTEMS

Mucocutaneous

Clearly, the cutaneous system is one of the most commonly affected, approaching 80% to 90%. In parallel with the myriad of signs and symptoms of SLE itself, the skin and mucous membranes can be involved in a variety of ways (8). Notably, 4 of the 11 formal criteria can be fulfilled in this system alone. SLE-specific skin lesions are classified into three types—chronic, subacute, and

acute—based strictly on clinical appearance and duration, without considering the extracutaneous manifestations or laboratory features of the overall disease.

The most common form of chronic disease is discoid lupus [DLE; 15%–30%; Figure 15A-2(A)], which can occur as part of the systemic disease or exist in isolation in the absence of any autoantibodies (2%–10% will develop SLE). DLE lesions are discrete plaques, often erythematous, covered by scale that extends into dilated hair follicles. These lesions most typically occur on the face, scalp, in the pinnae, behind the ears, and neck. They can be seen in non–sun-exposed areas. The lesions can progress, with active indurated erythema at the periphery. Central atrophic scarring is very characteristic. Irreversible alopecia can result from follicular destruction. Albeit rare, prominent dermal mucin accumulation in the early course of DLE can result in the succulent, edematous lesions of tumid lupus. Lupus panniculitis-lupus profundus is a less common form of chronic disease. These lesions spare the epidermis and represent involvement of the deep dermis and subcutaneous fat. The lesions of lupus panniculitis are firm

306 JILL P. BUYON

FIGURE 15A-2

Cutaneous manifestations of systemic
lupus erythematosus. (A) Discoid
lesions are present on the face and
in the pinnae. (B, C) Examples of the
lesions of subacute cutaneous lupus
erythematosus on the back and arm.
(D) Classic malar rash. (E) Extensive
acute perforating ulcer on the upper
palate. (F) Erythematous lesions
consistent with cutaneous vasculitis
on the digits. (Photographs provided
by Dr. Andrew Franks, Associate
Professor of Clinical Dermatology,
New York University School of
Medicine.)

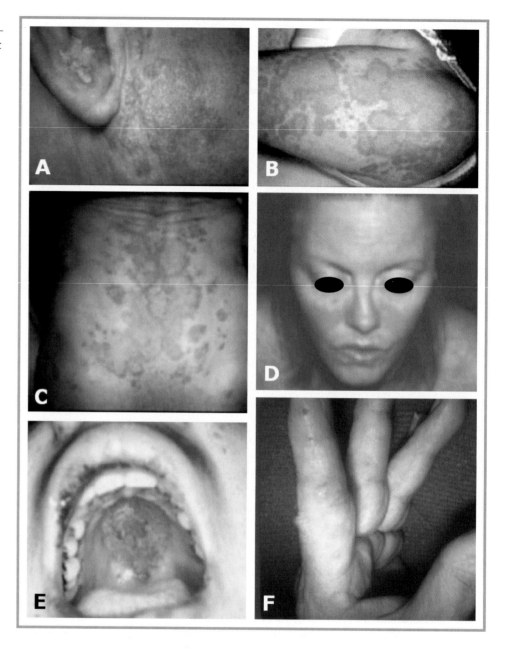

nodules generally without surface changes. In time, the
overlying skin becomes attached to the subcutaneous
nodular lesions and is drawn inward, resulting in deep
depressions.

Subacute cutaneous lupus erythematosus (SCLE)
lesions are seen in 7% to 27% of patients [Figure 15A-
2(B,C)]. SCLE primarily affects Caucasian females.
The lesions are typically symmetric, widespread, superficial, and nonscarring, and are most often present in
sun-exposed areas, for example, the shoulders, extensor
surfaces of the arms, upper chest, upper back, and neck.
The lesions begin as small, erythematous, scaly papules
or plaques that can evolve into papulosquamous (psoriasiform) or annular polycyclic forms. The latter often
coalesce to produce large confluent areas with central

hypopigmentation. Generally, both forms are nonscarring. Antibodies to SSA/Ro ribonucleoproteins are
commonly found in patients with SCLE.

Perhaps the most classic of all the rashes in SLE is
the malar or butterfly rash, which is categorized among
the acute rashes [Figure 15A-2(D)]. It occurs in 30% to
60% of all patients. This erythematous and edematous
eruption simulates the shape of a butterfly with its body
bridging over the base of the nose and wings spreading
out over the malar eminences. At times the same rash
can be seen on the forehead and chin but classically
spares the nasolabial folds. The absence of discrete
papules and pustules distinguishes it from acne rosacea.
The rash is abrupt in onset and can last for days. Postinflammatory changes are common, particularly in patients

with pigmented skin. The butterfly rash is often initiated and/or exacerbated by exposure to sunlight. However, patients can have a photosensitive erythematous rash elsewhere on the body in the absence of a butterfly rash. The criteria for photosensitivity and butterfly rash are thus independent of each other albeit coexistent in the majority of patients. The Systemic Lupus Erythematosus International Cooperating Clinics (SLICC), a group of internationally recognized experts in SLE, are working on a revision of the ACR classification criteria, and the assignment of photosensitivity based on history alone may likely prove to be an insensitive parameter. A more widespread, morbilliform or exanthemous eruption is another acute cutaneous manifestation of SLE.

Alopecia associated with SLE may be diffuse or patchy, reversible or permanently scarring as a result of discoid lesions in the scalp. The breakage of hairs at the temples—so-called lupus frizz—can be observed.

Mucosal lesions are also part of the clinical spectrum of SLE and can affect the mouth (most commonly), nose, and anogenital area. While oral lesions can be seen on the buccal mucosa and tongue, sores on the upper palate are particularly characteristic [Figure 15A-2(E)]. They are typically described as painless but need not be. Central depression often occurs and painful ulcerations develop.

Vasculitis is another component of skin disease in SLE. It may be manifest as urticaria, palpable purpura, nailfold or digital ulcerations, erythematous papules of the pulps of the fingers and palms, or splinter hemorrhages [Figure 15A-2(F)].

Because the skin can be an important marker of disease activity in SLE, the physical examination should always include inspection of often overlooked areas, the scalp, pinnae, behind the ears, palate, fingertips, and palms.

MUSCULOSKELETAL SYSTEM

Painful joints are the most common presenting symptom of SLE, with frequencies reported between 76% to 100%. In some cases the pain is more characteristic of arthralgia because it is unaccompanied by the traditional signs of inflammation. In others the classical signs of a true arthritis, such as swelling, erythema, heat, and decreased range of motion, are present. Notably, the patient's complaint of pain may be out of proportion to the degree of synovitis present on physical examination. Although arthritis can affect any joint, it is most often symmetrical with involvement of the small joints of the hands (proximal interphalangeal and metacarpal phalangeal), wrists and knees, but sparing the spine. The arthritis can be evanescent, resolving within 24 hours, or more persistent. Many of these features account for the initial diagnostic consideration of early rheumatoid arthritis (RA) in some patients. In contrast to RA, the arthritis in SLE is nonerosive and generally nondeforming. In those patients that do appear to have deforming features, such as ulnar deviation, hyperflexion, and hyperextension, the deformities are generally reducible (Figure 15A-3). These hypermobile digits with reducible deformities are secondary to involvement of para-articular tissues, such as the joint capsule, ligaments, and tendons, and are referred to as Jaccoud-like arthropathy. Exceptions are certainly possible and, when present, erosions may be clinically difficult to distinguish from RA; however, they are usually nonprogressive and

FIGURE 15A-3

(A) Swan neck deformity of the second and third digits. (B) Hyperextension of the first interphalangeal joint. (Courtesy of Dr. Harry Fischer, Beth Israel Medical Center, New York, NY.)

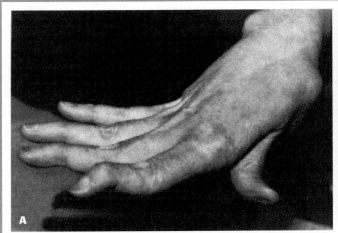
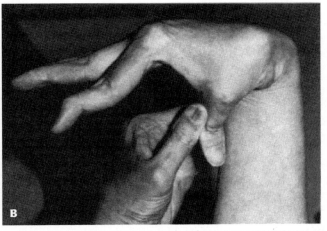

likely result from capsular pressure and an altered mechanical situation caused by subluxation.

Effusions tend to be modest. The synovial fluid is clear to slightly cloudy with good viscosity and mucin clot, reflecting the absence of major inflammation. Antinuclear antibodies can be present. White blood cell counts are usually <2000/mm^3 with a predominance of mononuclear cells. The fluid can be transudative or exudative. The serum/synovial fluid ratios of complement, total protein, and IgG can all be 1, indicating a proportional escape of proteins into the joint space, or >1 for complement levels only, indicating local consumption, not simply a reflection of decreased serum complement. Larger effusions with warmth should prompt the consideration of septic arthritis. Rheumatoid nodules can occur in SLE accompanied by the presence of rheumatoid factor, but this is not common.

Rheumatic complaints localized to the hips should raise serious consideration of osteonecrosis, the frequency of which has been reported to be 5% to 10%. Although the femoral head is the most common site of involvement, other sites include the femoral condyles, talus, humeral head, and, occasionally, the metatarsal heads, radial head, carpal bones, and metacarpal bones. Bilaterality is frequent but not necessarily simultaneous. Most cases are associated with the use of corticosteroids, but causality has also been attributed to Raynaud's, small vessel vasculitis, fat emboli, or the presence of antiphospholipid antibodies. Typically, patients with osteonecrosis complain of persistent painful motion localized to a single joint, and symptoms are relieved by rest.

Generalized myalgia and muscle weakness, frequently involving the deltoids and quadriceps, can be accompanying features of disease flares. Overt myositis with elevations of CPK occurs in <15% of patients. Electromyogram (EMG) and muscle biopsy findings range from normal to those seen in dermato/polymyositis. Exceptionally high levels of creatine kinase (CPK) are rare. Patients with SLE can develop myopathy as a consequence of glucocorticoids or antimalarials.

Renal

The kidney is considered by many to be the signature organ affected by SLE. Essentially all studies of prognosis have identified lupus nephritis as an important predictor of poor outcome. Renal disease is present in one half to two thirds of patients and, with rare exception, is diagnosed based on the presence of proteinuria (dipstick 2+, >500mg/24 hour). There is a spectrum of renal injury that can be assessed, in part on clinical grounds, and more definitively by biopsy (9). Initial categories of lupus nephritis were based on classification by the World Health Organization as assessed by histology and location of immune complexes (Table 15A-2) (10). Recently, this classification has been revised by the International Society of Nephrology and Renal Pathology Society (ISN/RPS; Table 15A-3) (11). The important difference is that this new classification is an attempt to stratify proliferative lesions—focal and diffuse (class III and IV, respectively)—as active versus chronic scarring, with the concept that the former is treatable. Furthermore, diffuse proliferative nephritis

TABLE 15A-2. WORLD HEALTH ORGANIZATION CLASSIFICATION OF LUPUS NEPHRITIS

CLASS	PATTERN	SITE OF IMMUNE COMPLEX DEPOSITION	Sediment	Proteinuria (24h)	Serum creatinine	Blood pressure	Anti-dsdna	C3/C4
					CLINICAL CLUES[a]			
I	Normal	None	Bland	<200mg	Normal	Normal	Absent	Normal
II	Mesangial	Mesangial only	RBC or bland	200–500mg	Normal	Normal	Absent	Normal
III	Focal and segmental proliferative	Mesangial, subendothelial, ± subepithelial	RBC, WBC	500–3500mg	Normal to mild elevation	Normal to elevated	Positive	Decreased
IV	Diffuse proliferative	Mesangial, subendothelial, ± subepithelial	RBC, WBC, RBC casts	1000–>3500mg	Normal to dialysis-dependent	High	Positive to high titer	Decreased
V	Membranous	Mesangial, subepithelial	Bland	>3000mg	Normal to mild elevation	Normal	Absent to modest titer	Normal

SOURCE: From Appel GB, Silva FG, Pirani CL (10), by permission of *Medicine*.
ABBREVIATIONS: RBC, red blood cells; WBC, white blood cells.
[a]These are only guidelines, and parameters may vary, substantiating the need for biopsy when precise diagnosis is required.

TABLE 15A-3. INTERNATIONAL SOCIETY OF NEPHROLOGY/RENAL PATHOLOGY SOCIETY (ISN/RPS) CLASSIFICATION OF LUPUS NEPHRITIS.

Class I	Minimal mesangial lupus nephritis
Class II	Mesangial proliferative lupus nephritis
Class III	Focal lupus nephritis
III (A):	Active lesions: focal proliferative lupus nephritis
III (A/C):	Active and chronic lesions
III (C):	Chronic inactive lesions with scars
Class IV	Diffuse lupus nephritis
IV-S (A):	Active lesions: diffuse segmental proliferative lupus nephritis
IV-G (A):	Active lesions: diffuse global proliferative lupus nephritis
IV-S (A/C):	Active and chronic lesions
IV-G (A/C):	Active and chronic lesions
IV-S (C):	Chronic inactive lesions with scars
IV-G (C):	Chronic inactive lesions with scars
Class V	Membranous lupus nephritis[a]
Class VI	Advanced sclerotic lupus nephritis

SOURCE: Adapted from Weening JJ, D'Agati VD, Schwartz MM, et al. (11), by permission of *J Am Soc Nephrol*.
[a]Class V may occur in combination with class II or IV, in which case both will be diagnosed.

was divided into those cases with predominantly segmental lesions and those with predominantly global lesions. To date it is not clear whether this histologic division will have clinical and prognostic impact. Class V/membranous is now purely membranous, and if there is evidence of a proliferative lesion, both classes are specified, for example, V + III or V + IV.

Renal biopsy is abnormal in most patients, especially when tissue is evaluated by electron microscopy and immunofluorescence. Diffuse proliferative nephritis and progressive forms of focal proliferative nephritis are associated with a poorer prognosis than membranous or mesangial disease.

Clinical evaluation initially includes urine dipstick and microscopic analysis. A baseline 24-hour urine for measurement of protein and creatinine, even in the presence of 1+ dipstick, is common practice, especially in a patient with antibodies to double-stranded DNA (dsDNA) and low complement levels. Given the inconvenience of obtaining a 24-hour urine collection, many physicians utilize the spot protein/creatinine ratio to gauge the extent of proteinuria. The sediment can be bland (consistent with mesangial or membranous) or active containing red blood cell casts (consistent with proliferative lesions). Persistent hematuria with >5 red blood cells per high power field (in the absence of other causes such as menstruation) and/or pyuria with >5 white blood cells per high power field (excluding infec-

tion) would each be an unusual reflection of lupus nephritis in the absence of proteinuria (unless pathology is limited to the mesangium in the case of red blood cells and interstitium in case of white blood cells). An elevated creatinine without concomitant proteinuria is unexpected unless advanced renal insufficiency is present. While renal disease is frequently insidious, symptoms which occur with progressive activity include swollen ankles, puffy eyes upon waking in the morning, and frequent urination. A low serum albumin is an indicator of persistent proteinuria. Isolated hypertension outside of the norms for age, race, and gender should raise suspicion of underlying renal disease.

Biopsies are not required to diagnose lupus nephritis but are extremely helpful in certain settings because clinical parameters are not absolute. Given the importance of identifying pathologic features suggestive of more aggressive disease, such as crescents, some clinicians believe kidney biopsy to be the fulcrum for therapeutic decisions. Thus, treatment with alkylating agents, such as cyclophosphamide, which can result in premature ovarian failure, becomes readily justified in circumstances where the clinical picture may have suggested a more favorable histology. For example, there are patients who have rapidly rising titers of anti-dsDNA and falling complements but only modest proteinuria (400 mg–1 g), bland sediment, normal creatinine, and no other systemic manifestations to warrant intense immunosuppression. Other patients may have nephrotic-range proteinuria and an active sediment yet serologic parameters are normal. Renal biopsies in these somewhat ambiguous situations can be quite informative. In contrast, the decision to withhold aggressive therapy is also important and may be appropriate for irreversible late-stage sclerotic disease. Renal biopsies should be performed when the result will make a clear difference in the approach and/or is required as part of a research study. Renal ultrasound is another helpful guide to therapy because the chances of successful treatment become smaller with decreased size and increased echogenicity of the kidneys.

Urine protein is a critical measurement of ongoing renal lupus activity. While new proteinuria of 500 mg is significant, patients with membranous nephropathy, in particular, can have continued proteinuria between 500 mg and 2 g and still be considered stable. In such cases, an exacerbation is best defined as at least a doubling of baseline proteinuria. It is essential to monitor blood pressure because hypertension can be a reflection of renal disease activity and, as such, accelerates functional impairment.

Renal transplantation in lupus has been successful. However, lupus nephritis can recur (~10%), even in the absence of clinical or serologic evidence of active SLE (12) but is not always associated with allograft loss. Clinical and serological activity in SLE may improve in patients who have end-stage renal disease (13), although this paradigm has recently been challenged (14).

Nervous System

Approximately two thirds of patients with SLE have neuropsychiatric manifestations. The pathophysiology of this broad clinical category is not well understood, which probably reflects the inaccessibility of the tissue involved. Proposed mechanisms include vascular occlusion due to vasculopathy, leukoaggregation or thrombosis, and antibody-mediated neuronal cell injury or dysfunction (15). Neuropsychiatric systemic lupus includes neurologic syndromes of the central, peripheral, and autonomic nervous systems, and psychiatric disorders in which other causes have been excluded. These manifestations may occur as single or multiple events in the same person. Symptoms can be present concomitantly with activity in other systems, or exist in isolation. While the formal ACR criteria for neuropsychiatric lupus include only seizures and psychosis, it has become increasingly clear that further descriptors might be important in diagnosis. In an effort to expand the criteria, an ACR Ad Hoc Committee has developed reporting standards, recommendations for laboratory and imaging evaluation, and case definitions for 19 neuropsychiatric syndromes observed in SLE (16).

A variety of psychiatric disorders are reported and include mood disorders, anxiety, and psychosis. Unequivocal attribution to lupus is difficult because such disorders may be related to the stress of having a major chronic illness, or be due to drugs, infections, or metabolic disorders. Patients can demonstrate significant cognitive defects, such as attention deficit, poor concentration, impaired memory, and difficulty in word finding. These abnormalities are best documented by neuropsychological testing and a decline from a higher former level of functioning. Another syndrome of diffuse neurologic dysfunction is termed *acute confusional state* and defined as disturbance of consciousness or level of arousal with reduced ability to focus, maintain, or shift attention, accompanied by cognitive disturbance and/or changes in mood, behavior, or affect. The syndrome often develops over a brief time frame, fluctuates over the day, and covers a wide spectrum ranging from mild alterations of consciousness to coma.

Inclusive in the neurologic manifestations of the central nervous system are seizures, which may be focal or generalized. Headache is a common complaint in patients but there is still debate as to whether this is a unique feature attributable to SLE. The lupus headache has been operationally defined as severe, disabling, persistent, and not responsive to narcotic analgesics. However, severe migraine in the absence of lupus may have these same characteristics. Benign intracranial

hypertension is also included in the case definition of headache. The term *lupoid sclerosis* has been used to describe a rare condition in which patients exhibit complex neurologic deficits similar to those observed in multiple sclerosis. Myelopathy and aseptic meningitis are rare. Chorea, albeit infrequent, is the most common movement disorder observed in SLE. This and cerebrovascular accidents have been related to the presence of antiphospholipid antibodies.

Disturbances of the cranial nerves can result in visual defects, blindness, papilledema, nystagmus or ptosis, tinnitus and vertigo, and facial palsy. Peripheral neuropathy may be motor, sensory, mixed motor–sensory, or mononeuritis multiplex. Transverse myelitis presenting with lower extremity paralysis, sensory deficits, and loss of sphincter control has been observed in a limited number of patients. An acute inflammatory demyelinating polyradiculoneuropathy (Guillain–Barre syndrome) has been described.

Examination of the cerebrospinal fluid is useful to rule out infection. However, with regard to neuropsychiatric lupus, often the findings are nonspecific with elevated cell counts, protein levels, or both, found in only about one third of patients. The fluid may be completely normal in the face of acute disease. Computerized tomography is sufficient for the initial diagnosis of most mass lesions and intracranial hemorrhages. The findings of magnetic resonance imaging (MRI) reflect the histopathologic findings of vascular injury and may involve the white or gray matter (17). Abnormalities on MRI are more likely with focal findings. Unfortunately, the correlation between MRI findings and clinical presentation is low.

Cardiovascular System

A variety of cardiac complications are seen in SLE but certainly the most common is pericarditis, occurring in 6% to 45%. The clinical picture is usually typical with the patient complaining of substernal or pericardial pain, aggravated by motion such as inspiration, coughing, swallowing, twisting, and bending forward. Symptoms may either be severe and last for weeks, or mild and last for hours. A pericardial rub may or may not be present and can be heard in an asymptomatic patient. Although the electrocardiogram may show the typical T-wave abnormalities, echocardiography is the best diagnostic test. Most effusions are small to moderate. The pericardial fluid is straw-colored to serosanguinous, exudative, and can have a high white blood cell count with a predominance of neutrophils. LE cells can be seen in the centrifuged cell sediment. Cardiac tamponade is rare as is constrictive pericarditis. Importantly, when a young woman presents with shortness of breath and pleuritic chest pain, the differential diagnosis must include SLE, and the patient should be tested for ANA.

Primary myocardial involvement in SLE is uncommon, <10%. The patient may have fever, dyspnea, palpitations, heart murmurs, sinus tachycardia, ventricular arrhythmias, conduction abnormalities, or congestive heart failure. Percutaneous endomyocardial biopsy may be helpful. It is now well recognized that hemodynamically and clinically significant valvular disease occurs and may require prosthetic valve replacement. Aortic insufficiency represents the most commonly reported lesion and may be the result of multiple factors, including fibrinoid degeneration, distortion of the valve by fibrosis, valvulitis, bacterial endocarditis, aortitis, and Libman–Sacks endocarditis. Libman–Sacks atypical verrucous endocarditis, the classic cardiac lesion of SLE, is comprised of verrucous vegetations ranging from 1 to 4mm in diameter, initially reported to be present on the tricuspid and mitral valves. Interestingly, it has been noted that neither the usual clinical and immunologic markers of lupus activity, nor its treatment, are temporally related to the presence of or changes in valvular disease (18). Prophylactic antibiotics for surgical and dental procedures have been recommended for all SLE patients.

Accelerated atherosclerosis has received considerable attention and is an important cause of morbidity and mortality in SLE. It has been established that the proportionate mortality from myocardial infarction is approximately 10 times greater in patients with SLE than in the general age- and sex-matched population (6,7,19). Autopsy studies support the clinical data, as severe coronary artery atherosclerosis is present in up to 40% of patients with SLE, compared with 2% of control subjects, matched for age at the time of death (20). Studies have identified hypercholesterolemia, hypertension, and lupus itself as risk factors in these patients (21). Glucocorticoid therapy contributes to the elevation of plasma lipids, while antimalarials may result in a reduction of plasma cholesterol, low-density lipoprotein (LDL), and very low-density lipoprotein (VLDL). Coronary arteritis is rare and may coexist with atherosclerotic heart disease. Studies of clinical outcomes for atherosclerotic disease, including angina and myocardial infarction, have shown a prevalence of 6% to 12% in a number of SLE cohorts (6,7,21). More sensitive investigations, including carotid plaque and intima-media thickness (IMT) measured by B-mode ultrasound, revealed that 40% of 175 women with SLE had focal plaque (22).

Two recent articles further link SLE and premature atherosclerosis. Roman and colleagues (23) performed carotid ultrasonography, echocardiography, and assessment for risk factors for coronary artery disease (CAD) in a cross-sectional study of 197 patients with SLE and 197 controls. Atherosclerosis occurred prematurely in patients with SLE and was independent of traditional risk factors for cardiovascular disease. Among patients with SLE, plaque was independently associated with age, longer disease duration, higher damage index, and less frequent use of cyclophosphamide and antimalarial drugs, as well as a lower prevalence of anti-Sm antibody. Asanuma and colleagues (24) used electron beam computer tomography (EBCT) to evaluate 65 patients with SLE and 69 controls. Patients with SLE had higher coronary calcium scores, independent of other atherosclerotic risk factors. Furthermore, on analysis within age strata, patients with SLE were found to have coronary artery calcification at younger ages than controls.

Pleura and Lungs

The lungs and contiguous structures involved in normal respiration are commonly affected in SLE, but are generally not as life threatening as the renal and central nervous system complications. Over 30% of patients have some form of pleural disease in their lifetime, either as pleuritis with chest pain or frank effusion. Pleurisy is a more common feature of serositis than pericarditis. The pain of pleuritis can be quite severe and must be distinguished from pulmonary embolus or infection. Pleural rubs are less common than either clinical pleurisy or radiographic abnormalities. Pleural effusions are most often small and bilateral. The fluid is usually clear, exudative with increased protein, normal glucose, white blood cell count <10,000, a predominance of neutrophils or lymphocytes, and decreased levels of complement.

Pulmonary involvement includes pneumonitis, pulmonary hemorrhage, pulmonary embolism, pulmonary hypertension, and shrinking lung syndrome. The term *acute lupus pneumonitis* has been applied to individuals with an abrupt febrile pneumonitic process in whom infection has been ruled out. Prominent features are pleuritic chest pain, cough with hemoptysis, and dyspnea. Diffuse alveolar hemorrhage is considered a manifestation of acute lupus pneumonitis and associated with a 50% mortality rate. It can occur in the absence of hemoptysis and is suggested by a falling hematocrit and pulmonary infiltrates. Rare patients (<10%) develop a more chronic syndrome characterized by progressive dyspnea, nonproductive cough, basilar rales, and diffuse interstitial lung infiltrates.

Pulmonary hypertension should be suspected in patients complaining of progressive shortness of breath and in whom the chest radiograph is negative and profound hypoxemia is absent. Pulmonary function studies show a restrictive pattern with a reduction in the diffusing capacity for carbon monoxide. Doppler ultrasound studies and cardiac catheterization confirm the diagnosis. Frequently, these patients also have Raynaud's phenomenon. Intrapulmonary clotting and/or multiple pulmonary emboli must be addressed, especially in the setting of antiphospholipid antibodies. Recent studies

15

suggest that pulmonary hypertension is gradually progressive over time and related to an increase in pulmonary resistance (25).

LESS COMMONLY INVOLVED ORGAN SYSTEMS

Gastrointestinal Tract and Liver

Involvement of the gastrointestinal tract can, as in other organ systems, be quite varied, but for most patients is not the source of any diagnostic criteria. The peritoneum is the least likely of the serosal linings to be affected in SLE. Symptoms include rebound tenderness, fever, nausea, vomiting, and diarrhea. Unfortunately, confusion with serious abdominal pathology or infection can prompt surgical intervention. Abdominal pain in SLE can also be caused by pancreatitis and bowel vasculitis. Rectal bleeding can be present in mesenteric vasculitis. Protein-losing enteropathy is quite uncommon but should be considered in the face of low serum albumin, pedal edema, and the absence of proteinuria.

Parenchymal liver disease as a result of SLE is rare. However, elevated transaminases can be encountered during periods of active disease and/or following the use of many medications prescribed to treat lupus, such as nonsteriodal anit-inflammatory drugs (NSAIDs), azathioprine, and methotrexate. In the absence of known offending drugs, persistent signs of hepatitis may require a liver biopsy. The term *lupoid hepatitis* was coined by Bearn in 1956 and initially believed to be a manifestation of SLE. However, an individual need not have lupus; it is defined serologically and histologically and is a subset of chronic, active hepatitis. It is seen in less than 10% of patients who fulfill the ACR criteria for SLE.

Ocular System

With regard to the eye itself, "cotton wool spots" in the retina are generally cited as being the most common lesion, followed in frequency by corneal and conjunctival involvement, with only rare patients exhibiting uveitis or scleritis. Although also quite uncommon, retinal damage from antimalarials used in treating SLE is probably a greater cause of visual loss than is retinal involvement occurring in the natural course of the disease. Cotton wool spots (an ophthalmologic term) are not pathognomonic for lupus and result from focal ischemia. They occur preferentially in the posterior part of the retina and often involve the optic nerve head. Each spot appears as a grayish-white soft, fluffy exudate, averaging about one third of a disc diameter in width.

Cytoid bodies refer to the histologic features of the cotton wool spot.

LABORATORY FEATURES
Hematologic Abnormalities

Each of the cellular elements of the blood can be affected in SLE. Accordingly, the complete blood count is a critical part of the initial and continued evaluation of all lupus patients. In the absence of offending medications, the "penias" are generally secondary to peripheral destruction, and not marrow suppression.

Autoimmune hemolytic anemia is present in <10% of patients. A Coombs test can be positive (both direct and indirect) without active hemolysis. A nonspecific anemia reflecting chronic disease is present in up to 80% of patients. Leukopenia is seen in over 50% of patients. Absolute lymphopenia is more common than neutropenia. Unfortunately, the criterion for lymphopenia (<1500/mm^3) is not very stringent and in most laboratories is not highlighted as abnormal. While leukopenia does represent some degree of disease activity and has been described as a signal of more systemic activity, there are clearly patients whose low white blood cell counts do not associate with disease flares in other organs and do not predispose them to infection. Thrombocytopenia can be modest (platelet counts of 50,000–100,000/mm^3), chronic and totally asymptomatic, or profound (<20,000/mm^3) and acute, with gum bleeding and petechiae. In some cases, thrombocytopenia is the sole manifestation of disease activity at a given point in time. Moreover thrombocytopenia can be the initial presentation of SLE, antedating the development of other symptoms or signs by years. Any young woman presenting with "idiopathic" thrombocytopenia should be evaluated for SLE. Fortunately, there are rarely qualitative defects in the platelets and therefore life-threatening bleeding is unusual. Analogous to the other cell lines, antiplatelet antibodies may be present without thrombocytopenia.

The erythrocyte sedimentation rate is frequently elevated in SLE and is generally not considered a reliable marker of clinical activity. A rise in the C-reactive protein may be an indicator of infection, but this has not proven to be absolute.

Hallmark Autoantibodies and Complement

Measurement of the so-called *serologic parameters* is an integral part of the baseline evaluation and follow-up of patients with SLE. The term simply refers to those tests performed using the serum component of whole blood, although testing for antibodies, but not functional assays of complement, can be obtained using plasma. For example, testing the ability of serum complement to lyse sheep red blood cells in the CH50 test (see below) cannot be done using plasma, because it is generally accepted that complement activation does not proceed in EDTA- and citrate-plasma because of calcium chelation by EDTA and citrate.

The presence of a positive ANA is clearly one of the most important abnormalities to identify at presentation because it establishes that the differential diagnosis includes autoimmunity. However, a positive ANA, particularly in young women, can be detected in about 2% of normals. This test should be considered a valuable guide but by no means diagnostic. Once documented, the continued measurement of the ANA is not useful as a gauge of disease activity. In contrast, the presence of antibodies to dsDNA [not single-stranded DNA (ssDNA)] is not only of major diagnostic significance but in select patients, particularly those with renal involvement (see below), a valuable means of predicting and assessing disease activity. Anti-Sm antibodies, which recognize determinants on proteins associated with small ribonucleoproteins involved in processing of messenger RNA, are of diagnostic importance but do not track disease. Antibodies reactive with SSA/Ro and SSB/La ribonucleoproteins, the latter involved in transcription termination, also do not correlate with activity, but are often seen in patients who may have one or more of the following: photosensitivity, dry eyes and dry mouth (secondary Sjögren's syndrome), subacute cutaneous lesions, risk of a child with neonatal lupus. Anti-SSA/Ro antibodies, depending on the methodology used for screening, can stain the cytoplasmic component of the cell and therefore account for some ANA-negative lupus. While ANA-negative lupus is considered, it is difficult to conceptualize a situation whereby an individual is said to have SLE, a prototypic autoimmune disease, yet has no detectable autoantibodies.

The frequency of various autoantibodies and their clinical relevance are summarized in Table 15A-4. A very recently described autoantibody in the sera of about 30% of lupus patients is directed against an epitope of the glutamate/N-methyl-D-aspartic acid (NMDA) receptor subunits NR2a and NR2b (highly expressed in human brain) (26). Albeit not unambiguously proven, access of this antibody across the blood–brain barrier may result in neuropsychiatric abnormalities.

Complement proteins, the bullets of the antibodies and intrinsic components of immune complexes, can be measured both functionally (CH50) and antigenically (C3, C4). Most laboratories measure the C3 and C4 because they are stable and do not require special handling as does the CH50. The CH50 reflects the function of serum complement to lyse sheep red blood cells (RBCs); its value is the reciprocal of the dilution of serum that lyses 50% of antibody-coated sheep RBCs. A reduction of the CH50 occurs when individual complement component(s) are deficient or consumed. In fact, none of these traditional measures of the complement system discriminate between accelerated consumption of complement or decreased synthesis. Such distinction requires measurement of the complement split products (e.g., C3a), which is still considered a research tool and is not readily available in most commercial laboratories.

A challenge in the management of patients with SLE is to identify parameters that will stratify those at risk for disease flares, particularly flares which might lead to permanent damage in major organs. The presumption is that earlier treatment in the high-risk patient might have an impact on subsequent morbidity and mortality. Interest in measurements of the complement system and anti-DNA antibodies to evaluate lupus patients originates from the longstanding observation that decreased complement levels and rising titers of anti-DNA are often associated with severe disease (27).

TABLE 15A-4. AUTOANTIBODIES AND CLINICAL FEATURES

ANTIBODIES	FREQUENCY	CLINICAL ASSOCIATIONS	RELATIONSHIP TO DISEASE ACTIVITY
ANA	>90%	Nonspecific	For diagnostic purposes only
Anti-dsDNA	40%–60%	Nephritis	May predict disease flare and associates with flare
Anti-RNP	30%–40%	Raynaud's, musculoskeletal	Does not track disease
Antiribosomal P	10%–20%	Diffuse CNS, psychosis, major depression	Does not track disease
Anti-SSA/Ro	30%–45%	Dry eyes and mouth, SCLE, neonatal lupus, photosensitivity	Does not track disease
Anti-SSB/La	10%–15%	Dry eyes and mouth, SCLE, neonatal lupus, photosensitivity	Does not track disease
Antiphospholipid	30%	Clotting diathesis	Varied

ABBREVIATIONS: CNS, central nervous system. SCLE, subacute cutaneous lupus erythematosus.

FIGURE 15A-4

Longitudinal clinical and autoantibody profile in a patient with a lupus flare. This patient demonstrates concordance of clinical and serologic activity with regard to anti-dsDNA and complements. Note that despite changes in disease activity, titers of anti-Ro/La (elevated throughout) and anti-Sm/RNP (absent throughout) remain stable.

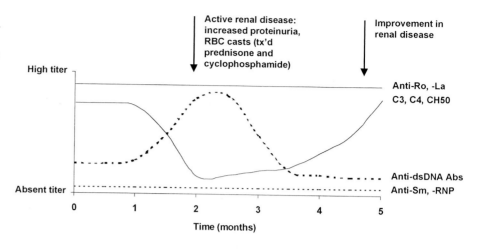

These findings are linked to the notion that immune complexes result in complement activation products that are present locally or in the circulation, and are capable of stimulating inflammatory cells with resultant vascular injury.

Measurements of anti-DNA antibodies and complement are an essential part of baseline evaluation, but treatment is dictated by the clinical picture, not necessarily the serologic one. Over time it should become obvious in an individual patient whether these parameters do predict and accompany disease flares. It is well appreciated that in certain patients low complements and elevated anti-DNA antibodies persist despite relative clinical quiescence. In contrast, there are patients who repeatedly demonstrate concordance of clinical and serologic activity (an illustrative case is provided in Figure 15A-4). In these individuals treatment may be considered solely on the basis of change in serologic parameters in advance of overt clinical disease, thus preventing relapse (28). These issues have been recently addressed in a prospective clinical trial to evaluate serologically active, clinically stable patients and determine whether anti-DNA, C3, C4, or the complement split product C3a are predictive of flare, and whether a short trial of glucocorticoids can avert major disease (29). Albeit a relatively small study, it appeared that preemptive therapy with glucocorticoids did prevent flares. At the very least it is probably prudent to increase the frequency of simple dipstick analysis of the urine in a patient with rising titers of anti-DNA and falling complement levels. It has been suggested that antinucleosome antibodies constitute a selective biologic marker of active SLE, specifically for lupus nephritis (30).

Current studies are aimed at evaluating specific biomarkers in the urine that might predict onset and type of glomerulonephritis. Recently published candidates include adiponectin, an adipocyte-derived cytokine that has anti-inflammatory properties (31); monocyte chemoattractant protein (MCP-1), a key chemokine involved in monocyte chemotaxis (32); and soluble endothelial protein C receptor (sEPCR), a protein that promotes both procoagulant and proinflammatory responses (33,34).

SPECIAL CONSIDERATIONS

Systemic Lupus Erythematosus and Pregnancy

Sterility and fertility fates for women with SLE are comparable to control groups without disease. However, increased disease activity can be associated with secondary amenorrhea. Moreover, menstrual irregularities have been noted in patients taking high doses of glucocorticoids, and age-dependent premature ovarian failure occurs in those receiving cyclophosphamide. Women with SLE have a higher rate of spontaneous abortion, intrauterine fetal death, and premature birth compared to otherwise healthy women.

In contrast to the rule of remission during pregnancies in women with RA, the influence of pregnancy on SLE disease activity is variable. There are two principal areas of concern. The first is that the clinical and serologic expression of SLE may be adversely altered by pregnancy. The second is that the placenta and fetus may become targets of specific attack by maternal autoantibodies, resulting in a generalized failure of the pregnancy or specific syndromes of passively acquired autoimmunity, such as neonatal lupus (see below).

Pregnancy outcome is optimal when disease is in complete clinical remission for 6 to 12 months (35,36). Not unexpectedly, the most recent study to address the effect of SLE clinical status on pregnancy outcome identified that high lupus activity in the first and second trimesters led to a threefold increase in pregnancy loss (miscarriages and perinatal mortality) (37). Whether flare rates increase during or after pregnancy is still unsettled, because individual patient series vary in the characteristics of patients accepted for study and in the definitions of flare. Current definitions of flare are imprecise, and accepted instruments used to measure disease activity—such as the Systemic Lupus Erythematosus Disease Activity Index (SLEDAI), British Isles Lupus Activity Group (BILAG), and Systemic Lupus Activity Measurement (SLAM)—do not account for the physiologic adaptations of pregnancy and have not been validated for pregnant lupus patients (38). Suggestions for valid criteria attributable to a flare are characteristic dermatologic involvement, arthritis, fever not secondary to infection, lymphadenopathy, leukopenia, alternative-pathway hypocomplementemia, and rising titers of antibodies to DNA. In contrast, invalid markers of disease activity include alopecia, facial or palmar blush, arthralgia, musculoskeletal aching, mild anemia, and fatigue, each of which may be present as part of the normal physiologic changes of pregnancy. Additionally, thrombocytopenia and proteinuria emerge in the setting of preeclampsia and cannot be attributed unambiguously to active lupus. In one major study comparing pregnant and nonpregnant women with SLE, the flare rates for both groups were similar (39). Despite a high overall flare rate in one series approaching 60% (35), recorded flares were usually not severe. In general, if all possible abnormalities are presumed due to SLE, disease exacerbation occurs in approximately 25%, and if only SLE-specific abnormalities are considered, disease exacerbation occurs in <13% (40).

In counseling a patient about the maternal risks of a prospective pregnancy, major issues include the presence of active nephritis and/or deterioration of renal function, neither likely in the absence of prior involvement. However, newly diagnosed lupus nephritis in the first trimester is associated with a poor fetal outcome. In a patient with established membranous nephritis, the normal increase in glomerular filtrate rate may result in protein excretion greater than 300mg/24 hours, the upper limit accepted for an otherwise normal pregnancy. In some cases there will be coexistent hypertension which then must be differentiated (if possible) from preeclampsia, especially if it first becomes evident in the third trimester. In other patients, proteinuria will more clearly represent an exacerbation of lupus nephritis as suggested by cellular casts in the urinary sediment. Activation of the alternative complement pathway with a concomitant decrease in CH50 accompanies disease flares in SLE, a laboratory finding that may be useful in distinguishing active lupus nephritis from preeclampsia or pregnancy-induced hypertension (41). The presence of active lupus nephritis and/or preeclampsia increases the risk for pre-term delivery and fetal death. Encouragingly, women in whom renal disease is stable (serum creatinine <1.5 and 24-hour protein <2g) prior to pregnancy can experience an uncomplicated course during pregnancy, despite a history of severe histopathologic changes and heavier proteinuria in the past. Additionally reassuring are the results of a recent Canadian study comparing 53 pregnant and 78 nonpregnant patients with lupus nephritis, which found that changes in renal disease activity and progression were similar in the two groups (42).

Neonatal Lupus

This illness of the fetus and neonate is considered a model of passively acquired autoimmunity, in which immune abnormalities in the mother lead to the production of anti-SSA/Ro-SSB/La antibodies that cross the placenta and presumably injure fetal tissue (43). The most serious manifestation is damage to the cardiac conducting system resulting in congenital heart block (CHB), which is most often third degree although less advanced blocks have been observed. CHB is generally identified between 16 and 24 weeks of gestation. The mortality rate is ~20% and the majority of children require pacing. Cutaneous involvement (erythematous and often annular lesions with a predilection for the eyes, face and scalp, frequently photosensitive) and, to a lesser extent, hepatic and hematologic involvement are also associated with maternal anti-SSA/Ro-SSB/La antibodies and are grouped under the heading of Neonatal Lupus Syndromes. Neonatal lupus—so termed because the dermatologic lesions of the neonate resembled those seen in SLE—is a misnomer in that less than a third of mothers of affected children actually have SLE (many are asymptomatic) and the neonatal disease is frequently only manifest as heart block, a problem rarely reported in adults with lupus. To date, complete block is irreversible. In contrast, the noncardiac manifestations are transient, resolving at about 6 months of life coincident with the disappearance of maternal autoantibodies from the neonatal circulation.

The incidence of neonatal lupus in an offspring of a mother with anti-SSA/Ro antibodies is estimated at 1% to 2%. No serologic profile is unique to mothers of affected children, but compared with mothers of healthy children, anti-SSA/Ro antibodies are usually of high titer (frequently anti-52kD SSA/Ro positive by immunoblot) and associated with anti-SSB/La antibodies (44). Reports of discordant dizygotic and monozygotic twins, and relatively low recurrence rates of CHB [in our series, 18 of 101 (18%) next pregnancies following the birth of a child with CHB] indicate that factors (likely fetal) in addition to anti-SSA/Ro and SSB/La antibodies contribute to the development of neonatal lupus (45). A Research Registry for Neonatal Lupus was established in 1994; with its current enrollment of 361 mothers and their 423 affected children, this database (along with available serum and DNA) provides a valuable resource for basic researchers and clinicians (43,45).

15

Antiphospholipid Antibody Syndrome

Antiphospholipid antibodies, ascertained by a variety of different assays, are associated with the risk of clotting. The clinical consequences include venous and arterial thromboses and placental insufficiency resulting in recurrent fetal loss. Except for manifestations of active SLE, lupus patients with antiphospholipid antibodies do not appear to have different pregnancy courses than patients with the primary antiphospholipid syndrome. Paradoxically, thrombocytopenia can also be part of the clinical spectrum because the surfaces of activated platelets display the anionic phospholipid target antigens. Patients who have antiphospholipid antibodies and one of the above clinical features in the absence of any other manifestations of SLE are classified as having primary antiphospholipid syndrome (APS), as outlined in Table 15A-5; 46,47). Alternatively a patient can have these antibodies in the context of SLE (secondary APS).

Currently, assessment of antiphospholipid antibodies is done by enzyme-linked immunosorbent assay (ELISA) to measure reactivity with cardiolipin, or by prolonged clotting in an in vitro system which is not corrected by mixing studies. The latter test is paradoxical because the readout is the inability to form a clot due to interference with proper assembly of the clotting factors, yet in vivo these antibodies are thrombogenic. Experimental data suggest that "antiphospholipid" antibodies are not directed against anionic phospholipids, as initially hypothesized, but are part of a larger group of autoantibodies that recognize phospholipid-binding proteins. At present, the best-characterized antigenic target is beta2-glycoprotein I (beta 2GPI) (48), which has been shown to possess multiple inhibitory functions in coagulation pathways. Although the measurement of antiphospholipid antibodies by ELISA is now well standardized, these new observations on beta 2GPI will require large-scale testing, the outcome of which may substantially alter current recommendations.

TABLE 15A-5. PRELIMINARY CLASSIFICATION CRITERIA FOR ANTIPHOSPHOLIPID SYNDROME (APS)*

CLINICAL CRITERIA

Vascular thrombosis
- ≥ 1 arterial, venous, or small-vessel thrombosis in any tissue or organ,

AND
- Confirmation by imaging or Doppler studies or histopathology (not SVT)

Pregnancy morbidity:
- ≥ 1 unexplained death(s) of normal fetus at ≥ 10 weeks gestation,

OR
- ≥ 1 premature birth(s) of normal neonate at ≤ 34 weeks gestation due to severe preeclampsia or placental insufficiency,

OR
- ≥ 3 unexplained consecutive spontaneous abortions < 10 weeks gestation (exclude anatomic, hormonal, or chromosomal abnormality)

LABORATORY CRITERIA

- Anticardiolipin antibody of IgG and/or IgM isotype
  - medium or high titer (15–80 GPL, 6–50 MPL)
  - on ≥ 2 occasions at least 6 weeks apart
  - measured by standard ELISA for beta2-glycoprotein I-dependent anticardiolipin antibodies

OR
- Lupus anticoagulant (LAC)
  - on ≥ 2 occasions at least 6 weeks apart

SOURCE: Adapted from Derksen RH, Khamashta MA, Branch DW (46), by permission of *Arthritis Rheum.*
ABBREVIATION: APS, antiphospholipid syndrome.
*APS considered definite if at least one clinical and one laboratory criteria are met.

Drug-Related Lupus

The term *drug-related lupus* (DRL) refers to the development of a lupuslike syndrome which follows exposure to chlorpromazine, hydralazine, isoniazid, methyldopa, minocycline, procainamide, or quinidine. In addition to these definitively associated drugs, there is a long list of other potential offending agents, such as diphenylhydantoin, penicillamine, and gold salts (49). There are no specified ACR criteria for DRL, but in general these patients present with fewer than four SLE criteria. A temporal association (generally a matter of weeks or months) between ingestion of an agent and development of symptoms is required. Following removal of the offending agent, there should be rapid resolution of the clinical features although autoantibodies may persist for 6 months to a year. Drugs capable of causing DRL do not seem to aggravate idiopathic SLE. The demographic features of DRL tend to reflect those of the diseases for which the offending drug has been prescribed. Accordingly, DRL occurs more frequently in the elderly, occurs only slightly more frequently in females than males, and is more common in Caucasians than African Americans.

Drug-related lupus patients frequently present with constitutional symptoms such as malaise, low grade fever, and myalgia, which may occur acutely or insidiously. Articular complaints are present in over 80%, with arthralgia being more common than arthritis. Pleuropulmonary disease and pericarditis are present most often in procainamide-related lupus. Other clinical manifestations of idiopathic SLE, such as dermatologic, renal, and neurologic, are rare in DRL. ANAs should be present in order to diagnose DRL. However, the development of an ANA without accompanying clinical features is insufficient for the diagnosis and not reason by itself to discontinue medication. Typically the ANA is a diffuse-homogenous pattern, which represents binding of autoantibodies to chromatin that consists of

DNA and histones. Anti-dsDNA and anti-Sm are not characteristic of DRL.

CONCLUSIONS

Systemic lupus erythematosus is a composite of clinically unrelated manifestations often accumulated over time which are unified, with rare exception, by the presence of antibodies directed against one or more self components of the nucleus, cytoplasm, and/or cell membrane. Greater awareness of the clinical features and advances in the laboratory evaluation of autoantibodies have facilitated diagnosis and eliminated much of the frustration previously experienced both by the patient and physician. In many patients flares are mimetic, but new manifestations can always be a threat. Physicians caring for patients with lupus should maintain high vigilance for the unexpected. The accurate prediction of flares and preemptive treatment in clinically quiescent patients is likely to result in longer periods of remission. Accordingly, the search for biomarkers to predict future morbidity and mortality offers unparalleled promise.

REFERENCES

1. Tan EM, Cohen AS, Fries JF, et al. The 1982 revised criteria for the classification of systemic lupus erythematosus. Arthritis Rheum 1982;25:1271–1277.
2. Hochberg MC. Updating the American College of Rheumatology revised criteria for the classification of systemic lupus erythematosus [letter]. Arthritis Rheum 1997;40:1725.
3. Gladman DD. Systemic lupus erythematosus: Clinical features. In: Klippel JH, Weyand CM, Wortmann RL, eds. Primer on the rheumatic diseases. 11th ed. Atlanta: Arthritis Foundation; 1997:267–272.
4. Ginzler EM, Schorn K. Outcome and prognosis in systemic lupus erythematosus. Rheum Dis Clin North Am 1988;14:67–78.
5. Boumpas DR, Fessler BJ, Austin HA, Balow JE, Klippel JH, Lockshin MD. Systemic lupus erythematosus: emerging concepts. Part 2: Dermatologic and joint disease, the antiphospholipid antibody syndrome, pregnancy and hormonal therapy, morbidity and mortality, and pathogenesis. Ann Int Med 1995;123:42–53.
6. Urowitz MB, Bookman AAM, Koehler BE, et al. The bimodal mortality in systemic lupus erythematosus. Am J Med 1976;60:221–225.
7. Urowitz MB, Gladman DD. Accelerated atheroma in lupus—background. Lupus 2000;9:161–165.
8. Mimouni D, Nousari CH. Systemic lupus erythematosus and the skin. In: Lahita R, ed. Systemic lupus erythematosus. 4th ed. New York: Elsevier/Academic Press; 2004:855–876.
9. Hill GS, Delahousse M, Nochy D, et al. A new morphologic index for the evaluation of renal biopsies in lupus nephritis. Kidney Int 2000;58:1160–1173.
10. Appel GB, Silva FG, Pirani CL. Renal involvement in systemic lupus erythematosus (SLE): a study of 56 patients emphasizing histologic classification. Medicine 1978;75:371–410.
11. Weening, JJ, D'Agati VD, Schwartz MM, et al. Classification of glomerulonephritis in systemic lupus erythematosus revisited. J Am Soc Nephrol 2004;15:241–250.
12. Stone JH, Millward CL, Olson JL, Amend WJ, Criswell LA. Frequency of recurrent lupus nephritis among ninety-seven renal transplant patients during the cyclosporine era. Arthritis Rheum 1998;41:678–686.
13. Nossent HC, Swaak TJG, Berden JHM. Systemic lupus erythematosus: analysis of disease activity in 55 patients with end-stage renal failure treated with hemodialysis or continuous ambulatory peritoneal dialysis. Am J Med 1990;89:169–174.
14. Krane NK, Burjak K, Archie M, O'Donovan R. Persistent lupus activity in end-stage renal disease. Am J Kidney Dis 1999;33:872–879.
15. Boumpas DR, Austin HA, Fessler BJ, Balow JE, Klippel JH, Lockshin MD. Systemic lupus erythematosus: emerging concepts. Part 1: renal, neuropsychiatric, cardiovascular, pulmonary and hematologic disease. Ann Int Med 1995;122:940–950.
16. ACR Ad Hoc Committee on Neuropsychiatric Lupus Nomenclature. The American College of Rheumatology nomenclature and case definitions for neuropsychiatric lupus syndromes. Arthritis Rheum 2000;42:599–608.
17. West SG, Emlen W, Wener M, Kotzin BL. Neuropsychiatric lupus erythematosus: a 10-year prospective study on the value of diagnostic tests. Am J Med 1995;99:153–163.
18. Roldan CA, Shively BK, Crawford MH. An echocardiographic study of valvular heart disease associated with systemic lupus erythematosus. N Engl J Med 1996;335:1424–1430.
19. Rosner S, Ginzler EM, Diamond HS, et al. A multicenter study of outcome in systemic lupus erythematosus. II. Causes of death. Arthritis Rheum 1982;25:612–617.
20. Haider YS, Roberts WC. Coronary arterial disease in systemic lupus erythematosus: quantification of degree of narrowing in 22 necropsy patients (21 women) aged 16 to 37 years. Am J Med 1981;70:775–781.
21. Petri M. Detection of coronary artery disease and the role of traditional risk factors in the Hopkins Lupus Cohort. Lupus 2000;9:170–175.
22. Manzi S, Selzer F, Sutton-Tyrrell K, et al. Prevalence and risk factors of carotid plaque in women with systemic lupus erythematosus. Arthritis Rheum 1999;42:51–60.
23. Roman MJ, Shanker BA, Davis A, et al. Prevalence and correlates of accelerated atherosclerosis in systemic lupus erythematosus. N Engl J Med 2003;349:2399–2406.
24. Asanuma Y, Chung CP, Oeser A, et al. Increased concentration of proatherogenic inflammatory cytokines in systemic lupus erythematosus: relationship to cardiovascular risk factors. J Rheumatol 2006;33:539–545.
25. Winslow TM, Ossipov MA, Fazio GP, Simonson JS, Redberg RF, Schiller NB. Five-year follow-up study of the prevalence and progression of pulmonary hypertension in systemic lupus erythematosus. Am Heart J 1995;129:510–515.

26. DeGiorgio LA, Konstantinov KN, Lee SC, Hardin JA, Volpe BT, Diamond B. A subset of lupus anti-DNA antibodies cross-reacts with the NR2 glutamate receptor in systemic lupus erythematosus. Nature Med 2001;7:1189–1193.

27. Schur PH, Sandson J. Immunologic factors and clinical activity in systemic lupus erythematosus. N Engl J Med 1968;278:533–538.

28. Bootsma H, Spronk P, Derksen R, et al. Prevention of relapses in systemic lupus erythematosus. Lancet 1995;345:1595–1599.

29. Tseng CE, Buyon JP, Kim M, et al. The effect of moderate-dose corticosteroids in preventing severe flares in patients with serologically active, but clinically stable, systemic lupus erythematosus: findings of a prospective, randomized, double-blind, placebo-controlled trial. Arthritis Rheum 2006;54:3623–3632.

30. Amoura Z, Koutouzov S, Chabre H, et al. Presence of antinucleosome autoantibodies in a restricted set of connective tissue diseases. Antinucleosome antibodies of the IgG3 subclass are marker of renal pathogenicity in systemic lupus erythematosus. Arthritis Rheum 2000;43:76–84.

31. Rovin BH, Song H, Hebert LA, et al. Plasma, urine, and renal expression of adiponectin in human systemic lupus erythematosus. Kidney Int 2005;68:1825–1833.

32. Li Y, Tucci M, Narain S, et al. Urinary biomarkers in lupus nephritis. Autoimmun Rev 2006;5:383–438.

33. Sesin CA, Yin X, Esmon CT, Buyon JP, Clancy RM. Shedding of endothelial protein C receptor contributes to vasculopathy and renal injury in lupus: in vivo and in vitro evidence. Kidney Int 2005;68:110–120.

34. Rivera TL, Izmirly PM, Buyon JP, Clancy RM. Contribution of vasculopathy to lupus nephritis: endothelial protein C receptor levels and genotype [abstract]. Arthritis Rheum 2006;54:S824–S825.

35. Petri M, Howard D, Repke J. Frequency of lupus flares in pregnancy. The Hopkins Lupus Pregnancy Center experience. Arthritis Rheum 1991;34:1538–1545.

36. Urowitz MB, Gladman DD, Farewell VT, Stewart J, McDonald J. Lupus and pregnancy studies. Arthritis Rheum 1993;36:1392–1397.

37. Clowse ME, Magder LS, Witter F, Petri M. The impact of increased lupus activity on obstetric outcomes. Arthritis Rheum 2005;52:514–521.

38. Buyon J, Kalunian K, Ramsey-Goldman R, et al. Assessing disease activity in SLE patients during pregnancy. Lupus 1999;8:677–684.

39. Lockshin MD, Reinitz E, Druzin ML, Murrman M, Estes D. Lupus pregnancy. Case control prospective study demonstrating absence of lupus exacerbation during or after pregnancy. Am J Med 1984;77:893–898.

40. Lockshin MD. Pregnancy does not cause systemic lupus erythematosus to worsen. Arthritis Rheum 1989;32:665–670.

41. Buyon JP, Tamerius J, Ordorica S, Abramson SB. Activation of the alternative complement pathway accompanies disease flares in systemic lupus erythematosus during pregnancy. Arthritis Rheum 1992;35:55–61.

42. Tandon A, Ibanez D, Gladman DD, Urowitz MB. The effect of pregnancy on lupus nephritis. Arthritis Rheum 2004;50:3941–3946.

43. Buyon JP, Hiebert R, Copel J, et al. Autoimmune-associated congenital heart block: Mortality, morbidity, and recurrence rates obtained from a national neonatal lupus registry. J Am Coll Cardiol 1998;31:1658–1666.

44. Buyon JP, Winchester RJ, Slade SG, et al. Identification of mothers at risk for congenital heart block and other neonatal lupus syndromes in their children: comparison of ELISA and immunoblot to measure anti-SSA/Ro and anti-SSB/La antibodies. Arthritis Rheum 1993;36:1263–1273.

45. Buyon JP, Clancy RM. Neonatal lupus. In: Wallace DJ, Hahn, BH, eds. Dubois' lupus erythematosus. 7th ed. Philadelphia: Lippincott Williams & Wilkins; 2006:1058–1080.

46. Derksen RH, Khamashta MA, Branch DW. Management of the obstetric antiphospholipid syndrome. Arthritis Rheum 2004;50:1028–1039.

47. Miyakis S, Lockshin MD, Atsumi T, et al. International consensus statement on an update of the classification criteria for definite antiphospholipid syndrome (APS). J Thromb Haemost 2006;4:295–306.

48. McNeil HP, Simpson RJ, Chesterman CN, Krilis SA. Antiphospholipid antibodies are directed against a complex antigen that includes a lipid-binding inhibitor of coagulation: beta2-glycoprotein I (apolipoprotein H). Proc Natl Acad Sci U S A 1990;87:4120–4124.

49. Mongey A-B, Hess EV. Drug and environmental systemic lupus erythematosus: clinical manifestations and differences. In: Lahita R, ed. Systemic lupus erythematosus. 4th ed. New York: Elsevier/Academic Press; 2004:1211–1240.

50. Lahita R, ed. Systemic lupus erythematosus. 4th ed. New York: Elsevier/Academic Press; 2004.

51. Wallace DJ, Hahn BH, eds. Dubois' lupus erythematosus. 7th ed. Philsdelphia: Lippincott Williams & Wilkins; 2006.

Systemic Lupus Erythematosus
B. Epidemiology, Pathology, and Pathogenesis

DAVID S. PISETSKY, MD, PHD

- Systemic lupus erythematosus (SLE) is primarily a disease of young women, though it can be seen in both pediatric and older patients where the sex ratio is more balanced.
- The pathologic findings of SLE occur throughout the body and are manifested by inflammation, blood vessel abnormalities that encompass bland vasculopathy and vasculitis, and immune-complex deposition.
- Autoantibodies can occur in the absence of clinical lupus, but pathogenic autoantibodies are important contributors to tissue damage in the kidney as well as in other involved organs.

- Autoantibodies in lupus may be driven by self-antigens implicating a more generalized immune cell dysfunction. which promotes B-cell hyperactivity.
- Genetic susceptibility to lupus is likely polygenic, as exemplified by multiple types of genes associated with lupuslike diseases in mice.
- Triggering events for disease initiation and flares may include may environmental exposures, such as hormones, infectious agents, diet, sunlight, toxins (including drugs), and others.

EPIDEMIOLOGY

Systemic lupus erythematosus (SLE) is a prototypic autoimmune disease with diverse clinical manifestations in association with autoantibodies to components of the cell nucleus. SLE primarily is a disease of young women, with a peak incidence between the ages of 15 and 40 and a female:male ratio of 6 to 10:1. The age at onset, however, can range from infancy to advanced age; in both pediatric- and older-onset patients, the female:male ratio is approximately 2:1. In a general outpatient population, SLE affects approximately one in 2000 individuals, although the prevalence varies with race, ethnicity, and socioeconomic status (1).

Like other autoimmune diseases, SLE can display familial aggregation, with a higher frequency among first-degree relatives of patients. The disease occurs concordantly in approximately 25% to 50% of monozygotic twins and 5% of dizygotic twins. Moreover, in extended families, SLE may occur with other autoimmune conditions, such as hemolytic anemia, thyroiditis, and idiopathic thrombocytopenia purpura. Despite the influence of heredity, most cases of SLE appear sporadic.

IMMUNOPATHOLOGY

The pathologic findings of SLE occur throughout the body and are manifested by inflammation, blood vessel abnormalities that encompass bland vasculopathy and vasculitis, and immune-complex deposition. The best-characterized pathology involves the kidney, which displays increases in mesangial cells and mesangial matrix, inflammation, cellular proliferation, basement membrane abnormalities, and immune-complex deposition. These deposits are comprised of IgM, IgG, and IgA, as well as complement components. On electron microscopy, the deposits can be seen in the mesangium and the subendothelial and subepithelial sides of the glomerular basement membrane (Figure 15B-l). Renal pathology is classified according to two systems to provide information for clinical staging (see Chapter 15A) (2,3). With either system, lupus nephritis exhibits marked variability, differing in severity and pattern among patients, as illustrated in Figure 15B-2.

Skin lesions in SLE demonstrate inflammation and degeneration at the dermal–epidermal junction, and the basal or germinal layer is the primary site of injury. In these lesions, granular deposits of IgG and complement

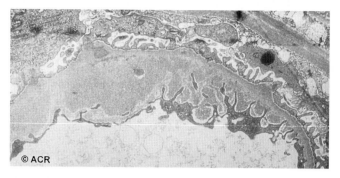

FIGURE 15B-1

Immune deposits in lupus nephritis. This electron micrograph illustrates large granular subendothelial immune deposits, as well as smaller subepithelial and intramembranous deposits. Broadening and fusion of the foot processes also are present. (Reprinted from the Revised Clinical Slide Collection on the Rheumatic Diseases, with permission of American College of Rheumatology.)

components occur in a bandlike pattern as observed by immunofluorescence microscopy. Necrotizing vasculitis also may cause skin lesions. Other organ systems affected by SLE usually display nonspecific inflammation or vessel abnormalities, although pathologic findings sometimes are minimal. For example, despite the severity of central nervous system (CNS) involvement, the typical findings are cortical microinfarcts and a bland vasculopathy with degenerative or proliferative changes; inflammation and necrosis indicative of vasculitis are found only rarely.

The heart may show nonspecific foci of inflammation in the pericardium, myocardium, and endocardium, even in the absence of clinically significant manifestations. Verrucous endocarditis, known as Libman–Sacks endocarditis, is a classic pathologic finding of SLE and is manifested by vegetations, most frequently at the mitral valve. These vegetations consist of accumulations of immune complexes, inflammatory cells, fibrin, and necrotic debris.

Occlusive vasculopathy with venous and arterial thrombosis is a common pathologic finding in SLE. Although coagulation can result from inflammation, autoantibodies also may trigger thrombotic events. These autoantibodies represent a spectrum of specificities designated as antiphospholipid antibodies, anticardiolipin antibodies, or lupus anticoagulants (4). Although some of these antibodies bind lipid antigens, others are directed to the serum protein beta$_2$-glycoprotein 1, a protein that can form complexes with lipids. Vessel abnormalities in SLE may also result from increases in endothelial cell adhesiveness by a mechanism analogous to the Schwartzman reaction triggered by Gram-negative bacteria.

Other pathologic findings prominent in SLE have an uncertain relationship to inflammation. Patients, including women without the usual risk factors for cardiovascular disease, frequently develop accelerated atherosclerosis and have an increased risk of stroke and myocardial infarction. It is unclear whether these lesions result from corticosteroid-induced metabolic abnormalities, hypertension, or vascular changes caused by a chronic burden of inflammation. Similarly, osteonecrosis, as well as neurodegeneration in people with chronic severe disease, may arise from vasculopathy, drug side effects, or persistent immunologic insults.

FIGURE 15B-2

(Left) Signs of "active" lupus nephritis showing glomerular proliferation, crescents, abundant inflammatory cell infiltration, and interstitial cell infiltrates (hematoxylin–eosin stain). (Right) Signs of "chronic" lupus nephritis showing glomerular cirrhosis, vascular thickening, tubular atrophy, and interstitial fibrosis (periodic acid, Schiff stain).

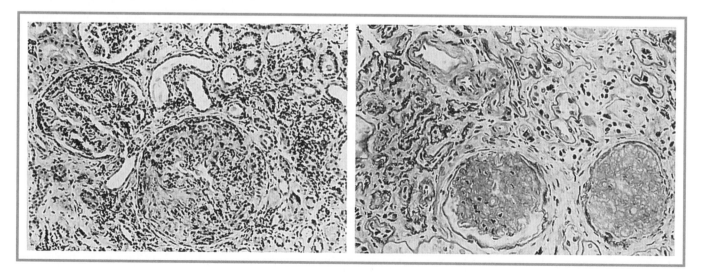

IMMUNOPATHOGENESIS OF ANTINUCLEAR ANTIBODIES

The central immunologic disturbance in SLE is autoantibody production. These antibodies are directed to a host of self-molecules found in the nucleus, cytoplasm, or surface of cells. In addition, SLE sera contain antibodies to such soluble molecules as IgG and coagulation factors. Because of the wide range of its antigenic targets, SLE is classified as a disease of generalized autoimmunity.

Among autoantibodies found in patient sera, those directed against components of the cell nucleus (antinuclear antibodies, or ANA) are the most characteristic of SLE and are found in more than 95% of patients (5). These antibodies bind DNA, RNA, nuclear proteins, and protein/nucleic acid complexes (Table 15B-1). As a group, the molecules targeted by ANA are highly conserved among species, serve important cellular functions, and exist inside cells as part of complexes (e.g., nucleosomes). Furthermore, these molecules, depending upon context (e.g., presence in immune complexes), display intrinsic immunological activity. This activity results from stimulation of the innate immune system via receptors known as the Toll-like receptors (TLR). The TLRs can recognize a diverse array of foreign and self-molecules, with DNA, single-stranded RNA and double-stranded RNA all TLR ligands (6).

Antibodies to certain nuclear antigens (e.g., DNA and histones) frequently occur together, a phenomenon known as linkage. Linkage suggests that a complex, rather than the individual components, serves as the target of autoreactivity, as well as its driving antigen.

Among ANA specificities in SLE, two appear unique to this disease. Antibodies to double-stranded (ds) DNA and a nuclear antigen called Sm are essentially found only in people with SLE, and are included as serologic criteria in the classification of SLE (see Appendix I). Although both anti-DNA and anti-Sm are serologic markers, they differ in their pattern of expression and clinical associations. Whereas anti-DNA levels can fluctuate markedly over time, anti-Sm levels remain more constant. The anti-Sm and anti-DNA responses also differ in the nature of their target antigens. The Sm antigen is designated an snRNP (small nuclear ribonucleoprotein) and consists of uridine-rich RNA molecules complexed with proteins. In contrast to anti-DNA antibodies, which react to a nucleic acid determinant, anti-Sm antibodies target snRNP proteins and not RNA.

Perhaps the most remarkable feature of the anti-DNA response is its association with immunopathologic events in SLE, especially glomerulonephritis. This role has been established by correlating anti-DNA serum levels with disease activity, isolating anti-DNA in enriched form from glomerular eluates of patients with active nephritis, and inducing nephritis by administering anti-DNA antibodies to normal animals. The relationship between levels of anti-DNA and active renal disease is not invariable; some patients with active nephritis may lack serum anti-DNA, and others with high levels of anti-DNA are clinically discordant and escape nephritis (7).

The occurrence of nephritis without anti-DNA may be explained by the pathogenicity of other autoantibody specificities (e.g., anti-Ro or anti-Sm). The converse situation of clinical quiescence despite serologic

TABLE 15B-1. PRINCIPLE ANTINUCLEAR ANTIBODIES IN SYSTEMIC LUPUS ERYTHEMATOSUS.

SPECIFICITY	TARGET ANTIGEN	FUNCTION
Native DNA	dsDNA	Genetic information
Denatured DNA	ssDNA	Genetic information
Histones	H1, H2A, H2B, H3, H4	Nucleosome structure
Sm	snRNP proteins B, B', D, E	Splicesome component, RNA processing
U1RNP	snRNP proteins, A, C, 70K	Splicesome component, RNA processing
SSA/Ro	60- and 52-KDa proteins, complexed with Y1-Y5 RNAs	Unknown
SSB/La	48-kDa protein complexed with various small RNAs	Regulation of RNA polymerase-3 transcription
Ku	86- and 66-kDa proteins	DNA binding
PCNA/cyclin	36-kDa protein	Auxiliary protein of DNA polymerase alpha
Ribosomal RNP	38-, 16-, 15-kDa phosphoproteins, associated with ribosomes	Protein synthesis

SOURCE: Modified from Tan EM, Adv Immunol 1989;44:93–151, with permission of *Advances in Immunology*.
ABBREVIATIONS: ss, double-stranded; ss, single-stranded; snRNP, small nuclear ribonucleoprotein.

activity suggests that only some anti-DNA provoke glomerulonephritis. Antibodies with this property are denoted as pathogenic or nephritogenic. Features promoting pathogenicity may include isotype, charge, ability to fix complement, and capacity to bind glomerular preparations (7). In this regard, anti-DNA antibodies appear to be a subset of pathogenic antibodies that bind to nucleosomes, the likely form of DNA in the circulation as well as in immune deposits. Unless the full range of antinucleosomal antibodies is assessed, the presence of nephritogenic antibodies may be missed.

In addition to their direct role in nephritis, antibodies to DNA may promote immune system disturbances that potentiate inflammation systemically as well in the kidney. Thus, immune complexes containing DNA can promote the expression of interferon alpha (IFN-alpha) by a specialized population of dendritic cells known as plasmacytoid dendritic cells. This response requires the presence of both antibody and DNA in an immune complex and depends upon Fc receptors. While the basis of this response is not well understood, stimulation may involve the TLRs as well as other non-TLR signaling systems that respond to internalized nucleic acids. Antibodies to other nuclear antigens, including RNP complexes, can also stimulate this response, raising the possibility that immune complexes, in addition promoting organ damage, can contribute to the overall disturbance in the immune system in patients (8).

In addition to anti-DNA, other autoantibodies may have a clinical impact because of effects on organ-specific manifestations. Associations of other autoantibodies with disease events include antibodies to ribosomal P proteins (anti-P) with neuropsychiatric disease and hepatitis; antibodies to Ro with neonatal lupus and subacute cutaneous lupus; antibodies to phospholipids with vascular thrombosis, thrombocytopenia, and recurrent abortion; and antibodies to blood cells with cytopenias.

The contribution of ANAs to clinical events in SLE has been difficult to understand because the intracellular location of the target antigens should protect them from antibody interactions. The location of these antigens may not be fixed, however, and some antigens may translocate to the membrane and become accessible to antibody attack either during development or during apoptosis. Thus, during cardiac development, a molecule bound by anti-Ro appears on the surface of myocytes and, in the presence of complement, lead to local inflammation and damage to the conducting system (9).

Because of the impact of kidney disease on morbidity and mortality, nephritis has been the clinical event in SLE most intensively studied mechanistically. Clinical observations strongly suggest that SLE renal disease results from the deposition of immune complexes containing anti-DNA, because active nephritis is marked by elevated anti-DNA levels with a depression of total hemolytic complement. Because anti-DNA shows preferential renal deposition, these findings suggest that DNA/anti-DNA immune complexes are a major pathogenic species. DNA in these complexes likely is in the form of nucleosomes, suggesting that antibodies to other components of this structure may participate in immune-complex formation.

Although immune complexes may provoke renal injury in SLE, the amounts of such complexes in the serum appear limited. This finding has suggested that complexes may form in situ, rather than within the circulation. According to this mechanism, immune complexes assemble in the kidney on DNA or other nucleosomal components adherent to the glomerular basement membrane. Another mechanism for nephritis in SLE is the direct interaction of autoantibodies with glomerular antigens. Many anti-DNA antibodies are polyspecific and interact with molecules other than DNA. The binding of anti-DNA to these molecules could activate complement and inciting inflammation.

The pathogenesis of other SLE manifestations is less well understood, although immune-complex deposition at relevant tissue sites generally has been considered a likely mechanism. Indeed, the frequent association of depressed complement levels and signs of vasculitis with active SLE suggests that immune complexes are important agents for initiating or exacerbating organ damage. These considerations do not exclude the possibility that tissue injury results from either cell-mediated cytotoxicity or direct antibody attack on target tissues. Consistent with the operation of such a mechanism, a cross-reactive population of antibodies to the NMDA receptor may CNS disturbances by inducing excitotoxic damage (10).

DETERMINANTS OF DISEASE SUSCEPTIBILITY

Studies of patients suggest that SLE is caused by genetically determined immune abnormalities that can be triggered by exogenous or endogenous factors. Although the predisposition to disease is hereditary, it is likely multigenic and involves different sets of genes in different individuals (see Chapter 5). Analysis of genetic susceptibility has been based primarily on the search for gene polymorphisms occurring with greater frequency in people with SLE than in control populations. The study of genetic factors predisposing to SLE also has involved genomewide scans of siblings with SLE or multiplex families. Although this approach has led to the identification of chromosomal regions that contain genes potentially relevant to pathogenesis, the identities of these genes are not yet known definitively. Furthermore, the regions associated with disease may differ depending upon racial and ethnic group (11).

Of genetic systems that could predispose to autoimmunity, the major histocompatibility complex (MHC) has been most intensively scrutinized for its contribution to human SLE. Using a variety of MHC gene markers, population-based studies indicate that the susceptibility to SLE, like many other autoimmune diseases in humans, involves class II gene polymorphisms. An association of human leukocyte antigen (HLA)-DR2 and HLA-DR3 (and various subspecificities) with SLE has been commonly observed, with these alleles producing a relative risk of disease that ranges approximately from 2 to 5. This analysis of MHC gene associations is complicated by the existence of extended HLA haplotypes in which class II genes are in linkage disequilibrium with other potential susceptibility genes. Because the MHC is rich in genes for immune-system elements, the association of disease with a class II marker does not denote a specific functional abnormality promoting pathogenesis.

Among other MHC gene systems, inherited complement deficiencies can influence disease susceptibility. Like class I and II molecules, complement components, in particular C4a and C4b, show striking genetic polymorphism, with a deficiency of C4a molecules (null alleles) a common occurrence in the population. As many as 80% of people with SLE have null alleles irrespective of ethnic background, with homozygous C4a deficiency conferring a high risk for SLE. Because C4a null alleles are part of an extended HLA haplotype with the markers HLA-B8 and HLA-DR3, the influence of these class I and class II alleles of disease susceptibility may reflect linkage disequilibrium with complement deficiency. SLE also is associated with inherited deficiency of Clq, Clr/s, and C2 (12).

An association of SLE with inherited complement deficiency may seem surprising because of the prominence of immune-complex deposition and complement consumption during disease. However, a decrease in complement activity could promote disease susceptibility by impairing the clearance of foreign antigen or apoptotic cells. Apoptosis, or programmed cell death, is associated with the breakdown of DNA, the rearrangement of intracellular constituents, and the release DNA and RNA into external milieu where these molecules, alone or in the context of immune complexes, could stimulate the immune system by the TLRs.

As shown in in vitro and in vivo systems, the clearance of apoptotic cells, a process called *efferocytosis*, involves diverse cellular and humoral pathways, including the complement system. Clq, for example, binds to apoptotic cells, initiating complement's role in clearance. In the absence of complement, apoptotic cells may persist and stimulate immune responses. The importance of complement deficiency to autoimmunity is illustrated by the features of mice in which C1q has been eliminated by genetic knockout techniques. C1q-deficient mice have elevated anti-DNA levels, glomerulonephritis, and increased apoptotic cells in the tissue (13). Impairment of other aspects of the clearance system (e.g., IgM and DNase) can also provoke immune system abnormalities, including the stimulation of interferon by dead and dying cells and their constituents.

GENETICS OF MURINE SYSTEMIC LUPUS ERYTHEMATOSUS

Several strains of inbred mice with inherited lupuslike disease have been studied as models to elucidate the human disease. These mice mimic human SLE in ANA production, immune complex glomerulonephritis, lymphadenopathy, and abnormal B-cell and T-cell function. These strains differ in the expression of certain serologic and clinical findings (e.g., anti-Sm, hemolytic anemia, and arthritis), as well as in the occurrence of disease among males and females. Among various lupus strains described (NZB, NZB/NZW, MRL-lpr/lpr, BXSB, and C3H-gl/lgld), the development of a full-blown lupus syndrome requires multiple unlinked genes (11).

In mice, single mutant genes (lpr, gld, and Yaa) can promote anti-DNA production and abnormalities in the number and function of B and T cells. In lpr and gld mice, these abnormalities result from mutations in proteins involved in apoptosis. Apoptosis plays a critical role in the development of the immune system, as well as in the establishment and maintenance of tolerance. The lpr mutation leads to the absence of Fas, a cell-surface molecule that triggers apoptosis in lymphocytes, and gld affects a molecule that interacts with Fas, the Fas ligand. These gene defects appear to operate in peripheral, in contrast to central, tolerance and allow the persistence of autoreactive cells. Among humans, while mutations of Fas can lead to lymphoproliferation and autoantibody production, clinical and serologic findings of SLE are uncommon, suggesting that in humans, as in the mouse, SLE requires more than one gene.

The interaction of genes in SLE also occurs in New Zealand mice. NZB/NZW F1 mice develop an SLE-like illness that results from genes contributed by both NZB and NZW parents. Among these genes, an interferon inducible gene called Ifi202 contributes powerfully to the development of autoimmunity, providing additional evidence between the link between the interferon system and SLE (8). In the NZM2410 model, extensive genetic studies have shown that genes that can promote as well as suppress autoimmunity. Individually, genes that promote autoimmunity (denoted sle1, sle2, sle3) lead to distinct immune disturbances, including expression of ANA. When these genes are co-expressed because of genetic crosses, the clinical and serologic features of SLE occur. Importantly, other genes can suppress the development of SLE in mice, indicating complexity in the genetic predisposition for disease (11).

Among lupus mice, New Zealand strains have an MHC-linked deficiency in the expression of the proinflammatory cytokine tumor necrosis factor alpha (TNF-alpha). This deficiency may be pathogenic because administration of TNF-alpha to mice with low endogenous production ameliorates disease. In humans, TNF blockers have not been extensively used to treat patients because of concerns that it can potentiate autoreactivity; in small clinical trials, however, such therapy did not exacerbate disease (14). A role of TNF-alpha in the pathogenesis of autoimmunity is also suggested by the development of anti-DNA antibodies in patients with rheumatoid arthritis treated with TNF blockers, although the full development of SLE is very uncommon in this setting.

A variety of new SLE models have been created using molecular genetic techniques. These models reflect aberrant patterns of gene expression that occur in mice in which specific genes are eliminated by knockout techniques or enhanced by transgene expression. Studies of these mice suggest that a variety of genetic abnormalities may predispose to autoimmunity and genes regulating immune cell life span or signaling threshold may lead to autoantibody production. These genetic defects may affect the establishment of tolerance or the persistence of autoreactive cells.

IMMUNE CELL DISTURBANCES

Autoantibody production in SLE occurs in the setting of generalized immune cell abnormalities that involve the B cell, T cell, and monocyte lineages. These immune cell disturbances appear to promote B-cell hyperactivity, leading to hyperglobulinemia, increased numbers of antibody-producing cells, and heightened responses to many antigens, both self and foreign. Another consequence of B-cell and T-cell disturbance in SLE may be abnormal tolerance. In healthy individuals, anti-DNA precursors are tolerated by anergy or deletion; however, people with SLE or animals with SLE models may retain such precursors, which can be stimulated to generate high affinity autoantibody responses (15).

While these immune cell disturbances can affect multiple cell types and lineages, the appearance of an interferon signature is a prominent feature in peripheral blood cells of patients. As shown using microarray and related molecular techniques, peripheral blood cells of SLE patients demonstrate patterns of gene expression consistent with stimulation by IFN-alpha. Furthermore, this signature appears to be associated with antibodies to DNA or RNP antigens, consistent with stimulation of this cytokine by the nucleic acid components of immune complexes impacting on Toll-like receptors (TLR) or other receptors (see Chapter 4) (16,17). In view of the broad effects of the type I interferons on the immune system, a host of nonspecific functional abnormalities could result from the presence of high levels of this cytokine.

Although nonspecific immune activation can provoke certain ANA responses, it does not appear to be the major mechanism for inducing pathogenic autoantibodies, especially anti-DNA. Levels of these antibodies far exceed the extent of hyperglobulinemia. In addition, anti-DNA antibodies have features indicative of in vivo antigen selection by a receptor-driven mechanism. These features include variable-region somatic mutations that increase DNA binding activity and specificity for dsDNA. The generation of such responses also may be affected by the composition of the pre-immune repertoire and the content of precursors that can be mutated under influence of self-antigen drive.

The ability of DNA to drive autoantibody production in SLE contrasts with the poor immunogenicity of mammalian DNA when administered to normal animals. This discrepancy suggests that SLE patients either have a unique capacity to respond to DNA or are exposed to DNA in a form with enhanced immunogenicity (e.g., surface blebs on apoptotic cells or nucleosomes). Although serologic profiles of people with SLE and mice with murine models of SLE point to nucleosomes as the driving antigen, bacterial or viral DNA may stimulate this response. Bacterial DNA, because of characteristic sequence motifs, can stimulate a TLR directly and has potent adjuvant properties. As a result, bacterial DNA is immunogenic and may be able to elicit anti-DNA autoantibodies in a genetically susceptible host (18).

The specificity of ANA directed to nuclear proteins supports the hypothesis that these responses are antigen driven, because these antibodies bind multiple independent determinants found in different regions of these proteins. The pattern of ANA binding minimizes the possibility that molecular mimicry is the exclusive etiology for autoimmunity in SLE. This type of cross-reactivity has been hypothesized for many different autoimmune diseases, and it has been suggested for SLE because of the sequence similarity between certain nuclear antigens and viral and bacterial proteins. However, if SLE autoantibodies resulted from molecular mimicry, they would be expected to bind self-antigen only at sites of homology with foreign antigen, rather than throughout the entire molecule. While self-antigen can sustain ANA production, a cross-reactive response to a foreign antigen can initiate it. A role of infection in SLE is suggested by the finding that people with SLE are infected more commonly with Epstein–Barr virus than are control populations (19).

Studies analyzing the genetics of SLE and the pattern of ANA production both strongly suggest that T cells are critical to disease pathogenesis. In murine models of lupus, the depletion of helper T cells by monoclonal antibody treatment abrogates autoantibody production and clinical disease manifestations. The basis of T-cell help in autoantibody responses may differ, however, from conventional responses because of the nature of the antigens. Most SLE antigens exist as complexes, such as nucleosomes, containing multiple protein and nucleic acid species. Because these antigens may trigger B-cell activation by multivalent binding, T-cell help for autoimmune responses could be delivered by nonspecifically activated T cells. Alternatively, T-cell reactivity to these antigens could be elicited to only one protein on a complex, allowing a single helper T cell to collaborate with B cells for determinants.

TRIGGERING EVENTS

Although inheritance and the hormonal milieu may create a predisposition toward SLE, the initiation of disease and its temporal variation in intensity likely result from environmental and other exogenous factors. Among these potential influences are infectious agents, which could induce specific responses by molecular mimicry and perturb overall immunoregulation; stress, which can provoke neuroendocrine changes affecting immune cell function; diet, which can affect production of inflammatory mediators; toxins, including drugs, which could modify cellular responsiveness and the immunogenicity of self-antigens; and physical agents, such as sunlight, which can cause inflammation and tissue damage. The impingement of these factors on the predisposed individual is likely to be highly variable, providing a further explanation for the disease's heterogeneity and its alternating periods of flare and remission.

Because many patients with SLE can show serological abnormalities years in advance of clinical disease manifestations (20), mechanistically, disease may develop sequentially, with one step leading to autoantibody expression, and another step leading to clinical manifestation. The second triggering event could lead, for example, to the release of self-antigen and allow the formation of immune complexes to drive cytokine production. The separation of these events could also explain the phenomenon of serologically active, clinical quiescent lupus and the occurrence of remission in some patients following a flare.

REFERENCES

1. Ward MM, Pyun E. Studenski S. Long-term survival in systemic lupus erythematosus. Patient characteristics associated with poorer outcomes. Arthritis Rheum 1995; 38:274–283.
2. Weening JJ, D'Agati VD, Schwartz MM, et al. The classification of glomerulonephritis in systemic lupus erythematosus revisited. Kidney Int 2004;65:521–530.
3. Austin HA III, Boumpas DT, Vaughan EM, Balow JE. Predicting renal outcomes in severe lupus nephritis: contributions of clinical and histologic data. Kidney Int 1994;45:544–550.
4. Roubey RA. Immunology of the antiphospholipid antibody syndrome. Arthritis Rheum 1996;39:1444–1454.
5. Tan EM. Antinuclear antibodies: diagnostic markers for autoimmune diseases and probes for cell biology. Adv Immunol 1989;44:93–151.
6. Iwasaki A, Medzhitov R. Toll-like receptor control of the adaptive immune responses. Nat Immunol 2004;5: 987–995.
7. Pisetsky DS. Antibody responses to DNA in normal immunity and aberrant immunity. Clin Diagn Lab Immunol 1998;5:1–6.
8. Rönnblom L, Eloranta M-L, Alm GV. The type I interferon system in systemic lupus erythematosus. Arthritis Rheum 2006;54:408–420.
9. Clancy RM, Kapur RP, Molad Y, et al. Immunohistologic evidence support apoptosis, IgG deposition, and novel macrophage/fibroblast crosstalk in the pathologic cascade leading to congenital heart block. Arthritis Rheum 2004; 150:173–182.
10. Huerta PT, Kowal C, DeGiorgio LA, et al. Immunity and behavior: antibodies alter emotion Proc Natl Acad Sci U S A 2006;103:678–683.
11. Lauwerys BR, Wakeland EK. Genetics of lupus nephritis. Lupus 2005;14:2–12.
12. Manderson AP, Botto M, Walport MJ. The role of complement in the development of systemic lupus erythematosus. Ann Rev Immunol 2004;22:431–456.
13. Botto M, Dell'Agnola C, Bygrave AE, et al. Homozygous C1q deficiency causes glomerulonephritis associated with multiple apoptotic bodies. Nat Genet 1998;19: 56–59.
14. Aringer M, Graninger WB, Stein G, Smolen JS. Safety and efficacy of tumor necrosis factor α blockade in systemic lupus erythematosus: an open-label study. Arthritis Rheum 2004;50:3161–3169.
15. Yurasov S, Wardemann H, Hammersen J, et al. Defective B cell tolerance checkpoints in systemic lupus erythematosus. J Exp Med 2005;202:341–344.
16. Baechler E, Batliwalla FM, Karypis G, et al. Interferon-induction gene expression signature in peripheral blood cells of patients with severe lupus. Proc Natl Acad Sci U S A 2003;100:2610–2615.
17. Kirou KA, Lee C, George S, Louca K, et al. Activation of interferon-α pathway identifies a subgroup of systemic lupus erythematosus patients with distinct serologic features and active disease. Arthritis Rheum 2005;52:1491–1503.

18. Gilkeson GS, Pippen AMM, Pisetsky DS. Induction of cross-reactive anti-dsDNA antibodies in preautoimmune NZB/NZW mice by immunization with bacterial DNA. J Clin Invest 1995;95:1398–1402.

19. James JA, Kaufman KM, Farris AD, Taylor-Albert E, Lehman TJA, Harley JB. An increased prevalence of Epstein-Barr virus infection in young patients suggests a possible etiology for systemic lupus erythematosus. J Clin Invest 1997;100:3019–3026.

20. Arbuckle MR, McClain MT, Rubertone MV, et al. Development of autoantibodies before the clinical onset of systemic lupus erythematosus. N Engl J Med 2003;349: 1499–1500.

Systemic Lupus Erythematosus
C. Treatment and Assessment

SUSAN MANZI, MD, MPH
AMY H. KAO, MD, MPH

- Global management of systemic lupus erythematosus (SLE) importantly includes education, photoprotection, maintaining good physical conditioning, appropriate immunization, and identifying and treating risk factors for cardiovascular disease.
- Many traditional treatments are available for the nonorgan manifestations of SLE, including nonsterio-

dal anti-inflammatory drugs (NSAIDs), corticosteroids, and antimalarials.
- Treatment of severe organ involvement typically requires immunosuppressive agents.
- Targeted biologic therapies are under development that may change treatment algorithms in the future.

The significant improvement in survival and quality of life in patients with systemic lupus erythematosus (SLE) is the result of major advances over the past half century in the management of SLE. Milestones in the treatment of lupus include the discovery and use of corticosteroids in the 1950s, renal dialysis in the 1960s, and cyclophosphamide in the 1970s. However, there has been a drought of almost 40 years when it comes to new therapeutic agents for lupus. Corticosteroids, hydroxychloroquine, and aspirin are the only three drugs currently approved by the US Food and Drug Administration (FDA) for treatment of SLE. Novel therapeutics with more specific targets directed toward the autoimmune aspects of SLE are on the horizon. The goals of therapy are the reduction of both autoimmunity and target organ damage from inflammation and injury. In addition, side effects of therapy must be addressed as part of the management of SLE. It is crucial to recognize the wide spectrum of clinical manifestations in SLE. The treatment should be tailored based on the clinical manifestations in an individual patient because SLE manifests a unique disease profile in everyone afflicted.

GENERAL MANAGEMENT

Patient education directed toward understanding of the disease and therapy is fundamental in management of any chronic illness. Many patients may already have begun their own investigation through the information

highway, primarily the Internet. It is the duty of the physicians and health care providers to clarify the confusion and alleviate the fear caused by learning about the worst-case scenarios of SLE through the means of Internet, friends, and family members.

Fatigue is very common in patients with SLE. The cause may be multifactorial, and include other comorbid conditions, such as hypothyroidism, depression, fibromyalgia, and deconditioning from chronic illness. Thus, therapy relies on identifying the underlying etiologies. Patients with photosensitivity can also develop fatigue and disease flare following exposure to ultraviolet light. Photoprotection includes avoidance of excess sunlight during mid-day, routine sunscreen/sunblock, and photoprotective clothing. Window films and fluorescent light shields reduce ultraviolet light exposure and can minimize the risk of lupus flare due to photosensitivity. Patients also need to be cautioned regarding drug-induced photosensitivity, commonly seen with antibiotics. Sedentary lifestyle resulting from chronic illness, depression, or fibromyalgia is another prominent feature in patients with SLE. This problem can lead to obesity and poor physical and cardiac health. SLE patients have been found to have diminished aerobic capacity (1). Low impact aerobic exercise, such as aquatic therapy, and walking exercise should be considered part of the nonpharmacologic regimen in patients with SLE.

Infections are common in SLE due to the intrinsic immune dysregulation and chronic immunosuppressive use. Patients should be advised to seek medical attention for unexplained fevers and not immediately attribute these fevers to lupus flares. Judicious use of corticosteroids and immunosuppressive agents and appropriate immunization with influenza and pneumococcal vaccines can minimize the risk of infection.

Patients with SLE are at increased risk of premature cardiovascular disease (CVD). It is important to reduce modifiable risk factors including tobacco use, obesity, sedentary lifestyle, dyslipidemia, and hypertension. The disease and its treatment can exacerbate these known CVD risk factors. Smoking cessation, weight reduction by dietary and exercise modalities, good blood pressure control, and annual monitoring of fasting lipid profiles are ways that may reduce the CVD risk in SLE patients. Similarly, osteoporosis is quite common, especially in patients that require prolonged corticosteroid therapy. Several studies have demonstrated that the heightened risk of bone loss in lupus is seen in all ethnicities, including African American women, who are normally less susceptible. Calcium plus vitamin D supplementation and antiresorptive agents (bisphosphonate) should be instituted appropriately. The safety of bisphosphonates in young individuals and those in childbearing age remains unclear. Because of recent evidence to support a high prevalence of vitamin D deficiency in SLE, it is advisable to check levels of 25-hydroxy vitamin D as a part of routine health maintenance.

Women with SLE may be at increased risk for cervical dysplasia and cervical cancer, in part due to the chronic infection from human papilloma virus. Similarly, a recent international collaborative study reported an increased risk of malignancy, particularly non-Hodgkin's lymphoma, in patients with lupus (2). Whether this increased risk is related to the underlying disease or the drugs used to treat lupus is unclear. Age-appropriate health maintenance, including gynecological and breast examination, and colonoscopy is recommended.

CURRENT THERAPY

The key to selecting appropriate therapies relies on the careful assessment of the organ involvement and the severity of lupus disease activity. Because most medications have potential adverse reactions, Table 15C-1 outlines the strategies for toxicity monitoring of medications commonly used in SLE.

Nonsteroidal Anti-Inflammatory Drugs

Nonsteroidal anti-inflammatory drugs (NSAIDs) are effective in pain relief and are widely used in patients for diverse manifestations including arthritis, myalgia,

serositis, and headaches. The choice of NSAID is determined by cost, effectiveness, and side effects. The effectiveness of these agents varies among individual patients and also can change in the same patient over time. In patients with renal impairment from lupus nephritis, both selective and nonselective NSAIDs should be avoided because the inhibition of cyclooxygenase (COX) by NSAIDs can further impair the renal blood flow and the maintenance of tubular transport through the reduction of both prostaglandins and prostacyclins. Side effect profiles for renal, hepatic, and central nervous system (CNS) toxicities are similar in nonselective COX inhibitors and selective COX-2 inhibitors. These side effects may be confused with SLE activity. Mild and reversible increases in hepatic enzymes are common side effect of NSAIDs. Similarly, aseptic meningitis, headache, confusion, cognitive dysfunction, and even psychosis may be seen in patients using NSAIDs. Selective COX-2 inhibitors reduce the gastrointestinal side effects, namely peptic ulcers and bleeding. However, due to the increased risk of cardiovascular events in selective COX-2 users, these agents should generally be avoided in patients with known coronary heart disease. Only one selective COX-2 inhibitor (celecoxib) remains in the current market. The antiplatelet effect of nonselective COX inhibitors can increase the risk of bleeding during surgical procedures and with concomitant use of anticoagulants; thus, nonselective COX inhibitors should be discontinued prior to surgery and should be used judiciously in the setting of anticoagulation. NSAIDs should be discontinued towards the third trimester in pregnant patients, due to the risk of premature closure of ductus arteriosus.

Corticosteroids

Corticosteroids are effective in the treatment of various inflammatory rheumatic diseases; they can also provide immediate relief of many manifestations of SLE. Topical corticosteroids are frequently used for local treatment of mucocutaneous disease. Systemic corticosteroids ranging from 5 mg to 30 mg equivalent dose of prednisone in single or divided doses given daily are effective in treatment of mild-to-moderate SLE disease, including cutaneous disease, arthritis, and serositis. More severe organ involvement, specifically nephritis, pneumonitis, hematologic abnormalities, CNS disease, and systemic vasculitis, require high dosages of corticosteroids in oral or parental preparations in equivalent dosages of prednisone of 1 to 2 mg/kg/day. Intravenous pulse methylprednisolone (1 g) can be given for three consecutive days when these severe manifestations of SLE are life threatening.

Systemic corticosteroids can act as bridging therapy for the slower-acting immunomodulatory agents (discussed later). Corticosteroids can then be tapered when

TABLE 15C-1. RECOMMENDED MONITORING FOR TOXICITIES OF DRUGS USED IN SYSTEMIC LUPUS ERYTHEMATOSUS.

DRUG	ADVERSE REACTIONS	PREGNANCY	Baseline evaluation	MONITORING Routine evaluation	Annual evaluation
NSAIDs	GI bleeding, hepatotoxicity, nephrotoxicity, hypertension, headache, aseptic meningitis	Discontinue in third trimester	CBC, creatinine, urinalysis, AST, ALT	Creatinine, AST, ALT every 6 months	CBC
Corticosteroids	Cushingoid features (hypertension, dyslipidemia, hyperglycemia), cataracts, osteonecrosis, osteoporosis	Safe but keep to the lowest dose	Fasting lipid profile, DXA, glucose, blood pressure	Blood pressure, glucose	DXA and fasting lipid profile
Antimalarials	Retinopathy, GI complaints, rash, myalgia, headache; hemolytic anemia in patients with G6PD deficiency	Safe	Eye exam in patients over 40 years old or with previous eye diseases; G6PD level in high risk patients;	Fundoscopic and visual field exams every 6–12 months	
Dapsone	Hemolytic anemia in patients with G6PD deficiency; methemoglobinemia	Discontinue 4 weeks before delivery	CBC, platelets, creatinine, AST, ALT; G6PD level in high-risk patients	CBC and platelet every 1–2 weeks with changes in dose (every 1–3 months afterwards)	
Azathioprine	Myelosuppression, hepatatoxicity, lymphoproliferative disorders	Safe	CBC, platelets, creatinine, AST, ALT, hepatitis B and C serology	CBC and platelet every 1–2 weeks with changes in dose and then AST, ALT every 1–3 months afterwards	Pap test and age-appropriate routine health maintenance
Methotrexate	Mucositis, myelosuppression, hepatatoxicity, cirrhosis, pneumonitis, pulmonary fibrosis	Teratogenic	CBC, platelets, creatinine, AST, ALT, hepatitis B and C serology	CBC and platelet, AST, ALT, albumin, creatinine every 1–2 months	Pap test and age-appropriate routine health maintenance
Mycophenolate mofetil	Myelosuppression, GI complaints, myalgia	Limited data (avoid)	CBC, platelets, creatinine, AST, ALT, hepatitis B and C serology	CBC and platelet, AST, ALT, albumin, creatinine every 1–2 months	Pap test and age-appropriate routine health maintenance
Cyclosporine	Myelosuppression, gingival hypertrophy, hepatotoxicity, nephrotoxicity, dyslipidemia, hyperuricemia	Safe	CBC, platelets, creatinine, AST, ALT, hepatitis B and C serology, urinalysis	CBC and platelet, AST, ALT, albumin, creatinine, urinalysis every 1–2 months	Fasting lipid profile; Pap test and age-appropriate routine health maintenance
Cyclophosphamide	Myelosuppression, hemorrhagic cystitis, lymphoproliferative disorders, malignancy, infertility	Teratogenic	CBC, creatinine, AST, ALT, hepatitis B and C serology, urinalysis	CBC and platelet, AST, ALT, creatinine, urinalysis monthly	Urine cytology; Pap test and age-appropriate routine health maintenance

ABBREVIATIONS: ALT, alanine transaminases; AST, aspartate transaminases; CBC, complete blood cell count; DXA, bone densitometry; G6PD, glucose-6-phosphate dehydrogenase; GI, gastrointestinal; Pap, Papanicolaou.

15

the immunomodulator begins to take effect. Once the disease activity is under control, corticosteroids are tapered to none or minimal daily (prednisone ≤5 mg/day) or alternate-day dosing for maintenance therapy. The goal of successful tapering of the corticosteroids is to reduce the numerous potential but common side effects of prolonged corticosteroid therapy while avoiding disease relapse or exacerbation. Common side effects of systemic corticosteroids include emotional lability, glaucoma, cataracts, peptic ulcer disease, osteoporosis, osteonecrosis, increased infection risk, and Cushingoid features (central obesity, striae, hypertension, diabetes mellitus, and dyslipidemia).

Topical Agents

Similar to minimizing the use of systemic corticosteroids, topical corticosteroids can be tapered to discontinuation or on an as-needed basis once the slower-acting immunomodulators or immunosuppressive agents are instituted. Clobetasol (high potency) in the preparation of solution or foam can be used to treat alopecia caused by SLE-associated rashes. The use of high potency or fluorinated topical corticosteroids should be avoided on the face and intertriginous areas due to the increased risk of developing skin atrophy and telangiectasias. In addition, topical corticosteroids should not be used continuously due to the development of tachyphylaxis. Typically, patients can apply the topical corticosteroids on weekdays and none on weekends. Other steroid-sparing topical agents, such as tacrolimus or pimecrolimus, can be given during "steroid-drug" holidays. Intralesional triamcinolone may be administered in hypertrophic lupus lesions. Both topical tacrolimus and pimecrolimus ointments are FDA approved for atopic dermatitis. They inhibit T-cell proliferation and release of cytokines. Unlike corticosteroids, they do not affect keratinocytes, endothelial cells, and fibroblasts, and thus do not induce skin atrophy. Topical retinoids, including tretinoin and tazarotene, have both anti-inflammatory and immunosuppressive effects and have been used successfully for the treatment of chronic cutaneous lupus. Common side effects include local skin irritation.

Antimalarials

Antimalarial agents are the most common background therapy for SLE. Hydroxychloroquine (HCQ) is the agent most frequently prescribed in the United States, followed by chloroquine and quinacrine. The antimalarials are commonly used as the first-line immunomodulatory agents in the treatment of mild SLE disease manifestations, including constitutional, cutaneous, and musculoskeletal. HCQ is usually initiated at 200 mg/day dosage and eventually increased to 200 mg twice daily or 400 mg/day (5–6.5 mg/kg/day). The response of HCQ is very slow and typically occurs after 6 weeks; its peak efficacy may not be reached for 4 months. Hydroxychloroquine demonstrated clinical efficacy in a randomized withdrawal trial when patients who discontinued HCQ were 2.5 times more likely to develop mild lupus flare than those who maintained the treatment (3). Long-term follow-up of this study suggested a trend towards reduction in flares in those who remained on HCQ, although this reduction was not statistically significant (4). In addition, HCQ use appeared to predict renal remission within 1 year in lupus patients treated with mycophenolate mofetil for membranous glomerulonephritis (5). Two studies have shown that cigarette smoking may interfere with the efficacy of antimalarials in treating patients with discoid lupus and subacute cutaneous lupus (6,7). Smokers were found to be less responsive to the antimalarial therapy than nonsmokers with a dose effect, meaning patients who smoked the most had the least response to antimalarials (7). In addition, improvement of skin lesions occurred once the patients stopped smoking while remaining on antimalarial therapy.

Chloroquine is used at 250 mg/day (3.5 mg/kg/day) with effects seen within 3 to 4 weeks, sooner than that of HCQ. Quinacrine, which has a rapid onset of action similar to chloroquine, is usually dosed at 100 to 200 mg/day (2.5 mg/kg/day). Combination therapy with HCQ (or chloroquine) and quinacrine is commonly used with success when one agent alone is not effective.

Gastrointestinal side effects are the most common. They are often transient and reduced by lowering the dose of the antimalarials or administering brand rather than generic. Most common complaints include crampy abdominal pain, nausea, vomiting, bloating, or diarrhea. Chloroquine less frequently causes gastrointestinal reactions followed by hydroxychloroquine and quinacrine. Chloroquine has a higher incidence of retinal toxicity causing visual field defects than HCQ. Therefore, HCQ and chloroquine should be used together with caution because the risk of retinopathy is high with this combination. Other visual symptoms include blurred distance vision, difficulty in reading, photophobia, and flashing lights. The risk of retinal toxicity can be minimized when the total daily recommended dose of HCQ is kept ≤6.5 mg/kg/day, chloroquine ≤3 to 4 mg/kg/day, and quinacrine ≤2.5 mg/kg/day. A long-term follow-up study demonstrated a very low incidence of HCQ-related retinopathy (0.5%) in 400 patients who were treated with the recommended dosages for >6 years (8). Despite the rarity of retinal toxicity, patients receiving antimalarials should have ophthalmologic evaluations at baseline and then at 6- to 12-month intervals. This evaluation should include a fundoscopic examination, visual field, and visual acuity testing. Antimalarials may cause hyperpigmentation on nails, anterior legs, face, and, rarely mucous membranes, predominantly on sun-exposed areas. Bluish-gray to dark purple discoloration is associated with HCQ therapy, while yellow discoloration with quinacrine. Hypopigmented lesions that involve mainly the hair or lentigines may occur with chloroquine therapy. These cutaneous lesions can gradually resolve after discontinuation of the drug. Rare but serious cardiotoxicity from HCQ and chloroquine with the presentation of myocardial dysfunction has been reported, although less than half of the cases were biopsy proven (9–12). Histologic findings of the endomyocardial biopsy may reveal myeloid and curvilinear bodies (lipid-rich structures representing abnormal lysosomes) with variable myofiber atrophy and necrosis (13). Older women with long duration of antimalarial therapy appeared to be in greater risk for this cardiotoxicity. Drug-induced myopathy from HCQ has also been reported with the presence of curvilinear bodies in skeletal muscle biopsy.

Hydroxychloroquine has hypoglycemic properties that could improve glycemic control in patients with poorly controlled type 2 diabetes (14). In addition, HCQ may lower the insulin requirement in patients with type 2 diabetes on insulin therapy, thereby placing these patients at greater risk for hypoglycemic events. Thus, patients should be aware of the hypoglycemic effects of HCQ. Another precaution of antimalarials is the risk of hemolytic anemia in patients with glucose-6-phosphate dehydrogenase (G6PD) deficiency. G6PD deficiency is more common in the Mediterranean regions, Middle East, Africa, and the Indian subcontinent. Physicians need to be aware of this increased risk in patients of these descents. HCQ has been shown to be safe during pregnancy (15). No retinal toxicity or otoxicitiy in children born to women on HCQ has been reported. The safety of HCQ, chloroquine, and quinacrine in breastfeeding has not been established.

Dapsone

Dapsone is a sulfone antibiotic used in the treatment of leprosy and for the prophylaxis of *Pneumocystis jirovecii* pneumonia (previously known as *Pneumocystis carinii* pneumonia). Dapsone has additional immunomodulatory properties, particularly effective against neutrophil-mediated processes, and is used to treat various bullous disorders, erythema nodosum, pyoderma gangrenosum, Sweet's syndrome, cutaneous vasculitis, and cutaneous lupus. Dapsone (100 mg/day) alone or in combination with systemic corticosteroids/antimalarials, is the drug of choice for bullous SLE as well as for cutaneous lesions involving the small dermal vessels, such as leukocytoclastic vasculitis.

The most serious but rare side effect is the hypersensitivity syndrome, characterized by fever, rash, lymphadenopathy, hepatitis, and hepatosplenomegaly.

Another serious adverse effect is bone marrow suppression, which appears to be an idiosyncratic reaction to dapsone that is exacerbated by the concomitant use of a folate antagonist. Similar to antimalarials, patients with G6PD deficiency are at increased risk of developing hemolytic anemia while taking dapsone. Although dapsone is not teratogenic, it can increase the risk of methemoglobinemia and cyanosis in neonates as observed in adults (16). Discontinuation of dapsone therapy 1 month before the expected date of delivery to minimize the theoretical risk of kernicterus is recommended (17). Breastfeeding by mothers taking dapsone should be cautioned because this drug is secreted in breast milk and can place the infants at risk of developing hemolytic anemia.

Azathioprine

Azathioprine (2–2.5 mg/kg/day) is frequently used as a steroid-sparing agent in patients with mild-to-moderate disease activity, and as an alternative maintenance therapy to cyclophosphamide in patients with lupus nephritis and other organ-threatening manifestations. This agent is a purine analog and a mercaptopurine immunosuppressant that inhibits nucleic acid synthesis and thus affects both cellular and humoral immune function. Azathioprine can be used during pregnancy in women who may require an immunomodulator stronger than the antimalarials can provide. Azathioprine passes into breast milk; thus mothers on azathioprine should not breastfeed their infants.

The main adverse reaction of azathioprine is acute myelotoxicity, manifesting as pancytopenia in patients who are deficient in the enzyme thiopurine methyltransferase (TPMT) that inactivates azathioprine. Drug interaction between azathioprine and allopurinol (used in the treatment of gout) can also cause acute pancytopenia. This combination should be avoided. The other common side effect is gastrointestinal toxicity similar to the antimalarials. Azathioprine requires regular monitoring of renal and liver functions because of the hepatic metabolism and renal excretion. Dosage should be adjusted in patients with renal or hepatic dysfunction.

Methotrexate

Methotrexate has been the standard therapy of rheumatoid arthritis, with extensive data demonstrating its efficacy and safety in this disease. However, there are only a few prospective randomized trials of methotrexate therapy for SLE, with conflicting results. Numerous case series and few retrospective studies have demonstrated success in the treatment of active cutaneous and/or articular involvements, allowing corticosteroid taper.

Methotrexate is an analog of dihydrofolic acid, which inhibits dehydrofolate reductase, and has immunomodulatory effects at low doses without the cytotoxic or antiproliferative effects seen in the very high doses that are typically given in chemotherapy. Side effects are common and include gastrointestinal complaints, mucositis, alopecia, hepatic enzyme elevations, and infections, especially when the dosage is high. These side effects may be minimized if the methotrexate is given in the range of 7.5 to 15 mg/week. Addition of daily folate or weekly folinic acid supplementation may alleviate the common side effects of oral ulcers and alopecia. Injectable administration of methotrexate can improve the bioavailability of this medication and may also minimize the gastrointestinal complaints (nausea, vomiting, diarrhea, and abdominal cramps). Abnormal liver function tests are of concern if the elevations persist; however, they are often poor predictors of the severity of hepatotoxicity by histopathology. Patients taking methotrexate should be advised against regular alcohol consumption because the combination of methotrexate and alcohol can further increase the risk of hepatotoxicity. A rare but potentially life-threatening pulmonary complication is methotrexate-induced pneumonitis. This adverse reaction can develop early as well as late in the course of the treatment and needs to be distinguished from infectious pneumonia and lupus pneumonitis. Discontinuation of methotrexate is warranted when either pneumonia or methotrexate-induced pneumonitis is suspected. The teratogenicity of methotrexate is well established. Methotrexate should therefore be discontinued 6 months prior to pregnancy, regardless of the patient's gender.

Cyclosporine

Cyclosporine primarily inhibits the proliferation of T lymphocytes and selectively inhibits T-cell–mediated responses, such as interleukin 2 (IL-2), IL-3, and interferon gamma (IFN-gamma), and other cytokines at the transcriptional level from naive T cells. Although SLE has been thought to arise from B-cell–mediated autoimmunity with autoantibody production and immune-complex formation, there is evidence that indicates a primary role for T cells. In murine models of SLE, depletion of CD4+ T cells prevents disease onset (18) and athymic mice do not develop SLE (19). Dosages of cyclosporine ranging from 2.5 to 5 mg/kg/day are generally well tolerated, with reduction of corticosteroid dosage and improvement in disease activity, proteinuria, leukopenia, thrombocytopenia, and complement levels (20). Limited pregnancy data primarily from the transplant patients showed no increased in adverse outcomes in pregnancy. This medication is not teratogenic in animals. Cyclosporine can be continued in pregnant patients with SLE if the benefits outweigh the risks. Mothers taking cyclosporine are advised against breastfeeding because cyclosporine passes into breast milk.

Most side effects are dose dependent and reversible. They include hypertension, elevations in serum creatinine and hepatic enzymes, tremor, hypertrichosis, gingival hypertrophy, parathesis, gastrointestinal complaints, and infections. Cyclosporine can also cause hyperkalemia, dyslipidemia, and worsen hyperuricemia that can lead to a gouty flare. Although cyclosporine appears to be effective in treatment of refractory nephrotic syndrome or membranous glomerulonephritis (WHO class V), long-term therapy can result in structural changes in the kidneys, such as interstitial fibrosis and tubular atrophy. Therefore, regular monitoring of renal function and blood pressure are advised.

Cyclophosphamide

Cyclophosphamide is an alkylating and cytotoxic agent, which cross-links DNA and DNA-associated proteins. It is reserved for the treatment of severe SLE, including lupus nephritis, central nervous system disease, pulmonary hemorrhage, and systemic vasculitis. The results of the landmark randomized trial by the National Institutes of Health (NIH) in 1986 set the gold standard for treatment of patients with diffuse proliferative glomerulonephritis (21). In this study, patients treated with corticosteroids and intermittent cyclophosphamide (intravenous bolus regimens of 0.5–1 g/m² body surface area) had significantly better renal survival than those treated with corticosteroids alone. However, no significant difference in renal survival was found between this regimen and the one with azathioprine. The traditional cyclophosphamide regimen for diffuse proliferative glomerulonephritis is 6 to 7 monthly pulse of cyclophosphamide alone or with pulse methylprednisolone in the induction, and then quarterly pulse cyclophosphamide for 2 years. The intravenous administration of cyclophosphamide has the advantage over oral formulations in that the bladder can be protected by intravenous infusion of mesna (mercapto-ethanesulphonic acid) along with rigorous hydration to prevent hemorrhagic cystitis and bladder cancer from acrolein, a toxic metabolite of cyclophosphamide. Variations of shorter duration and/or lower dose of cyclophosphamide therapy have been studied with varying results; however, due to the toxicity of an extended cyclophosphamide regimen, attempts to reduce exposure by changing to alternate treatments are an active area of investigation.

Adverse effects of cyclophosphamide include nausea and vomiting, alopecia, bone marrow suppression, increased risk of infections, and bladder carcinoma. Cyclophosphamide has been associated with increased risk for cervical dysplasia and cervical intraepithelial neoplasia (22,23). Nausea and vomiting can be prevented with anti-emetic drugs such as ondansteron and dolasetron, given on a regular schedule during the first

24 hours and then as needed afterwards. A dose-dependent nadir leukocyte count should be checked 8 to 12 days after intravenous cyclophosphamide therapy. Infertility due to gonadal toxicity from cyclophosphamide is one of the most concerning side effects. The two key factors associated with the risk of ovarian failure in women are older age at the start of treatment and higher cumulative dose of cyclophosphamide. Use of cyclophosphamide during pregnancy and lactation is prohibited.

Mycophenolate Mofetil

Mycophenolate mofetil (MMF) is an inactive prodrug of mycophenolic acid (MPA), which inhibits inosine monophosphate dehydrogenase, lymphocyte proliferation, and both T- and B-cell function. MMF has been widely used to prevent renal allograft rejection. Many case series and small controlled trials have suggested the effectiveness of MMF in treatment of lupus nephritis. A recent randomized, open-label, noninferiority trial supports the notion that MMF appeared to be as effective as intravenous cyclophosphamide in inducing short-term remission of lupus nephritis with a better safety profile (24). The role of MMF in improving long-term outcomes of lupus nephritis remains unknown. An ongoing larger, multicenter, randomized, controlled trial will examine effectiveness of MMF compared to intravenous cyclophosphamide during induction, and MMF compared to azathioprine during the maintenance phase. MMF is a promising addition to the armamentarium of treatment of lupus nephritis, particularly in young women of childbearing potential when there are concerns of infertility. Pregnancy safety data of MMF is limited; thus, it should be avoided during pregnancy and lactation.

Mycophenolate mofetil is generally well tolerated at the dosing range from 500 mg to 1500 mg twice daily. Side effects include gastrointestinal complaints (nausea, bloating, and diarrhea), cytopenias, and increased risk of infections. The gastrointestinal reactions can be minimized with gently escalating dosing of MMF or the use of a preparation that comes in 250 mg capsules.

Leflunomide

Leflunomide is effective in the treatment of rheumatoid arthritis. It inhibits dihydro-orotate dehydrogenase, a key enzyme in de novo pyrimidine synthesis, and thus decreases T- and B-cell proliferation. A few small studies of short duration showed that leflunomide was well tolerated in patients with SLE (25,26). Due to the relative lack of renal toxicity, and mainly hepatic and gastrointestinal metabolism, leflunomide appears to be more favorable than cyclosporine or methotrexate in those with renal impairment. Larger and long-term prospective studies are needed to provide more information on the efficacy and safety of leflunomide in treatment of SLE.

The most common adverse reaction is diarrhea, which is usually transient or improves with dose reduction. Other common side effects include elevation in hepatic enzymes, hypertension, and transient leukopenia. Subacute cutaneous lupus precipitated by leflunomide has been reported (27). Leflunomide is teratogenic. Because the half-life of leflunomide is quite long (~15 days) due to enterohepatic circulation, its use is contraindicated in patients who are pregnant or who plan to have a child. Breastfeeding is not advised while taking leflunomide. Before pregnancy is considered, plasma concentration of its active metabolite (A77 1726) should be <0.2 mg/L on two occasions ≥2 weeks apart. In the event of pregnancy or toxicity, leflunomide can be eliminated by administering 8 g cholestyramine three times daily for 11 days. Therefore, use of leflunomide may not be recommended in young SLE patients of childbearing age.

Hormonal Therapy

Dehydroepiandrosterone (DHEA) is an adrenal steroid with mild androgenic activity that has shown some promise for the treatment of mild-to-moderate SLE disease activity in several clinical trials. Preliminary results from a recent randomized, controlled trial showed that prasterone (DHEA) preserved bone mineral density (BMD) and significantly improved the BMD in women with SLE receiving chronic corticosteroids (28). However, the findings were not considered robust enough for approval by the FDA. This drug is well tolerated, with acne being the most frequent adverse effect. Another hormonal therapy studied in SLE is bromocriptine, a dopamine analog and a selective inhibitor of anterior pituitary secretion of the immune-stimulatory hormone prolactin. Bromocriptine has shown benefit in improving disease activity in SLE patients with and without hyperprolactinemia (29). However, bromocripine therapy remains experimental. Danazol, a weak androgen, has been shown to be effective in the treatment of autoimmune cytopenias, particularly thrombocytopenia and hemolytic anemia (30).

Thalidomide

Much of the controversy associated with the use of thalidomide concerns its well-recognized teratogenicity. Thalidomide is an immunomodulator with anti-angiogenic effects. It is highly effective at dosage ranging from 50 to 400 mg/day for treatment of refractory chronic cutaneous lupus although the precise mechanism remains unclear. There is a high rate (~68%) of relapse off the drug (31). Another common adverse effect is peripheral neuropathy, reported in up to 50% of patients,

15

although there is a wide range of incidence rates (32). The neuropathy is not felt to be dose related and can be irreversible if the drug is not discontinued or the dose is not reduced promptly. An important complication of thalidomide is deep venous thrombosis, which occurs in up to 30% of patients with malignancy and has also been reported in patients with SLE (33,34).

Intravenous Immunoglobulin

High dose intravenous immunoglobulin (IVIG) has been used in the treatment of hypogammaglobulinemia, refractory thrombocytopenia, and Kawasaki's disease. The mechanisms of action are thought to include the blockade of Fc receptors, complement inhibition, and immunomodulation of T- and B-cell functions. Improvement in thrombocytopenia, arthritis, nephritis, and immunologic parameters have been reported after treatment with IVIG. Because IVIG provides protection against infections in immunodeficient patients, it is a favorable treatment alternative in acutely ill patients with SLE when there is a concern for a commitment infection. IVIG can be administered in the usual dose of 2 g/kg, divided into 2 to 5 daily doses. Common side effects of IVIG include fever, myalgia, arthralgia, and headache. Rarely, aseptic meningitis and thromboembolism can occur. Patients with IgA deficiency will develop serious anaphylactic reactions to IVIG infusion; thus, its use is contraindicated in these patients. Quantitative immunoglobulins should be checked for IgA deficiency prior to the IVIG therapy. Patients with a hypercoagulable state, such as antiphospholipid syndrome, should be cautioned against the use of IVIG therapy due to the increased risk of thromboembolism.

Plasmapheresis

Plasma exchange or plasmapheresis is an effective but costly therapy to rapidly remove circulating autoantibodies and immune complexes. It also comes with the price of heightened risk of infection and anaphylaxis. The most common indications for plasmapheresis in SLE include thrombotic thrombocyptopenic purpura (TTP), catastrophic antiphospholipid syndrome, pulmonary hemorrhage, cryoglobulinemia, and hyperviscosity syndrome. Other life-threatening complications of SLE may also be treated with plasmapheresis if conventional therapy has failed.

Immunoablation with Autologous Stem Cell Transplantation

In severe cases of SLE, cyclophosphamide is the mainstay of therapy with its dose limited by myelosuppression. The rationale behind immunoablation with cyclophasmide followed by stem cell transplantation is to rescue bone marrow of the patient with autologous stem cell transplantation after receiving a high myeloablative dose of cyclophosphamide. In addition, a high dose cyclophosphamide regimen is purported to reset the naive immune response in the bone marrow stem cells by destroying the autoreactive lymphocytes. In the retrospective analysis of 53 patients with refractory SLE who underwent immunoablation and autologous stem cell transplantation, a European group found a remission rate based on a reduction of SLE disease activity index (SLEDAI) to less than 3 in 66% of these patients (35). However, 1-year transplant related mortality was high at 12%. A recent open-label study demonstrated a reduction in disease activity by nonmyeloablative autologous hematopoietic stem cell transplantation in patients with refractory SLE (36). There is a heightened infection and mortality risk associated with immunoablation therapy.

Immunoablation Without Stem Cell Transplantation

High dose cyclophosphamide without stem cell transplantation is another approach that can lead to rapid hematopoietic reconstitution through granulocyte cell stimulating factor (G-CSF) therapy and clinical improvement in patients with refractory SLE. Durable complete remission of SLE has been reported in some patients with treatment-refractory moderate-to-severe disease (37). These studies are not randomized and thus are still preliminary. These approaches require further validation by controlled randomized studies.

Renal Dialysis and Transplantation

The availability of renal dialysis and transplantation has improved survival of patients with SLE. Aside from an increased risk of infection, SLE patients generally do well with dialysis. For those patients who undergo renal transplantation, long-term patient and renal graft survival are similar to those transplant patients without SLE (38). However, the risk for thrombotic complications, such as early graft thrombosis, may be greater in SLE patients, particularly those with positive antiphospholipid antibodies. The outcome of kidney transplantation largely depends on the clinical condition at the time of transplantation. The risk of recurrence of lupus nephritis in the transplanted kidneys ranges between 2% and 30% (39).

NOVEL THERAPIES

Moving away from global immunosuppression by traditional drug therapies for SLE, designed therapeutics of the future provide improved efficacy and lower toxicity

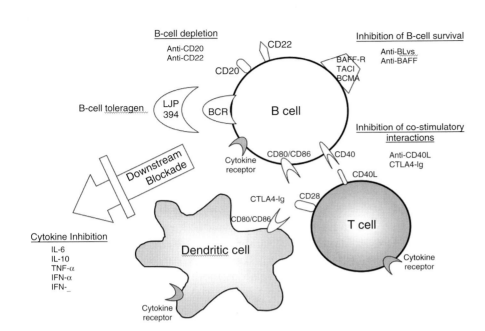

FIGURE 15C-1

Targets for novel therapies in systemic lupus erythematosus. Abbreviations: BCR, B-cell receptor; BAFF-R, B-cell activating factor receptor; TACI, transmembrane activator and cyclophilin ligand interactor; BCMA, B-cell maturation activator; IL, interleukin; TNF, tumor necrosis factor; CTLA4-Ig, cytotoxic T-lymphocyte antigen-4 Ig.

by targeting specific steps in the pathogenesis of SLE while preserving immunocompetence. Many of the novel therapeutics are being developed and studied currently in clinical trials. Some of the promising novel therapies are discussed in the following overview. Figure 15C-1 depicts the specific targets for the novel therapies.

B-Cell Depletion

Rituximab and epratuzumab are two antibody-based agents, which target a specific cell-surface antigen on B cells and result in B-cell depletion. Rituximab is a chimeric monoclonal antibody that binds CD20 on the surface of B cells. It is the first monoclonal antibody therapy approved by the FDA for the treatment of non-Hodgkin's lymphoma. Rituximab is currently approved for use in rheumatoid arthritis that is refractory to anti–tumor necrosis factor (TNF) alpha therapy. In small anecdotal and clinical studies, rituximab has been shown to be beneficial in the treatment of patients with SLE. Various dosing regimens have been used to achieve complete B-cell depletion. A multicenter, randomized, placebo-controlled (phase II/III) trial has begun to study the efficacy of rituximab in patients with moderate-to-severe lupus flares. Another similar phase III trial will study the efficacy of rituximab in the treatment of lupus nephritis in adult patients.

Epratuzumab is a human monoclonal antibody that targets CD22 on B cells. In an open-label phase II trial, epratuzumab showed efficacy in patients with SLE, despite causing only modest B-cell depletion. Two ongoing phase III clinical trials of epratu-

zumab will validate its safety and efficacy in patients with SLE.

B-Cell–Specific Toleragen

Abetimus sodium (LJP 394) is a tetramer of double-stranded oligonucleotides that can bind to DNA-reactive B cells and induce B-cell anergy or apoptosis, resulting in reduction of circulating double-stranded DNA antibodies. Results of a clinical trial in SLE patients with renal disease showed that abetimus was well tolerated and potentially effective in preventing renal flares in a subset of patients with sustained reductions in anti–double-stranded DNA (anti-dsDNA) antibodies.

Inhibition of B-Cell Survival

B-cell activating factor (BAFF)/B-cell stimulator (BlyS) modulates B-cell survival and maturation, and is a member of the TNF superfamily. Belimumab is a human BAFF monoclonal antibody that recognizes BlyS and reduces B-cell proliferation and differentiation in animal models. A phase II clinical trial failed to demonstrate efficacy. However, in a subset of SLE patients with elevated anti-dsDNA antibodies and low serum C3, there was a significant reduction in disease activity. Thus, a phase III trial may be needed for further validation.

Inhibition of Costimulatory Interactions

Dendritic or antigen presenting cells link innate to adaptive immunity and thus play an important role in both initiating and maintaining inflammatory and immune responses. These cells also possess costimulatory potential, sufficient to activate naive T cells. Abatacept is a fusion protein of CTLA4-Ig that binds to B7 molecules (CD80/CD86) on dendritic cells and blocks the binding of costimulatory molecules CD80 and CD86 with CD28 on T cells, thereby interrupting signals required for the activation of naive T cells and their downstream effects on B-cell activation. This drug has been approved by the FDA for the treatment of rheumatoid arthritis. Multicenter clinical trials of two available compounds, abatacept and RG2077, are currently under way in SLE.

The interaction of CD40 on B cells and CD40 ligand (CD40L) on T cells is also essential for B-cell activation and antibody production. The therapeutic blockade of the CD40–CD40L interaction has been studied extensively in animal models. However, clinical trials of two such monoclonal antibodies (IDEC-131 and BG9588) against CD40L that interrupts the CD40–CD40L interaction revealed disappointing results. IDEC-131 was shown to be safe but ineffective, whereas BG9588 was associated with a high incidence of thromboembolic events unacceptable for clinical use, despite limited data demonstrating potential efficacy.

Cytokine Blockade

Tumor necrosis factor alpha inhibitors (etanercept, infliximab, and adalimumab) have been very successful in treatment of rheumatoid arthritis and psoriatic arthritis. A small open-label study of infliximab in SLE showed significant improvement in patients with refractory nephritis, despite a parallel increase in levels of anti-dsDNA antibodies (40). However, anti–TNF-alpha therapy has been associated with autoantibody production, specifically anti-dsDNA antibodies, in patients with various autoimmune conditions. Although this autoantibody production may be common in RA patients on this therapy, it is not frequently associated with a lupuslike syndrome. Anti–TNF-alpha therapy has also been associated with several cases of demyelinating disease. Controlled clinical trials are needed to determine the long-term safety and efficacy of this therapy in SLE. The potent anti-inflammatory effects of anti–TNF-alpha therapy may make it suitable for short-term induction therapy in lupus nephritis without the concern of long-term effects on autoantibody production.

Interleukin 10 (IL-10) is a cytokine that may participate in the pathogenesis of SLE. A small open-label study of six SLE patients using murine monoclonal antibody against IL-10 showed improvement of cutaneous and articular symptoms (41). However, all of the patients developed antibodies to the murine monoclonal antibodies.

Interleukin 6 (IL-6) is another proinflammatory cytokine secreted predominantly by macrophages and T cells and has a wide range of biologic activities that mediate immune regulation and inflammation in autoimmune diseases like SLE. It also induces terminal differentiation of B lymphocytes into antibody-forming plasma cells and the differentiation of T lymphocytes into effector cells. IL-6 is highly expressed in lupus nephritis (42). In murine models, IL-6 promotes disease activity whereas IL-6 blockade delays the development of lupus nephritis (43). Tocilizumab is a humanized monoclonal antibody against IL-6 receptor (IL-6R) that suppresses IL-6 signaling mediated by both membranous and soluble IL-6R. An open-label trial of IL-6 blockade is currently under way.

Elevated serum levels of IFN-alpha are found in patients with SLE. IFN-alpha has been associated with B-cell lymphopenia, germinal center differentiation, generation of antibody-forming plasma cells, and activation of dendritic cells, findings relevant to the immunologic characteristics of SLE. The concept of disease pathogenesis by IFN-alpha is supported by the finding of patients with lupuslike illness on IFN-alpha therapy. More recent studies showed a striking IFN-alpha signature on gene expression in peripheral blood mononuclear cells of patients with SLE compared with those of controls (44). IFN-alpha modulation may be another promising therapeutic target for use in the treatment of SLE.

This is an exciting time for drug development in SLE, and several of these novel biologic agents appear to be promising. The complexity of lupus and the wide range of severity in different organ systems will likely translate into the need for a variety of therapeutic options.

REFERENCES

1. Keyser R, Rus V, Cade W, et al. Evidence for aerobic insufficiency in women with systemic lupus erythematosus. Arthritis Rheum 2003;49:16–22.
2. Bernatsky S, Boivin J, Joseph L, et al. An international cohort study of cancer in systemic lupus erythematosus. Arthritis Rheum 2005;52:1481–1490.
3. The Canadian Hydroxychloroquine Study Group. A randomized study of the effect of withdrawing hydroxychloroquine sulfate in systemic lupus erythematosus. N Engl J Med 1991;324:150–154.
4. Tsakonas E, Joseph L, Esdaile J, et al. A long-term study of hydroxychloroquine withdrawal on exacerbations in systemic lupus erythematosus. The Canadian Hydroxychloroquine Study Group. Lupus 1998;7:80–85.

5. Kasitanon N, Fine D, Haas M, et al. Hydroxychloroquine use predicts complete renal remission within 12 months among patients treated with mycophenolate mofetil therapy for membranous lupus nephritis. Lupus 2006;15: 366–370.

6. Rahman P, Gladmann D, Urowitz M. Efficacy of antimalarial therapy in cutaneous lupus in smokers versus nonsmokers. J Rheumatol 1998;25:1716–1719.

7. Jewell M, McCauliffe D. Patients with cutaneous lupus erythematosus who somke are less responsive to antimalarial treatment. J Am Acad Dermatol 2000;42:983–987.

8. Mavrikakis I, Sfikakis P, Mavrikakis E, et al. The incidence of irreversible retinal toxicity in patients treated with hydroxychloroquine: a reappraisal. Ophthalmology 2003;110:1321–1326.

9. Nord J, Shah P, Rinaldi R, et al. Hydroxychloroquine cardiotoxicity in systemic lupus erythematosus: a report of 2 cases and review of the literature. Semin Arthritis Rheum 2004;33:336–351.

10. Keating R, Bhatia S, Amin S, et al. Hydroxychloroquine-induced cardiotoxicity in a 39-year-old woman with systemic lupus erythematosus and systolic dysfunction. J Am Soc Echocardiogr 2005;18:981.

11. Reuss-Borst M, Berner B, Wulf G, et al. Complete heart block as a rare complication of treatment with chloroquine. J Rheumatol 1999;26:1394–1395.

12. Costedoat-Chalumeau N HJ, Amoura Z, Delcourt A, et al. Cardiomyopathy related to antimalarial therapy with illustrative case report. Cardiology 2006;107:73–80.

13. Ardehali H, Qasim A, Cappola T, et al. Endomyocardial biopsy plays a role in diagnosing patients with unexplained cardiomyopathy Am Heart J 2004;147:919–923.

14. Gerstein H, Thorpe K, Taylor D, et al. The effectiveness of hydroxychloroquine in patients with type 2 diabetes mellitus who are refractory to sulfonylureas—a randomized trial. Diabetes Res Clin Pract 2002;55:209–219.

15. Costedoat-Chalumeau N, Amoura Z, Duhaut P, et al. Safety of hydroxychloroquine in pregnant patients with connective tissue diseases: a study of one hundred thirty-three cases compared with a control group. Arthritis Rheum 2003;48:3207–3211.

16. Brabin B, Eggelte T, Parise M, et al. Dapsone therapy for malaria during pregnancy: maternal and fetal outcomes. Drug Safety 2004;27:633–648.

17. Thornton Y, Bowe E. Neonatal hyperbilirubinemia after treatment of maternal leprosy. South Med J 1989;82;668.

18. Wofsy D, Seaman W. Successful treatment of autoimmunity in NZB/NZW F1 mice with monoclonal to L3T4. J Exp Med 1985;161(Suppl 2):378–391.

19. Mihara M, Ohsugi Y, Saito K, et al. Immunologic abnormality in NZB/NZW F1 mice: thymus independent occurrence of B cell abnormality and requirement for T cells in the development of autoimmune disease, as evidenced by an analysis of the athymic nude individuals. J Immunol 1998;141:85–90.

20. Griffiths B, Emery P. The treatment of lupus with cyclosporin A. Lupus 2001;10:165–170.

21. Austin H, Klippel J, Balow J, et al. Therapy of lupus nephritis: controlled trial of prednisone and cytotoxic drugs. N Engl J Med 1986;314:614–619.

22. Bateman H, Yazici Y, Leff L, et al. Increased cervical dysplasia in intravenous cyclophosphamide-treated patients iwth SLE: a preliminary study. Lupus 2000;9: 542–544.

23. Lima F, Guerra D, Sella E, et al. Systemic lupus erythematosus and cervical intraepithelial neoplasia. Arthritis Rheum 1998;41(Suppl):S66.

24. Ginzler E, Dooley M, Aranow C, et al. Mycophenolate mofetil or intravenous cyclophosphamide for lupus nephritis. N Engl J Med 2005;353:2219–2228.

25. Tam L-S, Li EK, Wong C-K, et al. Double-blind, randomized, placebo-controlled pilot study of leflunomide in systemic lupus erythematosus. Lupus 2004;13: 601–604.

26. Tam L, Li E, Wong C, et al. Safety and efficacy of leflunomide in the treatment of lupus nephritis refractory or intolerant to traditional immunosuppressive therapy: an open label trial. Ann Rheum Dis 2006;65:417–418.

27. Chan S, Hazleman B, Burrows N. Subacute cutaneous lupus erythematosus precipitated by leflunomide. Clin Exp Dermatol 2005;30:724–725.

28. Mease P, Ginzler E, Gluck O, et al. Effects of prasterone on bone mineral density in women with systemic lupus erythematosus receiving chronic glucocorticoid therapy. J Rheumatol 2005;32:616–621.

29. Walker S. Bromocriptine treatment of systemic lupus erythematosus. Lupus 2001;10:762–768.

30. Avina-Zubieta J, Galindo-Rodriguez G, Robledo I, et al. Long-term effectiveness of danazol corticosteroids and cytotoxic drugs in the treatment of hematologic manifestations of systemic lupus erythematosus. Lupus 2003;12: 52–57.

31. Pelle M, Werth V. Thalidomide in cutaneous lupus erythematosus. Am J Clin Dermatol 2003;4:379–387.

32. Clemmensen O, Olsen P, Andersen K. Thalidomide neurotoxicity. Arch Dermatol 1984;120:338–341.

33. Rodeghiero F, Elice F. Thalidomide and thrombosis. Pahthophysiol Haemost Thromb 2003;33(Suppl 1):15–18.

34. Flageul B, Wallach D, Cavelier-Balloy B, Bachelez H, Carsuzaa F, Dubertret L. Thalidomide and thrombosis. Ann Dermatol Venereol 2000;127:171–174.

35. Jayne D, Passweg J, Marmont A, et al. Autologous stem cell transplantation for systemic lupus erythematosus. Lupus 2004;13:168–176.

36. Burt R, Traynor A, Statkute L, et al. Nonmyeloablative hematopoietic stem cell transplantation for systemic lupus erythematosus. JAMA 2006;295:559–560.

37. Petri M, Jones R, Brodsky R. High-dose cyclophosphamide without stem cell transplantation in systemic lupus erythematosus. Arthritis Rheum 2003;48:166–173.

38. Moroni G, Tantardini F, Gallelli B, et al. The long-term prognosis of renal transplantation in patients with lupus nephritis. Am J Kidney Dis 2005;45:903–911.

39. Ponticelli C, Moroni G. Renal transplantation in lupus nephritis. Lupus 2005;14:95–98.

40. Aringer M, Graninger W, Steiner G, et al. Safety and efficacy of tumor necrosis factor alpha blockade in systemic lupus erythematosus: an open-label study. Arthritis Rheum 2004;50:3161–3169.

41. Llorente L, Richaud-Patin Y, García-Padilla C, et al. Clinical and biologic effects of anti-interleukin-10 monoclonal antibody administration in systemic lupus erythematosus. Arthritis Rheum 2000;43:1790–1800.
42. Aringer M, Smolen J. Cytokine expression in lupus kidneys. Lupus 2005;14:189–191.
43. Ryffel B, Car B, Gunn H, et al. Interleukin-6 exacerbates glomerulonephritis in (NZB×NZW)F1 mice. Am J Pathol 1994;144:927–937.
44. Kirou K, Lee C, George S, et al. Coordinate overexpression of interferon-alpha-induced genes in systemic lupus erythematosus. Arthritis Rheum 2004;50:3958–3967.

CHAPTER 16

Antiphospholipid Syndrome

Michelle Petri, MD, MPH

- An acquired cause of hypercoagulability; 50% of antiphospholipid syndrome (APS) patients have systemic lupus erythematosus (SLE).
- Antiphospholipid syndrome predisposes to both venous and arterial thrombosis. The most common venous thrombosis is deep venous thrombosis; the most common arterial thrombosis is stroke.

- Antiphospholipid syndrome predisposes to miscarriage and other pregnancy morbidity.
- Antiphospholipid syndrome may cause thrombocytopenia.
- Antiphospholipid syndrome is diagnosed by persistent antiphospholipid antibody: lupus anticoagulant; anticardiolipin; and anti–beta 2 glycoprotein I.

Antiphospholipid antibodies (aPL) are autoantibodies directed against negatively charged phospholipid/plasma proteins. The most common plasma protein target is beta 2 glycoprotein I. The three most important antiphospholipid antibodies are the lupus anticoagulant, anticardiolipin, and anti–beta 2 glycoprotein I.

Antiphospholipid syndrome (APS) is one of the most common acquired causes of hypercoagulability. Fifty percent of APS patients have systemic lupus erythematosus (SLE). APS presents in two major ways: thrombosis (venous or arterial) and pregnancy loss. Thrombocytopenia, present in about 20% of cases, can be an important clue.

EPIDEMIOLOGY

Antiphospholipid antibodies (aPL) occur in 1% to 6% of the general population (1). The estimated relative risk of venous thromboembolism with anticardiolipin is 2 and with the lupus anticoagulant is 10 (2). APL also increase the risk of an initial myocardial infarction, initial stroke, recurrent stroke, and death. In patients presenting with a deep venous thrombosis, up to 30% will have the APS. In a person under age 50 with a stroke, up to 46% will have APS.

If APS occurs in a patient without SLE or other connective tissue disease, it is termed *primary APS*. About 8% of primary APS patients later develop SLE (3). In SLE patients, about 30% have anticardiolipin and about 25% have the lupus anticoagulant. The term *secondary APS* is used for SLE patients who have aPL and have had thrombosis or pregnancy losses. The risk of venous thrombosis in a SLE patient

with the lupus anticoagulant is 50% by 20 years after diagnosis.

CLINICAL FEATURES

The most common cutaneous finding in APS patients is livedo reticularis, a purplish lacelike reticular pattern, especially apparent on the extremities. Other cutaneous signs include splinter hemorrhages, superficial thrombophlebitis, cutaneous necrosis, digital gangrene, and leg ulcers (4).

Venous thrombosis in APS usually presents as a deep venous thrombosis of the lower extremities. Other possible sites of venous thrombosis include pulmonary emboli, Budd–Chiari syndrome, and dural sinus thrombosis.

The most common site of arterial thrombosis is the brain. Although strokes can occur from in situ thrombosis, about one third of patients with primary APS have cardiac valve vegetations or valve thickening that can lead to emboli. Rarely, a destructive valvulitis occurs requiring valve replacement. Other sites of arterial thrombosis include myocardial infarction, retinal thromboses, renal artery thrombosis, glomerular capillary thrombi, and digital gangrene. Pregnancy losses from APS can occur in the first trimester or as late fetal deaths. Severe placental insufficiency can occur. HELLP syndrome (hemolysis, elevated liver enzymes, low platelets) has been reported in APS, as well, but the true relationship between the HELLP syndrome and APS is unclear.

Some nonthrombotic neurologic presentations of APS include chorea and transverse myelitis.

Approximately 20% of APS patients have thrombocytopenia, usually in the range of 50 to 140,000/mm^3.

The antiphospholipid syndrome. Boca Raton, FL: CRC Press; 1996:13–28.

2. Bates SM, Ginsberg JS. Clinical practice. Treatment of deep-vein thrombosis. N Engl J Med 2004;351:268–277.

3. Gomez-Puerta JA, Martin H, Amigo MC, et al. Long-term follow-up in 128 patients with primary antiphospholipid syndrome: do they develop lupus? Medicine (Baltimore) 2005;84:225–230.

4. Frances C, Niang S, Laffitte E, Pelletier F, Costedoat N, Piette JC. Dermatologic manifestations of the antiphospholipid syndrome: two hundred consecutive cases. Arthritis Rheum 2005;52:1785–1793.

5. Asherson RA, Cervera R, de Groot PG, et al. Catastrophic antiphospholipid syndrome: international consensus statement on classification criteria and treatment guidelines. Lupus 2003;12:530–534.

6. Nachman RL, Silverstein R. Hypercoagulable states. Ann Intern Med 1993;119:819–827.

7. Miyakis S, Lockshin MD, Atsumi T, et al. International consensus statement on an update of the classification criteria for definite antiphospholipid syndrome (APS). J Thromb Haemost 2006;4:295–306.

8. Holers VM, Girardi G, Mo L, et al. Complement C3 activation is required for antiphospholipid antibody-induced fetal loss. J Exp Med 2002;195:211–220.

9. Cowchock FS, Reece EA, Balaban D, Branch DW, Plouffe L. Repeated fetal losses associated with antiphospholipid antibodies: a collaborative randomized trial comparing prednisone with low-dose heparin treatment. Am J Obstet Gynecol 1992;166:1318–1323.

10. Schulman S, Svenungsson E, Granqvist S, the Duration of Anticoagulation Study Group. Anticardiolipin antibodies predict early recurrence of thromboembolism and death among patients with venous thromboembolism following anticoagulant therapy. Am J Med 1998;104:332–338.

11. Crowther MA, Ginsberg JS, Julian J, et al. A comparison of two intensities of warfarin for the prevention of recurrent thrombosis in patients with the antiphospholipid antibody syndrome. N Engl J Med 2003;349:1133–1138.

12. Finazzi G, Marchioli R, Brancaccio V, et al. A randomized clinical trial of high-intensity warfarin vs. conventional antithrombotic therapy for the prevention of recurrent thrombosis in patients with the antiphospholipid syndrome (WAPS). J Thromb Haemost 2005;3:848–853.

Systemic Sclerosis
A. Clinical Features

Maureen D. Mayes, MD, MPH

■ Systemic sclerosis (scleroderma; SSc) is divided further into limited cutaneous disease and diffuse cutaneous disease on the basis of the extent of skin thickening.

■ Limited disease is defined as skin thickening that only affects the extremities below the elbows and/or below the knees. Diffuse cutaneous disease is defined as skin thickening proximal to the elbows and/or knees in addition to distal extremity involvement. Truncal skin may also be involved in diffuse cutaneous systemic sclerosis (dcSSc).

■ The face can be involved in both forms and has no bearing on subset designation.

■ The clinical manifestations of SSc may be considered the result of three pathological processes: (1) a small vessel non-inflammatory obliterative vasculopathy; (2) the pathological accumulation of collagen in skin and other organs (fibrosis); and (3) autoimmunity.

■ The obliterative small vessel vasculopathy is responsible for Raynaud's phenomenon, scleroderma renal crisis, and pulmonary artery hypertension.

■ The fibrosing process results in thickened skin, pulmonary parenchymal disease, and gastrointestinal dysmotility.

■ Tendon friction rubs, caused by an inflammation in the tendon sheath, are usually palpable on examination and sometimes cause pain with motion.

■ A variety of autoantibodies occur in SSc, including those anti–topoisomerase III antibodies and anticentromere antibodies.

■ Raynaud's phenomenon, usually the first manifestation of SSc, may precede the development of other features by months to years.

■ Pulmonary disease is now the leading cause of death in SSc. Pulmonary fibrosis occurs in many SSc patients, with 20% ultimately requiring supplemental oxygen.

■ Scleroderma renal crisis, the most common cause of death in SSc prior to the introduction of angiotensin-converting enzyme (ACE) inhibitors, remains an important source of patient morbidity in SSc.

From a clinical point of view, scleroderma is usually divided into two main forms, localized scleroderma and systemic scleroderma or systemic sclerosis (Figure 17A-1). Localized scleroderma includes the disease entities of morphea (one or more patches of thickened skin), linear scleroderma (a line of thickened skin affecting one or more extremities), and scleroderma en coup de sabre, which is a distinct subset of linear disease that affects the forehead and face [for review, see Piette (1)]. Although atrophy of the subcutaneous tissue underlying the lesions typically occurs in localized scleroderma, there is usually no associated internal organ or systemic involvement.

Systemic sclerosis (SSc), on the other hand, almost always has an element of internal organ disease (2). SSc is divided further into limited cutaneous disease (lcSSc) and diffuse cutaneous disease (dcSSc) on the basis of the extent of skin thickening. The terms *limited sclero-derma* and *localized scleroderma* cause linguistic confusion, but these terms refer to very different conditions. In spite of a few reported cases of localized and systemic

disease occurring in the same patient, this is a rare event and the two conditions should be thought of as two separate diseases with very different clinical pictures and prognosis.

For rheumatologists, scleroderma is synonymous with systemic disease. Only SSc will be considered in the remainder of this chapter. In broad terms, the clinical manifestations of SSc may be considered the result of three pathological processes: (1) a small vessel non-inflammatory obliterative vasculopathy; (2) the pathological accumulation of collagen in skin and other organs (fibrosis); and autoimmunity (3). The mechanisms by which these three processes are linked are unclear.

VASCULOPATHY

The obliterative small vessel vasculopathy is responsible for Raynaud's phenomenon, scleroderma renal crisis, and pulmonary artery hypertension. In contrast, the

FIGURE 17A-1

Scleroderma is usually divided into two main forms, and then further subdivided.

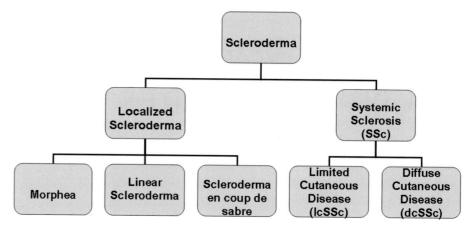

fibrosing process results in thickened skin, pulmonary parenchymal disease, and gastrointestinal dysmotility. Some patients have an associated inflammatory component manifested by tendon friction rubs and synovitis. Other features such as calcinosis are less well understood.

Raynaud's phenomenon is caused by vasospasm of the small vessels of the hands on cold exposure. This vasospasm, in turn, results in blanching, cyanosis, and then reactive hyperemia (rubor) as the affected area rewarms (4). An episode of Raynaud's phenomenon can be triggered by emotional stress, but the association with cold exposure must be present to make the diagnosis. Of the three phases—pallor, cyanosis, and rubor—rubor is the least frequent. The diagnosis is usually made on the basis of a compelling history rather than on attempts to recreate an episode under observation. This condition is common in the general population; approximately 5% to 10% or more of American adults will experience episodes of Raynaud's phenomenon (5,6). Most of these individuals have primary Raynaud's disease, not with a connective tissue disease. Primary Raynaud's disease does not result in tissue damage.

Thus, digital ulcers or gangrene should not result from primary Raynaud's phenomenon.

Secondary Raynaud's phenomenon due to SSc, on the other hand, frequently results in irreversible tissue loss. In addition to the cold-induced vasospasm that occurs in such patients, the caliber of the blood vessels at baseline becomes narrowed by a vasculopathy. Chronic ischemia leads to reduction of the finger pad substance with consequent tapering of the fingers. Tender digital pitting scars are the result of more ischemia, leading to losses of small areas of tissue. Digital ulcers and digital gangrene are caused by even more severe degrees of ischemia [Figure 17A-2(A,B)]. Ulcers that spontaneously occur on the fingertips are due almost exclusively to ischemia, whereas those over the extensor surfaces of the proximal interphalangeal (PIP), metacarpophalangeal (MCP), ulnar styloid, and elbow joints are due to a combination of poor perfusion in areas of stretched skin and repeated minor trauma (Figure 17A-3).

Raynaud's phenomenon, usually the first manifestation of SSc, may precede the development of other features by months to years. In some cases, the delay

FIGURE 17A-2

(A, B) Digital ulcers and digital gangrene are caused by severe degrees of ischemia.

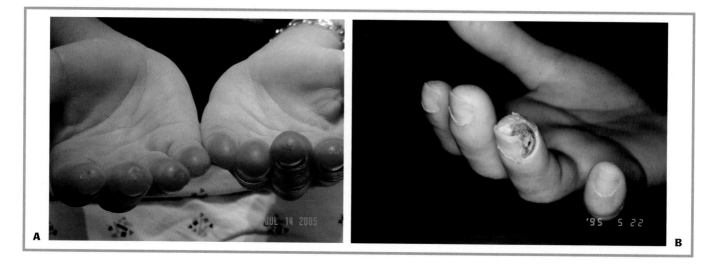

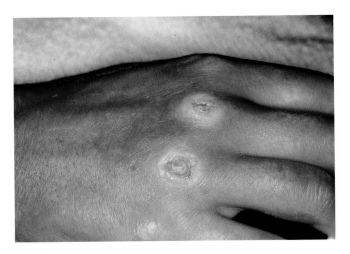

FIGURE 17A-3

Metacarpophalangeal ulcers are due to poor perfusion in areas of stretched skin or in areas of repeated minor trauma.

in diagnosis is due to the absence of full-blown SSc manifestations. In others, the diagnosis is delayed by the failure to realize that mild sclerodactyly (skin thickening limited to the fingers), gastroesophageal reflux, and other symptoms or signs of SSc are incipient indications of a broader systemic illness. Antinuclear antibodies (ANA) are usually present at the time of Raynaud's phenomenon onset. Indeed, the finding of a positive ANA in a patient with Raynaud's phenomenon suggests the need for further scrutiny of a possible connective tissue disorder.

The 1980 classification criteria for SSc, established by the American Rheumatism Society (now the American College of Rheumatology), consist entirely of clinical features (7). The single major criterion is the presence of thickened skin proximal to the MCP joints. There are three minor criteria, including sclerodactyly, permanent ischemic changes of the fingertips (loss of finger pad substance, digital pitting scars, or digital ulcers), and bibasilar pulmonary fibrosis. Classification of SSc is considered correct if proximal skin thickening is present, or if two of the three minor criteria are met. These classification criteria have a specificity of 98% and a sensitivity of 97%. However, this system may miss individuals who clearly have SSc by our current understanding. For example, individuals with only the CREST features (calcinosis, Raynaud's phenomenon, esophageal dysmotility, sclerodactyly, and telangiectasias) do not meet this definition (8).

The division of SSc into limited cutaneous or diffuse cutaneous disease subsets has important prognostic implications and can be accomplished in a straightforward, clinically applicable approach. Limited disease is defined as skin thickening that only affects the extremities below the elbows and/or below the knees (8). Diffuse cutaneous disease (dcSSc) is defined as skin thickening proximal to the elbows and/or knees in addition to distal extremity involvement. Truncal skin may also be involved in dcSSc. The face can be involved in both forms and has no bearing on subset designation.

Limited cutaneous disease (lcSSc) typically begins with Raynaud's phenomenon, followed by the gradual development of other scleroderma-associated signs and symptoms including heartburn on a frequent, often daily, basis; tender digital pitting scars or ulcers; and thickening of the skin of the fingers, which may progress to include the dorsum of the hands and forearms. Later features include dyspnea related to pulmonary fibrosis; telangiectasias (initially on the hands and face); and, much later, the development of dyspnea related to pulmonary arterial hypertension.

In contrast, dcSSc has a more rapid onset, with skin changes shortly after or coincidental with the onset of Raynaud's phenomenon, and with internal organ involvement occurring during the first 2 years of disease. Skin involvement usually progresses over the first 1 to 5 years, then stabilizes, and can gradually improve but seldom totally resolves. Even if the extent and severity of skin disease recede with time, the designation of diffuse disease remains relevant because the course of the internal organ involvement does not parallel skin improvement. Fibrosis in the pulmonary, cardiac, and gastrointestinal (GI) systems fibrosis does not resolve. Individuals with dcSSc are at risk for progressive involvement in these organs. In addition, early dcSSc patients, especially in the phase of skin worsening, are at the highest risk of developing scleroderma renal crisis (SRC).

Inflammatory features are also prominent in this group of patients with early, diffuse disease. Such features include inflamed, reddened, and intensely pruritic skin, tendon friction rubs, and synovitis (which may be difficult to appreciate due to the thickened overlying skin). Although prednisone can provide symptomatic relief, doses of 15 mg per day or higher have been linked to the development of SRC.

In general, poor prognostic factors include diffuse skin involvement, late age of disease onset, African- or Native-American race, a diffusing capacity <40% of the predicted value, the presence of a large pericardial effusion, proteinuria, hematuria, renal failure, anemia, elevated erythrocyte sedimentation rate, and abnormal electrocardiogram (9,10).

Autoantibody status is also helpful in considering prognosis (11). Nearly all SSc patients are ANA positive. Those with a centromere pattern ANA usually have limited disease and a relatively good prognosis but are at an increased risk of developing pulmonary arterial hypertension, primary biliary cirrhosis, and severe digital ischemia. Antitopoisomerase antibodies (also known as anti–Scl 70) identify individuals with an increased risk of severe pulmonary fibrosis. Antibodies to RNA-polymerase (not to be confused with anti-RNP antibodies) are associated with increased risk of SRC.

TABLE 17A-1. KEY CLINICAL FEATURES OF SYSTEMIC SCLEROSIS.

Diffuse cutaneous systemic sclerosis (dcSSc)
- Proximal skin thickening involving the trunk, upper arms and thighs, in addition to symmetrical involvement of the fingers, hands, arms, and face/neck
- Rapid onset of disease following the appearance of Raynaud's phenomenon
- Significant visceral disease: lungs, heart, gastrointestinal, and/or kidneys
- Absence of anticentromere antibodies
- Variable disease course but overall poor prognosis, with survival 40% to 60% at 10 years

Limited cutaneous systemic sclerosis (lcSSc)
- Symmetrical skin thickening limited to the areas below the elbows and knees and involving the face/neck
- Progression of disease typically months or years after the onset of Raynaud's phenomenon
- Later and less severe development of visceral disease
- Late development of pulmonary arterial hypertension
- Association with anticentromere antibodies
- Relatively good prognosis with survival >70% at 10 years

Overlap syndromes
- Diffuse or limited systemic sclerosis with typical features of one or more of the other defined connective tissue diseases
- Mixed connective tissue disease: features of systemic lupus erythematosus, systemic sclerosis, and polymyositis in the presence of anti-U_1 RNP antibodies

Table 17A-1 provides a summary of key clinical features of the subsets of SSc. Although the recognition of limited and diffuse disease subsets is useful, SSc is a highly variable disorder. Severe internal organ disease can occur even in those in the lcSSc group.

SKIN MANIFESTATIONS

The hallmark feature of SSc is thickened skin. However, skin manifestations also include swollen hands (and sometimes feet), pruritus, hyper- and/or hypopigmentation, telangiectasias, calcinosis, dermal ulcers, digital tip pitting scars, and digital tip gangrene (12). Frequently, the first symptom following the onset of Raynaud's phenomenon is that of puffy hands; patients find that their rings no longer fit. This is followed by thickening of the skin beginning distally and progressing proximally, affecting the upper extremities more than the lower. Pruritus, a common feature, usually affects those with early diffuse disease and frequently predates clinically apparent skin thickening. Occasionally patients complain of sharp fleeting pains and superficial skin tenderness. Both the pruritus and the skin pain tend to be early symptoms and usually improve as the fibrosis becomes well established.

Diffuse hyperpigmentation is believed to be due to chronic inflammation in the skin. In time, the skin may develop a spotty hypopigmentation known as a salt-and-pepper appearance, caused by maintenance of pigment at the base of hair follicles but the loss of pigment in the surrounding skin. As time progresses, areas of pigment loss coalesce and may become quite extensive over the hands, face, and chest.

Telangiectasias most commonly occur over the fingers, palms, dorsum of the hands, and face (Figure 17A-4). By definition, telangiectasias blanch with pressure. The lesions, initially ≤1 mm in diameter, can enlarge over time and affect the upper extremities and trunk, as well as the vermilion border of the lips and oral mucosa. For reasons that are not clear, telangiectasias rarely affect the lower extremities. These lesions are cosmetically disturbing for many patients. When telangiectasias involve the GI tract extensively, they may be associated with significant blood loss. Otherwise, telangiectasias do not cause clinical problems.

Digital tip pitting scars, ulcers, and gangrene caused by ischemia are invariably painful. Ulcers over bony prominences (PIPs, MCPs, elbows, malleoli) are due to a combination of stretched and thickened skin, poor circulation in the microvasculature, and repetitive minor trauma. Although infection is not the primary cause of these ulcers, the areas can become secondarily infected due to their chronicity. Digital tip gangrene can occur suddenly and may require surgical intervention. Whenever possible from the standpoint of pain management, however, unsalvageable digital tissue should be allowed to undergo autoamputation rather than surgical

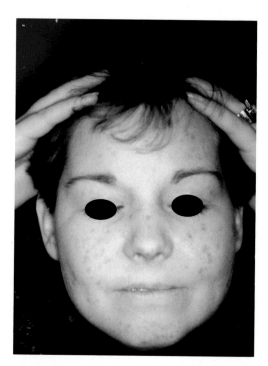

FIGURE 17A-4

Telangiectasias most commonly occur over the fingers, palms, dorsum of the hands, and face.

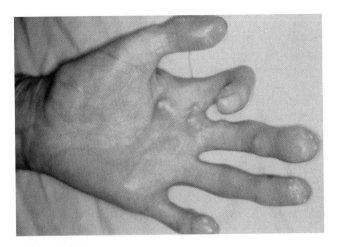

FIGURE 17A-5

Calcinosis can occur in the hands as well as in the forearms, elbows, knees, and legs.

removal, as surgical interventions generally lead to the loss of more tissue.

Calcinosis cutis, usually a late manifestation of SSc, occurs more frequently in limited disease but can occur in late diffuse disease, as well. Calcinosis can occur in the hands as well as in the forearms, elbows, knees, and legs (Figure 17A-5). These deposits can erupt through the skin, become secondarily infected, and pose major problems in management.

Although more than 95% of SSc patients have evidence of skin thickening, a small proportion will have scleroderma sine sclerosis, characterized by Raynaud's phenomenon, typical GI signs and symptoms, positive autoantibodies, and/or telangiectasias (13). The prognosis for these individuals, who have an increased risk for pulmonary arterial hypertension late in their course, is similar to those with limited cutaneous SSc. The diagnosis of SSc is usually quite delayed for this subtype due to the lack of thickened skin.

GASTROINTESTINAL MANIFESTATIONS

Next to skin involvement, the GI system is most commonly affected (14). Depending on the extent of involvement, signs and symptoms can include frequent heartburn, dysphagia, esophageal stricture formation, mucosal dysplasia (Barrett's esophagus), erosive esophagitis, gastritis, gastric antral vascular ectasia (GAVE or watermelon stomach), postprandial bloating, early satiety, weight loss, constipation, flatulence, and malabsorptive diarrhea.

The severity of GI tract disease is highly variable among individual patients. Most have some evidence of gastroesophageal reflux disease (GERD) due to lowered pressure of the gastroesophageal sphincter, but only a few develop severe GI dysmotility to the extent that hyperalimentation is required.

Gastrointestinal symptoms are related to dysmotility which, in turn, is related to smooth muscle atrophy and fibrosis. One current theory regarding SSc in the GI tract attributes gut dysfunction to early neural involvement with secondary muscular atrophy. In this scenario, fibrosis is a repair mechanism rather than the primary process (15).

Initially, there is incoordination of peristaltic waves in the esophagus. Over time, the esophagus may become totally aperistaltic. The sensation of dysphagia can occur on the basis of an esophageal stricture due to chronic reflux, or on the basis of disordered peristalsis such that food hangs up in one area, requiring several swallows to clear the material.

Chronic GERD can lead to mucosal erosions, dysplasia, stricture formation, and reactive airway disease due to nocturnal aspiration. GAVE, which is seen on upper endoscopy, is due to the thinning of the gastric mucosa such that the underlying parallel blood vessels in the antrum resemble the stripes of a watermelon. This condition, sometimes associated with blood loss, is amenable to endoscopic laser coagulation. Mucosal telangiectasias, which late in disease can develop throughout the GI tract, sometimes lead to occult, difficult-to-control blood loss.

Gastroparesis and small bowel dysmotility leads to early satiety, bloating, and flatulence. Bacterial overgrowth in the small intestine may cause malabsorption and diarrhea, requiring intermittent or rotating antibiotics. Decreased motility in the large bowel is associated with constipation, which can be severe. Radiographic contrast studies demonstrate wide-mouthed diverticuli as well as pneumotosis cystoides intestinalis. These latter two features are rarely of clinical consequence. Decreased pressure of the anal sphincter can also be seen in SSc, leading to stool incontinence.

Primary biliary cirrhosis (PBC) occurs in a small proportion of patients but at a rate that is greater than expected in the general population (16).

PULMONARY AND PULMONARY VASCULAR DISEASE

Pulmonary disease is now the leading cause of death in SSc (9). Pulmonary fibrosis occurs in many SSc patients, with 20% ultimately requiring supplemental oxygen. Patients with dcSSc are at higher risk of developing significant lung fibrosis compared to those with lcSSc. However, this distinction is not absolute, and pulmonary function test (PFT) monitoring is recommended for both groups. Early lung disease is frequently asymptomatic. Dry cough, a later symptom, is not specific for lung

17

disease and may be related to chronic GERD. Dyspnea on exertion may be a consequence of multiple factors.

Pulmonary function test that show a restrictive pattern is the most sensitive test for pulmonary parenchymal disease. Periodic testing is suggested. Decreases in the vital capacity, lung volumes, and/or diffusing capacity for carbon monoxide (DLCO) are indicative of restrictive changes. An isolated decrease in DLCO may also indicate pulmonary hypertension.

Computed tomography (CT) scans of the lung are more sensitive than radiographs for the detection of early fibrotic changes. High resolution CT views are required to detect a ground glass appearance, which is believed to represent inflammation or alveolitis. Bronchoalveolar lavage (BAL) showing neutrophils and/or eosinophils is suggestive of active inflammation. Patients who are positive for antitopoisomerase antibodies are at an increased risk for clinically significant pulmonary fibrosis, but this complication is not confined solely to this autoantibody subgroup.

Pulmonary hypertension can occur on the basis of two main pathologic processes: (1) those primarily involving destruction or obliteration of lung vasculature, such as pulmonary fibrosis, recurrent thromboembolic disease, or scleroderma vasculopathy; or (2) those associated with decreased cardiac output, for example, diastolic dysfunction, congestive heart failure, or valvular disease. *Pulmonary arterial hypertension* (PAH) is a term used to describe the first group of conditions.

As noted, PFTs in patients with PAH show an isolated decrease in DLCO with other parameters being normal, or a DLCO that is decreased out of proportion to the other measures. An echocardiogram is helpful in making the diagnosis, particularly if the right ventricular systolic pressure and/or the velocity of the regurgitant jet of the tricuspid valve are high. However, the echocardiogram is less reliable in borderline cases. In addition, the echocardiogram does not provide a measure of pulmonary capillary wedge pressure. Right heart catheterization should therefore be performed in patients suspected of PAH to confirm the diagnosis and obtain an accurate measurement of both the pulmonary artery and pulmonary capillary wedge pressures. Chronic thromboembolic disease must be excluded in patients with PAH.

In terms of symptoms, PAH is initially silent. Early symptoms can be nonspecific, for example, a sense of generalized weakness on exertion. Dyspnea is a later symptom and can be attributed to multiple other factors. PAH in SSc typically develops late in the course of patients with lcSSc. Many SSc patients with PAH are anticentromere antibody positive. However, in individuals with restrictive lung disease of mild or moderate severity, it is difficult to distinguish which patients have PAH secondary to their lung fibrosis and which patients have a combination of scleroderma lung disease with scleroderma pulmonary vasculopathy. The mortality risk in SSc patients with the combination of pulmonary

fibrosis and PAH is similar to that of patients with isolated PAH and worse than those with pulmonary fibrosis alone (17).

The prevalence of PAH in the SSc patient population when measured by right heart catheterization is 8% to 12% (18,19). The prevalence of PAH by echocardiogram alone is more than double this figure (20) and emphasizes the point that right heart catheterization is necessary to confirm the diagnosis.

As echocardiography is being done more frequently in the SSc population, it is becoming clear that this condition is more common than believed previously, and that it can affect both lcSSc and dcSSc patients. Risk factors for progression to severe pulmonary hypertension include older age, limited skin disease, and elevated pulmonary artery pressures at the time of initial evaluation (21).

CARDIAC INVOLVEMENT

If cardiac involvement in SSc is defined as any change in the electrocardiogram (EKG), pericardium, or cardiac function, then heart disease in SSc is common (22). However, clinically apparent cardiac disease, usually a late finding associated with a poor prognosis, is relatively uncommon. When present, SSc cardiac disease is manifested by disturbances in the conduction system of the heart, arrhythmias, left ventricular or global heart failure, and pericarditis. Patchy fibrosis throughout the myocardium is the typical histological picture in SSc. Contraction band necrosis, characteristic of ischemia/reperfusion injury, has been described.

Asymptomatic small or moderate-sized pericardial effusions are frequently found, but tamponade is rare. Large pericardial effusions, however, are associated with a poor prognosis (23).

RENAL DISEASE AND SCLERODERMA RENAL CRISIS

Scleroderma renal crisis (SRC) was the most common cause of death in SSc prior to the introduction of angiotensin-converting enzyme (ACE) inhibitors (24). SRC still occurs, typically in the setting of early diffuse disease (<4 years from onset). In SRC, malignant hypertension can occur suddenly in individuals with previously normal blood pressure values. Clinical signs and symptoms are those of severe hypertension and can include headaches, stroke, and heart failure. The creatinine is elevated and urinalysis shows proteinuria and microscopic hematuria. Changes of microscopic angiopathy can be seen with anemia and thrombocytopenia, which resolve on normalization of the blood pressure. If treated early and aggressively with ACE inhibition (combined if necessary with other antihypertensives), the outcome is favorable, with return to normal or near normal renal function within several days of blood pressure normalization. Good outcomes are dependent on lowering of the blood pressure to truly normal levels.

Factors predictive of SRC include diffuse skin disease, rapid progression of skin involvement, disease duration <4 years, anti-RNA polymerase III antibody, new anemia, new cardiac events, and antecedent high dose corticosteroid usage. In addition, prior use of cyclosporine has been linked to SRC.

Poor prognostic factors in SRC include a creatinine level >3 mg/dL at the time of diagnosis of SRC, delay in blood pressure normalization >3 days, male sex, older age, and presence of congestive heart failure. In one study, 55% of patients who initially required dialysis were able to discontinue dialysis at a mean of 8 months. It is therefore important to continue ACE inhibition and blood pressure control even after dialysis is initiated.

Normotensive renal crisis, characterized by a slow rise in creatinine in the absence of significant blood presssure elevation and without a microangiopathic picture, also has been described in SSc. Other causes for renal failure must be investigated thoroughly, and ACE inhibitors employed empirically.

MUSCULOSKELETAL DISEASE

Characteristics of musculoskeletal involvement include joint contractures, tendon friction rubs, myopathy, myositis, bone resorption, cutaneous calcifications, synovitis, and compression neuropathies (25).

In the absence of inflammatory synovitis, joint contractures are due to involvement of overlying skin that restricts motion. The degree of contractures reflects the extent of skin involvement. The hands, wrists, and elbows are the most commonly affected joints. Upper extremity involvement can interfere with normal hand and arm activities. Range of motion may also be reduced at the shoulders, hips, knees, and ankles. Lower extremity involvement can lead to marked gait impairment.

Tendon friction rubs, caused by an inflammation in the tendon sheath, are usually palpable on examination and sometimes cause pain with motion. If a patient complains of pain over the tendon with joint motion and no rub is palpated, it can usually be heard with the stethoscope. The most commonly affected tendon sheaths are those of the ankle dorsiflexors, the finger extensors, and the knee extensors. Tendon friction rubs may also be detected around the shoulders, wrists, and other joints.

In SSc, both a myopathy and a myositis can occur. Scleroderma myopathy is characterized by a relatively nonprogressive course; mild proximal muscle weakness; normal or slight elevations of creatine phosphokinase (CPK); and poor response to corticosteroids (26). Muscle biopsy shows replacement of muscle fibers with fibrosis, and lymphocytic infiltrates (if present) are scanty. In contrast, true myositis—a less common clinical finding—is characterized by progressive proximal muscle weakness, elevation of CPK, and typical electromyographic changes of inflammatory muscle disease. True myositis usually responds to immunosuppression.

Osteolysis or bone resorption of the digital tufts, seen in 40% to 80% of patients, is believed to be on the basis of chronic ischemia. Osteolysis of other bones is also seen but is much less common than digital tuft resorption. These sites include the ribs, the mandible, the distal clavicle, the humerus and the cervical spine.

Inflammatory synovitis of the peripheral joints, particularly those of the hands and wrists, is a frequent finding early in the disease course. Joint swelling can be difficult to appreciate under the thickened and taut scleroderma skin. The arthritis of SSc is nonerosive, usually responsive to anti-inflammatory agents (including methotrexate), and can resolve after several months.

In contradistinction to the above situation, some patients have an overlap of SSc and rheumatoid arthritis with positive rheumatoid factor, erosive joint disease, and progressive articular destruction. Treatment is the same as the treatment of idiopathic rheumatoid arthritis.

The most common compression neuropathy in SSc is carpal tunnel syndrome. This frequently occurs in the edematous phase of early disease. Other compression neuropathies, such as ulnar neuropathy, can occur as the skin becomes thickened and taut and as flexion contractures develop.

SCLERODERMA-LIKE DISORDERS

Several SSc-like disorders have been described (27). The most clinically relevant today include nephrogenic systemic fibrosis (NSF, previously called nephrogenic fibrosing dermopathy), eosinophilic fasciitis, scleredema, and scleremyxedema.

Nephrogenic systemic fibrosis (NSF) occurs in the setting of chronic renal insufficiency, usually but not always affecting individuals on dialysis (28). Features that distinguish this from SSc are the following: The fibrosis affects the lower extremities more than the upper extremities, occurs relatively rapidly, and tends to spare the hands. Raynaud's phenomenon is not associated with NSF, and renal transplantation has been reported to cause regression of this disease. Although the mechanism is not fully established, it is thought that circulating fibrocytes, derived from the bone marrow, are recruited to the skin, become activated and result in fibrosis.

Eosinophilic fasciitis (Shulman's disease) is characterized by fairly rapid onset of skin and fascial thickening with the early development of flexion contractures, particularly at the elbow. The skin has an orange peel or puckered appearance, sparing the hands and fingers. A deep biopsy that extends to the underlying fascia needs to be done in order to make the diagnosis. An eosinophilic infiltrate is seen on biopsy affecting the fascia which is thickened. Peripheral eosiniphilia, unusual to any substantial degree in SSc, is common in eosinophilic fasciitis.

Scleredema (or scleredema diabeticorum) occurs, as its name suggests, as a complication of diabetes mellitus and causes induration and thickening of the skin of the neck, shoulder girdle area, proximal upper extremities, and back. The distribution is contrasts with the distal involvement of SSc and there is no Raynaud's phenomenon. A biopsy shows excess mucin as well as collagen. Scleredema can also be associated with a paraprotein or with multiple myeloma. Paraproteins are usually not demonstrated in the skin.

Scleromyxedema, on the other hand, is characterized by a more generalized cutaneous induration than that seen in scleredema. Scleromyxedema can involve the hands but there is also the presence of mucinous papules and nodules. This condition is also associated with a paraprotein. It can be distinguished by the presence of folded and pendulous skin, rather than the tight, hidebound character of SSc skin.

REFERENCES

1. Piette WW. Morphea or localized scleroderma. In: Clements PJ, Furst DE, eds. Systemic sclerosis. Philadelphia: Lippincott Williams & Wilkins; 2004:29–37.
2. Medsger TA Jr. Classification, prognosis. In: Clements PJ, Furst DE, eds. Systemic sclerosis. Philadelphia: Lippincott Williams & Wilkins; 2004:17–28.
3. Korn JH. Pathogenesis of systemic sclerosis. In: Koopman WJ, Moreland LW, eds. Arthritis and allied conditions. Philadelphia: Lippincott Williams & Wilkins; 2005:1621–1632.
4. Boin F, Wigley FM. Understanding, assessing and treating Raynaud's phenomenon. Curr Opin Rheumatol 2005;17:752–760.
5. Fraenkel L, Zhang Y, Chaisson CE, et al. Different factors influencing the expression of Raynaud's phenomenon in men and women. Arthritis Rheum 1999;42:306–310.
6. Suter LG, Murabito JM, Felson DT, Fraenkel L. The incidence and natural history of Raynaud's phenomenon in the community. Arthritis Rheum 2005;52:1259–1263.
7. Subcommittee for Scleroderma Criteria of the American Rheumatism Association Diagnostic and Therapeutic Criteria Committee: preliminary criteria for the classification of systemic sclerosis (scleroderma). Arthritis Rheum 1980;23:581–590.
8. LeRoy EC, Black C, Fleischmajer R, et al. Scleroderma (systemic sclerosis): classification, subsets, and pathogenesis. J Rheumatol 1988;15:202–205.
9. Steen VD, Medsger TA Jr. Severe organ involvement in systemic sclerosis with diffuse scleroderma. Arthritis Rheum 2000;43:2437–2444.
10. Bryan C, Knight C, Black CM, Silman AJ. Prediction of five-year survival following presentation with scleroderma: development of a simplet model using three disease factors at first visit. Arthritis Rheum 1999;42:2660–2665.
11. Cepeda EJ, Reveille JD. Autoantibodies in systemic sclerosis and fibrosing syndromes: clinical indications and relevance. Curr Opin Rheumatol 2004;16:723–732.
12. Clements PJ, Medsger TA Jr, Feghali CA. Cutaneous involvement in systemic sclerosis. In: Clements PJ, Furst DE, eds. Systemic sclerosis. Philadelphia: Lippincott Williams & Wilkins; 2004:129–150.
13. Poormoghim H, Lucas M, Fertig N, Medsger TA Jr. Systemic sclerosis sine scleroderma: demographic, clinical, and serologic features and survival in forty-eight patients. Arthritis Rheum 2000;43:444–451.
14. Weinstein WM, Kadell BM. The gastrointestinal tract in systemic sclerosis. In: Clements PJ, Furst DE, eds. Systemic sclerosis. Philadelphia: Lippincott Williams & Wilkins; 2004:293–308.
15. Goldblatt F, Gordon TP, Waterman SA. Antibody-mediated gastrointestinal dysmotility in scleroderma. Gastroenterology 2002;123:1144–1150.
16. Mackey RI. Autoimmunity and primary biliary cirrhosis. Baillieres Best Pract Res Clin Gastroenterol 2000;14:519–533.
17. Chang B, Wigley FM, White B, Wise RA. Scleroderma patients with combined pulmonary hypertension and interstitial lung disease. J Rheumatol 2003;30:2398–2405.
18. Hachulla E, Gressin V, Guillevin L, et al. Early detection of pulmonary arterial hypertension in systemic sclerosis: a French nationwide prospective multicenter study. Arthritis Rheum 2005;52:3792–3800.
19. Mukerjee D, St George D, Coleiro B, et al. Prevalence and outcome in systemic sclerosis associated pulmonary arterial hypertension: application of a registry approach. Ann Rheum Dis 2003;62:1088–1093.
20. Wigley FM, Lima JAC, Mayes M, McLain D, Chapin JL, Ward-Able C. The UNCOVER study: prevalence of undiagnosed pulmonary arterial hypertension in subjects with connective tissue disease at the secondary healthcare level of community-based rheumatologists. Arthritis Rheum 2005;52:2125–2132.
21. Chang B, Wigley FM, White B, Wise RA. Scleroderma patients with combined pulmonary hypertension and interstitial lung disease. J Rheumatol 2006;33:269–274.
22. Follansbee WP, Marroquin OC. Cardiac involvement in systemic sclerosis. In: Clements PJ, Furst DE, eds. Systemic sclerosis. Philadelphia: Lippincott Williams & Wilkins; 2004:195–220.
23. Smith JW, Clements PJ, Levisman J, Furst D, Ross M. Echocardiographic features of progressive systemic sclerosis (PSS): correlation with hemodynamic and postmortem studies. Am J Med 1979;66:28–33.
24. Steen VD. Renal involvement in systemic sclerosis. In: Clements PJ, Furst DE, eds. Systemic sclerosis. Philadelphia: Lippincott Williams & Wilkins; 2004:279–292.
25. Pope JE. Musculoskeletal involvement in scleroderma. Rheum Dis Clin North Am 2003;52:391–405.
26. Clements PJ, Furst DE, Campion DS, et al. Muscle disease in progressive systemic sclerosis: diagnostic and therapeutic consideration. Arthritis Rheum 1978;21:62–71.
27. Mori Y, Kahari VM, Varga J. Scleroderma-like cutaneous syndromes. Curr Rheumatol Rep 2002;4:113–122.
28. Cowper SE, Boyer PJ. Nephrogenic systemic fibrosis: an update. Curr Rheumatol Rep 2006;8:151–157.

Systemic Sclerosis
B. Epidemiology, Pathology, and Pathogenesis

John Varga, MD

- Systemic sclerosis (SSc) is a chronic, multisystem disease of unknown etiology characterized by autoimmunity and inflammation, functional and structural abnormalities in small blood vessels, and progressive fibrosis of the skin and visceral organs.
- Estimates of its incidence in the United States range from 9 to 19 cases per million per year. The only community-based survey of SSc yielded a prevalence of 286 cases per million population.
- SSc is more common in females, with women-to-men ratios of 3 to 5:1.
- African Americans have a higher incidence than whites, and disease onset occurs at an earlier age. Furthermore, African Americans are more likely to have the diffuse cutaneous form of the disease with interstitial lung involvement and worse prognosis.
- Some SSc patients (1.6%) have a first-degree relative with the disease [relative risk (RR) = 13], indicating an important genetic contribution to disease susceptibility.
- Among environmental factors, infectious agents (particularly viruses), exposure to environmental and occupational toxins, and drugs have been suspected of playing a role in the etiology of SSc.
- The distinguishing pathological hallmark of SSc is an obliterative vasculopathy of small arteries and arterioles, combined vascular and interstitial fibrosis in target organs. In patients with established SSc, these lesions occur in the absence of inflammation.
- In relatively early-stage disease, perivascular cellular infiltrates are detected in many organs prior to the appearance of fibrosis.
- The organs most prominently affected by obliterative vasculopathy are the heart, lungs, kidneys, and intestinal tract.
- Fibrosis is prominent in the skin, lungs, gastrointestinal tract, heart, tendon sheath, perifascicular tissue surrounding skeletal muscle, and in some endocrine organs, such as the thyroid gland.
- Multiple cell types and their products interact in the processes that underlie the diverse clinical manifestations of SSc.
- An integrated view of the pathogenesis of SSc must incorporate the development of vasculopathy, activation of the cellular and humoral immune responses, and progressive fibrosis of multiple organs.
- Autoimmunity, altered endothelial cell function, and vascular reactivity may be the earliest manifestations of SSc, leading to Raynaud's phenomenon years before other disease features are present. Complex interplay among these processes initiates, amplifies, and sustains aberrant tissue repair and fibrosis.

Systemic sclerosis (SSc) is a chronic, multisystem disease of unknown etiology characterized by autoimmunity and inflammation, functional and structural abnormalities in small blood vessels, and progressive fibrosis of the skin and visceral organs. The pathogenesis of SSc is highly complex and incompletely understood. Multiple cell types and their products interact in the processes that underlie the diverse clinical manifestations of SSc.

EPIDEMIOLOGY

Systemic sclerosis, an acquired, sporadic disease with worldwide distribution, affects all races. Estimates of its incidence in the United States range from 9 to 19 cases per million per year. Prevalence rate estimates range from 28 to 253 cases per million. The only community-based survey of SSc yielded a prevalence of 286 cases per million population (1). It is estimated that some

100,000 people in the United States have SSc, although this number may be significantly higher if patients who may have milder disease and do not meet formal classification criteria are also included. There does not appear to be a difference in incidence between warmer and colder climates within the United States. Studies from England, Australia, and Japan have shown lower rates compared to the United States (2).

Age, gender, and ethnicity are important factors determining disease susceptibility. Like other connective tissue diseases, SSc is more common in females, with women-to-men ratios of 3 to 5:1. The female predominance, most striking among patients aged 15 to 40 years, declines after menopause. The most common age of onset is in the 30 to 50 years range, and in contrast to localized forms of scleroderma, SSc is rare in children. African Americans have a higher incidence than whites, and disease onset occurs at an earlier age. Furthermore, African Americans are more likely to have the diffuse cutaneous form of the disease with interstitial lung involvement and worse prognosis. Increased disease severity and mortality of SSc in African Americans may be related to the greater frequency of severe disease subtypes and subtype-specific autoantibodies such as those directed against topoisomerase I (Scl-70) and U3-RNP (3).

Associations of SSc with specific human leukocyte antigen (HLA) haplotypes are generally weak. In contrast, specific autoantibodies are associated with particular HLA alleles. For instance, antitopoisomerase I antibodies show strong association with the HLA-DRB1*1101-1104 alleles in white and black Americans, and with DRB1*1502 in Japanese. Certain antibody–HLA associations differ among different ethnic groups. Among whites with SSc, the HLA-DQB1 molecule is associated with anticentromere antibodies.

GENETIC FACTORS

Systemic sclerosis is not inherited in a Mendelian fashion. Furthermore, monozygotic and dizygotic twin pairs show a similarly low rate of disease concordance (4). On the other hand, 1.6% of SSc patients have a first-degree relative with the disease [relative risk (RR) = 13], indicating an important genetic contribution to disease susceptibility. The risk of other autoimmune diseases, including systemic lupus erythematosus (SLE) and rheumatoid arthritis, is also increased in first-degree relatives of SSc patients. Among Choctaw Native Americans from Oklahoma, the prevalence of SSc may be as high as 4690 per million. Moreover, affected individuals in the Choctaw population display striking homogeneity of disease phenotype, with diffuse cutaneous involvement, pulmonary fibrosis, and antitopoisomerase I antibodies. Genetic investigations in SSc have focused on polymorphisms of candidate genes, particularly those involved in regulation of immunity and inflammation, vascular function, and connective tissue homeostasis. Weak associations of single nucleotide polymorphisms (SNPs) with SSc have been reported in genes encoding angiotensin-converting enzyme (ACE), endothelin 1, nitric oxide synthase, B-cell markers (CD19), chemokines (monocyte chemoattractant protein 1) and chemokine receptors, cytokines (interleukin 1 alpha, IL-4, and tumor necrosis factor alpha), growth factors and their receptors (connective tissue growth factor [CTGF] and transforming growth factor beta [TGF-beta]), and extracellular matrix proteins (fibronectin, fibrillin, and SPARC). The list continues to grow.

ENVIRONMENTAL FACTORS

The relatively low rates of twin concordance for SSc suggest the importance of environmental factors in disease susceptibility. Infectious agents (particularly viruses), exposure to environmental and occupational toxins, and drugs have been suspected. Patients with SSc have increased serum antibodies to human cytomegalovirus (hCMV), and antitopoisomerase I autoantibodies recognize antigenic epitopes that are present on the hCMV-derived UL94 protein. Because antibodies to UL94 induce endothelial cell apoptosis and activation of dermal fibroblasts—two of the pathophysiologic hallmarks of SSc—molecular mimicry may be a possible mechanistic link between hCMV infection and SSc. Other studies have implicated hCMV infection in the allograft vasculopathy that follows solid organ transplantation. This vasculopathy is characterized by vascular neointima formation and smooth muscle proliferation, reminiscent of the obliterative vasculopathy of SSc. Demonstration that hCMV can directly induce CTGF production in infected fibroblasts lends further rationale to the hypothetical connection between hCMV and SSc. Human parvovirus B19 infection has also been postulated to have a link with SSc.

Several reports of apparent geographic clustering of SSc cases suggest shared environmental exposures, but careful investigations have failed to substantiate these clusters. In the past two decades, two epidemics of multisystemic illnesses reminiscent of SSc have been reported. One of these, the toxic oil syndrome, was linked to contaminated rapeseed cooking oils in Spain. The other, eosinophilia–myalgia syndrome, was caused by the ingestion of a dietary supplement (L-tryptophan) in the United States. Both of these apparently novel syndromes, each of which affected more than 10,000 individuals, were characterized by chronic scleroderma-like skin fibrosis. Yet both showed clinical and pathological features that clearly distinguished them from

SSc. Some observers have noted an increased incidence of SSc among men with occupational exposure to silica, such as miners. Other occupational exposures tentatively linked with SSc include polyvinyl chloride, epoxy resins, and aromatic hydrocarbons (e.g., toluene and trichloroethylene). Drugs implicated in SSc-like illnesses include bleomycin, pentazocine, cocaine, and appetite suppressants (primarily derivatives of fenfluramine) associated with pulmonary hypertension. The occurrence of SSc in some women with silicone breast implants raised concern regarding a possible association, but careful epidemiologic investigations found no evidence of increased risk of SSc (5).

PATHOLOGY

The distinguishing pathological hallmark of SSc is an obliterative vasculopathy of small arteries and arterioles combined with interstitial fibrosis in target organs. In patients with established SSc, these lesions occur in the absence of inflammation. In relatively early-stage disease, however, perivascular cellular infiltrates are detected in many organs prior to the appearance of fibrosis. Cutaneous infiltrates are composed primarily of CD4+ T lymphocytes (6). In addition, CD8+ T cells, monocytes/macrophages, plasma cells, mast cells, and occasionally B cells are detected. In contrast to skin, the majority of T cells infiltrating the lungs are CD8+. Evidence of eosinophil degranulation is found in lesional skin and lungs in the absence of intact eosinophils.

The vascular lesion of SSc, characterized by bland intimal proliferation in the small and medium-sized arteries, results in luminal narrowing. The organs most prominently affected by obliterative vasculopathy are the heart, lungs, kidneys, and intestinal tract. Fibrosis is prominent in the skin, lungs, gastrointestinal tract, heart, tendon sheath, perifascicular tissue surrounding skeletal muscle, and in some endocrine organs, such as the thyroid gland. SSc-associated fibrosis is characterized by homogeneous-appearing connective tissue composed of type I collagen, fibronectin, proteoglycans, and other structural macromolecules. The process leads to progressive replacement of normal tissue, disruption of architecture, functional impairment, and (frequently) organ failure. In the skin, fibrosis is preceded by inflammatory cell accumulation. This causes massive dermal expansion with obliteration of the hair follicles, sweat glands, and other appendages (Figure 17B-1). Collagen accumulation is most prominent in the reticular dermis, and the fibrotic process invades the subjacent adipose layer with entrapment of fat cells. The epidermis is atrophic, and the rete pegs are effaced.

Pathological changes can be found in any part of the gartrointestinal tract, from the mouth to the rectum. The striated muscle in the upper third of the esophagus

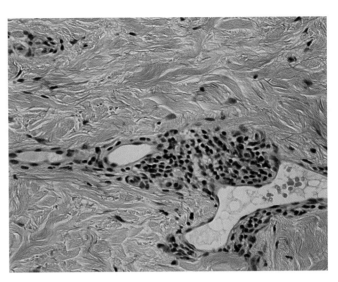

Figure 17B-1

Inflammation and fibrosis in the skin. This skin lesion from a patient with early systemic sclerosis shows a focal perivascular infiltrate composed on monocytes and lymphocytes, surrounded by densely packed collagen fibers in the deep layer of the dermis. Adnexal structures are encased by connective tissue. (Hematoxylin and eosin). (From Varga J, Abraham D. Systemic sclerosis: a prototypic multisystem fibrotic disorder, by permission of *J Clin Invest* 2007 117:557–67.)

is generally spared. The lower esophagus is frequently involved, with prominent fibrosis of the lamina propria and submucosa, characteristic vascular lesions, and atrophy of the muscular layers. Lower esophageal dysfunction leads to gastroesophageal reflux in a high percentage of patients. Chronic reflux is associated with esophageal inflammation, ulcerations, and stricture formation, and may lead to Barrett's esophagus. Replacement of the normal intestinal tract architecture results in disordered peristaltic activity, dysmotility, and small bowel obstruction.

In the lungs, patchy infiltration of the alveolar walls with CD8+ lymphocytes, macrophages, and eosinophils is prominent in early disease. With disease progression, fibrosis and vascular damage dominate the pathological picture in diffuse SSc, often coexisting within the same lesions. In patients with limited cutaneous disease, vascular lesions predominate with little or no fibrosis. Intimal thickening of the pulmonary arteries, best seen with elastin stain, underlies pulmonary hypertension. At autopsy in such cases, multiple pulmonary emboli and evidence of myocardial fibrosis are often found. Pulmonary fibrosis is characterized by expansion of the alveolar interstitium, with accumulation of collagen and other connective tissue proteins. This pattern is classified histopathologically as nonspecific interstitial pneumonitis (NSIP). Progressive thickening of the alveolar septae results in obliteration of the air spaces and honeycombing, as well as loss of pulmonary blood vessels

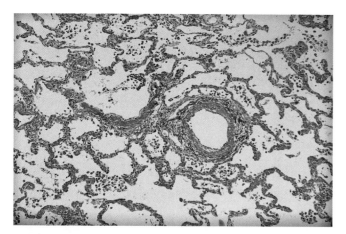

Figure 17B-2

Pulmonary artery. There is thickening of the intimal layer of a small pulmonary artery, leading to occlusion of vascular lumen. (Hematoxylin and eosin).

(Figure 17B-2). This process impairs gas exchange and contributes to worsening pulmonary hypertension.

The heart is frequently affected, with prominent involvement of the myocardium and pericardium. The characteristic arteriolar lesions of intimal proliferation and luminal narrowing are accompanied by contraction band necrosis, reflecting ischemia-reperfusion injury, and patchy myocardial fibrosis. The electrical system of the heart (bundle of His, Purkinje fibers) may be involved, leading to conduction disturbances.

In the kidneys, lesions of the interlobular arteries predominate. Glomerulonephritis is not characteristic of SSc. Chronic renal ischemia is associated with shrunken glomeruli. Patients with scleroderma renal crisis show dramatic changes in small renal arteries: reduplication of elastic lamina, marked intimal proliferation and narrowing of the lumen, and often thrombosis and microangiopathic hemolysis. The renal lesion in scleroderma renal crisis may be identical histopathologically to that of thrombotic thrombocytopenic purpura. Other organs may also be affected. Synovitis may be found in patients with early SSc, but with progression the synovium becomes fibrotic, as do tendon sheaths and fascia, producing audible tendon friction rubs. Inflammatory myositis and muscle fibrosis are common findings.

PATHOGENESIS

An integrated view of the pathogenesis of SSc must incorporate the development of vasculopathy, activation of the cellular and humoral immune responses, and progressive fibrosis of multiple organs (Figure 17B-3).

Autoimmunity, altered endothelial cell function, and vascular reactivity may be the earliest manifestations of SSc, leading to Raynaud's phenomenon years before other disease features are present. Complex interplay between these processes initiates, amplifies, and sustains aberrant tissue repair and fibrosis (7).

ANIMAL MODELS OF DISEASE

No animal model reproduces all three cardinal features of human SSc (vascular damage, autoimmunity, and fibrosis), but some models recapitulate selected disease characteristics. The tight skin mouse (Tsk1/+) is a naturally occurring model of SSc characterized by spontaneous development of scleroderma-like skin changes. The mutation responsible for the mouse phenotype, an in-frame duplication in the gene responsible for Marfan's disease (fibrillin-1), results in defective matrix assembly and altered TGF-beta activation. However, corresponding mutations have not been found in human SSc. A chronic condition with fibrosis in the skin and lungs can be induced in mice by chemical exposure (bleomycin injections) or by transplantation of HLA-mismatched bone marrow or spleen cells (sclerodermatous graft versus host disease). Increasingly, manipulation of mice via mutagenesis or targeted genetic modifications such as knockout models or transgenesis have created new approaches to studying SSc and dissecting the roles of individual molecules in the underlying processes. For instance, genetic targeting of Smad3, an intracellular mediator for TGF-beta, and of the chemokine MCP-1, both resulted in mice that were resistant to bleomycin-induced scleroderma.

VASCULOPATHY

Vascular involvement is widespread in SSc and has important clinical implications. Raynaud phenomenon, an early disease manifestation, is characterized by an altered blood flow response to cold challenge. This initially reversible abnormality is due to alterations in the autonomic and peripheral nervous systems, with impaired production of neuropeptides, such as calcitonin gene-related peptide (from sensory afferent nerves) and heightened sensitivity of alpha 2-adrenergic receptors (on vascular smooth muscle cells). While primary Raynaud's phenomenon is a relatively benign, nonprogressive condition, in SSc irreversible morphological and functional changes in the circulation develop, leading to endothelial injury. Within the endothelium, there is altered production of and responsiveness to endothelium-derived factors that mediate vasodilatation (nitric oxide and prostacyclin) and vasoconstriction (endothelin 1). Microvessels show increased

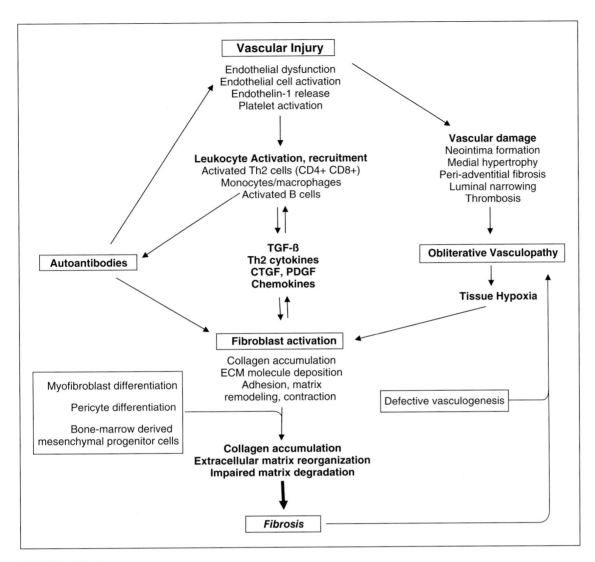

FIGURE 17B-3

Schematic representation of the complex pathogenesis of systemic sclerosis. Initial vascular injury in genetically susceptible individuals leads to functional and structural vascular alterations, inflammation, and the generation of autoimmunity. The inflammatory and immune responses then initiate and sustain fibroblast activation and differentiation, resulting in pathological fibrogenesis and irreversible tissue damage. CTGF, connective tissue growth factor; PDGF, platelet-derived growth factor; ECM, extracellular matrix.

permeability, enhanced transendothelial leukocyte diapedesis, activation of coagulation and fibrinolytic cascades, and platelet aggregation. These processes culminate in thrombosis. Endothelial cells show increased expression of intercellular adhesion molecule 1 (ICAM-1) and other surface adhesion molecules. Vasculopathy affects capillaries, arterioles, and even large vessels in many organs. Smooth muscle cell-like myointimal cells proliferate, the basement membrane is thickened and reduplicated, and adventitial fibrosis develops.

Progressive vascular luminal occlusion due to intimal and medial hypertrophy and adventitial fibrosis, combined with persistent endothelial cell damage and apoptosis, establish a vicious cycle. Angiograms of the hands and kidneys of patients with late-stage disease reveal a striking absence of blood vessels. Damaged endothelium promotes platelet aggregation and release of thromboxane, a potent vasoconstrictor, and platelet-derived growth factor (PDGF). Vascular compromise is aggravated further by defective fibrinolysis. Oxidative stress due to ischemia-reperfusion is associated with generation of free radicals that further contribute to endothelial damage through peroxidation of membrane lipids. Paradoxically, the process of revascularization that normally re-establishes blood flow to ischemic tissue appears to be defective in SSc. Failure of vasculogenesis occurs in the setting of elevated levels of angiogenic factors, such as vascular endothelial growth factor (VEGF). In patients with SSc, the number of bone marrow–derived CD34+ CD133+ endothelial progenitor cells circulating in the system is reduced markedly; moreover, their differentiation in vitro into mature endothelial cells is impaired (8). Thus, widespread obliterative vasculopathy and failure to replace damaged vessels are hallmarks of SSc.

CELLULAR AND HUMORAL AUTOIMMUNITY

In the early stages of the disease, activated T cells and monocytes/macrophages accumulate in lesional skin, lungs, and other affected organs. Infiltrating T cells express activation markers such as CD3, CD4, CD45, and HLA-DR, and display restricted receptor signatures indicative of oligoclonal expansion in response to unknown antigens. Circulating CD4+ T cells also have elevated levels of chemokine receptors and express alpha 1 integrin (an adhesion molecule), accounting for their enhanced ability to bind to endothelium and to fibroblasts. Endothelial cells express ICAM-1 and other adhesion molecules that facilitate leukocyte diapedesis. Activated macrophages and T cells show a Th2-polarized response, and secrete interleukin 4 and interleukin 13. Both of these Th2 cytokines can induce TGF-beta, a powerful modulator of immune regulation and matrix accumulation (Table 17B-1). Because it can

induce its own production, as well as that of CTGF (also termed CCN2) and other cytokines, TGF-beta establishes sustained autocrine/paracrine loops for activation of fibroblasts and other effector cells. DNA microarray studies of global gene expression in CD8+ T cells in bronchoalveolar lavage fluids from patients with SSc have demonstrated an activated Th2 pattern of gene expression, characterized by increased levels of IL-4 and IL-13, and reduced production of interferon gamma (IFN-gamma). Th2 cytokines promote collagen synthesis and other profibrotic responses. IFN-gamma inhibits collagen synthesis and blocks cytokine-mediated fibroblast activation.

Circulating autoantibodies are detected in virtually all patients with SSc. These mutually exclusive autoantibodies are highly specific for SSc, and show strong association with individual disease phenotypes and genetically determined HLA haplotypes. Autoantibody levels correlate with disease severity and their titers fluctuate to some degree with disease activity, albeit the precise temporal relationships between antibody titer and disease activity is imperfect. Some SSc-specific autoantibodies are antinuclear and directed against proteins involved in mitosis, such as topoisomerase I and the RNA polymerases. Others are directed against cell surface antigens or secreted proteins. The concordance rates for positive ANA in twin pairs in which one sibling has SSc are 85% (monozygotic) and 60% (dizygotic), indicating a major role for genetics in the SSc-specific immune response.

Although autoantibodies have well-established clinical utility as diagnostic and prognostic markers, their role in clinical manifestations of SSc remains uncertain. Topoisomerase I autoantibodies in SSc patients can directly bind to fibroblasts, and autoantibodies to fibroblasts, endothelial cells, fibrillin-1, and matrix metalloproteinase enzymes have all been described. Some of these autoantibodies may have direct pathogenic roles as mediators of tissue damage. Multiple potential mechanism(s) have been proposed to account for autoantibody generation in SSc. According to one theory, in SSc patients specific self-antigens undergo novel modifications, such as structural alterations due to proteolytic cleavage, increased expression level, or changes in subcellular localization, resulting in their recognition by the immune system. For example, cytotoxic T cells release the protease granzyme B, which cleaves autoantigens, generating novel fragments with potential neo-epitopes that break immune tolerance. Recent studies implicate B cells in both autoimmunity and fibrosis in SSc. In addition to their well-recognized role in antibody production, B cells can present antigen, produce cytokines, such as IL-6 and TGF-beta, and modulate T-cell and dendritic-cell function. B cells from SSc patients show intrinsic abnormalities, with elevated expression of the CD19 B-cell receptor, expansion in the naive B-cell

TABLE 17B-1. SOLUBLE MEDIATORS OF FIBROBLAST ACTIVATION ELEVATED IN SYSTEMIC SCLEROSIS.

MOLECULE	CELLULAR SOURCE
TGF-beta	Inflammatory cells, platelets, fibroblasts
PDGF	Platelets, macrophages, fibroblasts, endothelial cells
CTGF	Fibroblasts
Insulinlike growth factor 1	Fibroblasts
IL-4, IL-13	Th2 lymphocytes, mast cells
IL-6	Macrophages, B cells, T cells, fibroblasts
Chemokines (MCP-1, MCP-3)	Neutrophils, epithelial cells, endothelial cells, fibroblasts
Fibroblast growth factor	Fibroblasts
Endothelin 1	Endothelial cells

ABBREVIATIONS: CTGF, connective tissue growth factor; IL, interleukin; PDGF, platelet-derived growth factor; TGF-beta, transforming growth factor beta. MCP, monocyte chemotactic protein.

compartment, and reduced numbers of memory B cells and early plasma cells (9). Gene expression profiling of SSc skin biopsies has identified mRNA expression signatures characteristic of activated B cells.

FIBROSIS: CELLULAR AND MOLECULAR COMPONENTS

Fibrosis affecting multiple organs is a prominent hallmark, distinguishing SSc from other connective tissue diseases. Fibrosis is thought to be a consequence of autoimmunity and vascular damage. The process is characterized by progressive replacement of normal tissue architecture with dense acellular connective tissue, and accounts for substantial morbidity and mortality in SSc.

Fibroblasts and related mesenchymal cells are normally responsible for the functional and structural integrity of connective tissue in parenchymal organs. When activated by TGF-beta and related cytokines (Table 17B-2), fibroblasts proliferate, migrate, elaborate collagen and other matrix macromolecules, secrete growth factors and cytokines and express surface receptors for them, and differentiate into myofibroblasts. Together, these fibroblast responses facilitate effective repair of tissue injury. Under physiologic conditions, the fibroblast repair program is self-limited, terminating upon completion of healing. In pathological fibrotic responses however, fibroblast activation is sustained and amplified, resulting in exaggerated matrix remodeling and scar formation. Dysregulated fibroblast activation and matrix accumulation are the fundamental pathogenetic alterations underlying tissue fibrosis in SSc.

In addition to locally derived connective tissue fibroblasts, circulating mesenchymal progenitor cells of bone marrow origin also participate in fibrogenesis. Peripheral blood mononuclear cells expressing CD14 and CD34 have been shown to differentiate into collagen-producing alpha-smooth muscle actin-positive fibrocytes in vitro. This process is enhanced by TGF-beta (10). The factors that regulate the production of mesenchymal progenitor cells in the bone marrow and their trafficking from the circulation into lesional tissue, and promote their differentiation in situ into matrix-producing adhesive and contractile fibrocytes, remain unknown. Epithelial to mesenchymal cell transition (EMT), a process implicated in the development of fibrosis following injury in the lungs and kidney, may also be involved in organ fibrosis in SSc. Fibroblasts can differentiate into smooth muscle–like myofibroblasts. Both EMT and myofibroblast differentiation are mediated by TGF-beta. Although myofibroblasts can be transiently detected during normal wound healing, their persistence in tissue, possibly due to apoptosis resistance, indicates dysregulated repair during pathological fibrogenesis. Myofibroblasts contribute to scar formation via their ability to produce collagen and TGF-beta, and to generate contractile forces on the surrounding matrix, converting it into dense scar.

Fibroblasts explanted from lesional SSc tissues display an abnormal phenotype indicative of autonomous activation. Compared to normal fibroblasts, SSc fibroblasts in culture are characterized by variably increased rates of type I collagen gene transcription. Furthermore, they have smooth muscle actin stress fibers, enhanced synthesis of various extracellular matrix molecules, expression of chemokine receptors and cell surface adhesion molecules, secretion of PDGF, Akt-mediated resistance to apoptosis, and autocrine TGF-beta signaling. This abnormal scleroderma phenotype persists during serial passage in vitro. The mechanisms underlying the acquisition of the autonomously activated phenotype are unknown; persistent fibroblast activation via autocrine stimulatory loops involving TGF-beta, selection of activated fibroblast subpopulations driven by hypoxia or immune factors, intrinsic abnormalities in SSc fibroblasts, and altered cell–matrix interaction are some of the mechanisms under investigation. Recent reports indicate that intracellular blockade of TGF-beta signaling can abrogate the activated phenotype in SSc lesional fibroblasts, resulting in their partial normalization. Autocrine TGF-beta signaling, therefore, contributes to the persistence of the fibrogenic phenotype of SSc fibroblasts. Results from global transcriptome analyses of SSc fibroblasts show

TABLE 17B-2. PROFIBROGENIC ACTIVITIES OF TRANSFORMING GROWTH FACTOR BETA POTENTIALLY IMPORTANT IN SYSTEMIC SCLEROSIS.

Recruits monocytes

Stimulates fibroblast synthesis of collagens, extracellular matrix, inhibitors of proteolytic enzymes; suppresses matrix metalloproteinase enzymes

Stimulates fibroblast proliferation, chemotaxis

Induces fibrogenic cytokine production: CTGF; autoinduction; blocks synthesis and activity of interferon gamma

Induces fibroblast mitogenic responses to PDGF

Promotes fibroblast–myofibroblast differentiation

Promotes monocyte–fibrocyte differentiation

Promotes epithelial–mesenchymal transition

Inhibits fibroblast apoptosis

ABBREVIATIONS: CTGF, connective tissue growth factor; PDGF, platelet-derived growth factor.

differential expression of many ECM genes, including collagens, fibronectin, and fibrillins (11). A majority of the abnormally expressed genes could be mechanistically linked to TGF-beta responses, but other fibrogenic signaling pathways also operate in SSc.

Autocrine/paracrine TGF-beta and its intracellular signaling pathways play pivotal roles in the initiation and propagation of the fibrotic response in SSc. Intracellular TGF-beta signaling is a complex and cell type–specific process involving multiple primary and accessory receptors, stimulatory and inhibitory members of the Smad family of signal transducer proteins and other transcriptional factors, coactivators and repressors. Lesional fibroblasts secrete TGF-beta and exhibit TGF-beta hyper-responsiveness due to elevated expression of TGF-beta receptors and activation of latent TGF-beta. Inappropriate activation of the intracellular TGF-beta signal transduction pathways due to constitutive Smad3 phosphorylation and defective Smad-7–dependent negative feedback loops have been described in SSc. The nuclear coactivator protein p300 facilitates Smad-mediated collagen transcription and is an important locus of integration for multiple extracellular signals modulating fibroblast function. The cellular abundance of p300 appears to control the magnitude of its response to TGF-beta (12). Abnormalities in the expression, function, and interactions of Smads, p300, and other cellular proteins account for the persistence and progression of the scleroderma fibrogenic process by modulating target gene transcription.

REFERENCES

1. Maricq HR, Weinrich MC, Keil JE, et al. Prevalence of scleroderma spectrum disorders in the general population of South Carolina. Arthritis Rheum 1989;32:998–1006.
2. Mayes MD, Lacey JV Jr, Beebe-Dimmer J, et al. Prevalence, incidence, survival, and disease characteristics of systemic sclerosis in a large US population. Arthritis Rheum 2003;48:2246–2255.
3. Kuwana M, Kaburaki J, Arnett FC, Howard RF, Medsger TA Jr, Wright TM. Influence of ethnic background on clinical and serologic features in patients with systemic sclerosis and anti-DNA topoisomerase I antibody. Arthritis Rheum 1999;42:465–474.
4. Feghali-Bostwick C, Medsger TA Jr, Wright TM. Analysis of systemic sclerosis in twins reveals low concordance for disease and high concordance for the presence of antinuclear antibodies. Arthritis Rheum 2003;48:1956–1963.
5. Janowsky EC, Kupper LL, Hulka BS. Meta-analyses of the relation between silicone breast implants and the risk of connective-tissue diseases. N Engl J Med 2000;342:781–790.
6. Prescott RJ, Freemont AJ, Jones CJ, Hoyland J, Fielding P. Sequential dermal microvascular and perivascular changes in the development of scleroderma. J Pathol 1992;166:255–263.
7. Abraham DJ, Varga J. Scleroderma: from cell and molecular mechanisms to disease models. Trends Immunol 2005;26:587–595.
8. Kuwana M, Okazaki Y, Yasuoka H, Kawakami Y, Ikeda Y. Defective vasculogenesis in systemic sclerosis. Lancet 2004;364:603–610.
9. Sato S, Fujimoto M, Hasegawa M, Takehara K. Altered blood B lymphocyte homeostasis in systemic sclerosis: expanded naive B cells and diminished but activated memory B cells. Arthritis Rheum 2004;50:1918–1927.
10. Abe R, Donnelly SC, Peng T, Bucala R, Metz CN. Peripheral blood fibrocytes: differentiation pathway and migration to wound sites. J Immunol 2001;166:7556–7562.
11. Whitfield ML, Finlay DR, Murray JI, et al. Systemic and cell type-specific gene expression patterns in SSc skin. Proc Natl Acad Sci U S A. 2003;100:12319–12324.
12. Bhattacharyya S, Ghosh AK, Pannu J, et al. Fibroblast expression of the coactivator p300 governs the intensity of profibrotic response to transforming growth factor beta. Arthritis Rheum 2005;52:1248–1258.

Systemic Sclerosis
C. Treatment and Assessment

Maya H. Buch, MBchB, MRCP
James R. Seibold, MD

- Systemic sclerosis (SSc; scleroderma) targets several aspects of disease pathophysiology: vascular features that are currently highly treatable; inflammatory features that are currently partly amenable to therapy; fibrotic features for which therapies of modest efficacy (at best) exist; and atrophic, end organ damage for which only supportive therapy is available.
- The extent of skin involvement is neither a robust primary outcome measure for clinical trials nor a reliable guide to the therapy of individual patients.
- Regular pulmonary function testing is a cornerstone of assessment.
- Continuous intravenous epoprostenol, subcutaneous or intravenous treprostinil, and bosentan all have important roles in selected patients with pulmonary arterial hypertension.
- Early recognition of scleroderma renal crisis (SRC) and prompt treatment with angiotensin-converting enzyme (ACE) inhibitors has improved outcomes in SRC dramatically.
- Cyclophosphamide is a cornerstone of interstitial lung disease treatment in SSc, but the therapeutic gains from this agent are relatively small.
- Long-term proton-pump inhibition is highly effective in treating the gastroesophageal reflux. High doses, sometimes two to three times the normal therapeutic dose, are required to alleviate symptoms.

Systemic sclerosis (SSc, scleroderma) has one of the highest mortality rates among all connective tissue disorders. To date, no effective therapy that addresses the underlying disease process exists. Significant strides have been made in improving survival, however, largely through therapies directed at the treatment of specific organ complications. State-of-the-art management entails organ-based therapy with particular attention to lung and renal involvement, the major causes of morbidity and mortality. This strategy emphasizes the role of early detection of internal organ involvement, and the timely implementation of treatment. In simple terms, SSc includes vascular features that are eminently treatable; inflammatory features that are at least partly amenable to therapy, as well; fibrotic features for which therapies of modest efficacy (at best) exist; and atrophic, end organ damage for which only supportive therapy is available.

ASSESSMENT OF DISEASE

The extent of skin involvement is the basis for SSc subset classification and a major indicator of risk for certain internal organ complications. Unfortunately, skin involvement is neither a robust primary outcome measure for clinical trials nor a reliable guide to the therapy of individual patients. Monitoring for lung involvement with regular pulmonary function testing is a cornerstone of assessment, particularly in patients with early diffuse scleroderma. Reduction in forced vital capacity suggests the presence of interstitial lung disease, which is usually confirmed then by the demonstration of reticular or alveolar parenchymal disease on high resolution computed tomography (CT) of the chest.

Isolated or disproportionate reduction in diffusing capacity suggests pulmonary vascular pathology; namely, pulmonary arterial hypertension (PAH).

Doppler echocardiography can provide estimates of pulmonary artery pressures and is useful in serial follow-up, but right heart catheterization remains the gold standard for confirmation of that diagnosis (1).

Measures of renal function and blood pressure serve as prime indicators of scleroderma renal crisis in early diffuse disease. Creatinine phosphokinase and aldolase levels are sensitive indicators of myositis/myopathy. Specific serologies, including antitopoisomerase and anti-U1RNP antibodies, predict diffuse disease. In contrast, anticentromere antibodies predict limited SSc. Not all patients with scleroderma are positive for one of these autoantibodies (see Chapter 17A).

TREATMENT

When treating individual complications, a core set of principles applies, regardless of patients' subset and stage. Certain targeted treatment approaches may also address individual organ system components of disease. Disease subset and stage, however, are key in guiding initial treatment. Progression of skin changes in early, diffuse SSc signals the need for aggressive management to limit internal organ damage. The precise choice of therapy depends upon the specific organ system manifestations.

The natural tendency for skin involvement to improve by the second to third year complicates the assessment of treatment efficacies. Therapeutic strategies have evolved rapidly in recent years, but still permit relatively few evidence-based approaches (see Figure 17C-1). The next sections focus in turn on treatments of the vascular, inflammatory, and fibrotic components of scleroderma.

Vascular Therapy

Complications of scleroderma that result clearly from vascular dysfunction include PAH, scleroderma renal crisis (SRC), and Raynaud's phenomenon (RP). Treatment approaches to these disease manifestations are evolving rapidly (2).

Pulmonary Arterial Hypertension

The endothelial dysfunction of PAH leads to increased endothelin and reduced nitric oxide and prostacyclin. Continuous intravenous epoprostenol (Flolan) and subcutaneous or intravenous treprostinil (Remodulin), both US Food and Drug Administration (FDA)–approved therapies, are consensus first-line treatments for PAH patients with World Health Organization (WHO) class IV disease. The delivery systems (indwelling catheters), associated risks (line infection), and

FIGURE 17C-1

A summary of organ-directed treatment in limited and diffuse scleroderma. Treatments in bold: FDA-approved. Cyclophosphamide*: Confirmed efficacy over placebo in a randomized, double-blind study in patients with interstitial lung disease. MMF^x: No controlled studies. Abbreviations: ACEI, angiotensin-converting enzyme inhibitor; ARB, angiotensin receptor blocker; CTGF, connective tissue growth factor; GAVE, gastric antral venous ectasia; GERD, gastroesophageal reflux disease; MCP-1, macrophage chemoattractant protein 1; MMF, mycophenylate mofetil; MTX, methotrexate; NTG, nitroglycerin; OT/PT, occupational therapy/physical therapy; PAH, pulmonary arterial hypertension; PDE-5, type 5 phosphodiesterase; RP, Raynaud's phenomenon; SRC, scleroderma renal crisis; SSRI, specific serotonin receptor uptake inhibitor; Stem cell Tx, stem cell transplantation; TGF-β, transforming growth factor beta.

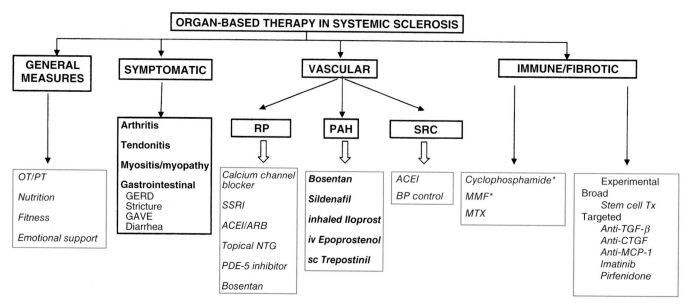

other side effects (infusion site pain) have forced a search for alternative therapies.

The selectivity of prostacyclin's effects on pulmonary vasculature provided the rationale behind the development of inhaled therapy for PAH, which have the added potential advantage of avoiding some systemic side effects. Repeated inhalation of iloprost (Ventavis) has been shown to improve function and hemodynamics, and to slow the rate of clinical decline. The role of endothelin 1 in idiopathic PAH and SSc-PAH pathophysiology has led to the development of endothelin receptor antagonists (ERA). Bosentan (Tracleer), an oral, nonselective ERA, is considered a first-line therapy in WHO class III patients. Regular monitoring is required for possible abnormal liver function.

Other ERA therapies are under investigation. Type V phosphodiesterase (PDE-5) metabolizes cyclic guanine monophosphate (cGMP). Inhibition of cGMP metabolism with the PDE-5 inhibitor sildenafil (Viagra) enhances pulmonary vasodilation. Side effects include axial muscle cramps. To date, long-term studies examining mortality as the primary outcome are not available for any agent. Combination therapies using agents from each of the different classes are under active investigation.

Scleroderma Renal Crisis

Development of accelerated to malignant hypertension with microangiopathic hemolytic anemia is the definition of SRC. Until the availability of angiotensin-converting enzyme (ACE) inhibitors, the treatment of SRC was extraordinarily difficult despite the use of other antihypertensive approaches, and the onset of SRC nearly always signaled a terminal phase of the illness.

Early recognition of SRC and the prompt institution of ACE inhibition (at the maximum tolerable dose) has improved outcomes in SRC dramatically. Deaths from SRC are now decidedly rare, and fewer than 50% of patients in SRC progress to end-stage renal disease (ESRD) (3). If patients do progress to ESRD, ACE inhibition should be continued into the phase of dialysis; some patients demonstrate renal recovery even after several months of dialysis.

For patients with diffuse scleroderma—the subset at highest risk for SRC—prophylactic treatment with an ACE inhibitor is advisable. Although not yet tested in a rigorous fashion, angiotensin receptor blockade (ARB) therapies are also probably efficacious in SRC.

Raynaud's Phenomenon

A growing number of treatments are now available for RP. A cornerstone of the therapy of this complication, however, is the maintenance of a warm core body temperature. In addition to gloves, handwarmers, and other approaches to warming the extremities, patients are strongly advised to several layers of clothing over their entire bodies, particularly during cold months.

Calcium-channel blockers, such as amlodipine, nifedipine, or felodipine, are the initial medical treatment for RP. Low dose selective serotonin reuptake inhibitors (SSRIs) are also used because of their allegedly salubrious effects on platelet aggregation and activation. Among the SSRIs, fluoxetine (Prozac; Symbyax; Sarafem) is the best studied. Despite their striking effectiveness in SRC, ACE inhibitors and ARBs are not particularly effective for RP.

Digital ischemia and ulceration are often managed with intermittent intravenous iloprost, particularly during the winter months. In addition, therapies introduced originally for the management of PAH now are being applied to the treatment of recalcitrant RP. Two large, multicenter, controlled trials of bosentan confirmed a reduction in the development of new digital ulcers compared to placebo (4). Case series and reports have suggested improved RP control with the use of sildenafil. Despite the improved options for the treatment of RP now, therapy is expensive, access often limited, and the responses (albeit dramatic in some patients) frequently inconsistent.

Anti-Inflammatory Treatments

In addition to the vascular nature of some scleroderma-related problems, other manifestations of this disease, for example, interstitial lung disease and myositis, have clear inflammatory components. At the present time, anti-inflammatory therapies for scleroderma are less targeted than are those for vascular problems. An approach involving the use of nonspecific, broadly immunosuppressive agents assumes that immunological activation influences both the fibrotic and vascular components.

Cyclophosphamide

Cyclophosphamide (CYC) has been used as the primary therapeutic agent for interstitial lung disease in scleroderma. In a recent controlled trial (5), cyclophosphamide improved forced vital capacity (FVC) by only 2.9% compared to placebo. Although the demonstration of a modest benefit of CYC supports its continued use, the small effect suggests the need for a more targeted approach.

Autologous Stem Cell Transplantation

Immunoablation with immune reconstitution using autologous peripheral stem cells has been considered for severe diffuse scleroderma. Pilot studies have suggested robust effects on skin and patient function and neutral effects on internal involvement (6). Ongoing studies comparing stem cell transplantation with CYC treatments will determine the appropriateness of this strategy.

TABLE 18A-1. IDIOPATHIC INFLAMMATORY MYOPATHIES.

CRITERIA	SUBSETS
1. Symmetric proximal muscle weakness	Polymyositis
2. Muscle biopsy evidence of myositis	Dermatomyositis
3. Increase in serum skeletal muscle enzymes	Myositis with an associated collagen vascular disease
4. Characteristic electromyographic pattern	Cancer-related myositis Juvenile dermatomyositis
5. Typical rash of dermatomyositis	Inclusion body myositis

esophageal dysmotility and dysphagia. If weight loss persists or is severe, an associated malignancy should be considered.

Skeletal Muscle

Typically, skeletal muscle involvement develops insidiously, is bilateral and symmetric in distribution, affects proximal muscles much more than distal muscles, and is painless. An exception is IBM, in which an asymmetric distribution, distal weakness, or atrophy can occur alone or in combination with proximal weakness. In polymyositis and dermatomyositis, the lower extremity (pelvic girdle) is often affected causing difficulty walking up steps or arising from a seated position. Walking on level ground may be fairly normal, but the patients are prone to falls. Upper extremity (shoulder girdle) symptoms, which may lag behind those of the lower extremity, include difficulty raising their arms overhead or combing their hair. Neck flexor weakness may also occur. When myalgias are present, they are more common with exercise. Proximal dysphagia, with nasal regurgitation of liquids and pulmonary aspiration, is a poor prognostic sign and indicates pharyngeal striated muscle involvement. Pharyngeal weakness also results in hoarseness or dysphonia and a nasal quality voice. Ocular or facial muscle weakness is very uncommon in IIM, and their presence should prompt consideration of another diagnosis.

Physical examination using manual muscle testing confirms weakness of individual muscles or muscle groups. In JDM, the Childhood Myositis Assessment Scale has been shown to be reliable and valid for assessing physical function, muscle strength, and endurance. Muscle atrophy and joint contractures are sequelae of disease damage and are late findings in chronic muscle inflammation.

Skin

The skin rash of dermatomyositis may precede, develop simultaneously with, or follow symptoms of myopathy (4). Gottron's papules and the heliotrope rash on eyelids are considered pathognomonic features. Gottron's papules are scaly, erythematous, or violaceous papules and plaques located over bony prominences, particularly over the small joints of the hands, elbows, knees, and ankles. Gottron's sign is a macular erythema that occurs in the same distribution. Photosensitivity with rash on the face or anterior chest, termed the *V sign*, may also be seen. Pruritus is common, particularly in the scalp. Other cutaneous changes include a rash located over the upper back and across both shoulders (the shawl sign), rash on the lateral surface of the thighs and hips (holster sign), erythroderma, cuticular hypertrophy, and periungual erythema. Capillary changes are often present proximal to the cuticles in patients with Raynaud's phenomenon. Cracking, fissuring, or both, of the lateral and palmar digital skin pads is termed *mechanic's hands*. Later in the disease course, skin lesions may become shiny, atrophic, and hypopigmented with telangiectasias. Characteristic changes seen in JDM that are rare in adults include cutaneous necrosis, lipodystrophy, and subcutaneous calcifications.

Joints

Arthralgias or arthritis, if they occur, usually develop early in the disease course. They tend to be rheumatoid-like in distribution and are generally mild. Joint findings are more common with overlap syndromes and in childhood dermatomyositis.

Lung

The lung is the most common extramuscular target in IIM (5,6). Dyspnea may result from interstitial lung disease as well as nonparenchymal problems, such as ventilatory (diaphragmatic and intercostal) muscle weakness or cardiac dysfunction. Pulmonary function testing reveals restrictive physiology, with reduced lung volumes, for example, total lung capacity and forced vital capacity and a parallel decrease in the diffusion capacity for carbon monoxide.

The presence of a "ground glass" appearance on high resolution computed tomography (CT) indicates alveolitis, a potentially treatment-responsive inflammatory condition with a more favorable prognosis. In contrast, the presence of "honeycombing" usually indicates fibrosis (7). The progression of interstitial lung disease is unpredictable but the more favorable histologies include nonspecific interstitial pneumonitis (NSIP) and the organizing pneumonias. In contrast, the finding of usual interstitial pneumonitis (UIP) or diffuse alveolar damage (DAD) portends a more ominous course.

Patients with progressive interstitial lung disease can develop secondary pulmonary arterial hypertension. Diffuse alveolar hemorrhage with pulmonary capillaritis and pneumomediastinum are rare associations.

Heart

Cardiac involvement is common in IIM but is seldom symptomatic (8). The most common finding is a rhythm disturbance. More ominous complications, such as congestive heart failure and pericardial tamponade, are quite rare.

Gastrointestinal Tract

Swallowing problems (upper dysphagia) manifest as difficulty in the initiation of deglutition or nasal regurgitation of liquids. If severe, aspiration of oral contents leads to chemical pneumonitis. Cricopharyngeal muscle dysfunction is more common in inclusion body myositis, but also occurs in other IIM. This can also cause dysphagia, with the complaint of a "blocking" sensation with swallowing. Patients note a retrosternal "sticking" sensation on swallowing bread or meat and heartburn (reflux) with esophageal body and gastroesophageal sphincter involvement, respectively. Gastrointestinal mucosal ulceration and hemorrhage are rare.

Malignancy and Myositis

There has been considerable controversy regarding the validity and magnitude of the relationship between malignancy and inflammatory myopathy (9). Recent reports strongly support an increased risk of cancer in patients with polymyositis and an even greater risk with dermatomyositis. Amyopathic dermatomyositis patients also have an increased risk of malignancy (10). Patients with pulmonary fibrosis, circulating myositis-specific autoantibodies, or an associated connective tissue disease have a decreased likelihood of cancer. The overall risk of cancer is greatest in the first 3 years after the diagnosis of myositis, but an increased risk of malignancy persists through all years of follow-up, emphasizing the importance of continued surveillance.

In general, the sites of origin of malignancy are typical for the age of the patient (11). The strongest associations are with ovarian, lung, pancreatic, stomach, and colorectal cancer and with non-Hodgkin's lymphoma. However, many other types of cancer occur with myositis, including genitourinary malignancies and melanoma. Ovarian cancer is over-represented in some series. Asian and Chinese patients with dermatomyositis have a clear increase in nasopharyngeal carcinoma.

INVESTIGATIONS

Serum Muscle Enzymes

Enzymes that leak into the serum from injured skeletal muscle include the CK, aldolase, AST, ALT, and LDH (12,13). Which enzymes are elevated and which one is the best to follow varies from patient to patient. Some feel that the CK is the most reliable enzyme to use in routine patient care and best reflects disease activity. The CK is elevated at least at some time during the course of illness in patients with an IIM. Lower values are often seen late in the disease course, in IBM, and in cancer-related myositis. The myocardial fraction of CK (CK-MB) may be increased in myositis without any cardiac involvement because this isoform is also released from regenerating myoblasts.

In contrast, elevated CK levels do not necessarily evidence active inflammation. Previously damaged muscle membranes may remain permeable to CK after the disease has been controlled, resulting in elevated serum levels. In addition, many non–disease-related factors, such as race, may cause an elevated CK (see Chapter 18C for more information on CPK).

Electromyography

Electromyography is a sensitive but nonspecific method of evaluating muscle for evidence of inflammation. Of the 90% of patients with active myositis who have an abnormal EMG, about half show the classic findings of inflammation of fibrillation potentials, complex repetitive discharges, positive sharp waves, and complex motor unit potentials of low amplitude and short duration. In addition to aiding in the diagnosis, EMG is helpful in the selection of a site for muscle biopsy. When this is the case, the study should be performed unilaterally and a contralateral muscle chosen for biopsy to avoid confusion with inflammation artifact that can result from injury caused by the needle.

Later in the course, EMG examination may be helpful for the detection of low grade myositis in the setting of chronic damage from fibrosis or fatty infiltration. It may also be useful in differentiating active inflammation from steroid myopathy.

Muscle Biopsy

Muscle histology remains the gold standard for confirming the diagnosis of an IIM (14). Despite the characteristic features described below, some patients with active myositis have a normal biopsy. Because the disease is patchy in distribution, sampling error precludes 100% sensitivity. Furthermore, the changes in some biopsies may be too nonspecific.

The most characteristic changes in polymyositis include degeneration and regeneration of muscle fibers

18

and CD8+ T lymphocytes invading non-necrotic fibers. In dermatomyositis, CD4+ T cells and B cells predominate in the perivascular areas and perifascicular atrophy, related to capillary depletion and dropout, is noted. The histology of IBM is characterized by the presence of lined or rimmed vacuoles. Otherwise IBM may appear identical to that of polymyositis, be essentially normal, or show triangulated cells with fiber-type grouping, changes considered to be indicative of a neuropathic process. In chronic myositis, macrophages are seen phagocytosing necrotic fibers and muscle is replaced by fibrous connective tissue or fat (see Chapter 18B for a more detailed discussion of the muscle pathology).

Magnetic Resonance Imaging

Magnetic resonance imaging techniques add an important dimension to our approach to patients with myopathy (15). MRI is noninvasive and can be used to visualize large areas of muscle. T1-weighted images provide excellent anatomic detail, with clear delineation of various muscle groups and are useful in assessing changes resulting from damage and chronicity. T2-weighted images with fat suppression or STIR (short tau inversion recovery) sequences can identify edema, which is indicative of active inflammation. Accordingly, MRI can be used to document myositis or a disease flare, distinguish chronic active from chronic inactive myositis, and noninvasively direct the site of biopsy.

Skin

The characteristic cutaneous histopathologic findings of dermatomyositis include vacuolar alteration of the epidermal basal layer, necrotic keratinocytes, vascular dilatation, and a perivascular lymphocytic infiltrate (4). The pattern is similar to that seen with systemic lupus erythematosus and closely resembles those of chronic graft-versus-host reaction. Vasculitis or vasculopathy may be found in small cutaneous vessels. Capillary changes proximal to the cuticles are often seen in patients with Raynaud's phenomenon (see Chapter 18B for a more detailed discussion of the skin pathology in IIM).

Lung

Chest radiographs may show fibrotic changes in patients with interstitial lung disease, but they are insensitive compared with high resolution CT (HRCT) (16,17). HRCT findings include ground-glass opacities typical of alveolitis and/or consolidation, subpleural lines or bands, traction bronchiectasis, and honeycombing indicating fibrosis. The most common HRCT pattern is a combination of reticular and/or ground glass opacities with or without consolidation and without honeycombing. When honeycombing is present on the initial HRCT, the prognosis is generally poor.

Pulmonary function testing is useful in assessing a variety of potential problems. Reduced ventilatory muscle strength is determined by measuring inspiratory pressures at the mouth. Impaired function results in a weak cough and an increased risk of aspiration. A forced vital capacity of less than 55% of normal predicts carbon dioxide retention that can result when ventilatory muscle function is compromised and interstitial disease is absent. Interstitial lung disease also causes restrictive physiology on pulmonary function testing but is typically accompanied by pulmonary fibrosis. More sensitive indicators of compromised gas exchange include a reduction in the diffusing capacity for carbon monoxide and a decrease in the alveolar–arterial oxygen gradient with exercise.

Heart

Clinically significant cardiac findings are uncommon in IIM. However, electrical disturbances are not uncommon. These include nonspecific ST-T segment changes and conduction system abnormalities. Using sensitive cardiac scintigraphic techniques, increased technitium-99m pyrophosphate uptake and indium-labeled anti-myosin binding have been reported.

Intestine

When pharyngeal muscles are involved, a barium swallow may show cricopharyngeal muscle spasm, poorly coordinated motion of the pharyngeal musculature, vallecular pooling of the dye, and, occasionally, aspiration of barium into the trachea (18). Cinesophagrams and manometry are best for evaluation of distal dysphagia resulting from distal esophageal hypomotility.

Serum Autoantibodies

Antinuclear or anticytoplasmic antibodies are present in the majority of patients with IIM, with the exception of IBM, where the frequency is low. Patients with myositis and an associated collagen vascular disease will manifest the antibodies characteristic of that disease [i.e., anti–double-stranded DNA (dsDNA) antibodies and SLE, anti–Scl 70 and scleroderma, etc]. In addition, some antibodies are termed *myositis-specific autoantibodies* (MSAs) because they are found exclusively in patients with features of an inflammatory myopathy (3). Although a few patients have more than one serum autoantibody, several MSAs are rarely detected in the same patient. A negative antinuclear antibody (ANA) test does exclude an MSA, as the latter antigens are cytoplasmic in location and the immunofluorescence staining pattern may be subtle. Testing for serum autoantibodies can both solidify the diagnosis of myositis in patients with atypical clinical features and provide prognostic information regarding the likelihood of future clinical complications.

Although the MSAs are relatively insensitive markers for myositis, the presence of one suggests that the patient will have certain associated features (see Table 18C-1). Anti–Jo 1 antibodies are directed against histidyl-tRNA synthetase. Anti–Jo 1 is the most common MSA and is one of a group of anti–aminoacyl-tRNA synthetases. The clinical associations of the antisynthetase antibodies have been termed the *antisynthetase syndrome*. The muscle involvement in this syndrome is often severe with multiple exacerbations, requiring immunosuppressive agents in addition to corticosteroids. Antibodies against signal recognition particle (anti-SRP) identify patients with polymyositis who may have cardiomyopathy and who often have severe, refractory disease. Anti–Mi 2 is an antinuclear antibody that is almost always associated with dermatomyositis and a good response to immunosuppression.

NATURAL HISTORY AND PROGNOSIS

The clinical course is quite variable among patients with IIM (19). In some, the illness is brief and is followed by remission that does not require continued treatment. That is more common in dermatomyositis than in polymyositis and most common in patients with an associated collagen vascular disease. Other patients with theses diseases experience exacerbations and remissions or persistent disease activity, necessitating chronic use of immunosuppressive drugs, with the frequency of clinical and biochemical relapse varying from 34% to 60% in different series. Patients with IBM do not respond to any known medications. This disease is characterized by a slow and gradual decline in muscle strength, although the level of weakness can plateau for some.

As long as the myositis is active, there is the potential for absolute loss of muscle mass and strength (20). In general, the best functional outcomes occur in dermatomyositis, whereas the worst are seen in IBM, myositis with anti-SRP antibody, cancer-related myositis, and patients with interstitial lung disease. In JDM, predictors of chronic active myositis include delay in diagnosis, failure to regain normal muscle strength after 4 months of corticosteroid treatment, continued increased serum muscle enzyme beyond 3 months, increased plasma von Willebrand factor antigen after 10 months of treatment, and anasarca with hypoalbuminemia.

Factors associated with poor survival include older age, malignancy, delayed initiation of corticosteroid treatment, pharyngeal dysphagia with aspiration pneumonia, ILD, myocardial involvement, and complications of corticosteroid or immunosuppressive treatment. Additional adverse risk factors for survival among patients with JDM are gastrointestinal vasculitis and sepsis.

REFERENCES

1. Bohan A, Peter JB. Polymyositis and dermatomyositis. N Engl J Med 1975;292:344–347, 403–407.
2. Lindsley CB. Juvenile dermatomyositis update. Curr Opin Rheumatol 2006;8:174–177.
3. Targoff IN. Myositis specific autoantibodies. Curr Opin Rheumatol 2006;8:196–206.
4. Santmyire-Rosenberger B, Dugan EM. Skin involvement in dermatomyositis. Curr Opin Rheumatol 2003;15:714–722.
5. Kang EH, et al. Interstitial lung disease in patients with polymyositis, dermatomyositis and amyopathic dermatomyositis. Rheumatology 2005;44:1282–1286.
6. Schnabel A, Hellmich B, Gross WL. Interstitial lung disease in polymyositis and dermatomyositis. Curr Rheum Rep 2005;7:99–105.
7. Bonnefoy O, et al. Serial chest CT findings in interstitial lung disease associated with polymyositis-dermatomyositis. Eur J Radiol 2004;49:235–244.
8. Yazici Y, Kagen LJ. Cardiac involvement in myositis. Curr Opin Rheumatol 2002;14:663–665.
9. Buchbinder R, Hill CL. Malignancy in patients with inflammatory myopathy. Curr Rheum Rep 2002;4:415–426.
10. Whitmore SE, et al. Dermatomyositis sine myositis: association with malignancy. J Rheumatol 1996;23:101–105.
11. Chen Y-J, Wu C-Y, Shen J-L. Predicting factors of malignancy in dermatomyositis and polymyositis: a case-control study. Br J Dermatol 2001;144:825–831.
12. Sultan SM. Clinical assessment in adult onset idiopathic inflammatory myopathy. Curr Opin Rheumatol 2004;16:668–672.
13. Targoff I. Laboratory testing in the diagnosis and management of idiopathic inflammatory myopathies. Rheum Dis Clin North Am 2002;28:859–890.
14. Grundtman C, Lundberg IE. Pathogenesis of idiopathic inflammatory myopathies. Curr Opin Rheumatol 2006;8:188–195.
15. Scott DL, Kingsley GH. Use of imaging to assess patients with muscle disease. Curr Opin Rheumatol 2004;16:678–683.
16. Arakawa H, et al. Nonspecific interstitial pneumonia associated with polymyositis and dermatomyositis: serial high-resolution CT findings and functional correlation. Chest 2003;123:1096–1103.
17. Tansey D, et al. Variations in histological patterns of interstitial pneumonia between connective tissue disorders and their relationship to prognosis. Histopathology 2004;44:585–596.
18. Marton K, et al. Evaluation of oral manifestations and masticatory force in patients with polymyositis and dermatomyositis. J Oral Pathol Med 2005;34:164–169.
19. Ponyi A, et al. Disease course, frequency of relapses and survival of 73 patients with juvenile or adult dermatomyositis. Clin Exp Rheum 2005;23:50–56.
20. Ponyi A, et al. Functional outcome and quality of life in adult patients with idiopathic inflammatory myositis. Rheumatology 2005;44:83–88.

18

Idiopathic Inflammatory Myopathies
B. Pathology and Pathogenesis

LISA G. RIDER, MD
FREDERICK W. MILLER, MD, PhD

- Major pathology consists of focal inhomogeneous inflammation with injury, death, and repair of muscle cells.
- Each subgroup of myositis has characteristic changes on microscopy and immunochemistry.

- Etiology is still unclear but selected environmental exposures in genetically predisposed hosts have been found.

PATHOLOGY AND IMMUNOPATHOLOGY

The characteristic skeletal muscle pathology in the idiopathic inflammatory myopathies (IIM) consists of chronic inflammation with infiltration by mononuclear cells, including lymphocytes, plasma cells, macrophages and dendritic cells, in the endomysium (between myocytes), perimysium (within fascicles), or perivascular (vessels in interstitium surrounding muscle fibers) areas (Figure 18B-1). The muscle fibers (myocytes), which may be necrotic or non-necrotic, show evidence of degeneration and regeneration, fiber hypertrophy or atrophy, and replacement by fibrosis or fat, and are often accompanied by increased connective tissue or fibrosis in the interstitial areas around the muscle cells (1).

These features collectively are characteristic of myositis, but each feature may be seen as part of the pathology of other muscle disorders, particularly muscular dystrophies. Macrophages may infiltrate to scavenge necrotic muscle as a secondary inflammatory process in dystrophies and other myopathies. Some features of other neuromuscular disorders, such as small angulated fibers, may also be present in myositis. A muscle biopsy is not always diagnostic of myositis. First, the inflammation is often focal and inhomogeneous. Inflammation is also diminished after the initiation of immunosuppressive therapy. A muscle biopsy should also not be

performed at the site of an electromyogram (EMG), due to artifactual changes from the EMG. In inclusion body myositis (IBM), the inclusions are not always apparent, either because of their patchy nature or because they may appear later in the course of illness. Paraffin processing also dissolves the vacuoles, so that a Gomori trichrome stain is needed for detection.

A muscle biopsy should be performed, processed, and evaluated by persons experienced in these procedures because careful attention to selection of the biopsy site, to collection of the tissue, and to rapid freezing and appropriate histochemistry is needed to obtain the most informative biopsies. Standard procedure should include hematoxylin and eosin and Gomori trichrome stains to highlight the cellular infiltrates as well as muscle architecture. Alkaline phosphatase positive connective tissue, even in the absence of cellular infiltrates, can also aid in the diagnosis of myositis. A portion of the frozen tissue block should be saved for enzymatic and metabolic stains, as well as immunohistochemistry or detection of muscle sarcolemmal proteins if needed for diagnosis (1).

Each subgroup of myositis has somewhat characteristic changes on routine microscopy and immunohistochemistry. In dermatomyositis (DM), the mononuclear cells are focused more along the vessel walls of perimysial arterioles and venules, with such changes more prominent in the juvenile form of DM (2,3). Vessel thrombosis may also occur. Infarcts from the perifascicular region to the center of the fascicle are

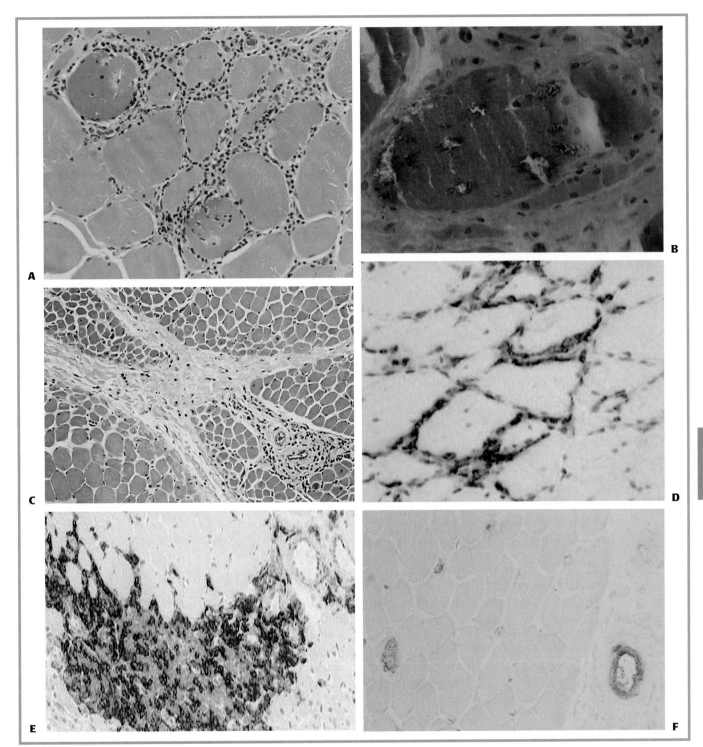

FIGURE 18B-1

Muscle pathology and immunopathology by light microscopy. Cross-sectional views of muscle biopsies showing characteristic changes in IIM. (A) Endomysial mononuclear cell infiltrates surrounding and invading myocytes in a patient with polymyositis (hematoxylin and eosin stain). (B) Similar findings are present in inclusion body myositis, with the exception of typical multiple reddish-rimmed vacuoles in myocytes on trichrome staining that define the inclusion bodies (trichrome stain). (C) Dermatomyositis and juvenile dermatomyositis show more prominent vascular changes, including perivascular mononuclear cell infiltration and vessel thrombosis, as well as perifascicular atrophy. (From Rider LG, Targoff IN. In: Lahita RG, Chiorazzi N, Reaves WH, eds. Textbook of autoimmune diseases. Philadelphia: Lippincott Raven; 2000.) (D) Immunohisto-chemistry demonstrating staining for CD8+ cells that are surrounding myocytes in polymyositis. (From Figarella-Branger D et al., Muscle Nerve 2003;28:659.) (E) Positive immunostaining for B cells in dermatomyositis. (From Figarella-Branger D et al., Muscle Nerve 2003;28:659.) (F) Staining for the C5–C9 membrane attack complex on capillaries and myocytes in dermatomyositis. (Courtesy of Dr. J.T. Kissel.)

18

particularly present in juvenile DM and less frequently in adult DM (3). Perifascicular atrophy with small fibers at the external rim of a fascicle is also characteristic of DM. In contrast, in polymyositis (PM) and IBM, the inflammatory cells invade non-necrotic muscle fibers in a primarily endomysial distribution (4,5).

Immunohistochemistry also implicates different pathogeneses in the various forms of myositis. In DM, more frequent in the juvenile than adult form, the earliest changes include activation of the complement cascade through C3, deposition of the complement C5b-9 membrane attack complex on the endomysial vasculature, with resultant capillary destruction, muscle ischemia, and dilatation of the remaining capillaries (high endothelial venule formation) (6–8). This leads to resulting inflammation, with the infiltrating cells consisting mainly of B lymphocytes and CD4+ helper T cells in perimysial areas around the muscle fascicles and small blood vessels. MHC class I antigen and intracellular adhesion molecule (ICAM) are upregulated on the cell surfaces of damaged fibers or in perivascular areas, respectively (9). In PM and IBM, the weight of evidence suggests a predominant cytotoxic T lymphocyte–mediated process with CD8+ T cells, accompanied by smaller numbers of macrophages, surrounding and invading otherwise normal-appearing myocytes in endomysial areas (10). MHC class I antigen is upregulated on the surface of the majority of muscle fibers, even those not affected by inflammation, although this is not specific to myositis (1). Necrotic muscle fibers may be scattered in the biopsy, particularly in PM.

In IBM, in addition to these inflammatory findings, there are vacuolated myofibers occurring in the center or periphery of muscle fibers, with wide variation in myofiber size, including scattered atrophic fibers, and prominence of central muscle nuclei. The vacuoles are rimmed by granular eosinophilic material, which on Gomori trichrome stains purple-red and on Congo red staining reveals amyloidlike deposits, including phosphorylated tau, ubiquitin, beta-amyloid, and presinilin 1 (9). Diffuse inflammatory infiltrates and ragged red fibers are sometimes seen. In IBM-characteristic tubulofilaments, 15 to 18 nm in diameter and seen most often in the cytoplasm and less often in the nuclei, are often visible by electron microscopy (1).

In terms of the pathologic features of other organs, the skin in DM demonstrates interface dermatitis, often with basement membrane thickening and mucin deposition. Many of the changes in muscle, including the types of infiltrating cells and the predominance of perivascular inflammation, are also evident in the skin. In the gastrointestinal tract, ischemic ulceration is a potentially life-threatening manifestation and may include a non-inflammatory acute endarteropathy with arterial and venous intimal hyperplasia and occlusion of intestinal vessels by fibrin thrombi in the submucosa, muscularis,

and serosal layers (3). A chronic endarteropathy characterized by narrowing or complete occlusion of multiple small and medium-sized arteries, subintimal foam cells, fibromyxoid neointimal expansion, and significant luminal compromise and infiltration of macrophages through the muscle layers into the intima may also be seen. The pathology of the interstitial lung disease most commonly is that of nonspecific interstitial pneumonitis (NSIP), but occasionally diffuse alveolar damage, usual interstitial pneumonitis (UIP), and bronchiolitis obliterans organizing pneumonia (BOOP) may be present. The myocardium may demonstrate myocarditis with subsequent fibrosis.

PATHOGENESIS

While the etiology and pathogenesis of the IIM remain unclear, a number of lines of investigation have suggested possible ways in which selected environmental exposures in genetically susceptible individuals may lead to chronic immune activation and the ultimate immunologic attack on muscle and other involved tissues (Figure 18B-2). A number of these mechanisms, which include upregulation of MHC class I on muscle fibers, immune activation, and activation of the endoplasmic reticulum stress response, are processes common to other myopathies besides myositis. While some of the mechanisms are found in all forms of myositis, others are likely unique to selected groups.

Genetic Factors

The finding of families in which two or more blood relatives have myositis and associations of myositis with particular genes support the hypothesis that myositis is at least in part inherited. Polymorphic alleles in the major histocompatibility locus (MHC) are the major immunogenetic risk and protective factors identified for the IIM. The A1-B8-Cw07-DRB1*0301-DQA1*0501 ancestral haplotype is the major immunogenetic risk factor for PM, as well as adult and juvenile DM in Caucasians, with the risk factor likely in the class II HLA region at or near human leucocyte antigen (HLA) DRB1*0301. For IBM, DRB1*0301 and its linked allele DQA1*0501 are risk factors along with the class I Cw*14 allele. HLA DQA1*0201 is protective for all forms of myositis, and other DRB1 or DQA1 alleles are protective for specific clinical groups (11). In the class III MHC region, the tumor necrosis factor alpha (TNF-alpha)-308A allele is a risk factor for adult and juvenile DM and PM in Caucasians, and may also be a severity factor, perhaps related to photosensitive rashes and the development of calcinosis. DMA*0103 and DMB*0102 are possible risk factors for juvenile DM. Outside the HLA region, the IL1 receptor antagonist VNTR A1

Environmental Risk Factor(s) Interact With Genetic Risk Factor(s)

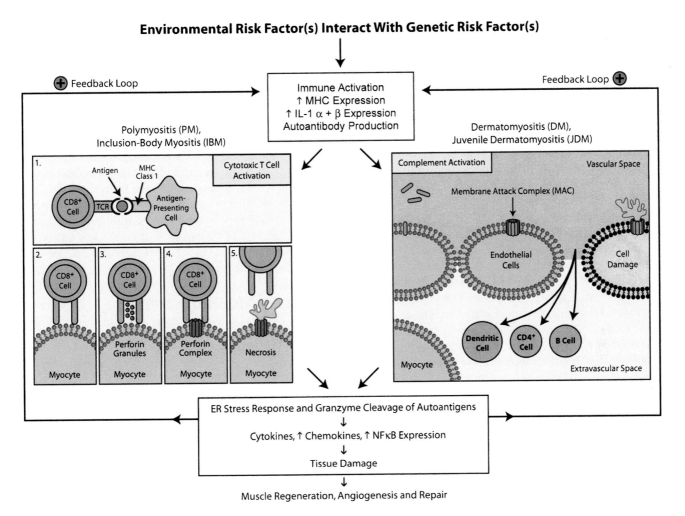

FIGURE 18B-2

Possible pathogenic mechanisms in IIM. All forms of myositis appear likely to involve immune activation following specific exposure to environmental risk factors in genetically susceptible individuals. Common immune activation processes in muscle and other tissues include upregulation of MHC expression and IL-1 alpha and beta, leading to autoantibody production prior to clinical disease onset. Following this, myocyte-directed cytotoxic T-cell mechanisms predominate in PM and IBM, while complement-mediated endothelial damage, leading to CD4, B-cell, and dendritic-cell infiltrations, predominate in DM and JDM. Other general mechanisms may involve hypoxia, activation of the endoplasmic reticulum stress response, and cleavage of autoantigens, resulting in cytokine and chemokine release and positive feedback loops that lead to further immune activation. Later processes include muscle regeneration, angiogenesis, and repair, and in some cases fibrotic changes and other damage in affected tissues.

allele is a risk factor for juvenile DM in Caucasians. The Gm allotypes, serologic markers on the heavy chains of IgG, rather than HLA alleles, are genetic risk or protective factors for myositis in Koreans and Mesoamericans, suggesting that genetics likely varies among ethnic groups (12).

Human leukocyte antigen risk factors are more strongly associated with specific autoantibodies (13). The ancestral haplotype A1-B8-Cw07-DRB1*0301-DQA1*0501 is a strong risk factor for patients with antisynthetase autoantibodies, including Jo1, in Caucasian patients. MHC class II alleles DRB1*0701 and DQA1*0201 are risk factors for Mi 2 autoantibodies. DQA1*0301 is a risk factor for p155, a myositis-associated autoantibody common in adult and juvenile DM.

Environmental Factors

The temporal association of exposure to a number of infectious and noninfectious agents prior to the onset of the IIM in certain individuals, as well as reports documenting temporal, seasonal, or geographic clustering of

IIM cases suggest a role for environmental factors in initiation of disease (12).

Epidemiologic investigations have also suggested a number of environmental factors which may be important in the development of IIM. Most are not proven environmental risk factors, but for some exposures, case-controlled epidemiologic studies, cases of de-challenge and re-challenge, and biomarker assays strengthen the association with illness onset. Of the infectious agents, Group A streptococcus and influenza have the strongest evidence of association with onset of juvenile IIM and toxoplasmosis with adult DM from case-controlled epidemiologic studies. With Group A streptococcus, peripheral blood T lymphocytes from juvenile DM patients react with streptococcal M5 protein and a myosin peptide with homology to M5. The evidence is mixed for coxsackie B virus, with reports of isolation of the virus from some affected muscles but a case-controlled study not supporting an association with onset of juvenile DM. Echoviruses, however, have been clearly associated with a DM-like illness in patients with agammaglobulinemia. Other infections temporally associated with onset of IIM which are not yet defined as definite risk factors for IIM include retroviruses, hepatitis viruses, *Borrelia burgdorferi*, and *Trypanosoma cruzi*. Parvovirus B19 is not associated with onset of juvenile DM in a case-controlled study. A search for viral genomes by sensitive molecular methodology in DM and PM biopsies has failed to identify consistently any viral nucleic acid, suggesting that known viruses are not contributing to the persistent inflammation (12).

Noninfectious agents, including ultraviolet light, physical exertion, psychological stress, medications, and vaccines have been suggested as possible triggers for some forms of IIM. Growing evidence suggests a role for ultraviolet radiation (UV) in the onset of DM. DM patients have a number of photosensitive rashes and, anecdotally, illness may exacerbate following sun exposure. Adult DM patients also have increased sensitivity to UVB as demonstrated by an abnormally low minimal erythema UVB dose. An increase in the proportion of DM relative to PM and an increase in the proportion of patients with the DM-associated Mi 2 autoantibody in areas of the world with higher surface UV radiation suggest that UV light exposure may modulate the clinical and immunologic expression of myositis. Keratinocytes damaged by UV radiation also undergo apoptosis, with increased autoantigen expression on the surface of such cells.

Case-controlled studies support a role for psychological stress, muscular exertion, and collagen implants in the onset of adult DM or PM (14). Exposure to D-penicillamine may induce myositis in 1% to 2% of patients and this has been associated with HLA B18, B35, and DR4 in Caucasians but with DQw1 in patients from India, which are genes distinct from those associ-

ated with IIM. Similarly, although there is no epidemiologic evidence from population studies confirming an association between silicone exposure and myositis, Caucasian women who develop myositis following silicone implants do not have the characteristic genetic features seen in IIM, but rather have an increased frequency of HLA DQA1*0102. Temporal associations of onset of the IIM with certain other drugs (including lipid-lowering agents, zidovudine, leuprolide, and local anesthetics), biologic therapies (such as interferon alpha and interleukin 2), and vaccines have been reported, but additional evidence is needed to confirm their potential associations (12). Certain alum-containing vaccines have also been associated with the distinct entity of macrophagic myositis, in which macrophages are the predominant infiltrating cell.

Cytotoxic Mechanisms in Polymyositis and Inclusion Body Myositis

Many lines of evidence suggest that cytotoxic mechanisms play a more important role in PM and IBM than adult or juvenile DM (15). First, as is the case for the quantitation of subsets of lymphocytes in the affected muscle, studies of peripheral mononuclear cells demonstrate that PM and IBM are virtually indistinguishable in showing higher numbers of circulating activated T cells. Second, peripheral blood cells from PM patients have an increased proliferative response to, and demonstrate cytotoxicity to, autologous muscle tissue in vitro. Third, T cells in PM and IBM contain perforin and granzyme granules that are directed towards the surface of the myofibers and that, on release, induce pores in the myocyte membranes (10). Fourth, based on restricted T-cell receptor usage, there is clonal expansion of muscle-infiltrating T cells selected for certain gene families in PM and IBM, implying an antigen-driven process, in contrast to a more polyclonal pattern of T-cell receptor usage in DM. Additionally, the CD8+ cells found in PM and IBM appear to preferentially target MHC class I–expressing myocytes, which would be required for their antigen-specific recognition of cellular targets. These findings, taken together, suggest that in PM and IBM, subpopulations of T cells are selected and expanded in response to as yet uncharacterized antigens and may explain some of the T-cell–mediated pathology seen in these diseases.

Humoral and Endothelial Mechanisms in Adult and Juvenile Dermatomyositis

Humoral and endothelial mechanisms appear to be more important for adult and juvenile DM compared to

PM and IBM (15). First, higher numbers of circulating B and CD4+ T lymphocytes are present in the periphery as well as in the affected muscle. Second, immunoglobulin and the terminal portion of complement are deposited on blood vessels in the earliest phases of illness (6), resulting in a decrease in the number of capillaries and muscle injury, including ischemia. From microarray experiments, in some cases confirmed by immunohistochemistry or real-time polymerase chain reaction (PCR), a number of promoters and inhibitors of angiogenesis are overexpressed in the affected muscle tissue (16,17). There is also increased expression of genes promoting endothelial differentiation and activation, as well as classical and alternative complement pathway regulators that facilitate angiogenesis in the muscle tissue of adult DM patients (16). In juvenile DM, a number of angiostatic ELR-chemokines are increased in expression and correlate with the degree of capillary loss (17). Upregulation of leucocyte adhesion molecules, particularly ICAM-1 on the muscle arterioles and venules in juvenile DM and somewhat in adult DM, results in the infiltration of B and CD4+ T lymphocytes, dendritic cells, and macrophages (9). Proinflammatory cytokines result in damage and further infiltration of cells.

Immune dysregulation is also a key part of the pathogenesis, with upregulation of interferon alpha/beta inducible genes and genes upregulated in a type I interferon response, as well as genes involved in antigen presentation, suggesting either viral initiation of disease or activation of plasmacytoid dendritic cells (18,19). Some of these factors are also angiostatic.

Cytokines, Chemokines, and Related Factors

A growing number of signaling molecules have been discovered to be important in regulating the movement of immune cells from the circulation into different tissues and in altering their subsequent function (9). Immunohistochemistry and array studies have suggested an increased expression of many types of these signaling molecules in the form of cytokines, chemokines, chemokine receptors, and related proteins in muscles of myositis patients. Cytokines frequently found in inflamed muscle include: proinflammatory cytokines, such as interleukin (IL) 1 and tumor necrosis factor alpha (TNF-alpha); cytokines involved in T-cell differentitation, including interferons (IFNs), IL-2, IL-5, and IL-10; and cytokines involved in fibrotic processes, such as transforming growth factor beta (TGF-beta). Chemokines—especially macrophage inflammatory protein-1 alpha (MIP-1 alpha, CCL3), monocyte chemoattractant protein-1 (MCP-1, CCL2) and CCL5 (RANTES)—as well as CXC-chemokine ligands (CXCL 9 and 10) and chemokine receptors (CCR1-5, CCR2A,

and CCR2B) are also upregulated in myositis, thus attracting monocytes, macrophages, and T lymphocytes to the inflammatory sites. The molecules that facilitate leukocyte migration from the vasculature into the tissues, including intercellular adhesion molecule 1 (ICAM-1), vascular cell adhesion molecule 1 (VCAM-1), CD142, and CD31 (which facilitate dendritic cell migration), have also been found to be increased in the muscle tissue of myositis patients compared to controls. ICAM-1 is upregulated on perimysial or perivascular areas in DM and on endomysial vessels in PM and IBM. Other studies demonstrate increased expression of interferon alpha/beta–inducible genes as one of the major features differentiating adult and juvenile DM from PM and IBM. Furthermore, an investigation of serial muscle biopsies from three DM and four IBM patients, before and after treatment with intravenous immunoglobulin, suggested decreases in selected chemokine and ICAM-1 genes in those DM patients who responded to therapy (20).

The cytokines present in the muscle biopsies of myositis subjects may be involved in regulating immune responses, but they may also have direct effects on muscle and other target tissues (9). For example, TNF-alpha has been shown to induce many changes in muscle from accelerated catabolism to contractile dysfunction. IL-1 alpha may play a role in direct myotoxicity via its influence on insulinlike growth factor, thereby leading to metabolic disturbances in nutrition supply, and by suppressing myoblast proliferation and fusion. Differences in methodology and patient populations under study, however, have made it difficult to determine if any of these signaling molecules are playing a primary or secondary role in pathogenesis and if there are critical differences in cytokine patterns in the different forms of IIM.

Major Histocompatibility Complex Overexpression and Sequelae

Increased MHC class I antigen expression occurs on scattered myocytes in all forms of IIM, and MHC class I molecules are present even on myocytes far removed from inflammation, suggesting that this may be an early event in pathogenesis (1). How specific this process is to IIM remains unclear because myocytes in muscle biopsies from some muscular dystrophies also show MHC class I expression. Nonetheless, additional evidence that overexpression of MHC class I may be related to myositis comes from an animal model where directed transgenic upregulation in skeletal muscle led to muscle inflammation as well as decreased muscle strength, even before detectable histological damage in the skeletal muscles of these mice (21). The increased MHC class I not only renders muscle a possible target for the recognition by cytotoxic T cells, but it may also

18

negatively impact cellular metabolism. When there is an imbalance between the load of proteins in the endoplasmic reticulum (ER) and the cell's ability to process that load, signaling pathways are activated that adapt cells to ER stress. This process is called the *ER stress response* and it can be provoked by a variety of conditions, including ischemia, viral infections, mutations that impair protein folding, and excess accumulation of proteins in the ER. The assembly and folding of MHC class I molecules in the ER involves a highly regulated process to assure their proper conformation and to prevent accumulation of unfolded proteins. When excess MHC class I molecules are present, this system can be overloaded to result in many cellular changes, including activation of the NF-κB pathway, as has been demonstrated in both IIM and the transgenic upregulated MHC class I animal model (22,23). This finding suggests that excess production of MHC class I molecules may lead to the ER stress response, which may play a role in IIM pathogenesis via activtaion of NF-κB, resulting in the induction of a number of cytokines, chemokines, adhesion molecules, and further MHC upregulation, thus initiating a self-sustaining positive feedback loop.

REFERENCES

1. Dalakas MC. Muscle biopsy findings in inflammatory myopathies. Rheum Dis Clin North Am 2002;28:779–798, vi.
2. Arahata K, Engel AG. Monoclonal antibody analysis of mononuclear cells in myopathies. I. Quantitation of subsets according to diagnosis and sites of accumulation and demonstration and counts of muscle fibers invaded by T cells. Ann Neurol 1984;16:193–208.
3. Crowe WE, Bove KE, Levinson JE, Hilton PK. Clinical and pathogenetic implications of histopathology in childhood polydermatomyositis. Arthritis Rheum 1982;25:126–139.
4. Engel AG, Arahata K. Monoclonal antibody analysis of mononuclear cells in myopathies. II: Phenotypes of autoinvasive cells in polymyositis and inclusion body myositis. Ann Neurol 1984;16:209–215.
5. Engel AG, Arahata K. Mononuclear cells in myopathies: quantitation of functionally distinct subsets, recognition of antigen-specific cell-mediated cytotoxicity in some diseases, and implications for the pathogenesis of the different inflammatory myopathies. Hum Pathol 1986;17:704–721.
6. Kissel JT, Mendell JR, Rammohan KW. Microvasculature deposition of complement membrane attack complex in dermatomyositis. N Engl J Med 1986;314:329–334.
7. Emslie-Smith AM, Engel AG. Microvascular changes in early and advanced dermatomyositis: a quantitative study. Ann Neurol 1990;27:343–356.
8. Estruch R, Grau JM, Fernandez-Sola J, Casademont J, Monforte R, Urbano-Marquez A. Microvascular changes in skeletal muscle in idiopathic inflammatory myopathy. Hum Pathol 1992;23:888–895.
9. Figarella-Branger D, Civatte M, Bartoli C, Pellissier JF. Cytokines, chemokines, and cell adhesion molecules in inflammatory myopathies. Muscle Nerve 2003;28:659–682.
10. Goebels N, Michaelis D, Engelhardt M, et al. Differential expression of perforin in muscle-infiltrating T cells in polymyositis and dermatomyositis. J Clin Invest 1996;97:2905–2910.
11. O'Hanlon TP, Carrick DM, Arnett FC, et al. Immunogenetic risk and protective factors for the idiopathic inflammatory myopathies: distinct HLA-A, -B, -Cw, -DRB1 and -DQA1 allelic profiles and motifs define clinicopathologic groups in Caucasians. Medicine (Baltimore) 2005;84:338–349.
12. Reed AM, Ytterberg SR. Genetic and environmental risk factors for idiopathic inflammatory myopathies. Rheum Dis Clin North Am 2002;28:891–916.
13. O'Hanlon TP, Carrick DM, Targoff IN, et al. HLA-A, -B, -DRB1 and -DQA1 allelic profiles for the idiopathic inflammatory myopathies: distinct immunogenetic risk and protective factors distinguish European American patients with different myositis autoantibodies. Medicine 2006;85:111–127.
14. Lyon MG, Bloch DA, Hollak B, Fries JF. Predisposing factors in polymyositis-dermatomyositis: results of a nationwide survey. J Rheumatol 1989;16:1218–1224.
15. Dalakas MC. Mechanisms of disease. Signaling pathways and immunobiology of inflammatory myopathies. Nat Clin Pract Rheumatol 2006;2:219–227.
16. Nagaraju K, Rider LG, Fan C, et al. Endothelial cell activation and neovascularization are prominent in dermatomyositis. J Autoimmune Dis 2006;3:2.
17. Fall N, Bove KE, Stringer K, et al. Association between lack of angiogenic response in muscle tissue and high expression of angiostatic ELR-negative CXC chemokines in patients with juvenile dermatomyositis: possible link to vasculopathy. Arthritis Rheum 2005;52:3175–3180.
18. Tezak Z, Hoffman EP, Lutz JL, et al. Gene expression profiling in DQA1*0501+ children with untreated dermatomyositis: a novel model of pathogenesis. J Immunol 2002;168:4154–4163.
19. Greenberg SA, Sanoudou D, Haslett JN, et al. Molecular profiles of inflammatory myopathies. Neurology 2002;59:1170–1182.
20. Raju R, Dalakas MC. Gene expression profile in the muscles of patients with inflammatory myopathies: effect of therapy with IVIG and biological validation of clinically relevant genes. Brain 2005;128:1887–1896.
21. Nagaraju K, Raben N, Loeffler L, et al. Conditional upregulation of MHC class I in skeletal muscle leads to self-sustaining autoimmune myositis and myositis-specific autoantibodies. Proc Natl Acad Sci U S A 2000;97:9209–9214.
22. Nagaraju K, Casciola-Rosen L, Lundberg I, et al. Activation of the endoplasmic reticulum stress response in autoimmune myositis: potential role in muscle fiber damage and dysfunction. Arthritis Rheum 2005;52:1824–1835.
23. Nogalska A, Engel WK, McFerrin J, Kokame K, Komano H, Askanas V. Homocysteine-induced endoplasmic reticulum protein (Herp) is up-regulated in sporadic inclusion-body myositis and in endoplasmic reticulum stress-induced cultured human muscle fibers. J Neurochem 2006;96:1491–1499.

Idiopathic Inflammatory Myopathies
C. Treatment and Assessment

CHESTER V. ODDIS, MD

- Precise diagnosis is essential and muscle biopsy may identify myositis not responsive to therapy.
- Autoantibodies define heterogeneous clinical subsets.

- Steroids are the main pillar of therapy with immunosuppressive drugs, such as methotrexate and azathioprine, utilized as steroid-sparing agents.
- A core set of measures has been developed for assessing disease activity.

ASSESSMENT OF INFLAMMATORY MYOPATHY

Given the rarity of idiopathic inflammatory myopathies (IIM) and the heterogeneity of the myositis syndromes, their management is difficult. There are few well-controlled clinical trials in IIM and many of the reported studies have not adequately distinguished muscle weakness as secondary to irreversible disease damage (muscle atrophy with fatty infiltrate and fibrosis) or disease activity (reversible inflammation) so that assessing treatment response in such reports is problematic. A systematic approach to the assessment and treatment of IIM is essential. This begins with accurately establishing the diagnosis of an immune-mediated myopathy and excluding the various mimics of myositis. This is especially important in polymyositis (PM), which lacks the hallmark cutaneous features of dermatomyositis (DM) that make the latter disease easier to diagnose. A consortium of myositis experts, the International Myositis Assessment and Clinical Studies Group (IMACS), has been organized to address many of these concerns. Recent efforts from this group include the (1) development of core set measures for assessing disease activity in myositis trials (1); (2) proposal of a preliminary definition of improvement in adult and juvenile myositis clinical trials (2); and (3) development of an international consensus document on the conduct of therapeutic trials in adult and juvenile myositis (3). The systematic assessment of the inflammatory myopathies will first be discussed and then a treatment approach will be outlined.

Routine Assessment Tools
Serum Muscle Enzymes

Serum creatine kinase (CK) is generally the most reliable muscle enzyme test to use in the routine care of adult myositis. It tends to predict clinical events as serum CK levels often increase weeks before overt muscle weakness develops during disease flares. Conversely, the CK often decreases to normal prior to an objective improvement in muscle strength. There are exceptions, as some patients with active biopsy-proven myositis (DM > PM and children > adults) have a normal CK. It has been suggested that in children with juvenile DM (JDM) the combination of lactate dehydrogenase (LDH) and aspartate aminotransferase (AST) are the best predictors of disease flare (4). There is considerable racial variation in CK concentrations as persons of Afro-Caribbean descent have an upper limit of normal CK that is higher compared to other ethnic subsets (5). Any form of exercise (anaerobic or aerobic) or trauma (sharp or blunt) can raise CK levels. Many medications and drugs (statins, alcohol, colchicine, cocaine, etc.) can cause increases. Finally, at different times, as many as 30% of people may have an asymptomatic hyper-CK-emia which is of no clinical significance.

In addition to the CK, other serum enzyme activity levels that may be elevated in myositis include the transaminases, alanine aminotransferase (ALT) and aspartate aminotransferase (AST), lactate dehydrogenase (LDH), and aldolase. When the CK is normal any one or a combination of these enzymes may be elevated and useful in following disease activity. Elevation of the AST and ALT can often lead to an erroneous diagnosis of liver disease because these enzymes are also released with hepatic injury. A muscle source should be considered when the alkaline phosphatase and gamma-glutamyl transferase (GGT) activity levels are concomitantly normal. From a practical standpoint, if ALT and AST levels do not fall with the CK during treatment, then investigations for hepatic disease should occur. The serum aldolase, although helpful in some patients, is not as specific as the CK. Aldolase is widely distributed and found in more tissue than CK and may be elevated with liver disease, hematologic and other disorders, and with specimen hemolysis.

Electromyography

Although electrical testing is a sensitive but nonspecific method of evaluating muscle inflammation, it allows for several muscle groups to be examined. The typical electromyographic features of myofibril irritability include fibrillation potentials, complex repetitive discharges, and positive sharp waves on needle insertion. Due to its sensitivity nearly all patients with active myositis will have an abnormal electromyography (EMG) such that a normal study indicates inactive disease. Electromyography is often used in the selection of a muscle for biopsy and it should be performed unilaterally to avoid confusion with inflammation artifact resulting from the needle itself. Due to disease symmetry, a contralateral muscle that is abnormal by EMG should be chosen for biopsy. Although corticosteroid myopathy is often difficult to clinically distinguish from active inflammatory disease, the presence of fibrillation potentials suggests active inflammation due to the disease process.

Muscle and Skin Biopsy

Muscle histology can confirm the diagnosis of IIM, but patchy changes within muscle or choosing the wrong muscle to biopsy can limit diagnostic sensitivity. Degeneration and regeneration of myofibrils is the most common finding, while a chronic inflammatory infiltrate in the perivascular and interstitial area is more specific for immune-mediated myositis. PM and inclusion body myositis (IBM) is histologically distinct from DM. The pathognomonic feature of PM (and occasionally IBM) is lymphocytic (cytotoxic T cell) invasion of non-necrotic myofibers. T-helper cells may also be found in the perivascular and perimysial areas but the vasculature is often spared. In contrast, B cells and the terminal component of complement (C5–C9, membrane attack complex) are found in the perivascular area in DM along with CD8+ and CD4+ T cells. The vasculature is commonly targeted in DM and perifascicular myofibril atrophy, likely secondary to an ischemic microangiopa-

thy is noted. Occasionally, overt vasculitis is found in DM. The characteristic cutaneous histopathologic findings of DM include vacuolar degeneration of the epidermal basal layer, vascular dilatation, and a perivascular lymphocytic infiltrate. This interface dermatitis may be similar to that seen with systemic lupus erythematosus (SLE). Microvascular injury is again mediated by the terminal components of complement as in the case of muscle (see Chapter 18B for more detailed discussion on muscle and skin pathology).

Radiographic Assessment of Myositis

The availability of magnetic resonance imaging (MRI) adds another assessment tool to adult and juvenile myositis. (6). MRI is noninvasive, which makes it particularly useful in children where electromyography is painful and poorly tolerated. Large areas of muscle (e.g., the thighs) can be studied and the results used to increase the diagnostic yield of muscle biopsy. The T1-weighted image provides excellent anatomic detail as normal tissue is homogeneously dark with a low signal, while fat (subcutaneous tissue and bone marrow) appears bright. Although muscle is darker on T2-weighted images, inflammation is bright on both T1 and T2 images. Utilizing techniques of fat suppression with short tau inversion recovery (STIR) sequencing with T2 imaging improves the detection of muscle inflammation by enhancing its bright signal and decreasing the darker fat signal. The indications for MRI include (1) documentation of myositis or disease flare in a patient with normal muscle enzymes or a normal EMG and biopsy; (2) confirmation of "amyopathic dermatomyositis" in a patient with normal serum enzymes, dermatologic features, and no apparent muscle involvement; (3) distinguishing chronic active disease from chronic inactive myositis (i.e., damage) where both groups of patients may have muscle weakness but the fat-suppressed technique will distinguish fatty changes from inflammation; (4) directing the site of muscle biopsy particularly in PM where mimics are more of a diagnostic problem; and (5) distinguishing PM from IBM as some useful distinguishing features have been noted in IBM (7). Limitations of MRI include the expense of the procedure and the nonspecificity of edema (even with STIR sequences and T2 imaging) that may be found in other inflammatory processes, toxic myopathies, or dystrophic conditions.

Extramuscular Organ Assessment

Idiopathic inflammatory myopathies are systemic connective tissue disorders and affect patients in ways well beyond the musculoskeletal system. Lung disease can be particularly devastating and patients with antibodies to the aminoacyl-transfer RNA synthetases (see Serum Autoantibodies section) are at risk for interstitial lung disease (ILD). Involvement of the respiratory musculature is less common but can occur in severe cases of muscle weakness. In the latter instance, reduced ventilatory muscle strength is determined by measuring inspiratory pressures at the mouth. ILD, however, shows restrictive physiology on pulmonary function testing and is accompanied by radiographic evidence of pulmonary fibrosis. Compromised gas exchange leads to a reduction in the diffusing capacity for carbon monoxide and a decrease in the alveolar–arterial oxygen gradient (desaturation) with exercise. The chest radiograph is insensitive compared with high-resolution CT (HRCT) scanning, which reveals "ground glass" opacities (alveolitis), consolidation, subpleural lines or bands, traction bronchiectasis, and honeycombing (fibrosis). Biopsy and autopsy studies of patients with myositis show an interstitial infiltrate of predominantly CD8+ T cells, while bronchoalveolar lavage (BAL) yields mostly CD8+ cells and a minor B-cell component (8). Clinically significant cardiac involvement is uncommon in IIM although autopsy studies detect a higher frequency of myocarditis. Electrical disturbances are commonly reported, including nonspecific ST-T segment changes and various conduction system abnormalities that can be monitored by electrocardiography. The myocardial fraction of CK (CKMB) is increased in patients with active myositis as regenerating myoblasts release this enzyme. However, cardiac troponin I is not influenced by skeletal muscle injury and elevations indicate myocardial damage. In myositis patients with proximal or distal dysphagia, the barium swallow may demonstrate cricopharyngeal hypertrophy or spasm in the case of IBM or poorly coordinated motion of the pharyngeal (striated) musculature, vallecular pooling, or aspiration of barium into the trachea in the case of severe PM or DM. Distal dysphagia reveals distal esophageal (smooth muscle) hypomotility on the cinesophagram or manometry, and occurs most frequently in patients with myositis in overlap with another connective tissue disorder.

Serum Autoantibodies

Antinuclear or anticytoplasmic autoantibodies are found in up to 90% of patients with PM or DM and are useful in defining clinically homogeneous subsets of patients (9). Myositis-specific autoantibodies (MSAs) have been previously reported to occur exclusively in IIM but the presence of MSAs without evidence of an inflammatory myopathy have being reported (10). It is rare for myositis patients to have more than one MSA. Autoantibodies seen in other connective tissue diseases may also be found in patients with myositis and are termed *myositis-associated autoantibodies*. Both groups of autoantibodies and their clinical associations are summarized in Table 18C-1. Although the frequency of autoantibody positivity is low with IBM, 18% (7/38) of

IBM patients in one European cohort had identifiable antibodies (10). A negative antinuclear antibody test does not exclude MSA because the antigens targeted by these autoantibodies may be cytoplasmic in location. Testing for serum autoantibodies is helpful and can solidify the diagnosis of myositis in patients with atypical clinical features and provide prognostic information because of the known clinical associations.

Anti–Jo-1 is the most common MSA but the clinical features of the various antisynthetase antibodies are similar, and have been described as comprising the "antisynthetase syndrome" characterized by fever, "mechanic's hands," Raynaud's phenomenon, inflammatory arthritis, ILD, and myositis. Patients with an antisynthetase autoantibody may not manifest all features of the syndrome and some will never develop myositis. For example, anti–PL-12 antibody-positive patients are more likely to have ILD without myositis. Antibodies against signal recognition particle (anti-SRP) comprise a separate subgroup of MSAs targeting a ribonucleoprotein involved in protein translocation. Most patients have PM with severe, refractory disease and the muscle biopsy often does not demonstrate the characteristic lymphocytic endomysial inflammation (11) that is commonly found in PM. Mi-2 is a multi-unit protein complex involved in transcription and, unlike the cytoplasmic location of the synthetases and SRP, anti-Mi-2 is an antinuclear antibody. In general, anti–Mi-2 is associated with the rash of DM and a good response to therapy but it has been observed in PM patients as well as JDM and in malignancy, where the rash can be severe (12).

Anti–polymyositis-Scl is an antinucleolar antibody associated with a good prognosis that can be seen in PM or DM alone, systemic sclerosis alone, or in patients with overlap syndromes. Anti–U1-RNP antibodies should be suspected in patients with a high-titer speckled pattern on routine antinuclear antibody testing and occur in patients with an overlap syndrome of "mixed connective tissue disease" where clinical findings include Raynaud's phenomenon and variable features of SLE, myositis, and/or systemic sclerosis. Antibodies to Ro/SSA are seen in at least 10% of myositis, especially those with antibodies to the aminoacyl-tRNA synthetases.

Malignancy and Myositis

Recent reports strongly support an increased risk of cancer in patients with PM and DM with the greatest risk in DM. In a pooled study from Sweden, Denmark, and Finland, 618 cases of DM were identified, 198 of whom had cancer (13). Fifty-nine percent of the 198 patients developed a malignancy after the diagnosis of DM was made and the most common cancers were ovarian, lung, pancreatic, stomach, colorectal, and non-Hodgkin's lymphoma. A lower but statistically increased

18

TABLE 18C-1. SERUM AUTOANTIBODIES IN POLYMYOSITIS AND DERMATOMYOSITIS.

AUTOANTIBODY	ANTIGENIC TARGET	FREQUENCY IN IDIOPATHIC INFLAMMATORY MYOPATHIES (%)	CLINICAL ASSOCIATIONS
MYOSITIS-SPECIFIC AUTOANTIBODIES			
Jo-1	Histidyl-tRNA synthetase	20	Antisynthetase syndrome (fever, interstitial lung disease, arthritis, Raynaud's and mechanic's hands and poor response to Rx)
PL-7	Threonyl-tRNA synthetase	2	Antisynthetase syndrome
PL-12	Alanyl-tRNA synthetase	2	Antisynthetase syndrome; lower frequency of myositis
OJ	Isoleucyl-tRNA synthetase	1	Antisynthetase syndrome
EJ	Glycyl-tRNA synthetase	1	Antisynthetase syndrome; DM > PM
KS	Asparaginyl-tRNA synthetase	<1	Rare; most patients have ILD
Mi-2	Nuclear helicase	5–10	DM (good response to Rx); PM only when ELISA used
SRP	Signal recognition particle	5	PM (with cardiomyopathy and unresponsive to Rx); rare cases of overlapping CTD
MYOSITIS-ASSOCIATED AUTOANTIBODIES			
PM-Scl	Exosome proteins; multiprotein complex	5–10	Overlap with limited systemic sclerosis; myositis less severe
U1RNP	U1 small nuclear ribonucleoprotein	5–10	"MCTD" or overlapping myositis syndromes
Ku	DNA binding complex	1	PM-SSc overlapping; occasionally SLE
Ro/SSA	Ro60 and Ro52	10–20	Sjögren's; seen with antisynthetases

ABBREVIATIONS: CTD, connective tissue disease; DM, dermatomyositis; ILD, interstitial lung disease; MCTD, mixed connective tissue disease; PM, polymyositis; SSc, systemic sclerosis.

risk of cancer was seen with PM and several case reports note that amyopathic DM may also be associated with malignancy. The overall risk of cancer is greatest in the first 3 years after the diagnosis of myositis, but an increased risk of malignancy continues, emphasizing the importance of ongoing surveillance. Serum CA-125 screening may be useful in women with DM. The presence of myositis-associated or specific serum auto-antibodies and/or another connective tissue disease decreases the likelihood of cancer. A cancer screening evaluation of high-risk patients may increase early detection and reduce mortality. In addition to a careful history and physical examination (including a gynecologic evaluation in women) with routine laboratory testing, it is appropriate to complete an age-specific malignancy evaluation given the distribution of tumors noted above. This would include chest, abdominal, and pelvic CT scans, along with colonoscopy and mammography (see Chapter 18A for further discussion of malignancy and myositis).

TREATMENT OF INFLAMMATORY MYOPATHY

General Rehabilitative Measures

After confirming the diagnosis, assessing for systemic involvement and defining the relative contribution of disease activity and damage treatment should commence. Although the timing and aggressiveness of physical therapy is controversial, the overall goal is to improve and preserve existing muscle function and prevent atrophy and muscle contractures. Patients with acute, severe muscle weakness should receive passive exercises including a stretching program to prevent contractures. As muscle strength improves to near 50% to 60% normal then an active, assisted program can be instituted including an isotonic and isometric component involving resistive bands of varying elasticity. A more aggressive approach with free weights and resistive machines can later be incorporated. Controlled studies utilizing strength training programs in patients with active but stable disease have shown that muscle enzymes do not increase and an improvement in muscle strength and well-being results.

Pharmacologic Therapy

Very few well-designed trials in IIM have been completed over the past 20 years. Although there are only a handful of randomized, blinded, and controlled studies, a pharmacologic approach can be recommended (14).

Corticosteroids

Although fraught with side effects, corticosteroids (CS) remain the agents of choice for the initial empiric treatment of inflammatory myopathy. The dosing depends on the disease severity and risk factors for toxicity because some patients with milder (i.e., overlapping syndromes) disease may benefit from lower CS doses. In general, patients should begin on daily, oral, divided-dose CS equivalent to 60 mg/day of prednisone. After normalization of the serum CK (often within 1–3 months), the prednisone can be consolidated to a once-daily dose and tapered by approximately 20% to 25% of the existing dose every 3 to 4 weeks to a daily morning dose of 5 to 10 mg. This dose should be maintained for several months depending on the clinical course, but patients often flare, necessitating an increase of CS to a previously effective (but not necessarily initial) dose. To evaluate treatment response, patients should be seen at least monthly with measurement of serum muscle enzymes and an assessment of manual muscle testing and functional status. With severe myositis or life-threatening extramuscular manifestations such as ILD, intravenous pulse methylprednisolone should be instituted to effect more rapid disease control. In IBM the use of steroids is controversial but in a patient with new-onset disease an acceptable regimen might include prednisone at 40 to 60 mg/day for 2 to 3 months. A favorable response would include a clear increase in muscle strength with or without a decrease in the serum CK because it is well known that the CK will drop in IBM without any clinical benefit. If improvement occurs, another immunosuppressive agent may be considered as a CS-sparing agent. However, assessing a response in IBM is difficult as the disease progresses insidiously and no studies in IBM have ever established the efficacy of any therapies.

Other Immunosuppressive Agents

Most myositis patients at least partially respond to CS and a complete lack of response in "PM" should prompt a reconsideration of that diagnosis. Methotrexate or azathioprine are often the first IS, steroid-sparing agents chosen and their combination has proven efficacious in refractory myositis (15). Methotrexate can be used in synthetase-positive patients if pulmonary function is carefully monitored. Cyclosporine is useful in both adult and childhood IIM in prospective and retrospective reports and another calcineurin inhibitor, tacrolimus, has efficacy for both myositis and ILD, particularly in Jo-1–positive patients (16). Mycophenolate mofetil has been increasingly reported in both PM and DM as well as the ILD associated with connective tissue diseases including myositis. The use of alkylating agents is controversial and should be reserved for refractory disease or severe systemic complications. In patients presenting with significant extramuscular manifestations or severe disease a CS-sparing agent should be concomitantly administered initially with prednisone. Immunosuppressive (IS) regimens in IBM have generally not been beneficial and treatment expectations with IBM patients should be different than with PM or DM given the greater "damage" at the time of diagnosis. Studies suggest that the inflammatory response in IBM may play a secondary role in disease pathogenesis and although corticosteroid treatment results in a decrease in inflammation in muscle biopsies and improved serum CK levels, muscle strength continues to deteriorate (17).

Intravenous Immune Globulin

Although the mechanism of action is unknown, several prospective trials of intravenous immune globulin (IVIG) have been efficacious in PM, DM, and IBM (18). This agent is often used in JDM early in the disease course in combination with CS and/or another IS agent. It can be utilized as bridge therapy but is unlikely to be helpful without concomitant disease-modifying therapy. It is also useful in the infected myositis where IS agents are contraindicated. IVIG can be administered for 2 consecutive days per month in conventional doses for 3 months and with a positive response, therapy may be continued for 6 months. Limitations include its expense and availability.

Other Therapies

Tumor necrosis factor alpha antagonists are anecdotally helpful and may be considered in the refractory patient but caution should be exercised as alveolitis has been reported with these agents in other rheumatic disease populations. Rituximab has been reported as effective in a small pilot study of DM (19) as well as other isolated cases of both PM and DM. Although one might postulate its improved efficacy in B cell-mediated DM, it is being studied in the largest clinical trial to date in adult and juvenile DM as well as PM.

18

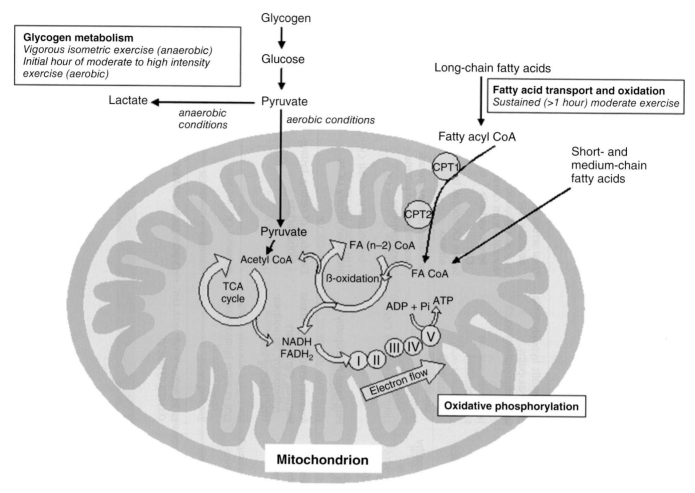

Glycogen metabolism
Vigorous isometric exercise (anaerobic)
Initial hour of moderate to high intensity exercise (aerobic)

Glycogen

Glucose

Long-chain fatty acids

Fatty acid transport and oxidation
Sustained (>1 hour) moderate exercise

Lactate ← Pyruvate

anaerobic conditions

aerobic conditions

Fatty acyl CoA

CPT1

Short- and medium-chain fatty acids

CPT2

Pyruvate

Acetyl CoA

FA (n–2) CoA

ß-oxidation

FA CoA

TCA cycle

ADP + Pi → ATP

NADH FADH₂

I II III IV V

Electron flow

Oxidative phosphorylation

Mitochondrion

FIGURE 19-1

Skeletal muscle bioenergetics. The primary muscle fuels are glucose and free fatty acids. At rest, muscle utilizes predominantly fatty acids. During a sudden, vigorous bout of exertion, energy is derived from anaerobic glycolysis. Glucose, derived primarily from the breakdown of muscle glycogen, is metabolized by the glycolytic pathway to yield pyruvate. In anaerobic conditions, the pyruvate is converted to lactate. During submaximal exercise, the utilization of muscle fuels depends on its relative intensity and duration. At higher intensities, aerobic metabolism of glycogen is an important source of energy. Pyruvate derived from glycolysis enters mitochondria and is metabolized by the tricarboxylic acid (TCA) cycle. At lower intensities, muscle energy is derived from both blood glucose and free fatty acids. With longer durations of low intensity exercise, free fatty acids become the primary fuel source. The free fatty acids enter the mitochondria, either via the carnitine shuttle (long-chain fatty acids) or by passive diffusion (short and medium chain fatty acids). The carnitine shuttle transports fatty acids into mitochondria as their acylcarnitine derivatives and involves the enzymatic activities of the carnitine palmitoyltransferases, CPT1 and CPT2. Within the mitochondria, the fatty acids are converted to their coenzyme A (CoA) derivative and then undergo successive cycles of beta-oxidation, their acyl chains shortening by two carbons with each cycle. Acetyl CoA, NADH, and FADH₂ are produced during each cycle of beta-oxidation; the acetyl CoA is then metabolized in the TCA cycle, yielding additional molecules of NADH and FADH₂. Electrons derived from these reduced flavoproteins are passed along the respiratory chain, releasing energy that is stored as a proton gradient across the mitochondrial inner membrane. This energy is used by the last component of the respiratory chain, adenosine triphosphate (ATP) synthase, to produce ATP from adenosine diphosphate (ADP) and phosphate.

estimated prevalence of 1 case per 100,000 persons (3). Symptoms develop during intense isometric exercise, such as weight lifting, and during the initial minutes of moderately intense exertion, such as walking uphill (2). Most affected persons are well at rest and can function without difficulty at low levels of exertion. Symptoms often begin during childhood, but significant problems, such as severe cramping or exercise-induced rhabdomyolysis, may not develop until the teenage years. Patients with myophosphorylase deficiency may first present in mid-adult life with a history of slowly progressive proximal muscle weakness. Patients commonly describe a "second wind" phenomenon. With the initial onset of exercise-induced symptoms, they must stop or reduce the level of exercise, but are often able to resume the same level of exercise with better endurance after a few minutes of rest. The second wind occurs as a result of increased availability of blood glucose and free fatty acids derived from nonmuscle sources.

Serum creatine kinase (CK) levels are commonly increased in the muscle glycogenoses. Electromyography (EMG) may be normal or show nonspecific myopathic changes. The forearm ischemic exercise test is a useful screening test for most of these disorders (4). In one version of the test, the patient squeezes a ball repeatedly for 2 minutes or to the point of exhaustion while arterial blood flow to the exercising arm is occluded by a blood pressure cuff inflated to above systolic blood pressure (5). The blood pressure cuff is then released. Levels of lactate and ammonia are measured in blood obtained from the antecubital vein of the exercising arm, both at baseline and then 2 minutes after the cessation of the anaerobic exercise. In individuals with a muscle glycogenosis (except in those with acid maltase, brancher enzyme, or phosphorylase b kinase deficiencies), plasma levels of ammonia increase at least threefold while those of lactate do not rise. False-positive results may result if the patient does not exercise with sufficient vigor to increase lactate production. The characteristic abnormality on muscle biopsy is PAS (periodic acid Schiff)-positive deposits of glycogen in the periphery of muscle fibers. The putative diagnosis can be confirmed by specific enzyme analysis of muscle tissue whenever it is suspected based on histology or ischemic exercise testing. Molecular genetic tests for the mutations that account for up to 90% of cases of myophosphorylase deficiency can also be performed using whole blood, thereby obviating the need for muscle biopsy (6).

Adult-onset myopathies may occur in debrancher deficiency. Four different clinical phenotypes are recognized: a generalized myopathy that may resemble polymyositis, a distal myopathy involving calves and peroneal muscles, a selective myopathy of respiratory muscles, and mild weakness accompanying severe liver involvement (7). Childhood hepatomegaly is an important historical feature.

Acid maltase (lysosomal alpha-1,4-glucosidase) deficiency has three modes of clinical presentation (8). The classic form, known as Pompe's disease, is characterized by a hypertrophic cardiomyopathy, progressive myopathy, and death by the age of 2 years. The nonclassic forms are dominated by skeletal muscle involvement (9). A childhood variant is characterized by severe proximal, truncal, and respiratory muscle weakness. Affected individuals usually die of respiratory insufficiency in their second or third decade of life. Acid maltase deficiency may also present in young adults with slowly progressive proximal muscle weakness, simulating polymyositis and limb-girdle muscular dystrophy. In contrast to other muscle glycogenoses, there are no exercise-related muscle symptoms. A minority of adult patients presents with respiratory insufficiency, manifested by dyspnea on exertion, excessive daytime somnolence, or morning headaches. Respiratory involvement eventually occurs in all adults and is the usual cause of death. CK levels are usually elevated. Adult acid maltase deficiency causes characteristic electromyographic changes of intense electrical irritability and myotoniclike discharges in the absence of clinical myotonia. Muscle biopsy shows a glycogen storage vacuolar myopathy. The diagnosis can be confirmed by demonstrating deficient alpha-glucosidase activity in muscle, leucocytes, or fibroblasts.

Management of patients with a muscle glycogenosis includes modification of their exercise and dietary regimens. A high-protein, low-carbohydrate diet is generally recommended for patients with myophosphorylase deficiency because branched chain amino acids may be an alternative to glycogen as a fuel source. Ingestion of sucrose before exercise can markedly improve exercise tolerance (3). Vitamin B_6 and creatine supplementation may also be beneficial. Patients with phosphofructokinase deficiency should avoid high-carbohydrate diets because these may provoke decreased exercise capacity, the so-called out-of-wind phenomenon (10).

Disorders of Lipid Metabolism

The disorders of lipid metabolism in muscle result from various biochemical defects in mitochondria. Some are caused by defective transport of fatty acids into the mitochondria and others by defects in their subsequent beta-oxidation. The mitochondrial myopathies result from defects in oxidative phosphorylation. Disorders of fatty acid transport and oxidation share common features. They present most commonly in the neonatal period or infancy with hypoketotic hypoglycemia and liver dysfunction. Older children and young adults typically present with exercise intolerance and myoglobinuria.

Carnitine is an amino acid that is required for the transport of long-chain fatty acids into mitochondria.

Carnitine deficiency causes a lipid storage myopathy. Primary and secondary types are distinguished. One primary form, inherited as an autosomal recessive trait, is related to mutations in OCTN2, an organic cation transporter (11). It affects multiple tissues and usually presents with a progressive cardiomyopathy in children between the ages of 2 and 4 years, with or without skeletal muscle weakness. Some affected children present at a younger age with recurrent episodes of hypoketotic hypoglycemia and hepatic encephalopathy, resembling Reye's syndrome. Another primary form affects skeletal muscle only (12). It presents in late childhood and through the early adult years as a progressive myopathy affecting the proximal limbs and occasionally the facial and respiratory muscles. The molecular basis for this form has not been defined. Carnitine deficiency may also occur in the setting of other metabolic disorders (fatty acid oxidation disorders, organic acidemias), pregnancy, long-term hemodialysis, end-stage cirrhosis, myxedema, adrenal insufficiency, and chronic treatment with valproate or pivampicillin.

Carnitine deficiency may be confused with polymyositis because serum CK concentrations may be increased and EMG may reveal myopathic changes. Measurement of carnitine levels in muscle and plasma is required to establish the diagnosis. In the systemic form of primary carnitine deficiency, both plasma and tissue carnitine levels are markedly reduced, while in the myopathic form, only carnitine levels in the muscle are reduced. The carnitine deficiency syndromes can be treated effectively with pharmacologic doses of oral carnitine.

Two distinct carnitine palmitoyltransferases (CPT) serve to transport long-chain fatty acids into mitochondria. CPT1 is located on the inner surface of the outer mitochondrial membrane and CPT2 is located on the inner side of the inner mitochondrial membrane. Deficiencies of both CPT1 and CPT2 occur, but muscle disease is confined to the latter. CPT2 deficiency is an autosomal recessive disorder with clinical presentations in juvenile or adult life (myopathic form), in infancy (hepato-cardio-muscular form) and at birth (hepatic form) (13). The myopathic form of CPT2 deficiency is the most common cause of hereditary recurrent myoglobinuria. It occurs most often in young men aged 15 to 30 years. Women are affected far less frequently, usually later in life and with a milder form of the disease. Paroxysmal rhabdomyolysis is the primary clinical feature of CPT2 deficiency and is usually precipitated by sustained exercise, ranging in vigor from strolling to mountain hiking (13). Other precipitants include fasting, infection, or exposure to cold. Stiffness, pain, and weakness of the exercising muscles are commonly experienced following prolonged exercise. True cramps do not occur. Muscle weakness is not present between attacks. Serum CK concentrations, EMG, and muscle histology are normal, except during episodes of symptomatic rhabdomyolysis or, often, after prolonged exercise or fasting. Molecular genetic testing, using whole blood, can detect known mutant alleles in approximately 80% of affected patients (1). The diagnosis may also be established by assaying muscle tissue for enzyme activity. Management of CPT2 deficiency includes avoidance of prolonged fasting and of exercise lasting more than 30 minutes. Consumption of small low-fat, high-carbohydrate meals throughout the day may reduce the frequency of attacks. If sustained exercise is anticipated, carbohydrate loading may prevent attacks. Dietary supplementation with medium chain triglycerides may be beneficial.

Defects in fatty acid beta-oxidation are rare causes of myopathies. Late-onset forms of very-long-chain acyl-coenzyme A dehydrogenase deficiencies may share the same clinical features as CPT2 deficiency (14). The multiple acyl-coenzyme A dehydrogenase deficiencies may present in late childhood or adulthood as lipid storage myopathies. One form, responsive to riboflavin supplementation, is characterized predominantly by respiratory and neck muscle weakness (14). Patients with mitochondrial trifunctional protein enzyme deficiency typically have episodic rhabdomyolysis and a peripheral neuropathy.

Mitochondrial Myopathies

The mitochondrial myopathies are a clinically heterogenous group of disorders that arise due to defects in mitochondrial respiratory chain function. Their varied clinical features and multisystemic nature reflect dysfunction of organs that are highly dependent on oxidative metabolism, such as skeletal muscle, brain, peripheral nerve, organ of Corti, heart, retina, endocrine glands, and renal tubules. Clinical features of these disorders include a proximal myopathy, strokelike episodes, seizures, ataxia, cognitive decline, axonal neuropathy, sensorineural hearing loss, hypertrophic cardiomyopathy, pigmentary retinopathy, diabetes mellitus, short stature, and renal tubular acidosis. A number of diverse syndromes are characterized by specific combinations of these clinical features (15). Predominant involvement of one organ system can also occur. The age at onset of symptoms ranges from birth to late life, but is usually childhood or early adult life (16). Most mitochondrial myopathies are caused by mutations in mitochondrial DNA (mtDNA) genes that encode polypeptide subunits of the respiratory chain or transfer or ribosomal RNAs that mediate the synthesis of entire mitochondrial proteins (15). These mtDNA mutations are usually inherited through maternal transmission and are thus expressed in a heteroplasmic fashion in cells and tissues. A minority of mitochondrial myopathies are caused by mutations of genes in the nuclear DNA that encode functional subunits or ancillary proteins of the respiratory chain, as well as factors involved in intergenomic communication. These nuclear DNA defects are inherited as autosomal recessive or dominant traits. Mitochondrial diseases have an estimated prevalence of 10 to 15 cases per 100,000 persons (15).

Muscle involvement is present in the majority of mitochondrial diseases and varied in its clinical presentation. Chronic progressive external ophthalmoplegia and eyelid ptosis often precede or accompany the skeletal muscle disease (16). Mild weakness of the proximal limb musculature is usually present and is made worse by exertion. Patients often note myalgias and premature fatigue during exercise. Headache and nausea may occur during strenuous activity. More severe defects of oxidative phosphorylation result in a disparity between oxygen delivery and oxygen utilization and a hyperdynamic cardiopulmonary response to exercise (17). Patients thus experience marked tachycardia and exertional dyspnea when they engage in submaximal exercise.

Serum CK levels are normal or only mildly elevated. Electromyography usually shows mild myopathic or neuropathic changes, or a combination of both. An elevated resting and fasting lactate level (>2.5 mmol/L) in the blood has high specificity but only modest sensitivity for the diagnosis (18). Exercise testing using a cycle ergometer typically shows a reduction in maximal whole body oxygen consumption due to a reduction in peripheral oxygen extraction and a disproportionately greater production of carbon dioxide relative to oxygen consumption (18). Muscle biopsy is required for specific diagnosis. The characteristic findings include ragged red fibers, evident with the modified Gomori trichrome stain, and/or muscle fibers with reduced or absent cytochrome c oxidase activity. Electron microscopy may also show mitochondria in increased numbers or with abnormal morphology or inclusions. Identification of the responsible mitochondrial defect requires biochemical assessment of respiratory chain function in muscle tissue, often coupled with molecular genetic studies (19).

Myoadenylate Deaminase Deficiency

Myoadenylate deaminase deficiency is the most common genetic abnormalitiy of skeletal muscle, affecting up to 2% of the population. The affected biochemical pathway normally metabolizes adenosine monophosphate (AMP), generated via the adenylate kinase reaction, to inosine monophosphate and ammonia. This serves to buffer increases in AMP that occur during strenuous exertion. Individuals with this deficiency do not have a measurable impairment in exercise energy metabolism (20) and are almost always asymptomatic. If an individual with this deficiency has muscle weakness, myalgia, or fatigue, another diagnosis should be sought to explain these symptoms. Patients with primary myoadenylate deaminase deficiency have normal serum CK concentrations, EMG, and muscle histology. However, the forearm ischemic exercise test is abnormal. In contrast to the muscle glycogenoses, levels of lactate, but not those of ammonia, increase several-fold in the blood after ischemic exercise.

SECONDARY METABOLIC MYOPATHIES

Proximal muscle weakness is the primary feature of the myopathies that may accompany Cushing's syndrome, hypothyroidism, hyperthyroidism, vitamin D deficiency, acromegaly, and hyperparathyroidism. Hypothyroidism may be associated with elevation of the serum CK and be misdiagnosed as polymyositis. Disorders that cause abnormally high or low concentrations of sodium, potassium, calcium, magnesium, or phosphorus can also cause weakness, fatigue, myalgias, or cramps. Zidovudine may induce a mitochondrial myopathy.

REFERENCES

1. Vladutiu GD. The molecular diagnosis of metabolic myopathies. Neurol Clin 2000;18:53–104.
2. DiMauro S, Lamperti C. Muscle glycogenoses. Muscle Nerve 2001;24:984–999.
3. Vissing J, Haller RG. The effect of oral sucrose on exercise tolerance in patients with McArdle's disease. N Engl J Med 2003;349:2503–2509.
4. Livingstone C, Chinnery PF, Turnbull DM. The ischaemic lactate-ammonia test. Ann Clin Biochem 2001;38:304–310.
5. Wortmann RL, DiMauro S. Differentiating idiopathic inflammatory myopathies from metabolic myopathies. Rheum Dis Clin North Am 2002;28:759–778.
6. Greenberg SA, Walsh RJ. Molecular diagnosis of inheritable neuromuscular disorders. Part II: application of genetic testing in neuromuscular disease. Muscle Nerve 2005;31:431–451.
7. Kiechl S, Kohlendorfer U, Thaler C, et al. Different clinical aspects of debrancher deficiency myopathy. J Neurol Neurosurg Psychiatry 1999;67:364–368.
8. Amato AA. Acid maltase deficiency and related myopathies. Neurol Clin 2000;18:151–165.
9. Winkel LP, Hagemans ML, van Doorn PA, et al. The natural course of non-classic Pompe's disease; a review of 225 published cases. J Neurol 2005;252:875–884.
10. Haller RG, Lewis SF. Glucose-induced exertional fatigue in muscle phosphofructokinase deficiency. N Engl J Med 1991;324:364–369.
11. Wang Y, Ye J, Ganapathy V, Longo N. Mutations in the organic cation/carnitine transporter OCTN2 in primary

19

carnitine deficiency. Proc Natl Acad Sci USA 1999;96: 2356–2360.

12. Cwik VA. Disorders of lipid metabolism in skeletal muscle. Neurol Clin 2000;18:167–184.

13. Deschauer M, Wieser T, Zierz S. Muscle carnitine palmitoyl-transferase II deficiency: clinical and molecular genetic features and diagnostic aspects. Arch Neurol 2005;62:37–41.

14. Olpin SE. Fatty acid oxidation defects as a cause of neuromyopathic disease in infants and adults. Clin Lab 2005; 51:289–306.

15. DiMauro S, Schon EA. Mitochondrial respiratory-chain diseases. N Engl J Med 2003;348:2656–2668.

16. Nardin RA, Johns DR. Mitochondrial dysfunction and neuromuscular disease. Muscle Nerve 2001;24:170–191.

17. Taivassalo T, Jensen TD, Kennaway N, DiMauro S, Vissing J, Haller RG. The spectrum of exercise tolerance in mitochondrial myopathies: a study of 40 patients. Brain 2003;126:413–423.

18. Tarnopolsky MA, Raha S. Mitochondrial myopathies: diagnosis, exercise intolerance, and treatment options. Med Sci Sports Exerc 2005;37:2086–2093.

19. Taylor RW, Schaefer AM, Barron MJ, McFarland R, Turnbull DM. The diagnosis of mitochondrial muscle disease. Neuromuscul Disord 2004;14:237–245.

20. Tarnopolsky MA, Parise G, Gibala MJ, Graham TE, Rush JW. Myoadenylate deaminase deficiency does not affect muscle anaplerosis during exhaustive exercise in humans. J Physiol 2001;533:881–889.

CHAPTER 20

Sjögren's Syndrome

Troy Daniels, DDS, MS

- Primary Sjögren's syndrome (pSS) is a systemic autoimmune disease with early and gradually progressive lacrimal and salivary dysfunction.
- Secondary SS occurs in association with other autoimmune disorders, the most common of which is rheumatoid arthritis.
- Minor salivary glands and lacrimal glands in SS exhibit a particular pattern of periductal lymphocytic infiltration known as focal lymphocytic sialadenitis.
- About 90% of patients with SS are women.
- Sjögren's syndrome is very common, with a community prevalence of pSS ranging from 0.1% to 0.6% of all individuals.
- The major eye problem in SS is keratoconjunctivitis sicca, leading to xerophthalmia. The principal oral manifestation of SS is decreased salivary gland production, leading to xerostomia and a predilection for dental caries.
- Extraglandular manifestations of SS include arthralgias, thyroiditis, renal involvement (leading to renal tubular acidosis), peripheral neuropathy, cutaneous vasculitis, and lymphoma.
- The risk of lymphoma in pSS is approximately 5%.
- Most patients with SS develop increased circulating polyclonal immunoglobulins and autoantibodies. These autoantibodies include two fairly specific antibodies directed against the Ro (SS-A) and La (SS-B) antigens.
- Anti-Ro and -La antibodies may be associated with fetal heart block during the pregnancies of women with SS.

Primary Sjögren's syndrome (pSS) is a systemic autoimmune disease with gradually progressive lacrimal and salivary dysfunction, which can be symptomatic or asymptomatic and include a variety of extraglandular conditions. Secondary Sjögren's syndrome (sSS) occurs when lacrimal and salivary dysfunction develop in patients with another autoimmune connective tissue disease (ACTD), most commonly rheumatoid arthritis. Because of the persistence and progression of secretory dysfunction, patients with either form of SS often experience significant misery. The community prevalence of pSS, using current diagnostic criteria, ranges from 0.1% to 0.6%, depending on the study design. Affected organs in patients with SS exhibit a particular pattern of chronic inflammation that is gradually progressive and uncommonly undergoes transformation to lymphoma. Patients with SS produce a variety of circulating autoantibodies, but no combination of these has yet been established as a satisfactory classification criterion for pSS, which requires multisystem diagnostic tests. Treatment of SS requires effective management of both ocular and oral secretory dysfunction, the prevention or treatment of disease sequelae, and therapy for any extraglandular conditions that occur. There is currently no single treatment that addresses all of the diverse manifestations of this disease.

EPIDEMIOLOGY

Women comprise the great majority (>90%) of patients with pSS. The mean age at onset is 45 to 55 years of age, but the disease affects a broad age range of individuals, including small numbers of children.

The prevalence and incidence of SS are defined rather poorly because reliable indicators of the disease for epidemiologic studies are not available and the various currently used diagnostic criteria give widely differing results (discussed below). Based on the widely used 1993 Preliminary European Community (EC) diagnostic criteria, the prevalence of pSS was estimated to be as high as 1% to 2% of the general population. However, more recent prevalence estimates of pSS range from 0.1% to 0.6%, based on the 2002 American–European Consensus criteria for pSS (1). There are traditional estimates that about 50% of patients with SS have the secondary form of the disease (sSS) and, in rheumatology clinics, approximately 25% of patients with rheumatoid arthritis (RA) or systemic lupus erythematosus (SLE) have objective evidence of sSS.

ETIOLOGY

The etiology of SS, also called *autoimmune exocrinopathy*, remains unknown. There is evidence of both genetic and nongenetic contributions. Families have been reported in which there is clustering of SS with other autoimmune diseases. There are also reports of similarity of specific SS phenotypes among affected twin pairs. Various associations between specific class II human leukocyte antigen (HLA)-DR and -DQ alleles, haplotypes, and patients with SS have been found, but regional and racial differences occur. More recently, the association between HLA and SS was found to be restricted to those patients with circulating anti-SS-A and/or -SS-B antibodies, while no such association was apparent in SS patients without those antibodies (2).

For many years, the possibility that a virus participates in the pathogenesis of SS has been considered, either in the context of an infectious agent inducing chronic inflammation, a source of exogenous antigen that triggers autoimmunity, or a molecular mimic of the candidate autoantigen. Viruses that have been considered include Epstein–Barr virus (EBV), Coxsackie virus, human immunodeficiency virus (HIV), and hepatitis C virus (HCV). The DNA of EBV, a highly prevalent virus latent in the majority of humans, has been identified in major and minor salivary glands. Latent EBV may serve as a cofactor in SS by contributing to chronic inflammation in salivary glands, but an etiologic role for this virus has not been established. RNA from Coxsackie virus B4 was found in minor salivary glands from pSS patients, but not from sSS patients and controls (3). This suggestion of an environmental trigger role for Coxsackie virus in pSS has not been confirmed.

Because HIV-infected adult patients occasionally present with mild salivary hypofunction, bilateral parotid enlargement, and focal lymphocytic infiltrates in minor salivary glands, HIV and other retroviruses have been theorized to have pathogenic roles in some cases of SS. In contrast to primary SS, however, salivary infiltrates in patients with HIV are composed of CD8+ lymphocytes, not memory CD4+ T cells and B cells (see below). Further, recent clinical trials of antiretroviral drugs in pSS patients did not show any significant changes in either the clinical or histopathological features of SS.

Because some HCV-infected patients develop clinical features similar to SS, an association of HCV with SS has been considered since the early 1990s. The SS-like clinical and immunological profiles of HCV patients are different from those of patients with pSS, however, and most patients with pSS do not have serological evidence of HCV infection. A recent multicenter study concluded that HCV infection should be considered as a cofactor in the development of a subset of patients with SS (4). The true relationship between HCV and SS (or a subset of SS patients), if any, requires further definition.

IMMUNOPATHOLOGY

Histopathology

Minor salivary glands and lacrimal glands in SS exhibit a particular pattern of periductal focal lymphocytic infiltration in otherwise normal-appearing glands. The severity of this inflammation, called *focal lymphocytic sialadenitis*, can be estimated by a semiquantitative "focus score" (described below), which correlates with the diagnosis and severity of keratoconjunctivitis sicca (5). This pattern must be distinguished from other commonly occurring patterns of chronic inflammation that are not associated with SS.

Cellular Immunopathology

The earliest lymphocytic infiltrates in salivary glands are composed of T cells—mostly of the CD45RO primed memory T-helper phenotype—and CD20+ B cells. Later, CD27+ (memory) and CD79a+ B cells join the infiltrates. Clusters of CD38+ plasma cells are present in normal salivary glands and at the periphery of T/B-cell infiltrates in SS (6). These infiltrates also may exhibit lymphoid follicle formation in various stages of development, including mostly CD20+ B cells and CD21+ follicular dendritic cells with a few CD4+ helper T cells, and immunoglobulin deposits (7).

T-helper (Th) cell infiltrates in SS elaborate both Th1 and Th2 cytokines. Th2 cytokines [interleukin (IL)-4, -5, and -13] predominate in early stages of SS, but shift towards a Th1 profile (interferon gamma and IL-2) in patients with more advanced disease (8). A newly identified B-cell activating factor (BAFF; also known as B lymphocyte stimulator, BLyS) promotes the survival and maturation of B cells. BAFF regulated by interferon gamma, is implicated in polyclonal activation of B cells. BAFF levels are elevated in SS serum, correlate with the levels of circulating autoantibodies (9), and may have a long-term role in development of lymphoma.

Autoantibodies

Most patients with SS develop increased circulating polyclonal immunoglobulins and autoantibodies. These autoantibodies include the highly nonspecific rheumatoid factor and antinuclear antibodies, and the more specific anti-Ro (SS-A) and anti-La (SS-B) antibodies, which are more highly associated with pSS and SLE. The roles of anti-Ro and anti-La antibodies in the pathogenesis of pSS itself remain unclear. In women who are pregnant, anti-Ro and anti-La antibodies may lead to particular pregnancy complications: after the 20th week of gestation, these antibodies may cross the placenta can cause inflammation within the conduction system of the fetal heart, leading in 1% to 2% of cases to congenital heart block. The likelihood of congenital heart block is higher in fetuses of women who have previously given birth to children with heart block.

Antibodies against alpha-fodrin, a protein in the cytoskeleton of most eukaryotic cells, are more prevalent than anti-Ro. Antifodrin antibodies are present in almost all pSS patients diagnosed by the San Diego diagnostic criteria (the most restrictive set), but are found in fewer patients diagnosed by the EC criteria. Antifodrin antibodies have been proposed as a specific diagnostic marker for pSS, but this remains controversial.

Antibodies against the M3 muscarinic acetylcholine receptor (M3R) have been identified in sera from patients with pSS. A possible role of anti-M3R in decreasing lacrimal and salivary secretions was supported by experiments showing that pSS sera inhibit aquaporin AQP-5 (a transmembrane protein affecting water transport in acinar cells) (10). The effects of anti-M3R on the receptor remain unclear, but in theory slowed gastric emptying and decreased bladder muscle contractility seen in pSS patients may relate at least in part to the effects of this antibody.

CLINICAL FEATURES AND ASSESSMENT

Ocular

The ocular component of SS, called keratoconjunctivitis sicca (KCS), was first described by Henrik Sjögren in 1933. KCS causes a prolonged but slowly progressive decrease in tear production and qualitative changes in the tear film, leading to decreased tear film stability. This, in turn, causes repeated dehydration of the ocular surface epithelium and ultimately results in keratinization. Bacterial infection, usually by *Staphylococcus aureus*, is an occasional result of KCS. The most characteristic symptoms of KCS are insidious onset of ocular foreign body sensation, burning, pain, inability to tear, or photophobia (Table 20-1). However, some patients with KCS are asymptomatic. The term *xerophthalmia* is occasionally, but inappropriately, used for SS because the term refers to the ocular manifestations of vitamin A deficiency, which are not the same as KCS.

TABLE 20-1. DRY EYE SYMPTOMS—DIFFERENTIAL DIAGNOSIS.

Sjögren's syndrome (keratoconjunctivitis sicca)
Conjunctival cicatrization:
Stevens–Johnson syndrome
Ocular cicatricial pemphigoid
Drug-induced pseudopemphigoid
Trachoma
Graft-vs.-host disease
Anticholinergic drug effects
AIDS-associated keratoconjunctivitis sicca
Trigeminal or facial nerve paralysis
Vitamin A deficiency (xerophthalmia)

SOURCE: Whitcher J, Gritz D, Daniels T. Int Ophthalmal Clin 1998;38:23–37, by permission of *International Ophthalmology Clinics*.
ABBREVIATION: AIDS, acquired immunodecifiency syndrome.

Clinical signs of KCS, best observed at the slit lamp, include scanty or absent tear meniscus, decreased tear breakup time, and characteristic staining of the cornea with fluorescein and conjunctiva with lissamine green. Fluorescein dye provides the basis for measuring tear breakup time, which assesses stability of the tear film and reveals corneal changes by the location and pattern of its staining. Lissamine green or rose bengal dyes can assess surface changes to the air-exposed conjunctiva, which are characteristic of KCS (Figure 20-1) (11). The use of lissamine green is preferred oral rose bengal, however, because rose bengal staining is painful to the patient in direct proportion to the severity of their KCS.

The quantity of tear production can be estimated with an unanesthetized Schirmer test (Schirmer I test) using sterile filter paper strips. Results of ≤5mm in 5 minutes indicate abnormal tear production; however, such a result is not specific to KCS and can be caused by other unrelated conditions.

Oral–Salivary

The salivary and oral components of SS are characterized by decreased saliva production and qualitative changes in the saliva and oral flora, called *salivary hypofunction or dysfunction*. Early in the course of SS, most patients complain of symptoms of dry mouth (xerostomia; Table 20-2). Others complain of difficulty chewing or swallowing food, difficulty wearing a lower denture, or oral burning symptoms (usually associated with chronic candidiasis). The onset of these symptoms is usually insidious. However, some patients with significant signs of salivary dysfunction do not complain of oral symptoms. The late stages of this salivary change in

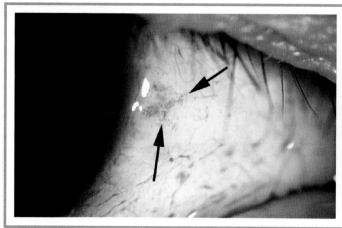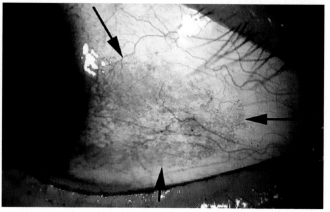

FIGURE 20-1

Lissamine green staining (*arrows*) of air-exposed conjunctiva, lateral to the cornea, in patients with mild (left) and severe (right) keratoconjunctivitis sicca. (Courtesy of Dr. K. Kitagawa.)

SS are similar to those experienced by patients undergoing radiation therapy to the head and neck for an oropharyngeal cancer.

The clinical signs of salivary dysfunction in SS include a reduced or absent salivary pool in the mouth floor, reduced mucosal lubrication, and a particular pattern of progressive dental decay. Dental caries in SS are located on the necks of teeth (next to the gingiva), the incisal edges of the anterior teeth, or the cusp tips of posterior teeth, patterns unusual for common diet-associated caries. Thickened or cloudy-appearing saliva may be expressible from the parotid or submandibular ducts. About one third of SS patients develop signs of chronic erythematous candidiasis (i.e., loss of filiform papillae from the dorsal tongue and symmetrical areas of mucosal erythema, with or without angular cheilitis; Figure 20-2).

About 20% to 30% of pSS patients experience prolonged bilateral enlargement of the parotid or submandibular glands, which are usually firm and nontender to palpation (Table 20-3). When examined by biopsy, these tumors are usually diagnosed as lymphoepithelial lesion (or lymphoepithelial sialadenitis), which is a benign reactive process. However, these chronic tumors may transform into MALT (mucosa-associated lymphoid tissue) lymphomas, which are usually indolent for many years but may later give rise to rapidly growing high-grade, large-cell lymphomas.

TABLE 20-2. DRY MOUTH SYMPTOMS—
DIFFERENTIAL DIAGNOSIS.

Chronically administered drugs (e.g., antidepressants, parasympatholytics, neuroleptics)
Sjögren's syndrome[a]
Sarcoidosis,[a] tuberculosis
HIV[a] or hepatitis C infection
Uncontrolled diabetes
Amyloidosis
Therapeutic radiation to head and neck
Graft-vs.-host disease

ABBREVIATION: HIV, human immunodeficiency virus.
[a] May also cause bilateral major salivary gland enlargement.

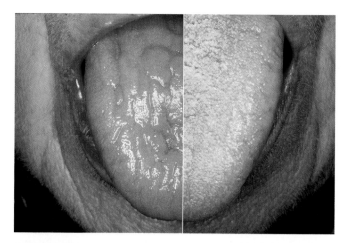

FIGURE 20-2

Chronic erythematous candidiasis in a 64-year-old woman, before (left) and after (right) treatment with an antifungal drug, accompanied by significant improvement in oral symptoms. The dorsal tongue (left) illustrates characteristic features: atrophy of filiform papillae, erythema, and fissuring, accompanied by intraoral areas of symmetrically distributed mucosal erythema and by angular cheilitis.

TABLE 20-3. BILATERAL SALIVARY GLAND ENLARGEMENT—DIFFERENTIAL DIAGNOSIS.

Sjögren's syndrome[a] (lymphoepithelial lesion)

Viral infections (mumps, CMV, HIV,[a] Coxsackie)

Granulomatous diseases[a] (e.g., sarcoidosis)

Sialadenosis[b] (associated with diabetes mellitus, acromegaly, gonadal hypofunction, hyperlipoproteinemia, hepatic cirrhosis, anorexia/bulimia, or pancreatitis)

Recurrent parotitis of childhood

ABBREVIATIONS: CMV, cytomeglovirus; HIV, human immunodeficiency virus.
[a] Associated with chronic salivary hypofunction.
[b] Affects parotid glands only; symmetrical enlargement that is soft and nontender to palpation; no symptoms or signs of salivary hypofunction; diagnosis by clinical presentation; biopsy unnecessary.

The most disease-specific assessment of the salivary component of SS is from a labial salivary gland (LSG) biopsy. This office procedure consists of local anesthetic infiltration, a 1.5 to 2.0 cm incision just through the lower lip mucosal epithelium, and careful dissection of 4 or 5 minor salivary glands, one at a time, from the subepithelial connective tissue (12). A LSG biopsy is not necessary for patients who have objective evidence of KCS and serum anti-Ro or anti-La antibodies. In patients with KCS and signs of salivary hypofunction who lack serum anti-Ro/La antibodies, however, a LSG biopsy demonstrating focal lymphocytic sialadenitis and a focus score ≥ 1 focus/4 mm^2 is required for the diagnosis of pSS.

Salivary function is assessed most easily by measuring whole unstimulated salivary flow for 5 to 10 minutes. This can also be accomplished by sequential salivary scintigraphy, but at greater expense. Functional assessments of salivary flow can quantify patients' salivary production as a severity measure or an assessment of disease progress. Various means of imaging salivary glands (e.g., contrast sialography, magnetic resonance imaging, ultrasound, or combinations of those) have been proposed to diagnose the salivary component of SS, but do not assess function and are not yet sufficiently disease-specific to replace LSG biopsy.

Extraglandular

Symptoms and signs of various diseases and conditions affecting other organ systems are observed in patients with pSS at higher rates than in the general population. Many of these conditions also have autoimmune mechanisms. The following descriptions of extraglandular conditions associated with pSS are derived from the comparisons of 10 pSS cohorts (13).

Arthralgias or signs of arthritis have been noted in 25% to 85% of pSS patients, usually in the form of tenderness or swelling in multiple peripheral joints. Raynaud's phenomenon was noted in 13% to 62% of patients.

Autoimmune thyroiditis was identified in 10% to 24% of pSS patients, usually in the form of Hashimoto's thyroiditis, characterized by goiter and the presence of antithyroglobulin antibodies. SS patients with thyroid disease are usually hypothyroid or euthyroid, and only rarely hyperthyroid.

Renal involvement, usually in the form of distal renal tubular acidosis (dRTA), has been reported in 5% to 33% of pSS patients. Risk factors for the development of dRTA include high levels of serum gamma globulin and beta 2 microglobulin. Glomerulonephritis occurs uncommonly in pSS.

Hepatic disease, usually in the form of autoimmune hepatitis or primary biliary cirrhosis, has been identified in 2% to 4% of pSS patients. In a recent study of pSS patients selected for liver biopsy, 47% had autoimmune hepatitis, 35% primary biliary cirrhosis, and 18% nonspecific chronic or acute hepatitis (14).

Symptoms of peripheral nerve dysfunction, such as paresthesias, numbness, or motor defects of the upper or lower limbs, have been reported in 2% to 38% of pSS patients. Central nervous system disease was reported in some patients with pSS, but it has not been established whether this occurs at a higher rate than in the general population.

Pulmonary disease, reported in 7% to 35% of pSS patients, may include persistent cough and/or dyspnea with chronic diffuse interstitial infiltrates, a restrictive pattern on pulmonary function studies, and evidence of pulmonary alveolitis or fibrosis.

Cutaneous vasculitis occurs in 9% to 32% of pSS patients. This usually takes the form of palpable purpura, urticarial lesions, or erythematous maculopapules. On biopsy, most lesions are shown to involve only small-sized blood vessels with a leucocytoclastic vasculitis (albeit lymphocytes sometimes predominate, as well). Involvement of medium-sized blood vessels in pSS-associated cutaneous vasculitis is unusual (15).

Patients with pSS have a substantially higher risk of developing non-Hodgkin's lymphoma than the general population. Patients undergoing malignant transformation of their disease may exhibit monoclonal immunoglobulins and/or loss or reduction of circulating autoantibodies. Tumors, which may occur in the salivary glands, gastrointestinal tract, or lungs, often begin as B-cell MALT lymphomas, or in lymph nodes as marginal zone lymphomas. Over time, either of these indolent tumors can progress to rapidly growing, high-grade large-cell lymphomas. Risk factors for development of lymphoma include hypocomplementemia, particularly low C4 levels, presence of palpable purpura, and prolonged salivary gland enlargement. Meta-analysis of five cohort studies, including a total of 1,300 pSS cases

20

in which lymphoma had developed, found a pooled standardized incidence rate of 18.8 (16).

Laboratory Features

Sjögren's syndrome patients often exhibit polyclonal increases in serum immunoglobulins and a variety of autoantibodies, consistent with chronic B-cell activation. The erythrocyte sedimentation rate is increased in SS, usually in proportion to increased gamma globulins. In a multicenter report of 400 pSS patients diagnosed according to the European Community Preliminary Criteria (1993), serology identified anti-Ro antibodies in 40%, anti-La antibodies in 26%, antinuclear antibodies in 74%, and rheumatoid factor in 38% (13). Hematological abnormalities (anemia, 20%), leukopenia (16%), and thromombocytopenia (13%) were also present in sizeable portions of the cohort (17). In pSS patients diagnosed using the recent American–European Consensus Criteria, hypocomplementemia was detected in 24%, including low levels of C3, C4, and/or CH50 activity (18).

DIAGNOSIS

Diagnosing pSS is more difficult than sSS because patients usually present with the three most common symptoms (dry eyes, dry mouth, and musculoskeletal pain) to different specialists. Furthermore, patients developing pSS are more likely not to be receiving regular medical attention during their gradual symptom onset, in contrast to patients with underlying connective tissue disorders, who normally are in periodic contact with a rheumatologist when SS symptoms develop. Each pSS symptom has its own differential diagnosis, and a specialist dealing with one SS complaint may not be familiar with common considerations relating to the others. When a patient has any of these symptoms, SS must be considered along with the probability that other organ systems are involved. Regardless of which specialist patient sees the patient first, interdisciplinary consultation early in the course of the disease is appropriate. Unfortunately, delay in diagnosis and failure to appreciate the full extent of patients' organ involvement remains the rule. A survey of more than 3000 SS patients reported that the average time between occurrence of their first symptoms and diagnosis of SS was 6.5 years (19).

Classification/Diagnostic Criteria

Since 1965, at least 10 diagnostic/classification criteria have been proposed for SS. Each uses different combinations of tests, therefore diagnosing different numbers of patients who have different clinical features. For example, the least restrictive (and most widely used)

TABLE 20-4. AMERICAN–EUROPEAN CONSENSUS GROUP CLASSIFICATION CRITERIA FOR SJÖGREN'S SYNDROME.

I. Ocular symptoms: a positive response to at least one of the following questions:
  1. Have you had daily, persistent, troublesome dry eyes for more than 3 months?
  2. Do you have a recurrent sensation of sand or gravel in the eyes?
  3. Do you use tear substitutes more than 3 times a day?

II. Oral symptoms: a positive response to at least one of the following questions:
  1. Have you had a daily feeling of dry mouth for more than 3 months?
  2. Have you had recurrently or persistently swollen salivary glands as an adult?
  3. Do you frequently drink liquids to aid in swallowing dry food?

III. Ocular signs: a positive result for at least one of the following two tests:
  1. Schirmer I test, performed without anesthesia ≤5 mm in 5 minutes)
  2. Rose bengal[a] score or other ocular dye score (≥4 on the van Bijstervled scale)

IV. Histopathology: In minor salivary glands (obtained through normal-appearing mucosa) focal lymphocytic sialadenitis, evaluated by an expert histopathologist, with a focus score ≥1, defined as a number of lymphocytic foci (which are adjacent to normal-appearing mucous acini and contain more than 50 lymphocytes) per 4 mm^2 of glandular tissue.

V. Salivary gland involvement: a positive result for at least one of the following tests:
  1. Unstimulated whole salivary flow ≤1.5 mL in 15 minutes)
  2. Parotid sialography showing the presence of diffuse sialectasis (punctate, cavitary, or destructive pattern), without evidence of major duct obstruction
  3. Salivary scintigraphy showing delayed uptake, reduced concentration, and/or delayed excretion of tracer

VI. Autoantibodies: presence in the serum of the following:
  1. Antibodies to Ro(SS-A) or La(SS-B) antigens, or both

Rules for Classification
For *primary SS*: In patients without any potentially associated disease
  a. Presence of any 4 of the 6 items indicates pSS as long as either item IV (histopathology) or VI (serology) is positive
  b. Presence of any 3 of the 4 objective criteria items (i.e., items III, IV, V, VI)
  c. The classification tree procedure (best used in clinical–epidemiological surveys)
For *secondary SS*: patients with a potentially associated disease (e.g., another well-defined connective tissue disease), the presence of item I or item II plus any 2 from among items III, IV and V.

Exclusion criteria: Past head and neck radiation treatment; hepatitis C infection; acquired immunodeficiency syndrome (AIDS); preexisting lymphoma; sarcoidosis; graft-vs.-host disease; use of anticholinergic drugs (since a time shorter than fourfold the half-life of the drug)

SOURCE: From Vitali C, Bombardieri, Jonsson R, et al. Ann Rheum Dis 2002;61:544–558, by permission of *Annals of the Rheumatic Diseases.*
[a] Rose bengal has now been replaced by lissamine green for this test.

criteria—the European Community Preliminary Criteria (20)—diagnose pSS in about five times as many patients as the most restrictive criteria (21). Subsequent analysis of the European Community Preliminary Criteria has led to several revisions, the most current of which are the American–European Consensus Group Classification Criteria (Table 20-4) (22).

TREATMENT

No cure for SS is available and no single treatment modality addresses the diverse symptoms of SS. However, a number of medications provide symptom relief and help prevent complications of many individual organ system manifestations of SS. Treatment requires separately managing the ocular and oral secretory dysfunction, preventing or treating their sequelae, and treating extraglandular conditions as they occur. Rheumatologists must develop and maintain therapeutic collaborations with other specialists in caring for patients with pSS or sSS.

Ocular

The treatment provided by ophthalmologists for patients with SS expands with increasing severity of the patient's KCS. Primary ocular treatment for all patients with KCS includes the use of preservative-free artificial tears during the day and preservative-free ointments at night. The selection of these and their frequency of use should be established by the ophthalmologist.

For patients with advanced disease, the ophthalmologist may consider occlusion of the lacrimal puncta. The performance of this procedure should be withheld until a patient's tear production has become sufficiently low that the patient will not experience tearing after closure of the puncta. Systemic cholinergic drugs, such as pilocarpine (5 mg t.i.d. to q.i.d.) or cevimeline (30 mg t.i.d.) may provide supplemental benefit but do not serve as primary treatment. The intermittent use of topical antibiotics for intermittent bacterial infections, topical mucolytic agents, and autologous serum eye drops may be useful on an as-needed basis. Weak solutions of cyclosporine (0.05%) have had mixed results in relieving patient discomfort in severe cases of KCS.

Oral

The oral treatment for patients with SS includes treating and preventing dental caries, reducing oral symptoms, improving oral function, and diagnosing and treating oral sequelae, such as chronic erythematous candidiasis.

Patients with chronic salivary hypofunction from SS, or from any other cause, are susceptible to a particular pattern of dental caries (described above) in direct proportion to the severity of their hypofunction. Appropriate dental care is therefore essential. The dentist must treat and prevent this pattern of caries in its early stages because once it begins to progress, arresting the process is extremely difficult. Loss of the affected tooth is the common result. When many teeth are affected concurrently, the results can be devastating because, among other negative outcomes, patients with severe salivary hypofunction are often unable to wear a lower denture. To prevent further dental caries, the dentist will include dietary control of sucrose, personal and professional oral hygiene procedures, regular topical fluoride applications in proportion to the patient's risk for decay (e.g., fluoride mouth rinse, home applications of fluoride gel in custom fitted trays, office applications of fluoride varnish), and control of oral flora that are particularly cariogenic through focused antibiotic therapy.

Reducing oral symptoms and improving oral function are often managed by the attending physician through increasing salivary secretion, selective use of saliva substitutes, and monitoring patients' systemic drugs to eliminate, if possible, those with significant anticholinergic effects.

- Patients with mild salivary dysfunction may benefit from regular gustatory stimulation with *sugar-free* lozenges. For other patients, prescription of cevimeline (30 mg t.i.d.) or pilocarpine (5 mg t.i.d. or q.i.d.) should be considered. The side-effect profiles of these drugs are usually mild.
- Frequent sips of water are helpful, but if too frequent can reduce the mucus film in the mouth and actually increase symptoms. If water consumption continues up to bedtime, it may initiate a pattern of sleep disruption from nocturia.
- Saliva substitutes (particularly a glycerate polymer preparation) can be helpful for patients with moderate-to-severe dysfunction, mainly when awakening at night, by using a small amount of substitute, in lieu of water when awakening from sleep, to reduce oral symptoms and prevent nocturia. Current saliva substitutes are seldom helpful for patients with only mild dysfunction.

About one third of patients with chronic salivary dysfunction develop chronic erythematous candidiasis, as described above. In such patients, who have observable saliva production (i.e., by noting pooled saliva in the mouth floor or examining the parotid or submandibular duct orifice while applying gentle pressure to the corresponding gland), fluconazole (100 mg q.d.) can be prescribed for 2 to 4 weeks. The treatment endpoint is resolution of mucosal erythema, return of filiform papillae on the dorsal tongue, and resolution of any oral mucosal "burning" symptoms. In those patients with

20

signs of erythematous candidiasis but no observable saliva production, systemically administered antifungal drugs may not reach therapeutic levels on the oral mucosa, necessitating topical treatment. All commercially available "oral" antifungal drugs in the United States contain cariogenic amounts of glucose or sucrose, making their use contraindicated for any patient with chronic salivary hypofunction and remaining teeth. Therefore, off-label topical antifungal treatment is needed, perhaps with the assistance of an oral medicine specialist.

Extraglandular

Treatment of the arthralgias/arthritis of SS is through appropriate use of anti-inflammatory medicines, discussed elsewhere in this book. Hydroxychloroquine has long been used empirically as an immunomodulating drug for patients with SS. The known anticholinesterase activity of hydroxychloroquine and increased cholinesterase levels in saliva from pSS patients (which may contribute to glandular hypofunction) offer a potential therapeutic mechanism, however (23). Outlining treatment for each of the other various extraglandular conditions occurring in SS is beyond the scope of this chapter.

PROGNOSIS

Both pSS and sSS are characterized by chronic courses and variable rates of progression. For any given patient, the glandular dysfunction can progress or plateau at various levels of severity. In pSS, there is a high probability of one or more extraglandular conditions occurring over time, but patients with pSS rarely develop another connective tissue disease. Patients with sSS generally have less severe ocular and oral problems than patients with pSS, but are prone to all of the potential problems associated with their underlying disorder.

The overall mortality rate in SS is not increased compared with that of the general population (24). However, in subgroups of pSS patients who have previously described risk factors for developing lymphoma, there is higher mortality. Lymphoma development in SS is relatively uncommon but as noted occurs at a much higher rate than in the general population. The mortality rate of patients with sSS would be the same as that associated with their primary connective tissue disease.

Acknowledgment. The author is grateful to Drs. Lindsey Criswell, Ken Sack, and Jack Whitcher for reading a draft version of this chapter and offering helpful suggestions. However, the author alone is responsible for the final content.

REFERENCES

1. Bowman S, Ibrahim G, Holmes G, Hamburger J, Ainsworth J. Estimating the prevalence among Caucasian women of primary Sjögren's syndrome in two general practices in Birmingham, UK. Scand J Rheumatol 2004;33: 39–43.
2. Gottenberg J, Busson M, Loiseau P, et al. In primary Sjögren's syndrome, HLA class II is associated exclusively with autoantibody production and spreading of the autoimmune response. Arthritis Rheumatol 2003;48:2240–2245.
3. Triantafyllopoulou A, Tapinos N, Moutsopoulos H. Evidence for Coxsackievirus infection in primary Sjögren's syndrome. Arthritis Rheumatol 2004;50:2897–2902.
4. Ramos-Casals M, Loustaud-Ratti V, DeVita S, et al. Sjögren syndrome associated with hepatitis C virus. A multicenter analysis of 137 cases. Medicine 2005;84:81–89.
5. Daniels T, Whitcher J. Association of patterns of labial salivary gland inflammation with keratoconjunctivitis sicca. Analysis of 618 patients with suspected Sjögren's syndrome. Arthritis Rheumatol 1994;37:869–877.
6. Larsson C, Bredberg A, Henriksson G, Manthorpe R, Sallmyr A. Immunohistochemistry of the B-cell component in lower lip salivary glands of Sjögren's syndrome and healthy subjects. Scand J Immunol 2005;61:98–107.
7. Prochorec-Sobieszek M, Wagner T, Loukas M, Chwaliska-Sadowska H, Olesiska M. Histopathological and immunohistochemical analysis of lymphoid follicles in labial salivary glands in primary and secondary Sjögren's syndrome. Med Sci Monit 2004;10:BR115–BR21.
8. Mitsias D, Tzioufas A, Veiopoulou C, et al. The Th1/Th2 cytokine balance changes with the progress of the immunopathological lesion of Sjögren's syndrome. Clin Exp Immunol 2002;128:562–568.
9. Mariette X, Roux S, Zhang J, et al. The level of BlyS (BAFF) correlates with the titer of autoantibodies in human Sjögren's syndrome. Ann Rheum Dis 2003;62: 168–171.
10. Li J, Ha Y, Ku N, et al. Inhibitory effects of autoantibodies on the muscarinic receptors in Sjögren's syndrome. Lab Invest 2004;84:1430–1438.
11. Whitcher J, Gritz D, Daniels T. The dry eye: a diagnostic dilemma. Int Ophthalmal Clin 1998;38:23–37.
12. Daniels T. Labial salivary gland biopsy in Sjögren's syndrome. Assessment as a diagnostic criterion in 362 cases. Arthritis Rheumatol 1984;27:147–156.
13. Garcia-Carrasco M, Ramos-Casals M, Rosas J, et al. Primary Sjögren's syndrome. Clinical and immunologic disease patterns in a cohort of 400 patients. Medicine 2002;81:270–280.
14. Matsumoto T, Morizane T, Aoki Y, et al. Autoimmune hepatitis in primary Sjögren's syndrome: pathological study of the livers and labial salivary glands in 17 patients. Pathol Int 2005;55:70–76.
15. Ramos-Casals M, Anaya JM, Garcia-Carrasco M, et al. Cutaneous vasculitis in primary Sjögren's syndrome. Classification and clinical significance of 52 patients. Medicine 2004;83:96–106.

16. Zintzaras E, Voulgarelis M, Moutsopoulos H. The risk of lymphoma development in autoimmune diseases. Arch Intern Med 2005;165:2337–2344.

17. Ramos-Casals M, Font J, Garcia-Carrasco M, et al. Primary Sjögren's syndrome. Hematologic pattern of disease expression. Medicine 2002;81:281–292.

18. Ramos-Casals M, Brito-Zern P, Yage J, et al. Hypocomplementaemia as an immunological marker of morbidity and mortality in patients with primary Sjögren's syndrome. Rheumatology 2005;44:89–94.

19. Sjögren's Syndrome Foundation. And the survey says . . . The Moisture Seekers 2006;24:1–3.

20. Vitali C, Bombardieri S, Moutsopoulos H, et al. Preliminary criteria for the classification of Sjögren's syndrome. Results of a prospective concerted action supported by the European Community. Arthritis Rheumatol 1993;36: 340–347.

21. Fox R, Robinson C, Curd J, Kozin F, Howell F. Sjögren's syndrome. Proposed criteria for classification. Arthritis Rheumatol 1986;29:577–585.

22. Vitali C, Bombardieri, Jonsson R, et al. Classification criteria for Sjögren's syndrome: a revised version of the European criteria proposed by the American-European Consensus Group. Ann Rheum Dis 2002;61: 544–558.

23. Dawson L, Caulfield V, Stanbury J, Field A, Christmas S, Smith P. Hydroxychloroquine therapy in patients with primary Sjogren's syndrome may improve salivary gland hypofunction by inhibition of glandular cholinesterase. Rheumatology 2005;44:449–455.

24. Theander E, Manthorpe R, Jacobsson TH. Mortality and causes of death in primary Sjögren's syndrome. Arthritis Rheum 2004;50:1262–1269.

20

Vasculitides
A. Giant Cell Arteritis, Polymyalgia Rheumatica, and Takayasu's Arteritis

CORNELIA M. WEYAND, MD
JÖRG J. GORONZY, MD

- Giant cell arteritis (GCA) and Takayasu's arteritis (TA) are prototypes of large vessel vasculitis, tending to involve the aorta and its branches.
- Giant cell arteritis predominantly affects the second- to fifth-order aortic branches, often in the extracranial arteries of the head.
- Giant cell arteritis occurs exclusively among individuals who are 50 years of age or older. The mean age at diagnosis onset is approximately 72.
- In TA, the aorta and its major branches are the prime disease targets.
- Both GCA and TA are associated with granulomatous inflammation within the blood vessel wall.
- In both GCA and TA, clinical symptoms of vascular inflammation and vascular insufficiency are usually accompanied or preceded by a systemic inflammatory process.
- Visual loss is the most feared complication of GCA. Visual loss may occur through the syndrome of anterior ischemic optic neuropathy, caused by narrowing of the posterior ciliary artery and other vessels to the eye.
- The diagnosis of GCA is made usually by biopsy of the temporal artery.
- Polymyalgia rheumatica (PMR), a syndrome of muscle pain and stiffness in the neck, shoulders, and hips, often occurs with GCA but can occur independently.
- Glucocorticoids are the cornerstone of treatment for GCA, TA, and PMR. Isolated PMR requires a lower dose of prednisone for disease control.

Despite the spatial closeness of blood vessels and inflammatory cells, blood vessel walls are infrequently targeted by inflammation. Giant cell arteritis (GCA) and Takayasu's arteritis (TA) are characterized by inflammation directed against the vessel wall. GCA and TA display stringent tissue tropism and affect defined vascular territories in a preferential manner. GCA predominantly affects the second- to fifth-order aortic branches, often in the extracranial arteries of the head. The aorta itself may also be affected in GCA, albeit less often than other regions. In contrast, in TA, the aorta and its major branches are the prime disease targets.

In both GCA and TA, clinical symptoms of vascular inflammation and vascular insufficiency are usually accompanied or preceded by a systemic inflammatory process not localizable to a single tissue or organ. Systemic inflammation is also characteristic of polymyalgia rheumatica (PMR), a syndrome of muscle pain and stiffness in the neck, shoulders, and hips. PMR can accompany, precede, or follow GCA, but it also occurs independently. In a subset of PMR patients, GCA is present but not clinically evident.

GIANT CELL ARTERITIS

Epidemiology

Giant cell arteritis is the most common primary form of vasculitis among adults in the United States and Europe. The disease occurs almost exclusively in individuals aged 50 years and older, and its incidence increases progressively with age (1). Women are more likely to be affected than men. The prevalence is highest in Scandinavian countries and in regions settled by people of Northern European descent, with incidence rates reaching 15 to 25 cases per 100,000 persons aged 50 years and older. GCA occurs much less frequently in Southern Europeans (6 cases per 100,000 individuals) and is rare in blacks and Hispanics (1–2 cases per 100,000 individuals).

The Vasculitic Lesion

The histological hallmark of GCA is a mononuclear cell infiltrate dominated by T lymphocytes and macrophages. The inflammatory infiltrate penetrates all layers of the arterial wall (Figure 21A-1). The infiltrates can be granulomatous with the accumulation of histiocytes and multinucleated giant cells. Granuloma formation is most likely to be observed in the media. Although the presence of multinucleated giant cells inspired the name of the disease, they are often absent, and the mononuclear infiltrates lack a complex organization. If present, giant cells lie in close proximity to the fragmented internal elastic lamina. Their presence correlates with increased risk for ischemic complications. GCA can also present with perivascular cuffing of vasa vasorum or T cell–macrophage infiltrates in the adventitia, sometimes arranged along the external elastic lamina. This finding is consistent with recent studies suggesting that the adventitia is a critical site in the disease process.

The inflammation causes a series of structural changes to the arterial wall. Among the first pathologic changes observed is the finding of a lymphoplasmacytic infiltrate in the adventitia. With progress of the inflammatory process, the media of the arterial wall becomes thinner. As the medial smooth muscle cell layer loses thickness,

the intima becomes hyperplastic, compromising or occluding the arterial lumen. Although the vessel lumen may become critically narrowed, thrombosis is not the central event. Hyperplasia of the intimal layer with scarring in the media and fragmentation of the elastic lamina are irreversible changes that persist beyond the stages of active arterial inflammation.

Fibrinoid necrosis is rare and should raise the suspicion for other forms of vasculitis. Polyarteritis nodosa, microscopic polyangiitis, and Wegener's granulomatosis, for example, are known to affect the temporal artery as well as other more typical vascular beds. When these forms of vasculitis affect the temporal artery, their first pathological manifestations may be lymphoplasmacytic infiltrates within the adventitia, indistinguishable at an early stage from GCA.

Pathogenesis
The Immune Response in the Arterial Wall

Experimental evidence supports a T-cell–mediated immunopathology of GCA (2). Humoral immunity does not appear to be important: B cells are not found within the arterial wall; no pathognomic antibodies have been identified; and hypergammaglobulinemia is absent. T cells enter the vessel wall from the vasa vasorum in the adventitia, not from the macroendothelium. Recruitment and activation of tissue-invading T cells is controlled by dendritic cells (DCs) in the adventitia. DCs are an indigenous cell population in normal medium-sized and large vessels. In the adventitia, they are typically localized at the outside of the external elastic lamina, close to the adventitia–media junction. Evidence suggests that these vascular DCs utilize Toll-like receptors (TLRs) to scan their environment for signs of infection, specifically for pathogen-related molecules.

In GCA and PMR, such adventitial DCs are strongly activated, produce chemokines, and express T-cell stimulatory ligands. This model is supported by experiments in human artery mouse chimeras. In these experiments, human temporal arteries from GCA patients are implanted into severe combined immunodeficiency mice. Depletion of either T cells or DCs from the implanted vascular lesions terminates the inflammatory response, with subsequent clearing of the inflammatory infiltrate. In contrast, administration of TLR ligands to chimeras implanted with normal temporal arteries followed by the adoptive transfer of T cells is sufficient to induce the initial steps of vasculitis (3).

Based on these studies, it has been proposed that the vessel wall, in its physiologic state, is an immunoprivileged site. In GCA, activation of vascular DCs by microbial products can break this immunoprivilege and lead to the recruitment and stimulation of T cells. The nature of the peptide antigens recognized by these T cells is

21

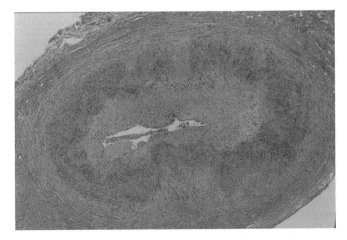

FIGURE 21A-1

Histomorphology of giant cell arteritis. A typical temporal artery biopsy specimen is shown. Characteristic changes include a panmural mononuclear infiltrate, destruction of the internal and external elastic laminae, and concentric intimal hyperplasia.

FIGURE 21A-3

Clinical spectrum of the giant cell arteritis/polymyalgia rheumatica syndrome.

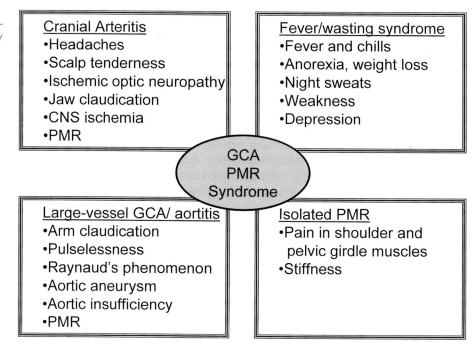

Cranial Arteritis
• Headaches
• Scalp tenderness
• Ischemic optic neuropathy
• Jaw claudication
• CNS ischemia
• PMR

Fever/wasting syndrome
• Fever and chills
• Anorexia, weight loss
• Night sweats
• Weakness
• Depression

GCA
PMR
Syndrome

Large-vessel GCA/ aortitis
• Arm claudication
• Pulselessness
• Raynaud's phenomenon
• Aortic aneurysm
• Aortic insufficiency
• PMR

Isolated PMR
• Pain in shoulder and pelvic girdle muscles
• Stiffness

Focal arteritic lesions in the ophthalmic artery produce the most feared complication of GCA: vision loss. The disease is an ophthalmological emergency, because prompt recognition and treatment can prevent blindness. Ischemia anywhere along the visual pathway can lead to visual loss, but anterior ischemic optic neuropathy is the most common cause. Visual loss is sudden, painless, and usually permanent. Amaurosis fugax, reported as fleeting visual blurring with heat or exercise or posture-related visual blurring and diplopia, may precede partial or complete blindness. On ophthalmologic examination, anterior ischemic optic neuropathy is recognized by optic disc edema, eventually followed by sectoral or generalized optic atrophy with optic disc cupping. Besides optic neuropathy, the spectrum of ophthalmic complications is wide, ranging from pupillary defects to orbital ischemia and from ocular motor ischemia to anterior and posterior segment ischemia.

A relatively disease-specific manifestation of GCA that is present in about half of the patients is jaw claudication: pain in the masseter or temporalis muscles caused by compromised blood flow in the extracranial branches of the carotid artery. Prolonged talking and chewing produce pain in the muscles of mastication. The onset of jaw claudication following the initiation of chewing is surprisingly swift. Cases of trismus have been described. Claudication of the tongue is less frequent, but tongue infarctions have been reported. Vaso-occlusive disease of the carotid and vertebrobasilar arteries results in ischemia of the central nervous system (CNS), manifesting as transient ischemic attacks or infarcts. Neurologic manifestations are increasingly

being recognized and can be expected in 20% to 30% of patients. True intraparenchymal CNS vasculitis in GCA is rare, but reported.

Occult presentations of GCA are common. GCA is the cause of fever of unknown origin in up to 15% of elderly individuals, for example. Nonspecific symptoms of pain in the face, neck, or throat are other warning signs of possible GCA. Chronic nonproductive cough can be an initial presentation of GCA. The involvement of cough receptors (present throughout the repiratory tree) by the vasculitic process is believed to be the cause of cough in GCA.

Giant Cell Arteritis Manifesting as Fever of Unknown Origin

Symptoms related to systemic inflammation are frequently present. Laboratory abnormalities are detectable in more than 90% of patients. In a subset of patients, the disease process is dominated by a systemic inflammatory syndrome. Fever of unknown origin with spiking temperatures and chills usually leads to diagnostic evaluations designed to exclude infections and malignancies. In less dramatic cases, malaise, anorexia, weight loss, low-grade fever, and fatigue eventually become severe enough to prompt medical attention. Physical examination of the scalp arteries is often negative, and symptoms of vascular insufficiency can be absent. Temporal artery biopsy, even if the artery is normal on clinical examination, remains the diagnostic procedure of choice.

Large Vessel Giant Cell Arteritis

In at least 10% to 15% of patients, GCA involves the large arteries in a clinically evident manner. (The percentage of cases with subclinical large vessel disease may be substantially higher.) Preferred vascular beds are the carotid, subclavian, and axillary arteries. Vasculitis of the femoral arteries is infrequent. The major clinical presentation is that of aortic arch syndrome, producing claudication of the arms, absent or asymmetrical pulses, paresthesias, and (rarely) symptoms of digital ischemia. Patients with the large vessel variant of GCA often lack evidence of cranial involvement; they do not complain about headaches, have normal temporal arteries on examination, and almost 50% of temporal artery biopsies are negative for vasculitis (12).

Aortitis in GCA can coexist with cranial arteritis. Whether the patient subset with subclavian–axillary GCA is distinct from the subset progressing to aortic involvement is not known. Overall, the risk of patients with GCA to develop thoracic aortic aneurysm is increased 17-fold (13). The elastic membranes supporting the aortic wall are destroyed and replaced by fibrotic tissue. The resulting histopathology can be indistinguishable from that of TA. Most cases of aortitis have been diagnosed several years after the initial diagnosis of GCA, raising the possibility that smoldering aortitis is more common than previously expected (14). The spectrum of clinical manifestations ranges from silent aneurysm to aortic dissection and fatal rupture.

Diagnosis

In 1990, the American College of Rheumatology (ACR) formulated classification criteria for GCA. These criteria, not intended for the purposes of establishing a clinical diagnosis of GCA, are shown in Appendix I.

The diagnosis of GCA should be considered in patients aged 50 years and older with recent onset of unexplained headache, signs of tissue ischemia in the extracranial vascular territory, loss of vision, symptoms of limb or jaw claudication, or polymyalgia rheumatica. Laboratory evidence of an acute phase response heightens concern about GCA. The diagnostic procedure of choice is the histological verification with the superficial temporal artery. In a recent meta-analysis, positive clinical predictors of a positive biopsy were jaw claudication, diplopia, and abnormalities of the temporal artery biopsy on physical examination (15). All other symptoms, including vision loss, elevated sedimentation rate, headaches, and constitutional symptoms, were not particularly helpful in predicting the results of temporal artery biopsies (i.e., in diagnosing GCA). The presence of synovitis was a negative predictor of GCA, indicative of the fact that most patients with true arthritis have another diagnosis, such as rheumatoid arthritis.

Even the most specific findings for history, physical examination, and routine laboratory testing have sensitivities of only (at best) 50%. In view of the fact that rendering the diagnosis of GCA commits a patient to long-term course of glucocorticoid therapy, confirmation of the diagnosis by temporal artery biopsy is essential whenever possible. True negative results are expected in more than 50% to 70% of all patients undergoing biopsies at most institutions. False-negative biopsies, which occur as frequently as 10% of the time, can be minimized by taking a sufficient length of biopsy, by examining serial sections, and by removing the contralateral temporal artery when the first biopsy is free of arteritis. Short-term glucocorticoid treatment (up to 2 weeks, or even significantly longer) is unlikely to interfere with the results of a temporal artery biopsy. Prednisone should therefore not be withheld if a biopsy cannot be performed immediately.

Laboratory Testing

A pathognomic laboratory test for GCA does not exist. Specific autoantibodies have not been identified. Highly elevated acute phase responses are typical for GCA but are not present in all patients. Although a high erythrocyte sedimentation rate (ESR) is usually considered a hallmark of GCA, in a recent study 25% of all patients with positive temporal artery biopsies had normal ESRs before the initiation of glucocorticoid therapy (16). Other markers of acute phase response, particularly C-reactive protein (CRP), may be more sensitive than ESR in some patients, but studies have not demonstrated this consistently. Some evidence indicates that the most sensitive serum marker for ongoing systemic inflammation in GCA (both before and after glucocorticoid therapy) is IL-6. IL-6, a strong inducer of acute phase reactants, probably functions upstream in the disease process. Unfortunately, reliable IL-6 measurements are not widely available, and knowledge about how (or if) to adjust therapy in the context of changing IL-6 levels remains incomplete. There is currently no evidence that treatment decisions should be predicated upon the results of laboratory tests—ESR, CRP, or IL-6—in the absence of clinical symptoms.

Other laboratory abnormalities in GCA include mild-to-moderate normochromic or hypochromic anemia. Elevated platelet counts are common. Liver function tests, particularly alkaline phosphatase, can be abnormal.

Imaging Studies

Precise mapping of the vaso-occlusive process still requires angiography. Angiography is also essential for patients with significant stenoses in vessels to all four extremities, for the purpose of measuring central aortic

21

therapy can provide a clue towards reevaluating the diagnosis of PMR.

Treatment

Polymyalgia rheumatica is dramatically responsive to glucocorticoid therapy. Currently there are no data documenting glucocorticoid-sparing effects of other medications. However, almost all patients with PMR can be safely managed with glucocorticoids; doses for long-term treatment are low and unlikely to cause serious side effects.

A critical decision in treating PMR is the dose of glucocorticoids required for successful suppression of symptoms and inflammation. The glucocorticoid requirements may differ quite markedly among patients. Two thirds of patients can be expected to respond with remission of pain and stiffness when started on 20 mg/day or less prednisone (25). Some patients will need doses as high as 40 mg/day for complete clinical control. Such patients may be at higher risk of full-blown GCA. Patients initially controlled on 20 mg/day of prednisone can usually taper the dose by 2.5 mg every 10 to 14 days. More protracted tapering may be necessary once daily doses of 7 to 8 mg prednisone are attained. Dose adjustments should be based mainly on clinical evaluation, not exclusively on laboratory abnormalities. In many patients, PMR can go into long-term remission, and prednisone can be discontinued. Occasionally, successful suppression of recurrent myalgias and stiffness may only be achieved by giving very low doses of prednisone over an extended period. Patients should be warned about the potential of PMR progressing to GCA and should be monitored for vascular complications, particularly when discontinuing glucocorticoid therapy.

Prognosis

The prognosis of patients with PMR is good. In the majority of patients, the condition is self-limited. A proportion of patients will eventually present with typical symmetrical polyarthritis, fulfilling the criteria for the diagnosis of seronegative rheumatoid arthritis. Such patients may require disease-modifying antirheumatic drug (DMARD) therapy.

TAKAYASU'S ARTERITIS

Takayasu's arteritis is a vasculitis of the large elastic arteries, specifically the aorta and its main branches. The disease may also affect the coronary and pulmonary arteries (28). Inflammatory injury to the vessel wall leads to patchy disappearance of the elastica and smooth muscle layer and subsequent intimal hyperplasia, resulting in vascular stenosis in virtually all patients and dila-

tation and aneurysm in about 25%. Complete occlusion of upper extremity arteries results in the loss of palpable pulses, which is why TA is also termed the *pulseless disease*. The preference for the aorta and its primary branches is signified in another alternative name, *aortic arch syndrome*. The ACR has developed a set of criteria to distinguish TA from other vasculitic syndromes (see Appendix I).

Epidemiology

Takayasu's arteritis is a rare disease that primarily affects adolescent girls and young women. The diagnostic criteria include an age of less than 40 years at disease onset; however, TA can start later in life, particularly in Asians (29). (In addition, the diagnosis is often not made until the patient is older than 40, but symptoms may have begun years before the diagnosis.) Incidence rates are highest in Asia (Japan, Korea, China, India, and Thailand), with estimates of approximately 1 case per 1 million persons annually. TA can occur in all races and geographic regions, but South American countries have recently been recognized as additional areas of relatively high incidence. An international survey among 20 countries has indicated differences in the clinical spectrum of TA in different ethnic groups.

Pathogenesis

Takayasu's arteritis is a granulomatous polyarteritis. The adventitia is characterized by striking thickening, often with intense perivascular infiltrates around the vasa vasorum. Granuloma formation and giant cells are predominantly found in the media of the large elastic arteries. The medial elastic smooth muscle cell layer is destroyed in a centripetal direction and replaced by fibrotic tissue, leading (in the aorta) to vessel wall dilatation and aneurysm formation. Smooth tapering, narrowing, or complete occlusion of the vascular lumen results from proliferation of the intima, occasionally with thrombosis.

The etiology of TA remains unknown. In view of the systemic features of the syndrome, microbial infections have been implicated, but no conclusive evidence for infectious organisms has been provided. CD8 T cells are a major component of vascular infiltrates, setting TA apart from GCA. Cytotoxic activities of tissue infiltrating CD8 T cells, mediated by the release of the pore-forming enzymes perforin and granzyme B, have been suspected of contributing to smooth muscle cell damage (30).

Support for a role of CD8 T-cell–mediated cytolytic tissue injury has come from the observation that selected HLA class I molecules, specifically HLA-B52, are overrepresented among TA patients (31). CD8 T cells recognize antigens when bound to HLA class I molecules.

The role of CD4 T-cell responses and the contribution of macrophage effector functions in the vascular lesions are not understood. The focus of lymphocytic infiltrates on the adventitia and accumulation of T cells around vasa vasorum makes it less likely that the macroendothelium has major involvement in the pathogenesis of TA.

Clinical Features

A generalized inflammatory syndrome with fever, night sweats, malaise, anorexia, weight loss, and diffuse myalgias often dominates initial manifestations of TA. These symptoms are frequently misdiagnosed as infection. The clinical pattern of ischemic complications that emerge—often years later—directly reflect the vascular territory targeted by the disease (Figure 21A-4).

Involvement of the carotid and vertebral arteries leads to neurologic and ophthalmologic symptoms, including dizziness, tinnitus, headaches, syncope, stroke, and visual disturbances. Atrophy of facial muscles and jaw claudication are mostly late manifestations. Occlu-sions of the brachiocephalic and subclavian arteries impair blood flow to the upper extremities, presenting as arm claudication, pulselessness, and discrepant blood pressures. The detection of bruits can be helpful in making the diagnosis.

Cardiac disease, including ischemic coronary disease, arrhythmia, and congestive heart failure, can be related to aortitis of the ascending aorta or severe hypertension. Aortic regurgitation, a serious complication requiring prompt clinical attention, is a consequence of aortic dilatation. Coronary arteries can be involved directly or indirectly, producing classical symptoms of myocardial ischemia. Progressively enlarging aneurysms and possible rupture are a major concern in patients with TA of the aortic arch and the descending thoracic aorta. Patients from India, China, and Korea often have lesions in the abdominal aorta and its branches (particularly the renal arteries, causing renovascular hypertension). The proximal ends of mesenteric arteries are less frequently affected, but gastrointestinal symptoms, such as nausea, vomiting, and ischemic bowel disease can be seen in patients with TA.

FIGURE 21A-4

Clinical spectrum of Takayasu's arteritis in relationship to vascular bed involvement.

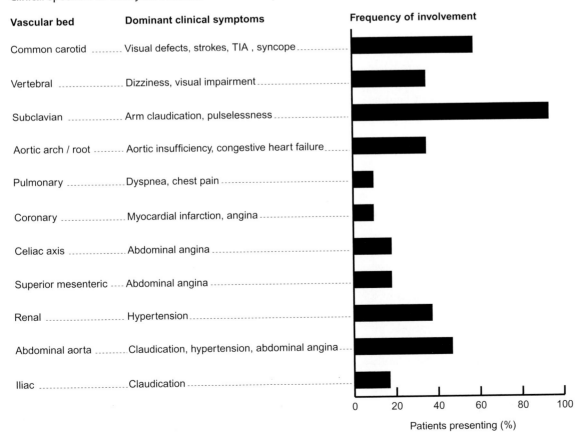

Diagnosis

A combination of vaso-occlusive disease and systemic inflammation in a young patient should immediately raise suspicion for TA. Typically, the diagnosis is made by characteristic findings on vascular imaging (32). Tissue is rarely available. The findings on conventional angiography can be diagnostic for TA in the proper clinical setting. Angiography reveals long, smooth taperings of involved vessels, with a remarkable web of collateral blood vessels in advanced cases. As in GCA, conventional angiography is essential in many patients with TA in order to measure accurately the central aortic blood pressure.

Several noninvasive imaging techniques are informative for assessing progression of occlusive disease, but currently lack standardization and are subject to investigator bias and experience. Far more problematic than assessing the degree of stenosis within a given blood vessel is the reliable assessment of inflammatory activity by imaging. MRI/A has largely replaced conventional angiography for serial assessments of the distribution and degree of vessel involvement, and also permits evaluations of the vessel wall as well as the lumen. MRI/A is particularly important in the longitudinal monitoring of TA although, as noted, the correct interpretation of all MRI/A findings is not always clear. MRI/A has clear utility in monitoring the progress or stability of vascular stenoses, provided that serial studies are compared carefully for changes. Doppler ultrasound provides a good assessment of cervical vessels. Computed tomography angiography can be used to survey the aorta and proximal vessels, but rigorous serial studies of its use in TA remain to be performed. The role of PET scanning in gauging the degree of ongoing inflammation (as opposed to uptake that might be related to a process of healing or fibrosis) has not been established.

Treatment

Although some patients with TA have disease that appears to "burn out," becoming quiescent after years of active disease, most patients have progressive or relapsing/remitting disease and require long-term immunosuppressive treatment (33). Glucocorticoids are the therapy of choice for management of TA. Recommendations of initial doses have varied, but 40 to 60 mg of prednisone may be necessary to control vascular as well as systemic inflammation. Monitoring of acute phase reactants (ESR, CRP) is only helpful in a subset of patients. In a National Institutes of Health (NIH) cohort, 50% of patients had active progressing disease despite nonelevated acute phase reactants (34). Prednisone doses are tapered as clinically indicated and tolerated, usually by 5 mg/day every 2 weeks until a maintenance dose of 10 mg/day is reached. Further dose reductions

must be tailored to the individual patient. Low-dose aspirin or other antiplatelet agents should complement glucocorticoid therapy. Methotrexate, given in weekly doses of up to 25 mg, has shown promise in improving remission rates and sparing glucocorticoids (35), but has never been tested in a randomized trial (the same is true for all other potential steroid-sparing agents). Azathioprine, mycophenolate mofetil, cyclosporine, and TNF-alpha blockers have been used with reported success in individual patients, but controlled studies are required. Contrary to other vasculitides, cyclophosphamide does not play a major role in this disease because of its toxicity and uncertain efficacy.

Stenotic lesions are irreversible. Surgical management and angioplasty or stent placement have a role in selected patients, but for most patients revascularization attempts of vessels to the extremities are not necessary because of the exuberant collateralization that develops in TA. When revascularization is necessary, bypass grafts are generally successful, while stenting appears to have a high rate of reocclusion (33). Angioplasty is reserved for short stenotic segments. Treatment of hypertension secondary to renal artery stenosis may or may not benefit from revascularization, depending on the location of the lesion leading to renovascular hypertension. Decisions about whether or not to attempt revascularization should be undertaken in consultation with experts accustomed to the management of complex hypertension cases.

Prognosis

For much of the past several decades, TA has been viewed as an inevitably devastating disease. The diagnosis was seldom made before damage from prolonged vascular inflammation was already extensive. More recently, the potential for earlier diagnosis, effective immunosuppressive therapy, and astute surgical management have led to an improved prognosis for many patients. Long-term follow up of almost 1000 Japanese patients found stable clinical conditions in two thirds of the patients and serious complications occurring in only 25% of affected individuals. Cardiac complications, including congestive heart failure and ischemic heart disease, have become the most common cause of death in Japanese patients with TA. Acceleration of atherosclerotic disease emerges as a critical factor in long-term outcome.

REFERENCES

1. Hunder GG. Giant cell arteritis and polymyalgia rheumatica. Med Clin North Am 1997;811:195–219.
2. Weyand CM, Goronzy JJ. Medium- and large-vessel vasculitis. N Engl J Med 2003;349:160–169.

3. Ma-Krupa W, Jeon MS, Spoerl S, et al. Activation of arterial wall dendritic cells and breakdown of self-tolerance in giant cell arteritis. J Exp Med 2004;1992:173–183.
4. Weyand CM, Wagner AD, Bjornsson J, et al. Correlation of the topographical arrangement and the functional pattern of tissue-infiltrating macrophages in giant cell arteritis. J Clin Invest 1996;987:1642–1649.
5. Rittner HL, Kaiser M, Brack A, et al. Tissue-destructive macrophages in giant cell arteritis. Circ Res 1999;849: 1050–1058.
6. Weyand CM, Tetzlaff N, Bjornsson J, et al. Disease patterns and tissue cytokine profiles in giant cell arteritis. Arthritis Rheum 1997;401:19–26.
7. Weyand CM, Goronzy JJ. Arterial wall injury in giant cell arteritis. Arthritis Rheum 1999;425:844–853.
8. Kaiser M, Weyand CM, Bjornsson J, et al. Platelet-derived growth factor, intimal hyperplasia, and ischemic complications in giant cell arteritis. Arthritis Rheum 1998;414: 623–633.
9. Kaiser M, Younge B, Bjornsson J, et al. Formation of new vasa vasorum in vasculitis. Production of angiogenic cytokines by multinucleated giant cells. Am J Pathol 1999;1553: 765–774.
10. Rittner HL, Hafner V, Klimiuk PA, et al. Aldose reductase functions as a detoxification system for lipid peroxidation products in vasculitis. J Clin Invest 1999;1037: 1007–1013.
11. Weyand CM, Goronzy JJ. Giant-cell arteritis and polymyalgia rheumatica. Ann Intern Med 2003;1396:505–515.
12. Brack A, Martinez-Taboada V, Stanson A, et al. Disease pattern in cranial and large-vessel giant cell arteritis. Arthritis Rheum 1999;422:311–317.
13. Nuenninghoff DM, Hunder GG, Christianson TJ, et al. Incidence and predictors of large-artery complication (aortic aneurysm, aortic dissection, and/or large-artery stenosis) in patients with giant cell arteritis: a population-based study over 50 years. Arthritis Rheum 2003;4812: 3522–3531.
14. Evans JM, O'Fallon WM, Hunder GG. Increased incidence of aortic aneurysm and dissection in giant cell (temporal) arteritis. A population-based study. Ann Intern Med 1995;1227:502–507.
15. Smetana GW, Shmerling RH. Does this patient have temporal arteritis? JAMA 2002;2871:92–101.
16. Weyand CM, Fulbright JW, Hunder GG, et al. Treatment of giant cell arteritis: interleukin-6 as a biologic marker of disease activity. Arthritis Rheum 2000;435:1041–1048.
17. Seo P, Stone JH. Large-vessel vasculitis. Arthritis Rheum 2004;511:128–139.
18. Salvarani C, Silingardi M, Ghirarduzzi A, et al. Is duplex ultrasonography useful for the diagnosis of giant-cell arteritis? Ann Intern Med 2002;1374:232–238.
19. Hayreh SS, Zimmerman B, Kardon RH. Visual improvement with corticosteroid therapy in giant cell arteritis. Report of a large study and review of literature. Acta Ophthalmol Scand 2002;804:355–367.
20. Hoffman GS, Cinta-Cid M, Hellmann D, et al. A multicenter placebo-controlled study of methotrexate (MTX) in giant cell ateritis (GCA). Arthritis Rheum 2000;43: S115.
21. Hoffman GS, Cinta-Cid M, Rendt KE, et al. Prednisone and infliximab for giant cell arteritis: a randomized, double-blind, placebo-controlled, multicenter study of efficacy and safety. Ann Int Med 2007;146:621–630.
22. Mazlumzadeh M, Hunder GG, Easley KA, et al. Treatment of giant cell arteritis: induction therapy with high dose glucocorticoids. Arthritis Rheum 2006;54:3310–3318.
23. Nesher G, Berkun Y, Mates M, et al. Low-dose aspirin and prevention of cranial ischemic complications in giant cell arteritis. Arthritis Rheum 2004;50:1332–1337.
24. Salvarani C, Cantini F, Boiardi L, et al. Polymyalgia rheumatica and giant-cell arteritis. N Engl J Med 2002; 3474:261–271.
25. Weyand CM, Hicok KC, Hunder GG, et al. Tissue cytokine patterns in patients with polymyalgia rheumatica and giant cell arteritis. Ann Intern Med 1994;1217: 484–491.
26. Weyand CM, Fulbright JW, Evans JM, et al. Corticosteroid requirements in polymyalgia rheumatica. Arch Intern Med 1999;1596:577–584.
27. Salvarani C, Cantini F, Olivieri I, et al. Proximal bursitis in active polymyalgia rheumatica. Ann Intern Med 1997; 1271:27–31.
28. Kerr GS. Takayasu's arteritis. Rheum Dis Clin North Am 1995;214:1041–1058.
29. Numano F. Differences in clinical presentation and outcome in different countries for Takayasu's arteritis. Curr Opin Rheumatol 1997;91:12–15.
30. Seko Y. Takayasu arteritis: insights into immunopathology. Jpn Heart J 2000;411:15–26.
31. Kimura A, Kitamura H, Date Y, et al. Comprehensive analysis of HLA genes in Takayasu arteritis in Japan. Int J Cardiol 1996;54(Suppl):S61–S69.
32. Kissin EY, Merkel PA. Diagnostic imaging in Takayasu arteritis. Curr Opin Rheumatol 2004;161:31–37.
33. Liang P, Hoffman GS. Advances in the medical and surgical treatment of Takayasu arteritis. Curr Opin Rheumatol 2005;171:16–24.
34. Kerr GS, Hallahan CW, Giordano J, et al. Takayasu arteritis. Ann Intern Med 1994;12011:919–929.
35. Langford CA, Sneller MC, Hoffman GS. Methotrexate use in systemic vasculitis. Rheum Dis Clin North Am 1997;234:841–853.

21

Vasculitides
B. Polyarteritis Nodosa

Keith T. Rott, MD, PhD

- Polyarteritis nodosa (PAN) primarily affects medium-sized arteries that supply the skin, gut, nerve, and kidney, but may involve multiple organs.
- Microaneurysms of arteries to or within the kidneys, liver, or gastrointestinal tract are highly characteristic of PAN.
- Polyarteritis nodosa is not associated with antineutrophil cytoplasmic antibodies (ANCA) directed against either proteinase-3 or myeloperoxidase.
- Mononeuritis multiplex, an asymmetric sensory and motor neuropathy due to ischemia and infarction of peripheral nerves, occurs frequently in PAN.
- In mononeuritis multiplex, nerve conduction studies of peripheral nerves reveal a distal, asymmetric, axonal neuropathy involving both motor and sensory nerves.
- Polyarteritis nodosa is characterized pathologically by patchy, transmural inflammation in medium- and small-sized muscular arteries, sparing large arteries, capillaries, and the venous system. The inflammation leads to fibrinoid necrosis, but is not associated with granulomatous features.
- High-dose glucocorticoids are the mainstay of therapy in PAN. In cases that are rapidly progressive or life- or organ-threatening, however, cyclophosphamide is added to glucocorticoid treatment.
- Most cases of idiopathic PAN do not recur once a sound remission has been achieved with 6 to 12 months of therapy.
- A minority of PAN cases (now >10%) are associated with acute hepatitis B infection. Cases associated with hepatitis B are treated with regimens emphasizing antiviral therapy and only short courses of immunosuppression and plasmapheresis.

Polyarteritis nodosa (PAN) is a vasculitis affecting predominantly medium-sized arteries. Clinically, PAN often presents insidiously with nonspecific, constitutional symptoms. The disease has a predilection for medium-sized arteries supplying skin, gut, nerve, and kidney, but may involve multiple organs. The majority of PAN cases have no known cause, but cases secondary to hepatitis B virus infection have been reported.

Described by Kussmaul and Maier in 1866 (1,2), PAN is often regarded as the first reported form of systemic vasculitis. In fact, earlier descriptions of Behcet's disease, Takayasu's arteritis, Henoch–Schönlein purpura, and even PAN itself exist in the medical literature. For nearly a century after the case reported by Kussmaul and Maier, however, most forms of systemic vasculitis were termed *periarteritis nodosa*, and forms of vasculitis recognized later were contrasted and classified in comparison to PAN. The patient described by Kussmaul and Maier was a 27-year-old male with fever, weight loss, abdominal pain, and a polyneuropathy that progressed over the period of 1 month to paralysis. An autopsy revealed microaneurysms ("whitish small tumors up to the size of poppy and hemp seeds") throughout medium-sized arteries, conspicuously sparing both the venous circulation and the lungs.

Before the delineation of vasculitis subsets and the formulation of definitions based principally on vessel size (3), PAN was used to describe two now-distinct forms of vasculitis: the classic PAN described by Kussmaul and Maier, and "microscopic PAN" (now called *microscopic polyangiitis*). According to current convention, and as described in this text, PAN is a vasculitis affecting medium-sized arteries. PAN is also not associated with antineutrophil cytoplasmic antibodies (ANCA), at least not those directed against proteinase-3 (PR3) or myeloperoxidase (MPO) that are such a distinctive feature of the majority of cases of Wegener's granulomatosis, microscopic polyangiitis, and, to a lesser extent, the Churg–Strauss syndrome. Although patients may be P-ANCA-positive on immunofluorescence testing, enzyme immunoassays for PR3- and MPO-ANCA are negative in PAN. Further, in contrast to the ANCA-associated vasculitides (see Chapter 21C), PAN does not involve either the lungs or blood vessels as small as the renal glomeruli (which are essentially capillaries).

Polyarteritis nodosa affects men and women approximately equally and has a broad age range of patients. Although the incidence of PAN varies according to the population studied, it is rare in all populations, with annual incidence rates generally ranging from 2 to 9 cases per million. Higher rates have been reported in populations with a high burden of hepatitis B virus infection, but with the availability of a vaccine, hepatitis B virus infection now accounts for less than 10% of PAN cases in developed countries (4). PAN has also been reported to occur in conjunction with hairy cell leukemia.

CLINICAL FEAURES

Polyarteritis nodosa can present with nonspecific constitutional symptoms such as fever, fatigue, malaise, myalgias, and arthralgias. This phase of the illness can last weeks or months. The more specific clinical manifestations of PAN are the direct results of inflammation in medium- and small-sized muscular arteries. PAN often has cutaneous involvement, a feature it shares with small vessel vasculitides such as the ANCA-associated disorders. This differentiates it from large vessel vasculitis (e.g., giant cell arteritis and Takayasu's arteritis), in which skin disease is very rare. However, unlike the ANCA-associated vasculitides, PAN is not associated with glomerulonephritis or pulmonary involvement. Common clinical features of PAN and their frequency are listed in Table 21B-1 (5).

In autopsy studies, the most frequently involved organ in PAN is the kidney. Involvement of the medium-sized arteries supplying the renal parenchyma can result

TABLE 21B-1. SELECTED CLINICAL AND DIAGNOSTIC FEATURES OF PAN AND THEIR FREQUENCY.

Clinical Features

Myalgias, general weakness, or leg muscle tenderness	69%
Weight loss ≥4 kg	67%
Mononeuropathy or polyneuropathy	65%
Azotemia (BUN > 40 mg/dL or Cr > 1.6 mg/dL)	40%
Hypertension (diastolic blood pressure >90 mm Hg)	37%
Testicular pain or tenderness	29%
Skin ulcers, infarction, or peripheral gangrene	27%
Livedo reticularis	25%
Abdominal angina or ischemic perforation	24%

Diagnostic Features

Visceral arteriogram with aneurysm or occlusion	73%
Biopsy of small- or medium-sized artery with granulocytes	48%
Abnormal arteriogram or characteristic biopsy	92%

SOURCE: From Lightfoot RW, et al. Arthritis Rheum 1990;33:1088–1093, by permission of *Arthritis and Rheumatism*.
ABBREVIATIONS: BUN, serum urea nitrogen; Cr, creatinine.

in hypertension due to renal ischemia; hypertension is mediated by the renin–angiotensin system. Renal insufficiency, another common manifestation of PAN, is due to ischemia resulting from the involvement of arteries the size of renal arteries and smaller. Microaneurysms, detectable by angiography [Figure 21B-1(A,B)], are a hallmark of PAN.

The gastrointestinal (GI) tract is involved in up to 50% of patients. Postprandial periumbilical pain, or intestinal angina, is the result of mesenteric ischemia. More severe disease can result in bowel infarction and perforation. Other GI symptoms can include nausea, vomiting, diarrhea, and bleeding. While the small intestine is most commonly involved, rare presentations involving ischemia of the gallbladder or appendix have

FIGURE 21B-1

Microaneurysms detected by angiography in polyarteritis nodosa. (A) Renal microaneurysms. (B) Mesenteric vessel microaneurysms. (Courtesy of Dr. John Stone.)

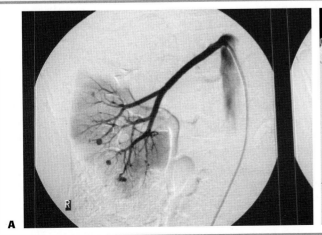
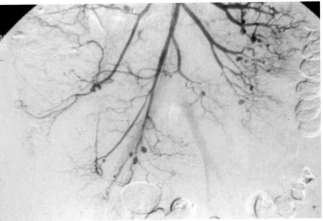

A   B

been described (6). Moderately elevated hepatic transaminases often betray liver involvement. Asymptomatic mircoaneurysms within the liver are common; these occasionally rupture.

Involvement of the peripheral nervous system is seen in 50% to 75% of patients, usually as an asymmetric sensory and motor neuropathy due to ischemia of peripheral nerves (7). Infarction of named nerves results in mononeuritis multiplex (Figure 21B-2). Progressive sensory neuropathy has been described less frequently. Central nervous system involvement is much less common, but has been reported in the form of cerebrovascular accidents.

Polyarteritis nodosa can have multiple cutaneous manifestations: livedo reticularis, nodules, ulcerations (Figure 21B-3), and frank ischemia of digits (8). A small group of patients have a form of disease termed *cutaneous PAN*, a variant limited ostensibly to the skin. These patients develop nodules and ulcerations, primarily of the lower legs, which can occur in crops and can be very painful. However, as with any other vasculitis, cutaneous manifestations should prompt a thorough evaluation for evidence of systemic disease.

As with Kawasaki's disease, the other medium vessel vasculitis described in this text, PAN can also involve the coronary arteries. Clinical proof of coronary disease during life is difficult. Myocardial infarction is uncom-

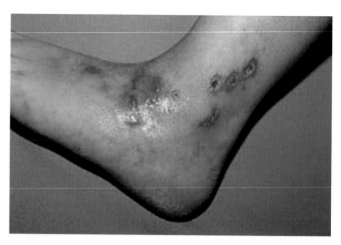

FIGURE 21B-3

Cutaneous ulcerations over both medial malleoli in polyarteritis nodosa. (Courtesy of Dr. John Stone.)

mon, and coronary involvement is usually only seen at autopsy. Contraction band necrosis, indicative of segmental ischemia, is a common finding in the myocardium at autopsy, attesting to the presence of vasculitis below the resolution of conventional angiography. PAN can involve other organs, such as the testicle, ovary, breast, and eye.

PATHOLOGY

Polyarteritis nodosa is characterized pathologically by patchy, transmural inflammation in medium- and small-sized muscular arteries, sparing large arteries, capillaries, and the venous system. There is a pleomorphic cellular infiltrate and fibrinoid necrosis in the vessel, but no features of granulomatous inflammation. Disruption of the elastic laminae of the vessel wall can lead to aneurysmal dilatation at the site of the lesion. PAN has a predilection for certain organs: arteries to the kidney are estimated to be involved 70% to 80% of the time, the GI tract is involved in 50% of cases, the peripheral nerves are involved in 50% of cases, and the central nervous system is involved in 10% of cases (9).

DIAGNOSIS

Polyarteritis nodosa is diagnosed based on characteristic symptoms, physical examination findings, and compatible laboratory, angiographic, and pathologic data. Because PAN is a rare disease and its treatment can result in serious adverse events, the diagnosis should be supported with either abdominal angiography or biopsy whenever possible. PAN must be differentiated from other forms of vasculitis, such as the ANCA-associated disorders, cryoglobulinemia, and Buerger's disease.

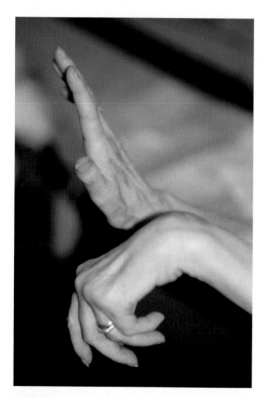

FIGURE 21B-2

Mononeuritis multiplex. (Courtesy of Dr. John Stone.)

TABLE 21B-2. AMERICAN COLLEGE OF RHEUMATOLOGY CRITERIA FOR CLASSIFICATION OF PAN.

At least 3 of 10 criteria:
1. Weight loss ≥4 kg
2. Livedo reticularis
3. Testicular pain or tenderness
4. Myalgias, weakness, or leg tenderness
5. Mononeuropathy or polyneuropathy
6. Diastolic blood pressure >90 mm Hg
7. Elevated serum nitrogen urea (>40 mg/dL) or creatinine (>1.5 mg/dL)
8. Hepatitis B virus infection
9. Arteriographic abnormality
10. Biopsy of small- or medium-sized artery containing polymorphonuclear neutrophils

SOURCE: From Lightfoot RW, et al. Arthritis Rheum 1990;33:1088–1093, by permission of *Arthritis and Rheumatism*.

Common vasculitis mimics, such as viral hepatitis, bacterial endocarditis, or other embolic diseases, should be excluded. Undiagnosed connective tissue diseases, such as systemic lupus erythematosus, rheumatoid arthritis, or systemic sclerosis, must be ruled out, as such diseases can be associated with systemic vasculitis or widespread vascular dysfunction that involves multiple organs. Atrophie blanche, a thrombotic disorder that may lead to lower extremity ulcerations, must be differentiated from PAN by skin biopsy.

The American College of Rheumatology criteria for the classification of PAN are listed in Table 21B-2 (5). The criteria were developed through the selection of clinical findings that identify PAN and distinguish it from other forms of vasculitis. Although the criteria are useful for classifying patients in clinical studies, they were not intended for use in diagnosing individual patients (10).

Laboratory Studies

Routine laboratory studies are often abnormal but nonspecific, such as elevated inflammatory markers (erythrocyte sedimentation rate or C-reactive protein), anemia, and thrombocytosis. The patient may have mild renal insufficiency, with an elevated blood urea nitrogen and creatinine. Non-nephrotic range proteinuria and mild hematuria are also seen, but active urine sediments are not a feature of PAN.

As not, PAN is not associated with ANCA. Indeed, there is no characteristic autoantibody for PAN—a fact that creates one of the diagnostic challenges in this disease. Electromyography/nerve conduction velocity (EMG/NCV) studies may be very useful in confirming patterns of nerve dysfunction consistent with mononeuritis multiplex; namely, a distal, asymmetric, axonal neuropathy involving both motor and sensory nerves.

Imaging

Imaging in a patient with suspected PAN should be guided by symptoms. In patients with abdominal pain, abdominal arteriography often reveals characteristic strictures and aneurysms (beading) of the mesenteric vessels [see Figure 21B-1(B)]. Similar findings can be seen in the renal vasculature.

Biopsy

As with imaging, biopsy should be guided by organ involvement. Blind biopsy of an asymptomatic organ, such as muscle or testicle, is not recommended. Skin biopsy is often the easiest way to confirm this diagnosis, with a biopsy from the center of a nodule or the edge of a vasculitic ulcer. Routine punch biopsy of involved skin reveals leukocytoclastic vasculitis and fibrinoid necrosis within the blood vessel wall. Because punch biopsy samples include only epidermis and superficial dermis, they do not capture medium-sized, muscular-walled arteries whose inflammation is characteristic of PAN. When PAN is suspected and skin biopsy is indicated, a full thickness skin biopsy that includes some subcutaneous fat should be performed (arteries within the fat lobules of subcutaneous tissue are often involved.)

Another option for confirming the diagnosis of PAN is a peripheral nerve biopsy. The sural nerve is biopsied most often because it does not mediate motor function. Whenever the sural nerve is biopsied, a muscle biopsy (of the gastrocnemius) should be performed simultaneously. Because of the highly vascular nature of muscle, biopsies of this organ may yield proof of vasculitis even in the absence of clinical indications of muscle involvement (Figure 21B-4).

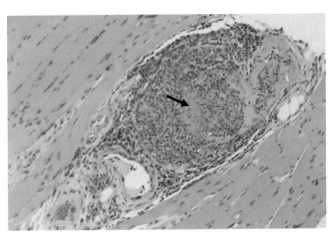

FIGURE 21B-4

Muscle biopsy showing fibrinoid necrosis within the wall of a medium-sized muscular artery. Although the patient had clinical symptoms of a neuropathy and nerve conduction studies were consistent with a mononeuritis multiplex, the nerve biopsy was negative. The diagnosis of polyarteritis was confirmed by the muscle biopsy. (Courtesy of Dr. John Stone.)

21

PROGNOSIS

Untreated PAN has a high mortality, with an estimated 5-year survival of 13% prior to the introduction of glucocorticoids. With current treatment, survival is greatly improved, approximately 80% at 5 years. In a population of 278 patients enrolled in prospective trials for PAN, MPA, and Churg–Strauss syndrome, approximately 75% of the deaths occurred during the first 18 months after the diagnosis was made and treatment initiated. Of the patients who died, 26% died from progression of their vasculitis, while 13% died of infectious complications related to treatment. No major differences were seen among the three vasculitides studied (11).

Not surprisingly, more severe disease is associated with increased mortality. A Five Factor Score has been used to classify disease severity (12). The five factors are (1) proteinuria >1 g/day, (2) renal insufficiency (Cr > 1.6 mg/dL), (3) cardiomyopathy, (4) gastrointestinal symptoms, and (5) CNS involvement. A Five Factor Score of 0 is associated with a 5-year mortality of only 13% (with not all deaths caused directly by PAN). Five Factor Scores of 1 and 2 or more are associated with mortalities of 26% and 46%, respectively (12).

TREATMENT

The treatment of PAN is guided by both the etiology of the disease (if known) and its severity. PAN cases associated with hepatitis B are treated with a short course of prednisone (1 mg/kg/day) to suppress the inflammation. Patients begin 6-week courses of plasma exchange (approximately three exchanges per week) simultaneously with the start of glucocorticoids. The dose of prednisone is tapered rapidly (over approximately 2 weeks), followed by the initiation of antiviral therapy (e.g., lamivudine 100 mg/day).

For idiopathic PAN, the mainstay of treatment is glucocorticoids, with an initial dose of approximately 1 mg/kg daily of prednisone. Intravenous glucocorticoids can be used in patients with difficulty taking oral medications due to GI involvement. Pulse doses (e.g., methylprednisolone 1 g intravenously each day times three) may be used in severe disease. Glucocorticoids alone may be enough to treat milder cases. Approximately half of all patients with PAN may be cured with glucocorticoids alone.

In cases of PAN that are rapidly progressive or life- or organ-threatening, cyclophosphamide is added to glucocorticoid treatment. Cyclophosphamide should be considered for any patient with a Five Factor Score of 1 or greater. In addition, severe peripheral neuropathy or mononeuritis multiplex is also a strong indication for cyclophosphamide. Although many clinicians still prefer daily oral cyclophosphamide to monthly pulsed intravenous cyclophosphamide, a meta-analysis comparing the two regimens in ANCA-associated vasculitis showed little difference (13). Therapy should be tailored to the individual patient's circumstances.

Most cases of idiopathic PAN do not recur after remission has been achieved and the patient has received 6 to 12 months of cyclophosphamide. Current regimens generally emphasize shorter courses of cyclophosphamide, with durations of therapy closer to 6 months than to 12. After treatment with 6 months of cyclophosphamide, patients in remission—the great majority—should be switched to another immunosuppressive agent for remission maintenance. As with the ANCA-associated vasculitides, azathioprine or methotrexate is often used. After a total treatment length of approximately 18 months, the remission maintenance agent can often be stopped, with a low relapse rate. Patients should continue to be monitored for evidence of recurrence.

Much potential morbidity in PAN relates to adverse events from inappropriate (or overly aggressive) treatment. Conversely, poor outcomes also result from undertreatment, for example, failure to employ cyclophosphamide in a patient clearly failing high-dose glucocorticoids. An important aspect of treatment is avoiding known side effects of agents used. This includes the use of calcium and vitamin D supplementation in all patients on glucocorticoids, along with use of a bisphosphonate in those at high risk for bone loss and monitoring of bone density. Patients on cyclophosphamide should have routine monitoring for cytopenias and hematuria and receive trimethoprim/sulfamethoxazole for prevention of *Pneumocystis jiroveci* (formerly *carinii*) pneumonia. Patients receiving pulsed intravenous cyclophosphamide are also candidates for MESNA (sodium-2-sulfanyl ethanesulfonate) for prevention of hemorrhagic cystitis. Premenopausal females on cyclophosphamide are candidates for leuprolide to suppress the GnRH axis and prevent premature ovarian failure; males may opt to bank sperm. Finally, as a teratogen, patients should not become pregnant or father children on cyclophosphamide.

REFERENCES

1. Kussmaul A, Maier R. Ueber eine bisher nicht beschriebene eigenthumliche arterienerkrankung (periarteritis nodosa), die mit morbus brightii und rapid fortschreitender allgemeiner muskellahmung einhergeht. Dtsch Arch Klin Med 1866;1:484–518.
2. Matteson EL. Polyarteritis nodosa: commemorative translation of the 130-year anniversary of the original article by Adolf Kussmaul and Rudolf Maier. Rochester, MN: Mayo Foundation; 1996.

3. Jennette J, Falk R, Andrassy K, et al. Nomenclature of systemic vasculitides. Proposal of an international consensus conference. Arthritis Rheum 1994;37:187–192.

4. Stone JH. Polyarteritis nodosa. JAMA 2002;288:1632–1639.

5. Lightfoot RW, Michel BA, Bloch DA, et al. The American College of Rheumatology 1990 criteria for the classification of polyarteritis nodosa. Arthritis Rheum 1990;33:1088–1093.

6. Levine SM, Hellman DB, Stone JH. Gastrointestinal involvement in polyarteritis nodosa (1986–2000): presentation and outcomes in 24 patients. Am J Med 2002;112:386–391.

7. Tervaert JWC, Kallenberg C. Neurologic manifestations of systemic vasculitides. Rheum Dis Clin North Am 1993;19:913–940.

8. Gibson LE, Su WP. Cutaneous vasculitis. Rheum Dis Clin North Am 1995;21:1097–1113.

9. Conn DL. Polyarteritis. Rheum Dis Clin North Am 1990;16:341–362.

10. Hunder GH, Arend WP, Bloch DA, et al. The American College of Rheumatology 1990 criteria for the classification of vasculitis. Arthritis Rheum 1990;33:1065–1067.

11. Gayraud M, Guillevin L, Le Toumelin P, et al. Long term follow up of polyarteritis nodosa, microscopic polyangiitis and Churg-Strauss syndrome. Analysis of four prospective trials including 278 patients. Arthritis Rheum 2001;44:666–675.

12. Guillevin L, Lhote F, Gayraud M, et al. Prognostic factors in polyarteritis nodosa and Churg-Strauss syndrome. A prospective study in 342 patients. Medicine (Baltimore) 1996;75:17–28.

13. De Groot K, Adu D, Savage COS. The value of pulse cyclophosphamide in ANCA-associated vasculitis: meta-analysis and critical review. Nephrol Dial Transplant 2001;16:2018–2027.

TABLE 21C-3. CLINICAL FEATURES OF THE PRIMARY ANTINEUTROPHIL CYTOPLASMIC ANTIBODIES–ASSOCIATED VASCULITIDES.

FEATURE	WEGENER'S GRANULOMATOSIS	MICROSCOPIC POLYANGIITIS	CHURG–STRAUSS SYNDROME
ANCA positivity	80%–90%	70%	50%
ANCA antigen specificity	PR3 > MPO	MPO > PR3	MPO > PR3
Fundamental histology	Leukocytoclastic vasculitis; necrotizing, granulomatous inflammation (rarely seen in renal biopsy specimens)	Leukocytoclastic vasculitis; no granulomatous inflammation	Eosinophilic tissue infiltrates and vasculitis; granulomas have eosinophilic necrosis
Ear/nose/throat	Nasal septal perforation; saddle-nose deformity; conductive or sensorineural hearing loss; subglottic stenosis	Absent or mild	Nasal polyps; allergic rhinitis; conductive hearing loss
Eye	Orbital pseudotumor, scleritis (risk of scleromalacia perforans), episcleritis, uveitis	Occasional eye disease: scleritis, episcleritis, uveitis	Occasional eye disease: scleritis, episcleritis, uveitis
Lung	Nodules, infiltrates, or cavitary lesions; alveolar hemorrhage	Alveolar hemorrhage	Asthma; fleeting infiltrates; alveolar hemorrhage
Kidney	Segmental necrotizing glomerulonephritis; rare granulomatous features	Segmental necrotizing glomerulonephritis	Segmental necrotizing glomerulonephritis
Heart	Occasional valvular lesions	Rare	Heart failure
Peripheral nerve	Vasculitic neuropathy (10%)	Vasculitic neuropathy (58%)	Vasculitic neuropathy (78%)
Eosinophilia	Mild eosinophilia occasionally	None	All

SOURCE: Reproduced with permission from Seo P, Stone JH. The antineutrophil cytoplasmic antibody-associated vasculitides. Am J Med 2004;117:39–50.
ABBREVIATIONS: ANCA, antineutrophil cytoplasmic antibody; MPO, myeloperoxidase; PR3, proteinase 3.

CLINICAL FEATURES

There is substantial overlap in many of the clinical features of the AAVs. In some cases, distinguishing among two or more of these diseases on the basis of clinical features alone is difficult (Table 21C-3).

Upper Respiratory Tract and Ears

Although patients with the CSS or MPA may experience substantial ear, nose, or sinus disease, this pattern of involvement is most characteristic of WG. More than 90% of patients with WG eventually develop upper airway or ear abnormalities. The nasal symptoms of WG include nasal pain and stuffiness, rhinitis, epistaxis, and brown or bloody crusts. Nasal inflammation may lead to septal erosions, septal perforation, or, in many cases, nasal bridge collapse—the "saddle-nose deformity" (Figure 21C-1). The distinction between active WG in the sinuses and secondary infections in the sinuses may be challenging (see Nonmedical Interventions section).

In 60% to 70% of patients with the CSS, allergic rhinitis is the earliest disease manifestation, typically appearing years before the development of full-blown

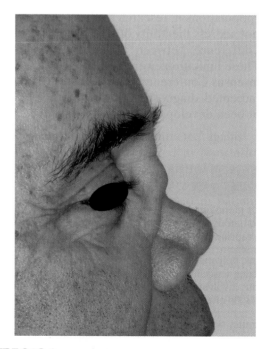

FIGURE 21C-1

Saddle-nose deformity in Wegener's granulomatosis.

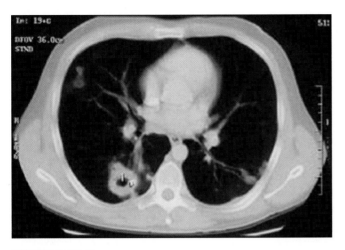

FIGURE 21C-2

Multifocal cavitary nodules in Wegener's granulomatosis.

systemic vasculitis. Rhinitis may be severe and may require serial polypectomies to relieve obstruction and sinusitis. Nasal crusting and conductive hearing loss (due to serous otitis or granulomatous middle ear inflammation) may also occur in the CSS.

Two principal categories of ear disease—conductive and sensorineural hearing loss—are typical of WG. The most common cause of conductive hearing loss may be Eustachian tube dysfunction due to nasopharyngeal disease. Inner ear disease in WG may be associated with sensorineural hearing loss, vestibular dysfunction, or both. In contrast to middle ear disease, the mechanism of inner ear disturbances in WG is poorly understood.

Trachea and Bronchi

Subglottic stenosis and stenotic lesions of the bronchi are potentially serious complications of WG. Subglottic involvement, often asymptomatic initially, becomes apparent as hoarseness, pain, cough, wheezing, or stridor. Thin-cut computed tomographic scans and often direct laryngoscopy are useful in assessing these airway narrowings.

Eyes

Scleritis may lead to necrotizing anterior scleritis (scleromalacia perforans) and blindness. Peripheral ulcerative keratitis may cause the corneal melt syndrome. Other ocular manifestations of AAV include conjunctivitis, episcleritis, and anterior uveitis. In WG, orbital masses termed *pseudotumors* occur in a retrobulbar location in 10% to 15% of patients, causing proptosis, diplopia, or visual loss. Nasolacrimal duct obstruction is most typical of WG.

Lungs

In WG, the pulmonary manifestations range from asymptomatic lung nodules and fleeting (or fixed) pulmonary infiltrates to fulminant alveolar hemorrhage. The nodules are usually multiple, bilateral (Figure 21C-2), and often cavitary. Infiltrates are often misdiagnosed initially as pneumonia.

Pulmonary capillaritis, equally likely to occur in WG and MPA, may lead to lung hemorrhage, hemoptysis, and rapidly changing alveolar infiltrates (Figure 21C-3). Patients with MPA may also develop interstitial fibrosis of the lungs.

Obstructive airway disease and fleeting pulmonary infiltrates are the hallmarks of the CSS. The majority of patients report the new onset of asthma months to years before the appearance of overt vasculitis. Following resolution of the vasculitic phase with treatment, many patients with CSS suffer from steroid-dependent asthma.

Kidneys

The most feared clinical presentation of renal disease among the AAVs is rapidly progressive glomerulonephritis. More than 75% of patients with WG will eventually develop renal involvement. The progression of the disease often appears to accelerate once kidney involvement is apparent. In MPA, renal disease may have a more indolent course, and renal biopsies typically demonstrate more sclerosis and fibrosis than do specimens from patients with WG. Severe renal disease in CSS is very rare. "Renal-limited" vasculitis is pauci-immune glomerulonephritis (see Pathology section) associated with ANCA, usually directed against MPO, without evidence of disease in other organs. ANCA-associated

21

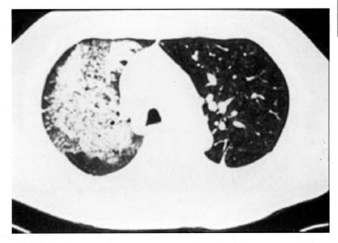

FIGURE 21C-3

Alveolar hemorrhage in microscopic polyangiitis.

renal disease may lead to fibrotic crescents and other scarring within the kidney. Subsequent disease flares and progression of renal dysfunction through hyperfiltration may lead to end-stage renal disease.

Arthritis/Arthralgias

Inflammatory joint complaints, often migratory and oligoarticular in nature, occur in at least 60% of patients with AAV. Joint problems are frequently the presenting complaint, but the diagnosis is seldom made until other symptoms are manifest. The combination of joint complaints, cutaneous nodules (frequently mistaken for rheumatoid nodules), and the high frequency of rheumatoid factor positivity among patients with AAV (approximately one third are rheumatoid factor positive) often lead to the misdiagnosis of rheumatoid arthritis early in the disease course. Arthralgias are more common than frank arthritis. The recurrence of musculoskeletal complaints in a patient in remission often marks the start of a disease flare.

Skin

In both the CSS and WG, cutaneous nodules may occur at sites that are also common locations for rheumatoid nodules, particularly the olecranon region (Figure 21C-4). Skin findings in the AAVs also include all of the potential manifestations of cutaneous vasculitis: palpable purpura, vesiculobullous lesions, papules, ulcers, digital infarctions, and splinter hemorrhages.

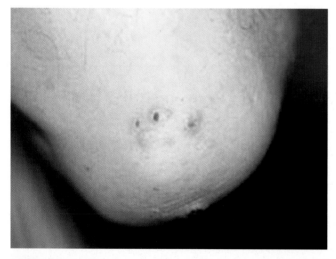

FIGURE 21C-4

Churg–Strauss granulomas, that is, cutaneous extravascular necrotizing granulomas, occurring over the elbow. These lesions may occur in both the Churg–Strauss syndrome and Wegener's granulomatosis, mimicking rheumatoid nodules.

Nervous System

Vasculitic neuropathy may lead to a devastating mononeuritis multiplex or a disabling sensory polyneuropathy. Mononeuritis multiplex occurs more commonly in the CSS [up to 78% of patients (11)] and MPA (up to 58%) than in WG. Central nervous system abnormalities occur in approximately 8% of patients with WG, usually in the form of cranial neuropathies, mass lesions, or pachymeningitis. The frequency of parenchymal brain involvement in AAV, though not yet known with certainty and generally regarded as rare, has been reported. Central nervous system disease generally occurs only when more typical disease manifestations are present elsewhere.

Heart

The CSS is the type of AAV that is most likely to involve the heart, usually in the form of rapid-onset heart failure. Cardiac complications in WG and MPA are both less common and more difficult to attribute with certainty to the underlying disease. Focal cardiac valvular lesions, valvular insufficiency, pericarditis, and coronary arteritis have been described in WG.

Gastrointestinal Tract

Eosinophilic gastroenteritis often precedes the frank vasculitic phase of the CSS. Among patients with either the CSS or MPA, unexplained abdominal pain occurs in up to one third of patients and may lead to ischemic bowel. Gastrointestinal involvement is less common in WG.

Blood

Eosinophilia (before treatment) is a sine qua non of the CSS. Eosinophil counts are usually sensitive markers of disease flares, but respond very quickly (within 24 hours) to treatment with high doses of glucocorticoids. Tissue infiltration by eosinophils, however, may remain. Mild eosinophilia (rarely more than 15% of the total white blood cell count) may also occur in WG. Most patients with CSS also have elevated serum immunoglobulin E levels. In addition to ANCA, nonspecific autoantibodies, such as antinuclear antibodies and rheumatoid factor, also occur in high percentages of patients with AAV.

Other

Antineutrophil cytoplasmic antibodies-associated vasculitides rarely affect the parotid gland, pulmonary artery, breast, or genitourinary organs. Involvement of these organs by AAV is usually an unexpected finding on biopsies performed to exclude other diseases, particularly cancer and infection.

PATHOLOGY

Fibrinoid necrosis, a pathological hallmark of AAV, may be found in a variety of vasculitic (and nonvasculitic) conditions, such as polyarteritis nodosa, scleroderma renal crisis, systemic lupus erythematosus, and malignant hypertension. Both vasculitic and necrotizing granulomatous features, which do not invariably coexist, may be confirmed in lung biopsy specimens. In addition, pulmonary WG frequently demonstrates an extensive, nonspecific inflammatory background. Coalescence of such neutrophilic microabscesses leads to extensive regions of "geographic" necrosis. Palisading granulomas, scattered giant cells, and poorly formed granulomas may also be found in WG.

Churg–Strauss syndrome typically evolves through three phases, with corresponding pathological findings. In the first phase, allergy, asthma, and other atopic symptoms predominate. In the second, eosinophilic infiltration occurs in the lung and other organs (eosinophilic pneumonia, eosinophilic gastroenteritis; Figure 21C-5). In the third phase, vasculitis ensues. Curiously, at the time the vasculitic phase begins, patients' asthma often improves significantly. The histopathological findings in CSS in the lung include eosinophilic infiltrates; extensive areas of necrosis (reminiscent of the geographic necrosis in WG); a granulomatous vasculitis of small arteries and veins, associated with striking eosinophilic infiltration. In contrast to WG and MPA, lymphadenopathy (with overwhelming eosinophilic infiltration into the lymph nodes), is frequently found in CSS.

The interstitial lung disease of MPA resembles usual interstitial pneumonitis (UIP), with the exception that necrosis of the alveolar septae and areas of hemorrhage can occur. More characteristic findings in MPA, however, reveal nonspecific infiltrates or alveolar hemorrhage. Vasculitis of the pulmonary capillaries may be difficult to prove.

Renal disease in the AAVs is associated with focal, segmental lysis of glomerular tufts, disruption of the basement membrane, and accumulation of fibrinoid material (i.e., fibrinoid necrosis). Crescents in Bowman's space develop as a result of spillage of inflammatory mediators across the ruptured glomerular capillaries, accumulation of macrophages, and epithelial cell proliferation. Thrombotic changes in the glomerular capillary loops are among the earliest histologic changes. Acute tubular necrosis and tubulointerstitial nephritis are also seen commonly. Immunofluorescence studies of renal biopsy specimens demonstrate scant deposition of immunoglobulin and complement, hence the term pauci-immune glomerulonephritis.

Tissue samples from involved areas of the upper respiratory tract (nose, sinuses, and subglottic region) in WG often reveal only acute and chronic inflammation. Nevertheless, these biopsies are easier to obtain than are biopsies of the lung and kidney. Moreover, the combination of these pathological findings (nondiagnostic in and of themselves) and compatible clinical features (e.g., pulmonary nodules and PR3-ANCA) may yield the diagnosis in some cases. Upper respiratory tract biopsies are therefore worth undertaking in patients with significant upper respiratory involvement.

FIGURE 21C-5

Eosinophilic infiltration of a salivary gland in a patient with the Churg–Strauss syndrome. The arrows in panel B indicate the formation of a Churg-Strauss granuloma, with multinucleated giant cells, palisading histiocytes, and scattered eosinophils.

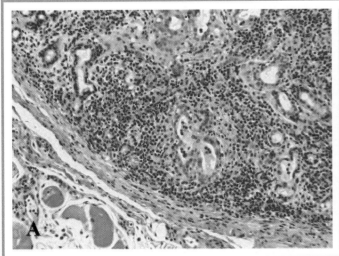
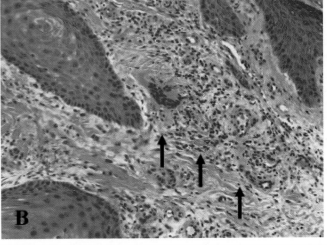

21

ANTINEUTROPHIL CYTOPLASMIC ANTIBODIES

The Antigens

Proteinase-3, a 29-kDa serine protease, is found in the azurophilic granules of neutrophils and peroxidase-positive lysosomes of monocytes. MPO, which constitutes nearly 5% of the total protein content of the neutrophil, is localized to the same cellular compartments as PR3. The protein is a covalently linked dimer with a molecular weight of 140 kDa. The autoantibodies directed against PR3 and MPO are directed against multiple epitopes. Sera from different patients may recognize different epitopes. All ANCA, however, recognize restricted epitopes of PR3 involving its catalytic site.

Clinical Testing for Antineutrophil Cytoplasmic Antibodies

Two types of assays for ANCA—immunofluorescence and enzyme immunoassay—are now in common use. Capture enzyme immunoassays may offer some advantages over the more widely available tests, but are currently performed only in specialty centers.

With immunofluorescence, three principal patterns of fluorescence are recognized: the cytoplasmic (C-ANCA), perinuclear (P-ANCA), and "atypical" patterns. In patients with vasculitis, the C-ANCA pattern usually corresponds to the detection of PR3-ANCA by enzyme immunoassay. The combination of a C-ANCA pattern on immunofluorescence testing and PR3-ANCA is associated most strongly with WG. The P-ANCA pattern, which usually corresponds to the presence of MPO-ANCA in vasculitis patients, occurs in approximately 10% of patients with WG, but is more typical of MPA, the CSS, and renal-limited vasculitis. The great majority of patients with drug-induced AAVs are P-ANCA positive, often with very high titers of MPO-ANCA.

Regardless of the immunofluorescence pattern, positive immunofluorescence assays should be confirmed by the performance of enzyme immunoassays for the specific antibodies associated with vasculitis: PR3- and MPO-ANCA. Even for C-ANCA, the positive predictive value for WG is only in the range of 45% to 50% (12,13).

Clinical Utility of Antineutrophil Cytoplasmic Antibody Serologies

Despite advances in ANCA testing techniques, the cornerstone of diagnosis in WG remains the rigorous interpretation of histopathological specimens within the overall clinical context. When biopsy specimens are nondiagnostic, ANCA assays provide an important adjunct to diagnosis (Table 21C-4).

In the proper clinical setting, a positive ANCA assay greatly increases the likelihood that a form of AAV is present. Most series indicate that up to 10% to 20% of patients with active, untreated WG are ANCA negative. For patients with limited WG, 30% or more of patients lack ANCA. Approximately 70% of patients with MPA and 50% of those with CSS (higher in some series) have ANCA.

TABLE 21C-4. CLINICAL UTILITY OF ANTINEUTROPHIL CYTOPLASMIC ANTIBODY TESTING.

Positive ANCA serologies are extremely useful in suggesting the diagnosis in the proper clinical setting.

Positive immunofluorescence assays without confirmatory enzyme immunoassays for anti-PR3 or anti-MPO antibodies are of limited utility.

Histopathology remains the gold standard for diagnosis in most cases.

Negative ANCA assays do not exclude ANCA-associated vasculitis because between 10% and 50% of patients with ANCA-associated vasculitis (depending on the particular disease) may be ANCA-negative.

Persistence of ANCA in the absence of clinical indications of active disease does not indicate a need for continued treatment.

In a patient who was ANCA-positive during active disease, persistent ANCA-negativity provides reassurance—but no guarantee—that the disease is not active. If disease flares occur in such patients, they are usually limited.

A patient who becomes ANCA-positive again following a period of clinical quiescence associated with negative ANCA assays may be at an increased risk for a disease flare. The temporal correlation between the return of ANCA and a disease flare, however, is poor.

Treatment of ANCA-associated vasculitis should never be predicated upon ANCA serologies or titers alone.

ABBREVIATIONS: ANCA, antineutrophil cytoplasmic antibody; MPO, myeloperoxidase; PR3, proteinase 3.

Utility of Antineutrophil Cytoplasmic Antibody Assays following Disease Activity and in Predicting Flares

In general, ANCA titers have imperfect correlations with disease activity. In one study, the positive predictive value of a rise in ANCA titers as measured by immunofluorescence was only 57% in a prospective study, compared with 71% for enzyme immunoassay (14). Moreover, among patients with an elevation of ANCA titers measured by enzyme immunoassay, only 39% suffered disease flares within 6 months. A more recent prospective study (15) showed that increases in PR3-ANCA levels did not predict disease relapses. The proportion of patients who relapsed within 1 year following an increase in ANCA levels was only 40%. Although some studies suggest that a rise in ANCA titer is a risk factor for a flare, the temporal relationship between a rise in ANCA titers and the development of disease activity requiring treatment is very poor, with months to years between these two events. Thus, the adjustment of immunosuppressive medications based solely on the rise or fall of ANCA titers is never justified.

PATHOPHYSIOLOGY

The AAVs are complex disorders mediated by the immune system in which tissue injury results from the interplay between an initiating inflammatory event and a highly specific pathogenic immune response (i.e., the production of ANCA) to previously shielded epitopes of neutrophil granule proteins. ANCAs produce tissue damage via interactions with primed neutrophils and endothelial cells. The hypothesis, supported strongly by in vitro evidence, is that the antibodies induce a necrotizing vasculitis by inciting a respiratory burst and degranulation of leukocytes (neutrophils and monocytes), leading to endothelial injury. The initial events in the process require the priming of leukocytes by cytokines and perhaps other stimuli, leading to the expression of PR3 and MPO on the cell surface. The effects of ANCAs are determined by the state of neutrophil activation. ANCAs may constitutively activate primed neutrophils and promote binding of the primed neutrophils to the vascular endothelium, degranulation, and the release of neutrophil chemoattractants, hence creating an autoamplifying loop.

There is now substantial evidence that ANCAs are directly involved in the widespread tissue damage that is the hallmark of the AAVs. Recombinant activating gene 2 (RAG-2)–deficient mice that receive anti-MPO antibodies develop clinical features consistent with AAV, including crescentic glomerulonephritis and systemic necrotizing vasculitis (16). In humans, the evidence is indirect. Propylthiouracil is known to accumulate within neutrophil granules and may lead to a drug-induced AAV (17), possibly by increasing the immunogenicity of MPO (leading to the characteristically high titers of MPO-ANCA seen in this disease).

In addition to ANCA, multiple other elements of the immune system participate in the pathophysiology of these diseases. If the autoantibody response leading to ANCA production follows the exposure of a cryptic epitope, epitope spreading may then generalize the antibody response to the rest of the molecule. This hypothesis implies a prominent role for the T cell in the pathogenesis of the AAVs. Moreover, most patients with AAVs produce isotype-switched IgG ANCA, implying a secondary immune response driven by T cells. Growing evidence, particularly data from clinical studies (18), now also implicates B cells as important participants in the inflammation of AAV. As the precursors of plasma cells (which produce ANCA), B cells now seem a logical therapeutic target in AAV. In addition to disrupting ANCA production, however, interference with B-cell function may also ameliorate AAV by disabling critical B cell/T cell interactions, by removing the antigen presenting function of B cells, and perhaps other mechanisms. B-cell depletion is the focus of ongoing randomized trials involving patients with WG and MPA.

The pathophysiology of CSS likely bears many similarities to that of WG and MPA, albeit ANCA are less common in CSS. In the CSS, however, relatively little is currently understood about the special role played by the eosinophil in that disease.

DIFFERENTIAL DIAGNOSIS

Because of their multiorgan system nature, the differential diagnosis of AAV is lengthy. One frequently challenging task is the differentiation of these diseases from other forms of vasculitis. Indeed, clear distinctions are often impossible between WG and MPA, because granulomatous inflammation is not detected on all biopsy specimens from patients with WG. Distinguishing the AAVs from other forms of vasculitis is often more critical because the specific treatments differ according to diagnosis. In addition, the AAVs must be distinguished from a host of other disorders associated with inflammation and multiorgan system dysfunction. The differential diagnosis of AAV is shown in Table 21C-5.

Churg–Strauss syndrome has an additional major branch of its differential diagnosis because of the eosinophilia associated with the disease. Allergic bronchopulmonary aspergillosis, chronic eosinophilic pneumonia, eosinophilic gastroenteritis, eosinophilic fasciitis, the hypereosinophil syndrome, and eosinophilic leukemias must all be excluded.

12. Stone JH, Talor M, Stebbing J, et al. Test characteristics of immunofluorescence and ELISA tests in 856 consecutive patients with possible ANCA-associated conditions. Arthritis Care Res 2000;13:424–434.

13. Boomsma MM, Stegeman CA, van der Leij MJ, et al. Prediction of relapses in Wegener's granulomatosis by measurement of antineutrophil cytoplasmic antibody levels: a prospective study. Arthritis Rheum 2000;43:2025–2033.

14. Finkielman JD, Merkel PA, Schroeder D, et al. Antineutrophil cytoplasmic antibodies against proteinase 3 do not predict disease relapses in Wegener's granulomatosis. Ann Intern Med 2007, (in press).

15. Xiao H, Heeringa P, Hu P, et al. Antineutrophil cytoplasmic autoantibodies specific for myeloperoxidase cause glomerulonephritis and vasculitis in mice. J Clin Invest 2002;110:955–963.

16. Choi HK, Merkel PA, Walker AM, et al. Drug-associated antineutrophil cytoplasmic antibody-positive vasculitis: prevalence among patients with high titers of antimyeloperoxidase antibodies. Arthritis Rheum 2000;43:405–413.

17. Keogh KA, Ytterberg SR, Fervenza FC, et al. Rituximab for refractory Wegener's granulomatosis: report of a prospective, open-label pilot trial. Am J Respir Crit Care Med 2006;173:180–187.

18. Wung PK, Stone JH. Therapeutics for Wegener's granulomatosis. Nat Clin Pract Rheumatol 2006;2:192–200.

19. WGET Research Group. Design of the Wegener's Granulomatosis Etanercept Trial (WGET). Control Clin Trials 2002;23:450–468.

20. Jayne D, Rasmussen N, Andrassy K, et al. A randomized trial of maintenance therapy for vasculitis associated with antineutrophil cytoplasmic autoantibodies. N Engl J Med 2003;349:36–44.

21. Langford CA, Talar-Williams C, Barron KS, et al. A staged approach to the treatment of Wegener's granulomatosis: induction of remission with glucocorticoids and daily cyclophosphamide switching to methotrexate for remission maintenance. Arthritis Rheum 1999;42:2666–2673.

22. The WGET Research Group. Etanercept in addition to standard therapy in patients with Wegener's granulomatosis. N Engl J Med 2005;352:351–361.

23. Stone JH, Holbrook JT, Tibbs A, et al. Solid malignancies in the Wegener's granulomatosis Etanercept trial. Arthritis Rheum 2006;54:1608–1618.

24. Hoffman GS, Thomas-Golbanov CK, et al. Treatment of subglottic stenosis, due to Wegener's granulomatosis, with intralesional corticosteroids and dilation. J Rheumatol 2003;30:1017–1021.

25. Booth AD, Almond MK, Burns A, et al. Outcome of ANCA-associated renal vasculitis: a 5-year retrospective study. Am J Kidney Dis 2003;41:776–784.

26. Seo P, Min Y-I, Holbrook JT, et al. Damage from Wegener's granulomatosis and its treatment: prospective data from the Wegener's Granulomatosis Etanercept Trial. Arthritis Rheum 2005;52:2168–2178.

Vasculitides
D. Immune Complex–Mediated Vasculitis

Philip Seo, MD, MHS

- Pathogenic immune complexes formed between antigen and antibodies tend to occur during periods of antigen excess. When the immune complexes precipitate into the tissues, they fix complement, leading to an intense immune reaction.
- In immune complex vasculitis, immune complexes deposit in the vascular endothelium or in capillary beds, such as those found in the skin, kidneys, or lungs.
- The most common skin manifestation of small vessel vasculitis is palpable purpura.
- Hypersensitivity vasculitis is characterized by immune complex deposition in capillaries, postcapillary venules, and arterioles. The usual causes are either

medications (e.g., penicillins, sulfonamides, or cephalosporins) or infections.
- Cryoglobulinemic vasculitis is usually caused by hepatitis C infections. The antigens involved in cryoglobulinemic vasculitis are portions of the hepatitis C virus (HCV) virion. The relevant antibodies are both IgG and IgM, leading to the designation "mixed" cryoglobulinemia.
- Henoch–Schönlein purpura is associated strongly with IgA deposition within blood vessel walls.
- Hypocomplementemic urticarial vasculitis has many features that overlap with systemic lupus erythematosus.

Exposure to a foreign antigen activates an adaptive immune response that leads to the production of antigen-specific antibodies. The combination of antibody with antigen creates immune complexes that neutralize the foreign antigen, and allow it to be cleared safely by the reticuloendothelial system. This complex system, however, contains within it the potential for failure. If the antibody response is just right, these immune complexes may escape early detection, and instead imbed themselves into joints and blood vessels. These immune complexes can then activate complement, leading to local inflammation. Immune complexes deposited in the kidneys, for example, create glomerulonephritis (1). Those deposited in the synovium lead to arthritis. If the immune complexes are found in the blood vessels, vasculitis is the result.

In pathology, the word *vasculitis* describes inflammation within blood vessel walls. This process frequently leads to cellular destruction, damage to the vascular structures, and compromise of blood flow to organs supplied by the involved vessels, resulting in organ compromise. Several forms of vasculitis are the direct result of immune complex deposition. This chapter outlines

several examples of immune complex–mediated vasculitis and highlights some common themes.

PATHOPHYSIOLOGY

In 1903, Maurice Arthus noted that intradermal injection of a rabbit with horse serum resulted in a cutaneous inflammatory reaction that evolved into localized tissue necrosis (2). The reaction was faster, he observed, if the animal had been previously exposed to horse serum. This response, now known as the Arthus reaction, forms the basis of our understanding of immune complex–mediated diseases. In the Arthus model, injection of the horse serum leads to immune complex formation that initiates complement activation and an influx of inflammatory cells. In the areas of most intense inflammation, in situ thrombosis formation can lead to tissue ischemia and hemorrhagic infarction.

In general, immune complexes are not pathogenic. Their immunogenicity is governed by a large number of factors, including antigen load, antibody response, the efficiency of the reticuloendothelial system in the clearance of immune complexes, physical properties of the blood vessels (including flow dynamics and previous endothelial damage), and the solubility of the immune complexes themselves.

Immune complex solubility is determined by the ratio of antibody to antigen. When antibody and antigen are present in equal proportion, large immune complexes are formed, which are identified easily and removed by the reticuloendothelial system. When there is an excess of antibody, small immune complexes are formed, which remain in solution, and do not elicit an immune response. When there is a slight excess of antigen, however, the immune complexes precipitate from solution, and become trapped in characteristic areas—either the capillary beds (such as those found in the skin, kidneys, or lungs), or the endothelium of medium-sized blood vessels previously damaged by turbulent blood flow.

When the immune complexes precipitate into the tissues, they fix complement, leading to an intense immune reaction. Complement fixation and local inflammation recruit neutrophils, which attempt to engulf the immune complexes. During this process, the neutrophils degranulate, releasing lysosomal enzymes and oxygen free radicals that cause tissue necrosis.

The inciting antigen can be from numerous sources. In infective endocarditis, the antibody response, formed against bacterial antigens, can lead to painful cutaneous lesions known as Osler nodes. In systemic lupus erythematosus (SLE), antibodies form against nuclear components (e.g., DNA and histones) that are released during tissue injury. Certain forms of malignancy can be associated with immune complex formation, with antibodies directed against tumor-associated antigens. Immune complexes may also form in response to a large number of drugs, including penicillin and sulfonamides.

CLINICAL SYNDROMES

Hypersensitivity Vasculitis

Definition

Hypersensitivity reactions were first noted in patients who were treated with antitoxin derived from horse serum. Such patients developed an antibody response to the horse antigens, which led to a characteristic syndrome of fever, joint pain, and rash now known as serum sickness.

Hypersensitivity vasculitis refers to a heterogeneous group of syndromes (including serum sickness and drug-induced vasculitis) characterized by immune complex deposition in capillaries, postcapillary venules, and arterioles. This is the most common form of vasculitis. Although multiple agents have been implicated, including penicillins, sulfonamides, and cephalosporins, the inciting agent cannot always be identified.

In 1990, the American College of Rheumatology proposed the following five criteria for the classification of hypersensitivity vasculitis in an adult (3):

- Age >16 years
- Use of a possible offending medication in temporal relation to the symptoms
- Palpable purpura
- Maculopapular rash
- Biopsy of a skin lesion showing neutrophils around an arteriole or venule

The presence of three or more criteria has a sensitivity of 71% and specificity of 84% for the diagnosis of hypersensitivity vasculitis.

Hypersensitivity vasculitis that occurs without systemic manifestations is sometimes referred to as cutaneous vasculitis or *cutaneous leukocytoclastic angiitis*. The term *serum sickness*, on the other hand, is reserved to describe a systemic illness, including rash and arthralgias, which occurs 1 to 2 weeks after exposure to a drug or foreign antigen.

Clinical Presentation

Most patients with hypersensitivity vasculitis will develop cutaneous manifestations, the most common of which is purpura (Figure 21D-1). These lesions are

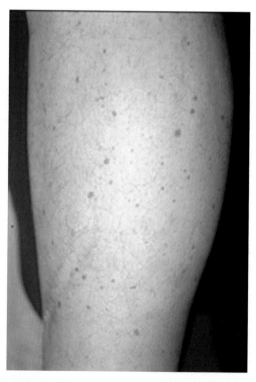

FIGURE 21D-1

Palpable purpura in a patient with hypersensitivity vasculitis. (Courtesy of Dr. John Stone.)

distributed usually in a symmetric fashion over dependent regions of the body, particularly the lower legs (and, in recumbent patients, over the buttocks) because of the increased hydrostatic pressure in such areas. Purpuric lesions are not always palpable to the touch. The term *palpable purpura* is essentially synonymous with small vessel vasculitis, but does not necessarily imply an immune complex–mediated pathophysiology; pauci-immune forms of vasculitis, such as Wegener's granulomatosis, microscopic polyangiitis, and the Churg–Strauss syndrome, for example, may present with identical skin findings (see Chapter 21C).

Diagnosis

Biopsy is the diagnostic method of choice. Cutaneous biopsies are associated with low morbidity, and are generally sufficient to confirm one's clinical suspicion. Light microscopy examination of a hematoxylin and eosin (H&E) preparation will demonstrate an inflammatory infiltrate primarily composed of mononuclear or polymorphonuclear cells, as well as telltale signs of small vessel vasculitis: leukocyte diapedesis, karyorrhexis, and leukocytoclasis. Although H&E preparations are adequate for confirming the presence of vasculitis, they often provide insufficient data for a precise diagnosis. In cases of immune complex–mediated vasculitis, direct immunofluorescence (DIF) studies on the biopsy demonstrate the types of immunoreactants (i.e., immunoglobulin and complement proteins) present at the site of disease. Although direct immunofluorescence requires a biopsy of a second cutaneous site, this procedure is critical in many cases to differentiating the array of conditions associated with cutaneous vasculitis. Biopsy is especially useful to exclude other causes of vascular injury, including embolism and hypercoagulability states, which may demonstrate evidence of erythrocyte extravasation but not immune complex deposition. Of course, the presence of small vessel vasculitis does not always confirm the presence of a primary autoimmune disease; malignancy, for example, can also be associated with leukocytoclastic vasculitis. All biopsies, therefore, must be evaluated in the appropriate clinical context.

Therapy

Removal of the inciting agent is the only reliable therapy. In patients who have been exposed to multiple medications, determining the inciting agent may be difficult, and may require withdrawal of multiple agents simultaneously until the syndrome clears, typically in 1 to 2 weeks. Immunosuppression with glucocorticoids should be reserved for patients with particularly fulminant disease, and may be discontinued usually within several weeks.

Prognosis

The prognosis for patients with hypersensitivity vasculitis depends on the nature of the inciting agent. In the case of drug-induced vasculitis, multiple agents may need to be discontinued and re-introduced gradually. Approximately half of cases of isolated cutaneous angiitis do not have an obvious cause. Many such cases are associated with a relapsing and remitting course, but remain restricted to the skin and do not mandate aggressive immunosuppressive therapy.

Cryoglobulinemic Vasculitis
Definition

In 1933, Wintrobe and Buell noted that when serum from a patient with a hyperviscosity syndrome due to multiple myeloma was held at temperatures less than 37°C, a protein precipitate formed (4). In 1947, this "cold precipitable serum globulin" was referred to for the first time as a "cryoglobulin." Cryoglobulins are immune complexes that are characterized by their tendency to precipitate from serum under conditions of cold. Cryoglobulins, detectable to a varying degree in a wide array of inflammatory conditions, are not invariably pathogenic. In some patients, however, cryoglobulins deposit in the small- and medium-sized blood vessels and activate complement, leading to cryoglobulinemic vasculitis (5).

Three major types of cryoglobulinemia are recognized, defined by the specific kinds of immunoglobulins with which they are associated. Type I cryoglobulinemia, characterized by a monoclonal gammopathy (generally IgG or IgM), can be associated with Waldenström's macroglobulinemia or, less frequently, multiple myeloma. Type I IgA cryoglobulinemia has also been described, although this is quite rare. In contrast to the monoclonal nature of type I cryoglobulinemia, type II and type III cryoglobulinemias are known as "mixed" cryoglobulinemias because they are comprised of both IgG and IgM. In most cases of type II cryoglobulinemia, more than 90% of which are caused by hepatitis C infections, the cryoproteins consist of monoclonal IgM and polyclonal IgG. Cases of type II cryoglobulinemia not associated with hepatitis C infections are sometimes termed "mixed essential" cryoglobulinemia. Such cases may be associated with a still undefined viral infection. Type III cryoglobulinemia, typically associated with polyclonal IgG and polyclonal IgM, is associated with many forms of chronic inflammation, including infection and autoimmune disease. Not every form of cryoglobulinemia fits neatly into this classification system; cryoglobulins can, for example, have an oligoclonal antibody component.

21

reveal florid IgA deposition. In the proper clinical setting, this finding is diagnostic of HSP. Other forms of small vessel vasculitis may have small quantities of IgA within blood vessels, but IgA is not the predominant immunoreactant in such cases.

Therapy

In mild cases of HSP, no specific therapy is necessary. Even for patients with glomerulonephritis, it has been difficult to demonstrate that treatment with glucocorticoids or immunosuppressive agents significantly alters outcomes. Despite this, it may be prudent to treat aggressive renal involvement with an immunosuppressive regimen, including high-dose glucocorticoids and another immunosuppressive agent such as cyclophosphamide, azathioprine, or mycophenolate mofetil, depending on disease severity (8). In patients with renal involvement, anecdotal evidence suggests that plasmapheresis and intravenous immunoglobulin may also be beneficial, particularly in patients who are refractory to standard immunosuppressive regimens.

Prognosis

Recurrences of skin disease, often comprised of multiple episodes occurring over many months, are not unusual. Generally, however, even in patients with recurrent disease, the rule is for the disorder to subside and to resolve completely over a few months to a year. In a minority of patients, some evidence of permanent renal damage persists in the form of proteinuria and hematuria. Only a small minority, probably well under 5%, develop renal failure as a result of HSP.

Hypocomplementemic Urticarial Vasculitis Syndrome

Definition

The study of urticaria is hampered by multiple terms that sound similar but describe different types of diseases. The word *urticaria* is most frequently used to describe *acute urticaria*, an IgE-mediated hypersensitivity reaction to a variety of stimuli, including medications, infection, and other triggers. Acute urticaria manifests as pruritic wheals that resolve days after the allergen is removed. *Chronic urticaria* is an autoimmune condition that is probably driven by an autoantigen. This form of urticaria may require immunosuppressive therapy in addition to antihistamines to prevent recurrence (9).

Urticarial vasculitis describes a form of small vessel vasculitis that is characterized by the appearance of urticarial wheals. *Normocomplementemic urticarial vasculitis* is most often simply an example of hypersensitivity vasculitis in which the principal skin manifestation is urticaria. Normocomplementemic urticarial vasculitis tends to be self-limited, as is the case with hypersensitivity vasculitis. In contrast, urticarial vasculitis associated with hypocomplementemia is much more likely to constitute a significant and persistent clinical problem.

Two categories of urticarial vasculitis associated with hypocomplementemia are recognized. The distinctions between these two categories are not always sharp, and both categories also share a number of features with systemic lupus erythematosus. The first category, known simply as hypocomplementemic urticarial vasculitis, refers to cutaneous vasculitis associated with low levels of serum complement (C3 and C4). The diagnosis of hypocomplementemic urticarial vasculitis is predicated upon the exclusion of other disorders that may present in a similar fashion, particularly cryoglobulinemia and SLE. The second category—a more specific but still loosely defined entity known as the *hypocomplementemic urticarial vasculitis syndrome* (HUVS)—consists of the constellation of low complement levels and urticaria for a period of at least 6 months, as well as some or all of the following: arthritis, glomerulonephritis, uveitis, angioedema, chronic obstructive pulmonary disease, pleurisy, or pericarditis.

Clinical Presentation

Although the lesions associated with chronic urticaria and urticarial vasculitis are similar in appearance, certain differences help differentiate these two conditions. In urticarial vasculitis, the urticaria typically have a purpuric quality, indicative of small blood vessel damage and red blood cell extravasation (Figure 21D-4). Unlike common urticaria, the lesions of urticarial vasculitis are frequently associated with moderate pain, burning, and

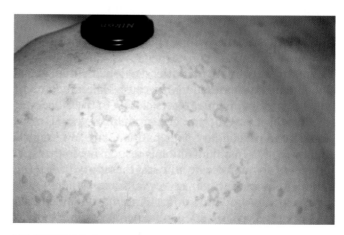

FIGURE 21D-4

Urticarial vasculitis. (Courtesy of Dr. John Stone.)

tenderness, in addition to pruritus. Whereas common urticaria typically resolve completely within 24 to 48 hours, the lesions of urticarial vasculitis may take days to resolve completely and often worsen without therapy. Arthralgias and myalgias are common in urticarial vasculitis. As noted above, patients with HUVS may also develop glomerulonephritis, pulmonary manifestations (particularly obstructive airway disease), and other findings. Gastrointestinal, cardiovascular, and neurologic manifestations are uncommon, but have been reported. There is striking overlap between HUVS and SLE, and patients will frequently have characteristics of both, although angioedema and COPD are more common in HUVS.

Diagnosis

Biopsy of an urticarial wheal in UV will demonstrate evidence of leukocytoclastic vasculitis, including injury to the endothelial cells of the postcapillary venules, erythrocyte extravasation, leukocytoclasis, fibrin deposition, and a perivascular neutrophilic (or less commonly, lymphocytic) infiltrate. Direct immunofluorescence demonstrates immune complex deposition around blood vessels in the superficial dermis and striking deposition of immunoglobulins and complement along the dermal–epidermal junction (Figure 21D-5). The "interface dermatitis" is identical to that observed in lupus—a histopathological finding termed the *lupus band test*. In the proper setting, these findings (interface dermatitis as well as immunoreactant deposition within blood vessels) are diagnostic of hypocomplementemic urticarial vasculitis. HUVS, in contrast, is a clinical diagnosis based not only on the presence of urticarial vasculitis but also the occurrence of typical features in extracutaneous organ systems.

Therapy

Some cases of hypocomplementemic urticarial vasculitis respond to therapies commonly used for the treatment of SLE, including low-dose prednisone, hydroxychloroquine, dapsone, or other immunomodulatory agents. There is anecdotal evidence that antihistamines, calcium channel antagonists, doxepin, methotrexate, indomethacin, colchicine, and pentoxifylline are effective in some cases. Serious cases, particularly those presenting with glomerulonephritis or other forms of serious organ involvement, may require treatment with high doses of glucocorticoids and cytotoxic agents. Both chronic obstructive pulmonary disease (COPD) and cardiac valvular abnormalities are associated with HUVS, and may require specific treatment as well.

Prognosis

The prognosis of HUVS is frequently linked to the disorder with which it is associated. SLE, COPD, angioedema, and valvular abnormalities are all known to occur in association with this disorder, and in such cases, may strongly influence both quality and quantity of life.

SUMMARY

The immune complex–mediated vasculitides are a clinically heterogeneous group of disorders linked by inefficient, defective, or dysregulated clearance of immune complexes by the reticuloendothelial system. Biopsy of an involved organ is frequently helpful in establishing the diagnosis. Direct immunofluorescence studies of involved blood vessels demonstrate characteristic patterns of immunoglobulin and complement deposition, which may be particularly useful in distinguishing these diseases. The prognosis of patients with immune complex–mediated vasculitis is tied closely to the ability to identify and to treat the underlying cause of the immune response.

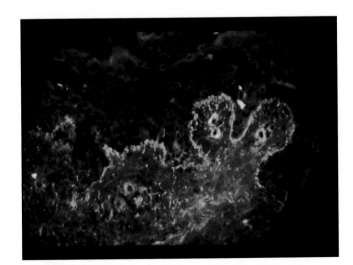

FIGURE 21D-5

Direct immunofluorescence of a skin biopsy in urticarial vasculitis. The immunostaining shows immunoreactant deposition within small blood vessels in the superficial dermis, and florid deposition along the dermal–epidermal junction. (Courtesy of Dr. John Stone.)

REFERENCES

1. Nangaku M, Couser WG. Mechanisms of immune-deposit formation and the mediation of immune renal injury. Clin Exp Nephrol 2005;9:183–191.
2. Arthus M. Injections repetees de serum de cheval cuez le lapin. Seances et Memoire de la Societe de Biologie 1903; 55:817–825.

3. Calabrese LH, Michel BA, Bloch DA, et al. The American College of Rheumatology 1990 criteria for the classification of hypersensitivity vasculitis. Arthritis Rheum 1990;33: 1108–1113.

4. Wintrobe MM, Buell MV. Hyperproteinemia associated with multiple myeloma: with report of a case in which an extraordinary hyperproteinemia was associated with thrombosis of the retinal veins and symptoms suggesting Raynaud's disease. Bulletin Johns Hopkins Hosp 1933; 52:156.

5. Ferri C, Mascia MT. Cryoglobulinemic vasculitis. Curr Opin Rheumatol 2006;18:54–63.

6. Mills JA, Michel BA, Bloch DA, et al. The American College of Rheumatology 1990 criteria for the classification of Henoch-Schönlein purpura. Arthritis Rheum 1990; 33:1114–1121.

7. Blanco R, Martinez-Taboada VM, Rodriguez-Valverde V, Garcia-Fuentes M, Gonzalez-Gay MA. Henoch-Schonlein purpura in adulthood and childhood: two different expressions of the same syndrome. Arthritis Rheum 1997;40:859–864.

8. Flynn JT, Smoyer WE, Bunchman TE, Kershaw DB, Sedman AB. Treatment of Henoch-Schonlein purpura glomerulonephritis in children with high-dose corticosteroids plus oral cyclophosphamide. Am J Nephrol 2001;21:128– 133.

9. Davis MD, Brewer JD. Urticarial vasculitis and hypocomplementemic urticarial vasculitis syndrome. Immunol Allergy Clin North Am 2004;24:183–213.

Vasculitides
E. Miscellaneous Vasculitis (Behçet's Disease, Primary Angiitis of the Central Nervous System, Cogan's Syndrome, and Erythema Elevatum Diutinum)

KENNETH T. CALAMIA, MD
CARLO SALVARANI, MD

- The prevalence of Behçet's disease is highest in countries of the eastern Mediterranean, the Middle East, and East Asia.
- Aphthous oral ulcers are usually the first and most persistent clinical feature of Behçet's disease. Aphthous ulcers also occur frequently on the genitals (e.g., the scrotum or vulva).
- Uveitis—either anterior or posterior—is common in Behçet's disease and a source of major morbidity.
- Many forms of central nervous system disease may occur in Behçet's disease. These include aseptic meningitis and white matter lesions in the brainstem.
- Human leukocyte antigen (HLA)-B51 is a strong risk factor for Behçet's disease.
- The diagnosis of primary angiitis of the central nervous system is predicated upon either biopsy evidence of vasculitis or angiographic findings suggestive of vasculitis in the setting of other compelling features, for example, strokes demonstrated by magnetic resonance imaging or the findings of a cerebrospinal fluid pleocytosis.

- The diagnosis of primary angiitis of the central nervous system should never be made on the basis of an angiogram alone.
- Patients with benign angiopathy of the central nervous system are predominantly female, tend to present acutely with headache (with or without focal symptoms), and have normal or near normal cerebrospinal fluid.
- Cogan's syndrome refers to the association of inflammation in both the eyes and ears: specifically, the occurrence of nonsyphilitic interstitial keratitis and immune-mediated inner ear disease, resulting in audiovestibular dysfunction.
- Any type of ocular inflammation may occur in Cogan's syndrome (e.g., scleritis, uveitis, orbital pseudotumor). The inner ear disease associated with this condition often leads to deafness.
- In erythema elevatum diutinum, skin lesions consist of purple, red, or brown plaques and often have an annular or nodular appearance. The skin lesions have a predilection for the extensor surfaces of the distal extremities and often overlie joints, but may be generalized.

BEHÇET'S DISEASE

Behçet's disease (BD) is a chronic inflammatory disorder of unknown cause. Its manifestations are thought to be caused by an underlying vasculitis. Although this disease is recognized worldwide, the prevalence is highest in countries of the eastern Mediterranean, the Middle East, and East Asia, thus the name Silk Road

disease. The disease tends to be more severe in areas where it is more common. Prevalence rates in all areas of the world are increasing, probably because of improved recognition and reporting.

Behçet's disease occurs primarily in young adults. The mean age at onset is between 25 and 30 years. The incidence of disease in males and females with the disease is approximately equal along the Silk Road, but in Japan, Korea, and Western countries the disease occurs more frequently in women. Familial aggregation and juvenile cases are not common. Case confirmation can be challenging because many patients labeled as having Behçet's disease have oral ulcers as the primary or sole manifestation.

Clinical Manifestations

Aphthous oral ulcers are usually the first and most persistent clinical feature of BD. Lesions occur in crops and some patients may have them during most of the course of the disease. Aphthae occur as ulcers that are 2 to 12 mm or larger. These are discrete, painful, round or oval red-rimmed lesions that affect mainly the nonkeratinized mucosa of the cheeks, the border of the tongue, the soft palate, and the pharynx (Figure 21E-1). Oral ulcers are identical to the lesions of recurrent aphthous stomatitis. The severity and behavior of the oral ulcers in BD often fit the description of complex aphthosis, in which multiple, recurrent, or persisting lesions result in a severe syndrome that may include perianal or genital ulceration.

Genital ulcers resemble oral aphthae but occur less frequently. They occur as single or multiple lesions of the vulva and in the vagina, or on the scrotum or penile shaft (Figure 21E-2). Genital lesions are usually painful

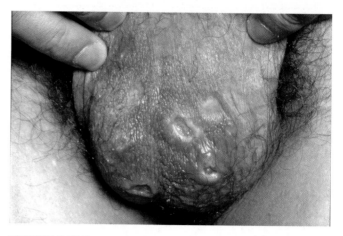

FIGURE 21E-2

Ulcers on the scrotum in a patient with Behçet's disease. (Courtesy of J.D. O'Duffy, MB.)

and may result in scarring, but vaginal ulcers may be asymptomatic or only produce a discharge. Perianal ulcers may occur.

Skin lesions are common in BD. The International Study Group (ISG) criteria for the diagnosis of BD (Table 21E-1) (1) include the presence of erythema nodosum, pseudofolliculitis, papulopustular lesions, or acneform nodules. Nodular lesions should be distinguished from superficial thrombophlebitis. A neutrophilic vascular reaction characterizes lesions typical of

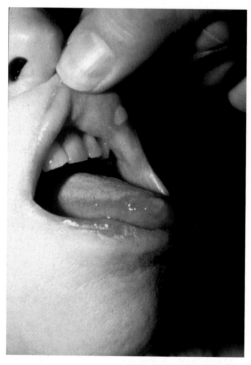

FIGURE 21E-1

Oral aphthous ulceration in Behçet's disease. (Courtesy of J.D. O'Duffy, MB.)

TABLE 21E-1. INTERNATIONAL STUDY GROUP CRITERIA FOR BEHÇET'S DISEASE.

Recurrent oral ulceration	Minor aphthous, major aphthous, or herpetiform ulceration observed by physician or patient, which recurred at least 3 times in one 12-month period[a]
Plus 2 of:	
Recurrent genital ulceration	Aphthous ulceration or scarring, observed by physician or patient[a]
Eye lesions	Anterior uveitis, posterior uveitis, or cells in vitreous on slit lamp examination; or retinal vasculitis observed by ophthalmologist
Skin lesions	Erythema nodosum observed by physician or patient, pseudofolliculitis, or papulopustular lesions; or acneform nodules observed by physician in postadolescent patients not receiving corticosteroid treatment[a]
Positive pathergy test	Read by physician at 24 to 48 hours

Source: From International Study Group for Behçet's Disease. Lancet 1990;335:1078–1080, by permission of *Lancet*.
[a] Findings applicable only in the absence of other clinical explanations.

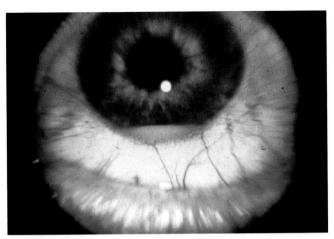

FIGURE 21E-3

Hypopyon in the anterior chamber of a patient with Behçet's disease, caused by anterior uveitis.

BD. A neutrophilic infiltrate is typical of other dermatoses occasionally seen with the disorder, including pyoderma gangrenosum and Sweet's syndrome.

Pathergy is an excessive skin response to trauma, reflecting neutrophil hyperreactivity, and is highly specific for BD. Pathergy is suggested if there is a history of red papules, pustules, or sterile abscesses after therapeutic injections, at intravenous catheter sites, or after minor skin trauma. Testing for pathergy can be done with a sterile 20-gauge needle, used to penetrate the cleansed skin perpendicularly to a depth of approximately one quarter of an inch, rotated briefly on its axis, and then removed. After 48 hours, the appearance of an erythematous papule or pustule at the puncture site constitutes a positive test. The volar forearm is usually chosen for the test and sensitivity is greater when three needle punctures are made. The positivity of the test may vary during the course of the disease and is more likely to be positive at times of active disease. The sensitivity of the test is lower in Western countries than in Silk Road countries, but a positive test adds great support for the diagnosis of BD.

Ocular inflammation typically follows mucocutaneous symptoms by a few years, but it often progresses with a chronic, relapsing course affecting both eyes. The ocular finding in Behçet's original patients was anterior uveitis associated with a hypopyon [the accumulation of an inflammatory cell infiltrate—essentially pus—in the anterior chamber (Figure 21E-3)]. Anterior uveitis that is not treated promptly with a mydriatic agent may result in synechiae formation between the iris and the lens and permanent papillary distortion. The ocular manifestations of Behçet's disease may also include a panuveitis, however, with posterior chamber involvement and retinal vasculitis, the complications of which may extend to visual loss. Retinal vasculitis, which leads to episodes of retinal occlusion and areas of ischemia, may be followed by neovascularization, vitreous hemorrhage and contraction, glaucoma, and retinal detachment. The earliest findings of retinal vasculitis may be detected with fluorescein angiography. Isolated optic disk edema in BD suggests cerebral venous thrombosis rather than ocular disease, but papillitis may occur with ocular inflammation and central nervous system disease. Cranial nerve palsies may result from brain stem lesions, and visual field defects may also be caused by intracranial disease involving the optic pathways.

With cerebral venous thrombosis, patients usually present with symptoms of intracranial pressure: headache, visual obscurations, and papilledema. Magnetic resonance imaging may be used to demonstrate acute or recent clot in the larger dural sinuses, but magnetic resonance venography is more reliable for recognizing clot in the cerebral venous system, especially in the smaller veins and older thromboses.

Central nervous system symptoms in BD may be due to aseptic meningitis or parenchymal lesions, resulting in focal or diffuse brain dysfunction. An increased protein concentration and lymphocytic pleocytosis in the cerebrospinal fluid (CSF) is supportive of the diagnosis. The clinical combination of stroke, aseptic meningitis with CSF pleocytosis, and mucocutaneous lesions can be diagnostic of BD. Focal or multifocal nervous system involvement reflects the predilection of the disease for diencephalon, midbrain, and brainstem (Figure 21E-4). In contrast to multiple sclerosis, there is

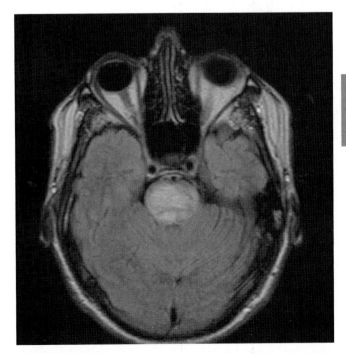

FIGURE 21E-4

Brainstem involvement in a patient with Behçet's disease.

21

no preference for the periventricular structures (2). Isolated headaches in BD are common but the cause is not well understood. These may represent secondary migraine or may not be related to the disease.

Large vessel involvement, which occurs in about one fourth of patients with BD, is a major cause of morbidity and mortality (3). Patients with vascular disease often have multiple lesions and involvement of both the arterial and venous systems (4). Deep venous thrombosis (DVT) is the most common large vascular lesion. Patients with recurrent DVTs are at risk for chronic stasis changes in the legs. Occlusions of the vena cava, hepatic, and portal veins, other recognized thrombotic complications in BD, are associated with an increased risk of mortality. Chest wall, abdominal, and esophageal varices may occur from deep-seated venous thrombosis. Right ventricular thrombi have been reported, usually in association with pulmonary vasculitis. No primary abnormality of the coagulation, anticoagulation, or fibrinolytic system explaining the thrombotic tendency in BD has been identified consistently.

Arterial complications occur in up to 7% of patients with BD (5). Stenoses, occlusions, and aneurysms occur in the systemic circulation or the pulmonary arterial bed. Arterial aneurysms, caused by vasculitis of the vasa vasorum, involve the aorta or its branches. The risk of rupture is high. Pulmonary artery aneurysms (6) may lead to fistulae between the pulmonary artery and bronchi, presenting with hemoptysis. Anticoagulant treatment for presumed pulmonary emboli can result in massive hemorrhage and death. Clinically apparent cardiac vascular involvement is unusual, but may result in myocardial infarction.

Gastrointestinal symptoms in BD include melena and abdominal pain. Colonoscopic lesions appear as single or multiple ulcerations involving primarily the distal ileum and cecum. Gastrointestinal lesions have a tendency to perforate or to bleed. The lesions in BD should be differentiated from those of Crohn's disease and those due to the use of nonsteroidal anti-inflammatory drugs.

An intermittent, symmetric oligoarthritis of the knees, ankles, hands, or wrists affects one half of the patients with BD; arthralgia is also common. An erosive or destructive arthropathy is unusual. Inflammatory cells of the synovium and synovial fluid are primarily polymorphonuclear leukocytes.

Epididymitis occurs in about 5% of affected patients. Glomerulonephritis and peripheral neuropathy occur much less frequently in BD than in other forms of systemic vasculitis. AA-type amyloidosis, presenting as nephrotic syndrome, can accompany BD. The occasional association of the disorder with ankylosing spondylitis [in human leukocyte antigen (HLA)-B27-positive patients] or relapsing polychondritis (MAGIC syndrome [mouth and genital ulcers with inflamed cartilage]) likely represents the simultaneous occurrence of two disorders.

No laboratory abnormality is diagnostic of BD. Acute-phase reactants may be increased, especially in patients with large vessel vasculitis, but they may be normal in other patients, even those with active eye disease. The histocompatibility antigen HLA-B51 is associated with BD in areas of high prevalence and in patients with ocular disease.

Diagnosis

The multiple manifestations of BD in the same patient may be separated in time, occasionally by several years. For definitive diagnosis, the manifestations must be documented or witnessed by a physician. The ISG criteria for the classification of BD (Table 21E-1) (1) are not meant to replace clinical judgment regarding the diagnosis in individual cases. For patients in Western countries, large vessel disease or acute central nervous system infarction in the setting of aphthosis should suggest the diagnosis (7).

The diagnosis of BD in patients with complex aphthosis requires the presence of other characteristic lesions and the exclusion of other systemic disorders. Inflammatory bowel disease, sprue, cyclic neutropenia or other hematologic disorders, herpes simplex infection, and acquired immune deficiency syndrome may cause similar lesions. Other disorders responsible for orogenital/ocular syndromes include erythema multiforme, mucous membrane pemphigoid, and the vulvovaginal–gingival form of erosive lichen planus. The differential diagnosis can be clarified with the aid of an experienced dermatologist and biopsy findings. In Reiter's disease, mucocutaneous lesions are nonulcerative and painless, and the uveitis is usually limited to the anterior chamber. Similarities between BD and Crohn's disease include gastrointestinal lesions, fever, anemia, oral ulcers, uveitis, arthritis, thrombophlebitis, and erythema nodosum. Granuloma formation in intestinal lesions is not typical in BD, and in Crohn's disease the iritis is typically confined to the anterior chamber. Genital ulcerations and central nervous system disease are rare in Crohn's disease.

Disease Activity

Frequent ophthalmologic examinations are essential for patients with ocular disease, and periodic monitoring of the eyes is recommended for all patients. A careful history and examination, with attention to the vascular and neurologic systems, should be part of the physician's assessment. Standardized forms for scoring disease activity and ocular inflammation have been developed for use in clinical trials and the care of individual patients (8).

Management

Aphthous lesions are treated with topical or intralesional corticosteroids. An empiric trial of dapsone or methotrexate may be appropriate in difficult cases. Colchicine is used in the treatment of mucocutaneous manifestations and as an adjunct in the treatment of more serious manifestations (0.6 mg three times daily may be required to achieve a therapeutic effect; many patients suffer gastrointestinal intolerance of the drug at that dose). The effectiveness of colchicine has been demonstrated for genital ulcers and erythema nodosum in females and for arthritis in both sexes (9). Thalidomide has been used for the treatment of mucosal and follicular lesions, but toxicity is a major concern. Short courses of prednisone are useful in the management of mucocutaneous disease in some patients. In others, low-dose prednisone as maintenance therapy is required.

Cyclosporine can be effective for the control of uveitis. A controlled study has demonstrated the value of azathioprine at a dose of 2.5 mg/kg per day in limiting the progression of ocular disease and preventing new eye disease in males. Combination treatment with cyclosporine and azathioprine can been used when single-agent treatment has failed. Azathioprine can have a beneficial effect on mucosal ulcers, arthritis, deep venous thrombosis, and long-term prognosis (10). Because young males are at the greatest risk for severe disease, especially uveitis, aggressive treatment is warranted in this disease subset. In open trials, interferon-alpha has been found useful for treating mucocutaneous lesions and arthritis and is emerging as an effective treatment for ocular disease (11). Etanercept, a tumor necrosis factor inhibitor, was shown to be beneficial for mucocutaneous manifestations in a controlled study (12). Reports of uncontrolled experience with infliximab for eye inflammation have been positive, but controlled data are lacking. Immunosuppression with chlorambucil or cyclophosphamide is used for uncontrolled ocular disease, central nervous system disease, and large vessel vasculitis, including recurrent deep venous thrombosis. Glucocorticoids are useful in suppression of inflammation in acute phases of the disease, but these agents are insufficient by themselves to treat such severe disease manifestations as posterior uveitis or parenchymal brain disease.

Because of the high risk of rupture, surgical treatment is indicated for systemic arterial aneurysms. Glucocorticoids and alkylating agents should also be used to minimize the high risk of anastomotic recurrences or continued disease. Pulmonary arterial aneurysms may respond to these same medications, but uncontrolled bleeding requires percutaneous embolization or surgical treatment. Cerebral venous thrombosis is treated with anticoagulation and corticosteroids. The treatment of Budd–Chiari syndrome has included anticoagulants or antiaggregants, colchicine, and glucocorticoids. Portocaval shunting should be considered if the inferior vena cava is patent.

Pathogenesis

In many geographic areas, genetic studies have shown a strong association with HLA-B51, but the exact role of this gene in the development of BD is uncertain. Neutrophilic hyperfunction is recognized in BD, in normal subjects with HLA-B51, and in HLA-B51 transgenic mice (13). Evidence also exists for antigen-driven immune mechanisms in the pathogenesis of BD. Cytokine analysis and cellular characterization suggest a T-helper cell (Th1) response by lymphocytes in BD. Molecular techniques have identified herpes simplex viral RNA and DNA in cells from patients with BD, and streptococcal antigens have been proposed as triggers of active disease. Activated gamma-delta T cells are increased in the circulation and in mucosal lesions, but the precise role of these cells in the pathogenesis of BD is uncertain. Peptides from mycobacterial heat shock protein (HSP) and homologous human peptides have been found to stimulate gd+ T cells from patients with BD in a specific fashion (14). Cross-reactivity and molecular mimicry between peptides from streptococcal or viral HSP, homologous human HSP, and mucosal antigens may result in selection of autoreactive T cells (15). More recently, similarities between BD and inflammatory disorders associated with autoimmunity have been recognized (16).

PRIMARY ANGIITIS OF THE CENTRAL NERVOUS SYSTEM

Primary angiitis of the central nervous system (PACNS) is a rare form of vasculitis limited to the brain and spinal cord. The term *granulomatosis angiitis* of the central nervous system was previously applied because of the histopathologic findings observed in arteries from early reported cases. However, an analysis of a larger number of cases supports varied mononuclear cell infiltrates, with fewer than 50% of cases showing granulomatous inflammation (17). Anatomically, the angiitis is multifocal and segmental in distribution and involves the small leptomeningeal and intracerebral arteries. In general, the arteries are involved much more frequently than the veins.

Clinical Manifestations

The disease predominantly affects males. Most patients are young or middle-aged, although patients of a broad age range are affected. Cases of PACNS in children have also been described. The clinical manifestations of PACNS are not distinctive. The most common symptom is headache. Because virtually every anatomic area of the central nervous system may be affected by the vasculitis, a wide range of neurologic presentations and deficits may be seen, including transient ischemic attacks (TIAs), cerebral infarction, paraparesis, quadriparesis, hemiparesis, ataxia, seizures, aphasia, and visual field defects, among others. Decreased cognitive function or fluctuating levels of consciousness are not uncommon. Progressive multifocal symptoms over time in a younger patient should suggest the possibility of PACNS, particularly in the absence of other risk factors. The spinal cord may occasionally be involved. Presentations with subarachnoid or intracerebral hemorrhage are rare.

Diagnosis

Timely diagnosis of PACNS is critical, before the occurrence of massive brain damage. Preliminary diagnostic criteria for PACNS have been proposed (18) but never validated. The diagnosis of PACNS is usually predicated upon either biopsy evidence of vasculitis or angiographic findings suggestive of vasculitis in the setting of other compelling features, for example, strokes demonstrated by magnetic resonance imaging or the findings of a cerebrospinal fluid pleocytosis (17). Histologic confirmation remains the most specific diagnostic procedure for PACNS, but the sensitivity of brain biopsy is limited because of the focal segmental distribution of the disease. A negative biopsy does not exclude the diagnosis of PACNS, but may be essential to excluding other disorders that mimic PACNS clinically.

In the absence of histologic confirmation, a cerebral angiogram typical of vasculitis in the appropriate clinical settings is frequently used to establish the diagnosis of PACNS. Suggestive angiographic findings include segmental narrowing, dilatation, or occlusion affecting multiple cerebral arteries in the absence of proximal atherosclerotic changes (Figure 21E-5). The findings of narrowing are, however, highly nonspecific, and can be caused by a host of nonvasculitic causes. Angiographic findings compatible with vasculitis are commonly encountered in conditions such as vasospasm, central nervous system infection, cerebral arterial emboli, intravascular lymphomatosis, and atherosclerosis. Furthermore, the sensitivity of angiography is limited if small vessels beyond its resolution are primarily involved. Cerebral angiography has been normal in some biopsy-proven cases.

General laboratory tests, including acute-phase reactants such as C-reactive protein and the erythrocyte sedimentation rate, are not useful in the diagnosis of PACNS. In addition to being nonspecific, in fact, acute-phase reactants are known often to be normal even in

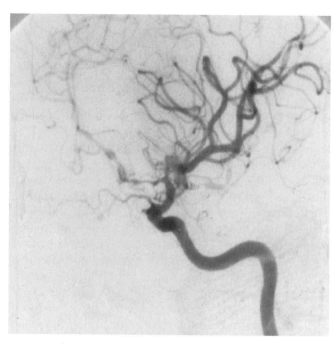

FIGURE 21E-5

Cerebral angiogram in a patient with central nervous system vasculitis. The angiogram reveals multiple segmental stenoses of the A1 and A2 segments of the anterior cerebral artery and the distal segments of the middle cerebral artery.

the setting of biopsy-proven active disease. Cerebrospinal fluid (CSF) analysis, however, is an essential part of the diagnostic workup of PACNS. The CSF findings are abnormal in 80% to 90% of cases documented pathologically. CSF findings are characterized by a modest pleocytosis and elevated protein levels. CSF analysis should include appropriate stains, cultures, and serologic tests to exclude for CNS infections.

Magnetic resonance imaging (MRI) is the most sensitive imaging study in the evaluation of PACNS. Only rare cases have no MRI abnormalities. The most common findings are multiple, bilateral, supratentorial infarcts distributed in the cortex, deep white matter, and/or leptomeninges, but the findings lack specificity. Magnetic resonance angiography (MRA) is limited in sensitivity in most cases of PACNS. Angiographically demonstrable lesions are often beyond the resolution of current MRA technology. Thus, a normal MRA does not rule out the disorder.

Management and Outcome

Primary angiitis of the central nervous system is considered a progressive disorder with a fatal course unless treated vigorously with a combination of high-dose glucocorticoids and a cytotoxic agent (usually cyclophosphamide). There are no controlled treatment trials on which to base this standard. The optimal duration of therapy is unknown, but in view of the substantial side effects associated with cyclophosphamide and the successful use of shorter courses of therapy in other forms of vasculitis, a 6-month course of cyclophosphamide followed by an additional 1 year of azathioprine appears reasonable. Prednisone should be discontinued in a tapering fashion over 6 to 9 months.

Benign Angiopathy of the Central Nervous System

The presence of a subset of patients with some features suggesting PACNS but demonstrating a more benign course has been suggested (19). This subset of patients is considered to have a disease entity known as benign angiopathy of the central nervous system (BACNS). BACNS patients are predominantly female, primarily present acutely with headache, with or without focal symptoms, and have normal or near normal CSF analysis. The diagnosis in these cases has been established angiographically and appeared to have a monophasic course with a favorable neurologic outcome. Most of these patients recover after only short-term glucocorticoid treatment, often supplemented by a calcium channel blocker to mitigate against vasospasm. Cytotoxic agents are not required for patients with BACNS.

The etiology of the vascular disease in this benign form has not been defined clearly, but could be the result of arteritis or reversible vasospasm. The existence of a benign, angiographically defined subset, however, remains controversial (20). Recently, we identified a subset of patients presenting with evidence of prominent leptomeningeal enhancement on MRI (21). These patients were characterized by normal cerebral angiography, brain biopsy evidence of vasculitis predominantly affecting the small leptomeningeal vessels, and a good response to corticosteroids and/or immunosuppressive therapy with a favorable neurologic course.

COGAN'S SYNDROME

Cogan's syndrome refers to the association of nonsyphilitic interstitial keratitis (Figure 21E-6) and immune-mediated inner ear disease, resulting in audiovestibular dysfunction. The disorder affects men and women equally at any age, but typically in their third and fourth decade. Presenting manifestations include sudden hearing loss, Ménière's-like vertigo and tinnitus, and ocular inflammation, alone or in any combination (22). Other features of the disease, if not present initially, usually follow within several months. Hearing loss is

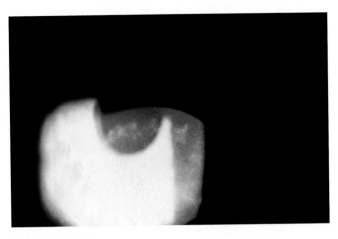

FIGURE 21E-6

Nonsyphilitic interstitial keratitis in a patient with Cogan's syndrome. Retroillumination image of the cornea with the slit lamp reveals a patchy, deep, granular corneal infiltrate characteristic of early Cogan's syndrome in the cornea. (Courtesy of Dr. Thomas J. Liesegang, Mayo Clinic College of Medicine.)

bilateral, shows a downsloping pattern on audiograms, and is often progressive and profound. Vestibular testing shows bilateral cochlear dysfunction, helping to distinguish this disorder from Ménière's syndrome. In comparison to Ménière's syndrome, the damage to hearing from Cogan's syndrome is typically more unremitting. Scleritis, uveitis, or other inflammatory conditions of the eye (Figure 21E-7) may be present initially but often patients will subsequently develop interstitial keratitis if not present initially. Systemic manifestations include headache, fever, arthralgia, and vasculitis, with or without aortitis. The critical evaluation and monitoring

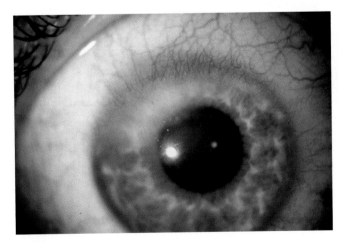

FIGURE 21E-7

Localized corneal edema in Cogan's syndrome. Direct corneal view of classic ocular Cogan's syndrome in an advanced stage. There is localized peripheral corneal edema, mild lipid infiltrate, and moderate vascularization extending from the corneal limbus. (Courtesy of Dr. Thomas J. Liesegang, Mayo Clinic College of Medicine.)

21

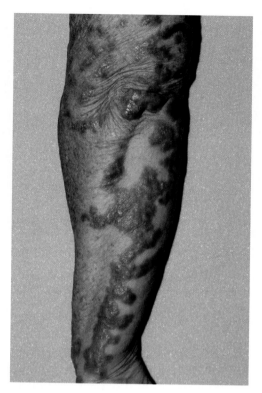

FIGURE 21E-8

Erythema elevatum diutinum.

of Cogan's patients requires the expertise and collaboration of the treating rheumatologist, otolaryngologist, and ophthalmologist (23).

There are no controlled studies on the treatment of Cogan's syndrome. Glucocorticoids are used topically for anterior eye disease and systemically for audiovestibular manifestations, unremitting ocular disease, or when the disorder is complicated by vasculitis or significant systemic manifestations. These agents should be started as soon as the disorder is recognized, in adequate doses (at least 1 mg/kg/day), and for a sufficient duration to initially control the disease or for relapse. Documented improvement in 2 to 3 weeks supports a therapeutic response and can be followed by gradual tapering of the dose and use of immunosuppressive agents if necessary for maintenance. The prognosis for hearing in these patients has been poor (22), but cochlear implants are used successfully in these patients with bilateral deafness.

ERYTHEMA ELEVATUM DIUTINUM

Erythema elevatum diutinum (EED) is an extremely rare, chronic, recurrent vasculitis with distinctive clinical and histopathologic features (24,25). The disorder affects both men and women in middle age. Individual lesions consist of purple, red, or brown plaques that often have an annular or nodular appearance. The skin lesions of EED have a predilection for the extensor surfaces of the distal extremities and often overlie joints, but may be generalized. Older lesions may be dense and coalesce (Figure 21E-8). Erupting lesions may be associated with stinging, burning, or tenderness, and may be accompanied by systemic symptoms. In early lesions, the pathology of EED is one of a leukocytoclastic vasculitis with a perivascular neutrophilic infiltrate. More mature lesions demonstrate perivascular or onion-skin–like fibrosis. Capillary proliferation and cholesterol-containing histiocytes may also be seen. The differential diagnosis includes other neutrophilic dermatoses, primarily Sweet's syndrome.

Erythema elevatum diutinum has been recognized to occur in association with infections diseases, including human immunodeficiency virus infection, hematologic disorders (particularly IgA gammopathies), and several immune-mediated inflammatory diseases, including rheumatoid arthritis. Treatment of any associated disorder may benefit EED. Dapsone (100 mg/day) has been reported to be successful in some patients.

REFERENCES

1. International Study Group for Behçet's Disease. Criteria for diagnosis of Behçet's disease. Lancet 1990;335:1078–1080.
2. Kural-Seyahi E, Fresco I, Seyahi N, et al. The long-term mortality and morbidity of Behcet syndrome: a 2-decade outcome survey of 387 patients followed at a dedicated center. Medicine (Baltimore), 2003;82:60–76.
3. Calamia KT, Schirmer M, Melikoglu M. Major vessel involvement in Behcet disease. Curr Opin Rheumatol 2005;17:1–8.
4. Le Thi Huong D, Wechsler B, Papo T, et al. Arterial lesions in Behçet's disease. A study in 25 patients. J Rheumatol 1995;22:2103–2113.
5. Hamuryudan V, Er T, Seyahi T, et al. Pulmonary artery aneurysms in Behcet syndrome. Am J Med 2004;117:867–870.
6. Borhani Haghighi A, Pourmand R, Nikseresht AR. Neuro-Behcet disease. A review. Neurologist 2005;11:80–89.
7. Schirmer M, Calamia KT. Is there a place for large vessel disease in the diagnostic criteria for Behçet's disease? J Rheumatol 1999;26:2511–2512.
8. Kaklamani VG, Vaiopoulos G, Kaklamanis PG. Behçet's Disease. Semin Arthritis Rheum 1998;27:197–217.
9. Yurdakul S, Mat C, Tuzun Y, et al. A double-blind trial of colchicine in Behçet's syndrome. Arthritis Rheum 2001;44:2686–2692.
10. Hamuryudan V, Ozyazgan Y, Hizli N, et al. Azathioprine in Behçet's syndrome: Effects on long-term prognosis. Arthritis Rheum 1997;40:769–774.

11. Kötter I, Zierhut M, Eckstein A, et al. Human recombinant interferon alfa-2a for the treatment of Behçet's disease with sight threatening posterior or panuveitis. Br J Ophthalmol 2003;87:423–431.

12. Melikoglu M, Fresco I, Mat C, et al. Short-term trial of etanercept in Behcet's disease: a double blind, placebo controlled study. J Rheumatol 2005;32:98–105.

13. Takeno M, Kariyone A, Yamasita M, et al. Excessive function of peripheral blood neutrophils from patients with Behçet's disease and from HLA-B51 transgenic mice. Arthritis Rheum 1995;38:426–433.

14. Hasan A, Fortune F, Wilson A, et al. Role of gamma delta T cells in pathogenesis and diagnosis of Behçet's disease. Lancet 1996;347:789–794.

15. Lehner T. The role of heat shock protein, microbial and autoimmune agents in the aetiology of Behçet's disease. Int Rev Immunol 1997;14:21–32.

16. Gul A. Behcet's disease as an autoinflammatory disorder. Curr Drug Targets Inflamm Allergy 2005;4:81–83.

17. Lie, JT. Primary (granulomatous) angiitis of the central nervous system: a clinicopathologic analysis of 15 new cases and a review of the literature. Hum Pathol 1992;23:164–171.

18. Calabrese LH, Mallek JA. Primary angiitis of the central nervous system. Report of 8 new cases, review of the literature, and proposal for diagnostic criteria. Medicine (Baltimore) 1988;67:20–39.

19. Calabrese LH, Gragg LA, Furlan AJ. Benign angiopathy: a distinct subset of angiographically defined primary angiitis of the central nervous system. J Rheumatol 1993;20:2046–2050.

20. Woolfenden AR, Tong DC, Marks MP, et al. Angiographically defined primary angiitis of the CNS: is it really benign? Neurology 1998;51:183–188.

21. Salvarani C, Hunder GG. Primary central nervous system vasculitis (PCNSV): Clinical features and outcome. Arthritis Rheum 2005(52 supplement):S650.

22. Gluth MB, Baratz KH, Matteson EL, et al. Cogan Syndrome: a retrospective review of 60 patients throughout a half century. Mayo Clin Proc 2006;81:483–488.

23. McCallum RM, St. Clair EW, Haynes BF. Cogan's Syndrome. In Hoffman GS, Weyand C, eds. Inflammatory Diseases of Blood Vessels. New York: Marcel Dekker, Inc.; 2002:491–509.

24. Wahl CE, Bouldin MB, Gibson LE. Erythema elevatum diutinum: clinical, histopathologic, and immunohistochemical characteristics of six patients. Am J Dermatopathol 2005;27:397–400.

25. Gibson LE, el-Azhary RA. Erythema elevatum diutinum. Clin Dermatol 2000;18:295–299.

21

Vasculitides
F. Kawasaki's Disease

BARRY L. MYONES, MD

- Kawasaki's disease (KD), once known as mucocutaneous lymph node syndrome, is a systemic inflammatory disorder occurring in children that is accompanied by vasculitis and a risk of coronary artery aneurysms.
- Other typical features of KD include spiking fevers, cervical lymphadenopathy, conjunctivitis, erythematous changes on the lips and in the oral cavity, dryness and cracking of the lips, a strawberry appearance to the tongue, and a polymorphous rash.
- Eighty percent of KD cases occur in children less than 5 years of age.

- Attempts to link KD definitively to some types of infection, particularly ones associated with superantigens, have thus far been unsuccessful.
- High dose aspirin and intravenous immune globulin (IVIG) are the cornerstones of therapy in KD. IVIG is essential to the prevention of coronary aneurysms.
- Years after KD has occurred during childhood years, some cases of myocardial infarction caused by thrombosis of coronary aneurysms have been reported.

Kawasaki's disease (KD) is a form of systemic vasculitis that occurs in young children and may be associated with the development of coronary arteritis and aneurysm formation (Figure 21F-1). KD is the leading cause of acquired heart disease of children in the United States. This illness, first recognized to be a new entity by Tomasaku Kawasaki in Japan in 1967 (1,2), was termed for *mucocutaneous lymph node syndrome* (MCLNS) until KD became the accepted designation for this disorder (3). Although the disorder was named after Kawasaki, at least one previous case exists in the medical literature (4). This case, recounted in detail below, is classic in its clinical features of KD.

A 5-year-old girl presented with a sore throat, a fever to 105°F, and an erythematous rash over her trunk, appearing "desperately and acutely ill" (4). Oropharyngeal lesions included an aphthous stomatitis, erythematous lesions of the hard palate, and prominent lingual papillae. On the fifth hospital day the hectic fevers ceased, but low-grade fevers and tachycardia to 140 beats per minute persisted. The skin of her fingers desquamated, but over the ensuing weeks she improved steadily. One month after admission, however, she developed acute chest pain, shortness of breath, and expired. A postmortem examination revealed blood and clots in the pericardial space, and several large aneurysms along the epicardial vessels. One aneurysm, the size of a large ripe cherry in the left coronary artery,

was the site of hemorrhage into the pericardium. Although the microscopic appearance of the disease was typical of periarteritis nodosa (i.e., PAN; see Chapter 21B), no hepatic or renal infarctions were present. Indeed, among the internal organs the heart alone was involved. The child's death was attributed to an atypical case of "infantile periarteritis nodosa," now recognized as KD.

CLINICAL FEATURES

Kawasaki's disease strikes quickly, runs a furious course over a few weeks, and then apparently resolves. In all 50 of the patients described initially by Kawasaki, the symptoms resolved without sequelae within 1 month. In subsequent years, however, mortality from cardiac complications (usually coronary artery thrombosis) was reported (5,6). Cardiac complications of KD result from a severe panvasculitis, leading to narrowing of the coronary lumina by the migration of myointimal cells from the media through the fragmented internal elastic lamina. Although catastrophic heart complications occur in only a small minority of patients (<5%), the preponderance of patients with KD appear to have at least some cardiac involvement. Heart lesions may include myocarditis, pericarditis, aneurysmal dilatation

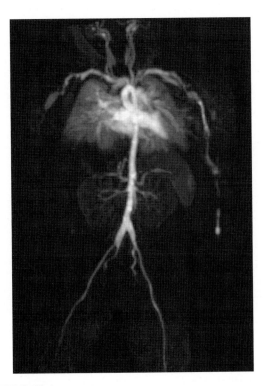

FIGURE 21F-1

Coronary and peripheral aneurysms in Kawasaki's disease (KD). Magnetic resonance angiogram in an infant with KD, revealing irregularities of the subclavian, axillary, and proximal brachial arteries, as well as fusiform dilatation of the right common iliac and right proximal internal iliac arteries. There is also a focal aneurysm of the left internal iliac artery.

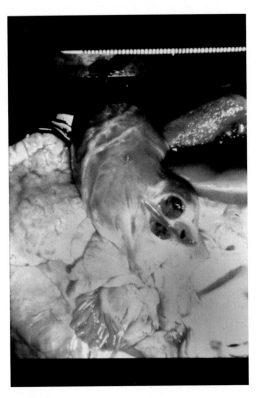

FIGURE 21F-2

Coronary artery thrombosis leading to death in Kawasaki's disease. [Reproduced with permission from the American College of Rheumatology collection, slide 124 (#9406010).]

and thrombosis of the coronary arteries (Figure 21F-2), and myocardial infarction. The tropism of the vascular inflammation for coronary arteries and its unusual propensity to cause aneurysm formation remain unexplained.

In addition to the cardiac findings, KD is associated with a number of other dramatic clinical findings (Table 21F-1). Spiking fevers may last for 5 days or more. The conjunctivae, generally inflamed in a nonpurulent manner, are accompanied by erythematous changes on the lips and in the oral cavity [Figure 21F-3(A)]. The lips become dry and cracked [Figure 21F-3(B)], with a diffuse reddening of the oropharyngeal area and a strawberry appearance to the tongue (Figure 21F-4). A polymorphous rash typically involves the trunk [Figure 21F-3(A)], and there may be extensive lymphadenopathy in the neck region. The palms and soles become erythematous and indurated, followed by desquamation in the skin of these areas during the healing phase (7–9).

The term *atypical KD* has been used to describe both older children and young infants presenting outside the typical age range of 2 to 5 years, as well as those presenting with features other than the classical criteria. *Incom-*

plete KD has been applied to any patient felt to have KD but who did not fulfill classical criteria. These are often diagnosed by echocardiogram findings of coronary aneurysms and often occur in the older children or young infants (10,11). Coronary aneurysms, in fact, are most likely to occur in infants <6 months of age. Because

TABLE 21F-1. PRINCIPAL CRITERIA FOR THE DIAGNOSIS OF KAWASAKI'S DISEASE (5 OUT OF 6 CRITERIA MET).[a]

Fever lasting 4 days or more

Bilateral nonpurulent conjunctival injection

Changes of the lips and oral cavity (including dry, fissured lips, strawberry tongue, diffuse reddening of the oropharyngeal mucosa)

Polymorphous rash primarily on the trunk

Acute nonpurulent swelling of a cervical lymph node to >1.5 cm

Changes of the peripheral extremities (including reddening of palms and soles, indurative edema of hands and feet, membranous desquamation from the fingertips)

[a] Illness not explained by any other known disease process.

21

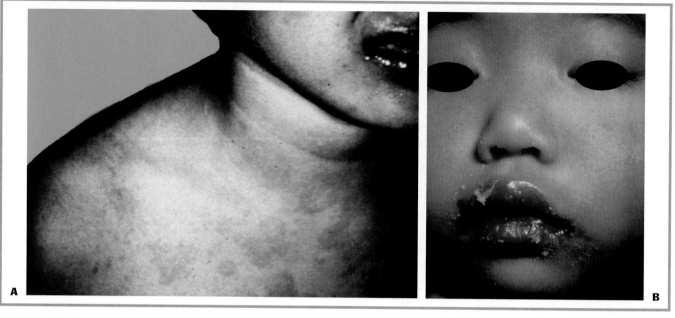

FIGURE 21F-3

Oral and cutaneous manifestations of Kawasaki's disease. (A) Erythema of the lips and an erythematous, annular rash on the skin. (B) Cracking and desquamation of the lips in a patient with Kawasaki's disease. [Reproduced with permission pending from the American College of Rheumatology slide collection. (A) Slide 93 (#9106110). (B) Slide 92 (#9106131).]

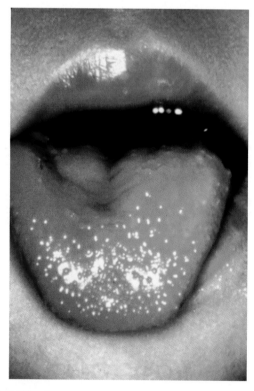

FIGURE 21F-4

Strawberry tongue in Kawasaki's disease. [Reproduced with permission pending from the American College of Rheumatology slide collection, Slide 95 (#9106120).]

of confusion (and often inappropriate use) surrounding disease terminology, there have been sentiments among KD experts to phase out the term *atypical* and to expand the term *incomplete*. Unusual disease features known to occur in KD include sterile pyuria and urethritis, arthral-

TABLE 21F-2. REVISED GUIDELINES FOR THE DIAGNOSIS AND TREATMENT OF KAWASAKI'S DISEASE.

Expanded epidemiologic case definition includes fever of at least 4 days and ≥4 principal criteria (Table 21F-1) without other explanation OR fever and <4 principal criteria if coronary artery abnormalities are detected by echocardiogram or coronary angiography

An echocardiogram should be performed in any patient ≤6 months of age if fever persists ≥7 days without other explanation and with laboratory measures of inflammation, even in the absence of any principal clinical criteria

The following laboratory parameters may be used to help with diagnosis and determine disease severity: CRP ≥3.0 mg/dL, ESR ≥40 mm/h, albumin ≤3.0 g/dL, anemia for age, ↑ ALT, platelets after 7 days ≥450,000, WBC ≥15,000, urine microscopic ≥10 WBC/high-powered field

SOURCE: From the scientific statement by the American Heart Association (AHA) Committee on Rheumatic Fever, Endocarditis, and Kawasaki Disease. Circulation 2004;110:2747–2771 and Pediatrics 2004;114:1708–1733.
ABBREVIATIONS: ALT, alanine aminotransferase; CRP, C-reactive protein; ESR, erythrocyte sedimentation rate; WBC, white blood cell count.

gia and arthritis, aseptic meningitis, diarrhea, abdominal pain, pericardial effusion, obstructive jaundice, and hydrops of the gallbladder.

Intravenous immune globulin (IVIG), a critical medication in the treatment of KD, is a limited resource in many parts of the world because of its expense. The American Heart Association (AHA), concerned about both the potential for overuse of IVIG as well as the failure to employ this medication in a timely manner in appropriate patients, issued guidelines on the diagnosis and treatment of KD (Tables 21F-2 through 21F-4) (12,13). In these guidelines, the epidemiologic case definition of KD included fever of at least 4 days and four or more principal criteria (Table 21F-1) without other explanation; or fever and less than four principal criteria if coronary artery abnormalities are detected by echocardiogram or coronary angiography.

EPIDEMIOLOGY

In Japan, the illness appears in late winter and spring. The peak age is 6 to 12 months, with 80% of cases occurring in patients younger than 5 years of age. The male: female ratio is 1.5:1. Except for three major pandemics (1979, 1982, 1985/6), the cases have reached a plateau of 5000 to 6000 per year. The endemic annual incidence is 67/100,000 children <5 years old, with a recurrence rate of 6%.

In the United States, there is also a seasonal variation in most places. The peak age is 18 to 24 months, and the illness accounts for 3000 hospitalizations/year. The recurrence rate is 1% to 3%. Data from Hawaii from 1971–1980 show ethnic incidence rate/100,000 children <8 years old per year of 33.6 in Japanese, 11.1 in Chinese, 9.2 in Hawaiians, 2.9 in Filipinos, 2.8 in Caucasians. In Los Angeles from 1980–1983, rates per 100,000 children

TABLE 21F-3. ECHOCARDIOGRAM CRITERIA INCLUDE ANY OF THE FOLLOWING THREE.

1. LAD[a] or RCA[b] z score ≥ 2.5

2. Japanese Ministry of Health Criteria (coronary artery diameter >3 mm in children <5 year or >4 mm in children ≥5 years, lumen diameter ≥1.5× an adjacent segment, coronary lumen is clearly irregular)

3. ≥3 suggestive features: (perivascular brightness, lack of tapering, ↓ left ventricular function, mitral regurgitation, pericardial effusion, LAD or RCA z scores = 2–2.5)

SOURCE: From the scientific statement by the American Heart Association (AHA) Committee on Rheumatic Fever, Endocarditis, and Kawasaki Disease. Circulation 2004;110:2747–2771 and Pediatrics 2004;114:1708–1733.
[a] Left anterior descending coronary artery.
[b] Right coronary artery.

TABLE 21F-4. KAWASAKI'S DISEASE: RECOMMENDED THERAPY.

Acute Stage
Aspirin 80–100 mg/kg/day in 4 divided doses until the 14th day of illness
+
IVIG 2 g/kg in 1 dose over 10–12 hours

Convalescent Stage (>14th illness day; afebrile patient)
ASA at 3–5 mg/kg/day in a single dose
Discontinue 6–8 weeks after onset of illness after verifying that no coronary abnormalities are present by echocardiography

Acute Coronary Thrombosis
Prompt fibrinolytic therapy with streptokinase, urokinase, or tissue plasminogen activator by a tertiary care center under the supervision of a cardiologist

Chronic Treatment for Patients with Coronary Aneurysms
ASA 3–5 mg/kg/day in a single dose
Some physicians add dipyridamole in selected patients deemed at high risk
Some physicians use warfarin or heparin in combination with antiplatelet therapy in patients with severe coronary findings or past evidence of coronary thrombosis

SOURCE: From the scientific statement by the American Heart Association (AHA) Committee on Rheumatic Fever, Endocarditis, and Kawasaki Disease. Circulation 1993;87:1776–1780 and Pediatrics 1979;63:175–179.

<14 years old per year include 23.0 in Asians, 2.3 in African Americans, and 1.6 in Caucasians and Hispanics (14–17).

ETIOLOGY

The epidemiology of KD is consistent with an infectious cause: clinical features that resemble infection (fever, lymphadenopathy), time/space clusters, epidemic occurrences, and alleged proximity of case foci to bodies of water. To date, however, no infectious etiology has been proven. There has been no culture or serologic evidence for conventional viral agents, Mycoplasmae, Rickettsiae, or bacterial agents (*Streptococcus, Staphylococcus*). Molecular biologic techniques have provided support, however, for a *Propionibacterium acnes* variant, retroviruses, Rickettsiae, parvovirus B19, Epstein–Barr virus, and coronavirus, as well as for the participation of the *S. aureus* toxin TSST-1 and other superantigens (e.g., *Yersinia pseudotuberulosis*).

Support exists for a superantigen-mediated process both from clinical studies (18–22) and from a murine model for coronary arteritis stimulated by *Lactobacillus casei* cell wall extracts (23). This hypothesis proposes that the etiologic agents—which may differ across geographic sites throughout the world—are capable of evoking immunologic responses via T-cell receptor V beta restriction. An oligoclonal response is supported by the discovery of IgA-secreting plasma cells within

21

the walls of the affected arteries. This finding lends credence to the hypothesis that the respiratory or gastrointestinal tract may be the portal of entry for the inciting organism, and that the process is antigen-driven (24,25).

PATHOGENESIS

The pathogenesis is characterized by immune activation. A host of immunologic irregularities have been described in KD, not all of which have been confirmed consistently: endothelial cell activation [particularly human leukocyte antigen (HLA)-DR expression on coronary endothelial cells]; autoantibody formation (e.g., anti-endothelial cell antibodies); complement activation and immune complex formation; abnormalities of immunoregulation (lymphocyte infiltration, activated CD4+ and B cells, activated monocyte/macrophages, T lymphopenia, polyclonal B-cell activation); adhesion molecule upregulation (soluble P-, E-, and L-selectins); increased vascular endothelial growth factor; and marked cytokine production with high levels of interferon-gamma, interleukins-1, -4, -6, and -10, and tumor necrosis factor (TNF)-alpha (18,26–28). In severe cases, this "cytokine storm" results in a macrophage activation syndrome (MAS).

TREATMENT

Following the initial recognition of KD, this illness was treated with salicylates, using the same doses of aspirin employed in the treatment of rheumatic fever. Because of the potential for impedance of aspirin absorption caused by vasculitic involvement of the gastrointestinal tract, however, the use of aspirin must be monitored carefully in this setting. If aspirin doses are too high (e.g., 100–150 mg/kg/day), improvement of intestinal absorption with therapy may lead to symptoms of toxicity. In Japan, doses of 30 to 50 mg/kg/day have been employed because of the high incidence of the slow-acetylator gene in the Japanese population. A combined US and Japanese multicenter study demonstrated that 30 to 50 mg/kg of aspirin plus IVIG (see below) was effective at preventing aneurysm formation in most cases (29). Current AHA guidelines, however, endorse aspirin doses of 80 to 100 mg/kg/day, in four divided doses (Table 21F-4).

Furusho studied the use of aspirin alone versus the combination of aspirin plus IVIG (0.4 mg/kg/day × 4 days), using a protocol then in use for immune thrombocytopenic purpura (30). A multicenter study demonstrated a decrease in the incidence of coronary artery abnormalities: only 4% (3 of 68) in the IVIG group, compared with 33% (38 of 119) in the aspirin-only arm

(31). No patients in the IVIG arm developed giant coronary artery aneurysms. In contrast, 6% of the aspirin-only group suffered this occurrence. This study established IVIG as the standard of care. Several years later, a follow-up trial compared a single dose of IVIG (2 g/kg) to the traditional 0.4 mg/kg/day × 4 schedule, confirming the superiority (a further lowering of the coronary aneurysm rate) of the single-dose regimen (32). Thereafter, the single-dose regimen became the standard of care recommendation by the AHA (Table 21F-4) (9,33).

The use of glucocorticoids in KD is, surprisingly, controversial. One retrospective study assessed the outcomes of five different treatment regimens, including aspirin alone, aspirin plus prednisolone, prednisolone alone, prednisolone plus warfarin, and no treatment aside from background antibiotic therapy (which all other treatment groups received, as well). Although aspirin alone reduced the aneurysm rate from 20% to 11% compared with the no-treatment group, treatment with prednisolone was associated with an increase in the percentages of patients who developed aneurysm to 67% (34). Of note, the seven patients treated with aspirin plus prednisolone—none of whom developed aneurysm—were not emphasized in the discussion. In addition, the patients in the prednisolone-only group were perhaps the most ill at baseline (and hence were treated with glucocorticoids, presumed empirically to be the most powerful therapy).

After the publication of this study's results, glucocorticoids for the treatment of KD fell into disfavor among pediatricians and in fact were viewed as contraindicated for this disease. More recent case series, evaluating the use of pulse methylprednisolone as rescue therapy for IVIG nonresponders, have been more encouraging with regard to the potential for a beneficial effect of glucocorticoids (35–37). Initial results from a multicenter trial (38) indicate no worsening in the coronary aneurysm rate among patients treated with glucocorticoids, and a decrease in fever, inflammatory markers, length of hospital stay, and IVIG side effects.

A consensus conference at the National Institutes of Health (18) was prompted by the recognition of an ongoing immune activation at microvascular levels in patients treated adequately by the current therapies. Outcome data from Japan with long-term (10–15 year) follow-up demonstrated persistence of disease in some cases, with intravascular ultrasound and ultrafast computed tomography studies demonstrating lingering coronary aneurysms and/or wall fibrosis. Of greatest alarm was the finding of such abnormalities in areas of the vasculature previously documented as normal by echocardiogram and even coronary angiography. Electron microscopy studies of endomyocardial biopsies up to 23 years after the KD episode showed ongoing microaneurysms and small vessel coagulopathy. In a small number of young adults who have experienced myocardial infarctions in the absence of known cardiac risk factors, angiograms have revealed giant coronary artery aneurysms compatible with old KD. The extent of active KD in such patients, if any, as opposed to the clinical sequelae occurring in arteries damaged years before, is not clear.

Newer treatment modalities have been utilized in selected patients and patient populations. Small studies and anecdotal reports of treatment with the antiglycoprotein IIb/IIIa monoclonal antibody (abciximab) or with low-molecular-weight heparin have suggested more rapid regression of aneurysms and perhaps endothelial cell remodeling. Noninvasive imaging modalities, such as magnetic resonance imaging studies of the chest and abdomen, have identified the extracardiac arterial aneurysms and dilatation (Figure 21F-1). The knowledge of the more widespread nature of the vasculitic involvement has prompted more aggressive and combination therapies (39).

Pentoxifylline, a phosphodiesterase inhibitor, has antiplatelet activity, vasodilatory effects, effects on red blood cell rheology, and the ability to inhibit TNF synthesis. A regimen of 20 mg/kg/day of pentoxifylline in three divided doses demonstrated an improvement in clinical features and the rate of aneurysm formation in KD (40). Further pharmacokinetic studies of a commercial liquid preparation of pentoxifylline demonstrated safety and a reduction in TNF levels in KD patients of 28% with doses up to 25 mg/kg/day (41). Anecdotal reports indicate tolerability of doses of 40 to 60 mg/kg/day in infants with KD. A multicenter trial of infliximab in KD is currently under way (42,43).

REFERENCES

1. Kawasaki T. Acute febrile mucocutaneous syndrome with lymphoid involvement with specific desquamation of the fingers and toes in children [in Japanese]. Arerugi 1967; 16:178–222.
2. Kawasaki T, Kosaki F, Okawa S, et al. A new infantile acute febrile mucocutaneous lymph node syndrome (MLNS) prevailing in Japan. Pediatrics 1974;54:271–276.
3. Takahashi M. Kawasaki syndrome (mucocutaneous lymph node syndrome). In: Emmanouilides GC, ed. Moss and Adams heart disease in infants, children, and adolescents: including the fetus and young adult. 5th ed. Baltimore: Williams & Wilkins, 1995:13909.
4. Spector S. Scarlett fever, periarteritis nodosa, aneurysm of the coronary artery with spontaneous rupture, hemopericardium. Arch Pediatr 1939;25:319.
5. Kato H, Ichinose E, Yoshioka F, et al. Fate of coronary aneurysms in Kawasaki disease: serial coronary angiography and long-term follow-up study. Am J Cardiol 1982; 49:1758–1766.
6. Kato H, Ichinose E, Kawasaki T. Myocardial infarction in Kawasaki disease: clinical analyses in 195 cases. J Pediatr 1986;108:923–927.
7. Japan Kawasaki Disease Research Committee. Diagnostic guideline of Kawasaki disease. Tokyo: Japan Kawasaki Disease Research Committee; 1984.
8. American Heart Association Committee on Rheumatic Fever, Endocarditis, and Kawasaki Disease. Diagnostic guidelines for Kawasaki disease. Am J Dis Child 1990; 144:1218–1219.
9. Dajani AS, Taubert KA, Gerber MA, et al. Diagnosis and therapy of Kawasaki disease in children. Circulation 1993;87:1776–1780.
10. Rowley AH, Gonzalez-Crussi F, Gidding SS, et al. Incomplete Kawasaki disease with coronary artery involvement. J Pediatr 1987;110:409–413.
11. Rosenfeld EA, Corydon KE, Shulman ST. Kawasaki disease in infants less than one year of age. J Pediatr 1995; 126:524–529.
12. Newburger JW, Takahashi M, Gerber MA, et al. Diagnosis, treatment, and long term management of Kawasaki disease. A statement for health professionals from the committee on rheumatic fever, endocarditis, and Kawasaki disease. Council on cardiovascular disease in the young. American Heart Association. Circulation 2004;110:2747–2771.
13. Newburger JW, Takahashi M, Gerber MA, et al. Diagnosis, treatment, and long term management of Kawasaki disease. A statement for health professionals from the committee on rheumatic fever, endocarditis, and Kawasaki disease. Council on cardiovascular disease in the young. American Heart Association. Pediatrics 2004;114: 1708–1733.
14. Taubert KA. Epidemiology of Kawasaki disease in the United States and worldwide. Prog Pediatr Cardiol 1997;6:181–185.
15. Mason WH, Takahashi M, Schneider T. Recurrence of Kawasaki disease in a large urban cohort in the United States. In: Takahashi M, Taubert K, eds. Proceedings of the Fourth International Symposium on Kawasaki Disease. Dallas: American Heart Association; 1993:21–26.
16. Taubert KA, Rowley AH, Shulman ST. A 10 year (1984–1993) United States hospital survey of Kawasaki disease. In: Kato H, ed. Kawasaki disease: proceedings of the 5th International Kawasaki Disease Symposium. New York: Elsevier; 1995:34–38.
17. Yanagawa H, Yashiro M, Nakamura Y, et al. Results of 12 nationwide epidemiological incidence surveys of Kawasaki disease in Japan. Arch Pediatr Adolesc Med 1995;149:779–783.
18. Barron KS, Shulman ST, Rowley A, et al. Report of the National Institutes of Health workshop on Kawasaki disease. J Rheumatol 1999;26:170–190.
19. Leung DY, Meissner HC, Shulman ST, et al. Prevalence of superantigen-secreting bacteria in patients with Kawasaki disease. J Pediatr 2002;140:742–746.
20. Leung DYM, Giorno RC, Kazemi LV, et al. Evidence for superantigen involvement in cardiovascular injury due to Kawasaki disease. J Immunol 1995;155:5018–5021.
21. Leung DY, Meissner HC, Fulton DR, et al. Toxic shock syndrome toxin-secreting *Staphylococcus aureus* in Kawasaki syndrome. Lancet 1993;342:1385–1388.

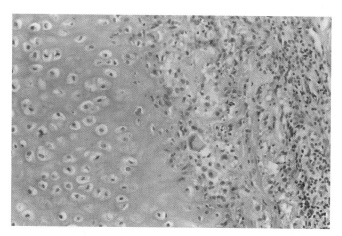

FIGURE 22-1

Histology of the fibrocartilagenous junction of the ear in a patient with relapsing polychondritis. Inflammatory mononuclear cells infiltrate this region with occasional polymorphonuclear leukocytes with damage to the cartilage. Hemotoxylin and eosin stain. Original magnification, ×200. (Courtesy of Dr. Lestor E. Wold.)

TABLE 22-1. Clinical manifestations of relapsing polychondritis.

MANIFESTATION	INITIAL (%)	TOTAL (%)
Auricular chondritis	40	85
Nasal cartilage	20	50
Hearing loss	9	30
Arthritis	35	50
Ocular	20	50
Larynotracheal–bronchial	26	48
Laryngotracheal stricture	15	23
Systemic vasculitis	3	10
Valvular dysfunction	0	6

SOURCE: Adapted from Isaak BL, Liesegang TJ, Michet CJ Jr. Ophthalmology 1986;93:681–689, by permission of *Ophthalmology*.

can be a clue to this involvement. Narrowing of the trachea, either localized or generalized, leads to inability to clear the throat, choking spells, and respiratory infections. These symptoms should be taken seriously because this is a potentially lethal complication. Respiratory symptoms of varying degree may be observed in up to 50% of patients (12).

CARDIOVASCULAR

Vasculitis of various varieties can be observed in about 10% of the patients. Small vessel involvement leading to a leukocytoclastic vasculitis, medium size vessel disease of the polyarteritis variety, and large vessel disease of the Takayasu's arteritis variety occur. Signs and symptoms depend upon the type of involvement as well as the associated disease. Inflammation of the root of the aorta can cause aortic valve dysfunction, including aortic incompetence. Myocarditis may manifest as arrhythmias or even heart block (13).

OCULAR

The ocular involvement is very variable with both intra- and extraocular disease. Intraocular changes seen include iridocyclitis and retinal vasculitis. Extraocular disease manifests as periorbital edema, extraocular muscle palsy, conjunctivitis, keratitis, scleritis, and episcleritis. Proptosis is observed rarely (11).

MUSCULOSKELETAL

A seronegative episodic inflammatory oligo- or polyarthritis can be observed in anywhere from 30% to 75% of the patients. This is generally nonerosive and nonde-

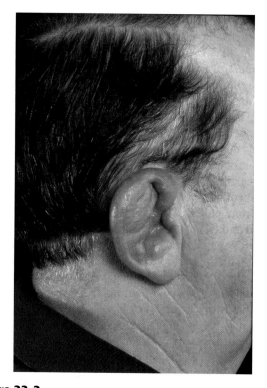

Figure 22-2

Acutely inflamed ear with sparing of the noncartilageneous lobule.

forming, affecting both the small and large joints. Articular cartilage damage can cause symmetrical joint space narrowing and costal cartilage damage may lead to a pectus excavatum deformity (14).

OTHER FEATURES

Segmental proliferative glomerulonephritis may be observed in approximately 10% of patients (15). Systemic features, including fever, weight loss, and fatigue, are commonly seen. Several cases of myelodysplastic syndrome have been described (16).

DIAGNOSIS

McAdam and colleagues (17) proposed that the diagnosis of RP require three or more of the following clinical criteria: (1) bilateral auricular chondritis, (2) nonerosive, seronegative inflammatory polyarthritis, (3) nasal chondritis, (4) ocular inflammation (conjunctivitis, keratitis, scleritis/episcleritis, uveitis), (5) respiratory tract chondritis (laryngeal and/or tracheal cartilages), and (6) cochlear and/or vestibular dysfunction (neurosensory hearing loss, tinnitus, and/or vertigo), and a compatible biopsy. The need for a biopsy has not been necessary in retrospective studies (4) and is not necessary in clinical practice if the patient has chondritis of both ears, or chondritis at multiple sites. If, however, the history is recent and the clinical picture unclear or confusing, a biopsy (see Figure 22-1) may be essential to make a diagnosis.

As with other inflammatory diseases there can be anemia of chronic disease, elevated sedimentation rate, and hypergammaglobulinemia. If macrocytosis is observed, the possibility of associated myelodysplasia should be investigated. An abnormal urinalysis generally reflects renal involvement and the possibility of glomerulonephritis should be investigated.

Respiratory involvement is always a serious complication and may go undiagnosed until complications develop. Thus, all patients should undergo pulmonary function tests, as well as inspiratory and expiratory flow volume curves (12). Radiologic assessment by tomography or computed tomography (CT) scan (3,18–20) has been helpful in delineating the inflammatory changes of the trachea and the bronchial tree and the presence of stricture/s (localized or diffuse) and calcification can be accurately assessed.

Echocardiogram may help assess involvement of the cardiac valves and CT/magnetic resonance angiography (MRA) may be necessary to look for large vessel disease. Other investigations depend upon the associated disease.

When faced with a patient with early RP, one is obligated to consider other diagnosis. Chondritis due to streptococcal infection, local fungal infections, syphilis, or leprosy need to be kept in mind. Local trauma may cause inflammatory changes that mimic chondritis. Nasal cartilage damage leading to collapse of the bridge can occur from trauma, infections, granulomatous diseases like Wegener's granulomatosis, as well as from neoplastic diseases. Vasculitis of large and small blood vessels from other connective tissue diseases should be considered.

MANAGEMENT

The management of patients with RP depends upon the manifestations of the disease. If the patients have mild disease with fever, ear cartilage and/ or nasal cartilage inflammation with arthalgias, then nonsteriodal anti-inflammatory drugs (NSAIDs) may be adequate. If, however, the symptoms are severe or resistant to NSAID therapy, then low-to-moderate doses of corticosteroids may be necessary. Presence of respiratory symptoms, renal disease, or vasculitis require high-dose corticosteroids. As the disease is better controlled the steroid dose can be reduced. Immunosuppressives may be necessary as steroid-sparing agents. Other drugs, for example, dapsone and cyclosporine, have been reported to be helpful in small numbers of patients and so have immunosupressive drugs, including azathioprine, methotrexate, chlorambucil, and cyclophosphamide. Recently, anti-CD4 antibodies and anti–tumor necrosis factor (TNF) agents have been used with mixed success. Because of the rarity of this illness, no controlled studies have been done. Involvement of the trachea is a serious complication and necessitates aggressive management, including tracheostomy, use of stents if there is tracheal collapse, high-dose corticosteroids, and immunosuppressives (21). Infection from respiratory compromise and immunosuppressed state, as well as systemic vasculitis have been increasingly common causes of death. Aortic valve disease can be successfully treated by surgery (22).

REFERENCES

1. Jaksch-Wartenhorst R. Polychondropathia. Wien Arch F Inn Med 1923;6:93–100.
2. Pearson CM, Kline HM, Newcomer VD. Relapsing polychondritis. N Engl J Med 1960;263:51–58.
3. Kent PD, Michet CJ, Luthra HS. Relapsing polychondritis. Curr Opin Rheumatol 2004;16:56–61.
4. Michet CJ Jr, McKenna CH, Luthra HS, O'Fallon WW. Relapsing polychondritis; survival and predictive role of early disease manifestations. Ann Int Med 1986;104:74–78.
5. Riccieri V, Spadaro A, Taccari E, Zoppini A. A case of relapsing polychondritis: pathogenetic considerations Clin Exp Rheumatol 1988;6:95–96.

22

6. Homma S, Matsumoto T, Abe H, Fukuda Y, Nagano M, Suzuki M. Relapsing polychondritis: pathological and immunological findings in an autopsy case. Acta Pathol Jpn 1984;34:1137–1146.

7. McKenna CH, Luthra HS, Jordan RE. Hypocomplementemic ear effusion in relapsing polychondritis. Mayo Clin Proc 1976;51:495–497.

8. Foidart J, Abe S, Martin GR, et al. Antibodies to type II collagen in relapsing polychondritis. N Engl J Med 1978; 299:1203–1207.

9. Herman JH, Dennis MV. Immunopathologic studies in relapsing polychondritis. J Clin Invest 1973;52:549–558.

10. Taneja V, Griffiths M, Behrens M, Luthra HS, David CS. Auricular chondritis in NOD.DQ8.A beta o (A(g7-/-)) transgenic mice resembles human relapsing polychondritis. J Clin Invest 2003;112:1843–1850.

11. Isaak BL, Liesegang TJ, Michet CJ Jr. Ocular and systemic findings in relapsing polychondritis. Ophthalmology 1986;93:681–689.

12. Krell WS, Staats BA, Hyatt RE. Pulmonary function in relapsing polychondritis. Am Rev Respir Dis 1986;133:1120–1123.

13. Delrosso A, Petix NR, Pratesi M, et al. Cardiovascular involvement in relapsing polychondritis. Semin Arthritis Rheum 1997;26:840–844.

14. O'Hanlon M, McAdam LP, Bluestone R, Pearson CM. The arthropathy of relapsing polychondritis. Arthritis Rheumatism 1976;19:191–194.

15. Chang-Miller A, Okamura M, Torres VE, et al. Renal involvement in relapsing polychondritis. Medicine 1987; 66:202–217.

16. Myers B, Gould J, Dolan G. Relapsing polychondritis and myelodysplasia: a report of two cases and review of the literature. Clin Lab Haematol 2000;22:45–48.

17. McAdam LP, O'Hanlon MA, Bluestone R, Pearson CM. Relapsing polychondritis: prospective study of 23 patients and a review of the literature. Medicine 1976;55:193–215.

18. Booth A, Dieppe PA, Goddard PL, Watt I. The radiological manifestations of relapsing polychondritis. Clin Radiol 1989;40:147–149.

19. Mendelson DS, Som PM, Crane R, Cohen BA, Spiera H. Relapsing polychondritis studied by computed tomography. Radiology 1985;157:489–490.

20. Davis SD, Berkmen YM, King T. Peripheral bronchial involvement in relapsing polychondritis: demonstration by thin-section CT. AJR Am J Roentgenol 1989;153:953–954.

21. Eng J, Sabanathan S. Airway complications of relapsing polychondritis. Ann Thorac Surg 1991;51:686–692.

22. Buckley LM, Ades PA. Progressive aortic valve inflammation occuring despite apparent remission of relapsing polychondritis Arthritis Rheum 1992;35:812–814.

CHAPTER 23

Adult-Onset Still's Disease

JOHN M. ESDAILE MD, MPH

- Diagnosis is one of exclusion and is suggested by the characteristic febrile pattern, evanescent rash, organomegaly, elevated white blood cell count, and a markedly elevated serum ferritin, serum IL-18 when available, and a reduced glycosylated fraction of ferritin.
- A predominance of T-helper cell (Th1) cytokines such as interleukin (IL)-2, IL-6, IL-18, interferon gamma,

tumor necrosis factor (TNF) alpha have been reported in persons with active adult Still's disease and therapy against these cytokines is an active area of investigation.
- Most have a chronic course with morbidity arising from a polyarthritis.

ADULT STILL'S DISEASE

The clinical features of adult Still's disease resemble the systemic form of juvenile rheumatoid arthritis. The disorder is rare, affects both genders equally, and exists worldwide. The majority of patients are 16 to 35 years of age (1).

Pathogenesis

The etiology of adult Still's disease is unknown. Studies of linkage to human leukocyte antigens (HLA) have been inconclusive (2). It has been suggested that immune complexes play a pathogenic role, but this suspicion has not been confirmed (1,2). The principal hypothesis is that Still's disease results from a virus or other infectious agent, but study results lack consistency (1). Pregnancy or use of female hormones have not been associated with the development of Still's disease (3). The possible role of stress as an inducing phenomenon has been raised, but lacks confirmation (3).

A predominance of T-helper (Th1) cytokines have been reported in the blood and tissues of persons with active adult Still's disease (4). Increased levels of interleukin (IL)-2, IL-6, IL-18, interferon gamma, and tumor necrosis factor (TNF) alpha have been described (1,4–6). Alterations in cytokines may be important in the pathogenesis of the disorder and in its future treatment.

Clinical, Laboratory, and Radiographic Findings

The clinical manifestations and laboratory findings of adult Still's disease (2,7) are summarized in Table 23-1. Usually the initial symptom is sudden onset of a high spiking fever. The fever spikes once daily (rarely, twice daily), usually in the evening, and the temperature returns to normal in 80% of patients untreated with antipyretics. Arthralgia and severe myalgia are universal. Arthritis is almost universal but may be mild and overlooked by a physician whose attention is drawn to more dramatic manifestations. Initially the arthritis affects only a few joints but may then evolve into polyarticular disease. The most commonly affected joints are the knee (84%) and wrist (74%). The ankle, shoulder, elbow, and proximal interphalangeal joints are involved in one half of patients and the metacarpophalangeal joints are involved in one third of patients. Involvement of the distal interphalangeal joints in one-fifth of patients is notable (2,8). Still's rash, present in more than 85% of patients, is almost pathognomonic. The rash is salmon pink, macular or maculopapular, frequently evanescent, and often occurs with the evening fever spike. Because the rash may not be noticed by the patient, a check during evening rounds can lead to the detection of this almost diagnostic finding. The rash is most common on the trunk and proximal extremities, but is present on the face in 15% of patients. It can be

TABLE 23-1. CLINICAL MANIFESTATIONS AND LABORATORY TESTS IN ADULT STILL'S DISEASE.[a]

CHARACTERISTIC[b]	PATIENTS POSITIVE/PATIENTS TOTAL	PERCENTAGE
Clinical manifestations		
Female	145/283	51
Childhood episode (≤15 years)	38/236	16
Onset 16−35 years	178/233	76
Arthralgia	282/283	100
Arthritis	249/265	94
Fever ≥ 39°C	258/266	97
Fever ≥ 39.5°C	54/62	87
Sore throat	57/62	92
JRA rash	248/281	88
Myalgia	52/62	84
Weight loss ≥ 10%	41/54	76
Lymphadenopathy	167/264	63
Splenomegaly	138/265	52
Abdominal pain	30/62	48
Hepatomegaly	108/258	42
Pleuritis	79/259	31
Pericarditis	75/254	30
Pneumonitis	17/62	27
Alopecia	15/62	24
Laboratory tests		
Elevated ESR	265/267	99
WBC ≥ 10,000 cells/mm³	228/248	92
WBC ≥ 15,000 cells/mm³	50/62	81
Neutrophils ≥ 80%	55/62	88
Serum albumin < 3.5 g/dL	143/177	81
Elevated hepatic enzymes[b]	169/232	73
Anemia (hemoglobin ≤ 10 g/dL)	159/233	68
Platelets ≥ 400,000/mm³	37/60	62
Negative antinuclear antibody test	256/278	92
Negative rheumatoid factor	259/280	93

ABBREVIATIONS: ESR, erythrocyte sedimentation rate; JRA, juvenile rheumatoid arthritis; WBC, white blood cell.
[a]Data from Pouchot and colleagues(2), including patients reviewed by Ohta and colleagues (J Rheumatol 1987;14:1139−1146). Data for fever ≥ 39.5°C, sore throat, myalgia, weight loss, abdominal pain, pneumonitis, alopecia, WBC ≥ 15,000 cells/mm³, neutrophils, and platelets are from Pouchot and colleagues only, as these data were likely underreported in early studies.
[b]Any elevated liver function test.

precipitated by mechanical irritation from clothing, rubbing (Koebner's phenomenon), or a hot bath. The rash may be mildly pruritic.

An elevated erythrocyte sedimentation rate is universal. Leukocytosis is present in 90% of cases, and in 80% the white blood cell count is 15,000/mm³ or more. The liver function tests may be elevated in up to three fourths of patients (1,2,9). Anemia, sometimes profound, is common. Rheumatoid factor and antinuclear antibody tests are generally negative and, if present, are of low titer. Synovial and serosal fluids are inflammatory with a predominance of neutrophils (2).

Radiographic findings at presentation are nonspecific. Early in the disease course, soft tissue swelling and periarticular osteoporosis may be found. With time, cartilage narrowing or erosion develop in most patients. Characteristic radiographic findings are typically found in the wrist, including nonerosive narrowing of the carpometacarpal and intercarpal joints, which progresses to bony ankylosis (2,10,11).

Diagnosis

Although several sets of diagnostic criteria have been proposed (8,12,13), the criteria of Cush and colleagues (8) are a practical guide (Table 23-2). It is important to note that most patients do not present with the full-blown syndrome. Fever is the most common first manifestation, and other features develop over a period of a couple of weeks or occasionally months. A patient with high daily fever spikes, severe myalgia, arthralgia, arthritis, Still's rash, and leukocytosis (frequently in combination with other manifestations outlined in Table

TABLE 23-2. CRITERIA FOR THE DIAGNOSIS OF ADULT STILL'S DISEASE.

A diagnosis of adult Still's disease requires the presence of all of the following:
    Fever ≥ 39°C (102.2°F)
    Arthralgia or arthritis
    Rheumatoid factor < 1:80
    Antinuclear antibody < 1:100

In addition, any two of the following are required:
    White blood cell count ≥ 15,000 cells/mm³
    Still's rash
    Pleuritis or pericarditis
    Hepatomegaly or splenomegaly or generalized
        lymphadenopathy

SOURCE: From Cush JJ, Medsger TA Jr, Christy WC, et al. Arthritis Rheum 1987;30:186–194, by permission of *Arthritis and Rheumatism.*

23-1) is unlikely to have anything other than adult Still's disease. Thus, this diagnosis should top the differential diagnosis list (Table 23-3). Most other diagnoses can be excluded on clinical grounds or by simple diagnostic tests. Recently, a markedly elevated serum ferritin and a reduced glycosylated fraction of ferritin has been proposed as suggesting Still's disease (12,14,15). The elevated ferritin likely results from the increased inflammatory cytokines and it has been suggested that IL-18 may be a better marker.

Disease Course and Outcome

Approximately one fifth of patients with Still's disease experience long-term remission within 1 year. One-third of patients have a complete remission followed by one or more relapses. The timing of relapse is unpredictable, although relapse tends to be less severe and of shorter duration than the initial episode (2,8). The remaining patients have a chronic disease course. The principal problem is chronic arthritis, and some patients with severe involvement of the hips and, to a lesser extent, the knees have required total joint replacement (2,8).

The presence of polyarthritis (four or more joints involved) or root joint involvement (shoulders or hips) has been identified as markers for a chronic disease course in a number of studies (2,8). A prior episode in childhood (which occurs in about 1 of 6 patients) and a need for more than 2 years of therapy with systemic corticosteroids may also be poor prognostic markers (8).

Overall, the prognosis is good. A recent controlled study noted that an average of 10 years after diagnosis, patients with adult Still's disease had significantly higher levels of pain, physical disability, and psychologic disability than their unaffected siblings of the same gender. However, the levels of pain and disability in patients

with adult Still's disease were lower than in other chronic rheumatic diseases. Educational attainment, occupational prestige, social functioning, and family income did not differ between the Still's patients and the controls (16). The results suggest that patients with Still's disease are remarkably resilient in overcoming handicaps. However, premature death may be slightly increased above that expected. Causes of fatality include hepatic failure, disseminated intravascular coagulation, amyloidosis, and sepsis, all of which were likely due to the Still's disease (1,2,7,8).

Treatment

Acute Disease

Nonsteroidal anti-inflammatory drugs (NSAIDs), including aspirin, are first-line treatment. Response to NSAIDs may be slow but responders usually have a good prognosis (2).

A major concern with NSAID therapy has been severe hepatotoxicity. Liver function test abnormalities, a common finding on presentation, are likely an integral part of the disease and may return to normal despite continued NSAID therapy (2). However, frequent

TABLE 23-3. DIFFERENTIAL DIAGNOSIS OF ADULT STILL'S DISEASE.

Granulomatous disorders
    Sarcoidosis
    Idiopathic granulomatosis hepatitis
    Crohn's disease

Vasculitis
    Serum sickness
    Polyarteritis nodosa
    Wegener's granulomatosis
    Thrombotic thrombocytopenic purpura
    Takayasu's arteritis

Infection
    Viral infection (e.g., hepatitis B, rubella, parvovirus, Coxsackie
        virus, Epstein–Barr, cytomegalovirus, human immunodefi-
        ciency virus)
    Subacute bacterial endocarditis
    Chronic meningococcemia
    Gonococcemia
    Tuberculosis
    Lyme disease
    Syphilis
    Rheumatic fever

Malignancy
    Leukemia
    Lymphoma
    Angioblastic lymphadenopathy

Connective tissue disease
    Systemic lupus erythematosus
    Mixed connective tissue disease

23

monitoring of liver function, even after hospital discharge, is mandatory for patients receiving NSAIDs. NSAIDs may also increase the risk of intravascular coagulopathy.

In patients who fail to respond to NSAIDs and those with severe disease require systemic intravascular coagulopathy, rising values on liver function tests during NSAID treatment, and individuals who do not respond to NSAIDs may require corticosteriod treatment. Generally, prednisone in a dose of 0.5 to 1.0 mg/kg/day is needed initially, but relapse can occur with tapering and continued treatment does not prevent progressive destructive arthropathy (1,2). Intravenous pulse methylprednisolone has been used for life-threatening acute disease (2).

Chronic Disease

No controlled studies of second-line agents for the treatment of Still's disease have been published. The most common cause of chronicity is arthritis. Low-dose weekly methotrexate in doses similar to that used in adult rheumatoid arthritis has been used to control both chronic arthritis and chronic systemic disease (1,17,18). While methotrexate is potentially hepatotoxic, this agent is being used increasingly. Approximately two thirds of patients will respond to methotrexate (17). Mild chronic systemic disease (e.g., fatigue, fever, rash, serositis) may also respond to hydroxychloroquine and this agent can be combined with methotrexate. Increased toxicity with sulfasalazine has been reported, thereby limiting its use (19).

Immunosuppressive agents, including azathioprine, cyclophosphamide, and, most recently, cyclosporin A (20), have been used in resistant cases. Intravenous immunoglobulin (21) has been used, alone (21) or in combination with mycophenolate mofetil (22), but its use is controversial.

Elevated serum levels of cytokines including TNF alpha, IL-6, interferon gamma, and especially IL-18 (1,4–6), although nonspecific, have suggested the possible benefit of anticytokine therapies. TNF-alpha blocking treatments, especially infliximab, appear effective (23,24), although a recent report noted that they were not continued in 17 of 20 patients because of adverse effects or loss of efficacy (25). Anakinra (100 mg subcutaneous daily) shows great promise as a treatment. It has been reported in a small number of cases to have dramatic benefits (1,26,27). A decade after disease onset, approximately one half of patients require second-line agents, and one third of these require low dose corticosteroids (16).

Adult Still's disease affects primarily young adults at a time when they are completing their education, starting a career, or starting a family, which can make it particularly devastating. Physiotherapists, occupational therapists, psychologists, or arthritis support groups may all be needed to care for individual patients. A knowledgeable, caring physician can make a tremendous difference. It is important to realize that Still's disease can remit even years after onset and that the vast majority of patients are leading remarkably full lives a decade after the onset of the disease.

REFERENCES

1. Efthimiou P, Paik PK, Bielory L. Diagnosis and management of adult onset Still's disease. Ann Rheum Dis 2006; 65:564–572.
2. Pouchot J, Esdaile JM, Sampalis J, et al. Adult Still's disease: manifestations, disease course, and outcome in 62 patients. Medicine 1991;70:118–136.
3. Sampalis JS, Medsger TA Jr, Fries JF, et al. Risk factors for adult Still's disease. J Rheumatol 1996;23:2049–2054.
4. Chen DY, Lan JL, Lin FJ, Hsieh TY, Wen MC. Predominance of Th1 cytokine in peripheral blood and pathological tissues of patients with active untreated adult onset Still's disease. Ann Rheum Dis 2004;63:1300–1306.
5. Hoshino T, Ohta A, Yang D, et al. Elevated serum interleukin 6, interferon-gamma, and tumor necrosis factor-alpha levels in patients with adult Still's disease. J Rheumatol 1998;25:396–398.
6. Kawashima M, Yamamura M, Taniai M, et al. Levels of interleukin-18 and its binding inhibitors in the blood circulation of patients with adult-onset Still's disease. Arthritis Rheum 2001;44:550–560.
7. Ohta A, Yamaguchi M, Tsunematsu T, et al. Adult Still's disease: a multicenter survey of Japanese patients. J Rheumatol 1990;17:1058–1063.
8. Cush JJ, Medsger TA Jr, Christy WC, Herbert D, Cooperstein LA. Adult-onset Still's disease: clinical course and outcome. Arthritis Rheum 1987;30:186–194.
9. Esdaile JM, Tannenbaum H, Lough JO, Hawkins D. Hepatic abnormalities in adult Still's disease. J Rheumatol 1979;6:673–679.
10. Medsger TA Jr, Christy WC. Carpal arthritis with ankylosis in late onset Still's disease. Arthritis Rheum 1976;19: 232–242.
11. Bjorkengren AG, Pathria MN, Sartoris DJ, et al. Carpal alterations in adult-onset Still's disease, juvenile chronic arthritis and adult-onset rheumatoid arthritis: a comparative study. Radiology 1987;165:545–548.
12. Yamaguchi M, Ohta A, Tsunematsu T, et al. Preliminary criteria for classification of adult Still's disease. J Rheumatol 1992;19:424–430.
13. Masson C, Le Loet X, Liote F, et al. Comparative study of 6 types of criteria in adult Still's disease. J Rheumatol 1996;23:495–497.
14. Fautrel B, Le Moel G, Saint-Marcoux B, et al. Diagnostic value of ferritin and glycosylated ferritin in adult onset Still's disease: J Rheumatol 2001;28:322–329.
15. Lambotte O, Cacoub P, Costedoat N, et al. High ferritin and low glycosylated ferritin may also be a marker of excessive macrophage activation. J Rheumatol 2003;30: 1027–1028.

16. Sampalis JS, Esdaile JM, Medsger TA Jr, et al. A controlled study of the long-term prognosis of adult Still's disease. Am J Med 1995;98:384–388.

17. Fujii T, Akizuki M, Kameda H, et al. Methotrexate treatment in patients with adult onset Still's disease – retrospective study of 13 cases. Ann Rheum Dis 1997;56:144–148.

18. Fautrel B, Borget C, Rozenberg S, et al. Corticosteroid sparing effect of low dose methotrexate treatment in adult Still's disease. J Rheumatol 1999;26:373–378.

19. Jung JH, Jun JB, Yoo DH, et al. High toxicity of sulfasalazine in adult-onset Still's disease. Clin Exp Rheumatol 2000;18:245–248.

20. Marchesoni A, Ceravolo GP, Battafarano N, Rossetti A, Tosi S, Fantini F. Cyclosporin A in the treatment of adult onset Still's disease. J Rheumatol 1997;24:1582–1587.

21. Vignes S, Wechsler B, Amoura Z, et al. Intravenous immunoglobulin in adult Still's disease refractory to nonsteroidal anti-inflammatory drugs. Clin Exp Rheumatol 1998;16:295–298.

22. Bennett AN, Peterson P, Sangle S, et al. Adult onset Still's disease and collapsing glomerulopathy: successful treatment with intravenous immunoglobulins and mycophenolate mofetil. Rheumatology 2004;43:795–799.

23. Kokkinos A, Iliopoulos A, Greka P, Efthymiou A, Katsilambros N, Sfikakis PP. Successful treatment of refractory adult-onset Still's disease with infliximab. A prospective, non-comparative series of four patients. Clin Rheumatol 2004;23:45–49.

24. Husni ME, Maier AL, Mease PJ, et al. Etanercept in the treatment of adult patients with Still's disease. Arthritis Rheum 2002;46:1171–1176.

25. Fautrel B, Sibilia J, Mariette X, Combe B. Tumour necrosis factor alpha blocking agents in refractory adult Still's disease: an observational study of 20 cases. Ann Rheum Dis 2005;64:262–266.

26. Fitzgerald AA, LeClercq SA, Yan A, Homik JE, Dinarello CA. Rapid response to anakinra in patients with refractory adults Still's disease. Arthritis Rheum 2005;52:1794–1803.

27. Vasques Godinho FM, Parreira Santos MJ, Canas da Silva J. Refractory adult onset Still's disease successfully treated with anakinra. Ann Rheum Dis 2005;64:647–648.

23

CHAPTER 24

Periodic Syndromes

JOHN G. RYAN, MB, MRCPI
DANIEL L. KASTNER, MD, PHD

- Hereditary periodic fever syndromes are autoinflammatory diseases characterized by episodes of fever with serosal, synovial, and/or skin inflammation.
- Familial Mediterranean fever (FMF) and hyperimmunoglobulinemia D with periodic fever syndrome (HIDS) are inherited in an autosomal recessive manner and tumor necrosis factor receptor–associated periodic syndrome (TRAPS), familial cold autoin-

flammatory syndrome (FCAS), Muckle–Wells syndrome (MWS), and neonatal-onset multisystem inflammatory disease (NOMID) are dominantly inherited.
- Colchicine and biologic therapies such as tumor necrosis factor alpha (TNF-alpha) and interleukin 1 beta (IL-1 beta) receptor agonists are successful in the treatment of some of these inherited diseases.

Several forms of arthritis may present with patterns of exacerbation and remission that may be considered periodic. This chapter focuses on six clinically distinct illnesses in which underlying genes have been identified, and in addition a group of disorders of unclear etiology.

HEREDITARY PERIODIC FEVER SYNDROMES

This group of diseases is characterized by episodes of fever with serosal, synovial, and/or cutaneous inflammation. Unlike the commonly recognized autoimmune diseases, there is a lack of either high titer autoantibodies or self-reactive T cells, and hence these conditions are sometimes referred to as *autoinflammatory* diseases (1). Based on clinical findings and patterns of inheritance, at least six distinct disorders have been grouped among the hereditary periodic fever syndromes (Table 24-1). Two of these illnesses, familial Mediterranean fever (FMF) and the hyperimmunoglobulinemia D with periodic fever syndrome (HIDS), are inherited in an autosomal recessive manner. The other diseases, tumor necrosis factor (TNF) receptor–associated periodic syndrome (TRAPS), familial cold autoinflammatory syndrome (FCAS), Muckle–Wells syndrome (MWS), and neonatal-onset multisystem inflammatory disease (NOMID, also known as chronic infantile neurologic cutaneous and articular syndrome, or CINCA), are dominantly inherited. Advances in molecular genetics

have identified four genes underlying these six clinical entities.

It should be noted at the outset that there are a number of patients with unexplained recurrent fevers who do not have demonstrable mutations in these four genes, and who may not meet clinical criteria for any of the six disorders described below. In children, the syndrome of periodic fever with aphthous stomatitis, pharyngitis, and cervical adenopathy (PFAPA) is relatively common (2). In addition to the cardinal manifestations making up the acronym, abdominal pain and arthralgia are also sometimes seen. Mutations in the known periodic fever genes are an exclusion criterion, and this condition almost uniformly abates in late adolescence or early adulthood.

Familial Mediterranean Fever

Familial Mediterranean fever is a recessively inherited disease most frequently observed in Jewish, Armenian, Arab, Turkish, and Italian populations (3), with a modest male predominance (4). FMF (entry 249100 of Online Mendelian Inheritance in Man, OMIM, at http://www.ncbi.nlm.nih.gov/entrez/query.fcgi?db=OMIM) is caused by mutations in *MEFV* (MEditerranean FeVer), a 10-exon gene encoded on the short arm of chromosome sixteen (5,6). To date, over 70 disease-associated *MEFV* mutations have been described, many clustered in exon 10. The online database of periodic fever mutations, INFEVERS (http://fmf.igh.cnrs.fr/infevers/), provides an updated listing of *MEFV* mutations and

TABLE 24-1. THE HEREDITARY PERIODIC FEVER SYNDROMES.

CLINICAL FEATURES	FAMILIAL MEDITERRANEAN FEVER	HYPER IGD SYNDROME	TNF RECEPTOR-ASSOCIATED PERIODIC SYNDROME	FAMILIAL COLD AUTOINFLAMMATORY SYNDROME	MUCKLE–WELLS SYNDROME	NEONATAL ONSET MULTISYSTEM INFLAMMATORY DISORDER/CINCA
Mode of inheritance	Autosomal recessive	Autosomal recessive	Autosomal dominant	Autosomal dominant	Autosomal dominant	Autosomal dominant
Underlying gene	MEFV, encoding pyrin (marenostrin)	MVK, encoding mevalonate kinase	TNFRS1A, encoding p55 TNF receptor	CIAS1, encoding cryopyrin (NALP3)	CIAS1, encoding cryopyrin	CIAS1, encoding cryopyrin (NALP3)
Usual ethnicity	Turkish, Armenian, Arab, Jewish, Italian	Dutch, other north European	Any ethnicity	Mostly European	Mostly European	Any ethnicity
Duration of attacks	12–72 hours	3–7 days	Days to weeks	12–24 hours	2–3 days	Continuous, with flares
Abdominal pain	Sterile peritonitis, constipation	Severe pain, vomiting, diarrhea, rarely peritonitis	Peritonitis, diarrhea, or constipation	Nausea	Abdominal pain, vomiting, diarrhea	Can occur
Pleural	Common	Rare	Common	Not seen	Rare	Rare
Arthropathy	Monoarthritis; rarely protracted arthritis in knee or hip	Arthralgia, symmetric polyarthritis	Arthritis in large joints, arthralgia	Polyarthralgia	Polyarthralgia, oligoarthritis, clubbing	Epiphyseal overgrowth, contractures, intermittent or chronic arthritis, clubbing
Cutaneous	Erysipeloid erythema on lower leg, ankle, foot	Diffuse maculopapular rash, urticaria	Migratory rash with underlying myalgia	Cold-induced urticarial rash	Urticarialike rash	Urticaria-like rash
Ocular	Rare	Uncommon	Periorbital edema, conjunctivitis	Conjunctivitis	Conjunctivitis, episcleritis	Progressive visual loss, uveitis, conjunctivitis
Neurologic	Rarely aseptic meningitis	Headache	Controversial	Headache	Sensorineural deafness	Headache, sensorineural deafness, chronic aseptic meningitis, mental retardation
Lymphatic	Splenomegaly, occasional lymphadenopathy	Painful cervical lymphadenopathy in children	Splenomegaly, occasional lymphadenopathy	Not seen	Rare	Hepatosplenomegaly, lymphadenopathy
Vasculitis	Henoch–Schönlein purpura (HSP), polyarteritis nodosa	Cutaneous vasculitis common, rarely HSP	HSP, lymphocytic vasculitis	Not seen	Not seen	Occasional
Systemic amyloidosis	Risk depends on MEFV and SAA genotypes, more common in Middle East	Rare	Occurs in 15%, risk increased with cysteine mutations	Rare	Occurs in ~25%	May develop in some patients, usually in adulthood
Treatment	Daily colchicine prophylaxis	Anti-TNF, statins investigational	Corticosteroids, etanercept	Anakinra (anti-IL1 receptor antagonist)	Anakinra (anti-IL1 receptor antagonist)	Anakinra (anti-IL1 receptor antagonist)

ABBREVIATIONS: TNF, tumor necrosis factor.

24

polymorphisms. Carrier frequencies in high risk populations can be as high as 1 in 3.

MEditerranean FeVer is expressed in polymorphonuclear leukocytes, the major cell found in FMF inflammatory infiltrates, as well as activated monocytes and synovial and peritoneal fibroblasts. *MEFV* codes for a 781 amino acid protein called pyrin (5), also known as marenostrin (6). The N-terminal 90 amino acids of pyrin are the prototype for a motif termed *the pyrin domain*, or PYD, found in over 20 human proteins involved in the regulation of inflammation and apoptosis. Through its PYD, pyrin associates with the apoptosis-associated specklike protein with a caspase recruitment domain (ASC), and thereby may regulate interleukin 1 beta (IL-1 beta) processing and leukocyte apoptosis (7). It is likely that pyrin variants in FMF lead to accentuated innate immune responses, and may have been selected by an as-yet unknown infectious agent.

Clinical and Laboratory Features

Familial Mediterranean fever is characterized by episodes of fever, usually lasting 1 to 3 days, with or without serositis, synovitis, or skin rash. Young children may present with fever alone. The first clinical episode usually occurs in childhood or adolescence, and 80% to 90% of patients experience their first episode by age 20. The time between attacks can vary for an individual patient, and may range from days to years. The magnitude of fever and type of attack (abdominal, pleural, or arthritic) may vary over time for any patient. During attacks, laboratory abnormalities in FMF include leukocytosis and elevated acute-phase reactants, including the erythrocyte sedimentation rate (ESR), C-reactive protein (CRP), fibrinogen, haptoglobin, and serum amyloid A (SAA).

Attacks comprised of fever and abdominal pain occur at some time in nearly all FMF patients. Abdominal pain may range from a dull ache to full-blown peritonitis, with rigid abdomen, absent bowel sounds, and rebound tenderness. Patients often undergo exploratory laparoscopy, which may reveal neutrophil-laden exudates. Repeated episodes of peritonitis may lead to adhesions. Constipation is common during attacks. Pleuritic episodes may occur without fever, and are usually unilateral. Other forms of serositis may occur. Pericarditis is uncommon; there have been rare reports of tamponade. Unilateral acute scrotal pain occurs in 5% of prepubertal boys, due to inflammation of the tunica vaginalis, an embryological remnant of the peritoneal membrane.

Joint involvement in FMF is particularly common in those with the M694V homozygous genotype (8). Acute monoarticular arthritis is most characteristic in FMF, particularly affecting the knee, ankle, or hip. These episodes of arthritis tend to last longer than serosal attacks, with large effusions, extreme pain, and inability to bear weight. Synovial fluid may appear septic, with as many as 100,000 polymorphonuclear leukocytes/mm^3, but is sterile. Nevertheless, erosive changes rarely develop. In the precolchicine era, up to 5% of patients developed chronic hip arthritis, with secondary osteoarthritis or osteonecrosis, requiring joint replacement. Chronic sacroiliitis may also occur in FMF, regardless of human leukocyte antigen (HLA)-B27 status or use of colchicine. Arthralgia is common in FMF, but nonspecific.

The most characteristic cutaneous lesion of FMF is *erysipeloid erythema*, a sharply demarcated, erythematous, tender swollen area occurring on the dorsum of the foot, ankle, or lower leg. FMF patients may rarely experience febrile myalgia, with excruciating muscle pain lasting up to several weeks; histologic features are suggestive of vasculitis. Other forms of vasculitis, including Henoch–Schönlein purpura and polyarteritis nodosum, are seen at increased frequency. Aseptic meningitis has been reported in FMF; however, a causal relationship has not been established.

The most serious complication of FMF is systemic amyloidosis (AA type), due to the deposition of a product of the acute phase reactant, SAA, in the kidneys, adrenal glands, intestine, spleen, lung, and testes. Risk factors for amyloidosis include M694V homozygous *MEFV* genotype (8), male gender, a positive family history for amyloidosis, and the SAA1 alpha/alpha genotype. Before the use of colchicine, renal failure due to amyloidosis was the most common cause of death. Amyloid deposition in the intestine may result in malabsorption. Cardiac involvement, neuropathy, and arthropathy are uncommon in the amyloidosis of FMF. Amyloidosis may rarely be the first manifestation of FMF (phenotype II). Urinalysis for protein is a rapid and inexpensive screen for amyloidosis. In patients with persistent proteinuria, amyloidosis can be evaluated directly by examination of a Congo red–stained rectal or renal biopsy specimen under polarized light.

In patients from high-risk ethnic groups with typical symptoms and a therapeutic response to colchicine, genetic testing is usually not considered necessary to confirm the diagnosis. Genetic testing may be a useful adjunct in atypical cases, or for physicians not familiar with FMF and related syndromes. Nevertheless, a significant fraction of patients with typical clinical findings of FMF have only one demonstrable *MEFV* mutation, rather than two, as would be expected in a recessive condition, and a small number of patients with clinical FMF may have no demonstrable mutations. These observations raise the possibility that there is a second FMF gene, or that *MEFV* mutations exist that are not accessible to current screening methods. Interpretation of genetic tests may be further complicated by the existence of complex alleles, where more than one mutation is identified on a single carrier chromosome, which at times appear sufficient to cause symptoms with a second normal allele. Thus, even in the era of molecular diagnostics, clinical judgment maintains a central role in the diagnosis of FMF.

Treatment

Daily oral cochicine therapy is the mainstay of treatment; it prevents both acute attacks and the development of amyloidosis. Over 75% of adults experience near-complete improvement in symptoms. The usual daily dose is 1.2 to 1.8 mg for adults, with children over 5 years of age requiring similar doses. In younger children, lower doses may be sufficient. In patients with amyloidosis, therapy should be aimed at reducing SAA levels below 10 mg/L. Diarrhea is a common side effect of colchicine, but may be minimized by starting at a low dose and gradually titrating upwards, by dividing the daily dose, and by taking appropriate measures should lactose intolerance develop. Neuropathy and myopathy are rare complications observed mainly in the elderly and those with renal impairment. There may be a slightly increased risk of trisomy 21 in the offspring of parents taking colchicine at the time of conception. The use of intravenous colchicine to abort acute episodes may cause severe toxicity in those taking daily oral colchicine. Patients with breakthrough attacks may benefit from subcutaneous interferon alpha, the IL-1 beta receptor antagonist anakinra, or biologic therapies targeted at TNF-alpha, although all of these approaches remain investigational. FMF patients with Henoch–Schönlein purpura or protracted febrile myalgia may require corticosteroids, and those with polyarteritis nodosa may require cyclophosphamide and high-dose corticosteroids.

Hyperimmunoglobulinemia D with Periodic Fever Syndrome

Hyperimmunoglobulinemia D with periodic fever syndrome (OMIM 260920) is a recessively inherited auto-inflammatory disorder described primarily in patients of Dutch or north European origin (9). In 1999, HIDS was shown to be caused by mutations in *MVK*, the gene encoding mevalonate kinase, an enzyme involved in cholesterol and nonsterol isoprene biosynthesis (10,11). As of this writing, over 50 disease-associated *MVK* mutations are listed on the INFEVERS website. HIDS mutations leave low levels of residual function of the enzyme, and lead to increased levels of the substrate, mevalonic acid, in the urine, especially during febrile attacks. Serum cholesterol levels are in the low–normal range. *MVK* mutations leading to complete loss of enzymatic activity cause mevalonic aciduria, a rare disease with mental retardation, cataracts, and failure to thrive,

in addition to features seen in HIDS. Current hypotheses on the pathogenesis of HIDS are based on the possible effects of isoprenoid deficiency or excess mevalonic acid on innate immune function. Elevated serum IgD is not thought to play a primary role in pathogenesis.

Clinical and Laboratory Findings

The first attack usually starts in infancy, often precipitated by childhood immunizations. The duration of attacks is between 3 and 7 days. Episodes may occur once or twice a month in childhood and adolescence, and may become less frequent or severe when the patient reaches adulthood. Minor infections, trauma, surgery, and menses may act as triggers.

The attacks of HIDS often begin with chills and headache. In children diffuse tender lymphadenopathy is common, and is considered a characteristic finding of HIDS. Abdominal pain is often present, but peritoneal irritation is less common than in FMF or TRAPS. Attacks are often accompanied by vomiting and diarrhea. A number of cutaneous manifestations have been described, including diffuse painful erythematous macules, urticaria, and a morbilliform rash. Unlike FMF there is no predilection for the lower limbs and the rash does not migrate. In as many as 70% of patients, HIDS may be associated with arthralgia or arthritis, and joint symptoms sometimes coincide with abdominal attacks. In contrast with the monoarticular arthritis of FMF, HIDS arthritis tends to be polyarticular. Large joints are usually affected, synovial fluid shows a predominance of granulocytes, and x-rays do not usually show erosions. Systemic amyloidosis is uncommon in HIDS.

During inflammatory attacks, HIDS patients present with leukocytosis and elevated acute-phase reactants. Prior to the identification of the underlying gene, HIDS was defined by polyclonal elevation of serum IgD (≥100 U/mL or >10 mg/dL) on two occasions at least 1 month apart in patients with a compatible history. While most *MVK* mutation-positive patients with recurrent fevers meet these criteria, a small percentage of mutation-positive patients have normal IgD levels despite clinical symptoms (HIDS sine hyperimmunoglobulinemia D). Serum IgD levels do not correlate with severity or frequency of attacks. Over 80% of patients also have elevated serum IgA levels (9). Urinary levels of mevalonic acid are markedly increased during attacks. The diagnosis of HIDS can be confirmed in patients with a typical history, with or without an elevated serum IgD, by finding increased urinary mevalonic acid during attacks or two mutations in *MVK* on genetic analysis. Patients with typical symptoms and increased serum IgD but without mutations or increased urinary mevalonate are sometimes said to have *variant HIDS*. It is likely that this latter category represents an etiologically heterogeneous group of patients.

Treatment

There has been no proven treatment for HIDS. Nonsteriodal anti-inflammatory drugs (NSAIDs) and intra-articular steroids may be of benefit in HIDS arthritis. Corticosteroids, cyclosporine, and intravenous immunoglobulin are not generally effective in HIDS. A modest benefit from HMGCoA reductase inhibitors such as simvastatin has been described (12). A study of etanercept, a TNF-alpha inhibitor, in two patients demonstrated marked improvement. Anecdotal evidence would suggest that some patients benefit from treatment with the IL-1 beta receptor antagonist, anakinra, or the leukotriene inhibitor montelukast. HIDS does not seem to have a major effect on longevity and attacks tend to ameliorate after adolescence.

Tumor Necrosis Factor Receptor–Associated Periodic Syndrome

Tumor necrosis factor receptor–associated periodic syndrome (OMIM 142680) is a dominantly inherited autoinflammatory disease caused by mutations in *TNFRSF1A*, a gene on the short arm of chromosome 12 that encodes the p55 receptor for TNF (1). Patients with TRAPS tend to have inflammatory episodes longer than those seen in FMF or HIDS, often lasting at least 1 week and sometimes as long as 4 to 6 weeks. Prior to the identification of causative *TNFRS1A* mutations, case reports described this condition under a number of clinical names, including familial Hibernian fever (13) and benign autosomal-dominant familial periodic fever. The recognition that this disorder may be seen in a wide range of ancestries has led to the introduction of the ethnically neutral TRAPS nomenclature, which emphasizes the pathogenesis of the disorder.

The TNFRSF1A protein, also known as the p55 TNF receptor, has four highly conserved extracellular cysteine-rich domains, a transmembrane domain, and an intracellular death domain. Five of the first six mutations identified were single-nucleotide differences causing amino acid substitutions at cysteines that participate in disulfide bonds that maintain the receptor's three-dimensional conformation. Other subsequently identified mutations have been shown to interfere with hydrogen bonding or to add or delete amino acids in the extracellular domains of the receptor. To date, over 50 mutations in the *TNFRSF1A* gene have been catalogued on the INFEVERS website, about half of which involve substitutions at conserved extracellular cysteine residues. Thus far no patients have been identified with transmembrane or intracellular mutations, null mutations (in which the protein is not expressed), or mutations in the p75 TNFRSF1B receptor, encoded on chromosome 1. Two particular TNFRSF1A variants, P46L and R92Q, are found at high frequency in the African-American and Caucasian populations, respectively, and are associated with a broader spectrum of clinical findings than cysteine mutations.

When *TNFRSF1A* mutations were first described, mechanistic studies suggested that TRAPS might be caused by a failure to shed mutant TNF receptors from the cell surface (1). Ordinarily, p55 receptors are cleaved by metalloproteases from leukocyte cell membranes upon cellular activation, thereby preventing repeated TNF signaling and creating a pool of soluble receptors that might compete for ligand with membrane-bound receptors. TRAPS patients have lower than normal levels of soluble p55 in the serum, and studies of leukocytes from three patients with the C52F mutation demonstrated impaired ectodomain cleavage upon activation. While this "shedding defect" was subsequently corroborated in patients with at least some other *TNFRSF1A* mutations, a number of other functional abnormalities in TRAPS-mutant receptors have been identified. These include reduced binding to TNF, decreased signaling for apoptosis, and impaired trafficking in the cell. This latter abnormality may lead to ligand-independent cellular activation through multiple pathways, and may account for the dominant inheritance of the TRAPS phenotype. It is interesting to note that, to date, it has been difficult to identify any effect of the R92Q TNFRSF1A variant on leukocyte function.

Clinical and Laboratory Features

In common with the other hereditary recurrent fever syndromes, TRAPS is characterized by episodes of fever and localized inflammation (14). Although there is a great degree of variability, attacks may last more than 1 month at a time. The cutaneous manifestations can be quite distinctive, the most characteristic of which is a migratory macular area of erythema that can occur on the torso (Figure 24-1), or on the limbs and migrate distally, with myalgia in the underlying muscle groups. Magnetic resonance imaging has demonstrated inflammatory changes extending into the muscle compartments (Figure 24-1). Ocular involvement is quite common in TRAPS, presenting with periorbital edema or conjunctivitis but rarely uveitis. The combination of prolonged attacks, characteristic rash, and ocular involvement, with more pronounced response to corticosteroids than to colchicines, are all suggestive of TRAPS.

Attacks of TRAPS are associated with a marked acute-phase response. Systemic AA amyloidosis may develop in approximately 15% of patients with TRAPS (Figure 24-1) and can result in renal failure. The risk of amyloidosis may be somewhat higher among those with a positive family history of amyloidosis and those with mutations causing substitutions at cysteine residues. The diagnosis of TRAPS should be considered in all patients with unexplained inflammatory episodes even when no

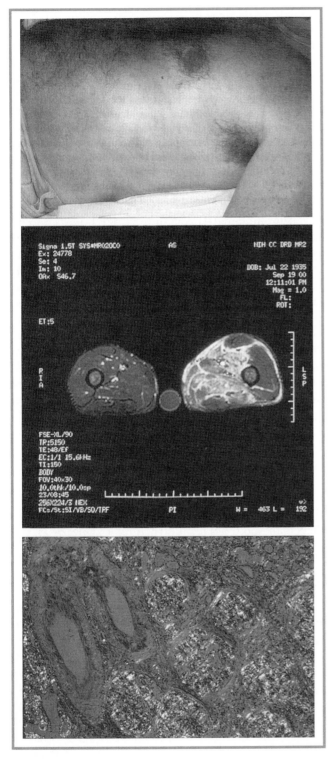

FIGURE 24-1

Clinical features of the tumor necrosis factor (TNF) receptor–associated periodic syndrome (TRAPS). (Top) Typical migratory erythematous rash on the trunk of a patient with the T50M mutation. (Center) Magnetic resonance image of a person with TRAPS (T50M) with skin rash and myalgia of the left thigh. The biopsy demonstrated fasciitis and panniculitis, but no myositis. (Bottom) Photomicrograph demonstrating amyloidosis in the kidney of a TRAPS patient with the C52F mutation. The kidney section was stained with Congo red and viewed under polarizing light.

family history has been elicited, as de novo *TNFRS1A* mutations have been reported. To make a diagnosis of TRAPS, the patient should have a documented *TNFRS1A* mutation and history suggestive of the disease. Patients with TRAPS-like illnesses who do not have mutations in *TNFRSF1A* have been described, but the molecular basis of their illness(es) remains unknown. Although TRAPS attacks are debilitating, they are self-limited. The prognosis of TRAPS is largely dependent on whether the patient develops amyloidosis.

Treatment

Daily colchicine neither prevents acute attacks nor prevents the development of amyloidosis. NSAIDs may be used in mild attacks, with corticosteroids reserved for more severe cases. Patients on corticosteroids frequently require increasing doses over the course of their illness with attendant increased adverse effects. Studies using etanercept, the p75 TNF receptor fusion protein, suggest a favorable response in clinical and laboratory parameters. It has been suggested that modifying the etanercept dose in response to normalized SAA levels may be important to prevent the development or progression of amyloidosis in patients at increased risk. Apropos of recent data suggesting a ligand-independent pathophysiology of TRAPS, there are anecdotal data indicating that TRAPS patients who cannot tolerate etanercept may respond to the IL-1 beta receptor antagonist, anakinra.

Cryopyrinopathies

The cryopyrinopathies include FCAS (OMIM 120100) (15), MWS (OMIM 191900) (16), and NOMID/CINCA (OMIM 607115) (17). These three disorders comprise a clinical spectrum, with FCAS the mildest and NOMID/CINCA the most severe, caused by dominantly inherited mutations in *CIAS1* (cold-induced autoinflammatory syndrome 1) (18,19). The protein encoded by *CIAS1,* denoted cryopyrin or NALP3, has an N-terminal PYD, thus establishing a relationship with the FMF protein pyrin, a central NACHT domain thought to be involved in nucleotide-binding and oligomerization, and a C-terminal leucine-rich repeat domain that may interact with microbial products. Nearly all of the over 50 disease-associated mutations in cryopyrin listed in the INFEVERS database reside in the NACHT domain, encoded by exon 3 of *CIAS1*.

The cryopyrin protein forms a macromolecular complex called the *inflammasome*, which activates caspase-1 and thereby cleaves IL-1 beta from its 31 kDa precursor to the biologically active 17 kDa fragment. Cryopyrin-deficient mice exhibit a number of immunologic abnormalities, most notably the inability to produce active IL-1 beta in response to certain bacteria

24

or bacterial products. Leukocytes from patients with the cryopyrinopathies exhibit accentuated IL-1 beta production at baseline or in response to various stimuli.

Clinical and Laboratory Features

Patients with the cryopyrinopathies usually present very early in life with fever, an urticarialike skin rash, and an intense acute-phase response. The rash is not true urticaria, in that there are infiltrates of granulocytes and lymphocytes rather than mast cells. The severity of joint and neurological involvement, along with the risk of amyloidosis, helps to distinguish among the three clinical disorders, although there is considerable overlap.

Familial cold autoinflammatory syndrome has a clear episodic quality, with attacks of rash, fever, polyarthralgia, and constitutional symptoms occurring 1 to 2 hours after generalized cold exposure. Amyloidosis is rare, and patients usually have normal life expectancy. In MWS, attacks occur with no clear relationship to cold exposure, and are manifested by fever, urticarial skin rash, limb pain, arthralgia, or arthritis, and sometimes abdominal pain, conjunctivitis, or episcleritis. Sensorineural hearing loss occurs in most patients, and AA renal amyloidosis may develop in about one quarter.

Patients with NOMID/CINCA usually present in infancy with nearly continuous clinical findings. These include fever, urticarial skin rash, and constitutional symptoms. Chronic aseptic meningitis also occurs, which can lead to headache, increased intracranial pressure, and intellectual impairment. Sensory organ involvement includes sensorineural hearing loss, conjunctivitis, and uveitis, sometimes leading to deafness and/or blindness. NOMID/CINCA patients may also develop a distinctive arthropathy with overgrowth of the epiphyses of the long bones. Untreated, about 20% die before reaching adulthood, and amyloidosis may occur later in life. Although all three disorders are dominantly inherited, NOMID/CINCA was not initially recognized as a genetic disease because of decreased reproductive fitness in patients carrying the diagnosis.

Genetic testing usually focuses on sequencing exon 3 of *CIAS1*. As is the case for FMF, TRAPS, and HIDS, there are patients who meet clinical criteria for the cryopyrinopathies who do not have identifiable mutations. This is particularly the case for NOMID/CINCA, where only about half of the patients carrying the clinical diagnosis have demonstrable *CIAS1* mutations. Nevertheless, the availability of genetic testing has markedly increased the awareness of these disorders.

Treatment

Promising results have been obtained with the IL-1 beta receptor antagonist, anakinra, in all three cryopyrinopathies. Patients with FCAS and MWS exhibit almost complete remission of all disease symptoms. In a trial involving 18 patients with NOMID/CINCA who had failed to respond to either corticosteroids or TNF blockers (20), treatment with daily subcutaneous injections of anakinra resulted in disappearance of rash and conjunctivitis within 3 days. In the 12 patients for whom cerebrospinal fluid (CSF) could be obtained, intracranial pressure, protein, and white cell counts decreased significantly. Vision remained stable in all patients, and hearing actually improved in one third. Complete remission of inflammation occurred in 10 of the 18 symptoms after 6 months of treatment. Magnetic resonance imaging demonstrated marked reduction in cochlear and leptomeningeal enhancement. These findings suggest that CNS as well as peripheral manifestations of NOMID/CINCA are mediated by an excess of IL-1 beta, and that these symptoms can be ameliorated by the administration of anakinra. The discontinuation of anakinra led to a relapse of symptoms within days, and re-treatment led to rapid improvement, thus supporting the need for continuous use of anakinra in NOMID/CINCA. Longer term follow-up will be required to determine whether IL-1 inhibition will prevent the intellectual sequelae of NOMID/CINCA, or the development of amyloidosis.

IDIOPATHIC INTERMITTENT ARTHROPATHIES

In contrast to the hereditary periodic fever syndromes, which are systemic diseases, these disorders primarily affect joints and adjacent structures (Table 24-2), and genetics appears to play a less important role.

Palindromic Rheumatism

Initially described in 1944, palindromic rheumatism (PR) describes intermittent, relatively brief episodes of typically monoarticular arthritis or periarthritis (inflammation of the soft tissues adjacent to the joint). The prevalence is roughly 20-fold less than that of rheumatoid arthritis (RA). The mean age of onset is approximately 45 years, with a relatively even gender balance. Occasional families have been reported with multiple cases of PR, or in which PR and RA have occurred together. Recent series suggest increased prevalence of the shared epitope DRB-0401 and DRB-0404 alleles in PR relative to controls (21). In the absence of laboratory and radiographic clues to the diagnosis, it is likely that PR represents a heterogeneous group of disorders.

Clinical and Laboratory Features

In PR, attacks occur suddenly, initially affect one joint, and last from hours to days. Recurrences can occur over

TABLE 24-2. IDIOPATHIC PERIODIC SYNDROMES.

FEATURE	PALINDROMIC RHEUMATISM	INTERMITTENT HYDRARTHROSIS	EOSINOPHILIC SYNOVITIS
Attacks	~2 days; monoarticular arthritis or periarticular soft tissue inflammation	3–5 days, monoarticular arthritis, large effusions	1–2 weeks, monoarthritis triggered by trauma
Joints involved	MCPs, PIPs, wrists, shoulders, MTPs, ankles	Knee to hip, ankle, elbow	Knee, MTP
Associated conditions	Familial aggregation with RA	Episodes may coincide with menses; heterozygous *MEFV* mutations?	Personal or family history of atopy, dermatographism
Prognosis	~50% persistent palindromic rheumatism, ~33% develop RA	Attacks often occur at predictable intervals; sometimes spontaneous remissions	Self-limited episodes, benign prognosis
Treatment	Injectable gold, antimalarials, sulfasalazine	NSAIDs, colchicine, intra-articular steroids, synovectomy	Symptomatic

ABBREVIATIONS: MCP, metacarpophalangeal joint; MTP, metatarsophalangeal joint; NSAID, nonsteriodal anti-inflammatory drug; PIP, proximal interphalangeal joint; RA, rheumatoid arthritis.

irregularly spaced intervals. The joints affected include the interphalangeal joints of the hands and feet, the wrists, shoulders, and ankles (22). Tender periarticular swelling, 2 to 4 cm in diameter, may accompany an attack, or occur independently. Small, sometimes painful subcutaneous nodules may develop near the elbows, wrists, or knees, with a particular predilection for the fingers. Periarticular swelling and nodule formation are usually transient.

During attacks, there is a mild-to-moderate acceleration of the ESR (22). Antibodies to cyclic citrullinated peptide (anti-CCP) and rheumatoid factor (RF) are positive in about half of patients with PR. Antinuclear antibodies are negative with normal complement levels. Synovial biopsies and fluid taken during an attack demonstrate polymorphonuclear leukocytes. Biopsies of subcutaneous nodules demonstrate inflammatory cells, and notably lack the areas of fibrinoid necrosis and palisading mononuclear cells seen in rheumatoid nodules.

Longitudinal data on patients with PR demonstrated that 33% eventually develop RA, the conversion heralded by conversion to seropositivity for RF, and development of more aggressive disease (22). A retrospective study identified RF positivity, female gender, and involvement of the wrist in proximal phalangeal joints as the greatest risk factors for the development of RA (23), and more recent data suggest that antibodies to CCP may be a better predictor than RF.

Treatment

Anecdotal evidence suggests a role for NSAIDs, injectable gold, antimalarials, or sulfasalazine. There have been no large randomized, controlled trials in the treatment of PR.

Intermittent Hydrarthrosis

Intermittent hydrarthrosis is characterized by periodic episodes of monoarticular or pauciarticular arthritis. Constitutional symptoms are rare. Attacks are notable for the periodicity of their nature, such that patients can accurately predict their next attack. Spontaneous remission occurs in some cases (24). Prevalence data are not available; however, it is a relatively rare condition. The usual age of onset is between 20 and 50, with a relatively even gender balance. There are cases in which attacks began at menarche, coincided with menses, and remitted during pregnancy and following menopause. Generally, familial clustering of this condition does not occur. Recently, three cases of intermittent hydrarthrosis with heterozygous *MEFV* mutations were reported from Spain, raising the intriguing possibility that this disorder might be a forme fruste of the more well-recognized autoinflammatory diseases.

Clinical and Laboratory Features

Attacks involve episodes of pain, swelling, and limitation of movement, usually affecting a single joint, although occasionally more than one joint may be affected. In most cases, attacks last 3 to 5 days, with massive joint effusions but no erythema or warmth. In an individual patient, a limited number of joints may be affected, the most commonly affected being the knee, with the hip, ankle, and elbow less frequently involved.

24

Laboratory findings during attacks demonstrate a normal ESR and leukocyte count. Synovial fluid is mildly inflammatory with less than 5000 white blood cells/mm^3. An inflammatory infiltrate with edema is present on synovial biopsy (24). Radiographs demonstrate soft tissue swelling but no erosions, even in patients with repeated attacks.

Treatment

A number of therapeutic interventions have been tried, including NSAIDs, colchicine, intra-articular corticosteroids, surgical synovectomy, and intra-articular radioactive gold.

Eosinophilic Synovitis

This rare condition is described in individuals with a history of atopy. Both genders are affected equally, and the typical age of onset is between 20 and 50 years (25). Minor trauma may trigger episodes of acute, painless monoarthritis. Synovial fluid demonstrates up to 50% eosinophils. Eosinophilic synovitis has been proposed to be the synovial equivalent of dermatographism. It has been speculated that trauma may trigger activation of mast cells, attracting eosinophils and thus producing an effusion (25). The knee is most commonly affected. Episodes are self-limiting, lasting up to 2 weeks, but require only symptomatic treatment.

Clinical and Laboratory Features

Swelling develops rapidly, usually over 12 to 24 hours, and lasts for 1 to 2 weeks. Although the effusions are large, there is little associated pain, warmth, or erythema. The ESR is not elevated. The peripheral white cell count, and in particular the eosinophil count, is normal, although some patients have elevated IgE levels. Synovial fluid shows mildly elevated leukocyte counts, with 16% to 52% eosinophils in the initial series (25). Charcot–Leyden crystals (bipyramidal, hexagonal-shaped protein crystals) are formed by products of intracellular lipases in eosinophils, and may be demonstrated following overnight incubation at 4°C. Synovial eosinophilia resolves following an attack. There are no long-term radiographic changes.

Numerous conditions are associated with synovial eosinophilia, including RA, psoriatic arthritis, rheumatic fever, infectious arthritidies including parasitic, tuberculous, and Lyme arthritis, and the hypereosinophilic syndrome. Synovial eosinophilia is also seen in patients with metastatic adenocarcinoma and following arthrography. Features suggestive of eosinophilic arthritis, in contrast to the wide differential mentioned, include a personal or family history of allergy and dermatographism (25).

REFERENCES

1. McDermott MF, Aksentijevich I, Galon J, et al. Germline mutations in the extracellular domains of the 55 kDa TNF receptor, TNFR1, define a family of dominantly inherited autoinflammatory syndromes. Cell 1999;97:133–144.
2. Thomas KT, Feder HM Jr, Lawton AR, Edwards KM. Periodic fever syndrome in children. J Pediatr 1999;135:15–21.
3. Aksentijevich I, Torosyan Y, Samuels J, et al. Mutation and haplotype studies of familial Mediterranean fever reveal new ancestral relationships and evidence for a high carrier frequency with reduced penetrance in the Ashkenazi Jewish population. Am J Hum Genet 1999;64:949–962.
4. Kastner DL, Aksentijevich I. Intermittent and periodic arthritis syndromes. In: Koopman WJ, Moreland LW, eds. Arthritis and allied conditions. 15th ed. Philadelphia: Lippincott Williams & Wilkins; 2005:1411–1461.
5. International FMF Consortium. Ancient missense mutations in a new member of the RoRet gene family are likely to cause familial Mediterranean fever. Cell 1997;90:797–807.
6. French FMF Consortium. A candidate gene for familial Mediterranean fever. Nat Genet 1997;17:25–31.
7. Chae JJ, Komarow HD, Cheng J, et al. Targeted disruption of pyrin, the FMF protein, causes heightened sensitivity to endotoxin and a defect in macrophage apoptosis. Mol Cell 2003;11:591–604.
8. Cazeneuve C, Sarkisian T, Pecheux C, et al. *MEFV*-gene analysis in Armenian patients with familial Mediterranean fever: diagnostic value and unfavorable renal prognosis of the M694V homozygous genotype-genetic and therapeutic implications. Am J Hum Genet 1999;65:88–97.
9. Drenth JP, Haagsma CJ, van der Meer JW. Hyperimmunoglobulinemia D and periodic fever syndrome. The clinical spectrum in a series of 50 patients. International Hyper-IgD Study Group. Medicine (Baltimore) 1994;73:133–144.
10. Drenth JP, Cuisset L, Grateau G, et al. Mutations in the gene encoding mevalonate kinase cause hyper-IgD and periodic fever syndrome. International Hyper-IgD Study Group. Nat Genet 1999;22:178–181.
11. Houten SM, Kuis W, Duran M, et al. Mutations in *MVK*, encoding mevalonate kinase, cause hyperimmunoglobulinaemia D and periodic fever syndrome. Nat Genet 1999;22:175–177.
12. Simon A, Drewe E, van der Meer JW, et al. Simvastatin treatment for inflammatory attacks of the hyperimmunoglobulinemia D and periodic fever syndrome. Clin Pharmacol Ther 2004;75:476–483.
13. McDermott EM, Smillie DM, Powell RJ. Clinical spectrum of familial Hibernian fever: a 14-year follow-up study of the index case and extended family. Mayo Clin Proc 1997;72:806–817.
14. Hull KM, Drewe E, Aksentijevich I, et al. The TNF receptor-associated periodic syndrome: emerging concepts of an autoinflammatory disorder. Medicine (Baltimore) 2002;81:349–368.
15. Wanderer AA, Hoffman HM. The spectrum of acquired and familial cold-induced urticaria/urticaria-like syn-

dromes. Immunol Allergy Clin North Am 2004;24:259–286.

16. Muckle TJ, Wells M. Urticaria, deafness, and amyloidosis: a new heredo-familial syndrome. Q J Med 1962;31:235–248.

17. Prieur AM, Griscelli C, Lampert F, et al. A chronic, infantile, neurological, cutaneous and articular (CINCA) syndrome. A specific entity analysed in 30 patients. Scand J Rheumatol Suppl 1987;66:57–68.

18. Hoffman HM, Mueller JL, Broide DH, Wanderer AA, Kolodner RD. Mutation of a new gene encoding a putative pyrin-like protein causes familial cold autoinflammatory syndrome and Muckle–Wells syndrome. Nat Genet 2001;29:301–305.

19. Aksentijevich I, Nowak M, Mallah M, et al. De novo *CIAS1* mutations, cytokine activation, and evidence for genetic heterogeneity in patients with neonatal-onset multisystem inflammatory disease (NOMID): a new member of the expanding family of pyrin-associated autoinflammatory diseases. Arthritis Rheum 2002;46:3340–3348.

20. Goldbach-Mansky R, Dailey NJ, Canna SW, et al. Neonatal-onset multisystem inflammatory disease responsive to interleukin-1b inhibition. N Engl J Med 2006;355:581–592.

21. Maksymowych WP, Suarez-Almazor ME, Buenviaje H, et al. *HLA* and cytokine gene polymorphisms in relation to occurrence of palindromic rheumatism and its progression to rheumatoid arthritis. J Rheumatol 2002;29:2319–2326.

22. Guerne PA, Weisman MH. Palindromic rheumatism: part of or apart from the spectrum of rheumatoid arthritis. Am J Med 1992;93:451–460.

23. Gonzalez-Lopez L, Gamez-Nava JI, Jhangri GS, Ramos-Remus C, Russell AS, Suarez-Almazor ME. Prognostic factors for the development of rheumatoid arthritis and other connective tissue diseases in patients with palindromic rheumatism. J Rheumatol 1999;26:540–545.

24. Ghormley RK, Weiner AD. Periodic benign synovitis; idiopathic intermittent hydrarthrosis. J Bone Joint Surg Am 1956;38A:1039–1055.

25. Brown JP, Rola-Pleszczynski M, Menard HA. Eosinophilic synovitis: clinical observations on a newly recognized subset of patients with dermatographism. Arthritis Rheum 1986;29:1147–1151.

24

Less Common Arthropathies
A. Hematologic and Malignant Disorders

ADEL G. FAM, MD, FRCP(C), FACP

- Recurrent hemarthrosis is the primary clinical manifestation of hemophilia.
- Hemophilia A (classic hemophilia) is a heritable, X-linked recessive disorder of blood coagulation, occurring almost exclusively in males. The disorder is associated with a deficiency of factor VIII.
- Hemophilia B (Christmas disease), somewhat rarer but essentially indistinguishable clinically from hemophilia A, is caused by factor IX deficiency.
- Sickle-cell hemoglobinopathies associated with chronic hemolytic anemia and rheumatic manifestations include both homozygous sickle-cell anemia (Hb SS) and the heterozygous states: sickle-beta thalassemia, sickle-C (S-C) disease, and sickle-D (S-D) disease.
- Sickle-cell disease results from a single nucleotide substitution of valine for glutamic acid in the beta globin gene.
- In SS disease, the painful crises, osteonecrosis, and dactylitis are the result of small blood vessel occlusion in the bone marrow by sickled red cells.
- Osteomyelitis in patients with Hb SS disease is due to a combination of ischemic bone infarction and impaired host immunity. *Salmonella* is the most common organism.
- Thalassemia is a group of inherited hemoglobin disorders characterized by defects in the synthesis of one or more of the alpha or beta subunits of Hb.
- In beta-thalassemia, the reduced or absent production of beta chains leads to the production of an imbalance between the numbers of alpha and beta chains. This leads, in turn, to unstable Hb molecules, precipitation of the unaffected chains during erythropoiesis, and hemolysis.
- Mechanisms by which cancer can cause musculoskeletal symptoms include direct tumor invasion of bones and joints, hemorrhage into the joint, secondary gout, and paraneoplastic syndromes.

Musculoskeletal manifestions of hematologic and malignant disorders are reviewed in this chapter. A list of these conditions is shown in Table 25A-1.

NONMALIGNANT HEMATOLOGIC DISORDERS

Hemophilia

Hemophilia A is a heritable, X-linked recessive disorder of blood coagulation, occurring almost exclusively in males (1 in 5000–10,000 male births). **Hemophilia A** (classic hemophilia) is due to factor VIII deficiency, whereas **hemophilia B** (Christmas disease) is caused by factor IX deficiency. Tissue factor–factor VIIa complex is important in initiating coagulation by activating small amounts of both factors X and IX in the environment of tissue factor–bearing cells. Factor Xa and factor IXa, formed in the initial reaction, then play a role in factor VIII activation, generation of thrombin on platelet surfaces, and blood clotting. Factor VIII is a 340,000 Da coagulant protein that activates factor X in the intrinsic coagulation pathway (1). In hemophilia, the extrinsic tissue-dependent pathway remains intact, and is probably the major hemostatic regulatory system. Gene deletions, insertions, or rearrangements have been implicated in the chromosomal abnormalities leading to hemophilia. These various genetic abnormalities lead to a range of disease severities in hemophilia. Identification of the gene for factor VIII, located on the X chromosome, facilitates both prenatal diagnosis of hemophilia and carrier detection for genetic counseling.

In mild hemophilia, the levels of factor VIII are 6% to 36% of normal, and bleeding generally occurs in response to minor trauma. In a moderately severe

TABLE 25A-1. LESS COMMON ARTHROPATHIES. HEMATOLOGIC AND MALIGNANT DISORDERS.

Nonmalignant hematologic disorders
    Hemophilic arthropathy
    Hemoglobinopathy-associated arthropathies
        Sickle-cell disease
        Thalassemia

Malignant disorders
    Metastatic (tumor invasion of joints)
        Metastatic carcinomatous arthritis
        Leukemic arthritis
        Lymphomatous arthritis
        Angioimmunoblastic T-cell lymphoma–associated arthritis
        Myelomatous arthritis
        Waldenstrom's macroglobulinemia
    Nonmetastatic (paraneoplastic)
        Hypertrophic osteoarthropathy (see Chapter 25F)
        Carcinoma polyarthritis
        Amyloid arthritis
        Secondary gout
        Miscellaneous: dermatomyositis, paraneoplastic vasculitis

hemophilia, the level ranges from 2% to 5% of normal. In severe hemophilia—two thirds of all patients—the level is 1% or less. Plasma levels of factor VIII of <5% of normal are associated with spontaneous hemarthrosis. The diagnosis of hemophilia can be confirmed by a coagulation screen, including bleeding time, platelet count, prothrombin time, plasma thromboplastin time, and determinations of the levels of factors VIII and IX.

Christmas disease (hemophilia B), due to factor IX deficiency, is less common than hemophilia A. The gene for factor IX is also located on the X chromosome. Hemophilia B, which occurs in approximately 1 in 30,000 to 100,000 male births, produces a clinical picture that is largely indistinguishable from that of hemophilia A. Factor IX is a 60,000 Da proenzyme that is converted to an active protease (factor IXa) by the tissue factor–VIIa complex. Factor IXa, in combination with activated factor VIII, subsequently activates factor X (2). In rare circumstances, deficiency of factors XI, VII, V, X, or II may be associated with hemarthrosis.

Recurrent hemarthrosis is the most common bleeding manifestation of hemophilia A, occurring in up to two thirds of patients (3). This may occur spontaneously or following minor trauma. The onset is rapid with pain, swelling, local tenderness, and limitation of joint movements. The rising intra-articular pressure eventually terminates bleeding, but resolution of the clot occurs slowly. The knee, elbow, and ankle are the most frequently affected joints. Bleeding into the hip joint can lead to osteonecrosis of the femoral head. Patients with factor VIII levels <5% of normal, who are inadequately treated, may develop a chronic arthritis with intermittent pain, stiffness, persistent synovial swelling, defor-

mity, instability, and secondary osteoarthritis. Chronic arthritis is less frequent and less severe in Christmas disease.

Hemophilic arthropathy is thought to be due to repeated intra-articular bleeding and excessive iron deposition in both the synovial membrane and articular cartilage. Because prothrombin and fibrinogen are absent in normal synovial fluid, the blood remains as a liquid. Plasma gradually resorbs while the remaining red cells are phagocytosed by synovial lining macrophages. Hemosiderin deposition in both synovial lining cells and subsynovial supporting tissue is associated with chronic proliferative synovitis and pannus formation. The synovitis results in the production of lysosomal enzymes, collagenase, catabolic cytokines [interleukin-1 (IL-1), tumor necrosis factor alpha (TNF-alpha)], superoxide anions, and hydroxyl radicals that can lead to cartilage breakdown and osteoarthritis.

Radiographs often show increased periarticular soft tissue swelling due to extensive iron deposition in the synovium. Widening or premature fusion of the epiphyses, enlargement of the femoral and humeral intercondylar notches (Figure 25A-1), "squaring" of the inferior patella, expansion of the radial head at the elbow, and secondary osteoarthritis may occur in later stages. Computed tomography (CT) scans are helpful in delineating the bone and soft tissue lesions. Magnetic resonance imagaing (MRI) is useful in demonstrating intra-articular hemorrhage, subsynovial or muscle hematomata, and chronic synovial hypertrophy.

Bleeding into muscles occurs less frequently and can lead to large bloody collections or "hemophilic pseudotumors" associated with muscle necrosis, cyst formation, and, sometimes, compartment syndromes. Compression femoral neuropathy may result from a retroperitoneal or psoas hematoma. Subperiosteal hemorrhage can result in a bone pseudotumor.

Septic arthritis is a rare complication of hemophilic arthropathy. *Staphylococcus aureus* is the most common organism; coincidental human immunodeficiency virus (HIV) infection appears to be an important contributing factor in this complication. Septic arthritis is suspected when an episode of hemarthrosis fails to respond promptly to treatment with factor VIII and joint immobilization, particularly in the presence of fever or leukocytosis.

Treatment

Since the 1960s, the widespread use of human donor plasma products, concentrated with factor VIII, including cryoprecipitate, has improved the care of patients with hemophilia by reducing the severity and frequency of the bleeding episodes and by permitting surgical procedures. Between 1980 and 1985, however, these products also led to the spread of HIV and viral hepatitis

FIGURE 25A-1

Elbow radiograph in a patient with chronic hemophilia A showing widening of the intercondylar notch and secondary osteoarthritis with joint space narrowing, marginal osteophytes, and intra-articular osseous bodies. Note increased periarticular swelling and density due to iron deposition in the synovium (*arrows*).

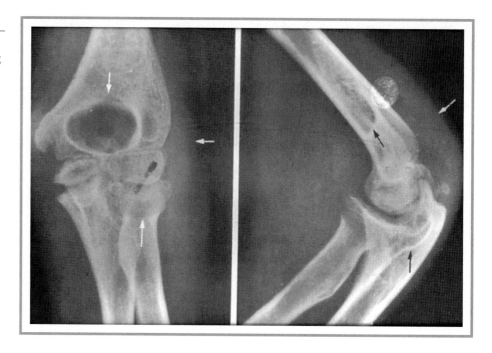

(hepatitis B and C) among hemophiliacs. Donor screening and purification of factor VIII concentrates with monoclonal anti–factor VIII antibody and heat lyophilization markedly reduced these infectious complications. The advent of recombinant factor VIII has completely eliminated the risk of infection. Replacement recombinant factor VIII therapy is administered prophylactically to children with severe hemophilia 1 to 3 years of age in order to maintain plasma factor levels >1% (3). This serves to reduce the frequency of spontaneous bleeding and prevent joint damage. Desmopressin (DDAVP), a synthetic analog of vasopressin, stimulates a transient increase in factor VIII levels, and can provide an alternative therapy for patients with mild or moderate hemophilia A (3). Inhibitor IgG antibodies to factor VIII develop in 5% to 10% of young patients with hemophilia A, but are less common in Christmas disease. Therapeutic options in these patients include plasmapheresis and treatment with oral glucocorticoids, azathioprine, cyclophosphamide, or porcine factor VIII concentrate. Factor IX is not present in cryoprecipitate or in factor VIII concentrates. Fresh frozen plasma is an effective therapy, but carries with it some risk of blood-borne infections. Virally inactivated factor IX concentrate and recombinant factor IX are preferred.

Acute hemarthrosis is treated with immobilization, ice packs, and prompt administration of factor VIII concentrate or recombinant factor VIII for approximately 48 hours. If the joint effusion is unusually tense or if infection is suspected, joint aspiration is recommended, preferably following factor VIII replacement. Short-term use of intra-articular or oral glucocorticoids may confer some additional benefit, but repeated use can lead to side effects. For subacute and chronic arthritis, nonsteroidal anti-inflammatory drugs (NSAIDs)—not including aspirin—are relatively safe and beneficial. Physical therapy is useful in preventing joint contractures and deformities (3).

Surgical synovectomy reduces the chronic synovitis and subsequent joint damage, but is associated with significant morbidity. Arthroscopic synovectomy, also effective, has fewer complications. Both chemical synovectomy (by injecting intra-articular osmic acid, rifampicine, or other sclerosing agent) and radiation synovectomy (using intra-articular radioisotope injections such as colloidal P 32 chromic-phosphate, 90-yttrium, or 186-rhenium) may be effective in the short term. The long-term efficacies of both chemical and radiation synovectomy, however, are less favorable (3). Total joint replacement is indicated for advanced osteoarthritis of the hip, shoulder, elbow, or ankle. Promising preliminary results with gene therapy have been reported in a small number of patients with severe hemophilia.

Hemoglobinopathy-Associated Musculoskeletal Manifestations

Sickle-Cell Disease

Sickle-cell hemoglobinopathies associated with chronic hemolytic anemia and rheumatic manifestations include both homozygous sickle-cell anemia (Hb SS) and the heterozygous states: sickle-beta thalassemia, sickle-C (S-C) disease, and sickle-D (S-D) disease. SS disease occurs mostly in Africans, but also in southern Italy, Greece, Turkey, Saudi Arabia, and India (4).

Sickle cell disease results from a single nucleotide substitution of valine for glutamic acid in the beta globin gene. The diagnosis can be confirmed by cellulose acetate Hb electrophoresis showing 76% to 100% Hb SS. Deoxygenation (hypoxia) results in polymerization of HbS, forming liquid crystals. This deforms the red cells from biconcave discs into elongated, rigid, crescent-shaped sickle cells, causing occlusion of the microcirculation and breakdown of red cells (hemolysis), leading in turn to further tissue hypoxia and sickling. Polymerization of HbS is influenced by intracellular concentrations of HbS, HbF, and HbC; blood oxygen saturation; and pH and temperature.

Once a sufficient number of rigid sickle cells is formed, microvascular occlusion will result. Hypoxia of tissues causes a secondary inflammatory reaction mediated by histamine, bradykinin, and prostaglandins, resulting in increased intramedullary pressure and bone pain (4). The painful crises, osteonecrosis, and dactylitis are the result of small blood vessel occlusion in the bone marrow by sickled red cells. These manifestations, most frequent in homozygous (SS) sickle-cell disease, may also occur under certain circumstances in the milder heterozygous sickle hemoglobinopathies such as HbS/beta-thalassemia ("sickle-thal disease") and S-C disease. Individuals with sickle-cell trait (HbAS), healthy carriers of the gene mutation, are free from musculoskeletal symptoms. Pure HbC disease, caused by substitution of lysine for glutamic acid in the beta chain, produces hemolysis. In contrast, Hb S-C disease results in features of both sickling and hemolysis (4). Recurrent painful crises mainly affect the juxta-articular areas of long bones, joints, spine, and ribs (5,6). The pain is often associated with local swelling and tenderness. The crises can be triggered by infection, dehydration, acidosis, cold exposure, traveling at high altitudes, and stress. The duration of crises is variable but usually no longer than 2 weeks. The "pain rate" (number of painful episodes per year) correlates with early death in patients with SS anemia. Hydroxyurea, which increases the levels of fetal Hb, reduces the pain rate and may ultimately improve survival (5,6).

Sickle-cell arthropathy, caused by microvascular ischemia and synovial infarctions, often affects large joints. Reaction to juxta-articular bone infarcts may also contribute to joint pain. Small, non-inflammatory synovial effusions are common.

Osteonecrosis (Figure 25A-2) affects the femoral head in approximately 33% of patients and the humeral head in 25%. Multiple joints, including the spine, may be involved (7). In the spine, the bony infarcts result in the characteristic biconcave or "Lincoln log" vertebrae. The risk of osteonecrosis is highest in those with frequent painful crises and in patients with Hb SS-alpha-thalassemia. Total replacement arthroplasty is recommended for those with advanced secondary osteo-

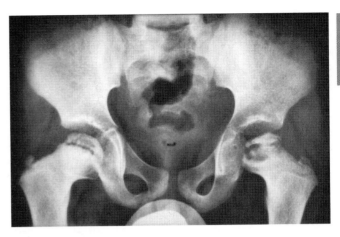

FIGURE 25A-2

Radiograph of the hips, showing bilateral osteonecrosis.

arthritis, but there is a high rate of perioperative complications and mechanical loosening (7).

Dactylitis typically occurs in children, and is characterized by acute, painful, nonpitting swelling of the hands and feet ("hand and foot syndrome") (4,6). Fever and leukocytosis, which may be the initial disease manifestations, occur in S-S, S-C, and S-thalassemia disease. Radiographs may show soft tissue swelling, periosteal new bone formation, or intramedullary sclerotic infarcts of the phalanges, metacarpals, and metatarsals. Scintigraphy and MRI are more sensitive in detecting bone infarcts. Symptoms usually resolve within 7 days, but recurrences are frequent. Osteonecrosis of the epiphyses can lead to digital shortening. Osteopenia, stress fractures, vertebral collapse, and growth abnormalities may also occur in sickle-cell disease (6).

Osteomyelitis in patients with Hb SS disease is due to a combination of ischemic bone infarction and impaired host immunity. *Salmonella* is the most common organism, followed by *Staphylococcus aureus* and Gram-negative bacilli. Osteomyelitis usually follows an episode of painful crisis and may affect multiple sites. Chronic sickling of the intestinal microvasculature may predispose the devitalized bowel to invasion by *Salmonella* and other enteric bacteria. Osteomyelitis should be suspected if symptoms of a painful crisis fail to respond after 1 to 2 weeks. The diagnosis is confirmed by radiography, bone scanning, and by cultures from the blood or bone (obtained through a CT-guided aspiration). MRI is more accurate in delineating the lesions. Septic arthritis is caused by the same organisms as osteomyelitis, often occurring in association with osteonecrosis or a painful vaso-occlusive crisis involving the same joint. A high index of suspicion and synovial fluid cultures are essential for early recognition.

Gout is a rare complication of sickle-cell disease. Hyperuricemia results from enhanced erythropoiesis secondary to chronic hemolysis, increased nucleic acid sythesis, and overproduction of uric acid. In addition, cumulative renal damage occurring by the third decade of life—the result of renal ischemia and microinfarctions—can lead to sustained hyperuricemia and gout.

Severe sickle-cell anemia is treated by blood transfusions and folic acid supplements (1–5 mg folic acid/day) (4). Enhanced erythropoietic activity secondary to chronic hemolysis may lead to folate deficiency through the depletion of folate stores. Measures to prevent painful crises include avoidance of stress, alcohol, over-exertion, swimming, and high altitudes. Treatment of the painful crises consists of acetaminophen or NSAIDs for mild episodes, and codeine or oxycodone for more severe attacks (4). Oral controlled-release morphine is as effective as continuous intravenous morphine for the management of painful episodes in children (8). Hydroxyurea enhances the production of HbF, which in turn reduces polymerization of Hb SS (9). Treatment with hydroxyurea has been shown to be both cost-effective and beneficial in reducing the rate of painful crises in adults with SS (9). Favorable results have been reported with bone marrow (stem cell) transplantation in children with SS disease.

Thalassemia

Thalassemia is a group of inherited hemoglobin disorders characterized by defects in the synthesis of one or more of the alpha or beta subunits of Hb. (Normally, alpha-globin proteins are equal to beta-globin proteins.) The reduced or absent production of beta chains in beta-thalassemia, for example, subunit leads to the production of an imbalance between the numbers of alpha and beta chain, unstable Hb molecules, and precipitation of the unaffected chains during erythropoiesis, resulting ultimately in hemolysis and the formation of Heinz bodies. In beta-thalassemia, the precipitated alpha-globin chains are particularly toxic, damaging red cell membranes and causing hemolysis, marrow erythroid hyperplasia, and often hypersplenism. In compensation for the decreased beta subunits, levels of both HbF and HbA2 are often elevated in these patients (10).

Thalassemia is especially common in persons of Mediterranean background. beta-Thalassemia major (also known as Cooley's anemia) is one of the most severe forms of congenital hemolytic anemia. These patients are typically transfusion-dependent and rarely survive into adulthood. Only beta-thalassemia major is associated with musculoskeletal manifestations. These result from expansion of the erythroid marrow, and include osteoporosis with wide medullary spaces, coarse trabeculae, and pathologic fractures. Epiphyseal deformities and leg shortening may also occur, but osteonecrosis is not a feature. Patients with HbS and

beta-thalassemia often have HbA2 and features of both SS disease and beta-thalassemia. beta-Thalassemia minor (trait) is a relatively common disorder that is rarely associated with clinical manifestations.

Blood transfusions are the main supportive treatment of beta-thalassemia major, but transfusion hemosiderosis is a common problem and chelation therapy with deferoxamine is often required (10). Splenectomy is indicated if 40% or greater increase in the transfusion requirements occur during a 1-year period. Allogeneic bone marrow (stem cell) transplantation and gene transfer is a promising new treatment in children.

MUSCULOSKELETAL SYMPTOMS AND CANCER

Malignant disease is associated with a number of musculoskeletal manifestations (Table 25A-2) (11). Mechanisms by which cancer can cause musculoskeletal symptoms include: (1) direct tumor invasion of bones and joints (skeletal metastases, metastatic carcinomatous arthritis, leukemic synovitis and lymphomatous arthritis); (2) hemorrhage into the joint (leukemia); (3) secondary gout (leukemia, polycythemia, lymphoma, myeloma, carcinoma); and (4) through remote, non-

TABLE 25A-2. CANCER AND RHEUMATIC DISEASE.

Direct tumor invasion of joints
  Metastatic carcinomatous arthritis
  Leukemic arthritis
  Lymphomatous arthritis
  Myelomatous arthritis

Nonmetastatic paraneoplastic rheumatic syndromes
  Articular
    Hypertrophic osteoarthropathy (Chapter 25F)
    Carcinomatous polyarthritis
    Amyloid arthritis
    Secondary gout
  Muscular
    Dermatomyositis and polymyositis
    Lambert–Eaton myasthenic syndrome
  Cutaneous
    Palmar fasciitis and arthritis
    Panniculitis and arthritis
    Eosinophilic fasciitis
  Vascular
    Paraneoplastic vasculitis
    Erythromelalgia
  Miscellaneous
    Multicentric reticulohistocytosis

Malignancy developing in a preexisting connective tissue disease
  Lymphoma developing in Sjögren's syndrome

Malignancy as a complication of therapy for rheumatic disorders
  Myelodysplastic syndrome after cyclophosphamide therapy

metastatic effects of the tumor (paraneoplastic syndromes), such as hypertrophic osteoarthropathy. There is an increased incidence of lymphoma in patients with Sjögren's syndrome, rheumatoid arthritis (RA), and systemic lupus erythematosus. Treatment of rheumatic disorders with immunosuppressive drugs may also result in malignancy. Conversely, chemotherapeutic drugs used in the treatment of neoplasms may cause rheumatic syndromes.

Direct Tumor Invasion of Joints

Metastatic Carcinomatous Arthritis

Metastatic carcinomatous arthritis, due to direct invasion of the joint or adjacent bones by metastases, is a rare form of arthritis (11,12). The arthritis may be the initial manifestation of malignant disease. Bronchogenic carcinoma is the most common primary tumor. Other sources include carcinoma of the breast, prostate, thyroid, kidney, and colon. The arthritis is often monoarticular and commonly affects the knee, hip, shoulder, elbow, or ankle. Metastases distal to the elbows and knees are uncommon and involvement of the joints of the hands and feet is rare.

Severe bone and joint pain, worse at night and with movements, is common. Joint effusions are commonly hemorrhagic and often re-accumulate rapidly after aspiration. The fluids are non-inflammatory with low cell counts characterized by mononuclear predominance. Using cytomorphologic techniques, tumor cells may be identified in synovial effusions (Figure 25A-3) (12). Radiographs commonly show juxta-articular osteolytic lesions and bone scanning may reveal metastases at

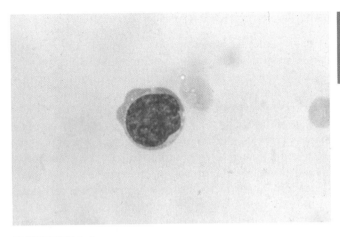

FIGURE 25A-4

Acute lymphoblastic leukemia, leukemic arthritis: cytocentrifuge preparation of synovial fluid from left elbow showing a cALLA-positive lymphoblast by immunocytology (Wright's stain, original magnification ×1000).

other sites. Carcinomatous invasion of the synovium can be demonstrated by arthroscopic or percutaneous needle synovial biopsy. Treatment with chemotherapy and radiotherapy is often palliative.

Leukemic Arthritis

Joint manifestations occur in about 14% of patients with leukemia (13,14). These are more common in acute leukemia, particularly acute lymphoblastic leukemia in children. Known mechanisms of arthritis in patients with leukemia include leukemic arthritis caused by direct invasion of articular tissues and juxta-articular bones by leukemic cells, joint infection, intra-articular hemorrhage, and gouty arthritis.

Leukemic arthritis is an asymmetric, painful polyarthritis of large joints, such as the knee, shoulder, or ankle. It may precede other manifestations of leukemia. Nocturnal bone pains and severe joint pains, often disproportionate to the apparent degree of arthritis, are characteristic. Hematologic and bone marrow abnormalities are inevitably present in leukemic arthritis. Radiographic findings include metaphyseal rarefaction, osteolytic lesions, and sometimes periosteitis. The diagnosis can be confirmed by demonstration of leukemic cells in synovial fluid and/or synovium (Figure 25A-4) (13,14). Immunocytological techniques employing indirect immunofluorescence and a panel of early B-cell and myeloid antigens (e.g., cALLA or acute lymphoblastic leukemia antigen) have been used to identify leukemic cells in joint effusions and in the synovium (13,14). Leukemic arthritis usually occurs in patients with widespread disease and the response to therapy is generally poor.

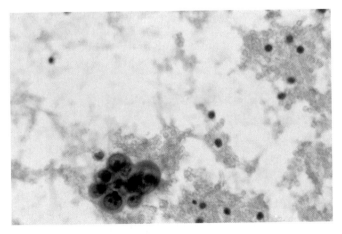

FIGURE 25A-3

Metastatic carcinomatous arthritis of right shoulder: synovial fluid cytology showing malignant cells (carcinoma of lung) with pleomorphic, eccentric, hyperchromatic nuclei and large irregular nucleoli.

Lymphoma and Arthritis

Musculoskeletal symptoms occur in up to 25% of patients with non-Hodgkin's lymphoma. Bone pain is the most common manifestation. Mechanisms of arthritis in patients with lymphoma include lymphomatous arthritis, hypertrophic osteoarthropathy (see Chapter 25F), joint infection, and secondary gout (15). Lymphomatous arthritis, due to invasion of juxta-articular bone or synovial tissue by lymphoma, is rare. Both polyarticular and monoarticular presentations have been described. Lymphoma is suspected in patients in whom severe constitutional symptoms appear out of proportion to the severity of arthritis, and in those with periarticular osteolytic lesions. The diagnosis can be confirmed by bone or synovial biopsy. A symmetric polyarthritis with fever has been described in patients with the rare intravascular lymphoma (intravascular lymphomatosis).

Angioimmunoblastic T-Cell Lymphoma–Associated Arthritis

Angioimmunoblastic T-cell lymphoma (AITL), previously termed *angioimmunoblastic lymphadenopathy*, is a rare type of non-Hodgkin's T-cell lymphoma characterized by fever, weight loss, lymphadenopathy, hepatosplenomegaly, urticaria or other skin eruption, vasculitis, serositis, hemolytic anemia, and polyclonal hypergammaglobulinemia (16).

A nonerosive, nondeforming, symmetric, seronegative polyarthritis may occur as initial manifestation of the disease or concurrent with other features. Joints of the hands are commonly affected. Synovial biopsies may show typical features of AITL. Synovial fluid leukocytosis with decreased number of CD8 lymphocytes may occur. The diagnosis is confirmed by lymph node biopsy showing proliferation of small blood vessels and replacement of normal lymph node architecture by plasma cells, immunoblasts, and eosinophils. Response to chemotherapy is often poor and only 30% of individuals survive 2 years (16).

Multiple Myeloma and Arthritis

Myeloma is a malignant bone marrow plasma cell tumor, occurring most commonly in the fifth and sixth decades. It is often associated with bone pains (particularly in the back and ribs), pathologic fractures, monoclonal serum protein abnormalities, and Bence–Jones proteinuria. Generalized osteopenia due to myeloma-secreted cytokines (IL-1 beta, TNF-beta, and IL-8) occurs in about a third of patients. Myelomatous arthritis, caused by invasion of the articular and juxta-articular bones by myeloma cells, is rare (17). More commonly, about 15% of patients with myeloma develop monoclonal light chain (AL amyloid) amyloidosis, associated with amyloid arthropathy. The arthritis typically affects the shoulder, wrists, and knees. It is often symmetrical and relatively painless, but may mimic RA. Amyloid infiltration of the synovium of the shoulders produces the characteristic "shoulder-pad sign." Synovial effusions are non-inflammatory with low total leukocyte counts ($<2000 \times 10^6$/L). Spun synovial fluid sediments often contain "amyloid bodies." These are synovial villi, laden with amyloid. Using Congo red stains, amyloid deposits in both the synovium and synovial fluid sediment demonstrate apple-green birefringence under polarized light. Other manifestations of AL amyloid in patients with myeloma include peripheral neuropathy, carpal tunnel syndrome, subcutaneous amyloid deposits, macroglossia, cardiomyopathy, nephropathy, and hepatosplenomegaly. The diagnosis of amyloid arthritis can be confirmed by bone marrow examination, serum and urine protein immunoelectrophoresis showing an M-protein, and by biopsy of the synovium, abdominal subcutaneous fat, or rectum. Management consists of therapy for the underlying myeloma, and symptomatic treatment of the arthritis with NSAIDs.

Osteosclerotic myeloma is a rare form of myeloma characterized by osteosclerotic rather than osteolytic solitary or multiple bone lesions (18). Other features include an indolent chronic course, polyneuropathy, organomegaly, endocrinopathy, M-protein, and skin changes (POEMS syndrome). Skin thickening, abnormal pigmentation, and, sometimes, a sclerodermatous appearance are common. Weight loss, fever, thrombocytosis, and arthritis may also occur.

Waldenstrom's Macroglobulinemia

Waldenstrom's macroglobulinemia is a neoplastic lymphoproliferative disorder associated with serum monoclonal IgM, lymphadenopathy, hepatosplenomegaly, purpuric skin lesions, and symptoms of hyperviscosity (headaches, visual changes). Direct tumor invasion of juxta-articular bone and joints is rare, but light chain amyloidosis and amyloid arthritis may occur (17).

Paraneoplastic Rheumatic Syndromes

Paraneoplastic symptoms, often bearing an only indirect relationship to tumor mass, are present at diagnosis in about 10% of patients with cancer. Up to 50% of patients with cancer develop paraneoplastic syndromes at some time during the course of their illness. One third of these are endocrine in nature; the remainder usually comprise hematological, rheumatic, and neuromuscular disorders. Among the paraneoplastic rheumatic syndromes, hypertrophic osteoarthropathy, carcinoma polyarthritis, myositis, and vasculitis are the most frequent (Table 25A-2). These disorders may coincide or follow the diagnosis of primary malignancy, but may precede the onset of cancer by as long as 2 years (11).

The clinical course of a paraneoplastic musculoskeletal syndrome generally parallels that of the primary tumor. Thus, radical treatment of the primary neoplasm usually, but not invariably, results in regression of the paraneoplastic syndrome. Conversely, recurrence of the tumor can lead to re-appearance of the musculoskeletal symptoms. Paraneoplastic manifestations may be mistaken for metastatic disease, leading to inappropriate therapies. On the other hand, symptoms of true metastases may be attributed to a paraneoplastic syndrome, thereby delaying therapy.

Carcinomatous Polyarthritis

Carcinomatous polyarthritis is an inflammatory, seronegative arthritis that may herald the presence of malignancy (11). Although its clinical presentation is variable, certain features suggest the possibility of an underlying malignancy and serve to distinguish this form of polyarthritis from RA. These include a late age of onset; an explosive onset of asymmetric oligoarthritis or polyarthritis; predominant involvement of the joints of the lower extremities; frequent sparing of the wrists and joints of the hands; and the absence of erosions, deformities, rheumatoid factor, nodules, or family history of RA. On rare occasions, the arthritis is symmetrical and may mimic RA.

The temporal relationship between the onset of carcinomatous polyarthritis and diagnosis of the tumor is usually a close one—typically less than 1 year. Exclusion of hypertrophic osteoarthropathy or metastatic invasion of the synovium or periarticular bone is critical for establishing the appropriate therapeutic approach. The arthritis typically occurs in women with carcinoma of the breast, and in men with carcinoma of the lung. Synovial effusions are mildly inflammatory and the erythrocyte sedimentation rate (ESR) is often elevated. There are no distinctive pathologic or radiographic abnormalities (11).

The pathogenesis of carcinoma polyarthritis is poorly understood. Broad possible mechanisms include: (1) an immune complex–mediated synovitis; (2) cross-reactivity of antigenic determinants on the synovium and neoplastic tissue; and (3) an abnormality of cell-mediated immunity, leading to the expression of both neoplasia and connective tissue disease. The most convincing evidence that carcinoma polyarthritis is a true paraneoplastic disorder is the frequent resolution of the arthritis following resection of the underlying neoplasm, and its reappearance with recurrence of the cancer. The arthritis may respond to NSAIDs and intra-articular glucocorticoids.

"Postchemotherapy rheumatism" is a rare, self-limited syndrome of unknown etiology, characterized by myalgias and migratory arthralgias of hands, feet, knees, and ankles, occurring in some patients with carcinoma of the breast, ovary, or non-Hodgkin's lymphoma, 1 to 3 months after treatment with cyclophosphamide, 5-fluorouracil, or methotrexate.

Gout is rare in patients with solid tumors until the tumor metastasizes widely. Clinically, secondary gout differs from idiopathic gout in that women are more commonly affected and a family history of gout is less frequent. In hematologic malignancies, gout may occur secondary to massive tumor lysis following the institution of chemotherapy. In many protocols, allopurinol is used routinely to prevent this complication of cancer therapy.

Erythromelalgia is an intense pain and erythema afflicting the palms and soles (palms > soles), typically in patients with either polycythemia vera or essential thrombocythemia. Erythromelalgia is exquisitely sensitive to aspirin, usually in doses not exceeding 325 mg/day. Miscellaneous paraneoplastic conditions include dermatomyositis (see Chapter 18A), paraneoplastic vasculitis, and panniculitis (11).

REFERENCES

1. Peake I. The molecular basis of haemophilia A. Haemophilia 1998;4:346–349.
2. Lillicup D. The molecular basis of haemophilia B. Haemophilia 1998;4:350–357.
3. Hilgartner MW. Current treatment of hemophilic arthropathy. Curr Opin Pediatr 2002;14:46–49.
4. Ballas SK. Sickle cell disease: clinical management. Baillieres Clin Hematol 1998;11:185–214.
5. Platt OS, Thorington BD, Brambilla DJ, et al. Pain in sickle cell disease. Rates and risk factors. N Engl J Med 1991;325:11–16.
6. Almeida A, Roberts I. Bone involvement in sickle cell disease. Br J Haematol 2005;129:482–490.
7. Vichinsky EP, Neumayr LD, Haberkern C, et al. The perioperative complication rate of orthopedic surgery in sickle cell disease: report of the national sickle cell surgery study group. Am J Hematol 1999;62:129–138.
8. Jacobson SJ, Kopecky EA, Joshi P, Babul N. Randomized trial of oral morphine for painful episodes of sickle-cell disease in children. Lancet 1997;350:1358–1361.
9. Moore RD, Charache S, Terrin ML, et al. Cost-effectiveness of hydroxyurea in sickle cell anemia. Am J Hematol 2000;64:26–31.
10. Perrine SP, Boosalis V. Thalassemia. In: Rakel RE, Bope ET, eds. Conn's current therapy. Philadelphia: Saunders (Elsevier); 2006:488–492.
11. Fam AG. Paraneoplastic rheumatic syndromes. Baillieres Clin Rheumatol 2000;14:515–533.
12. Fam AG, Kolin A, Lewis AJ. Metastatic carcinomatous arthritis and carcinoma of the lung. A report of two cases diagnosed by synovial fluid cytology. J Rheumatol 1980; 7:98–104.

13. Evans TL, Nercessian BM, Sanders KM. Leukemic arthritis. Semin Arthritis Rheum 1994;24:48–56.
14. Fam AG, Voorneveld C, Robinson JB, Sheridan BL. Synovial fluid immunocytology in the diagnosis of leukemic synovitis. J Rheumatol 1991;18:293–296.
15. Dorfman HD, Siegeel HL, Perry MC, Oxenhandler R. Non-Hodgkin's lymphoma of the synovium simulating rheumatoid arthritis. Arthritis Rheum 1987;30:155–161.
16. Tsochatzis A, Vassilopoulos D, Deutsch M, et al. Angiommunoblastic T-cell lymphoma-associated arthritis. Case report and literature review. J Clin Rheumatol 2005; 11:326–328.
17. Roux S, Fermand J-P, Brechignac S, et al. Tumoral joint involvement in multiple myeloma and Waldenstrom's macroglobulinemia – report of 4 cases. J Rheumatol 1996;23:1175–1178.
18. Fam AG, Rubenstein JD, Cowan DH. POEMS syndrome. Study of a patient with proteinuria, microangiopathic glomerulopathy and renal enlargement. Arthritis Rheum 1986;29:233–241.

Less Common Arthropathies
B. Rheumatic Disease and Endocrinopathies

PETER A. MERKEL, MD, MPH

- Musculoskeletal signs and symptoms frequently occur in endocrinopathies.
- A number of syndromes of limited joint mobility occur in people with diabetes mellitus, including diabetic hand syndrome (diabetic cheiroarthropathy), adhesive capsulitis (frozen shoulder, periarthritis), Dupuytren's contractures, trigger finger (flexor tenosynovitis), diffuse idiopathic skeletal hyperostosis (DISH syndrome), neuropathic arthritis (Charcot joints, diabetic osteoarthropathy), and diabetic muscle infarction.
- Hyperthyroidism may be associated with proximal myopathy, usually without serum creatine kinase (CK)

elevation; thyroid acropachy; and drug-induced vasculitis associated with antineutrophil cytoplasmic antibodies (ANCA), usually caused by propylthiouracil.
- Hypothyroidism may be associated with polyarthralgias, carpal tunnel syndrome, and proximal myopathy, with serum CK elevation.
- Hyperparathyroidism may cause osteoporosis, osteitis fibrosa cystica, chondrocalcinosis, and pseudogout.
- Other endocrinopathies that may lead to musculoskeletal complaints are hypoparathyroidism, acromegaly, and glucocorticoid-induced Cushing's syndrome.

Most endocrine disorders are associated with systemic manifestations caused by changes in the quantity or activity of various hormones. Musculoskeletal signs and symptoms are among the more frequent clinical sequelae of endocrinopathies. In some cases, the first clinical signs or symptoms of endocrine disease are rheumatic. Some rheumatic symptoms, such as myalgias, can be seen in a variety of different endocrinopathies; other rheumatic manifestations, such as Raynaud's phenomenon, are indicative of only one or two certain diseases. Various endocrinopathies also may be associated with specific rheumatic diseases.

Understanding the associations between endocrine and rheumatic diseases is important for several reasons. First, appreciating these clinical connections will help clinicians avoid misdiagnoses of primary rheumatic disease and can lead to prompt treatment of a primary endocrine disorder. Second, many of these rheumatic syndromes respond, in full or in part, to treatment of the underlying endocrinopathy. Third, some of the associations are sufficiently common or striking to justify screening for specific endocrine diseases when patients manifest certain rheumatic symptoms or signs. Finally, endocrine disorders may affect the disease activity of

established autoimmune diseases. Such findings have led to the investigation of pathophysiologic links between autoimmune and endocrine diseases.

RHEUMATIC SEQUELAE OF SPECIFIC ENDOCRINE DISEASES

Diabetes Mellitus

Diabetes mellitus is associated with a wide variety of musculoskeletal problems, some of which are unique to the disease (1,2). The spectrum of rheumatologic syndromes seen in people with diabetes is outlined in Table 25B-1. The nomenclature of these conditions can be confusing, with some having more than one name in the medical literature. Some of these manifestations are secondary to the microvascular disease, neuropathic complications, or proliferation of connective tissue seen in diabetes. These rheumatic syndromes affect people with either type I or type II diabetes, especially those with evidence of organ damage.

A number of syndromes of limited joint mobility occur in people with diabetes (3). Diabetic hand syn-

TABLE 25B-1. RHEUMATOLOGIC MANIFESTATIONS OF DIABETES MELLITUS.

Syndromes of limited joint mobility
  Diabetic hand syndrome (diabetic cheiroarthropathy)
  Adhesive capsulitis (frozen shoulder, periarthritis)
  Trigger finger (flexor tenosynovitis)
  Dupuytren's contractures

Osteoporosis

Diffuse idiopathic skeletal hyperostosis (DISH)

Neuropathies
  Neuropathic arthritis (Charcot joints, diabetic osteoarthripathy)
  Carpal tunnel syndrome
  Diabetic amyotrophy
  Reflex sympathetic dystrophy (multiple synonyms)
  Various other neuropathies

Diabetic muscle infarction

drome (diabetic cheiroarthropathy) is a condition stemming from alterations in the soft tissue of the hands and fingers, resulting in stiff, waxy skin and joint contractures. This condition can be confused with arthritis and the sclerodactyly seen in systemic sclerosis. Cheiroarthropathy is demonstrated when patients are asked to oppose the palmar surfaces of their hands and fingers (the prayer sign), and they are unable to fully touch these surfaces. Adhesive capsulitis (frozen shoulder, periarthritis) is a similar condition that leads to shoulder joint contractures, which often are severe. This condition frequently is bilateral and sometimes is accompanied by calcific deposits in the surrounding soft tissues (4). Physical therapy appears to be helpful, and spontaneous resolution may occur over months to years. Dupuytren's contractures and trigger finger (flexor tenosynovitis) are frequent, annoying, and potentially disabling conditions that are more common among people with diabetes. These finger problems may respond to glucocorticoid injection or surgical correction.

Two other common musculoskeletal diseases with an increased prevalence and generally younger age of presentation in people with diabetes are osteoporosis and diffuse idiopathic skeletal hyperostosis (DISH syndrome). Insulin-like growth factors are thought to play a pathogenic role in these diseases. Although the association between diabetes and osteoporosis has been questioned, the link between hyperostosis and diabetes is established more firmly. DISH is accompanied by ossification and calcification of spinal ligaments, but does not necessarily cause significant clinical problems.

Patients with diabetes mellitus may encounter several types of neuropathies that result in musculoskeletal symptoms or that may mimic rheumatic diseases. Neuropathic arthritis (Charcot joints, diabetic osteoarthropathy; see Chapter 25D), a destructive bone and joint

condition that is the consequence of peripheral neuropathy, most commonly affects the foot (5). Despite the resulting joint obliteration, ankylosis, and deformities, patients usually have little or no pain, and the diagnosis is based on radiographic appearance. Plain radiography, bone scintigraphy, and magnetic resonance imaging are useful imaging modalities for diagnosing diabetic osteoarthropathy and documenting the extent of disease. Similarly, the peripheral neuropathy of diabetes increases the incidence of foot infections and foreign body reactions, in which patients may be unaware of injury due to anesthetic feet; both of these conditions may lead to septic arthritis.

The incidence of carpal tunnel syndrome, a median nerve neuropathy, is increased in people with diabetes and may occur bilaterally. Similarly, reflex sympathetic dystrophy (causalgia) is more common among people with diabetes. Diabetic amyotrophy is characterized by painful, often bilateral, muscle weakness resulting from a mononeuropathy with non-inflammatory atrophy of type II muscle fibers (6). Spontaneous improvement may occur. Other neuropathies that can occur among people with diabetes may be central or peripheral, and include such conditions as mononeuritis multiplex and radiculopathies that mimic other musculoskeletal conditions.

Diabetic muscle infarction is a rare but increasingly recognized syndrome of acute infarction of multiple muscle areas in people with diabetes and organ damage (7). This condition usually occurs with severe pain in one extremity. Diabetic muscle infarction can be confused with pyomyositis or venous thrombosis. Magnetic resonance imaging (MRI) can be diagnostic, although biopsy may be needed in some cases. Although self-limited, this condition can recur. The etiology of diabetic muscle infarction is unclear but may be related to microvasculopathy and microthrombosis.

Improved glycemic control may not reverse the conditions outlined in Table 25B-l, but may help prevent future episodes. When these syndromes are present without an obvious explanation, it is appropriate to consider screening patients for undiagnosed diabetes mellitus by testing fasting glucose and glycosylated hemoglobin levels.

Thyroid Disease

Thyroid disease frequently is accompanied by various musculoskeletal problems (Table 25B-2) (8,9). Hyperthyroidism, hypothyroidism, and thyroxine replacement therapy, in particular, are associated with rheumatic disease. Some studies report that thyroid abnormalities are more common among people with various autoimmune syndromes, including rheumatoid arthritis, systemic lupus erythematosus, and systemic sclerosis. However, these associations have been questioned, and

TABLE 25B-2. RHEUMATOLOGIC MANIFESTATIONS OF THYROID DISEASE.

Hyperthyroidism
  Osteoporosis
  Myopathy
  Periarthritis
  Acropachy

Hypothyroidism
  Arthralgias
  Symmetrical polyarthritis
  Joint laxity
  Carpal tunnel syndrome
  Chondrocalcinosis and pseudogout
  Hyeruricemia and gout
  Myopathy

the perceived increased prevalence of thyroid disorders among patients with these autoimmune diseases may be confounded by the fact that thyroid diseases are common among women, and women account for 75% to 90% of people with these autoimmune diseases. Musculoskeletal problems may be the first, and sometimes only, clinical sign of thyroid disease.

Because thyroid diseases are easily diagnosed and highly responsive to treatment, screening for thyroid dysfunction among people with various rheumatic symptoms is essential. Achieving a euthyroid status improves many, but not all, of these conditions.

Hyperthyroidism

Hyperthyroidism is an important, reversible, and easily detected cause of osteoporosis. Administration of levothyroxine as replacement therapy or for suppression of thyroid nodules may lead to osteoporosis (10).

Thyrotoxicosis often causes a proximal myopathy that may be severe. Most patients with this myopathy do not have elevated creatinine kinase levels but do have electromyographic abnormalities. This myopathy almost always is reversible upon attainment of a euthyroid state. All patients presenting with weakness must be screened for thyrotoxicosis.

A shoulder periarthritis (often bilateral) may be seen in people with hyperthyroidism.

Thyroid acropachy, an unusual late manifestation of Graves' disease, involves painful soft tissue swelling of hands, fingers, and toes, with clubbing and periostitis. Although similar to hypertrophic osteoarthropathy, most patients with acropachy already have established exophthalmos, pretibial myxedema, and measurable levels of long-acting thyroid stimulator in the serum. Acropachy usually presents after treatment of hyperthyroidism and is thought to have an immunologic basis.

Although many drugs have been associated with vasculitis, some of these associations are poorly supported by the literature. However, the evidence is compelling that propylthiouracil and related thionamides used in the treatment of hyperthyroidism can cause vasculitis syndromes associated with antineutrophil cytoplasmic antibodies (11).

Hypothyroidism

Hypothyroidism in children or fetuses results in multiple skeletal abnormalities, as well as severe developmental problems. In adults, hypothyroidism can cause a series of musculoskeletal problems. Given the high prevalence of hypothyroidism in adults, this diagnosis must be considered in all patients presenting with the syndromes described in this section. The discovery of previously undiagnosed thyroid deficiency among people presenting with rheumatic symptoms is common.

Joint symptoms are extremely common among patients with hypothyroidism, and range from vague arthralgias to a symmetric polyarthritis that may be confused with rheumatoid arthritis. The joint effusions seen in hypothyroidism are non-inflammatory. Additionally, an increased incidence of joint laxity has been noted among people with myxedema. Carpal tunnel syndrome is associated with hypothyroidism and may be bilateral. When a euthyroid state is attained, these rheumatologic symptoms often remit fully.

There is an increased incidence of hypothyroidism among patients with crystal-induced arthritis. In particular, asymptomatic chondrocalcinosis and clinical pseudogout are associated with hypothyroidism. Similarly, there are reports linking hypothyroidism to asymptomatic hyperuricemia and gout.

Myopathy is a common feature of hypothyroidism and can include myalgias and weakness (especially proximally). The weakness usually is mild to moderate in severity and is accompanied by abnormal findings on electromyography. In contrast to the myopathy seen in hyperthyroidism, serum creatinine kinase levels are elevated in most patients with muscle disease associated with hypothyroidism. Muscle bulk is not changed appreciably, and biopsy specimens may demonstrate evidence of degeneration and regeneration of muscle fibers without inflammation. The myopathy reverses with treatment of the underlying thyroid disorder.

Parathyroid Disease

Table 25B-3 outlines the rheumatologic manifestations of parathyroid disease.

Hyperparathyroidism

A wide variety of bone and joint abnormalities have been associated with hyperparathyroidism. Some of these conditions have become less common due to the

Less Common Arthropathies
C. Hyperlipoproteinemia and Arthritis

ROBERT F. SPIERA, MD

- Several recognized heritable disorders of lipid metabolism result in a variety of clinical phenotypes, each of which may be associated with distinct musculoskeletal manifestations.
- Tendinous xanthomas are associated most often with the type II and type III hyperlipoproteinemias, known respectively as familial hypercholesterolemia and familial dysbetalipoproteinemia.
- Tendinous xanthomas characteristically occur on the dorsum of the hands over the digit extensor tendons, or on the heels at the Achilles tendon insertions.

- Osseous xanthomas, observed occasionally in type III hyperlipoproteinemia, can predispose patients to pathologic fractures, particularly in long bones.
- An episodic, acute, migratory inflammatory arthritis occurs in up to 50% of homozygotes with type II hyperlipoproteinemia. The joints are erythematous, warm, and swollen, and acute-phase reactants are elevated.
- Gout can be associated with hypertriglyceridemia in types I, IV, and V hyperlipoproteinemia.

Musculoskeletal problems can occur in association with hyperlipoproteinemia, a condition in which underlying genetic defects lead to overproduction or impaired removal of lipoproteins. The abnormalities, related either to the lipoprotein or its receptor, results in elevated levels of lipoprotein that contribute to the development of premature atherosclerosis. Recognition of these syndromes facilitates both the proper diagnosis and management of the musculoskeletal problem, and the appropriate treatment of a condition that poses significant long-term cardiovascular threats.

Several recognized heritable disorders of lipid metabolism result in a variety of clinical phenotypes (Table 25C-l) (1), each of which may be associated with distinct musculoskeletal manifestations. Hyperlipidemia also can occur secondary to other clinical contexts (e.g., the nephrotic syndrome, primary biliary cirrhosis, cigarette smoking). Arthritis and hyperlipidemia also may be linked because of a common risk factor (e.g., obesity as a risk factor for both osteoarthritis and hyperlipidemia). In this section, we will focus on musculoskeletal syndromes believed to be related directly to hyperlipidemia.

XANTHOMAS

Xanthomas can occur in any of the inherited hyperlipoproteinemias. Tendinous xanthomas are associated most often with the type II and type III hyperlipoproteinemias, known respectively as familial hypercholesterolemia and familial dysbetalipoproteinemia (1). Tendinous xanthomas characteristically occur on the dorsum of the hands over the digit extensor tendons, or on the heels at the Achilles tendon insertions (2). They have been described at other extensor surfaces as well, including the triceps, olecranon, or quadriceps insertions. Achilles tendon xanthomas are more strongly associated with type III hyperlipoproteinemia (1). Although patients with polygenic hypercholesterolemia can have similar lipid profiles, xanthomata are not seen in these patients.

Tendinous xanthomas often are noticeable but not necessarily symptomatic. Tendinitis or tenosynovitis can occur, however, particularly in the Achilles tendon, where the mass effect of the xanthoma contributes to local irritation by overlying footwear. Radiographic findings can include calcifications within the xanthomas, or

TABLE 25C-1. CLASSIFICATION OF HYPERLIPIDEMIA.

PHENOTYPE	LIPOPROTEIN ABNORMALITY	LIPID ABNORMALITY	MUSCULOSKELETAL MANIFESTATION
Type I	Chylomicrons increased	Markedly increased triglycerides	Eruptive xanthomas
Type IIa	LDL increased	Increased cholesterol	Tendinous, tuberous xanthomas; migratory, episodic polyarthritis; Achilles tendonitis
Type IIb	LDL and VLDL increased	Increased cholesterol and triglycerides	Tendinous, tuberous xanthomas, migratory, episodic polyarthritis; Achilles tendonitis
Type III	Chylomicrons and VLDL remnants increased	Increased cholesterol; increased to markedly increased triglycerides	Tendinous, tuberous, and plane xanthomas
Type IV	VLDL increased	Increased triglycerides	Eruptive tendinous and tuberous xanthomas; arthralgias
Type V	Chylomicrons and VLDL increased	Increased cholesterol, markedly increased triglycerides	Eruptive xanthomas

SOURCE: Modified from Fredrickson DS, Levy RI, Lees RS. N Engl J Med 1967;276:34–42, ff., by permission of *New England Journal of Medicine*.
ABBREVIATIONS: LDL, low-density lipoprotein, VLDL, very low-density lipoprotein.

even periarticular cortical erosions, presumably secondary to pressure effects of the enlarged tendons (3). Tendinitis preceding xanthoma formation or even spontaneous tendon ruptures are rare, but have been described in type IIa hyperlipoproteinemia (4,5). The tendinous xanthomas reside within the tendon fibers and move in conjunction with the tendon. Pathologic examination of such xanthomas reveals infiltrates of foam cells that seem to be macrophages congested with remnants of ingested (endocytosed) circulating lipoproteins.

Osseous xanthomas, observed occasionally in type III hyperlipoproteinemia, can predispose patients to pathologic fractures, particularly in long bones. Other locations include the small bones of the hands, skull, spine, and pelvis. Such xanthomas have the radiological appearance of well-defined, round, or oval lucencies (6). In a patient with type V hyperlipidemia, pathologic evaluation of a cystic femoral lesion revealed foamy histiocytes with granulomatous reaction around cholesterol clefts (7).

Tuberous xanthomas are subcutaneous masses generally found over extensor surfaces, including the elbows, knees, hands, or buttocks. They can be observed in types II, III, and IV hyperlipoproteinemias. Xanthomas on the palmar surfaces (xanthoma striata palmaris) occur in type III hyperlipoproteinemia (1).

Although xanthomas generally are associated with heritable disorders of lipid metabolism, other, rarer causes are recognized. Cerebrotendinous xanthomatosis is a rare autosomal recessive disorder in which accumulation of cholestanol or dihydrocholesterol in neural tissue or tendons results in clinical manifestations of disease, including ataxia, paresis, dementia, and tendon xanthomas (8). These manifestations can appear as early

as the second decade. Another disorder associated with tendinous xanthomas is beta-sitosterolemia, an autosomal recessive disorder in which there is hyperabsorption of cholesterol and plant sterols from the intestine (9). These disorders should be considered when a patient presents with tendinous xanthomas, particularly at a young age, in the absence of marked elevation of serum cholesterol. Xanthomata also can be seen in the secondary hypercholesterolemia associated with cholestatic liver disease, such as primary biliary cirrhosis.

ARTICULAR DISEASE

There is some controversy about the association of articular disease with familial hyperlipoproteinemias. Some arthropathies purported to be linked with hyperlipidemia based on descriptive case series (5,10,11) have not been borne out in all controlled studies (12,13), although some associations do appear to have been confirmed (14,15). Certain musculoskeletal presentations, however, are well-recognized. An episodic, acute, migratory inflammatory arthritis occurs in up to 50% of homozygotes with type II hyperlipoproteinemia (16,17). This condition primarily affects large peripheral joints, such as knees and ankles, but the small joints of the hands and feet can be involved. The joints are erythematous, warm, and swollen, and acute-phase reactants, such as sedimentation rate and plasma fibrinogen, are elevated. Distinction of this entity from acute rheumatic fever can be difficult, particularly because some of those patients may have valvular disease as a downstream effect of atherosclerosis. The presence of tendinous xanthomas, a markedly elevated cholesterol, and the absence of antecedent Streptococcal infection helps distinguish the entities. Generally, episodes are self-limited and resolve within 2 weeks. This pattern of arthritis is seen much less commonly (approximately 4%) in heterozygotes.

Self-limited episodes of acute mono- or oligoarthritis, often of the knee or ankle, can be seen in familiar hypercholesterolemia. In type IV hyperlipoproteinemia, a more chronic arthritis can occur. Patients complain of morning stiffness and a bland, often asymmetric, polyarticular arthritis. Both large and small joints may be involved, including proximal interphalangeal joints, metacarpophalangeal joints, wrists, knees, shoulders, and tarsophalangeal and metatarsophalangeal joints (18). Synovial fluid analysis reveals minimally inflammatory or non-inflammatory fluid, without crystals. Synovial biopsy has been described as revealing moderate synovial hyperplasia, with a modest infiltrate of mononuclear cells and foam cells. There may be a relationship between serum triglyceride level and joint complaints.

Even xanthomata, the hallmark physical finding in hyperlipoproteinemias, can be mistaken for other entities, such as gouty tophi in a person with oligoarthritis, or rheumatoid nodules in a person with polyarthritis. Clinicians caring for people with musculoskeletal complaints must therefore be aware of these hyperlipoproteinemia-related musculoskeletal syndromes and distinguish them from more common arthropathies.

CRYSTAL DISEASE

Gout, an eminently treatable form of arthritis related to hyperuricemia, can be associated with hypertriglyceridemia in types I, IV, and V hyperlipoproteinemia. When the clinical scenario is compatible with a microcrystalline disease, examination of the synovial fluid for crystals is essential. The presence of cholesterol crystals has been associated with a worse outcome for a joint affected by degenerative or inflammatory arthritis, and has been shown to maintain the inflammatory reaction in experimental animals (19). In people with primary hyperlipoproteinemia, however, cholesterol crystals have not been specifically implicated in acute or chronic arthritis. Crystals were found in a retrocalcaneal bursa adjacent to a xanthoma in a patient with type II hyperlipoproteinemia, but the significance of these crystals has not been determined (20).

MANAGEMENT

The acute migratory polyarthritis or oligoarthritis associated with type II hyperlipoproteinemia tends to be self-limited. Nonsteroidal anti-inflammatory drugs (NSAIDs) can be helpful, but recent concerns regarding the potential cardiovascular consequences of long-term NSAID use, particular with selective cyclooxygenase 2 inhibitors, must be considered in this high-risk group of patients (21). Treating the underlying dyslipidemia can lead to regression of tendinous xanthomas. Surgical excision also can be beneficial, particularly in the Achilles tendon, where mechanical irritation by footwear can cause pain and debility. Recurrences can occur. The arthropathy associated with type IV hyperlipidemia seems to wane with improved control of serum lipid levels.

REFERENCES

1. Fredrickson DS, Levy RI, Lees RS. Fat transport in lipoproteins: an integrated approach to mechanisms and disorders. N Engl J Med 1967;276:34–42, 94–103, 148–156, 215–225, 273–281.
2. Fahey JJ, Stark HH, Donovan WE, Drennan DB. Xanthoma of the Achilles tendon. J Bone Joint Surg Am 1973;55A:1197–1211.
3. Yaghami I. Intra- and extraosseous xanthomata associated with hyperlipidemia. Radiology 1978;128:49–54.
4. Shapiro R, Fallat RW, Tsang RC, Glueck CJ. Achilles tendinitis and tenosynovitis. Am J Dis Child 1974;128:486–490.
5. Glueck CJ, Levy R, Fredrickson DS. Acute tendinitis and arthritis. A presenting symptom of familial type II hyperlipoproteinemia. JAMA 1968;206:2895–2897.
6. Bardin T, Kuntz D. Primary hyperlipidemias and xanthomatosis. In: Klippel JH, Dieppe P (eds). Rheumatology. London: Times Mirror International Publishers Limited; 1994;27.1–27.4.
7. Siegelman SS, Schlossberg I, Becker NH, Sachs BA. Hyperlipoproteinemia with skeletal lesions. Clin Orthop 1972;87:228–232.
8. Truswell AS, Pfister PJ. Cerebrotendinous xanthomatosis. Br Med J 1972;1:353–354.
9. Shulman RS, Bhattacharyya AK, Connor WE, Fredrickson DS. Beta-sitosterolemia and xanthomatosis. N Engl J Med 1976;294:482–483.
10. Rooney PJ, Third J, Madkour MM, Spencer D, Dick WC. Transient polyarthritis associated with familial hyperbeta lipoproteinemia. Q J Med 1978;47:249–259.
11. Mathon G, Gagne C, Brun D, Lupien PJ, Moorjani S. Articular manifestations of familial hypercholesterolemia. Ann Rheum Vis 1985;44:599–602.
12. Welin L, Larsson B, Svardsudd K, Tibblin G. Serum lipids, lipoproteins and musculoskeletal disorders among 50- and 60-year-old men. Scand J Rheumatol 1977;1:7–12.
13. Struthers GR, Scott DL, Bacon PA, Walton KW. Musculoskeletal disorders in patients with hyperlipidemia. Ann Rheum Dis 1983;42:519–523.
14. Wysenbeek AJ, Shani E, Beigel Y. Musculoskeletal manifestations in patients with hypercholesterolemia. J Rheumatol 1989;16:643–645.

15. Klemp P, Halland AM, Majoos FL, Steyn K. Musculo-skeletal manifestations in hyperlipidemia: a controlled study. Ann Rheum Dis 1993;52:44–48.

16. Khachadurian AK. Migratory polyarthritis in familial hypercholesterolemia (type II hyperlipoproteinemia). Arthritis Rheum 1968;11:385–393.

17. Rimon D, Cohen L. Hypercholesterolemic (type II hyperlipoproteinemic) arthritis. Rheumatology 1989;16:703–705.

18. Buckingham RB, Bole GG, Bassett DR. Polyarthritis associated with type IV hyperlipoproteinemia. Arch Intern Med 1975;135:286–290.

19. Lazarevic MB, Skosey JL, Vitic J, et al. Cholesterol crystals in synovial and bursal fluid. Semin Arthritis Rheum 1993;23:99–103.

20. Schumacher HR, Michaels R. Recurrent tendinits and Achilles tendon nodule with positively birefringent crystals in a patient with hyperlipoprotenemia. J Rheumatol 1989;16:1387–1389.

21. Solomon DH, Avorn J, Stürmer T, Glynn RJ, Mogun H, Schneeweiss S. Cardiovascular outcomes in new users of coxibs and nonsteroidal antiinflammatory drugs. Arthritis Rheum 2006;54:1378–1389.

Less Common Arthropathies
D. Neuropathic Arthropathy

ANN K. ROSENTHAL, MD

- Neuropathic arthropathy, also known as a Charcot joint, is a destructive arthritis characterized by fracture, subluxation, and dislocation of the articular structures in the setting of neurologic damage to the involved joint or limb.
- Both central (upper motor neuron) and peripheral (lower motor neuron) lesions may lead to the development of neuropathic arthropathy.
- Diabetic neuropathy is now the most common cause of neuropathic arthropathy. Neuropathic arthropathy occurs in 7.5% of diabetic patients.
- The pathologic features of Charcot arthropathy include cartilage destruction, bone eburnation, osteophytosis, and loose body formation.
- Two major theories have been proposed to explain the development of neuropathic arthropathy: the neurovascular theory and the neurotraumatic theory.
- Neuropathic arthropathy typically presents as an acute or subacute monoarthritis with swelling, erythema, and variable amounts of pain in the affected joint.
- Two consistent clinical features of neuropathic arthropathy are the presence of a significant sensory deficit and a degree of pain that is less than would be expected considering the amount of joint destruction evident on radiographs.
- The differential diagnosis of neuropathic arthropathy includes osteomyelitis and other deep tissue infections, fracture, gout, calcium pyrophosphate dihydrate deposition disease, Milwaukee shoulder/knee syndrome, osteonecrosis, and osteoarthritis.
- Plain radiographs are extremely helpful in making the diagnosis of neuropathic arthropathy.
- Categorizing the disease into three clinical stages—acute, subacute, and remodeling—is a useful way to organize approaches to therapy.

Neuropathic arthropathy is a destructive arthritis characterized by fracture, subluxation, and dislocation of the articular structures in the setting of neurologic damage to the involved joint or limb. The concept of an association between sensory neurologic lesions and arthritis was described elegantly by Jean-Martin Charcot in 1868 (1). Consequently, the terms *Charcot arthropathy*, *neurotrophic arthropathy*, and *neuroarthropathy* are used synonymously with neuropathic arthropathy.

EPIDEMIOLOGY

Accurate figures on the incidence and prevalence of neuropathic arthropathy in the general population are difficult to ascertain. The presence of sensory neuropathy is the only established risk factor for neuropathic arthropathy. Both central (upper motor neuron) and peripheral (lower motor neuron) lesions may lead to the development of neuropathic arthropathy.

The neurologic diseases associated with neuropathic arthropathy have radically changed with time (Table 25D-1). In the pre-penicillin era, neuropathic arthropathy was most commonly seen in the setting of tabes dorsalis from tertiary syphilis. Diabetic neuropathy is now the most common cause of neuropathic arthropathy. Neuropathic arthropathy occurs in 7.5% of diabetic patients, with prevalence rates rising to 29% among diabetic patients with neuropathy (2). Syringomyelia, spina bifida, and spinal cord injuries may also result in neuropathic arthropathy. Less commonly encountered causes of neuropathic arthropathy include inflammatory or neoplastic lesions of the spinal cord or peripheral nerves, congenital neurologic abnormalities, and alcoholic neuropathies. Rarely, cases occur in which no neurologic abnormality is identifiable (3).

PATHOLOGY

The pathologic changes of neuropathic arthropathy are similar to those of advanced osteoarthritis: cartilage destruction, bone eburnation, osteophytosis, and loose body formation. The presence of *detritic synovium*,

TABLE 25D-1. NEUROLOGIC CONDITIONS ASSOCIATED WITH NEUROPATHIC ARTHROPATHY.

Diabetes mellitus
Syringomyelia
Spina bifida
Brain or spinal cord trauma
Peripheral nerve trauma
Syphilis
Multiple sclerosis
Charcot–Marie–Tooth disease
Riley–Day syndrome
Pernicious anemia
Congenital insensitivity to pain
Alcoholism
Amyloidosis
Thalidomide exposure
Polyneuropathy of Dejerine–Sottas
Leprosy
Yaws
Neurofibromatosis

defined as fragments of cartilage and bone embedded in the synovium, is characteristic of neuropathic arthropathy, but is also seen in severe osteoarthritis (3). As reflected radiographically, neuropathic arthropathy can cause exuberant bone and cartilage overgrowth as well as joint destruction. Usually both processes are seen, but one process often predominates.

PATHOPHYSIOLOGY

Two major theories have been proposed to explain the development of neuropathic arthropathy. The *neurovascular theory* postulates that joint denervation produces physiologic changes, such as increased blood flow from loss of sympathetic regulation, and upsets the balance between bone resorption and formation. The *neurotraumatic theory* proposes that repeated episodes of minor trauma to joints unprotected by the usual response to pain cause damage through further trauma and inadequate repair. The neurovascular hypothesis is supported clinically by reports of neuropathic arthropathy in patients at bedrest who could not have sustained trauma and the finding that demineral-

ization of the affected limb may precede the development of neuropathic arthropathy (4). In contrast, the observation that injury often accelerates or initiates neuropathic arthropathy supports the neurotraumatic hypothesis (5). Elements of both theories are probably correct.

CLINICAL FEATURES

Neuropathic arthropathy typically presents as an acute or subacute monoarthritis with swelling, erythema, and variable amounts of pain in the affected joint. The two most consistent clinical features of neuropathic arthropathy are the presence of a significant sensory deficit and a degree of pain that is less than would be expected considering the amount of joint destruction evident on radiographs. Abnormal sensation can be accurately detected with the Semmes–Weinstein monofilament test. When slowly progressive, neuropathic arthropathy often resembles osteoarthritis. When rapidly progressive and acute in onset, it mimics osteomyelitis. Initial examinations show swelling, erythema, effusions, and variable amounts of tenderness. With time, the neuropathic joint becomes deformed with large effusions, palpable osteophytes, and loss of range of motion. Categorizing the disease into three clinical stages—acute, subacute, and remodeling—is a useful way to organize approaches to therapy (see Management section, below) (6).

The pattern of joint involvement in neuropathic arthropathy depends on the location of the neurologic impairment and may involve small as well as large joints. In diabetes, the foot is most commonly involved. In spina bifida, the knee, hip, ankle, and lumbar spine are affected. Patients with syringomyelia typically demonstrate upper extremity involvement.

Neuropathic Arthropathy in the Diabetic Foot

Neuropathic arthropathy of the diabetic foot deserves special consideration. It typically occurs after the fifth decade of life in patients with longstanding diabetes, and may follow minor trauma or surgery. It is unilateral in 80% of patients. Five anatomic patterns have been described, including involvement of the toe joints, the tarsometatarsal joints, the midfoot, ankle, and calcaneus. Midfoot involvement is particularly common (Figure 25D-1) (2). During the acute stage, patients present with a swollen foot or ankle. Concurrent skin ulcers are common. The onset of symptoms and rate of destruction may be acute and dramatic with radiographic evidence of joint dissolution occurring within weeks (7). Involvement of the midfoot may result in

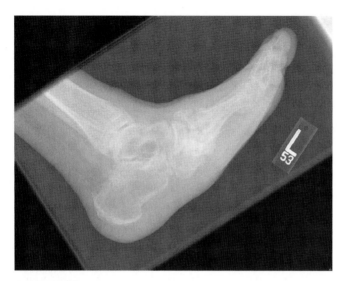

FIGURE 25D-1

Neuropathic arthropathy of the foot in a patient with diabetes. Note the midfoot collapse resulting in a "rocker bottom" deformity. (Courtesy of Dr. Daniel Toutant.)

reversal of the curve of the metatarsal arch and "rocker bottom" deformity. The possibility of osteomyelitis or soft tissue infection in the feet must always be considered in diabetic patients.

DIAGNOSIS

The diagnosis of neuropathic arthropathy can be made clinically. Helpful diagnostic tests include plain radiographs, bone scans, and indium-111–labeled white blood cell (WBC) scans. The differential diagnosis of neuropathic arthropathy includes osteomyelitis and other deep tissue infections, fracture, gout, calcium pyrophosphate dihydrate deposition (CPPD) disease, Milwaukee shoulder/knee syndrome, osteonecrosis, and osteoarthritis. The differentiation between osteomyelitis and acute neuropathic arthropathy in the diabetic foot is particularly challenging.

Plain radiographs are extremely helpful in making the diagnosis of neuropathic arthropathy (3). Early features include demineralization, joint space narrowing, and osteophyte formation. In established disease, bone fragmentation, periarticular debris formation, and joint subluxation occur (Figures 25D-1, 25D-2). Bone absorption, bone shattering, sclerosis and massive soft tissue swelling are seen in some patients. Neuropathic joints are often described radiographically as "disorganized," with chaotic bone destruction and repair. The presence of sharply defined articular surfaces in neuropathic arthropathy is helpful in differentiating radiographic changes of neuropathic arthropathy

from those of infection, where involved bone surfaces are indistinct. In neuropathic arthropathy of the diabetic foot, destruction with prominent fragmentation and loose body formation typically occurs in the tarsal bones, while absorptive changes may predominate in the metatarsals and forefoot (Figure 25D-2). In the spine, multilevel thoracic and lumbar involvement is common.

Bone scintigraphy with technetium 99m-MDP and indium-111–labeled WBC scans (8) demonstrate increased uptake of radiolabeled technetium in neuropathic arthropathy; unfortunately, uncomplicated neuropathy as well as infection both can produce similar findings (9). Magnetic resonance imaging should be interpreted with caution as bony changes in osteomyelitis can be difficult to differentiate from those of neuropathic arthropathy. A combined approach using multiple imaging techniques with or without bone cultures is often necessary to differentiate infection from neuropathic arthropathy.

Synovial fluid is typically non-inflammatory in neuropathic arthropathy. Fifty percent of synovial fluids from affected joints are hemorrhagic or xanthochromic. Effusions may be very large. CPPD crystals and basic calcium phosphate crystals have been identified in these joint effusions and may contribute to joint damage.

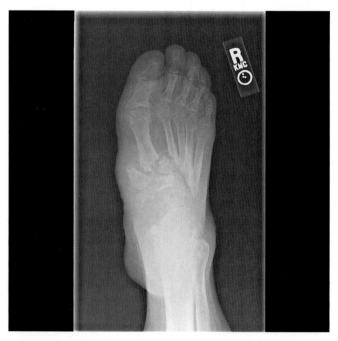

FIGURE 25D-2

Neuropathic arthropathy of the foot in a patient with diabetes. There is involvement of the forefoot and the midfoot. The typical combination of both resorptive and reparative processes results in a disorganized appearance of the involved bones. (Courtesy of Dr. Daniel Toutant.)

MANAGEMENT

There are no specific therapies for neuropathic arthropathy. The prognosis of affected patients is variable and depends on the severity of the condition and the response to treatment.

Standard management strategies for the acute phase (6) of neuropathic arthropathy include joint immobilization, usually achieved by casts, braces, orthotics, and restricted weight bearing. With immobilization, the average time to healing in neuropathic arthropathy of the diabetic foot is approximately 6 months (4). With early diagnosis and bracing, risks for amputation are 2.3%, but 23% will require bracing for 18 months, and 50% will have recurrent ulcers (10). There is some preliminary evidence for the efficacy of bisphosphonates in the early destructive phase of the disease (2).

Surgical treatments, another mainstay of therapy, are generally recommended in the remodeling phase of the disease (2). Goals are to improve pain, joint stability, and alignment, and to prevent or treat overlying skin ulceration. Arthrodesis is useful in the spine, foot, ankle, and knee. Removal of exostoses may restore some motion and decrease joint pain in patients with severe rocker bottom deformities of the foot. With current techniques, joint replacement may also be effective for selected patients.

Prevention is perhaps the best therapy. Prompt attention to any minor trauma to the diabetic foot or ankle may prevent the development of neuropathic arthropathy. Good control of blood glucose levels in diabetics decreases the incidence of neuropathy and thereby reduces the risk of neuropathic arthropathy.

References

1. Gupta A. A short history of neuropathic arthropathy. Clin Orthop 1993;296:43–49.
2. Lee L, Blume P, Sumpio B. Charcot joint disease in diabetes mellitus. Ann Vasc Surg 2003;17:571–580.
3. Resnick D. Neuropathic osteoarthropathy. In: Resnick D, ed. Diagnosis of bone and joint disorders. 3rd ed. Philadelphia: Saunders; 1995:3413–3442.
4. Sinacore D, Withrington N. Recognition and management of acute neuropathic (Charcot) arthropathies of the foot and ankle. J Orthop Sports Phys Ther 1999;29:736–746.
5. Fishco W. Surgically induced Charcot's foot. J Am Podiatr Med Assoc 2001;91:288–293.
6. Eichenholtz S. Charcot joints. Springfield: Thomas; 1966.
7. Sloman-Kovacs S, Braunstein E, Brandt K. Rapidly progressive Charcot arthropathy following minor joint trauma in patients with diabetic neuropathy. Arthritis Rheum 1990;33:412–417.
8. Lipman B, Collier B, Carrera G, et al. Detection of osteomyelitis in the neuropathic foot: nuclear medicine, MRI, and conventional radiography. Clin Nucl Med 1998;23:77–82.
9. Palestro C, Mehta H, Patel M, et al. Marrow versus infection in the Charcot joint: indium-111 leukocyte and technetium-99m sulfur colloid scintigraphy. J Nucl Med 1998;39:346–350.
10. Saltzman C, Hagy M, Zimmerman B, Estin M, Cooper R. How effective is intensive nonoperative intial treatment of patients with diabetes and Charcot arthropathy of the feet? Clin Orthop 2005;435:185–190.

Less Common Arthropathies
E. Dermatologic Disorders

JEFFREY P. CALLEN, MD

- Many rheumatologic diseases have prominent cutaneous findings.
- Careful examination of the skin may lead to prompt diagnoses, relatively noninvasive means of defining systemic disorders, and possibly better outcomes.
- Entities discussed in this chapter include the neutrophilic dermatoses (Sweet's syndrome,

pyoderma gangrenosum), panniculitis (e.g., erythema nodosum), the sclerosing/fibrosing diseases (e.g., morphea and scleromyxedema), pustular conditions, and a variety of cutaneous conditions with possible implications for rheumatic disease.

The skin often reflects the presence of disease involving internal organs. Consequently, careful examination of the skin may lead to prompt diagnoses, relatively non-invasive means of defining systemic disorders, and possibly better outcomes. Many rheumatologic diseases have prominent cutaneous findings. This chapter provides an overview of a group of conditions in which skin findings are a major component of systemic disease.

NEUTROPHILIC DERMATOSES

The neutrophilic dermatoses are noninfectious disorders characterized by infiltration of the skin by polymorphonuclear leukocytes (Table 25E-1) (1). Some of these disorders may be angiocentric, but typically they are not associated with the type of vessel wall destruction observed in vasculitis. The neutrophilic dermatoses include Sweet's syndrome, pyoderma gangrenosum, neutrophilic dermatosis of the dorsal hands, rheumatoid neutrophilic dermatosis, and the bowel-associated dermatosis–arthritis syndrome.

Sweet's syndrome (2), originally termed *acute febrile neutrophilic dermatosis*, is characterized by painful, erythematous plaques on almost any body surface (Figure 25E-1). The surface of the lesions, frequently tender, may be so edematous that the lesions appear vesicular. Subcutaneous nodules and dermal nodules are unusual manifestations of Sweet's syndrome. The characteristic histopathological findings of Sweet's syndrome are shown in Figure 25E-2. The patients are usually febrile, have a leukocytosis, and frequently

have arthralgias or arthritis. The process is more common in women. The disease may be classified further based upon its potential associations with malignancy, inflammatory disorders, infections, drugs, or a group of miscellaneous conditions. In approximately 15% to 20% of patients with Sweet's syndrome, myeloid malignancy or preleukemia occurs. Solid tumors are very rare in these patients. The diagnosis is confirmed by excluding other diseases, particularly cellulitis. Patients with Sweet's syndrome demonstrate pathergy—the occurrence of the characteristic skin lesions following minor trauma.

Patients with Sweet's syndrome often have antineutrophil cytoplasmic antibodies (ANCA) by immunofluorescence testing, but the ANCA specificity is not directed against either myeloperoxidase or proteinase-3 (the specificity observed in microscopic polyangiitis, Wegener's granulomatosis, and related vasculitides). No laboratory findings are pathognomonic of Sweet's syndrome. Patients with Sweet's syndrome secondary to myelodysplasia or leukemia, however, are frequently anemic or thrombocytopenic. Although generally confined to the skin, extracutaneous neutrophilic infiltration occurs in a small percentage of Sweet's syndrome patients, potentially affecting any organ (most commonly the lungs). Osteolytic bone lesions have also been reported. The entity known as *multifocal sterile recurrent osteomyelitis* might represent an orthopedic variant of Sweet's syndrome.

Therapy for Sweet's syndrome is directed toward any identified underlying condition, including cessation of drugs with the potential to trigger this condition.

TABLE 25E-1. ASSOCIATIONS WITH NEUTROPHILIC DERMATOSES.

DERMATOSIS	SWEET'S SYNDROME	PYODERMA GANGRENOSUM (PG)	RHEUMATOID NEUTROPHILIC DERMATOSIS	BOWEL-ASSOCIATED DERMATOSIS ARTHRITIS SYNDROME	NEUTROPHILIC DERMATOSIS OF THE DORSAL HANDS
Inflammatory bowel disease–Crohn's disease and ulcerative colitis	Some	20%–25%	No	Yes	Occasional
Rheumatoid arthritis	Occasional	10% for superficial forms, less for classical PG	Yes, occasionally seronegative	No, but joint disease may simulate RA	Occasional
Hematologic malignancies	25%–30%	15% for the superficial forms	No	No	15%
Solid tumors	Rare	Rare	No	No	Rare
Sjögren's syndrome	Possible	No	Possible	No	Possible
Drug-induced	Occasionally	No	No	No	Possible
Pregnancy	Occasionally	No	No	No	No

Medications known to be associated with Sweet's syndrome include granulocyte-monocyte colony-stimulating factor (GMCSF), granulocyte colony stimulating factor (GCSF), bortezomib, imatinib, minocycline, hydralazine, and oral contraceptives. For acute disease, a short course of oral prednisone tapered over 2 weeks is often sufficient. For recurrent disease without an associated condition, glucocorticoid-sparing agents such as dapsone, thalidomide, immunosuppressive agents, and tumor necrosis factor alpha (TNF-alpha) antagonists are often used. In patients with acute, idiopathic disease, the prognosis is generally good; many have only episode. However, the course of patients with underlying leukemia or myelodysplasia follows that of the associated disease. Absent disease remission or a cure, recurrences are common.

Pyoderma gangrenosum (PG) is a form of ulcerative skin disease. There are at least four clinical variants of PG: classical, atypical, peristomal, and mucosal (3). The classical lesion is a rapidly progressing, painful ulcer, most often on the leg, with a violaceous, undermined (overhanging) border (Figure 25E-3). Atypical PG occurs as a more superficial lesion, often on the dorsal hands (Figure 25E-4), extensor forearms, or face. The border of atypical PG may appear bullous, leading to clinical confusion with Sweet's syndrome. Peristomal PG occurs as a deep ulcer near the site of a stoma, usually created after gastrointestinal or genitourinary surgery. Finally, mucosal PG is associated with ulcerations that can resemble simple aphthae or vegetative lesions. Mucosal PG must be differentiated from Behçet's disease.

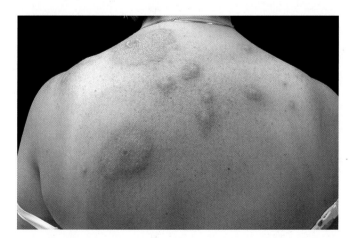

FIGURE 25E-1

Sweet's syndrome.

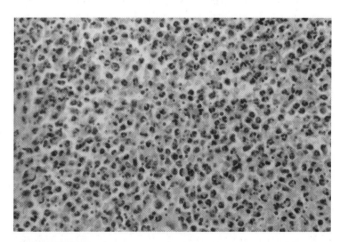

FIGURE 25E-2

Histopathological findings in Sweet's syndrome.

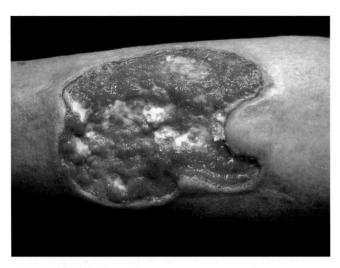

FIGURE 25E-3

Pyoderma gangrenosum in a patient without an associated disease.

Patients with PG also demonstrate pathergy. Thus, this condition has been reported following a variety of surgical procedures, for example, thoracotomy or fasciotomy. The systemic associations vary depending on the type of PG. Classical disease and peristomal PG are associated more frequently with inflammatory bowel disease and/or arthritis. Careful evaluation for inflammatory bowel disease is warranted in cases of peristomal PG, even when the stoma was created for other reasons (e.g., following cancer surgery). In contrast, atypical pyoderma gangrenosum is found more frequently in the setting of myelocytic leukemia or preleukemic conditions.

The diagnosis of PG is one of exclusion. Although biopsies should be performed to exclude other conditions, PG does not have a distinctive histopathology. Because of the importance of excluding disease mimickers—particularly infections—biopsy is almost always performed as part of the evaluation, despite the possibility that the ulcer will extend through pathergy. Culture of the lesions following skin biopsy is essential. Infectious mimickers are not common but include deep fungal infections; for example, blastomycosis, sporotrichosis, histoplasmosis, and coccidioidomycosis; as well as nocardiosis, tuberculosis, atypical mycobacteria; and herpes simplex virus. Following diagnosis, appropriate studies should be undertaken to exclude inflammatory bowel disease, rheumatoid arthritis (RA), systemic vasculitis, paraproteinemia, and other hematologic disorders. As with Sweet's syndrome, neutrophilic infiltration of organs other than the skin may sometimes occur in PG.

For cases of PG associated with an underlying disease (e.g., inflammatory bowel disease or RA), treatment of the primary condition often leads to improvement in PG. Prednisone (1 mg/kg/day) is generally the first line of therapy for idiopathic PG. Infliximab (3–5 mg/kg every 6 weeks following two initial doses 2 weeks apart) is also an effective therapy for PG, even in the absence of inflammatory bowel disease. Other therapies employed in PG include dapsone [100–200 mg/day (assuming normal levels of glucose-6-phosphate dehydrogenase; G6-PD)], thalidomide (100 mg/day), cyclosporine (5 mg/kg/day), azathioprine [2 mg/kg/day, assuming normal levels of thiopurine methyltransferase; (TPMT)], and mycophenolate mofetil (1.0–.5 g b.i.d.).

Neutrophilic dermatosis of the dorsal hands (NDDH) (4), considered by some to be a separate disease entity, is regarded more commonly as a variant of either Sweet's syndrome or atypical PG. NDDH is associated with the same underlying conditions as Sweet's syndrome and atypical PG, and the management considerations are identical.

Rheumatoid neutrophilic dermatosis, an unusual complication of RA, is characterized by symmetrical erythematous papules and plaques on the dorsal hands, elbows, and extensor surfaces of the forearms (5). Patients generally have active and often severe RA, but the condition has been reported in at least two patients with seronegative RA. In terms of histopathology, rheumatoid neutrophilic dermatosis resembles Sweet's syndrome. Treatments that have been suggested include glucocorticoids, dapsone (100–200 mg/day), and colchicine (0.6 mg b.i.d.); however, spontaneous resolution has been reported to occur.

Bowel-associated dermatosis–arthritis syndrome was first recognized in the 1970s following gastric bypass surgery for morbid obesity. Fortunately, because of major alterations in surgical technique, this syndrome is

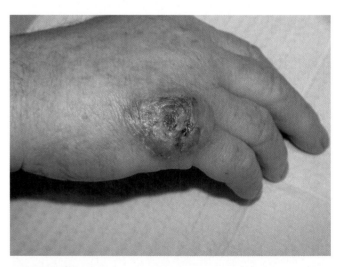

FIGURE 25E-4

Atypical pyoderma gangrenosum, also known as neutrophilic dermatosis of the dorsal hands.

rarely observed today. The former procedure involved the creation of a blind intestinal loop that frequently led to bacterial overgrowth, presumed responsible for the clinical manifestations. The bowel-associated dermatosis–arthritis syndrome was initially called *bowel bypass syndrome* until recognition of the fact that similar changes occurred in patients with ulcer surgery that created a blind loop.

The skin lesions of the bowel-associated dermatosis–arthritis syndrome are characterized by pustular lesions or erythematous papules and/or plaques. Lesions that simulate NDDH (see above) have also been reported. The joint manifestations consist of a symmetrical, nondeforming arthropathy, most often involving the small joints of the hands and feet. These patients often respond to antibiotic therapy, including tetracycline or metronidazole.

PANNICULITIDES

Panniculitis refers to inflammation of the subcutaneous fat (6,7). The process probably evolves from neutrophilic infiltration through lymphocytic and histiocytic infiltration to fibrosis. The classification of panniculitides is controversial, but several clear-cut entities are defined here.

Erythema nodosum, perhaps the most common form of panniculitis, is characterized histologically by septal inflammation (8). Erythema nodosum is most often characterized by red, tender subcutaneous nodules on the anterior leg (Figure 25E-5). The disorder is believed to be a reactive process commonly triggered by infections in the upper respiratory tract and/or lungs. The most common association is streptococcal pharyngitis, but tuberculosis, coccidioidomycosis, and psittacosis are other common infectious causes. Pregnancy, oral con-

traceptive use, inflammatory bowel disease, and sarcoidosis are other common causes of erythema nodosum. In sarcoidosis, erythema nodosum typically occurs in the setting of arthritis and hilar adenopathy, a syndrome known as Löfgren's syndrome. Löfgren's syndrome, self-limited in two thirds of cases, usually requires symptomatic treatment only.

Joint inflammation may accompany erythema nodosum, but at times the inflammatory reaction on the legs surrounds the joints, creating a "periarthritis" but not a true synovitis. Patients with erythema nodosum should be evaluated with a careful history and physical examination. Skin biopsies are required only for atypical presentations or persistent disease. Additional evaluation should include throat cultures, a streptozyme titer, and a chest radiograph. Treatment is often supportive, including gradient support stockings, elevation of the legs, and nonsteroidal anti-inflammatory agents. Other therapies that have been reported to be effective in single cases or small case series include potassium iodide, dapsone, antimalarial agents, colchicine, glucocorticoids, immunosuppressive agents, and TNF-alpha antagonists.

The existence of **Weber–Christian disease** as a distinct entity is controversial. The condition is characterized by recurrent, often multiple, tender subcutaneous nodules accompanied by fever. In contrast to erythema nodosum (a septal panniculitis), Weber–Christian disease is a lobular panniculitis. With regard to nomenclature, the issue is whether the lobular panniculitis associated with Weber–Christian disease occurs as a primary disorder or as a complication of another underlying illness. For example, a lobular panniculitis is known to occur in alpha-1-antitrypsin deficiency, pancreatic disease-associated panniculitis, and a wide array of other inflammatory disorders. Systemic involvement due to inflammation of fatty tissues other than the subcutis has also been reported in cases labeled Weber–Christian disease. There is no specific therapy for this entity, but suggested therapies include those for chronic erythema nodosum (see above).

Lupus panniculitis (also known as lupus profundus), a rare manifestation of systemic lupus erythematosus (SLE), is a form of chronic cutaneous lupus erythematosus. The histopathology of lupus profundus reveals both lobular and septal inflammation, sometimes demonstrating an interface dermatitis (deposition of immunoreactants such as immunoglobulins and complement proteins at the dermal/epidermal junction) that is characteristic of cutaneous lupus. Hydroxychloroquine [6.5 mg/kg (ideal body weight)/day in single or divided doses] is usually an effective first approach to therapy.

Lipodermatosclerosis, also known as sclerosing panniculitis, is characterized by tender, subcutaneous nodules most often over the medial malleolus, accompanied by hyperpigmentation, telangiectases, tortuous

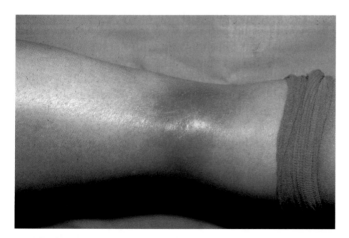

FIGURE 25E-5

Erythema nodosum.

TABLE 25E-2. *Continued*

DISEASE	CUTANEOUS MANIFESTATIONS	SYSTEMIC MANIFESTATIONS	EVALUATION	MANAGEMENT	COMMENTS
Scleromyxedema	Linear flesh-colored papules are an early change, but eventually induration occurs.	Monoclonal gammopathy and plasma cell dyscrasia is common.	Biopsy reveals increase in mucin in the dermis. SPEP, IEP, bone marrow aspiration or biopsy.	Stem-cell transplant has resulted in complete responses in patients with plasma cell dyscrasia. Systemic glucocorticoids or cytotoxic agents are used in patients without plasma cell dyscrasia.	
Nephrogenic fibrosing dermopathy/ nephrogenic systemic fibrosis	Acute onset of induration often follows anasarca. Usually affects the arms [Figure 25E-11(B)] and forearms, or the legs. Decrease in the range of motion of the hands [Figure 25E-11(A)] and feet lead to limitations of the patient's ability to function.	Renal disease of some sort is almost always present. Pulmonary fibrosis may occur. Calcifications may also compromise the process.	Tests of renal function. Monoclonal protein is absent. Biopsy looks identical to scleromyxedema.	Renal transplantation may improve process. Other therapies that have been reported to be effective include thalidomide, photopheresis, plasmapheresis, methotrexate, phototherapy, IVIG.	The process may be preceded by a surgical procedure, particularly vascular revision of hemodialysis shunt, or by a thrombotic event.
Graft-versus-host disease (GVHD)	Acute disease is associated with a morbilliform eruption. As the process becomes more chronic, lichen planus–like lesions may develop. Eventually sclerotic lesions, often with superficial features of lichen sclerosus occur. (Figure 25E-10).	Hepatic dysfunction and/or bowel dysfunction.	There is no test to determine whether a patient has GVHD. Biopsy in the late stages simulates morphea or lichen sclerosus, but there is often an interface dermatitis as well.	Topical superpotent glucocorticoids and/or calcineurin inhibitors for localized disease. Phototherapy, thalidomide, immunosuppressive agents for widespread or systemic disease.	

ABBREVIATIONS: ANA, antinuclear antibodies; Anti–ssDNA, anti–single-stranded DNA; IEP, immunoelectrophoresis; IVIG, intravenous immune globulin; PFT, pulmonary function tests; SPEP, serum protein electrophoresis; UV, ultraviolet.

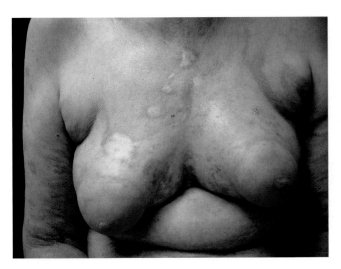

FIGURE 25E-7

Generalized morphea—this patient has widespread disease on her trunk and proximal extremities. Note the sparing of scleroderma on the nipples, which is a common feature of generalized morphea.

disease must also be excluded. Monoclonal gammopathies, particularly IgG lambda, are common in scleromyxedema, which may also be associated with multiple myeloma and amyloidosis. Treatment of patients with scleromyxedema is often difficult. Therapies that have been used include cytotoxic agents, including melphalan, thalidomide, and, most recently, autologous stem cell transplantation (13).

Nephrogenic systemic fibrosis (NSF; also termed **nephrogenic fibrosing dermopathy** or **nephrogenic fibrosing systemic disorder**) is a recently described process characterized by a rapid onset of skin thickening [14; Figure 25E-11(A,B)]. The process is accompanied by limited range of motion, particularly of the feet and hands. The biopsy is identical to the changes observed

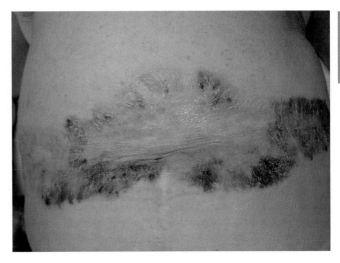

FIGURE 25E-9

Lichen sclerosus. Note the cigarette paper–like changes on the surface. Hemorrhage within the lesions is quite characteristic.

in scleromyxedema. Features that separate this entity from scleromyxedema are the lack of a monoclonal gammopathy and the presence of renal disease. Since its initial description, systemic fibrosis (particularly affecting the lungs) has been described in many patients, leading to debate over the appropriate name of the condition. Many patients improve with renal transplantation, while others have been treated with thalidomide, methotrexate, TNF antagonists, plasmapheresis, and photopheresis with variable success. NSF is now known to be associated strongly with the administration of gadolinium, a contrast agent used in magnetic resonance imaging, to patients with renel insufficiency.

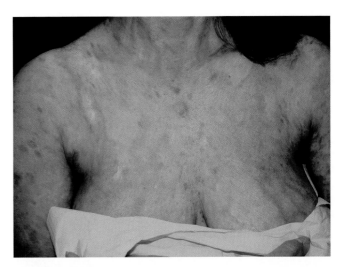

FIGURE 25E-10

Graft-versus-host disease (GVHD). Patients with chronic GVHD often have cutaneous manifestations. This patient demonstrates the widespread nature of the disease which simulates both morphea and lichen sclerosus.

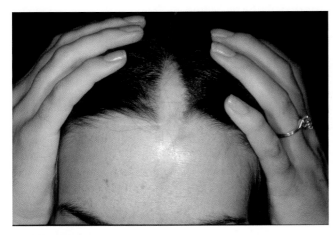

FIGURE 25E-8

Linear scleroderma.

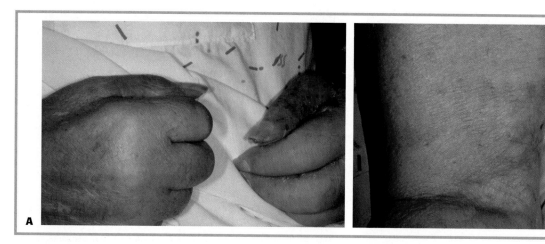

FIGURE 25E-11

(A, B) Nephrogenic systemic fibrosis in a patient with acute renal failure who underwent a magnetic resonance imaging study with gadolinium dialysis.

PUSTULAR CONDITIONS

The following disease entities, characterized by pustular lesions, demonstrate substantial overlap.

Generalized pustular psoriasis is a rare phenomenon, but pustular psoriasis localized to the palms and soles (Figure 25E-12) is relatively common. These diseases may be induced by various medications, including the withdrawal of systemic glucocorticoids in the case of generalized pustular psoriasis and the use of TNF antagonists in the case of palmoplantar pustular psoriasis (15). Generalized pustular psoriasis, a highly labile form of psoriasis, can be accompanied by systemic symptoms. Control with oral retinoids, methotrexate, or possibly infliximab is useful. Pustular lesions of the palms and soles are difficult to treat and can cause disability.

SAPHO syndrome is a rare disorder characterized by synovitis, acne, pustulosis of the palms and soles, hyperostosis of one of the bones of the chest wall, and sterile osteitis (16). These patients may also have psoriasis vulgaris or accompanying inflammatory bowel disease. The synovitis may involve either peripheral or axial joints. The osteitis is similar to chronic recurrent sterile osteomyelitis. The prevalence of human leukocyte antigen (HLA)-B27 is increased among patients with the SAPHO syndrome, leading some authorities to classify this entity as a spondyloarthropathy. SAPHO syndrome has considerable overlap with the other pustular conditions discussed in this section, however, as well as with the neutrophilic dermatoses discussed above. The pathogenetic mechanisms of all of these conditions remain incompletely defined. Treatment of SAPHO is often difficult. Drugs that have been reported to be effective in individual cases or small case series include nonsteriodal anti-inflammatory drugs (NSAIDs), colchicine, glucocorticoids, sulfasalazine, methotrexate, infliximab, and second generation bisphosphonates.

The **PAPA syndrome** is the occurrence of sterile pyogenic arthritis, pyoderma gangrenosum, and acne. Usually the acne is nodulocystic. The differentiation of this syndrome from SAPHO may be difficult.

Hidradenitis suppurativa is a disorder of apocrine glands. Patients present with pustules and draining sinus tracts in the axilla, under the breasts, within inguinal folds, and on the buttocks. Women appear to be affected more frequently than men. Hidradenitis may be associated with Crohn's disease in some patients. Oral antibiotics are frequently prescribed but often not fully effective. Oral isotretinoin is often suggested, but in this

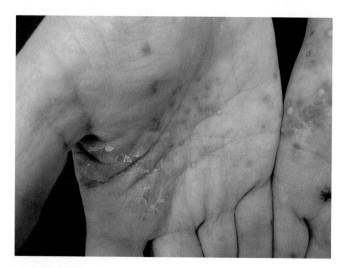

FIGURE 25E-12

Palmoplantar pustulosis—note the crusts accompanied by both large and small pustules on the palms of this patient.

author's opinion, it is rarely effective. Recent case reports and case series have documented responses to infliximab. Definitive therapy with surgical exenteration of the involved areas is curative.

Acne fulminans is a severe form of acne that is accompanied by systemic symptoms (17). It is explosive in its onset and most often occurs in adolescent boys. The face, chest, and upper back are the most common sites. The lesions may begin as mild typical acne, but they rapidly become markedly inflamed and coalesce into painful and oozing friable plaques with hemorrhagic crusts. Systemic involvement includes fever, arthralgia, myalgia, hepatosplenomegaly, and severe prostration. Erythema nodosum may occur in some patients with acne fulminans. Osteolytic bone lesions have also been reported. There is no specific laboratory abnormality associated with this process, but elevation of the erythrocyte sedimentation rate, leukocytosis, and anemia may occur. Therapy with oral glucocorticoids and isotretinoin is helpful. Oral dapsone has also been utilized as an adjunctive therapy. Residual scarring is common.

MISCELLANEOUS DERMATOLOGICAL CONDITIONS WITH POSSIBLE RHEUMATOLOGIC CONSEQUENCES

Scurvy, caused by vitamin C deficiency, frequently presents with purpura or ecchymoses and bone pain. It is more common in alcoholics. The purpuric lesions tend to be perifollicular (Figure 25E-13). Careful examination reveals corkscrew hairs that are also characteristic.

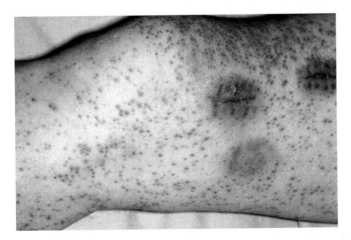

FIGURE 25E-13

Scurvy. Perifollicular purpura with corkscrew hairs. (Courtesy of Kenneth E. Greer, MD, Charlottesville, VA.)

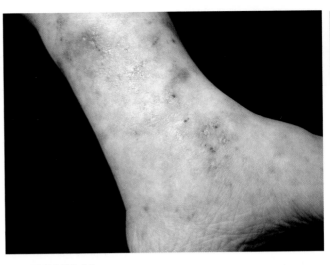

FIGURE 25E-14

Livedoid vasculopathy (also known as atrophie blanche).

Occasionally scurvy may masquerade as small vessel vasculitis. Reintroduction of vitamin C into the diet leads to resolution of the process.

Livedoid vasculopathy, also known as segmental hyalinizing vasculopathy, livedoid vasculitis, atrophie blanche, and livedo reticularis with summer ulcerations, is a clinical entity manifested by painful ulcerations of the distal legs, more commonly over the medial malleolus (Figure 25E-14). This process is not an inflammatory disease. On biopsy, the characteristic change is fibrin deposition within the vessel lumina. The process may represent an end result of a number of coagulation disorders, including cryofibrinogenemia, Factor V Leiden mutation, and other inherited thrombophilic conditions, and the antiphospholipid syndrome (18). Livedoid vasculopathy may mimic vasculitis or stasis dermatitis clinically. Therefore, a biopsy is helpful in directing the evaluation. Therapy should include smoking cessation and prevention of trauma, in addition to addressing any underlying coagulation disorder. Various platelet inhibitors and anticoagulants have been reported to be effective in individual cases or small case series.

Granuloma annulare is a relatively common cutaneous disease not generally associated with systemic conditions. The findings of granuloma annulare are flesh-colored or erythematous lesions that are annular (Figure 25E-15) and may occur on any surface of the body. The histopathology of granuloma annulare is a necrobiotic granuloma—essentially the same histopathological finding that occurs in necrobiosis lipoidica and rheumatoid nodules. Biopsies are frequently read as rheumatoid nodules by general pathologists; patients are then referred inappropriately for rheumatologic evaluations. Treatment of granuloma annulare with intralesional injections of triamcinolone acetonide in

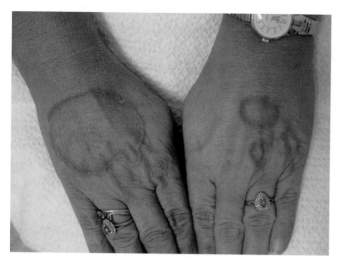

FIGURE 25E-15

Granuloma annulare on the dorsal hands.

dilute concentrations usually leads to resolution of the disorder.

Two variants of granuloma annulare are worth mentioning: the subcutaneous variant (19) and a recently described acute acral variant (20). Subcutaneous granuloma annulare often presents on the feet or hands and may be slightly tender (Figure 25E-16). Acute acral granuloma annulare is a process associated with the sudden onset of tender acral erythematous lesions, usually on the hands and fingers (Figure 25E-17). The acral variant, which often occurs in patients with a history of various forms of arthritis, is managed with topical glucocorticoids, oral antimalarial agents, oral dapsone, or (rarely) oral glucocorticoids.

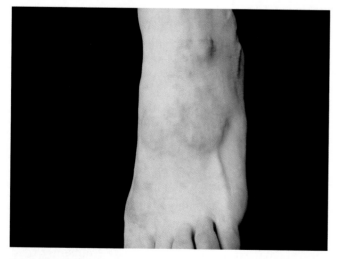

FIGURE 25E-16

Subcutaneous granuloma annulare. This patient was misdiagnosed as having rheumatoid arthritis after her initial biopsy was interpreted as a rheumatoid nodule.

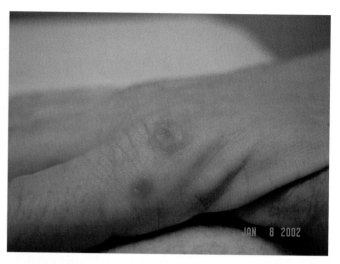

FIGURE 25E-17

Acute, acral granuloma annulare. This patient had disease which clinically mimicked Sweet's syndrome, but the histopathology demonstrated a necrobiotic granuloma.

Cutaneous extravascular necrotizing granulomas are known as the Churg–Strauss granulomas. The term *palisaded neutrophilic and granulomatous dermatitis with arthritis*, rheumatoid papules, superficial ulcerating rheumatoid necrobiosis, and interstitial granulomatous dermatitis with arthritis have also been used to describe this entity (21). Whether this is a distinct entity is controversial and the exact relationship to arthritis has been questioned. Patients present with symmetrical, annular, erythematous lesions, often favoring intertriginous sites. Recently multiple drugs have been linked to the development of interstitial granulomatous dermatitis, but even when a drug has appeared to trigger the cutaneous disease, it is likely that the patient has an underlying rheumatologic disease, particularly SLE, RA, Wegener's granulomatosis, or the Churg-Strauss syndrome. Treatment involves discontinuation of a drug in an appropriate setting and treatment of the associated condition.

Lichen planus is a common cutaneous disease characterized by pruritic, purple, polygonal papules and plaques (Figure 25E-18). The surface scale, when examined closely demonstrates a reticulated pattern known as "Wickham striae." Common areas of involvement include the wrists and mouth but any surface may be involved. Erosive oral and/or genital disease may lead to malignancy. Lichen planus is frequently associated with hepatitis C. A variant of lichen planus is caused by drugs and has occurred more commonly in patients treated with gold or penicillamine. Lichen planus–like lesions may be a manifestation of acute graft-versus-host disease. The disease is self-limited but may be treated with topical or systemic glucocorticoids.

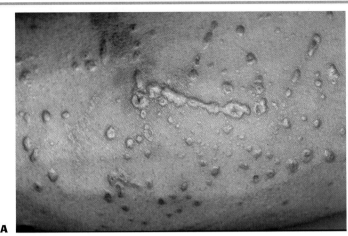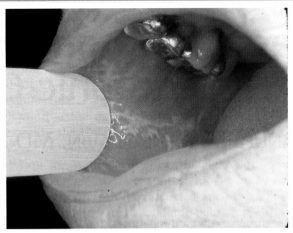

FIGURE 25E-18

Lichen planus lesions on the wrist (A) and in the mouth (B).

REFERENCES

1. Callen JP. Miscellaneous disorders that commonly affect both skin and joints. In: Sontheimer RD, Provost TT, eds. Cutaneous manifestations of rheumatic diseases. 2nd ed. Philadelphia: Lippincott Williams & Wilkins; 2004:221–241.
2. Cohen PR, Kurzrock R. Sweet's syndrome revisited: a review of disease concepts. Int J Dermatol 2003;42:761–778.
3. Jackson JM, Callen JP. Pyoderma gangrenosum. An expert commentary. Int J Dermatol 2006;41:916–918.
4. Walling HW, Snipes CJ, Gerami P, Piette WW. The relationship between neutrophilic dermatosis of the dorsal hands and sweet syndrome: report of 9 cases and comparison to atypical pyoderma gangrenosum. Arch Dermatol 2006;142:57–63.
5. Brown TB, Fearneyhough PF, Burruss JB, Callen JP. Rheumatoid neutrophilic dermatitis in a woman with seronegative rheumatoid arthritis. J Am Acad Dermatol 2001;45:596–600.
6. Requena L, Yus ES. Panniculitis. Part I. Mostly septal panniculitis. J Am Acad Dermatol 2001;45:163–183.
7. Requena L, Sanchez Yus E. Panniculitis. Part II. Mostly lobular panniculitis. J Am Acad Dermatol 2001;45:325–361.
8. Requena L, Requena C. Erythema nodosum. Dermatol Online J 2002;8:4.
9. Bruce AJ, Bennett DD, Lohse CM, Rooke TW, Davis MD. Lipodermatosclerosis: review of cases evaluated at Mayo Clinic. J Am Acad Dermatol 2002;46:187–192.
10. Ma L, Bandarchi B, Glusac EJ. Fatal subcutaneous panniculitis-like T-cell lymphoma with interface change and dermal mucin, a dead ringer for lupus erythematosus. J Cutan Pathol 2005;32:360–365.

11. Zulian F, Vallongo C, Woo P, et al. Localized scleroderma in childhood is not just a skin disease. Arthritis Rheum 2005;52:2873–2881.
12. Oyama N, Chan I, Neill SM, et al. Development of antigen-specific ELISA for circulating autoantibodies to extracellular matrix protein 1 in lichen sclerosus. J Clin Invest 2004;113:1550–1559.
13. Donato ML, Feasel AM, Weber DM, et al. Scleromyxedema: role of high-dose melphalan with autologous stem cell transplantation. Blood 2006;107:463–466.
14. Cowper SE, Boyer PJ. Nephrogenic systemic fibrosis: an update. Curr Rheumatol Rep 2006;8:151–157.
15. Sfikakis PP, Iliopoulos A, Elezoglou A, Kittas C, Stratigos A. Psoriasis induced by anti-tumor necrosis factor therapy: a paradoxical adverse reaction. Arthritis Rheum 2005;52:2513–2518.
16. Suei Y, Taguchi A, Tanimoto K. Diagnostic points and possible origin of osteomyelitis in synovitis, acne, pustulosis, hyperostosis and osteitis (SAPHO) syndrome: a radiographic study of 77 mandibular osteomyelitis cases. Rheumatology (Oxford) 2003;42:1398–1403.
17. Mehrany K, Kist JM, Weenig RH, Witman PM. Acne fulminans. Int J Dermatol 2005;44:132–133.
18. Hairston BR, Davis MDP, Pittelkow MR, Ahmed I. Livedoid vasculopathy: further evidence for procoagulant pathogenesis. Arch Dermatol 2006;142:1413–1418.
19. McDermott MB, Lind AC, Marley EF, Dehner LP. Deep granuloma annulare (pseudorheumatoid nodule) in children: clinicopathologic study of 35 cases. Pediatr Dev Pathol 1998;1:300–308.
20. Brey NV, Malone J, Callen JP. Acute-onset, painful acral granuloma annulare: a report of 4 cases and a discussion of the clinical and histologic spectrum of the disease. Arch Dermatol 2006;142:49–54.
21. Chu P, Connolly MK, LeBoit PE. The histopathologic spectrum of palisaded neutrophilic and granulomatous dermatitis in patients with collagen vascular disease. Arch Dermatol 1994;130:1278–1283.

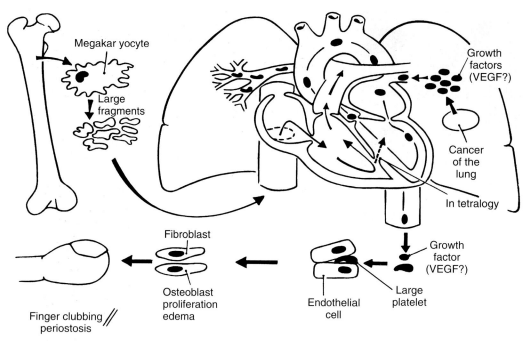

FIGURE 25F-2

The theoretical pathogenesis of hypertrophic osteoarthropathy.

one or two extremities. Such cases usually occur as a response to prominent endothelial injury to the involved limb, for example, damage caused by aneurysms or infective endarteritis. Alternatively, they may be associated with patent ductus arteriosus and reversal of the physiologic direction of blood flow. People with primary HOA may display a generalized skin hypertrophy called *pachyderma* (Figure 25F-3). This skin overgrowth roughens the facial features and can

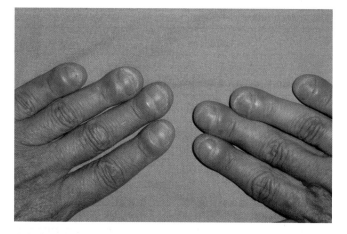

FIGURE 25F-3

Generalized skin hypertrophy in hypertrophic osteoarthropathy, known as pachyderma. Note also the clubbed fingers.

reach the extreme of *cutis verticis gyrata*, which is the most advanced stage of cutaneous hypertrophy. In addition, these patients often demonstrate glandular dysfunction of the skin that is manifested as hyperhidrosis, seborrhea, or acne (7).

LABORATORY FEATURES AND IMAGING

There are no distinctive clinical laboratory test abnormalities associated with HOA. However, an array of biochemical alterations that reflect the underlying illness may be found. Longstanding clubbing produces a prominent bone remodeling of the distal phalanges.

Periostosis evolves in an orderly manner, with symmetrical bone changes. Initially, periostosis affects the distal parts of the lower extremities and then evolves in a centripetal fashion (8). When mild it involves only few selected bones (usually the tibia and fibula). Moreover, periosteal apposition is limited to the diaphysis in mild cases, and has a monolayer configuration [Figure 25F-4(A)]. In contrast, severe periostosis affects all tubular bones, spreads to the metaphyses and epiphyses, and generates irregular configurations [Figure 25F-4(B)]. Typically, the joint space is preserved, and there are no erosions or periarticular osteopenia. Radionuclide bone scanning is a sensitive method for demonstrating periosteal involvement.

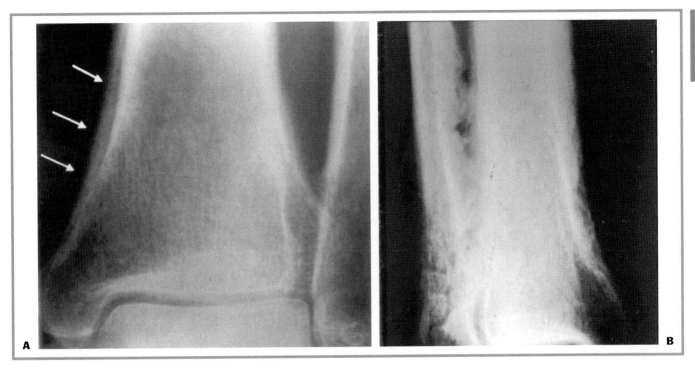

FIGURE 25F-4

Radiograph of the bones of the distal lower extremities in hypertrophic osteoarthropathy in mild (A) and severe (B) cases.

DIAGNOSIS

When HOA is fully expressed, the "drumstick" fingers are so unique that recognition poses no dilemma. The symptoms of HOA can be subtle. Nevertheless, in some patients with lung cancer, painful arthropathy may be the initial manifestation, occurring before clubbing is detectable. Such patients are sometimes misclassified as having an inflammatory arthritis. Patients with the exuberant skin hypertrophy of HOA may be misdiagnosed as having acromegaly.

The diagnosis of HOA requires the combined presence of clubbing and periostosis of the tubular bones (1). Synovial effusion is not essential for the diagnosis. An important feature that distinguishes HOA from inflammatory types of arthritis is that in HOA the pain involves not only the joint, but also the adjacent bones.

If a previously healthy individual develops any of the manifestations of HOA, a thorough search for underlying illness should be undertaken. Primary HOA should be diagnosed only after careful clinical scrutiny fails to disclose any of the internal illnesses listed in Table 25F-1. In an individual with a previous diagnosis of pulmonary fibrosis, cystic fibrosis, liver cirrhosis, or inflammatory bowel disease, the development of clubbing is usually a poor prognostic sign. Clubbing in a person with known rheumatic heart disease may indicate infective endocarditis. Similarly, clubbing in a patient with polyneuropathy of recent onset should lead to the suspicion of POEMS (polyneuropathy, organomegaly, endocrinopathy, M-protein, and skin changes) syndrome (see Chapter 25B) (9).

TREATMENT

Apart from the disfigurement, clubbing is usually asymptomatic and does not require therapy. Painful osteoarthropathy generally responds to analgesics or nonsteroidal anti-inflammatory drugs. Several uncontrolled case reports have described that pamidronate, an inhibitor of osteoclastic bone resorption, relieves the pain in cases of resistant painful osteoarthropathy (10). Interestingly, pamidronate and other biphosphonate compounds are potent VEGF inhibitors. Correction of a heart defect, removal of a lung tumor, or successful treatment of endocarditis produce rapid regression of the syndrome.

REFERENCES

1. Martínez-Lavín M, Matucci-Cerinic M, Pineda C, et al. Hypertrophic osteoarthropathy: consensus on its definition, classification, assessment and diagnostic criteria. J Rheumatol 1993;20:1386–1387.

2. Silveira L, Martínez-Lavín M, Pineda C, Navarro C, Fonseca MC, Nava A. Vascular endothelial growth factor in hypertrophic osteoarthropathy. Clin Exp Rheumatol 2000;18:57–62.

3. Vazquez-Abad D, Martínez-Lavín M. Macrothrombocytes in the peripheral circulation of patients with cardiogenic hypertrophic osteoarthropathy. Clin Exp Rheumatol 1991;9:59–62.

4. Olan F, Portela M, Navarro C, Gaxiola M, Silveira V, Martinez-Lavin M. Circulating vascular endothelial growth factor concentrations in a case of pulmonary hypertrophic osteoarthropathy. Correlation with disease activity. J Rheumatol 2004;31:614–616.

5. Atkinson S, Fox SB. Vascular endothelial growth factor (VEGF)-A and platelet-derived growth factor (PDGF) play a central role in the pathogenesis of digital clubbing. J Pathol 2004;203:721–728.

6. Vazquez-Abad D, Martínez-Lavín M. Digital clubbing: a numerical assessment of the deformity. J Rheumatol 1989; 16:518–520.

7. Martínez-Lavín M, Pineda C, Valdéz T, et al. Primary hypertrophic osteoarthropathy. Semin Arthritis Rheum 1988;17:156–162.

8. Pineda C, Fonseca C, Martínez-Lavín M. The spectrum of soft tissue and skeletal abnormalities in hypertrophic osteoarthropathy. J Rheumatol 1990;17:773–778.

9. Martínez-Lavín M, Vargas AS, Cabré J, et al. Features of hypertrophic osteoarthropathy in patients with POEMS syndrome. A metaanalysis. J Rheumatol 1997;24:2267–2268.

10. Guyot-Drouot MH, Solau-Grvais E, Cortet B, et al. Rheumatologic manifestations of pachydermoperiostosis and preliminary experience with bisphosphonates. J Rheumatol 2000;27:2418–2423.

CHAPTER 26

Complex Regional Pain Syndrome

GEOFFREY LITTLEJOHN, MD, MPH, MBBS[HON], FRACP, FRCP(EDIN)

■ Complex regional pain syndrome is an uncommon but long recognized and high-impact regional musculoskeletal pain disorder.

■ Current emphasis on pain sensitization mechanisms and earlier clinical recognition is facilitating management and improving outcomes.

Complex regional pain syndrome (CRPS) is a disorder of the musculoskeletal system that primarily relates to abnormal functioning of the sensory, sympathetic, and motor nerves. The clinical picture is varied, but the main components are those of regional pain and tenderness disproportionate to any inciting event and commonly coupled with vasomotor (swelling and color change), sudomotor (sweating), or motor abnormality (stiffness, weakness, tremor, or dystonia). There are a number of clinical presentations of CRPS, with milder forms being fairly common and having a good prognosis, but less common and more severe CRPS often responding poorly to treatment and being more persistent. Pain, emotional distress, and disability characterize this disorder.

EPIDEMIOLOGY

Criteria to define CRPS continue to evolve (1). Currently, most CRPS may be subclassified as CRPS type I, formerly called *reflex sympathetic dystrophy*, but when major nerve damage triggers the syndrome (around 10% of cases) it is subclassified as CRPS type II, formerly called *causalgia*. Both types are clinically identical. CRPS occurs in all races and geographical regions. It affects both sexes and may occur at any age, but most commonly between 40 and 60 years. In the adult presentation men slightly outnumber women but in the adolescent age group females predominate. Triggering factors associate with different age and sex distribution. For instance, CRPS following fall and fracture of the distal radius often occurs in osteoporotic women in the sixth decade.

The prevalence of CRPS is unclear (2). Minor forms are common after injury and might blend with clinical features which are part of the normal response to injury. Of 109 unselected patients with Colles' fracture, 25%

had two or more features of CRPS at 9 weeks and 62% still had residual features at 6 months (3). Between 1 in 20 and 1 in 200 people presenting to a trauma unit develop CRPS. Before intense mobilization of patients with myocardial infarction and hemiplegia became standard treatment, it was estimated that between 5% and 20% would develop CRPS (4,5).

CLINICAL FEATURES

Trauma precedes CRPS in around 50% of cases. Another 25% is associated with a variety of miscellaneous medical disorders. These include diseases of the central nervous system, such as hemiplegia, cerebral tumor, or meningitis, or disorders of the peripheral nerves, such as nerve injury from herpes zoster, nerve root impingement, or peripheral neuropathy. Medications, particularly barbiturates and isoniazide, as well as pregnancy, metastatic tumors, and prolonged immobilization of a limb, are also associated with CRPS. About 25% of CRPS occurs for no apparent reason. In this setting there may be a background history of overt or subtle psychosocial distress (6). Distress-associated psychological factors are also seen in individuals with the specific triggering factors named above. The link between psychological distress and the onset of CRPS remains unclear as the persistent pain of the disorder may result in emotional distress as part of the individual's adjustment to the disorder. Whether cause or effect, emotional distress is a characteristic clinical feature of CRPS.

Chronic regional pain syndrome usually affects a distal limb component, for example, patella, digit, hand, or foot, with the key symptom of being pain out of proportion to any tissue damage in the region (7). The majority have persistent spontaneous pain often described as tearing or burning in quality. Lancinating pain occurs in one third and activity-induced pain is

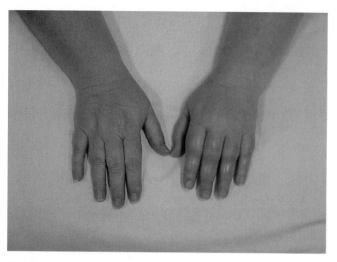

FIGURE 26-1

Chronic regional pain syndrome (CRPS) affecting left hand showing diffuse swelling, dusky discoloration, and shiny skin.

present in all. Many describe the painful area as "numb." Pain is associated with abnormal cutaneous sensitivity, manifesting as allodynia (whereby otherwise innocuous stimuli, such as touch, induce pain), and hyperalgesia (whereby pain perception is increased to a given painful stimulus, such as a pinprick). Unless there is a triggering nerve lesion, neurological examination of the painful and abnormally tender region will only show variable dysesthesia in a non-neuroanatomical distribution.

The most severe discomfort and allodynia is present distally, but the majority have abnormal tenderness present in the entire quadrant of the involved limb, including the low back or neck, as the case may be. The relevant spinal region is often stiff. Frozen shoulder may be a CRPS variant. In around 25% of cases, the opposite limb also develops similar but less marked clinical features.

Swelling of the involved area is common, usually diffuse and often associated with reticular or lividoid appearance over the skin of the involved part (Figure 26-1). Alteration in peripheral sympathetic tone may lead to other changes in skin color (cyanotic, pale, or red). Temperature may be decreased or increased, as may be sweating—there is no specific pattern. The distal involved limb of adolescents with CRPS tends to be cooler and those of adults warmer, but both may have temperature fluctuation over days and weeks. Finally, many patients have disorders of muscle function that might include peripheral weakness, proximal co-contraction and tightness, dystonia, spasm, tremor, or myoclonus. Tendon reflexes are usually normal or brisk. As time passes trophic changes may occur, but they are uncommon. Changes include unilateral differences in growth (more or less) of hair or nails and thinning of skin. A staging system for the progress of CRPS is now

little used due to poor correlation with mechanisms and outcomes (8).

Variants of CRPS include transient regional osteoporosis, which often affects the hip. Fairly rapid onset of pain and restricted movement, without cutaneous features, are characteristic and a combination of appropriate clinical assessment, plain x-ray, bone scan, and magnetic resonance imaging (MRI) are usually diagnostic (9). The duration of symptoms is shorter, possibly because mobilization is easier, and there is usually an absence of precipitating trauma. Good outcome is expected but there is a propensity for recurrent episodes as well as involvement of multiple regions, often termed *regional migrating osteoporosis*.

LABORATORY FEATURES

There are no specific abnormal features on investigation and clinical features remain the most important contributors to diagnosis (10). Acute-phase reactants are not elevated. Routine radiological imaging in the first weeks to months may show patchy osteopenia affecting adjacent bones in the involved region or diffuse osteopenia later. This has only moderate diagnostic predictive value. Fine-detailed radiography will show some degree of cortical bone resorption in around 80%. MRI shows more clear-cut abnormality with regional or diffuse bone loss and increased T2 bone signal affecting many adjacent bony areas. Three-phase technetium bone scans are abnormal in around 75% of patients with established CRPS, with regional change in blood flow in the early phase and increase in bone uptake in the late phase (Figure 26-2) (11). Diminished flow and uptake

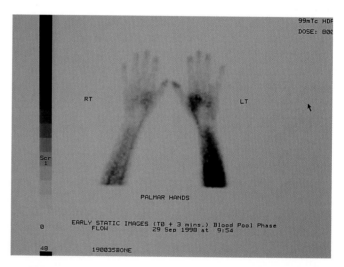

FIGURE 26-2

Technetium bone scan of patient with left forearm/hand chronic regional pain syndrome (CRPS) showing altered (increased) blood flow into involved part in early phase of study.

are more commonly seen in children and adolescents than in adults. Thermography may show significant changes compared to the unaffected side.

PATHOPHYSIOLOGY

The exact cause of CRPS remains unclear. However, the key pathophysiological abnormality lies in the change in function of peripheral sensory, autonomic, and motor nerves in the symptomatic region. This relates to both peripheral and central mechanisms. Increased activity in the two afferent nociceptor fiber types (the small diameter nonmyelinated C-fibers and myelinated A-delta fibers), the proprioception afferents (the large myelinated A-beta-fibers), and the sympathetic efferents appear to be mediators of many of the peripheral features (Table 26-1).

Enhanced sympathetic fiber activity, likely through release of norepinephrine will promote sensitization of peripheral nociceptors, decreasing threshold to mechanical and chemical stimuli. This may result in the hyperalgesia. In a minority subset of patients with CRPS, blockage of sympathetic nervous system inputs to the painful area will significantly modify clinical features, including pain. Release of proinflammatory neuropeptides, such as substance P, by activated C-fibers will likely contribute to regional neurogenic inflammation with increase in blood flow, edema, and other features such as synovitis and regional osteoporosis. The sensory peripheral nerves link to deeply placed pain transmission neurones located in the dorsal horn. In CRPS there is increased spontaneous activity of these neurones, called *central sensitization*. As a result of this process the large myelinated afferent A-beta fibers, which can also access these neurons, will now translate sensory mechanoreceptor function inputs into pain sensation.

Thus, movement and touch, which otherwise would be innocuous, activate pain and account for the key feature of allodynia. The pain transmission neurons are modulated by other inputs, including descending pathways from the mid-brain which involve the neurotransmitters norepinenephrine and serotonin. These pathways link in turn to higher cortical centers, including those that relate to the emotional part of the brain. Other brain changes in CRPS include expansion of pain-related limb areas, implying plasticity and significant functional changes within the cerebral cortex (12,13).

Where there is a painful triggering cause for the CRPS it is likely that the nociceptive pain input to the dorsal horn will activate the sensitization process. The resultant emotional response to the pain and the injury predicament may both increase sympathetic tone and also impact on spinal cord sensitization through a change in spinal cord pain modulation, as described above. Thus, a mixture of peripheral and central interactions, of differing degrees in different patients, may sensitize the spinal cord. The resultant cascade of downstream events leads to the typical clinical features.

TREATMENT

Appropriate management of CRPS requires early diagnosis. The key clinical predictors for the problem are regional pain occurring in an emotional context, particularly after injury. Pain which seems out of keeping with the original injury, particularly where it becomes more diffuse and persistent, coupled with swelling and vasomotor change are the usual early features. Not all people get all components of the syndrome. In others, the original injury triggering the problem may still be present and might require independent treatment and investigation. Preventive strategies thus include identification of clinical situations where this syndrome has been shown to be common. Early mobilization after myocardial infarction, cerebrovascular accident, hand surgery, or mild peripheral injury is essential. Appropriate reassurance and explanation of all patients in the post-traumatic setting is a part of routine treatment. Addressing anxiety and sleep disturbance with explanation, physical therapy, or medication is essential (14).

Chronic regional pain syndrome is a pain syndrome and hence holistic management is required. This should include a team of individuals, including relevant family members and health professionals, which could include an occupational therapist, physiotherapist, psychologist, and doctor, among others. Patient education about the nature of the problem and the expected good prognosis is essential.

In milder CRPS, particularly in children, exercise programs that include hydrotherapy can be very helpful. To achieve good exercise, adequate analgesia may be

TABLE 26-1. MECHANISMS OF CHRONIC REGIONAL PAIN SYNDROME CLINICAL FEATURES.

FEATURE	MECHANISM
Spontaneous pain	Peripheral nociceptor sensitization
Allodynia, movement	Mechanoreceptor input to sensitized dorsal horn transmission neuron
Swelling	Neuropeptide release from C-fibers, sympathetic neural effects
Sudomotor changes	
Vasomotor changes	
Bone, synovial changes	Neuropeptide and sympathetic effects
Dystrophy	Altered neural input to dermal structures

CHAPTER 27

Sarcoidosis

Edward S. Chen, MD

- Systemic inflammatory disorder with noncaseating granulomatous inflammation in affected organs, commonly involving the lungs, eyes, skin, joints, lymph nodes, and upper respiratory tract.
- Diagnosis attained via consensus between the clinical presentation and natural history, pattern of major organ involvement, confirmatory biopsy, and response to therapy.
- When treatment is indicated, glucocorticoids remain the only recognized effective therapy for active sarcoidosis.

Sarcoidosis is a systemic inflammatory disorder characterized by the presence of noncaseating granulomatous inflammation in affected organs (1). The etiology of sarcoidosis remains undetermined, the clinical manifestations of this disease are protean, and a diagnosis of sarcoidosis is often made by the exclusion of other processes. What helps distinguish sarcoidosis from other systemic disorders is a consideration of clinical presentation and natural history, confirmatory biopsy, and appropriate response to therapy. Although this disease most commonly affects the lungs, virtually any part of the body may be affected, and the presence and behavior of characteristic extrapulmonary manifestations may assist in supporting a diagnosis of sarcoidosis.

EPIDEMIOLOGY

The worldwide prevalence varies widely and has been reported to be 1 to 10 cases per 100,000 population in a diverse array of countries (Denmark, Belgium, Japan, Korea, Czechoslovakia). In Sweden, for reasons that are not clear, the prevalence is estimated to be between 60 to 80 per 100,000 (2,3). In the United States, the prevalence of sarcoidosis has been estimated to be 10 to 40 per 100,000. Studies using mass screening through chest radiography identify a significant number of asymptomatic patients with sarcoidosis (4,5). Other methods of case detection, for example, autopsy reports, generally conclude even higher rates of disease (6,7). Sarcoidosis tends to be diagnosed in younger adults (ages 20–40) although a second peak may be appreciated in Caucasian women over age 50. In the United States, the highest incidence of sarcoidosis is observed in young African-American women.

Genetic and Familial Associations in Sarcoidosis

Reports of families with more than one case of sarcoidosis support a genetic basis for this disease. The recently completed multicenter study in the United States—A Case Control Etiologic Study of Sarcoidosis (ACCESS) —estimated the relative risk for sarcoidosis to be approximately 5 among first-degree relatives of patients with sarcoidosis (8). In contrast to the higher annual incidence of sarcoidosis among African Americans (35.5 per 100,000) compared with Caucasians (10.9 per 100,000) (8), the relative risk of sarcoidosis among first-degree relatives of Caucasian patients may be substantially higher than that of first-degree relatives of African-American patients.

Many genetic associations have linked sarcoidosis with genes within the major histocompatibility complex (MHC) locus (9). Most recently, the novel gene BTNL2 (butyrophilinlike) (2) has been associated with sarcoidosis in a genomewide linkage analysis using a cohort of Caucasian patients (10). This finding was confirmed in a separate linkage analysis using a cohort of African-American patients from the Sarcoidosis Genetic Analysis (SAGA) consortium (11,12).

CLINICAL FEATURES

Sarcoidosis typically involves more than one organ. The frequency of involvement by organ system is shown in Table 27-1. Alternative diagnoses must always be excluded when considering rare and unusual presentations of sarcoidosis (13).

TABLE 27-1. CLINICAL FEATURES OF SARCOIDOSIS.

ORGAN SYSTEM	FREQUENCY OF CLINICALLY RELEVANT DISEASE (%)
Lung	70–90
Skin	20–30
Sinus and upper respiratory tract	5–10
Eye	20–30
Musculoskeletal	10–20
Abdominal	10–20
Hematological	20–30
Salivary/parotid	5–10
Cardiac	5–10
Neurological	5–10

Acute Sarcoidosis

Two acute presentations associated with eponyms are worth noting. First, Löfgren's syndrome consists of fever, erythema nodosum, bilateral hilar adenopathy, symmetric polyarthritis, and uveitis. Löfgren's syndrome is more common among Scandinavians. In most patients, the erythema nodosum and arthritis resolve after several weeks, often without specific therapy. Nonsteriodal anti-inflammatory drugs (NSAIDs) or low-dose glucocorticoids may be necessary in some patients. Once resolved, Löfgren's syndrome recurs in less than 30% of cases (14).

Second, lacrimal and salivary gland involvement causing glandular enlargement and the sicca syndrome may be a feature of an acute presentation of sarcoidosis, known as Heerfordt's syndrome ("uveoparotid fever"). Heerfordt's syndrome is a constellation of fever, granulomatous inflammation of the lacrimal and parotid glands, uveitis, bilateral hilar adenopathy, and cranial neuropathies.

Pulmonary Sarcoidosis

Lung involvement is detectable through chest radiographs in up to 90% of sarcoidosis patients. The most common symptoms include dyspnea and dry cough. Sputum production and hemoptysis are associated with fibrocystic pulmonary sarcoidosis and bronchiectasis. The physical examination is often unremarkable, with wheezes or crackles heard in less than 20% of patients.

A minority of patients may present with atypical chest pain. The etiology of this chest pain, which may occur either at rest or with activity, may be related to the presence of bulky mediastinal adenopathy. Most patients with mediastinal adenopathy, however, do not experience chest pain. The chest pain does not respond well to glucocorticoids, and the exclusion of cardiac, gastroesophageal, and musculoskeletal etiologies is important.

Pulmonary hypertension is a rare complication (<5%) of pulmonary sarcoidosis, usually found in patients with advanced lung disease (stage III or IV). Pulmonary hypertension is associated with higher rates of mortality. As with atypical chest pain, other potential contributors to pulmonary hypertension, for example, sleep apnea and thromboembolic disease, should be excluded.

Chronic Cutaneous Sarcoidosis

Skin lesions of various appearances may occur in up to one third of patients with sarcoidosis. The most common sarcoidosis skin lesions are hyperpigmented nodules, violaceous plaques, hypopigmented macules, and subcutaneous nodules (Figure 27-1). Such lesions most commonly occur over the extensor surfaces of the arms and legs and tend to resolve with scarring and retraction. Lupus pernio—a confusing name because the condition has nothing to do with systemic lupus erythematosus—refers to a particular type of sarcoidosis lesion that occurs on the face and scalp. Lupus pernio lesions (Figure 27-1) appear as violaceous plaques found on the nose, nasal alae, malar areas, eyelids, hairline, and scalp. They are indolent, but often difficult to treat.

Sinuses and Upper Respiratory Tract

Upper respiratory tract disease is common in sarcoidosis. Symptoms include severe nasal congestion and sinus pain. Hoarseness and stridor requires prompt evaluation by an otolaryngologist to document laryngeal involvement. A "saddle-nose deformity" may result from chronic disease or repeated surgical interventions. Mucocutaneous involvement is associated with other indolent manifestations, such as lupus pernio.

Ocular

A significant percentage of patients has ocular involvement. Nodular sarcoidosis lesions can involve all major compartments of the eye. Granulomatous conjunctivitis and conjunctival nodules are common findings that are sometimes accessible for biopsy. Intraocular sarcoidosis occurs more frequently in the anterior segment and can result in nodules on the pupilary margin, the surface of the iris, and the trabecular meshwork. Granulomatous

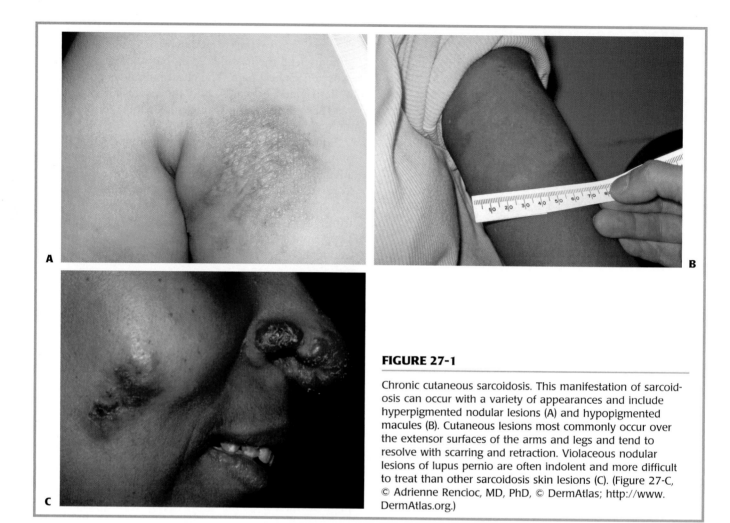

FIGURE 27-1

Chronic cutaneous sarcoidosis. This manifestation of sarcoidosis can occur with a variety of appearances and include hyperpigmented nodular lesions (A) and hypopigmented macules (B). Cutaneous lesions most commonly occur over the extensor surfaces of the arms and legs and tend to resolve with scarring and retraction. Violaceous nodular lesions of lupus pernio are often indolent and more difficult to treat than other sarcoidosis skin lesions (C). (Figure 27-C, © Adrienne Rencioc, MD, PhD, © DermAtlas; http://www. DermAtlas.org.)

uveitis of the anterior chamber can lead to keratic precipitates on the posterior surface of the cornea which, on slit-lamp examination, have the appearance of "mutton-fat" droplets. Intermediate uveitis can lead to suspended "snowball" or "string of pearl" vitreous opacities, also characteristic of sarcoidosis. Posterior segment uveitis is often associated with superficial "candle wax" exudates and deeper chorioretinal lesions that may require fluorescein angiography for detection. Posterior uveitis can be associated with neurological involvement, that is, optic neuritis, in up to one quarter of cases, which may be difficult to distinguish from posterior uveitis. Both kinds of posterior eye involvement can result in abrupt blindness. Rare extraocular manifestations include involvement of the lacrimal gland, tear duct system (dacrocystitis), ocular orbit (often unilateral), cornea, and scleritis. The range and potentially insidious nature of ocular findings in sarcoidosis make regular ophthalmologic evaluations an important part of care.

Musculoskeletal

Joint

As noted, frank arthritis tends to occur in patients with acute presentations of sarcoidosis (Löfgren syndrome). Arthralgias occur commonly in patients with chronic active sarcoidosis. Chronic sarcoid arthritis is a rare manifestation (<1%) that can result in joint deformities, and is associated with other chronic manifestations such as cutaneous sarcoidosis (15). Arthrocentesis reveals mild elevations in white blood cell counts (250–5000/ mL) with a mononuclear cell predominance. Synovial biopsy may reveal noncaseating granulomatous inflammation. Frank tenosynovitis and periarticular inflammation occur less frequently than arthralgias or arthritis, but periarthritis (inflammation around a joint rather than in it, sometimes difficult to discern from true synovitis) is well described in sarcoidosis. Other articular manifestations of sarcoidosis would include dactylitis, characterized by a violaceous swelling involving the

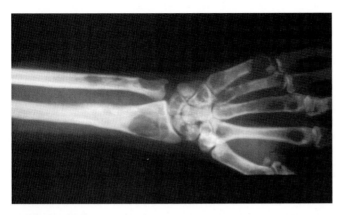

FIGURE 27-2

Osseous sarcoidosis. A 45-year-old woman with a 2- to 3-year history of cough, fevers, exertional dyspnea, and recurrent swelling and stiffness in both hands. A diagnosis of sarcoidosis was established by bronchoscopy. This plain film of the hand reveals multiple punched-out lesions that are characteristic of osseous sarcoidosis. (Johns Hopkins Arthritis Website, http://www.hopkins-arthritis.org., S. Levine, MD and W. Scott, MD.)

second or third fingers, sacroiliitis, and bilateral heel pain.

Bone

Cystic, punched-out lesions and lacey reticulations are commonly observed on plain radiographs or other imaging studies, often as incidental findings (Figure 27-2). Such lesions, typically located in the bones of the hands and feet, can also be found in the skull and vertebrae. Lesions involving the pelvis may be associated with pain that mimics sacroiliitis (16). Bone biopsies may be necessary in osseous sarcoidosis to exclude infections or cancers that may result in similar radiographic findings.

Myositis

Random muscle biopsies may reveal granulomas in 50% to 80% of cases, but muscle involvement in sarcoidosis is often asymptomatic. Muscle inflammation can also be detected incidentally by radiographic imaging using gallium scanning and magnetic resonance imaging (MRI). Glucocorticoid-induced myopathy should be considered in patients who develop acute-onset weakness following the initiation of treatment.

Abdominal

Granulomatous inflammation may be detected in more than 50% of liver biopsies in sarcoidosis, but clinically significant liver disease is present in not more than 10% of all cases. Elevated liver enzymes often resolve spontaneously or with therapy with glucocorticoids. Chronic

granulomatous hepatitis may progress to cirrhosis, however, particularly if severe and left untreated (17). The constellation of hepatosplenomegaly, abdominal adenopathy, hepatosplenomegaly, and hypercalcemia (and often bone marrow involvement) is often referred to as *abdominal sarcoidosis.*

Involvement of the gastrointestinal tract is rare. It is often associated with pain and dysmotility and does not respond well to glucocorticoids. In patients where this is the sole or principal manifestation of sarcoidosis, then other causes of inflammatory bowel disease (Crohn's disease, ulcerative colitis) should be excluded.

Other Important Manifestations

A wide range of hematological manifestations may be found in up to one third of patients with sarcoidosis (18). Peripheral adenopathy occurs commonly at time of disease presentation, and bulky adenopathy may persist in ~10% of cases. Massive splenomegaly may be present in 5% of cases. Anemia, lymphopenia, and leucopenia may be observed in 30% to 50% of all cases and is more common than thrombocytopenia. A polyclonal gammopathy is also frequently seen (~25%) in many patients with active sarcoidosis. Common variable immunodeficiency (CVID) should be suspected in patients who lack elevations in serum globulin fraction or develop an increased frequency of infections, both of which are unusual in sarcoidosis (19).

Cardiac sarcoidosis is a rare but important manifestation that can lead to heart block, malignant arrhythmias, and cardiomyopathy. Autopsy series suggest that the incidence of cardiac sarcoidosis may be as high as 25%, but clinical diagnoses of this condition are made in <10% of patients. Endomyocardial biopsy detects granulomatous inflammation in less than 25% of cases (20). The diagnosis is frequently rendered indirectly in a patient with biopsy-proven sarcoidosis at other sites and a compatible myocardial imaging study, such as nuclear medicine stress test, cardiac MRI with gadolinium contrast, or positron emission tomography (PET).

Presentations of neurosarcoidosis can be placed into three major groups. The most common form would be neuropathies involving cranial nerves II (optic neuritis), V, VII, IX, or XII. Cranial neuropathies, usually associated with an aseptic basilar meningitis, tend to recur intermittently. A second presentation of neurosarcoidosis is encephalopathy or myelopathy associated with either a mass or an enhancing lesion on MRI. Such patients benefit from prolonged courses of immunosuppression. Finally, the third presentation of neurosarcoidosis is peripheral neuropathy. This complication is potentially disabling and often unresponsive to glucocorticoids. A small fiber neuropathy has been implicated recently as a significant cause of chronic pain and fatigue in sarcoidosis (21).

27

RADIOGRAPHIC FEATURES

Chest radiographs detect abnormalities in ~ 90% of all patients with sarcoidosis (22). Chest radiograph abnormalities are assigned a category (stage) according to the Scadding system: 0, normal; I, bilateral hilar lymphadenopathy (BHL); II, BHL + interstitial infiltrates; III, interstitial infiltrates only; IV, fibrocystic lung disease (Figure 27-3). Computed tomography scans of the chest reveal that the pulmonary infiltrates of sarcoidosis are typically nodular in appearance, and tend to distribute themselves along bronchovascular structures (Figure 27-4).

The presence of inflammation suggesting active sarcoidosis can be identified in the brain, cranial nerves, spinal cord, heart, or other soft tissue organs using MRI with gadolinium contrast or PET scanning. Cardiac sarcoidosis can also be inferred from gated thallium scanning. Classic findings associated with sarcoidosis revealed by 67-gallium scanning include uptake in the parotid and lacrimal glands ("panda sign") and uptake in bilateral hilar and right paratracheal lymph nodes ("lambda sign"). Although these radiographic findings are highly typical of sarcoidosis, a biopsy is still required to confirm diagnosis.

LABORATORY FEATURES

Routine bloodwork consisting of comprehensive metabolic panel and complete blood count is useful to screen for abnormalities (renal function, kidney function, anemia, lymphopenia, hypercalcemia, hypergammaglobulinemia) associated with extrapulmonary sarcoidosis. No biomarkers are useful in predicting outcomes or guiding treatment decisions. Serum levels of angiotensin-converting enzyme and the active form of vitamin D (1,25-dihydroxy vitamin D_3) are elevated in some patients with active sarcoidosis, but these test results have poor specificity and little utility in either the diagnosis or management of sarcoidosis (23).

PATHOLOGY

Sarcoidosis is associated with well-formed epithelioid granulomas in the absence of other known causes of granulomatous disease, such as infection and malignancy. These granulomas are typically noncaseating, although fibrinoid necrosis can occasionally be seen. In the lung, the granulomas tend to occur along bronchovascular structures.

FIGURE 27-3

Pulmonary sarcoidosis (A, B). Chest radiograph (A) compatible with Scadding stage I, demonstrating bilateral hilar and right paratracheal adenopathy without significant parenchymal infiltrates. This patient presented with constitutional symptoms (fevers, unintentional weight loss), arthralgias, and a cough. A transbronchial biopsy revealed noncaseating granulomatous inflammation. In another patient (B), the presence of both adenopathy and pulmonary infiltrates signifies a Scadding stage III radiograph.

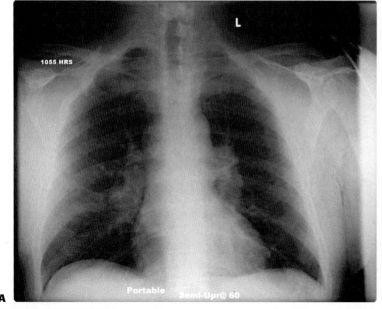
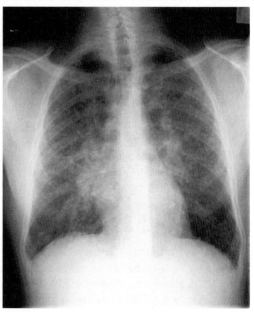

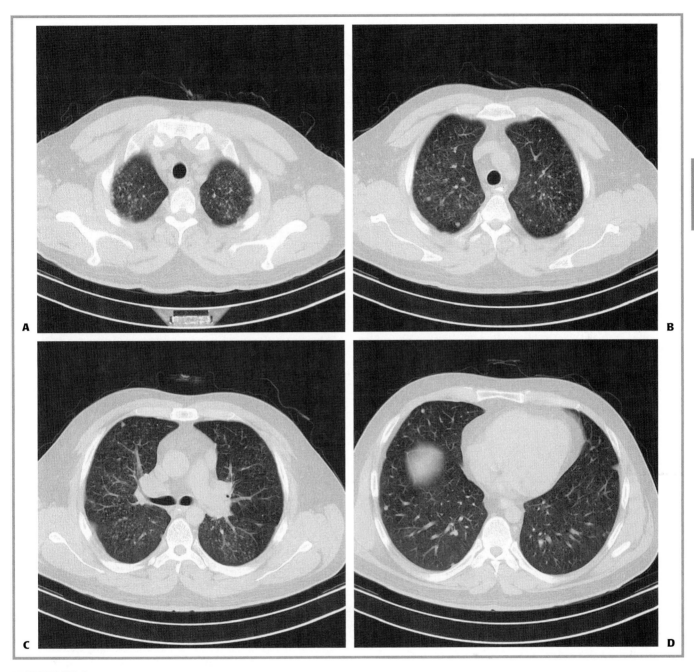

FIGURE 27-4

(A–C) Pulmonary sarcoidosis. Computed tomography scans of the chest, revealing patchy, diffuse reticulonodular infiltrates predominantly involving the upper and middle lung fields with a bronchovascular distribution. If observed on a chest radiograph, such findings would be comparable with a Scadding stage II (Scadding stages are based upon radiographs, not computed tomography scans).

PATHOGENESIS

The cause of sarcoidosis remains uncertain. The active granulomatous inflammation of sarcoidosis is associated with a dominant expression of T-helper (Th)1 cytokines [interferon gamma (IFN-gamma), interleukin (IL)-12, IL-18] and tumor necrosis factor (TNF) (24).

Oligoclonal expansion of T cells bearing a limited set of T-cell receptors in the lung, skin, and other sites of disease support the hypothesis that sarcoidosis involves an antigen-driven response (25). The most compelling example of this is the over-representation of T cells bearing the V alpha 2.3 T-cell receptor subunit reported in a significant portion of Scandinavian patients (26).

One prevailing hypothesis is that an exposure, possibly of microbial origin, triggers the development of sarcoidosis. Recent laboratory studies suggest that sarcoidosis may be associated with a previous exposure to microbial antigens (27,28), although sarcoidosis does not represent an active infection. The large multicenter ACCESS study failed to identify a dominant environmental or occupational exposure associated with an increased risk for developing sarcoidosis (29).

TREATMENT

Clinical Course and Prognosis

Nearly all patients with sarcoidosis experience one of two clinical courses: (1) sustained clinical remission or (2) chronic active disease that does not remit. Thus, sarcoidosis differs from many rheumatological diseases in that waxing and waning courses with intermittent flares and remissions are unusual. The major exception to this rule is the neurosarcoidosis presentation of optic neuritis and cranial neuropathies, which may recur several years after apparent remission.

Most patients who achieve remission do so within the first 2 to 3 years of diagnosis. Acute sarcoidosis (Löfgren syndrome) is associated with a high rate of remission (>70%). Unremitting, chronic active disease is associated with a greater burden of lung disease (stage III or IV), sinus and upper respiratory tract involvement, lupus pernio, neurosarcoidosis, cardiac involvement—organ system manifestations characterized by indolent presentations. Careful follow-up for at least several years (>2–3) is necessary to confirm whether a patient has remitting or chronic active sarcoidosis. Long-term follow-up is also important to ensure that patients with chronic active disease receive adequate treatment to minimize progressive impairment of organ function from chronic inflammation.

Although sarcoidosis is a systemic disorder, the extent of organ involvement is largely defined at presentation. The recent ACCESS study found that less than 25% of patients developed new organ involvement within 2 years of follow-up (30).

Therapy

The first step in deciding upon a treatment course is to exclude the presence of immediately life-threatening disease manifestations. In patients with limited cutaneous disease or the Löfgren syndrome, NSAIDs may be sufficient to control symptoms. Local steroid injections may be considered for isolated skin lesions. Patients with critical organ involvement (heart, central nervous system) should be treated aggressively with high doses of systemic glucocorticoids. In all cases, the selection of tangible endpoints (pulmonary function tests, chest radiograph, bloodwork, MRI studies) rather than subjective symptoms (fatigue, cough, localized pain) is essential to good therapeutic decision making. Although sarcoidosis is often considered a restrictive lung disease (low forced vital capacity or total lung capacity), changes in airway obstruction (FEV_1) and/or diffusion capacity (DLCO) may herald clinical deterioration in some patients with lung involvement.

For patients who require systemic therapy, glucocorticoids remain the only uniformly effective medication for active inflammation. Topical glucocorticoids (inhaled, ointment) are ineffective except for some instances of ocular involvement. In general, patients should be treated for an initial period of 8 to 12 months before attempting to discontinue glucocorticoids (tapering of the daily dose to a tolerable level, however, is essential). Patients with Löfgren syndrome generally have a good prognosis and earlier attempts to curtail systemic glucocorticoids can be considered. Patients who have chronic active disease should be treated with a stable maintenance regimen of low-dose glucocorticoids rather than repeated aggressive tapering regimens on and off glucocorticoids. End-stage changes (scarring) are not amenable to any treatment. Most patients demonstrate a lower limit for prednisone dosing, below which their disease will flare.

Untreated patients initially require higher doses of glucocorticoids (prednisone 20–40 mg/day) to control active disease, which can be tapered gradually after the first month, by 5-mg intervals every 2 weeks down to 20 mg/day, then more gradually below this dose with smaller increments (2.5 mg) and longer intervals (1–2 months). If symptoms recur or pulmonary function deteriorates with interval dose reduction, the patient should resume the previously effective dose of prednisone and the addition of a steroid-sparing agent should be considered. The average maintenance dose of sarcoidosis for most patients tends to be 5 to 15 mg/day. Patients with neurosarcoidosis or cardiac sarcoidosis may benefit from even higher doses of glucocorticoids in combination with steroid-sparing immunosuppressants.

Steroid-Sparing Agents

A variety of steroid-sparing immunosuppressants and immunomodulating agents are recommended to help minimize the maintenance dose of glucocorticoids (ideally ≤15 mg/day). However, most potential steroid-sparing agents have not been tested rigorously in randomized clinical trials. In contrast to glucocorticoids, which induce responses within several days to a few weeks, steroid-sparing agents may require a few months of therapy (2–6) before any clinical benefit is evident.

Antimalarial drugs (hydroxychloroquine, chloroquine) and synthetic tetracyclines (minocycline, doxycycline), medications with few serious side effects, are used primarily to help control mucocutaneous disease. Pentoxifylline and thalidomide may be useful in a small subset of patients, but may have more significant side effects. Other immunosuppressive agents (methotrexate, mycophenolate mofetil, azathioprine, cyclophosphamide) have been used in conjunction with glucocorticoids to treat more severe manifestations of sarcoidosis that cannot be managed with lower doses of glucocorticoids alone or when intolerable glucocorticoid-related side effects occur. A recently completed phase II trial demonstrated that patients treated with infliximab, a monoclonal antibody targeted against TNF, experienced mild improvement in pulmonary function (31). Etanercept, a soluble TNF inhibitor, was shown to be ineffective in a randomized clinical trial (32). Further evaluation is necessary to determine the role of anti-TNF agents such as infliximab (and an analogous agent, adalimumab) in the treatment of sarcoidosis.

REFERENCES

1. Hunninghake GW, Costabel U, Ando M, et al. ATS/ERS/WASOG statement on sarcoidosis. American Thoracic Society/European Respiratory Society/World Association of Sarcoidosis and other Granulomatous Disorders. Sarcoidosis Vas Diffuse Lung Dis 1999;16:149–173.

2. Kitaichi M. Prevalence of sarcoidosis around the world. Sarcoidosis Vas Diffuse Lung Dis 1998;15:16–18.

3. Siltzbach LE, James DG, Neville E, et al. Course and prognosis of sarcoidosis around the world. Am J Med 1974;57:847–852.

4. Nelson RS. Sarcoidosis in the armed forces. Am J Med Sci 1953;226:131–138.

5. Pietinalho A, Hiraga Y, Hosoda Y, Lofroos AB, Yamaguchi M, Selroos O. The frequency of sarcoidosis in Finland and Hokkaido, Japan. A comparative epidemiological study. Sarcoidosis 1995;12:61–67.

6. Hagerstrand I, Linell F. The prevalence of sarcoidosis in the autopsy material from a Swedish town. Acta Med Scand 1964;425:171–174.

7. Reid JD. Sarcoidosis in coroner's autopsies: a critical evaluation of diagnosis and prevalence from Cuyahoga County, Ohio. Sarcoidosis Vas Diffuse Lung Dis 1998; 15:44–51.

8. Rybicki BA, Major M, Popovich J Jr, Maliarik MJ, Iannuzzi MC. Racial differences in sarcoidosis incidence: a 5-year study in a health maintenance organization. Am J Epidemiol 1997;145:234–241.

9. Schurmann M, Reichel P, Muller-Myhsok B, Schlaak M, Muller-Quernheim J, Schwinger E. Results from a genome-wide search for predisposing genes in sarcoidosis. Am J Respir Crit Care Med 2001;164:840–846.

10. Valentonyte R, Hampe J, Huse K, et al. Sarcoidosis is associated with a truncating splice site mutation in BTNL2. Nat Genet 2005;37:357–364.

11. Rybicki BA, Hirst K, Iyengar SK, et al. A sarcoidosis genetic linkage consortium: the sarcoidosis genetic analysis (SAGA) study. Sarcoidosis Vas Diffuse Lung Dis 2005; 22:115–122.

12. Rybicki BA, Walewski JL, Maliarik MJ, Kian H, Iannuzzi MC. The BTNL2 gene and sarcoidosis susceptibility in African Americans and Whites. Am J Hum Genet 2005; 77:491–499.

13. Moller DR. Rare manifestations of sarcoidosis. In: Drent M, Costabel U, eds. Sarcoidosis. Vol 10. Wakefield, UK: European Respiratory Society Journals, Ltd.; 2005:233–250.

14. Gran JT, Bohmer E. Acute sarcoid arthritis: a favourable outcome? A retrospective survey of 49 patients with review of the literature. Scand J Rheumatol 1996;25:70–73.

15. Kaplan H. Sarcoid arthritis. A review. Arch Intern Med 1963;112:924–935.

16. Wilcox A, Bharadwaj P, Sharma OP. Bone sarcoidosis. Curr Opin Rheumatol 2000;12:321–330.

17. Kennedy PT, Zakaria N, Modawi SB, et al. Natural history of hepatic sarcoidosis and its response to treatment. Eur J Gastroenterol Hepatol 2006;18:721–726.

18. Lower EE, Smith JT, Martelo OJ, Baughman RP. The anemia of sarcoidosis. Sarcoidosis 1988;5:51–55.

19. Fasano MB, Sullivan KE, Sarpong SB, et al. Sarcoidosis and common variable immunodeficiency. Report of 8 cases and review of the literature. Medicine (Baltimore) 1996;75:251–261.

20. Ardehali H, Howard DL, Hariri A, et al. A positive endomyocardial biopsy result for sarcoid is associated with poor prognosis in patients with initially unexplained cardiomyopathy. Am Heart J 2005;150:459–463.

21. Voorter CE, Drent M, Hoitsma E, Faber KG, van den Berg-Loonen EM. Association of HLA DQB1 0602 in sarcoidosis patients with small fiber neuropathy. Sarcoidosis Vasc Diffuse Lung Dis 2005;22:129–132.

22. Johns CJ, Michele TM. The clinical management of sarcoidosis. A 50-year experience at the Johns Hopkins Hospital. Medicine 1999;78:65–111.

23. Sharma OP. Vitamin D, calcium, and sarcoidosis. Chest 1996;109:535–539.

24. Chen ES, Moller DR. Cytokines and chemokines in sarcoidosis. In: Baughman R, ed. Sarcoidosis. Vol 210. New York: Taylor & Francis Group; 2006:123–161.

25. Forman JD, Klein JT, Silver RF, Liu MC, Greenlee BM, Moller DR. Selective activation and accumulation of oligoclonal V beta-specific T cells in active pulmonary sarcoidosis. J Clin Invest 1994;94:1533–1542.

26. Grunewald J, Janson CH, Eklund A, et al. Restricted V alpha 2.3 gene usage by CD4+ T lymphocytes in bronchoalveolar lavage fluid from sarcoidosis patients correlates with HLA-DR3. Eur J Immunol 1992;22:129–135.

27. Song Z, Marzilli L, Greenlee BM, et al. Mycobacterial catalase-peroxidase is a tissue antigen and target of the adaptive immune response in systemic sarcoidosis. J Exp Med 2005;201:755–767.

28. Ebe Y, Ikushima S, Yamaguchi T, et al. Proliferative response of peripheral blood mononuclear cells and levels of antibody to recombinant protein from Propionibacterium acnes DNA expression library in Japanese patients with sarcoidosis. Sarcoidosis Vasc Diffuse Lung Dis 2000; 17:256–265.

29. Newman LS, Rose CS, Bresnitz EA, et al. A case control etiologic study of sarcoidosis: environmental and occupational risk factors. Am J Respir Crit Care Med 2004;170: 1324–1330.

30. Judson MA, Baughman RP, Thompson BW, et al. Two year prognosis of sarcoidosis: the ACCESS experience. Sarcoidosis Vas Diffuse Lung Dis 2003;20:204–211.

31. Baughman RP, Drent M, Kavuru M, et al. Infliximab therapy in patients with chronic sarcoidosis and pulmonary involvement. Am J Respir Crit Care Med 2006;174: 795–802.

32. Utz JP, Limper AH, Kalra S, et al. Etanercept for the treatment of stage II and III progressive pulmonary sarcoidosis. Chest 2003;124:177–185.

CHAPTER 28

Storage and Deposition Diseases

Duncan A. Gordon, MD, FRCPC, MACR

■ Some unusual arthropathies are caused by deposition of normal material, such as metal ions, or storage of abnormal material, such as lipids.

■ Hemochromatosis, ochronosis, and Wilson's disease are characterized by cellular deposition of the normal metal ions: iron, calcium, and copper, respectively.

■ In Gaucher's disease, Fabry's disease, Farber's disease, and multicentric reticulohistiocytosis, rheumatic manifestations result from cellular storage of abnormal lipids.

This chapter covers a number of unusual arthropathies that are caused by deposition of normal material, such as metal ions, *or* storage of abnormal material, such as lipids (1). Hemochromatosis, ochronosis, and Wilson's disease are characterized by cellular deposition of the normal metal ions: iron, calcium, and copper, respectively. In the case of Gaucher's disease, Fabry's disease, Farber's disease, and multicentric reticulohistiocytosis, rheumatic manifestations result from cellular storage of abnormal lipids. In hemochromatosis, arthralgias may be the first indication of a systemic disorder, but arthritis evolves as a predominant feature in ochronosis, Gauchers's disease, and multicentric reticulohistiocytosis.

HEMOCHROMATOSIS

Hemochromatosis is a common inherited autosomal recessive disorder affecting as many as 5 per 1000 white persons of European extraction. It is characterized by excessive body iron stores and the deposition of hemosiderin, which cause tissue damage and organ dysfunction (2). The disorder rarely appears before age 40 unless there is a family history, and men are affected 10 times more frequently than women, who are protected by menstruation. Increased intestinal iron absorption and visceral deposition can lead to the phenotypic features of hepatic cirrhosis, cardiomyopathy, diabetes mellitus, pituitary dysfunction (including hyogonadism), sicca syndrome, and skin pigmentation mostly of melanin (2). In a survey of 2851 patients with hemochromatosis, symptoms had been present for an average of 10 years before the diagnosis was made. Arthralgia (44%) was among the most common and most troublesome complaints (3).

The gene for hemochromatosis (HFE, *HLA-H*) was discovered in 1996 by positional cloning methods near the human leukocyte antigen (HLA)-A locus on chromosome 6 (4). More than 90% of typical patients possess the C282Y mutation of the *HFE* gene. Homozygous and heterozygous genotypes correlate with major or minor disease expression, respectively. The association of hemochromatosis with arthritis is most common in homozygotes with the heaviest iron overload. The C282Y mutation is most common in whites, and most C282Y homozygotes have elevations in serum ferritin levels and transferrin saturation. However, the absence of C282Y mutation does not account for high mean serum ferritin levels and transferrin values in nonwhites (5).

Prolonged excessive iron ingestion and repeated blood transfusion in chronic hypoproliferative anemia and thalassemia may also result in iron deposition. If iron overload occurs without tissue damage, the disorder is known as *hemosiderosis*. With tissue damage, it is called *secondary hemochromatosis*. The iron deposition in macrophages in secondary hemochromatosis is associated with less tissue damage and end-organ dysfunction compared with the idiopathic form.

Yersinia septic arthritis or septicemia is an unusual complication that may occur in people with hemochromatosis because of a microbial requirement for an iron-rich environment. Hepatitis B and C viral infection may accelerate liver damage in people with hemochromatosis (6).

Clinical Features

Chronic progressive arthritis, predominantly affecting the second and third metacarpophalangeal (MCP) and proximal interphalangeal (PIP) joints, is the presenting

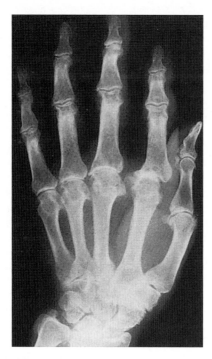

FIGURE 28-1

Radiograph of hand with hemochromatosis. Note the joint space narrowing, cystic subchondral lesions, joint space irregularity, mild subluxation, bony sclerosis, and small osteophytes in the metacarpophalangeal joints. Chondrocalcinosis is present in the ulnar carpal joint, and soft tissue has calcified around the interphalangeal joint of the thumb. (Courtesy of Dr. H.R. Schumacher, Jr.)

feature in about one half of cases (Figure 28-1). Involvement of the MCP joints is typically the most common rheumatologic feature at the time of diagnosis (7). The dominant hand may be solely or more severely affected. The finger joints and wrists are mildly tender with limited motion. Larger joints, such as the shoulders, hips, and knees, may also be affected. Hemochromatotic arthropathy of the hips or shoulders may, at times, be rapidly progressive. True morning stiffness is not a feature of hemochromatosis.

Individuals heterozygous for the C282Y *HFE* mutation may be at increased risk for hand osteoarthritis (8). Therefore the detection of an osteoarthritislike disease that involves MCP and wrist joints, particularly in men during the fifth and sixth decade of life, should signal the possibility of underlying hemochromatosis. Arthropathy may also be seen in juveniles and may affect individuals as young as 26 before any other manifestations of the disease develop.

Radiographic Features

The radiologic changes of hemochromatosis resemble osteoarthritis, except that in hemochromatosis there is less osteophytosis. Ulnar styloid erosion may suggest rheumatoid diseases, but the irregular joint narrowing and sclerotic cyst formation are more indicative of a degenerative process. Although the distal interphalangeal joints may be affected, the carpometacarpal joint changes of generalized osteoarthritis are not a feature. Somewhat similar MCP changes can occur in calcium pyrophosphate dehydrate crystal deposition without hemochromatosis. Some degree of diffuse osteoporosis may be present, presumably due to hypogonadism, but a direct effect of iron on bone is also possible. Chondrocalcinosis is characteristic of the arthropathy and is a late complication in about 50% of patients; it may be the sole abnormality (7). The hyaline cartilage of the shoulder, wrist, hip, and knee, and the fibrocartilage of the triangular ligament of the wrist and symphysis pubis may be affected. Superimposed attacks of calcium pyrophosphate dihydrate crystal synovitis occur in these cases. The finding of chondrocalcinosis should always suggest the possibility of hemochromatosis.

Laboratory Features

Synovial fluid has good viscosity, with leukocyte counts below 1000 cells/mm³. During acute episodes of pseudogout, synovial fluid leukocytosis with calcium pyrophosphate crystals can be found. Except for such episodes, the erythrocyte sedimentation rate is usually normal. In patients with chronic liver disease, rheumatoid factor tests may be positive.

The diagnosis may be suspected by a raised serum iron and high ferritin concentration with increased saturation of the plasma iron-binding protein transferrin (2). The latter, however, is more specific and should be regarded as the cornerstone test for diagnosis (2). For population screening, the simpler unbound *iron* binding capacity (UIBC) showed higher sensitivity and fewer false positives. Needle biopsy of the liver provides definitive evidence of iron overload in hemochromatosis, but nowadays it is usually reserved for cases in diagnostic doubt, or more often to assess the severity of liver damage associated with fibrosis, cirrhosis, or hepatoma.

In idiopathic hemochromatosis, iron deposits affect parenchymal hepatic cells, whereas reticuloendothelial cells are most affected in secondary forms. In hemochromatosis, synovial biopsy shows iron deposition in the type B synthetic lining cells of synovium. In rheumatoid arthritis, traumatic hemarthrosis, hemophilia, and villonodular synovitis, deposits are in the deeper layers or in the phagocyte type A lining cells. Hemosiderin deposits may also be found in the chondrocytes. Further evidence of iron may be found in biopsies of skin and intestinal mucosa, or in bone marrow, buffy coat, or urine sediment. The amount of iron excreted in the urine after administration of the iron-chelating agent deferoxamine correlates with the presence of parenchymal hepatic iron in hemochromatosis. Where available, direct noninvasive magnetic measurements of hepatic iron stores provide a quantitative method for early detection of iron overload or rapid evaluation of treatment.

The pathogenesis of the arthritis is unknown, as degenerative joint changes do not necessarily develop in relation to synovial iron. The low frequency of chondrocalcinosis in people with hemophilia and rheumatoid arthritis weighs against synovial hemosiderin as a cause of chondrocalcinosis. It is speculated that ionic iron might inhibit pyrophosphatase activity and lead to a local concentration of calcium pyrophosphate in the joint. The deposition of calcium in cartilage appears to predispose to inflammatory and degenerative joint disease (2).

Treatment

Following the diagnosis of hemochromatosis in any patient, it is imperative to obtain biochemical screening of at least first-degree relatives for medical preventive reasons. Screening may be done by measuring serum iron-binding transferrin or the UIBC test. Genotyping for the C282Y mutation of the *HFE* gene is a useful diagnostic aid and helpful in counseling and predicting the risk of disease in healthy relatives (2). However, it gives no indication of iron stores or prognosis.

Aggressive phlebotomy therapy promotes longevity and can prevent or reverse much organ damage. Weekly phlebotomies are generally needed until iron is depleted and mild anemia is present. Venesection may not prevent the progression of arthritis in hemochromatosis, but in some cases arthritis may improve after this therapy. It has been suggested that prophylactic phlebotomy should be considered on the basis of genetic predisposition. Iron-chelating therapy with intravenous deferoxamine is generally effective but impractical because of the expense and the need for intravenous administration. Arthritis symptoms may be difficult to control even with nonsteroidal anti-inflammatory drugs (NSAIDs). Agents requiring hepatic metabolism, such as diclofenac or nabumetone, should be avoided. Prosthetic hip, knee, and shoulder arthroplasties can be performed when required.

ALKAPTONURIA (OCHRONOSIS)

Alkaptonuria (AKU), a rare autosomal recessive inherited disorder, results from a complete deficiency of the enzyme homogentisic acid oxidase (HGO) (9). In six reported pedigrees it was mapped to chromosome 3q2. Since then a Spanish group has reported the cloning of the human HGO gene and established that it is the gene responsible for AKU (10). This *HGO* gene harbors misuse mutation(s) that represent a loss of function. This defect causes accumulation of homogentisic acid, a normal intermediate in the metabolism of phenylalanine and tyrosine, which is excreted in the urine. Alkalization and oxidation of this acid cause the urine to turn black. The homogentisic acid retained in the body is deposited as a pigmented polymer in the cartilage and, to a lesser degree, in skin and sclerae. The darkening of tissues parts by this pigment is designated *ochronosis*.

The pigment, which is found in the deeper layers of the articulator cartilage, is bound to collagen fibers, causing this tissue to lose its normal resiliency and become brittle and fibrillated. The erosion of this abnormal cartilage leads to denuding of subchondral bone and the penetration of tiny shards of pigmented cartilage into the bone, synovium, and joint cavity (11). It is likely that these pigmented cartilage fragments become a nidus for the formation of osteochondral bodies.

Clinical Features

A progressive degenerative arthropathy develops, with symptoms usually beginning in the fourth decade of life (9). Features include arthritis of the spine (ochronotic spondylosis) and larger peripheral joints, with chondrocalcinosis, formation of osteochondral bodies, and synovial effusions (ochrontonotic peripheral arthropathy). Initially, the spinal column is affected with pigment found in the annulus fibrosus and nucleus pulposus of the intervertebral discs (Figure 28-2). Later, the knees, shoulders, and hips deteriorate; the small peripheral joints are spared. In adults, the first sign of spondylosis may be an acute disc syndrome. Eventually, it clinically resembles ankylosing spondylitis, with progressive lumbar rigidity and loss of stature.

Disability is common and severe, with stiffness and loss of joint mobility predominant and pain less prominent (9). Knee effusions, crepitus, and flexion contractures are common, but other signs of articular inflammation are ordinarily lacking. Fragments of darkly pigmented cartilage can occasionally be found floating in the joint fluid. Osteochondral bodies, which form in response to the deposition of cartilaginous fragments in the synovium, are often palpable in and around the knee joint and may reach several centimeters in diameter.

Nonarticular features of ochronosis include bluish discoloration and calcification of the ear pinnae, triangular pigmentation of the sclera, and pigmentation over the nose, axillae, and groin. Prostatic calculi are common in men, and cardiac murmurs may develop from valvular pigment deposits.

28

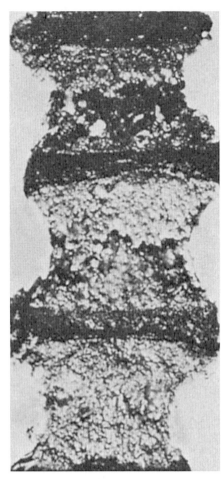

FIGURE 28-2

Part of a lumbar vertebral column of a 49-year-old woman with alkaptonuria who died of real failure (ochronotic nephrosis). Blackened intervertebral discs are thin and focally calcified. This patient had incapacitationg pain since age 36, with progressive limitation of back motion. Microscopic examination of the discs, which splintered easily, revealed nonrefractile granular pigment. (Reprinted from Cooper J, Moran TJ. Studies on ochronosis. I. Report of case with death from ochronotic nephrosis. Arch Pathol 1957;61:46–53.)

Radiographic Features

The earliest features visible on roentgenograms are multiple vacuum discs of the spine. Eventually, the entire spine shows ossification of the discs with narrowing, collapse, and fusion. Chondrocalcinosis may affect the symphysis pubis, costal cartilage, and ear helix. In contrast to ankylosing spondylitis, the sacroiliac and apophyseal joints are not affected. The roentgenographic appearance of the peripheral joints resembles that in primary osteoarthritis, with loss of cartilage space, marginal osteophytes, and eburnation of the subchondral bone. Unlike primary osteoarthritis, however, degeneration of the shoulders and hips is more severe, and osteochondral bodies are seen.

Laboratory Features

The diagnosis of AKU is suspected when the patient gives a history of passing dark urine, or when fresh urine turns black on standing or on alkalinization. In individuals lacking this history, the diagnosis is made only after the detection of a false-positive test for diabetes mellitus or the onset of arthritis. Dark pigmented synovium may be seen on arthroscopy. A specific enzymatic method permits quantitation of homogentisic acid in urine and blood and molecular cloning of the HGO gene makes detection of heterozygotic carriers possible (10).

Synovial fluid is usually clear, yellow, and viscous and does not darken with alkalinization. At times the fluid may be speckled with many particles of debris resembling ground pepper (Figure 28-3). Leukocyte counts of a few hundred cells are predominantly mononuclear. Occasionally, the cytoplasm of mononuclear and polymorphonuclear cells contains dark inclusions of phagocytosed ochronotic pigment.

Centrifugation and microscopic examination of synovial fluid sediment may show fragments of pigmented cartilage. Effusions may contain calcium pyrophosphate dihydrate crystals and show no inflammation. Pigmented cartilage fragments are embedded in synovium and are often surrounded by giant cells (11).

No effective treatment is available for the underlying metabolic disorder, but the herbicide nitisinone, an enzyme inhibitor, can deplete and markedly reduce urinary excretion of homogentisic acid in persons with

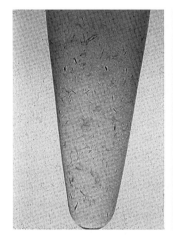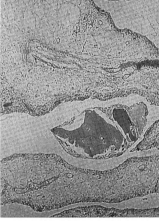

FIGURE 28-3

Ochronosis: synovial fluid and synovium (gross and microscopic). On the left, the synovial fluid reveals numerous dark particles and shards having the appearance of ground pepper. On the right, a low-power microscopic view of the synovium shows fragments of darkly pigmented cartilage (hemotoxylin and eosin stain). (Reprinted with permission from Hunter T, Gordon DA, Ogryzlo MA. The ground pepper sign of synovial fluid: a new diagnostic feature of ochronosis. J Rheumatol 1974;1:45–53.)

AKU. Limited trials with low doses of it suggest the possibility of preventing joint destruction and providing relief of pain. However, side effects may preclude its long-term use (12). Surgical removal of osteochondral loose bodies from the knee joint is warranted when these interfere with motion. Prosthetic joint replacement may be helpful.

WILSON'S DISEASE

Wilson's disease (hepatolenticular degeneration) is a rare metabolic disorder in which deposition of copper leads to dysfunction of the liver, brain, and kidneys. It is inherited as an autosomal recessive trait affecting about 1 in 30,000 persons in most populations. It becomes symptomatic for individuals aged 6 to 40 years. A defective gene and related mutations mapped to chromosome 13 provide some explanation for the wide phenotypic variation seen in Wilson's disease (13).

Clinical Features

Total body copper is increased. The accumulation of copper in the liver leads to cirrhosis; in the cornea, to characteristic Kayser–Fleischer rings; in the basal ganglia, to lentricular degeneration and movement disorders; in the kidneys, renal tubular damage (13). An arthropathy may develop in as many as 50% of affected adults, but arthritis is rare in children (14). Patients usually develop hepatic or neurologic symptoms in childhood or adolescence. Liver disease is the most common presentation between ages 8 and 16, with symptoms of jaundice, nausea, vomiting, and malaise. Acute hepatic failure may rarely develop. Neurologic symptoms are rare before age 12. Dysarthria and decreased coordination of voluntary movements are the most common complaints. Other presenting symptoms include acute hemolytic anemia, arthralgias, renal stones, and renal tubular acidosis. The arthropathy is characterized by mild premature osteoarthritis of the wrists, MCP joints, knees, or spine. Occasionally, joint hypermobility also may be found (14). Ossified bodies of the wrists may be associated with subchondral cysts. Chondromalacia patellae, osteochondritis dissecans, or chondrocalcinosis of the knee may be associated with mild knee effusions. Arthropathy tends to be mild in patients treated early in life, but it may be more severe in patients with untreated disease of longer duration. A few patients show acute or subacute polyarthritis that resembles rheumatoid arthritis and may be associated with a positive rheumatoid factor. These seropositive cases are possibly a result of penicillamine therapy.

The pathogenesis of the arthropathy is unclear, and its presence does not correlate with neurologic, hepatic, or renal disease. Although chondrocalcinosis has been observed in patients with Wilson's disease, light and transmission electron microscopy have failed to detect crystals containing calcium in synovial fluids or in cartilage and synovial biopsies. Copper has been found in the articular cartilage by elemental analysis of a few patients with Wilson's disease and could theoretically cause tissue damage mediated by oxygen-derived free radicals (14). Although the arthropathy is generally milder than that seen in hemochromatosis, its cause may be similar and it may involve deposition of calcium pyrophosphate dehydrate and the development of chronic arthritis.

Radiographic Features

Radiologic features may include subchondral cysts, joint space narrowing, sclerosis, marked ostophyte formation, and multiple calcified loose bodies, especially at the wrist. Unlike hemochromatosis, involvement of the hip and MCP joints is uncommon.

Periostitis at the femoral trochanters and other tendinous insertions, periarticular calcifications, and chondrocalcinosis have been reported. Changes in the spine are seen mainly in the mid-thoracic to lumbar areas and include squaring of the vertebral bodies, intervertebral joint space narrowing, osteophytes, and osteochondritis.

Skeletal manifestations of Wilson's disease include generalized osteoporosis in as many as 50% of patients. The osteoporosis is usually asymptomatic, unless spontaneous fractures occur (14). Osteomalacia, Milkman pseudofractures, and renal rickets have been reported. Some cases are from areas where nutritional deficiencies may also affect skeletal abnormalities.

Laboratory Features

Although Kayser–Fleischer corneal rings are pathognomonic of Wilson's disease, the diagnosis is established by laboratory investigations. Low serum copper and decreased serum ceruloplasmin levels occur in most cases, and in symptomatic patients urinary copper excretion is increased. Biliary excretion of copper is also markedly decreased. Microchemical evidence of copper deposition may be obtained from needle biopsy of the liver, but histochemical methods are unreliable. In doubtful cases, specialized studies with radioactive copper may be necessary.

Synovial biopsies show hyperplasia of synovial lining cells with mild inflammation. Neither calcium pyrophosphate nor copper are seen by standard methods. Limited data are available concerning morphologic changes in joints. Microvilli formation, initial cell hyperplasia, chronic inflammatory infiltrates, and vascular changes have been reported in synovium. Joint fluids have had low leukocyte counts.

Treatment

Copper chelation with penicillamine along with dietary copper restriction is the treatment of choice. Whether penicillamine can control the arthropathy is unclear, but contemporary series suggest that the arthropathy is milder because of earlier diagnosis with more intensive chelation therapy. Side effects from penicilamine reported in people with Wilson's disease rarely include acute polyarthritis, polymyositis, or a syndrome resembling systemic lupus erythematosus. Trientine or tetrathiomolybate are chelating agents available for patients intolerant of penicillamine. Liver transplantation is the only treatment option available for acute hepatic failure or longstanding cirrhosis where penicillamine or trientine are not options. Otherwise, symptomatic measures suffice to control arthritis symptoms.

GAUCHER'S DISEASE

Gaucher's disease is a *lysosomal glycolipid* storage disease in which glucocerebroside accumulates in the reticuloendothelial cells of the spleen, liver, and bone marrow (15). It is an autosomal recessive disorder caused by subnormal activity of the hydrolytic enzyme glucocerebrosidase. The gene for Gaucher's disease is located on chromosome 1 in the q21 region. Modern DNA technology has led to the cloning of the glucocerebroside genes and identification of their mutations. All the cells of the body are deficient in glucocerebroside activity in Gaucher's disease, but it is the glycolipid-engorged macrophages that account for all the non-neurologic features of the disease.

Fortunately, the most severe forms of Gaucher's disease are extremely rare, whereas milder forms are encountered frequently, particularly in the Jewish population. Gaucher's disease has been classified into clinical subdivisions. Type I, the most common form, is the adult or chronic type that accounts for more than 99% of cases. It is a common familial disorder in Ashkenzi Jews while other types occur in all ethnic groups. It is defined by the lack of neurologic involvement, and affected adults present with accumulation of glucocerebroside in the reticuloendothelial system causing organomegaly, hypersplenism, conjunctival pingueculae, skin pigmentation, and osteoarticular disease. It has the best prognosis, but may be mistaken for juvenile rheumatoid arthritis.

Clinical Features

Some patients with type I disease have few or no clinical manifestations. In these cases the condition may be discovered only when bone marrow is examined for some other reason, or if mild thrombocytopenia is investigated.

Type 2, infantile, is a fulminating disorder with severe brain involvement and death within the first 18 months of life. Type 3, the intermediate or juvenile form, begins in early childhood and shows many features of the chronic form, with or without central nervous system dysfunction.

Skeletal involvement is characteristic of type 1 and to a lesser extent type 3, but not type 2 disease. Musculoskeletal involvement occurs in the adult and juvenile forms, but it is rarely the first symptom. Patients usually present with lymphadenopathy, hepatosplenomegaly, or signs and symptoms of hypersplenism. Nevertheless, rheumatic complaints may appear early in the disease course. Pain in the hip, knee, or shoulder is caused by disease of adjacent bone. In young individuals, the most common complaint is chronic aching around the hip or proximal tibia. This may last a few days but is usually recurrent. Another complaint is excruciating pain (bone crisis) involving the femur and tibia with tenderness, swelling, and erythema. Monoarticular hip or knee degeneration is typical, and unexplained migratory polyarthritis sometimes occurs. Bony pain tends to lessen with age. Other skeletal features include pathologic long bone fractures, vertebral compression, and osteonecrosis of the femoral or humeral heads or proximal tibia. The osteonecrosis can develop slowly, or can appear rapidly with bone crisis. These crises usually affect only one bone area at a time. Because acute-phase reactants and bone scans are usually positive, the clinical picture of acute osteomyelitis is mimicked (pseudo-osteomyelitis). Surgical drainage in these cases commonly leads to infection and chronic osteomyelitis. Due to this increased susceptibility to infection, conservative management of bony lesions is recommended.

Radiographic Features

Asymptomatic radiologic areas of rarefaction, patchy sclerosis, and cortical thickening are common. Osteonecrosis of bone, particularly of the hips, and pathologic fractures of the femur and vertebrae are the most serious and deforming features of Gaucher's disease. Involvement of the femur is thought to be a "barometer" of bone symptoms. Widening of the distal femur with the radiologic appearance of an Erlenmeyer flask is a frequent finding, but flaring of the bones can occur in the tibia and humerus as well.

Laboratory Features

When bone pain or other articular symptoms appear, the serum acid phosphatase and the angiotensin-converting enzymes are usually elevated. However, the most reliable method for diagnosing Gaucher's disease is the determination of leukocyte beta-glucosidase. Diagnosis has been confirmed by examination of bone marrow aspirate for the Gaucher cell, a large lipid storage histiocyte. This cell should be differentiated from globoid cells of another lysosomal storage disorder, Krabbe's disease (galactocerebrosidosis). However, histologic diagnosis of Gaucher's disease is unnecessary and can be misleading. Moreover, bone biopsy is not recommended because of the risk of secondary infection. Needle biopsy of the liver for assay of glucocerebroside may be performed, but washed leukocytes and extracts of cultured skin fibroblasts are easily obtained for glucocerebrosidase testing. These assays may also be used to detect heterozygous carriers. Amniocentesis has been used for the prenatal detection of diseased fetuses. When the diagnosis is established, genetic counseling for family members or prospective parents is recommended. Although enzyme assays are useful for genetic screening, DNA analysis using the polymerase chain reaction is much more precise (15).

Treatment

Until recently, therapy of Gaucher's disease was mostly symptomatic, based on control of pain and infection. In adults, splenectomy may control hypersplenism, but bone disease may then accelerate. Bisphosphonates have been effective in treating bone disease in Gaucher's disease. Intermittent intravenous pamidronate with oral calcium has been effective in the treatment of a few patients with type I Gaucher's disease with severe bone involvement. Partial splenectomy has been recommended as protection against postsplenectomy infection, and for its hepatic and bone-sparing effect. Arthroplasty and complete joint replacement is often necessary, but loosening of prostheses occurs more often than in other disorders. Bleeding can be an operative problem.

With the commercial availability of replacement enzyme, the modified glucocerebroside (Ceredase), effective but costly treatment of Gaucher's disease has become a reality, but not without its limitations (16). Periodic intravenous infusions of the enzyme over many months commonly results in regression of the features of Gaucher's disease (15). However, alternatives to enzyme replacement therapy include substrate reduction, active site-specific chaperone therapy, and gene therapy (17). The latter involves using retroviral vector constructs for coding the gene for glucocerebrosidase into hematopoietic progenitors.

FABRY'S DISEASE

Fabry's disease is a lysosomal lipid storage disease in which glycosphingolipids accumulate widely in nerves, viscera, skin, and osteoarticular tissues. It is a sex-linked inherited disease caused by a deficiency of the enzyme alpha-galactosidase A. The gene and its mutations responsible for expression of this enzyme have been localized to the middle of the long arm of the X chromosome.

Clinical Features

As a slowly progressive disorder predominately affecting males, clinical features are widespread and nonspecific; thus, diagnosis is often missed or delayed. In childhood, the deposition is particularly marked in and around blood vessels, giving rise to the characteristic rash of dark blue or red angiokeratomas or angiectases around the buttocks, thighs, and lower abdomen. When diffuse, it is referred to as *angiokeratoma corgoris diffusum* and is almost always associated with hypohydrosis.

The kidneys are the main target organ and proteinuria gradually develops in childhood or adolescence, with abnormal urinary sediments including birefringent lipid crystals (Maltese crosses). Progressive renal disease leads to renal failure. Cardiovascular and cerebrovascular deposition of the sphingolipid parallels the renal disease, with vascular insufficiencies such as cryptogenic stroke or death in young persons. Ocular changes are severe. A characteristic corneal opacity seen by slit-lamp examination occurs early and can be helpful in diagnosis even in heterozygous women.

Some patients experience the insidious development of polyarthritis with degenerative changes and flexion contractures of the fingers, particularly of the distal interphalageal joints. Foam cells have been described in the synovial vessels and connective tissues. Radiographs may show infarctlike opacities of bone and osteoporosis of the spine. Osteonecrosis of the hip and talus have been described. Eighty percent of children or young adults undergo painful crises of burning paresthesias of the hands and feet and later of whole extremities. These attacks are associated with fever and elevations of the erythrocyte sedimentation rate.

Genetic counseling should be offered to affected families. Measurement of alpha-galactosidase to alpha-galactosidase activity ratios in leukocytes and fibroblasts provide reasonable discrimination between carriers and noncarriers. Identification by DNA studies is reserved for subjects showing equivocal results.

Treatment

Treatment has not been satisfactory. However, the prospect of effective gene therapy using recombinant adenovirus AxCAG alpha-gal to provide enzyme replacement has been reported in a randomized, controlled trial (18). Antiplatelet medication may suppress vascular damage. Burning paresthesias may benefit from phenytoin or carbamazepine. Without dialysis or transplantation most affected males succumb to renal failure before age 50.

FARBER'S DISEASE

Farber's disease is a lysosomal lipid storage disease in which a glycolipid ceramide accumulates widely in many tissues, including the skin and musculoskeletal system (19). It is an autosomal recessive disorder caused by a deficiency of the enzyme acid ceramidase. Affected children show disease manifestations by the age of 4 months and die before the age of 4 years.

A hoarse cry from thickened vocal cords or swollen painful joints may be the first feature. The appearance of tender, subcutaneous nodules follows and the early occurrence of nodules correlates with shortened survival. All the extremities may be swollen and tender, but this gives way to more localized joint swelling with nodules around the fingers, wrists, elbows, and knees. Joint contractures, especially affecting the fingers and wrists, develop later. The gastrointestinal, cardiovascular, and nervous systems gradually become involved, and death results from respiratory disease. Diagnosis can be confirmed by demonstrating a deficiency of ceramidase both in leukocytes and fibroblasts.

LIPOCHROME HISTIOCYTOSIS

Lipochrome histiocytosis is an extremely rare lysosomal storage disease associated with pulmonary infiltrates, splenomegaly, hypergammaglobulinemia, polyarthritis, and increased susceptibility to infection (20). The disorder is familial. Histiocytes show lipochrome pigment granulation and peripheral blood leukocytes exhibit impaired activity.

MULTICENTRIC RETICULOHISTIOCYTOSIS

Multicentric reticulohistiocytosis is a rare dermatoarthritis of unknown cause or familial association. It is characterized by the cellular accumulation of glycolipid-laden histocytes and multinucleated giant cells in skin and joints (21). The most common presentation is a painful destructive polyarthritis resembling rheumatoid arthritis, for which affected persons may be mistakenly treated. The joint manifestations precede the appearance of skin lesions in most patients, but the appearance and location of the skin nodules are not entirely characteristic of rheumatoid arthritis (Figure 28-4). Although a self-limited form may be seen in childhood, adult multicentric reticulohistiocytosis predominantly affects middle-aged women.

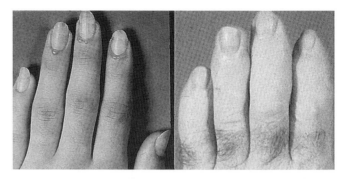

FIGURE 28-4

The fingers of a 16-year-old girl (left) with multicentric reticulo-histiocytosis reveal multiple, reddish-brown, tender papulonodules that are periungual in distribution. On the right is another patient with multiple nodules in the fingers. These nodules are firm, can fluctuate in size, and may disappear spontaneously. (Reprinted from Revised Clinical Slide Collection on the Rheumatic Diseases, with permission of the American College of Rheumatology.)

Clinical Features

Disease onset is insidious and is characterized by polyarthritis, skin nodules, and, in many cases, xanthelasma. Small papules and beadlike clusters around the nailfolds are characteristic, with skin nodulation of the face and hands. Varying sizes of skin nodules are yellowish, purple, and occur over the hands (Figure 28-5), elbows, face, and ears. Oral, nasal, and pharyngeal mucosa

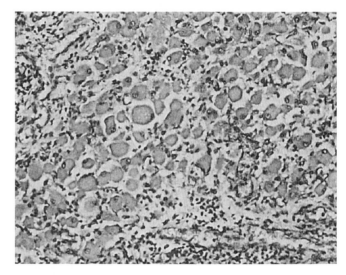

FIGURE 28-5

Photomicrograph of synovium (knee) from a 54-year-old woman with multicentric reticulohistiocytosis shows numerous histiocytes and multinucleated giant cells that contain large amounts of periodic acid-Schiff (PAS)-positive material. (Reprinted from McCarthy DJ, Koopman WJ. Arthritis and allied conditions. Philadelphia: Lea & Febiger; 1993.)

involvement sometimes with ulceration is seen in one fourth of patients. Various visceral sites may also be affected.

Symmetric polyarthritis resembles rheumatoid disease when PIP joints are affected, and psoriatic arthritis when involvement of distal interphalangeal joints predominates. Tenosynovial involvement may also occur. Remission of polyarthritis may be seen after many years of progressive disease.

Early radiographs early on show "punched out" bony lesions resembling gouty tophi. Severe joint destruction will be seen in later radiographs. Spinal involvement with erosions and subluxations including atlanto-axial damage may occur.

Laboratory Features

No specific laboratory abnormality has yet been demonstrated, and the diagnosis is established by examination of biopsies of affected tissues. Both the skin and synovium (Figure 28-5) are infiltrated by large, multinucleated giant cells. The cytoplasm has a "ground glass" appearance and stains positively for lipids and glycoproteins with periodic acid-Schiff stain (PAS positive). Definitive analysis of these cell contents has not been made, but it is probably a glycolipid. Triglycerides, cholesterol, and phosphate esters appear to be present in the lesion, suggesting either that histiocytes are stimulated to produce these substances or that this is a form of lipid storage disease. A lymphocytic origin for the giant cells has been proposed because of the presence of T-cell markers, but multicentric reticulocytosis cells also stain for macrophage markers (21). A monocyte/macrophage origin for these cells has also been suggested because of the detection of macrophage-activated cytokines of IL-1 beta, IL-12, and tumor necrosis factor alpha (TNF-alpha). The distribution of TNF-alpha appears similar to that for rheumatoid synovial cell proliferation. Synovial fluid leukocyte counts range from 220 to 79,000 cells/mm^3, with mononuclear cells predominating. Scanning the synovial fluid Wright-stained smear or wet preparation may reveal giant cells or large, bizarre macrophages.

The foregoing specific histologic picture of multicentric reticulohistiocytosis is quite different from the myofibroblast cells in a collagen matrix characteristic of the cutaneous nodules and polyarthritis of fibroblastic rheumatism (22).

Although the pathogenesis is unknown, hidden malignancy and tuberculosis have been implicated. Rheumatoid factor does not occur. Some patients develop positive reactions to tuberculin (PPD positive). There are case descriptions with associated Sjögren's syndrome and polymyositis. Multicentric reticulohistiocytosis has also been implicated with a variety of malignancies (21). Death due to the disease itself has not been reported, but patients may be left with severe joint disability.

Treatment

Spontaneous remission of skin and arthritis occurs in some cases, especially in childhood. In the remainder, corticosteroids or topical nitrogen mustard may improve the skin lesions. In cases with severe skin and joint disease combinations of corticosteroid, methotrexate (MTX) plus cyclophosphamide or cyclosporine, and bisphosphonates have been effective. Low-dose MTX alone has shown prolonged effect, and MTX plus hydroxychloroquine has also been beneficial. The presence of synovial TNF-alpha in the disease indicates that, in addition to MTX, dramatic clinical and serologic improvement may occur with TNF-alpha inhibition (23).

REFERENCES

1. Rooney PJ. Hyperlipidemias, lipid storage disorders, metal storage disorders and ochronosis. Curr Opin Rheumatol 1991;3:166–171.
2. Pietrangelo A. Hereditary hemochromatosis—a new look at an old disease. N Engl J Med 2004;350:2383–2397.
3. McDonnell SM, Preston BL, Jewell SA, et al. A survey of 2,851 patients with hemochromatosis: symptoms and response to treatment. Am J Med 1999;106:619–624.
4. Feder JN, Gnirke A, Thomas W, et al. A novel MHC class I-like gene is mutated inpatients with hereditary hemochromatosis. Nat Genet 1996;13:399–408.
5. Adams PC, Reboussin DM, Barton JC, et al. Hemochromatosis and iron-overload screening in a racially diverse population. N Engl J Med 2005;352:1769–1778.
6. Piperno A, Fargion S, D'Alba R, et al. Liver damage in Italian patients with hereditary hemochromatosis is highly influenced by hepatitis B and C virus infection. J Hepatol 1992;16:364–368.
7. Mathews JL, Williams HJ. Arthritis in hereditary hemochromatosis. Arthritis Rheum 1987;30:1137–1141.
8. Ross JM, Kowalchuk RM, Shaulinsky J, et al. Association of heterozygous hemochromatosis C282Y gene mutation with hand osteoarthritis. J Rheumatol 2003;30:121–125.
9. Perry MB, Suwannarat P, Furst GP, et al. Musculoskeletal findings and disability in alkaptonuria. J Rheumatol 2006;33:2280–2285.
10. Fernandez-Canon JM, Grandadino B, Beltram-Valero de Bernabe D, et al. The molecular basis of alkaptonuria. Nat Genet 1996;14:19–24.
11. Gaines JJ, Tom GD, Khan Khanian N. The ultrastructural and light microscopic study of the synovium in ochronotic arthropathy. Hum Pathol 1987;8:1160–1164.
12. Suwannarat P, Obrien K, Perry MB, et al. Use of nitisinone in patients with alkaptonuria. Metabolism 2005;54:719–728.
13. Gow PJ, Smallwood RA, Angust PW, et al. Diagnosis of Wilson's disease: an experience over three decades. Gut 2000;46:415–419.

28

14. Memerey KA, Eider W, Brewer GJ, et al. The arthropathy of Wilson's disease: clinical and pathologic features. J Rheumatol 1988;15:331–337.

15. Pastores GM, Meere PA. Musculoskeletal complications associated with lysosomal storage disorders: Gaucher disease and Hurler-Scheie syndrome (mucopolysaccharidosis type 1). Curr Opin Rheumatol 2005;17:70–78.

16. Grabowski GA. Enzyme therapy is not enough. Lancet 2001;358(Suppl):S29.

17. Brady RO. Emerging strategies for the treatment of hereditary metabolic storage disorders. Rejuvenation Res 2006;9:237–244.

18. Schiffmann R, Kopp JB, Austin HA 3rd, et al. Enzyme replacement therapy in Fabry Disease: a randomized controlled trial. JAMA 2001;285:2743–2749.

19. Chanoki M, Ishii M, Fukaik, et al. Farber's lipogranulomatosis in siblings: light and electron microscopic studies. Br J Dermatol 1989;121:779–785.

20. Rodey GE, et al. Defective bacteriocidel activity of peripheral blood leukocytes in lipochrome histiocytosis. Am J Med 1970;49:322–327.

21. Gorman JD, Danning C, Schumacher HR, et al. Multicentric reticulohistiocytosis: case report with immunochemical analysis and literature review. Arthritis Rheum 2000;43:930–938.

22. Romas E, Finlay M, Woodruff T. The arthropathy of fibroblastic rheumatism. Arthritis Rheum 1997;40:183–187.

23. Shannon SE, Schumacher HR, Self S, Brown AN. Multicentric reticulohistiocytosis responding to tumor necrosis factor-alpha inhibition in a renal transplant patient. J Rheumatol 2005;32:565–567.

CHAPTER 29

The Amyloidoses

PASHA SARRAF, MD, PHD

JONATHAN KAY, MD

- The prevalence of amyloid diseases varies in different geographic areas. Alzheimer's disease is the most common form of localized amyloidosis, while AL amyloidosis is the most common systemic form of amyloidosis in the United States, while AA amyloidosis is the most common form worldwide.
- Amyloid fibrils resemble a woven cable and are deposited in tissues depending of the specific causative protein. Amyloid deposits do not cause an inflammatory reaction, but interfere with the function of surrounding tissues.

- Clinical manifestations vary according to the type of amyloid disease.
- Diagnosis is made by recognition of deposits with a characteristic "apple green" birefringence under polarizing microscopy and the specific subunit protein by immunohistochemistry.
- Treatment is directed toward reducing production of aberrant proteins or surgical removal of amyloid deposits or affected organs.

The amyloid diseases involve a wide variety of proteins that share in common the property of forming fibrils (1). Deposition and accumulation of these fibrils in various tissues, ultimately interfering with normal organ function, results in the clinical entity known as amyloidosis. The amyloidoses can occur either as isolated localized processes or as systemic disorders involving multiple organ systems. Furthermore, amyloidosis may occur as a primary disease process or as a secondary consequence of other diseases. Both light and heavy chain (formerly known as primary) amyloidosis and familial amyloidosis belong to the former group, whereas serum amyloid A protein and beta$_2$-microglobulin (dialysis-associated) amyloidosis belong to the latter group. In the United States, primary (idiopathic) amyloidosis is the most common form of amyloid disease, while serum amyloid A-associated amyloidosis occurs more commonly in other countries. Alzheimer's disease and prion deposition disease are the only forms of localized amyloid fibril deposition which often lead to serious illness; other forms of localized amyloid deposition usually lead only to mechanical interference and generally are considered to be benign.

The name *amyloidosis* is preserved in deference to Rudolph Virchow, who first used histochemical stains in 1854 to characterize amyloid deposits in pathologic specimens of brain (2). Whereas all other structures in his brain sections stained yellow after the application of iodine and sulfuric acid, the corpora amylacea stained pale blue with iodine and brilliant violet upon subse-

quent acidification. Because this pattern of staining was characteristic of plant cellulose, Virchow concluded that the corpora amylacea was composed of a celluloselike substance that he labeled "amyloid." The term *amyloid*, derived from the Greek word *amylon*, refers to materials that contain or resemble starch. This is a misnomer, however, as it now is known that amyloid deposits contain mainly protein, even though some carbohydrate-containing substances may associate with the proteins. The study of amyloid has focused mainly on its protein composition.

The understanding of the protein structure of amyloid has been advanced by the observation that Congo red, an aniline textile dye, stains amyloid deposits. Congo red molecules deposit and align perpendicular to the long axis of amyloid fibrils, markedly enhancing the anisotropy of these fibrils and appearing as "apple green" birefringence under polarizing microscopy. Independent of their protein of origin, by definition, all amyloid proteins share three common characteristics: a cross-beta-pleated sheeted structure, an organized fibrillar ultrastructure, and congophilia producing "apple green" birefringence.

Amyloid deposits are amorphous and consist of a number of components (3). The wide array of proteins that may result in amyloidosis are not derived from common precursors and do not have any particular genetic homology. However, each protein, in the proper setting, can form amyloid fibrils. Other components of amyloid deposits include the serum amyloid P component and proteoglycans which, although not part of the fibrils themselves, may contribute to amyloid formation in situ.

Amyloid nomenclature is based on the name of the primary subunit protein: all amyloid fibril proteins are named "protein A-" with a suffix that identifies the specific subunit protein (e.g., protein AL for light chain amyloidosis and protein AA for serum amyloid A amyloidosis). Both the amyloid type and the resulting disease are named for the protein. Thus, *AA amyloidosis* replaces the label *secondary amyloidosis*, and *AL amyloidosis* replaces the names *primary amyloidosis* and *myeloma-associated amyloidosis*. Currently, 24 amyloid proteins that can cause clinically apparent amyloidosis have been identified. However, most of these types of amyloidosis are quite rare and occur primarily as hereditary diseases with clustering of cases in families.

PATHOGENESIS

The structure of an amyloid fibril resembles that of a woven cable, in which three to six filaments wrap around one another to form a fibril (4). Individual filaments have a lamellar beta sheet structure that is composed of thousands of individual, noncovalently associated peptide subunits. This higher ordered structure facilitates the binding of certain small molecules, such as Congo red, and macromolecules, such as proteoglycans and serum amyloid P component.

The initiation and progression of amyloidogenesis is entirely dependent on the causative protein, but generally follows one of three pathogenetic processes: overproduction and deposition of wild-type protein, deposition of a mutated variant of a protein, or deposition of protein fragments that have been generated by aberrant endoproteolytic cleavage. The first scenario results in AA or senile ATTR amyloidosis, in which serum amyloid A protein or transthyretin is overproduced and deposited. The second scenario, in which a mutation destabilizes the wild-type protein and confers amyloidogenic properties on the new variant protein, results in hereditary types of amyloidosis such as familial ATTR or AGel amyloidosis. The third scenario is illustrated by AL amyloidosis, in which normal immunoglobulin light chains undergo limited proteolysis that yields the amyloidogenic form. The unfolded proteolytic cleavage products then self-associate by a mechanism known as *seeded polymerization* to form a superstructure called a *seed*, the formation of which is rate-limiting. Once produced, the seed acts as a template for the rapid addition of new monomers, thus accelerating the assembly of an amyloid fibril.

Amyloid fibrillogenesis can occur both in vivo and in vitro. Virtually any protein can form amyloid fibrils in vitro, but only a limited repertoire of molecules form detectable deposits of amyloid in vivo. The reasons for this discrepancy are unknown, but likely are related to modifying influences of the affected individual. These include, but are not limited to, the presence and specificity of endoproteolytic enzymes, the presence of inherited single nucleotide polymorphisms that counteract the effect of the amyloidogenic mutation, and the amount of amyloidogenic protein synthesized. Factors such as these determine the timing of disease onset and the rapidity of its progression.

The presence of detectable amyloid is the sine qua non for expression of disease in patients. Although the extent and rapidity of organ damage and disease expression varies between patients, even in those with similar types of amyloid proteins, the whole body burden of amyloid correlates directly with the extent of disease. Thus, reducing the total amount of amyloid may stabilize or improve clinical manifestations of disease.

Amyloid deposits do not elicit a significant inflammatory reaction in vivo. This is consistent with the observation that amyloid fibrils prepared ex vivo do not induce a systemic acute-phase response or an inflammatory reaction when administered to experimental animals. In the absence of significant inflammation, it might be assumed that amyloid fibrils result in clinical disease because of a direct cytotoxic effect on surrounding cells. In Alzheimer's disease, oligomers of amyloid-beta protein interfere with cognition in experimental animals by causing cytopathic changes in neurons. However, there is no evidence that other amyloid proteins are directly cytopathic to surrounding tissues in vivo. Rather, the clinical course of amyloidosis suggests that physical interference of amyloid deposits with normal organ function is the primary mechanism of disease pathogenesis. In cardiac amyloidosis, the intrinsic contractility of heart muscle is not affected by amyloid deposition; instead, amyloid fibril deposition in the myocardium alters the elastic properties of cardiac muscle and causes a restrictive cardiomyopathy with reduced filling. Similarly, retinal cells are not affected by transthyretin deposition in the vitreous humor, as years of blindness can be reversed by replacing the vitreous fluid. Furthermore, patients with familial amyloidosis who undergo organ transplantation to restore function of failing organs do not exhibit recurrent organ dysfunction until many years after transplantation, when amyloid deposits once again become clinically evident. These observations suggest that the clinical manifestations of the amyloid diseases result from interference with normal organ and tissue architecture that causes predictable patterns of progressive organ dysfunction over time. Thus, it is critical to intervene to inhibit amyloid formation and deposition, as quickly as possible, so as to prevent disease progression.

EPIDEMIOLOGY

The prevalence of the amyloid diseases varies in different geographic locations (5). Although in the United States and throughout the world, Alzheimer's disease is the most frequent form of amyloidosis, this chapter will focus primarily on the most commonly encountered systemic forms of the disease. In the United States, AL is the most common form of systemic amyloidosis. The stable population of Olmstead County, Minnesota, has provided reliable data regarding the disease prevalence between 1950 and 1989, suggesting that approximately 1 in 100,000 people will develop AL amyloidosis (6). Of the Mayo Clinic patients with AL amyloidosis, 18% had a diagnosis of multiple myeloma and 16% had a prior diagnosis of monoclonal gammopathy of unknown significance. Among all patients with multiple myeloma, approximately 20% will develop AL amyloidosis.

Worldwide, AA is the most common form of systemic amyloidosis. In industrialized countries, inflammatory conditions are the leading cause of AA amyloidosis, whereas systemic or chronic infections are responsible for the majority of cases of AA amyloidosis in developing countries.

Of the hereditary forms of amyloidosis, those due to transthyretin (TTR) mutations occur most frequently, causing either systemic ATTR amyloidosis or isolated senile cardiac amyloidosis. The TTR mutation V122I is the most common amyloid-associated TTR variant worldwide and occurs in 3.9% of African Americans and in over 5% of the population in some areas of Western Africa. TTR V122I is the most frequently identified subunit protein in patients with isolated senile cardiac amyloidosis.

CLINICAL FEATURES

Amyloidosis can present as either a systemic or a localized disease. There are four classes of systemic amyloidosis: AL, AA, ATTR, and $A\beta_2M$ (Table 29-1). Numerous forms of localized amyloidosis have been identified. Alzheimer's disease and isolated laryngeal and urinary tract amyloid deposits are the most common forms of localized amyloidosis.

With the exception of Alzheimer's disease, where direct cellular cytotoxicity in the brain is observed, the clinical presentation of the other amyloidoses is caused by mechanical disruption of normal physiologic function as previously described. The clinical presentation of amyloidosis depends on the amyloid subunit protein involved. Table 29-2 summarizes the amyloid proteins, their associated clinical syndromes, and the distribution of organ involvement in the localized amyloid diseases. In the following sections, the most common acquired

TABLE 29-1. SYSTEMIC AMYLOIDOSIS.

TYPE	ASSOCIATION	HC CR	SAP	IMMUNOHISTOLOGY λ/κ	SAA	β_2M	TTR
AL	Plasma cell dyscrasia	+	+	+	−	−	−
AA	Chronic inflammation	+	+	−	+	−	−
$A\beta_2M$	Chronic dialysis	+	+	−	−	+	−
ATTR	Familial	+	+	−	−	−	+

ABBREVIATIONS: λ/κ, lambda and kappa light chains; β_2M, beta$_2$-microglobulin; CR, Congo red; HC, histochemistry; SAA, serum amyloid A protein; SAP, serum amyloid P component; TTR, transthyretin.

This table illustrates the histochemical and immunohistochemical properties of the main systemic amyloidoses. Tissue may be stained with Congo red (CR) to demonstrate presence of amyloid deposits and may subsequently be immunostained for the specific amyloid subunit protein to determine the specific type of the amyloid deposit.

Listing of the human amyloidoses and their precursor proteins. The amyloid diseases and their subunit proteins have been divided broadly into systemic and localized disease. It should be noted that some of the proteins may have overlapping disease presentations: for example, AL amyloidosis may present in a localized form, as well as in a systemic form (see text), and AGel amyloidosis may present in a systemic form as a neuropathy, as well as in a localized form. This has been indicated by "L" (localized) or "S" (systemic) under the heading: "Main Clinical Setting."

29

systemic amyloid diseases (AL, AA, ATTR, and $A\beta_2M$) are reviewed.

AL Amyloidosis

The clinical manifestations of AL amyloidosis are protean (7). The kidney, heart, and liver are the organs that are most frequently and most prominently involved; however, all organs other than the central nervous system may be affected. In the kidney, AL amyloid deposits primarily in the glomerulus, causing nephrotic syndrome that usually manifests as proteinuria with initial daily urine protein excretion of more than 2 g. Not infrequently, in more advanced disease, daily urine protein excretion may be as high as 5 to 15 g.

Cardiac involvement develops insidiously. By the time most patients with AL amyloidosis present with clinically apparent cardiac disease secondary to amyloidosis, significant myocardial damage already has occurred. Supraventricular tachyarrhythmias may occur as a result of atrial enlargement. The restrictive cardiomyopathy can result in significant orthostatic hypotension due to restricted ventricular filling, compounded by autonomic dysfunction caused by peripheral nervous system involvement.

Bleeding and motility disorders are the most common presentations of AL amyloid deposition in the gastrointestinal tract. Early satiety, caused by delayed gastric

with familial Mediterranean fever (FMF) who have subclinical elevation of SAA and other acute-phase reactants, but who are otherwise asymptomatic. These patients eventually may progress to systemic amyloidosis. Because many of these patients with FMF have lived in developing countries, environmental exposures, such as endemic infections, may potentiate this presentation by causing chronic inflammation, thereby increasing their risk of developing AA amyloidosis.

Serum amyloid A, a highly conserved acute-phase protein, is produced primarily in the liver. There are four SAA genes: *saa1* and *saa2* are under acute physiologic regulation, *saa3* is a pseudogene and is not expressed, and *saa4* is expressed at a continuous basal level. Although each SAA protein has been identified as an apolipoprotein component of the high-density lipoprotein (HDL) particle, only the SAA4 protein appears to function in this capacity, under physiological conditions, and does not appear to be involved in the pathogenesis of amyloid disease. SAA1 and SAA2, which are mainly responsible for the pathogenesis of AA amyloidosis, also can be found in the HDL particle at low levels. However, serum levels of both of these proteins increase dramatically in response to glucocorticoids and to proinflammatory cytokines, such as interleukin 1 and interleukin 6. Therefore, the broad conservation of these proteins across species and the tightly regulated acute control of their expression suggest a more important role for these SAA proteins in the control of inflammation. Thus, it is thought that chronic inflammation results in continuous overproduction of these proteins, which, over time, lead to form amyloid fibrils and deposit in tissues.

Full-length SAA1 and SAA2, each 104 amino acids, are cleaved at their N-termini by endoproteases in the liver to produce fragments of 76 amino acids. Both the full-length proteins and the cleaved products are found in serum and in AA amyloid deposits. In AA amyloidosis, both SAA1 and SAA2 can form amyloid fibrils; however, SAA1 usually contributes much more to fibril formation than does SAA2. The reason for this is unclear. Furthermore, the *saa1* gene has single nucleotide polymorphisms that define three haplotypes: 1.1 (1.alpha), 1.2 (1.beta), and 1.3 (1.gamma). Caucasian patients with the 1.1/1.1 (1.alpha/1.alpha) genotype have a three- to sevenfold increased risk of developing AA amyloidosis (12).

Treatment of AA amyloidosis is directed towards controlling the underlying inflammatory disease process. The clinical outcome of AA amyloidosis is more favorable when the serum SAA concentration remains below 10mg/L (11). For more advanced disease, renal transplantation effectively restores renal function in patients with AA amyloidosis. However, unless the underlying inflammatory process is suppressed, AA amyloid may deposit in the transplanted kidney.

ATTR Amyloidosis

The hereditary amyloidoses are caused by a variety of unrelated proteins (Table 29-2). These syndromes exhibit autosomal dominant inheritance with varying degrees of penetrance. Even though the gene mutation is present at birth, clinical features of disease usually do not manifest until after the third decade of life. These syndromes share clinical features, typically presenting with cardiomyopathy, nephropathy, and polyneuropathy. However, each amyloidogenic protein should be considered to cause a discrete disease entity, with other unique clinical features. The vast majority of the hereditary amyloidoses are caused by deposition of transthyretin (TTR) variants, with more than 100 mutations having been identified (13). TTR is also known as prealbumin, because it runs faster than does albumin on gel electropheresis. Transthyretin is a plasma protein that carries about 20% of thyroxine in plasma, as well as vitamin A associated with retinol binding protein. TTR is synthesized in the liver as a single polypeptide and, in plasma, forms a tetramer that consists of four identical monomers. The wild-type protein has significant beta sheet structure; a single amino acid substitution contributes to its aggregation and fibril formation.

Not all TTR-related amyloidosis is due to mutations in TTR. Fragments of wild-type TTR may form amyloid fibrils that deposit in the heart, causing senile cardiac amyloidosis. This nonheritable disorder affects about 25% of individuals over the age of 80 years.

Most TTR-related amyloidoses present initially with peripheral neuropathy. This often is a sensorimotor neuropathy involving the distal lower extremities that progresses proximally to involve the proximal extremities. Carpal tunnel syndrome may be the initial presentation in 20% of cases, with ATTR amyloid deposits compressing the median nerve. Autonomic neuropathy can cause gastrointestinal symptoms, such as alternating constipation and diarrhea, or genitourinary symptoms, such as incontinence or impotence.

Although peripheral nervous system disease is associated with significant morbidity, cardiomyopathy and renal disease are the predominant causes of mortality among patients with ATTR amyloidosis. The majority (60%) of deaths are due to cardiomyopathy, whereas renal disease accounts for only 5% to 7% of deaths. Vitreous amyloid deposits occur in 20% of patients with ATTR amyloidosis. These are thought to arise from TTR that is secreted by the choroid plexus and that forms amyloid fibrils, which accumulate in the vitreous.

ATTR amyloidosis is diagnosed by using genetic techniques to identify TTR mutations: the majority of mutations in ATTR occur in exons 2 through 4. The use of polymerase chain reactions to identify restriction fragment length polymorphisms has become commonplace to diagnose affected patients and to identify carriers of the mutant gene among their family members.

ATTR amyloidosis is treated by replacing the liver and other affected organs. Liver transplantation results in synthesis of wild-type (normal) TTR, with rapid disappearance of the variant transthyretin from the circulation. Combined liver/kidney transplantation has been performed in patients with ATTR amyloidosis with significant renal involvement. In patients affected by ATTR amyloidosis, it is important to intervene before severe malnutrition or cardiomyopathy develops, because transplant survival declines rapidly in those affected individuals. Amyloid deposition may continue, even after organ transplantation, perhaps related to the presence of small deposits of abnormal protein that serve as a nidus for the subsequent deposition of normal proteins. Because of this, patients with earlier presentations of ATTR amyloidosis may require repeat organ transplantation.

Aβ₂M Amyloidosis

Aβ₂M amyloid deposits predominantly in osteoarticular tissue (14). The presence of shoulder pain, carpal tunnel syndrome, and irreducible flexion contractures of the fingers in a patient undergoing long-term hemodialysis is highly suggestive of Aβ₂M (beta₂-microglobulin or dialysis-related) amyloidosis. Signs and symptoms of Aβ₂M amyloidosis are infrequently observed in patients with chronic renal failure who have not yet received dialysis treatment.

Axial skeletal involvement, which occurs in about 10% of patients undergoing long-term hemodialysis, presents as a destructive spondyloarthropathy, the radiographic features of which include narrowing of the intervertebral disk spaces and erosion of the vertebral endplates without appreciable formation of osteophyte. The lower cervical spine is most often affected; however, similar changes may also occur in the dorsal and lumbar spine. Cystic deposits of Aβ₂M amyloid within the odontoid process and the vertebral bodies of the upper cervical spine and peri-odontoid soft tissue masses of Aβ₂M amyloid, termed *pseudotumors*, have also been demonstrated. Although neurologic compromise occurs infrequently, significant myelopathy has resulted from Aβ₂M amyloid deposits in the cervical and lumbar spinal canal, especially in patients who have received hemodialysis for 20 years or longer.

Cystic bone lesions may develop in the appendicular skeleton of patients undergoing long-term hemodialysis. Subchondral amyloid cysts, most commonly found in the carpal bones, may also occur in the acetabulum and in long bones, such as the femoral head or neck, the humeral head, the distal radius, and the tibial plateau. Unlike brown tumors of hyperparathyroidism, these bone cysts typically occur adjacent to joints and increase

in number and enlarge with time. Pathologic fractures, especially of the femoral neck, may occur through areas of bone weakened by amyloid deposits.

Visceral deposits of Aβ₂M amyloid also have been identified in patients receiving long-term dialysis, most for 10 years or longer. Although gastrointestinal tract and cardiovascular complications have been reported, visceral Aβ₂M amyloid deposits usually do not cause symptoms.

Beta₂-microglobulin, the subunit protein in Aβ₂M amyloidosis, is the light chain of class I major histocompatibility antigens. Normally present in most biologic fluids, it is filtered by glomeruli and catabolized after proximal tubular reabsorption. Because the rate of beta₂-microglobulin synthesis exceeds the rate of its removal by different dialysis modalities, serum beta₂-microglobulin levels are elevated up to 60-fold in patients undergoing dialysis.

Current theories regarding the pathogenesis of Aβ₂M amyloidosis implicate the role of advanced glycation end product (AGE) modification of proteins, which confers on the proteins resistance to proteolysis, increased affinity for collagen, and the ability to stimulate activated mononuclear leukocytes to release pro-inflammatory cytokines such as tumor necrosis factor alpha (TNF-alpha), interleukin 1 beta (IL-1 beta), and interleukin 6 (IL-6). AGE-modified proteins are poorly cleared by dialysis modalities (14,15). Thus, patients undergoing dialysis have elevated levels of these modified proteins, as compared with individuals with normal renal function or functioning renal allografts. AGE-modified beta₂-microglobulin has been identified in amyloid deposits of patients receiving long-term hemodialysis and may play a significant role in the development of Aβ₂M amyloidosis. The propensity for Aβ₂M amyloid to deposit in osteoarticular tissue may be due to the enhanced binding of AGE-modified proteins to collagen. Surgery may be necessary for symptomatic patients with large deposits of Aβ₂M amyloid. Over the past decade, hemodialysis with newer, more permeable membranes appears to have postponed the onset of carpal tunnel syndrome and bone cysts and reduced the incidence of Aβ₂M amyloidosis. Aβ₂M amyloid deposits do not progress and may regress in patients who have undergone successful renal transplantation. Patients with Aβ₂M amyloidosis who undergo successful renal transplantation experience a marked reduction in joint pain and stiffness. Thus, early renal transplantation in appropriate candidates, before significant Aβ₂M amyloid deposition has occurred, may be the most effective preventive measure currently available for this condition.

Localized Amyloidosis

The localized forms of amyloidosis can involve many organ systems including the eye, the genitourinary tract, the endocrine system, and the respiratory tract (Table 29-2). With the exception of Alzheimer's disease, these types of amyloidosis are rare and challenging to diagnose. The pathophysiologic principles governing disease expression in the localized forms of amyloidosis are similar to those for the systemic forms. The most frequently occurring forms of localized amyloidosis affect the genitourinary and respiratory tracts (13).

Localized genitourinary amyloidosis may involve the entire tract, but more frequently involves the bladder and urethra and causes hematuria or signs of obstruction. The responsible amyloid subunit protein often is immunoglobulin light or heavy chain, but occasionally may be SAA. The localized finding of AL or AH amyloid deposits may prompt an exhaustive search for systemic disease, often with negative results. However, localized AL or AH amyloidosis usually is self-limited and does not portend a severe prognosis. Treatment consists of excision of the localized amyloid deposits.

In the respiratory tract, AL amyloid deposition often produces localized forms of disease. Three forms of localized amyloidosis affect the respiratory tract: tracheobronchial amyloidosis, which accounts for half of cases, nodular parenchymal amyloidosis, which accounts for about 45% of cases, and diffuse parenchymal amyloidosis, which accounts for about 5% of cases. In tracheobronchial amyloidosis, there is either localized or diffuse involvement of the tracheobronchial tree with submucosal deposition of amyloid. Computed tomography (CT) scanning demonstrates nodules or plaques of amyloid, sometimes with calcification, or circumferential thickening of the trachea, main bronchus, and lobar or segmental bronchi with luminal narrowing. In nodular parenchymal amyloidosis, CT scanning demonstrates nodules with sharp and lobulated margins in a peripheral, subpleural location. The nodules vary in size from micronodular to up to 15 cm in diameter; calcification is seen in half of the cases. In diffuse parenchymal or alveolar septal amyloidosis, amyloid deposition is widespread, involving both small vessels and the parenchymal interstitium; multifocal small nodules of amyloid also may be present. High-resolution CT scanning demonstrates abnormal reticular opacities, interlobular septal thickening, small (2–4 mm diameter) nodules, and confluent consolidated opacities predominantly in the subpleural regions (16). This pattern of localized amyloidosis sometimes is indistinguishable from systemic amyloidosis. Patients with this form of diffuse parenchymal pulmonary amyloidosis are more likely to die from respiratory failure than are patients with tracheobronchial or nodular parenchymal amyloidosis..

Localized amyloid deposition limited to the respiratory tract may be excised to cure this form of limited amyloidosis. Other amyloid subunit proteins may also deposit in the respiratory tract, but these are rare and generally do not result in significant pathology.

DIAGNOSIS

Imaging

Scintigraphy using ^{123}I-serum amyloid P component has been used to identify the systemic distribution of amyloid deposits (17). Serial imaging has demonstrated both progression and regression of amyloid deposition. However, this technique is limited in that it exposes patients to radioactive allogeneic protein and it is availability only in specialized centers.

The only widely available imaging technique that yields information specific for the diagnosis of systemic amyloidosis is echocardiography (18,19). Specific echocardiographic features of amyloidosis include atrial enlargement, reduced left ventricular size, biventricular and atrial septal thickening, and increased myocardial echogenicity. In more advanced disease, restrictive filling patterns become more evident. Unfortunately, by the time a patient has echocardiographic manifestations of amyloidosis, median survival is only 6 months. Also, echocardiography does not demonstrate regression of amyloid disease, even after successful therapy.

Cardiac magnetic resonance imaging (MRI) is a rapidly advancing field and has supplemented echocardiography in the diagnosis of cardiac amyloidosis (20). Cardiac MRI, using gadolinium enhancement, provides high spatial resolution (approximately 2 mm) and tissue contrast, differentiating diseased tissue from normal myocardium. In patients with amyloid involving the heart, cardiac MRI demonstrates qualitative global and subendocardial enhancement after intravenous administration of gadolinium. Although there are no sine qua non MRI findings for cardiac amyloidosis, future studies may elucidate a combination of noninvasive tools that could be used to select patients for definitive, more invasive, endomyocardial biopsy, as well as to follow the natural history of cardiac amyloid disease.

Because there are no findings specific for systemic amyloidosis, imaging should be used as an adjunct to physical examination and appropriate laboratory testing to evaluate symptomatic patients. Although the gastrointestinal tract is almost always involved in systemic amyloidosis, radiographic manifestations of gastrointestinal amyloidosis are infrequently seen. Ischemia and resulting edema, due to amyloid deposition in vessels, may cause symmetrical thickening of mucosal folds that appear as target lesions on abdominal CT scanning.

Ultrasound or CT scanning may reveal enlargement of the kidneys in early stages of amyloidosis. Ultrasonography usually demonstrates diffusely increased echogenicity of the renal parenchyma with preservation of the corticomedullary contrast, because the cortical architecture remains grossly normal in early disease. As disease progresses, the kidneys may appear contracted with substantial cortical thinning.

Histopathology

Once amyloidosis is suspected, its diagnosis is confirmed by a biopsy that demonstrates the characteristic "apple green" birefringence under polarizing microscopy and the specific subunit protein by immunohistochemistry. The biopsy may be taken from either an involved or an uninvolved organ. The latter approach usually is preferred because of the high risk of complications and discomfort associated with biopsy of internal organs. Three types of screening biopsies typically are performed to diagnose amyloidosis: gastrointestinal tract (rectal or gastroduodenal) biopsy, subcutaneous abdominal fat aspiration, and labial salivary gland biopsy (5).

Rectal biopsy, performed by sigmoidoscopy or proctoscopy, is the preferred gastrointestinal tract biopsy because of the accessibility of this site (5). The biopsy specimen must include submucosal blood vessels, which are more likely to contain amyloid deposits than are those in the mucosa or muscularis layers. Although the data are most robust for rectal biopsy, gastric or duodenal biopsies can be diagnostic of amyloidosis if the tissue specimen contains blood vessels of the appropriate size.

Abdominal fat aspiration was first performed after it was observed that specimens taken at autopsy of patients with amyloidosis often contained amyloid deposits around adipocytes; the highest density of amyloid deposits was in the adipose tissues isolated from the scalp and the abdominal wall (21). The reported sensitivity of abdominal fat aspiration varies between 55% and 75%, but is similar to that of rectal biopsy. This technique is useful for the diagnosis of AA, AL, and ATTR amyloidosis; however, because of the limited organ distribution of $A\beta_2M$ amyloid deposits, abdominal fat aspiration cannot reliably be used to diagnose $A\beta_2M$ amyloidosis.

Labial salivary gland biopsy samples the accessory salivary glands in the labial mucosa (22). Previously, gingival biopsy had been used to detect amyloid deposition, but was found to be of low sensitivity. In AA, ATTR, and AL amyloidosis, labial salivary gland biopsy has sensitivity comparable to that of rectal biopsy or abdominal fat aspiration.

If the suspicion for amyloidosis is high and one of the above techniques does not yield a positive finding, an involved organ should be biopsied. In the setting of renal involvement, a kidney biopsy usually provides diagnostic information. The organs predominantly involved in ATTR and AL amyloidosis, the heart and the bone marrow, should be biopsied in these forms of the amyloidosis to confirm the diagnosis. Although the sural nerve may be involved in the amyloid diseases, sural nerve biopsy is less desirable because it usually is painful and slow to heal and may leave a residual sensory deficit. Furthermore, the patchy distribution of amyloid deposits renders sural nerve biopsy less sensitive than biopsy of other involved organs.

Three points are essential to consider in the diagnosis of the amyloid diseases (23). (1) The pretest probability of a biopsy for amyloid is determined by the patient's clinical presentation. To determine pretest probability, it is critical to consider the patient's history (including a thorough family history), in the context of a complete physical examination and laboratory evaluation that includes a serum and urine protein electrophoresis and urinalysis to assess for proteinuria. (2) Immunohistochemistry should always be performed on tissue specimens that are being evaluated for amyloid deposits to identify the specific amyloid subunit protein. Occasionally, a patient with an inflammatory disorder may develop AL disease or a patient with a serum monoclonal protein may develop AA amyloidosis. Because the treatment of these diseases differ dramatically, it is imperative to establish a definite diagnosis. (3) Deposits of AA amyloid in abdominal fat are not uncommon in patients with inflammatory diseases, such as rheumatoid arthritis or ankylosing spondylitis. However, even after long-term follow-up, most of these patients do not have evidence of organ dysfunction. Thus, not all patients who have AA amyloid deposits have AA amyloid disease; biopsy results should be interpreted with caution.

SUMMARY

Rheumatologists play an important role in the recognition and treatment of the amyloid diseases. The amyloidoses occur and progress insidiously, taking years to cause clinically apparent organ damage. Delay in diagnosis may result in an increased burden of amyloid fibrils and may reduce the opportunity to effectively deliver therapy and improve prognosis. Each of the amyloidoses presents with a unique constellation of findings which, although not pathognomonic, may lead an astute physician to follow appropriate diagnostic algorithms and intervene expeditiously in the disease process. Finally, although the amyloid diseases are very heterogeneous, the clinical approach to their diagnosis and treatment is straightforward and an earnest understanding of the pathogenetic principles that contribute to disease expression should guide the rational management of the patient.

REFERENCES

1. Sipe JD, Cohen AS. Review: history of the amyloid fibril. J Struct Biol 2000;130:88–98.
2. Majno G, Joris I. Extracellular pathology. In: Cells, tissues, and disease: principles of general pathology. Oxford: Oxford University Press; 2004:250–267.

29

3. Pepys MB. Amyloidosis. Annu Rev Med 2006;57:223–241.
4. Merlini G, Bellotti V. Mechanisms of disease: molecular mechanisms of amyloidosis. N Engl J Med 2003;349:583–596.
5. Buxbaum J. The amyloidoses. In: Klippel JH, Dieppe PA, eds. Rheumatology. Mosby yearbook. 1998;8.27.1–8.27.10.
6. Kyle RA, Linos A, Beard CM, et al. Incidence and natural history of primary systemic amyloidosis in Olmsted County, Minnesota, 1950 through 1989. Blood 1992;79:1817–1822.
7. Kyle RA, Gertz MA. Primary systemic amyloidosis: clinical and laboratory features in 474 cases. Semin Hematol 1995;32:45–59.
8. Skinner M, Anderson J, Simms R, et al. Treatment of 100 patients with primary amyloidosis: a randomized trial of melphalan, prednisone, and colchicine versus colchicine only. Am J Med 1996;100:290–298.
9. Kyle RA, Gertz MA, Greipp PR, et al. A trial of three regimens for primary amyloidosis: colchicine alone, melphalan and prednisone, and melphalan, prednisone, and colchicine. N Engl J Med 1997;336:1202–1207.
10. Comenzo RL. Amyloidosis. Curr Treat Options Oncol 2006;7:225–236.
11. Gillmore JD, Lovat LB, Persey MR, Pepys MB, Hawkins PN. Amyloid load and clinical outcome in AA amyloidosis in relation to circulating concentration of serum amyloid A protein. Lancet 2001;358:24–29.
12. Booth DR, Booth SE, Gillmore JD, Hawkins PN, Pepys MB. SAA1 alleles as risk factors in reactive systemic AA amyloidosis. Amyloid 1998;5:262–265.
13. Benson MD. Amyloidosis. In: Koopman WJ, Moreland LW, eds. Arthritis and allied conditions: a textbook of rheumatology. Philadelphia: Lippincott Williams & Wilkins; 2005:1933–1960.
14. Kay J. β_2-microglobulin amyloidosis. Int J Exp Clin Invest 1997;4:187–211.
15. Miyata T, Inagi R, Iida Y, et al. Involvement of beta 2-microglobulin modified with advanced glycation end products in the pathogenesis of hemodialysis-associated amyloidosis. Induction of human monocyte chemotaxis and macrophage secretion of tumor necrosis factor-alpha and interleukin-1. J Clin Invest 1994;93:521–528.
16. Georgiades CS, Neyman EG, Barish MA, Fishman EK. Amyloidosis: review and CT manifestations. Radiographics 2004;24:405–416.
17. Hawkins PN, Lavender JP, Pepys MB. Evaluation of systemic amyloidosis by scintigraphy with 123I-labeled serum amyloid P component. N Engl J Med 1990;323:508–513.
18. Shah KB, Inoue Y, Mehra MR. Amyloidosis and the heart: a comprehensive review. Arch Intern Med 2006;166:1805–1813.
19. Falk RH, Plehn JF, Deering T, et al. Sensitivity and specificity of the echocardiographic features of cardiac amyloidosis. Am J Cardiol 1987;59:418–422.
20. Maceira AM, Joshi J, Prasad SK, et al. Cardiovascular magnetic resonance in cardiac amyloidosis. Circulation 2005;111:186–193.
21. Westermark P, Stenkvist B. A new method for the diagnosis of systemic amyloidosis. Arch Intern Med 1973;132:522–523.
22. Hachulla E, Janin A, Flipo RM, et al. Labial salivary gland biopsy is a reliable test for the diagnosis of primary and secondary amyloidosis. A prospective clinical and immunohistologic study in 59 patients. Arthritis Rheum 1993;36:691–697.
23. Comenzo RL, Zhou P, Fleisher M, Clark B, Teruya-Feldstein J. Seeking confidence in the diagnosis of systemic AL (Ig light-chain) amyloidosis: patients can have both monoclonal gammopathies and hereditary amyloid proteins. Blood 2006;107:3489–3491.

CHAPTER 30

Neoplasms of the Joint

ANDREW J. COOPER, MD
JAMES D. REEVES, MD
SEAN P. SCULLY, MD, PHD

- The most common primary neoplasms of the joint are pigmented villonodular synovitis and synovial chondromatosis and a diagnosis is best made using magnetic resonance imaging (MRI).
- Other primary lesions are rare and include lipoma arborescens, synovial hemangiomas,

intracapsular chondromas, and synovial chondrosarcomas.
- Secondary neoplasms of the joint are synovial sarcoma and giant cell tumors.
- The malignancies that metastasize to bone also may invade the articular space.

Although some neoplasms originate in the joint, others penetrate or metastasize to it. Pigmented villonodular synovitis and synovial chondromatosis are the most common proliferative disorders arising from within the joint. Other primary lesions are rare and include lipoma arborescens, synovial hemangiomas, intracapsular chondromas, and synovial chondrosarcomas. Synovial sarcoma and giant cell tumors are neoplasms that tend to extend into the joint. The malignancies that metastasize to bone also may invade the articular space.

PRIMARY NEOPLASMS OF THE JOINT

Pigmented Villonodular Synovitis

Pigmented villonodular synovitis (PVNS) is a rare proliferative disorder of unknown etiology that affects the synovial lining. PVNS does not exhibit cellular atypia, but there is recent evidence of cytogenetic abnormalities. Yet the presence of synovitis suggests an inflammatory process. The etiology of PVNS remains unresolved. Regardless, it is characterized by inflammation and deposition of hemosiderin in the synovium (1). It occurs in three forms: an isolated lesion involving the tendon sheaths (giant cell tumor of the tendon sheath); a solitary intra-articular nodule (localized PVNS); and a diffuse villous and pigmented lesion involving synovial tissue (diffuse PVNS) (2,3). This section focuses on the latter two forms.

The typical presentation is a 20- to 40-year-old patient who complaints of a traumatic swelling of a single joint (4–9). The knee is involved 80% of the time. Some patients may experience pain, warmth, and stiffness in the joint (7,8,10). Mechanical symptoms, such as locking and instability, may develop, particularly if the joint contains a large pedunculated nodule (11). The symptoms typically are episodic or slowly progressive (7). Results of laboratory studies, such as a complete blood count and erythrocyte sedimentation rate, are within normal limits and can help exclude infection and rheumatoid arthritis. Aspiration of the joint reveals a brown, red, or yellow fluid (7,9,12).

During the initial stages, plain radiographs reveal periarticular synovial swelling, absence of synovial calcification, normal bone density, and preservation of the cartilage space (13). Bone changes develop in the later stages. Recent evidence suggests that tissue expression of matrix metalloproteinases in PVNS contributes to the destruction of bone and cartilage often seen in PVNS (14). In joints with small synovial volumes (e.g., the hip), the synovial villi may abut the bone and cause subtle erosions. As the villi grow, pressure within the joint capsule increases. The villi then invade the bone and juxta-articular cysts appear (15,16). If the disorder is not diagnosed and treated, joint destruction can ensue.

Due to deposition of hemosiderin, a magnetic resonance image (MRI) typically will show nodular foci of decreased signal on both T1 and T2 images (Figures 30-1, 30-2) (12). Additionally, low signal on fast field

nonmineralized cartilage. Bony erosions may be seen, secondary to focal pressure. During the second and third stages, multiple juxta-articular calcifications or loose bodies are seen (Figure 30-4). These nodules typically are of a similar size and uniformly scattered. Joint space narrowing, osteophytes, sclerosis, and abundant calcified loose bodies represent end-stage disease (26).

If osteonecrosis, rheumatoid arthritis, post-traumatic arthritis, or degenerative arthritis is noted, a diagnosis of secondary synovial chondromatosis must be considered. This diagnosis is especially likely if the presence of the disorder preceded the diagnosis of chondromatosis. In contrast to the primary form, secondary synovial chondromatosis shows fewer ostechondral bodies, which vary more in size, and does not recur or show histologic atypia (11,26,27).

Magnetic resonance imaging can help define the location of the cartilaginous nodules and is the best noninvasive study to confirm a diagnosis of synovial chondromatosis. An intermediate density on T1 sequences and an intermediate-to-high density on T2 sequences characterize the immature nodules (Figure 30-5). Calcified and ossified areas appear hypointense on both T1 and T2 images. The exception occurs when a loose body contains marrow fat, which appears as a hyperintense area on T1 (26–29).

Synovial chondromatosis is treated by removal of the loose bodies and excision of all abnormal synovium. Stiffness may occur, and recurrence rates have been

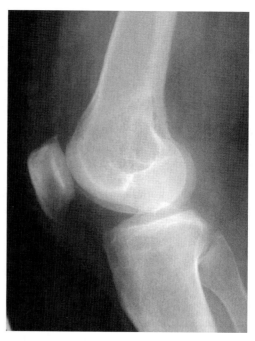

FIGURE 30-5

A lateral radiograph demonstrating a radiolucency involving the distal femoral epiphysis. Biopsy demonstrated tissue consistent with a giant cell tumor of bone.

reported as high as 11% after open treatment. In rare cases, the lesion may transform into a chondrosarcoma (25–27). Synovial chondromatosis of the hip can be treated arthroscopically assisted. The use of the arthroscope to address the intra-articular component of the disease avoids dislocation of the hip and is less invasive. Arthroscopically assisted synovectomy and removal of loose bodies has been shown effective by some surgeons (30). Similarly, arthroscopy for chondromatosis of the shoulder has been used with anticipated advantages of more complete removal of loose bodies, decreased postoperative pain, and enhanced rehabilitation (31). Dysregulation of the hedgehog signaling pathway has been implicated in the many benign cartilaginous tumors. Increased expression of the hedgehog transcription factor in mice recreates synovial chondromatosis. Medication-induced blockage of the hedgehog signaling pathway may be a future treatment option (28).

Other Primary Joint Tumors

A solitary intra-articular lipoma may occur but is extremely rare. More commonly, excessive intra-articular adipose tissue is due to lipoma arborescens. This entity involves fatty synovial villi and often is associated with osteoarthritis, rheumatoid arthritis, and trauma. It usually occurs in the knee and causes joint swelling and pain (29). Synovectomy often is curative.

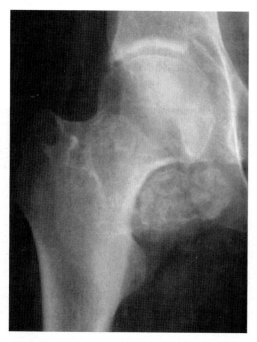

FIGURE 30-4

Plain radiograph of synovial chondromatosis showing calcified cartilage in the hip joint.

Synovial hemangiomas usually occur in children and young adults and almost exclusively involve the knee. Plain films often show the pathognomonic phleboliths. Histologically, it is identical to the soft tissue hemangiomas. Both the localized and diffuse forms can cause pain and hemarthrosis. This benign vascular neoplasm is treated by surgical excision (29,32).

Intracapsular solitary chondromas, like extra-articular chondromas, are benign cartilaginous neoplasms that may calcify. They may present as firm intra-articular mass.

Synovial chondrosarcomas are exceptionally rare and may be primary or secondary to synovial chondromatosis. Treatment is wide surgical resection (27).

SECONDARY JOINT NEOPLASMS

Synovial Sarcoma

Synovial sarcoma is an uncommon, highly malignant tumor involving mesenchymal cells. It typically occurs near tendon and fascial planes, although, on rare occasions, it may arise within or adjacent to a joint (22,33). The lower extremities are affected most frequently and the incidence is highest among those between the ages of 15 and 40 years (32). Although synovial sarcoma suggests a relationship to normal synovium, the disease is rarely found intra-articularly. However, there have been case reports of solely intra-articular involvement of synovial sarcoma (34).

Patients typically present complaining of a slowly growing soft tissue mass. Approximately 50% of the time, the lesion is described as painful. Plain radiographs often reveal a large, lobulated, juxta-articular mass. Calcification is seen in up to one third of cases and often has a diffuse speckled appearance. MRI shows nonspecific characteristics, but can narrow the diagnosis and define the lesion's anatomic location (29).

A biopsy often is required to confirm the diagnosis and will show the sarcoma to be one of the three types. The biphasic form is the most common and involves obvious epithelial and mesenchymal differentiation. The plump cuboidal or tall columnar epithelial cells line mucin-filled clefts and cystlike spaces. The round and oval epithelial cells form nests and cords. The fibroblasts are spindle-shaped and may be arranged in a manner similar to that seen in fibrosarcoma. Sometimes the field is dominated largely by either the epithelial cell (rarely) or the fibroblast (more commonly). The lesion then is categorized as monophasic. The monophasic form can be confused with other neoplasms of fibrous or epithelial origin and is thought by some to carry a worse prognosis. A rare, poorly differentiated type, represented histologically by numerous mitotic round cells, also has been described. Rapid growth and a very poor prognosis characterize this form (22,32,35).

SYT-SSX2 is the fusion product of translocation (X,18) found in a vast majority of synovial cell sarcomas. The fusion product has now been identified to regulate beta-catenin recruitment to the nucleus which subsequently regulates cell adhesion. Identification of the fusion product by molecular diagnostics in synovial sarcoma is becoming a standard (36).

Once synovial sarcoma is diagnosed, wide surgical resection with removal of any affected lymph nodes is indicated (32). Although adjuvant radiation and chemotherapy have improved the overall prognosis, the risk of regional and pulmonary metastasis remains high. Reports have shown the 5- and 10-year survival rates to be 55% and 40%, respectively (37). Increased age, tumor size greater than 5 cm, and 10 or more mitotic figures per 10 high-powered fields are thought to increase the risk of metastasis and/or death (33).

Giant Cell Tumor

Giant cell tumor is a benign, but locally aggressive, tumor of unknown origin that most commonly affects 20- to 40-year-olds. This lesion involves the knee (distal femur and proximal tibia) 50% of the time (32), and the distal radius and proximal humerus are the next most common sites. Plain radiographs show a purely lytic lesion that begins in the epiphysis and abuts the articular surface (22). It frequently extends into the joint (Figure 30-6) (36), tends to recur, and, 1% to 2% of the time, it will become malignant and metastasize to the lungs. The addition of phenol, bone graft, and methylmethacrylate to marginal resection can decrease the recurrence rate and allow the joint to be preserved. The use of a high speed burr also can decrease the rate of

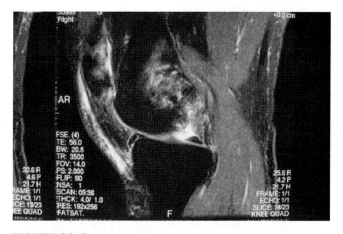

FIGURE 30-6

A sagittal fast spin echo (FSE) image of the distal femur demonstrating a distal femoral giant cell tumor of bone extending into the articular space along the cruciate ligaments.

recurrence. Radiation therapy should be reserved for inoperable tumors, as it is associated with malignant transformation (32).

REFERENCES

1. Tyler WK, Vidal AF, Williams RJ, Healey JH. Pigmented villonodular synovitis. J AAOS 2006;14:376–385.
2. Rao AS, Vigorita VJ. Pigmented villonodular synovitis (giant cell tumor of the tendon sheath and synovial membrane): a review of eighty-one cases. J Bone Joint Surg Am 1984;66:76–94.
3. Granowitz SP, D'Antonio J, Mankin HL. The pathogenesis and long term end results of pigmented villonodular synovitis. Clin Orthop 1976;114:335–351.
4. Docken WP. Pigmented villonodular synovitis: a review with illustrative case reports. Semin Arthritis Rheum 1979;9:1–22.
5. Dorwart RH, Genant HK, Johnston WH, Morris JM. Pigmented villonodular synovitis of synovial joints: clinical, pathologic, and radiologic features. AJR Am J Roentgenol 1984;143:877–885.
6. Bravo SM, Winalski CS, Weissman BN. Pigmented villonodular synovitis. Radiol Clin North Am 1996;34:311–326.
7. Byers PD, Cotton RE, Deacon OW, et al. The diagnosis and treatment of pigmented villonodular synovitis. J Bone Joint Surg Br 1968;50:290–305.
8. Flandry F, Hughston JC. Pigmented villonodular synovitis. J Bone Joint Surg Am 1987;69:942–949.
9. Flandry F, Hughston JC, Jacobsen KE, Barrack RL, McCann SB, Kurtz DM. Surgical treatment of diffuse pigmented villonodular synovitis of the knee. Clin Orthop 1994;300:183–192.
10. Wu KK, Ross PM, Guise ER. Pigmented villonodular synovitis: a clinical analysis of twenty-four cases treated at Henry Ford Hospital. Orthopedics 1980;3:751–758.
11. Jaffe HL. Tumor and tumorous conditions of the bone and joints. Philadelphia: Lea and Febiger; 1958.
12. Michael RH. Pigmented villonodular synovitis. Orthop Nurs 1997;16:66–68.
13. Lewis RW. Roentgen diagnosis of pigmented villonodular synovitis and synovial sarcoma of knee joint. Radiology 1947;49:26.
14. Uchibori M, Nishida Y, Tabata I, et al. Expression of matrix metalloproteinases and tissue inhibitors of metalloproteinases in pigmented villonodular synovitis suggests their potential for joint destruction. J Rheumatol 2004;31:110–119.
15. Schwartz HS, Unni KK, Pritcherd DJ. Pigmented villonodular synovitis. A retrospective review of affected large joints. Clin Orthop 1989;247:243–255.
16. Scott PM. Bone lesions in pigmented villonodular synovitis. J Bone Joint Surg Br 1968;50:306–311.
17. Cheng XG, You YH, Liu W, Zhao T, Qu H. MRI features of pigmented villonodular synovitis (PVNS). Clin Rheumatol 2004;23:31–34.
18. Goldman AB, DiCarlo EF. Pigmented villonodular synovitis: diagnosis and differential diagnosis. Radiol Clin North Am 1988;26:1327–1347.
19. Jaffe HL, Lichtenstein L, Sutro CJ. Pigmented villonodular synovitis, bursitis, and tenosynovitis. Arch Pathol 1941;31:731–765.
20. De Ponti A, Sansone V, Malchere M. Results of arthroscopic treatment of pigmented villonodular synovitis of the knee. Arthroscopy 2003;19:602–607.
21. Blanco CE, Leon HO, Guthrie TB. Combined partial arthroscopic synovectomy and radiation therapy for diffuse pigmented villonodular synovitis of the knee. Arthroscopy 2001;17:527–531.
22. Enneking WF. Clinical musculoskeletal pathology. 3rd ed. Gainesville, FL: University of Florida Press; 1990:243–250, 255–259, 312–317, 439–441.
23. Milgram JW. Synovial osteochondromatosis. J Bone Joint Surg Am 1977;59:792–801.
24. Trias A, Quintana O. Synovial chondrometaplasia: review of world literature and a study of 18 Canadian cases. Can J Surg 1976;19:151–158.
25. Coles MJ, Tara HH. Synovial chondromatosis: a case study and brief review. Am J Orthop 1997;26:37–40.
26. Crotty JM, Monu JU, Pope TL. Synovial osteochondromatosis. Radiol Clin North Am 1996;34:327–342.
27. Wuisman PI, Noorda RJ, Jutte PC. Chondrosarcoma secondary to chondromatosis. Report of two cases and a review of the literature. Arch Orthop Trauma Surg 1997;116:307–311.
28. Hopyan S, Nadesan P, Yu C, Wunder J, Alman BA. Dysregulation of hedgehog signaling predisposes to synovial chondromatosis. J Pathol 2005;206:143–150.
29. Laorr A, Helms CA. MRI of musculoskeletal masses. A practical text and atlas. New York: Igaku-Shoin; 1997:159–161, 275–280, 329–345.
30. Chen CY, Chen AC, Chang YH, Fu TS, Lee MS. Synovial chondromatosis of the hip: management with arthroscope-assisted synovectomy and removal of loose bodies: report of two cases. Chang Gung Med J 2003;26:208–214.
31. Fowble VA, Levy HJ. Arthroscopic treatment for synovial chondromatosis of the shoulder. Arthroscopy 2003;19:E2.
32. Campanacci M. Bone and soft tissue tumors. New York: Springer-Verlag; 1981:99–135, 1109–1126, 1243–1252, 1289–1306.
33. Kaakaji Y, Valle DE, McCarthy KE, Nietzschman HR. Case of the day. Case 4: synovial Sarcoma. AJR Am J Roentgenol 1998;171:868–870.
34. Namba Y, Kawai A, Naito N, Morimoto Y, Hanakawa S, Inoue H. Intraarticular synovial sarcoma confirmed by SYT-SSX fusion transcript. Clin Orthop 2002:221–226.
35. Machen KS, Easley KA, Goldblum JR. Synovial sarcoma of the extremities. A clinicopathologic study of 34 cases, including semi-quantitative analysis of spindles, epithelial, and poorly differentiated areas. Am J Surg Pathol 1999;23:268–275.
36. Pretto D, Barco R, Rivera J, Neel N, Gustavson MD, Eid JE. The synovial sarcoma translocation protein SYT-SSX2 recruits beta-catenin to the nucleus and associates with it in an active complex. Oncogene 2006;25:3661–3669.
37. Enzinger FM, Weiss SW. Soft tissue tumors. 2nd ed. St. Louis: Mosby; 1988:638–688, 861–881.

CHAPTER 31

Heritable Disorders of Connective Tissue

REED EDWIN PYERITZ, MD, PhD

- The genes that specify the hundreds of proteins involved in connective tissue have been mapped.
- The heritable disorders of connective tissue (HDCT) show both considerable variability within and among families and genetic heterogeneity.

- Phenotypes used: (1) disorders of fibrous elements, such as osteogenesis imperfecta and Marfan's syndrome, (2) disorders of proteogylcan metabolism, such as mucopolysaccharidoses, (3) dysostoses and osteochondrodysplasias, such as achondroplasia, and (4) inborn errors of metabolism, such as homocystinuria.

The molecular composition and organization of connective tissue, known as the *extracellular matrix*, are extraordinarily complex. Much remains unknown about the number, structure, map location, and regulation of genes that control synthesis, organization, and metabolism of this ubiquitous tissue. However, the genes that specify several hundred proteins involved in connective tissue metabolism and skeletal development have been mapped (1). Mutations in the genes for these proteins cause a variety of disorders. The heritable disorders of connective tissue (HDCT) follow Mendel's laws, but like many such disorders, show both considerable variability within and among families and genetic heterogeneity (2,3).

Some common disorders, such as osteoarthritis, osteoporosis, and aortic aneurysms, involve predominantly connective tissue and are mendelian in occasional families. For the majority of cases, however, multiple genes and other factors likely are important in cause and pathogenesis (4).

The phenotypic characterization of the HDCT, crude as it sometimes is, still outstrips biochemical or genetic understanding (5). More than 200 conditions are called HDCT. The more familiar ones have prevalences of 1 in 3000 to 1 in 50,000; many are less prevalent. More refined classification of the HDCT is unsatisfactory, and ultimately must be based on pathobiology. But several phenotypic groupings traditionally are used: (1) disorders of fibrous elements, such as osteogenesis imperfecta; (2) disorders of proteoglycan metabolism, including the mucopolysaccharidoses; (3) dysostoses and osteochondrodysplasias, such as achondcoplasia (see Chapter 35);

and (4) inborn errors of metabolism that secondarily affect connective tissue, such as homocystinuria and alkaptonuria. However, most of the features of Marfan syndrome, one of the preeminent disorders of a fibrous element, are now recognized as due to dysregulation of signaling because of impaired interaction between the latent transforming growth factor beta (TGF-beta) complex and the extracellular microfibril.

MARFAN SYNDROME

People with Marfan syndrome (MFS) have abnormalities in multiple organs and tissues, especially the skeletal, ocular, cardiovascular, pulmonary, and central nervous systems. Diagnosis is based primarily on clinical features and the autosomal dominant inheritance pattern (6). The basic defect in all cases studied is in fibrillin 1, the principal constituent of extracellular microfibrils (7). The locus (*FBN1*) for this protein maps to 15q21. Microfibrils are ubiquitous, 10 to 14 nm structures that, in conjunction with tropoelastin, form elastic fibers. Thus, fibrillin is a functionally important molecule in any organ containing elastic fibers, such as arteries, ligaments, and lung parenchyma. In other tissues, such as the zonular fibers of the eye, at the epidermal–dermal junction, and in the perichondrium, microfibrils are not associated with elastin. Thus, defective fibrillin is consistent with the pleiotropic manifestations of MFS.

In the past few years, considerable progress was made to understand the molecular and cellular pathogenesis of each manifestation in MFS, and to understand the cause and pathogenesis of other disorders related to MFS. Autosomal dominant ectopia lentis, autosomal dominant aortic aneurysm, and autosomal dominant tall stature are caused by mutations in *FBN1* in the absence of MFS (8). Congenital contractural arachnodactyly is due to mutations in *FBN2* on chromosome 5, a locus that specifies another member of the fibrillin family of proteins. Many of the features of MFS in a mouse model engineered with a human *FBN1* mutation are due to overexpression of TGF-beta during both development and growth (9,10). The latent TGF-beta–binding complex is held in check by normal microfibrils; mutant fibrillin 1 leads to dysregulation. Ectopia lentis may be the one feature that is indeed due to an abnormality of tensile strength of microfibrils.

Skeletal manifestations of MFS include excessive stature (11); abnormal body proportions with a long arm span and an abnormally low ratio of the upper segment to the lower segment (dolichostenomelia); elongated digits (arachnodactyly); anterior thoracic deformity (pectus excavatum, carinatum, or an asymmetric combination); abnormal vertebral column curvature (scoliosis, excessive kyphosis, or loss of thoracic kyphos resulting in "straight back"); hyperextensibility or, less often, congenital contractures of appendicular joints; protrusio acetabulae; and pes planus with a long, narrow foot. Most patients have myopia, and approximately half have subluxation of the lenses (ectopia lentis). The ascending aorta, beginning in the sinuses of Valsalva, gradually dilates in association with fragmentation of the medial elastic fibers; aortic regurgitation and dissection result and are the main causes of death. Mitral valve prolapse occurs in a majority and leads to severe mitral regurgitation in some, occasionally in childhood. Hernias are frequent; apical bullae lead to pneumothorax in 5%; and striae atrophicae over the pectoral, deltoid, and lumbar areas are a helpful diagnostic sign. Dural ectasia producing erosion of lower lumbar and sacral vertebrae usually is an incidental finding on computed tomography (CT) or magnetic resonance imaging (MRI), but may lead to pelvic meningoceles or radicular problems (12,13).

Management is both palliative and preventive. The size of the ascending aorta should be followed by echocardiography. beta-Adrenergic blockade is advisable to reduce stress on the aortic wall, and repair of the aortic root should be undertaken when the aortic diameter is greater than 50% expected (about 45–50 mm in the adult) (14,15). Scoliosis should be managed aggressively with bracing in the child and adolescent; when curvature exceeds about 40°, surgical stabilization should be considered (16). Hormonal advancement of pubarche can modulate excessive stature and reduce the time when vertebral curvature can worsen; this

therapy has been used occasionally in young girls, but rarely in boys. Most patients do not dislocate joints, but in those who do, the patella is the most common dislocation. People with MFS may be predisposed to develop degenerative arthropathy and osteoporosis in middle age. Women with MFS are at increased risk of aortic dissection and rupture during pregnancy; an aortic root diameter greater than 40 mm is a contraindication to pregnancy.

The mouse model of MFS responds in strikingly positive ways to the drug losartan, which in addition to its angiotensin receptor blocking action interferes with the action of TGF-beta (17). Clinical trials of losartan are underway in humans.

HOMOCYSTINURIA

Homocystinuria usually refers to an inborn error in the metabolism of methionine due to deficient activity of the enzyme cystathionine beta-synthase. Clinical features are similar superficially to those of MFS and include ectopia lentis, tall stature, dolichostenomelia, arachnodactyly, and anterior chest and spinal deformity (18). Generalized osteoporosis, "tight" joints, arterial and venous thrombosis, malar flush, mental retardation, and autosomal recessive inheritance are features of homocystinuria not consistent with MFS, whereas aortic aneurysm and mitral prolapse are not features of homocystinuria. Back pain and vertebral collapse due to osteoporosis occur in some patients. Most patients have no specific arthropathy.

The pathogeneses of the three cardinal manifestations—mental retardation, connective tissue disorder, and thrombosis—are not understood. One hypothesis holds that sulfhydryl groups of homocysteine and methionine interfere with collagen cross-linking. If true, this is a form of thiolism such as occurs from prolonged administration of penicillamine, a compound structurally similar to homocysteine. Fibrillin is rich in cysteine, and intra- and interchain disulfide bonds are crucial to the formation and function of microfibrils. Some of the phenotypic resemblance of homocystinuria to MFS may be due to disruption of microfibrils by the reactive sulfhydryl moiety of homocysteine (19).

Approximately one half of patients respond biochemically and clinically to large doses of vitamin B_6 (usually more than 50 mg pyridoxine per day), an obligate cofactor for cystathionine beta-synthase. Adequate levels of folate and vitamin B_{12} are required for therapeutic and biochemical response. Preexisting mental retardation and ectopia lentis are not reversed by pyridoxine treatment in patients who show biochemical correction, emphasizing the need for early diagnosis and therapy. Early diagnosis is feasible because many states include testing for elevated blood methionine as part of newborn screening. Unfortunately, some pyridoxine responders may escape detection in the typical screening protocols. In pyridoxine nonresponders, a low methionine diet and oral betaine therapy (to stimulate remethylation of homocysteine to methionine) are the usual treatments; this approach can be successful if the diet and vitamin are tolerated.

STICKLER SYNDROME

Stickler syndrome is a relatively common, autosomal dominant condition with severe, progressive myopia; vitreal degeneration; retinal detachment; progressive sensorineural hearing loss; cleft palate; mandibular hypoplasia; hyper- and hypomobility of joints; epiphyseal dysplasia; and potential disability from joint pain, dislocation, or degeneration (20). This condition, also called *progressive arthroophthalmopathy*, is underdiagnosed, in part due to patients often not having the full syndrome and in part due to the clinician's failure to obtain a detailed family history that might suggest a hereditary condition. The diagnosis should be strongly considered in any infant with congenitally enlarged ("swollen") wrists, knees, or ankles, particularly when associated with the Robin anomalad (hypognathia, cleft palate, and glossoptosis); any young adult with degenerative hip disease; and anyone suspected of MFS who has hearing loss, degenerative arthritis, or retinal detachment. The Stickler syndrome can be caused by mutations in at least four genes, three of which have been identified (21). Mutations in the alpha l(II) or the alpha 1(XI) procollagen loci (*COL2A1* and *COL11A2*, respectively) cause classic Stickler syndrome. These two genes are expressed in cartilage and the vitreous, in which both types II and XI collagen are prominent. A form of Stickler syndrome in which ocular features are absent is due to mutations in alpha 2(XI) procollagen (*COL11A2*); this protein is a component of type XI collagen only in cartilage and not in the vitreous. About two thirds of patients have mutations in *COL2A1*, typically ones that cause premature chain termination. Some families show genetic linkage to none of these three genes. Variability in clinical features among families is much more extensive than within a family, which likely reflects the genetic heterogeneity.

EHLERS–DANLOS SYNDROMES

The Ehlers–Danlos syndromes (EDS) are a group of disorders whose wide phenotypic variability is due largely to extensive genetic heterogeneity. The cardinal features relate to the joints and skin: hyperextensibility of skin, easy bruisability, increased joint mobility, and abnormal tissue fragility (22). Internal manifestations tend to occur only in specific types of EDS. Six main EDS types are accepted, based on phenotypic and inheritance characteristics (Table 31-1), but numerous other clinical types occur (23). Within individual types, however, biochemical studies have demonstrated considerable heterogeneity. Extensive phenotypic and biochemical characterization nonetheless fails the clinician as often as it helps; approximately one half of patients who have at least one "cardinal" feature defy categorization.

Ehlers–Danlos, Classical Type

People with classical type EDS (formerly, types I and II) have generalized hyperextensibility of joints and skin; bruisability and fragility of the skin, with gaping wounds from minor trauma; and poor retention of sutures. Congenital dislocation of the hips in the newborn, habitual dislocation of joints in later life, joint effusions, clubfoot, and spondylolisthesis are all consequences of loose jointedness. Hemarthrosis and "hemarthritic disability" have been described and are analogous to the bruisability of the skin in this syndrome. Scoliosis sometimes is severe. This type of EDS is inherited as an autosomal dominant trait with wide variability. Management of classical EDS stresses prevention of trauma and great care in treating wounds. Pregnancies of fetuses with EDS are prone to premature rupture of membranes. This form of EDS is genetically heterogenous, with mutations in *COL5A1* and *COL5A2* causing the phenotype in one half of cases (24). Heterozygosity for mutations in *COL1A1* can cause a classic EDS phenotype, often with mild features of osteogenesis imperfecta. Rare individuals with mutations in both *COL1A1* alleles have classic EDS with severe cardiovascular involvement.

Ehlers–Danlos, Hypermobility Type

Hypermobility type EDS (formerly type III) has less marked skin involvement than the classical form; joint hyperextensibility ranges from extreme to moderate. Many people with mild joint laxity and without joint instability are labeled as having this type, particularly if relatives show a similar manifestation (25). In some cases, such labeling does more harm than good, unless it is made quite clear that little disability, if any, is likely. A wide variety of biochemical and molecular abnormalities, including in type I and III collagen and tenascin-X, have been reported in patients with this broad phenotype (26).

Ehlers–Danlos, Vascular Type

Vascular type EDS (formerly type IV) is by far the most serious type because of a propensity for spontaneous

31

TABLE 31-3. MUCOPOLYSACCHARIDOSES.

DISORDER OMIM NUMBER[a] EPONYM	CLINICAL MANIFESTATIONS	GENETICS	URINARY MPS	ENZYME DEFICIENCY	LOCUS
MPS I 252800		AR	Dermatan sulfate; heparin sulfate	alpha-L-iduronidase; IDUA	4p16.3
MPS IH Hurler	Coarse facies; severe DM; clouding of cornea; progressive MR; death usually before 10 years				
MPS IS Scheie	Stiff joints; cloudy cornea; aortic valve disease; normal intelligence; survival to adulthood				
MPS IH/S Hurler–Scheie	Intermediate phenotype				
MPS II 309900		XL	Dermatan sulfate; heparin sulfate	Iduronate 2-sulfatase; IDS	Xq28
Hunter, severe	No corneal clouding, otherwise similar to MPS IH; death before 15 years				
Hunter, mild	Stiff joints; survival to 30s–60s; fair intelligence				
MPS IIIA 252900 Sanfilippo A	Mild physical features and DM; severe progressive MR	AR	Heparan sulfate	Heparan N-sulfatase (sulfamidase)	17q25.3
MPS IIIB 252930 Sanfilippo B	Indistinguishable from MPS IIIA	AR	Heparan sulfate	N-acetyle-alpha-D-glucosamindase; NAGLU	SGSH 17q21
MPSIIIC 252930 Sanfilippo C	Indistinguishable from MPS IIIA	AR	Heparan sulfate	Acetyl-CoA-alpha-glucosaminide; N-acetyltransferase; MPS3C	14
MPS IIID 252940 Sanfilippo D	Indistinguishable from MPS IIIA	AR	Heparan sulfate	N-acetylglucosamine-6-sulfate sulfatase; GNS	12q14
MPS IVA 253000 Morquio A	Severe, distinctive bone changes; cloudy cornea; aortic regurgitation; thin enamel	AR	Keratan sulfate	Galactosamine-6-sulfate; GALNS	16Q24.3
MPS IVB 253010 Morquio B (O'Brien–Arbisser)	Mild bone changes; cloudy cornea; hypoplastic odontoid; normal enamel	AR	Keratan sulfate	beta$_1$-galactosidase; GLB1	3p21.33
MPS V	No longer used				
MPS VI 253200 Maroteaux–Lamy		AR	Dermatan sulfate	Arylsufatase B (N-acetyl-galactosamine 4-sulfatase	5q11–q13
Severe	Severe DM and corneal clouding; valvular heart disease; striking WBC inclusions; normal intellect; survival to 20s				
Intermediate	Same spectrum as severe, but milder				
Mild	Same spectrum as severe, but mild				
MPS VII 253230	DM; progressive MR; WBC inclusions; hepatosplenomegaly	AR	Dermatan sulfate; heparin sulfate	beta$_1$-glucuronidase; GUSB	7q21.11
MPS VIII 253230	No longer used				
MPS IX 601492	Short stature; progressive soft tissue and periarticular accumulations of hyaluroran	AR	Hyaluroran	Hyaluronidase; HYAL1	3p21.3–p21.2

ABBREVIATIONS: AD, autosomal dominant; AR, autosomal recessive; DM, dysostosis multiplex; MR, mental retardation; OMIM, Online Mendelian Inheritance in Man; WBC, white blood cell; XL, X-linked.
[a] Entry in Online Mendelian Inheritance in Man (1).

defect in degradation of mucopolysaccharides. Both are autosomal recessive and genetically heterogeneous. The basic biochemical defect is an enzyme responsible for posttranslational modification of lysosomal enzymes. This defect results in multiple enzyme deficiencies and accumulation in tissues of both mucopolysaccharides and mucolipids.

Mucopolysacchariduria can be identified by one of several standard screening tests, at least one of which is part of the standard battery performed when a metabolic screen is ordered. Fractionation and characterization of the urinary mucopolysaccharides are useful in separating the several types of disorders, but enzymatic assay may be needed for diagnostic confirmation. Prenatal diagnosis by biochemical or molecular genetic methods is possible.

Like other lysosomal disorders, the mucopolysaccharide and mucolipid disorders have distinctive characteristics: (1) intracellular storage occurs; (2) storage material is heterogeneous because the degradative enzymes are not strictly specific; (3) deposition is vacuolar on electron microscopy; (4) many tissues are affected; and (5) the disorders are clinically progressive. Therapy by replacing the enzyme that is deficient is possible, but technically difficult and of transient benefit. Bone marrow transplant is effective in the disorders lacking central nervous system involvement, and it is being investigated in patients with mental retardation (43). Enzyme replacement therapy is available for MPS type I (44) and is in clinical trials for several other types.

REFERENCES

1. Online Mendelian Inheritance in Man OMIM. McKusick-Nathons Institute for Genetic Medicine, Johns Hopkins University (Baltimore), and National Center for Biotechnology Information, National Library of Medicine (Bethesda, MD). Available at: http://www.ncbi.nlm.nih.gov/omim.
2. Royce PM, Steinmann B, eds. Connective tissue and its heritable disorders: molecular, genetic and medical aspects. 2nd ed. New York: Wiley-Liss; 2001.
3. Rimoin DR, Connor JM, Pyeritz RE, Korf BR, eds. Principles and practice of medical genetics. 5th ed. New York: Elsevier; 2007.
4. Pyeritz RE. Common structural disorders of connective tissue. In: King RA, Rotter JI, Motulsky AG, eds. The genetic basis of common diseases. 2nd ed. New York: Oxford University Press; 2001.
5. Beighton P, de Paepe A, Danks D, et al. International nosology of heritable disorders of connective tissue, Berlin, 1986. Am J Med Genet 1988;29:581–594.
6. DePaepe A, Deitz HC, Devereux RB, Hennekem R, Pyeritz RE. Revised diagnostic criteria for the Marfan syndrome. Am J Med Genet 1996;62:417–426.
7. Loeys B, Nuytinck L, Delvaux I, et al. Genotype and phenotype analysis of 171 patients referred for molecular study of the fibrillin-1 gene FBN1 because of suspected Marfan syndrome. Arch Intern Med 2001;161:2447–2454.
8. Pyeritz RE. Marfan syndrome and other disorders of fibrillins. In: Rimoin DL, Connor JM, Pyeritz RE, Korf B, eds. Principles and practice of medical genetics. 5th ed. New York: Elsevier; 2007, Chapter 149.
9. Neptune ER, Frischmeyer PA, Arking DE, et al. Dysregulation of TGF-beta activation contributes to pathogenesis in Marfan syndrome. Nat Genet 2003;33: 407–411.
10. Ng CM, Cheng A, Myers LA, et al. TGF-beta-dependent pathogenesis of mitral valve prolapse in a mouse model of Marfan syndrome. J Clin Invest 2004;114:1543–1546.
11. Erkula G, Jones KB, Sponseller PD, Dietz HC, Pyeritz RE. Growth and maturation in Marfan syndrome. Am J Med Genet 2002;109:100–115.
12. Pyeritz RE, Fishman EK, Bernhardt BA, Siegelman SS. Dural ectasia is a common feature of the Marfan syndrome. Am J Hum Genet 1988;43:726–732.
13. Foran JR, Pyeritz RE, Dietz HC, Sponseller PD. Characterization of the symptoms associated with dural ectasia in the Marfan patient. Am J Med Genet A 2005;134: 58–65.
14. Gott VL, Greene PS, Alejo DE, et al. Replacement of the aortic root in patients with Marfan's syndrome. N Engl J Med 1999;340:1307–1313.
15. Miller DC. Valve-sparing aortic root replacement in patients with the Marfan syndrome. J Thorac Cardiovasc Surg 2003;125:773–778.
16. Sponseller PD, Hobbs W, Riley LH III, Pyeritz HE. The thoracolumbar spine in Marfan syndrome. J Bone Joint Surg Am 1995;77:867–876.
17. Habashi JP, Judge DP, Holm TM, et al. Losartan, an AT1 antagonist, prevents aortic aneurysm in a mouse model of Marfan syndrome. Science 2006;312:117–121.
18. Pyeritz, RE. Homocystinuria. In: Beighton P, ed. McKusick's heritable disorders of connective tissue. 5th ed. St. Louis: Mosby; 1993:137–178.
19. Majors A, Pyeritz RE. Deficiency of cysteine impairs deposition of fibrillin-1: implications for the pathogenesis of cystathionine β-synthase deficiency. Mol Genet Metab 2000;70:252–260.
20. Rose PS, Levy HP, Liberfarb RM, et al. Stickler syndrome: clinical characteristics and diagnostic criteria. Am J Med Genet 2005;138A:199–207.
21. Richards AJ, Baguley DM, Yates JR, et al. Variation in the vitreous phenotype of Stickler syndrome can be caused by different amino acid substitutions in the X position of the type II collagen Gly-X-Y triple helix. Am J Hum Genet 2000;67:1083–1094.
22. Byers PH. The Ehlers-Danlos syndromes. In: Rimoin DL, Connor J, Pyeritz RE, Korf B, eds. Principles and practice of medical genetics. 5th ed. New York: Elsevier; 2007, Chapter 149.
23. Beighton P, De Paepe A, Steinmann B, Tsipouras P, Wenstrup RJ. Ehlers-Danlos syndromes: revised nosology, Villefranche, 1997. Am J Med Genet 1998;77:31–37.
24. Malfait F, Coucke P, Symoens S, et al. The molecular basis of classic Ehlers-Danlos syndrome: a comprehensive study of biochemical and molecular findings in 48 unrelated patients. Hum Mutat 2005;25:28–37.

31

25. Grahame R. Time to take hypermobility seriously (in adults and children). Rheumatology 2001;40:485–487.

26. Zweers MC, Dean WB, van Kuppevelt TH, et al. Elastic fiber abnormalities in hypermobility type Ehlers-Danlos syndrome patients with tenascin-X mutations. Clin Genet 2005;67:330–334.

27. Pepin M, Schwarze U, Superti-Furga A, Byers PH. Clinical and genetic features of Ehlers-Danlos syndrome type IV. The vascular type. N Engl J Med 2000;342:673–680.

28. Malfait F, De Coster P, Hausser I, et al. The natural history, including orofacial features of three patients with Ehlers-Danlos syndrome, dermatosparaxis type (EDS type VIIC). Am J Med Genet 2004;131A:18–28.

29. Horton WA, Collins DL, DeSmet AA, Kennedy JA, Schmike RN. Familial joint instability syndrome. Am J Med Genet 1980;6:221–228.

30. Sillence D. Osteogenesis imperfecta. In: Rimoin DL, Connor JM, Pyeritz RE, Korf B, eds. Principles and practice of medical genetics. 5th ed. New York: Elsevier; 2007, Chapter 149.

31. Hartikka H, Kuurila K, Korkko J, et al. Lack of correlation between the type of COL1A1 or COL1A2 mutation and hearing loss in osteogenesis imperfecta patients. Hum Mutat 2004;24:147–154.

32. Rauch F, Plotkin H, Travers R, et al. Osteogenesis imperfecta types I, III, and IV: effect of pamidronate therapy on bone and mineral metabolism. J Clin Endocr Metab 2003;88:986–992.

33. Zeitlin L, Rauch F, Plotkin H, Glorieux FH. Height and weight development during four years of therapy with cyclical intravenous pamidronate in children and adolescents with osteogenesis imperfecta types I, III, and IV. Pediatrics 2003;111:1030–1036.

34. Lindsay R. Modeling the benefits of pamidronate in children with osteogenesis imperfecta. J Clin Invest 2002;110:1239–1231.

35. Horowitz EM, Gordon PL, Koo WK, et al. Isolated allogeneic bone marrow-derived mesenchymal cells engraft and stimulate growth in children with osteogenesis imperfecta: implications for cell therapy of bone. Proc Natl Acad Sci U S A 2002;99:8932–8937.

36. Uitto J. Inherited abnormalities of elastic tissue. In: Rimoin DL, Connor JM, Pyeritz RE, Korf B, eds. Principles and practice of medical genetics. 5th ed. New York: Elsevier; 2007, Chapter 149.

37. Bergen AA, Plomp AS, Schuurman EJ, et al. Mutations in ABCC6 cause pseudoxanthoma elasticum. Nat Genet 2000;25:228–231.

38. Miksch S, Lumsden A, Guenther UP, et al. Molecular genetics of pseudoxanthoma elasticum: type and frequency of mutations in ABCC6. Hum Mutat 2005;26:235–248.

39. Smith R, Athanasou NA, Vipond SE. Fibrodysplasia (myositis) ossifans progressiva: clinicopathological features and natural history. QJM 1996;89:445–446.

40. Shore EM, Xu M, Feldman GJ, et al. A recurrent mutation of the BMP type I receptor ACVR1 causes inherited and sporadic fibrodysplasia ossificans progressive. Nat Genet 2006;38:525–527.

41. Neufeld EE, Muenzer J. The mucopolysaccharidoses. In: Scriver CR, Beaudet AL, Sly WS, Valle D, eds. Metabolic basis of inherited disease. 8th ed. New York: McGraw-Hill; 2001:3421–3452.

42. Kornfield S, Sly WS. I-cell disease and pseudo-hurler polydystrophy: disorders of lysosomal enzyme phosphorylation. In: Scriver CR, Beaudet AL, Sly WS, Valle D, eds. The metabolic and molecular bases of inherited disease. 8th ed. New York: McGraw-Hill; 200l.

43. Staba SL, Escolar ML, Poe M, et al. Cord-blood transplants from unrelated donors in patients with Hurler's syndrome. N Engl J Med 2004;350:1960–1969.

44. Kakkis ED, Muenzer J, Tiller GE, et al. Enzyme-replacement therapy in mucopolysaccharidosis I. N Engl J Med 2001;344:182–188.

CHAPTER 32

Bone and Joint Dysplasias

William A. Horton, MD

- Chondrodysplasias are inherited disorders of cartilage that affect its function as a template for bone growth.
- Problems common to many chondrodysplasias are respiratory distress, osteoarthritis of the weight-bearing joints, dental crowding, obesity, obstetrical difficulties, and psychological issues due to short stature.
- The osteochondroses are a heterogeneous group of disorders in which localized non-inflammatory arthropathies result from regional disturbances of skeletal growth.

Bone dysplasias are a broad group of conditions in which skeletal development and function are disturbed. They include the chondrodysplasias and osteochondroses discussed in this chapter, as well as osteodysplasias, such as osteogenesis imperfecta syndromes (discussed in Chapter 31), and many others that are either extremely rare or of little relevance to rheumatology.

CHONDRODYSPLASIAS

The term *chondrodysplasia*—literally, abnormal (*dys*) cartilage (*chondro*) growth (*plasia*)—is used to designate inherited disorders of cartilage that affect its function as a template for bone growth (1). The clinical picture is typically dominated by varying degrees of dwarfism and bone and joint deformities. However, because the genes that harbor chondrodysplasia mutations are often not specific to bone growth, the clinical manifestations frequently extend to other cartilages, such as articular cartilage, and to other tissues (1–3).

Pathogenesis

Most bones develop and grow through the process of endochondral ossification, in which cartilage serves as a template for bone formation. In postembryonic growing bone, ossification occurs in the growth plate residing near the ends of bones (4). Growth plates have a leading and trailing edge. In essence, template cartilage is synthesized de novo at the leading edge, whereas it is degraded and replaced by an expanding front of bone at the trailing edge. Endochondral ossification accounts for linear bone growth from mid-gestation through the end of puberty.

The chondrodysplasias result from mutations in genes that encode the structural proteins of cartilage matrix and proteins that regulate growth plate function, including growth factors, receptors, and transcription factors. These proteins, which contribute to different aspects of endochondral ossification, are required for bone growth to proceed in a normal fashion (4,5). Although poorly understood, the different types of chondrodysplasias reflect the functional consequences of disturbances in these proteins with regard to bone growth and other clinical manifestations.

Classification

Well over 100 clinical forms of chondrodysplasia are currently recognized. Based on their differences in clinical presentation, characteristic appearances of skeletal radiographs, growth plate histology, and pattern of inheritance, these disorders have been grouped over the past decade into classes which correspond in many instances to a common gene that is mutated (1,6). A well-defined chondrodysplasia class, such as the achondroplasia or spondyloepiphyseal dysplasia (SED) class, typically contains a group of disorders ranging in severity from lethal at or around birth to very mild, often blending into the normal (nonchondrodysplasia) population. The current classification scheme is based primarily on molecular genetics, but the genetic basis of many disorders has yet to be determined. Consequently, the scheme continues to evolve.

Diagnosis

A few conditions, such as achondroplasia, can be diagnosed simply by seeing a patient. However, the

TABLE 32-1. SALIENT FEATURES OF SELECTED CHONDRODYSPLASIAS.

CLASS AND DISORDER	OMIM	INHERITANCE	GENE LOCUS	OVERALL SEVERITY	RHEUMATOLGIC COMPLICATIONS
Achondroplasia					
Thanatophoric dysplasia	187600/187610	AD	FGFR3	Lethal	
Achondroplasia	100800	AD	FGFR3	++/+++	Arthralgias
Hypochondroplasia	146000	AD	FGFR3	+	
Spondyloephiphyseal dysplasia (SED)					
Achondrogenesis type II	200610	AD	COL2A1	Lethal	
Hypochondrogenesis	14600	AD	COL2A1	Lethal	
SED congenita	183900	AD	COL2A1	+++	Precocious OA
Kniest dysplasia	156550	AD	COL2A1	+++	Contractures, precocious OA
Stickler dysplasia	108300	AD	COL2A1	++	Precocious OA
Stickler-like dysplasia	184840	AD	COL11A1	++	Precocious OA
Stickler-like dysplasia	184850	AR	COL11A2	++	Precocious OA
SED late onset		AD	COL2A1	+	Precocious OA
SED tarda	313400	XLR	SEDL	+	Precocious OA
Multiple epiphyesal dysplasia (MED)/pseudoachondroplasia					
MED	600969	AD	COMP	+++	Arthralgias, precocious OA
Pseudoachondroplasia	177170	AD	COMP	+++	Arthralgias, precocious OA
Diastrophic dysplasia					
Achondrogenesis type 1B	600972	AR	DTDST	Lethal	
Ateleosteogenesis type II	256050	AR	DTDST	Lethal	
Diastrophic dysplasia	222600	AR	DTDST	+++	Precocious OA, contractures
Metaphyseal chondrodysplasia					
Jansen type	156400	AD	PTHR1	+++	Contractures
Schmid type	156500	AD	COL10A1	++	
McKusick type	250250	AR	RMPR	+++	
Metatropic dysplasia					
Metatropic dysplasia	250600	AD	Unknown	+++	Contractures
Chondrodysplasia punctata					
Rhizomelic type	215100	AR	ACDPA	Lethal	Contractures
X-linked recessive type (CDPX1)	302950	XLR	ARSE	+++	
X-linked dominant type (CDPX2)	302960	XLD	EBP	++/+++	Contractures
Brachyolmia					
Hobaek type	271530	AR	Unknown	++	Arthralgia, stiffness in hip, back
Maroteaux type		AR	Unknown	++	Arthralgia, stiffness in hip, back
Autosomal dominant type	113500	AD	Unknown	++	Arthralgia, stiffness in hip, back

ABBREVIATIONS: *ACDPA,* acetyl-CoA dihydroxyacetone phosphate acetyltransferase; AD, autosomal dominant; AR, autosomal recessive; *ARSE,* arylsulfatase E; *COL10A1,* type X collagen alpha I chain; *COL11A1,* type XI collagen alpha I chain; *COL11A2,* type XI collagen alpha 2 chain; *COL2A1,* type II collagen alpha I chain; *COMP,* cartilage oligomeric matrix protein; *DTDST,* diastrophic dysplasia sulfate transporter; *EBP,* delta(8)-delta(7) sterol isomerase emopamil-binding protein; FGFR3, fibroblast growth factor receptor 3; OA, osteoarthritis; *PTHR1,* parathyroid hormone–related protein receptor 1; *RMPR,* RNA component of mitochondrial RNA processing endoribonuclease; XLD, X-linked dominant; XLR, X-linked recessive.
OMIM refers to Online Mendelian Inheritance of Man, which provides extensive references (http://www.ncbi.nlm.nih.gov/omim).

diagnosis is usually based on recognizing a unique combination of clinical, radiographic, and genetic features (1–3,7). Because the clinical features typically evolve over time, the natural history must be taken into account when patients are evaluated. The most useful information usually comes from skeletal radiographs; specific radiologic diagnostic criteria have been developed (7–10). Like the clinical picture, radiographic characteristics change with age. Films taken before puberty are usually more informative because the radiographic hallmarks of many disorders disappear after closure of the epiphyses. In fact, it is often difficult to make a specific diagnosis from postpubertal radiographs. Because many patients are the first and only known case in a family, a pedigree may be of little help as the inheritance pattern cannot be determined. Nevertheless, a family history sometimes provides critical clues toward a diagnosis.

Historically, laboratory tests have not been useful in diagnosing chondrodysplasias. However, as the mutations are being better defined, genetic testing may be helpful in disorders caused by a recurrent mutation in the population, as is the case with achondroplasia and perhaps in some forms of late-onset SED associated with precocious osteoarthritis. Although histologic evaluation of growth plate specimens often reveals characteristic changes, biopsy is seldom warranted as the diagnosis can usually be made by other means.

Salient features of the more common chondrodysplasias are summarized in Table 32-1 (6), and additional information can be found in several recent reviews (1,2,5,7,11). The most up-to-date information and references are available through the Online Mendelian Inheritance in Man, developed by McKusick and colleagues (http://www.ncbi.nlm.nih.gov/omim/).

CLASSIFICATION OF CHONDRODYSPLASIAS

Achondroplasias

This class of autosomal dominant disorders includes the following: thanatophoric dysplasia, the most common chondrodysplasia lethal in the perinatal period; achondroplasia, by far the most common nonlethal chondrodysplasia; and hypochondroplasia. Although the three differ substantially in severity, the features of each are qualitatively similar. Heterozygous mutations of the gene encoding fibroblast growth factor receptor 3 (FGFR3) have been identified in all three conditions.

Achondroplasia

The prototype of short-limb dwarfism, achondroplasia is recognizable at birth by a long narrow trunk, short limbs (especially proximally), and a large head with prominent forehead and hypoplasia of the mid-face. Most joints are hyperextensible, especially the knees, but elbow mobility is limited. The most serious problems are related to a small spinal canal, especially at the foramen magnum level. This anomaly contributes to hypotonia, failure to thrive, developmental delay, apnea, and even quadriparesis and sudden death in some infants. Common childhood problems include middle-ear infections, dental crowding, and bowing of the legs.

The lifespan is normal in the absence of life-threatening neurologic problems in early life. In adulthood, men reach an average height of 132 cm (about 45 inches) and women, 124 cm (about 40 inches). Pain is common in weight-bearing joints, probably due to misalignment of bones aggravated by physical activity and by obesity, which is common. However, people with achondroplasia rarely develop osteoarthritis. Stenosis of the lumbar spine may cause paresthesias, claudication and numbness of the legs, and bowel and bladder dysfunction.

Pregnant women with achondroplasia need to be monitored carefully and delivered by cesarean section. Because of the high prevalence of heterozygous achondroplasia in the short-stature community, people with this condition often marry; their offspring have a 25% risk for inheriting the much more severe homozygous achondroplasia.

Hypochondroplasia

Not usually recognized until mid- to late childhood, patients with hypochondroplasia appear to have "mild" achondroplasia with short limbs (mostly the proximal segments), a stocky build, and a normal or slightly enlarged head. The natural history is usually unremarkable other than for mild short (approximately 5' or less) stature. The true incidence of hypochondroplasia is unknown; because its features are mild, it may often escape detection.

Spondyloepiphyseal Dysplasias

Spondyloepiphyseal dysplasia (SED) is a large, diverse class of autosomal dominant disorders with clinical features that reflect varying degrees of dysfunction of type II collagen, the principal structural protein of cartilage. In severe forms, many types of cartilage and other tissues containing type II collagen are affected, whereas in milder forms, only articular cartilage is involved.

Spondyloepiphyseal Dysplasia Congenita

This form of dysplasia is the prototype of short trunk dwarfism. Neonates with SED congenita have a short

32

neck, a short barrel-shaped trunk, and sometimes cleft palate and club foot. The proximal limbs are short, but the hands, feet, head, and face appear to be normal in size. The shortening becomes more prominent with time. Scoliosis commonly develops in childhood and may cause respiratory compromise. Odontoid hypoplasia may predispose to cervicomedullary instability and spinal cord compression, but sudden death is uncommon. Osteoarthritis, especially of the hips and knees, typically appears in the third decade. Severe myopia is common, and retinal detachment may occur in older children and adults. Adults range in height from 95 to 128 cm (about 35 to 50 inches).

Kniest Dysplasia

At birth, infants with Kniest dysplasia have a short trunk and limbs and a flat face with prominent eyes. Their fingers are long and knobby, and many have club foot and cleft palate. The most debilitating aspect is the progressive enlargement of joints during childhood, which is associated with painful contractures and, eventually, with osteoarthritis. Hearing loss is common, as is severe myopia that is often complicated by retinal detachment.

Stickler Dysplasia

The clinical picture of Stickler dysplasia is dominated by ocular problems. Severe myopia is usually present at birth, together with cleft palate and a small jaw. Retinal detachment may occur during childhood, as may choroidoretinal and vitreous degeneration. Sensorineural hearing loss often develops during adolescence. Osteoarthritis typically begins during the second or third decade of life. Short stature is not a feature of Stickler dysplasia; indeed, some patients exhibit a Marfan-type habitus and joint laxity. A dysplasia similar to Stickler dysplasia may arise from mutations of genes encoding type XI collagen.

Late-Onset Spondyloepiphyseal Dysplasia

Some type II collagen mutations manifest primarily as precocious osteoarthritis of weight-bearing joints. Radiographs usually reveal subtle changes of SED, but many of these patients are of normal stature and have no other abnormalities. The term *familial* (or *autosomal dominant*) *osteoarthritis* is sometimes used to describe this syndrome. Recurrent mutations of the type II collagen gene have been observed in a few instances of familial osteoarthritis. Mutations of an X-linked gene encoding a protein termed "sedlin" can produce a similar but distinct clinical picture in males, which is called SED tarda.

Multiple Epiphyseal Dysplasia and Pseudoachondroplasia

Multiple epiphyseal dysplasia (MED) and pseudoachondroplasia are classified together because mutations in the cartilage oligomeric matrix protein (COMP) gene have been found in both disorders.

The Fairbank type of MED is usually diagnosed in childhood because of moderately short limbs, a waddling gait, and painful joints. Radiographs show generalized epiphyseal involvement. The Ribbing type of MED may not be detected until adolescence. Because involvement is typically restricted to the proximal femurs, the Ribbing type is often confused with bilateral Legg–Calvé–Perthes disease. Both types of MED are associated with moderately short stature (145–170 cm) and osteoarthritis of weight-bearing joints.

Pseudoachondroplasia typically presents in the second or third year of life with a dramatic slowing of bone growth accompanied by a waddling gait and generalized joint laxity. The head and face appear normal, but the hands are short and broad, and ulnar deviation occurs. The growth deficiency worsens with age. Major complications are related to excessive joint mobility, most notably involving the knees, where it produces various deformities. Osteoarthritis of the hips and knees is common.

Diastrophic Dysplasia

Diastrophic dysplasia is usually apparent at birth. Infants display very short extremities and distinctive hands with short digits and proximal displacement of the thumb (hitchhiker thumb). There may be bony fusion of metacarpophalangeal joints producing symphalangism and ulnar deviation of the hands. Cleft palate and club foot are common. The external ears often become inflamed soon after birth; healing results in small, fibrotic ears (cauliflower deformity). Scoliosis and multiple joint contractures usually begin during childhood and are typically progressive and severe. Adult height varies from 105 to 130 cm (40–44 inches).

Metaphyseal Chondrodysplasias

The metaphyseal chondrodysplasias (MCDs) are a heterogeneous group of disorders that share radiographic involvement of the metaphyses. However, studies have shown that they do not share a common genetic basis.

Jansen Metaphyseal Chondrodysplasias

Severely shortened limbs, prominent forehead, and small jaw are present at birth. Some infants have club foot and hypercalcemia. Joints enlarge and become restricted during childhood. Flexion contractures at the hips and knees often result in a bent-over posture.

Schmid Metaphyseal Chondrodysplasias

This disorder usually becomes apparent at age 2 to 3 years because of mild shortening of the limbs, especially the legs (which are bowed), a waddling gait, and sometimes hip pain. Adults are of mildly short stature and have few problems.

McKusick Metaphyseal Chondrodysplasias

Also called cartilage–hair hypoplasia, the McKusick type MCD manifests at age 2 to 3 years as growth deficiency. It is characterized by short limbs, bowed legs, and flaring of the lower rib cage. Hands and feet are short and broad, and fingers are short and stubby. Ligamentous laxity is marked. The hair tends to be blond and thin, and the skin is lightly pigmented. Some patients have associated problems, including immune deficiency, anemia, Hirschsprung's disease, and malabsorption. Adults exhibit marked dwarfism and are predisposed to certain infections and malignancies of the skin and lymphoid tissue.

Metatropic Dysplasia

Newborn infants with metatropic dysplasia have short limbs and a long narrow trunk. Kyphoscoliosis, which starts during late infancy or early childhood, may cause cardiorespiratory problems. Odontoid hypoplasia is common. Most joints become large and have restricted mobility, and contractures often develop at the hips and knees.

Chondrodysplasia Punctata

Disorders classified as chondrodysplasia punctata (CDP) share the radiographic finding of stippled epiphyses, but specific features differ substantially.

Rhizomelic Chondrodysplasia Punctata

At birth, rhizomelic CDP is evidenced by severe and symmetric shortening of limbs, multiple joint contractures, cataracts, ichthyosiform rash, absent hair, microcephaly, and flat face with hypoplasia of the nasal tip. These infants fail to thrive and usually die during the first year.

X-Linked Chondrodysplasia Punctata

Chondrodysplasia punctata may be X-linked dominant or recessive. The recessive form, CDPX1, is symmetric and severe, whereas the dominant form, CDPX2 is relatively mild and asymmetric in distribution. Varying degrees of contractures, cataracts, skin rash, and hair loss are found in CDPX2. The asymmetry may worsen and scoliosis may develop over time, but patients with CDPX2 usually have a normal life span.

Brachyolmia

Three types of brachyolmia are recognized, all of which have similar clinical features (Table 32-1). They present in early to mid-childhood with mildly short stature mainly involving the trunk. Back and hip pain typically arise during adolescence and continue into adulthood. Back stiffness is common and some patients develop scoliosis.

JUVENILE OSTEOCHONDROSES

The juvenile osteochondroses summarized in Table 32-2 are a heterogeneous group of disorders in which localized non-inflammatory arthropathies result from regional disturbances of skeletal growth (12,13). Children may present with painless limitation of movement

TABLE 32-2. JUVENILE OSTEOCHONDROSES.

REGION AFFECTED	EPONYM	TYPICAL AGE AT PRESENTATION	SEX PREDILECTION
Capital femoral epiphysis	Legg–Calvé–Perthes disease, coxa plana	3–12 years	Male
Tibial tubercle	Osgood–Schlatter disease	10–16 years	None
Os calcis	Sever's disease	6–10 years	None
Head of second metatarsal	Freiberg's disease	10–14 years	None
Vertebral bodies	Scheuermann's disease	Adolescence	Male
Medial aspect of proximal tibial epiphysis	Blount disease, tibia vara	Infancy or adolescence	None
Subchondral areas of diarthroidal joints (particularly knee, hip, elbow and ankle)	Osteochondritis dissecans	10–20 years	Male

of affected joints (such as in Legg–Calvé–Perthes disease and Scheuermann's disease) or with local pain and sometimes tenderness and swelling (such as in Freiberg's disease, Osgood–Schlatter disease, and osteochondritis dissecans). Bone growth may be altered to produce deformities, such as bowing of the tibia in Blount's disease.

The diagnosis of juvenile osteochondrosis can usually be confirmed radiographically, and magnetic resonance imaging is sometimes useful to define the lesions. The pathogenesis is thought to involve ischemic necrosis of primary or secondary endochondral ossification centers. Some cases may be related to stress and injury. Most of these disorders occur sporadically, but familial forms have been described.

MANAGEMENT OF BONE AND JOINT DYSPLASIAS

No definitive treatment is available to counter defective bone growth for any of the bone and joint dysplasias. Consequently, management is directed at prevention and correction of skeletal deformities and preventing nonskeletal complications. Management is guided by knowledge of the natural history of these disorders, so that disorder-specific problems can be anticipated and treated early.

A number of problems are common to many chondrodysplasias, including respiratory distress, osteoarthritis of weight-bearing joints, dental crowding, obesity, obstetrical difficulties, and psychological problems related to short stature. General recommendations can be made to address these problems (1,3). For example, most patients with a chondrodysplasia should avoid contact sports and other activities that traumatize or stress joints. Joint replacement is often necessary for progressive osteoarthritis. Dietary control should be instituted during childhood to prevent obesity in adulthood. Dental care should be started in early childhood to manage crowding and misalignment effectively. Because of their small pelvic bones, pregnant women with most chondrodysplasias should be managed in high-risk prenatal clinics and, in many instances, have their babies delivered by cesarean section. Intelligence is usually normal in the nonlethal chondrodysplasias, but because patients are so easily recognized as being "different" from their peers, they and their families often benefit from support provided by lay groups, such as the Little People of America and the Human Growth Foundation, and from publications directed to the lay population (11). Useful lay information is also available through websites such as http://www.lpaonline.org/.

REFERENCES

1. Horton WA, Hecht JT. The chondrodysplasias: general concepts and diagnostic and management considerations. In: Royce PM, Steinman B, eds. Connective tissue and its heritable disorders. 2nd ed. New York: Wiley-Liss; 2002: 641–676.
2. Rimoin D, Lachman R, Unger S. Chondrodysplasias. In: Rimoin DS, Connor JM, Pyeritz RE, Korf BR, eds. Emery and Rimoin's principles and practice of medical genetics. 4th ed. London: Churchill Livingstone; 2002:4071–4115.
3. Sponseller PD, Ain MC. The skeletal dysplasias. In Morrissy RT, Weinstein SL, eds. Lovell & Winter's pediatric orthopaedics. 6th ed. Philadelphia: Lippincott Williams & Wilkins; 2006:205–250.
4. Morris NP, Keene DR, Horton WA. Biology of extracellular matrix: cartilage. In Royce PM, Steinman B, eds. Connective tissue and its heritable disorders. 2nd ed. New York: Wiley-Liss; 2002:41–66.
5. Horton WA. Molecular genetic basis of the human chondrodysplasias. Endocrinol Metab Clin North Am 1996;25: 683–697.
6. Hall CM. International nosology and classification of constitutional disorders of bone (2001). Am J Med Genet 2002;113:65–77.
7. Spranger J, Maroteaux P. The lethal osteochondrodysplasias. Adv Hum Genet 1995;19:1–103.
8. Spranger JW, Brill PW, Poznanski A. Bone dysplasias, an atlas of genetic disorders of skeletal development. 2nd ed. New York: Oxford University Press; 2002.
9. Wynne-Davies R, Hall CM, Apley AG. Atlas of skeletal dysplasias. Edinburgh: Churchill Livingstone; 1985.
10. Tabyi H, Lachman RS. Radiology of syndromes, metabolic disorders, and skeletal dysplasias. 4th ed. St. Louis: Mosby; 1996.
11. Scott CI Jr, Mayeux N, Crandall R, Weiss J. Dwarfism, the family and professional guide. Irvine, CA: Short Stature Foundation & Information Center, Inc.; 1994.
12. Sharrard WJW. Abnormalities of the epiphyses and limb inequality. In: Paediatric orthopaedics and fracture. 3rd ed. Oxford: Blackwell Scientific Publications; 1993:719–814.
13. Herring JA, ed. Disorders of the knee/Disorders of the leg/Disorders of the foot [three chapters]. In: Tachdjian's pediatric orthopedics, 3rd ed. Philadelphia: Saunders; 2002:789–838, 839–890, 891–1038.

Osteonecrosis

THORSTEN M. SEYLER, MD
DAVID MARKER, BS
MICHAEL A. MONT, MD

- Osteonecrosis or vascular necrosis refers to the final result of a number of different pathways leading to bone death and ultimately to joint destruction. The femoral head is the most common site of osteonecrosis.
- Osteonecrosis develops bilaterally in more than 80% of cases. Besides the hip, the most common sites for necrosis are knees, shoulders, ankles, and elbows.
- The most common risk factors for osteonecrosis are glucocorticoid use, excessive alcohol consumption, and cigarette smoking.
- The first symptom associated with the disease is typically a deep, throbbing groin pain. This pain, usually intermittent and of gradual onset, occasionally appears abruptly.

- A variety of non-operative treatment interventions are available at some centers, including vasodilators, lipid-lowering agents, prostacyclin analogues, various types of anticoagulants, bisphosphonates, hyperbaric oxygen therapy, and extracorpeal shock wave therapy. Rigorous data on the efficacy of these approaches are currently not available.
- There are currently four general categories of operative treatment options aimed toward preserving the femoral head and delaying (or preventing) total arthroplasty: (1) core decompression; (2) osteotomy; (3) nonvascularized bone grafting; and (4) vascularized bone grafting.
- Many patients eventually undergo total joint arthroplasty or resurfacing arthroplasty.

Osteonecrosis (ON), also often termed *avascular necrosis*, is a disease that leads pathologically to dead bone. There are many direct and indirect causes of ON, which may be multifactorial and lead to joint destruction. ON of the femoral head, the most common location for this disease, is the focus of this chapter. In more than 10% of cases, symptomatic ON of the hip also involves the knee and shoulder. In approximately 3% of patients, more than three anatomic sites are involved. Between 10,000 and 20,000 patients are diagnosed with this disease each year, and approximately 10% of the hip replacements performed in the United States are related to ON. The disease usually occurs in the fourth decade of life, but the age range of patients is wide. Because of the relative youth of many patients with ON, joint replacements in many cases are unlikely to last the full life expectancy of the patient. Thus, much effort has been aimed at preserving the femoral head.

Rheumatologists are often the first medical practitioners to encounter these patients, whose major risk factor is frequently long-term glucocorticoid use. The key to joint preservation in ON is early diagnosis. ON was previously a disease that inevitably failed non-operative treatments and ultimately required surgical intervention. However, a number of new non-operative approaches have shown early success rates, confirming the importance of early diagnosis. The following section details the risk factors and pathophysiology of ON. We then describe the staging of this disease in relationship to the latest non-operative and operative treatment methods.

RISK FACTORS AND PATHOGENESIS

Recent advances in the understanding of ON have led to identification of a number of risk factors for this disease. The most common ones include: glucocorticoid use, excessive alcohol consumption, and cigarette smoking. Other risk factors and associated conditions are shown in Table 33-1. In approximately 15% of patients, the occurrence of ON must still be considered idiopathic, as no clear cause may be identified. Risk factors for ON are not mutually exclusive. Each increases the likelihood of establishing the appropriate pathological milieu for ischemic bone events and subsequent bone

TABLE 33-1. RISK FACTORS AND CLINICAL CONDITIONS ASSOCIATED WITH OSTEONECROSIS.

Direct causes

Fracture
Dislocation
Pregnancy
Radiation
Chemotherapy
Organ transplantation
Hypersensitivity reactions
Myeloproliferative disorders (Gaucher's disease, leukemia)
Sickle-cell disease
Coagulation deficiencies (thrombophilia, hypofibrinolysis)
Systemic lupus erythematosus
Gaucher's disease
Thalassemia
Dysbarism
Liver dysfunction
Gastrointestinal disorders
Caisson disease

Indirect causes

Glucocorticoids
Alcohol
Smoking
Idiopathic
Genetic factors

necrosis to occur. The location of these physiological abnormalities can be either intra- or extraosseous, and also either intra- or extravascular. The pathogenic mechanisms associated with these etiological factors can be grouped into two categories, direct and indirect.

Direct Causes

Direct causes of ON include trauma, nitrogen bubbles (caisson disease, a consequence of deep-sea diving), various myeloproliferative disorders that lead to an expanded bone marrow, sickle cell disease, and pathological entities leading to direct bone cell injury (e.g., radiation). The cause-and-effect relationship between trauma and ON is readily apparent in cases involving dislocations or fractures of the hip. In one study, ON was associated with 16% of nondisplaced subcapital fractures and 27% of displaced subcapital fractures (1).

Traumatic occlusion of vessels is the most direct cause of bone ischemia. Fractures and dislocations may directly injure both intra- and extraosseous vessels supplying blood to a specific bone such as the hip. Although the initial injury leads to ON, the healing process itself may also exacerbate the problem. Results of animal studies are consistent with the hypothesis that ON of the femoral head stems from the failed attempt to replace dead bone with new tissue (2). Similarly, arteriographic studies reveal extraosseous blockage of the superior retinacular arteries and poor revascularization in weight-bearing regions, suggesting that occlusion does not fully occur until after the healing process (3).

Arterial and venous abnormalities are relatively common in cases of ON. In the case of venous abnormalities, it remains unclear whether they are causative or simply a result of the ON. Studies on a rat model of ON showed that Legg–Calve–Perthes disease led to secondary mechanical instability of the femoral epiphyseal plate, collapse of this segment, and ultimately to blood supply compromise in a manner similar to that of traumatic-induced ischemia (4).

Mechanical occlusion of vessels can also be caused by embolic events. These emboli may be composed of fat, sickled red blood cells, or nitrogen bubbles (in the context of caisson disease or dysbarism). Thrombophilia, hypofibrinolysis, and heritable coagulation disorders are more common among patients with ON than among controls (5).

Other disorders strongly associated with ON are Gaucher's disease (see Chapter 28), leukemia, and myeloproliferative disorders. These disorders are linked to intraosseous marrow displacement and increased pressure in the bony compartment of the femoral head and neck (6). Because it cannot expand, the bone involved cannot compensate for increased pressure, resulting in vascular collapse, ischemia, and cell damage.

Another direct cause of ON is cellular toxicity caused by radiation, chemotherapy, and thermal injuries. In each of these cases, the external stimulus results in osteocyte and marrow cell damage or death, and ultimately in ON. Although even moderate amounts of alcohol are toxic to osteocytes, no in vitro studies have indicated direct cytotoxic effects of alcohol when consumed at physiologically tolerated concentration. Similarly, although glucocorticoids have been shown to increase fat accumulation and result in bone cell death, animal models have been unsuccessful in demonstrating collapse that is similar to the human conditions associated with ON.

Indirect Causes

Although glucocorticoid use, alcohol consumption, and smoking are found in more than 80% of ON cases, the pathogenic mechanism for these risk factors is not clear. For glucocorticoids, doses of >2 g of prednisone (or its equivalent) within 2 to 3 months are considered to raise the risk of ON (7). The onset of ON following the start of glucocorticoid use has been documented as being between a mean of 3 and 5 months (8). For both alcohol and cigarette smoking, the risk of ON rises with the level of exposure.

A mutation in a type II collagen gene was identified in three families demonstrating autosomal dominant inheritance of femoral head ON (9). Other genetic studies have reported an association between ON and certain polymorphisms involving alcohol-metabolizing enzymes and the drug transport protein P-glycoprotein. Further studies of genetic risk factors are needed, but this approach may serve one day as a tool for identifying patients at high risk for ON. This, in turn, may have implications for non-operative treatment to delay disease progression.

PATHOLOGY

Despite all the different causes and associated factors with this disease, the pathology is similar in all cases. A number of factors, including the size and location of the ON lesion, may influence the rate of progression. In some cases, small lesions may be stabilized by the healing response. More than 90% of patients with ON, however, demonstrate ineffective repair and progression of the disease (6). Early lesions typically demonstrate histological signs such as hemorrhage and necrosis, surrounded by areas of normal fatty marrow. Loss of hematopoietic elements and microvesicular changes of the marrow adipocytes are evident. The lesions then progress and lead to extensive necrosis of the hematopoietic and fatty bone marrow elements. This necrosis is accompanied by histiocytic phagocytosis of debris. Without revascularization, the necrotic zone remains acellular and the surrounding tissue alternates between repair and necrosis. Larger lesions cannot be repaired and progress to more advanced stages of ON. Advanced stages are characterized by a wedge or conically shaped area of dead bone that contains disorganized trabeculae and fatty tissue, later replaced by granular, reticular, or amorphous tissue. This region, known as the sequestrum, is characterized by an osteochondral fracture beneath the subchondral plate. This fracture ultimately leads to the death of the medullary bone, marrow, and cortex.

When healing is unsuccessful, revascularization and repair are prevented as fibrous scar tissue forms and separates the necrotic bone from healthy tissue. After the formation of this scar, the lesion often progresses and the mechanical stability of the necrotic region becomes compromised. Stress-induced fractures of the necrotic trabeculae lead to collapse of the subchondral bone, cartilage disintegration, and deformity of the femoral head. Collapse of the femoral head leads to substantial cartilage breakdown and induces additional degenerative changes to the joint.

CLINICAL PRESENTATION

The clinical manifestations of ON may follow the inciting injury or pathological conditions by months or years. The first symptom associated with the disease is typically a deep, throbbing groin pain. This pain, usually intermittent and of gradual onset, occasionally appears abruptly. This pain may correlate with movement and weight bearing, but later may advance to rest pain. The relationship between symptom manifestations and radiologic findings is imperfect. Some patients remain relatively asymptomatic despite advanced radiographic changes. As patients reach end-stage clinical symptoms, however, the pain worsens and range of motion becomes increasingly limited. The time course for ON varies according to individual patients, ranging from months to years between initial symptom onset and the development of end-stage ON.

RADIOGRAPHIC STAGING

Patients at risk for ON who have any groin pain should be evaluated radiographically as soon as possible. Patients diagnosed with ON should also be evaluated for potential bilateral presentation of the disease, as well as the involvement of other joints. ON develops bilaterally in more than 80% of cases. Besides the hip, the most common sites for necrosis are knees, shoulders, ankles, and elbows.

The most accurate imaging modalities for diagnosing ON are roentgenograms and magnetic resonance imaging (MRI). Other modalities such as bone scans, bone biopsies, computed tomography (CT) scans, and positron emission tomography (PET) scans are not necessary for the diagnosis of this disease and for formulating a treatment plan. One major obstacle to studying ON is the absence of a universally accepted method for classifying disease severity and determining prognosis. Authors classify the stages of ON variably, according to institutional practice, confounding comparisons of data across studies. Sixteen major classification systems are used currently to describe the various radiographic findings of ON. Four of these systems—the Ficat and Arlet, University of Pennsylvania, ARCO (Association Research Circulation Osseous), and Japanese Orthopaedic Association classifications—account for more than 85% of all published studies since 1985 (10). The stages for each system are shown in Table 33-2. In a systematic analysis of classification systems (10), the following parameters were found to be the most useful for uniform data collection:

- With regard to the femoral head, lesions should be classified by pre- or postcollapse status. Precollapse lesions have better prognoses.
- The size of the necrotic segment must be assessed. Smaller lesions have better prognoses.
- The amount of femoral head depression must be assessed. Lesions with <2 mm of depression have more favorable outcomes.
- Acetabular involvement, if present, should be characterized. Any sign of osteoarthritis will limit treatment options.
- The presence or absence of a crescent sign (Figure 33-1), indicative of femoral head collapse, should be noted.
- Diffuse sclerosis and the presence of cysts should be noted.

33

TABLE 33-2. RADIOGRAPHIC CLASSIFICATION OF OSTEONECROSIS OF THE FEMORAL HEAD.

STAGE	DESCRIPTION
	Ficat and Arlet
I	Normal
II	Sclerotic or cystic lesions, without subchondral fracture
III	Crescent sign (subchondral collapse) and/or step-off in contour of subchondral bone
IV	Osteoarthritis with decreased articular cartilage, osteophytes
	University of Pennsylvania System of Staging
I, II	First two stages are the same as Ficat and Arlet
III	Crescent sign only
IV	Step-off in contour of subchondral bone
V	Joint narrowing or acetabular changes
VI	Advanced degenerative changes
	Each lesion is divided into A, B, and C depending on the magnetic resonance imaging (MRI) size of the lesion (small, moderate, large)
	ARCO
0	None
1	X-ray and computed tomography (CT) normal; at least one other technique is positive
2	Sclerosis, osteolysis, focal porosis
3	Crescent sign and/or flattening of articular surface
4	Osteoarthritis, acetabular changes, joint destruction
	Japanese Investigation Committee
1	Demarcation line
	Subdivided by relationship to weight-bearing area (from medial to lateral)
	1A
	1B
	1C
2	Early flattening without demarcation line around necrotic area
3	Cystic lesions
	Subdivided by site in the femoral head
	3A (Medial)
	3B (Lateral)

FIGURE 33-1

Anteroposterior (A) and lateral (B) radiographs demonstrating advanced osteonecrosis of the femoral head. The lateral view (B) delineates a crescent sign (*arrow*) that is the result of a subchondral fracture, indicating biomechanical compromise of the femoral head.

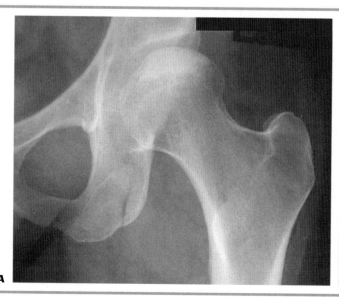
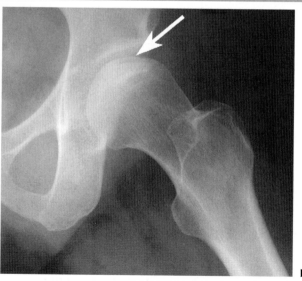

TABLE 33-3. PHARMACOLOGICAL TREATMENT OPTIONS AND REPORTED CLINICAL OUTCOMES.

PHARMACOLOGICAL AGENTS	AUTHOR	YEAR	FOLLOW-UP (MONTHS)	CLINICAL OUTCOME
Lipid-lowering drugs[a]	Pritchett (15)	2001	90 (60–132)	Three (1%) out of 284 patients taking high-dose glucocorticoids as well as statins developed osteonecrosis
Bisphosphonates[b]	Agarwala (16)	2005	12 (3–60)	Six (10%) out of 60 patients had disease progression and required surgery
	Lai (17)	2005	>24	Two (7%) out of 29 hips demonstrated loss of femoral head integrity which required further intervention
Prostacyclin analogues[c]	Disch (18)	2005	25 (11–37)	All 17 patients demonstrated improvement in Harris hip scores, range of extension, flexion and rotation, pain reduction, and patient satisfaction
Anticoagulants[d]	Glueck (19)	2005	161 (108–216)	In 19 (95%) out of 20 hips, disease progression was retarded

[a] Reduce elevated lipid levels associated with diseases such as systemic lupus erythematosus and osteonecrosis.
[b] Decrease osteoclastic resorption of bone and promote new bone growth.
[c] Inhibit platelet aggregation and alleviate hypertension to further enhance vascularization of ischemic bone areas.
[d] Reverse coagulation pathologies associated with hypofibrinolysis and/or thrombophilia.

NON-OPERATIVE TREATMENT OPTIONS

Osteonecrosis diagnosed in the early stages may be amenable to non-operative treatment modalities, but the precise stages at which specific interventions may be successful have not been established yet. Historically, non-operative treatment options consisted largely of assisted weight-bearing modalities such as canes or crutches. The rationale for these approaches was that the reduced stress would slow the progression of the disease enough to allow for procedures that might preserve the femoral head. This approach has proven unsuccessful: more than 80% of cases progressed to femoral head collapse by 4 years after diagnosis (11).

In response to the poor prognosis of previous non-operative treatment options, several non-operative treatment modalities are under study. The most common of these modalities are pharmacological measures, hyperbaric oxygen treatment, extracorporeal shock wave therapy, and various types of electrical stimulation (direct current, pulsed electromagnetic field therapy). The basic requirement for all of these treatment options is that they must be administered prior to biomechanical collapse of the femoral head (evidence of collapse with a crescent sign).

Pharmacological measures are intended to ameliorate one or more pathophysiological features of ON while allowing revascularization and bone growth. The most common drugs employed for this purpose are vasodilators, lipid-lowering agents, prostacyclin analogues, various types of anticoagulants, and bisphosphonates. Table 33-3 lists these pharmacological agents with their desired physiological outcomes and provides results of related studies using some of these novel drugs. Additional clinical work is necessary to determine the true effectiveness of these measures.

The concept of hyperbaric oxygen treatment is based on the notion that increased oxygenation will prevent any additional bone necrosis and promote healing. Pulsed electromagnetic field therapy, direct current electrical stimulation, and shock wave therapy are all designed to stimulate osteoblast activity and lead to new bone growth, in the theory that this will prevent collapse and promote healing. Among these modalities, extracorpeal shock wave therapy appears the most promising. Conflicting studies of pulsed electromagnetic field therapy and direct current electrical stimulation promote continued skepticism by some experts.

OPERATIVE TREATMENT OPTIONS

Multiple operative treatment options are available to treat ON prior to collapse of the femoral head. Some surgeons have begun to use these procedures in conjunction with non-operative modalities described above. The impetus for these strategies is the poor prognosis for patients treated with protected weight-bearing alone. There are currently four general categories of operative treatment options aimed toward preserving the femoral head and delaying (or preventing) total arthroplasty: (1) core decompression; (2) osteotomy; (3) nonvascularized bone grafting; and (4) vascularized bone grafting. Some of these methods can also be combined with each other; for example, core decompression may be combined with ancillary bone grafting.

Core Decompression

Core decompression appears to preserve the femoral head in many cases when ON is diagnosed at early stages (before femoral head collapse). Some authors have reported femoral head salvage rates of 70% to 90% at follow-ups ranging from 5 to 10 years (12). Techniques for core decompression continue to evolve (13). Preferences among different surgeons vary as to what procedure follows drilling of the initial core tract. Some surgeons leave the site alone, while others prefer to fill it with bone graft. There is also interest in using various bone growth factors, stem cells, and pro-osteogenic mediators simultaneously with the core decompression to enhance the long-term outcome of the procedure.

Osteotomy

Proximal femoral osteotomies, technically challenging to perform, have shown poor-to-moderate success with the exception of studies in Japan. This difference may be in part due to differences in the pattern of vascular anatomy found in the specific patient populations. The objective of an osteotomy is to redistribute forces to healthy bone by moving necrotic tissue away from areas which are weight-bearing. To increase the effectiveness of this procedure, surgeons have begun utilizing bone growth factors.

Nonvascularized Bone Grafting

The purpose of bone grafts is to provide structural support to the subchondral bone and articular cartilage. Grafts harvested from healthy bone are remodeled to the site of necrotic bone. The graft may be inserted through a trap door window in either the femoral head or neck. Surgeons have also begun to use growth and differentiation factors to improve the outcome of this procedure.

Vascularized Bone Grafting

Vascularized bone grafting was suggested as an alternative to nonvascularized bone grafting after initial results suggested there was not adequate vascularization following the procedure. Similar to nonvascularized bone grafting, growth factors and osteogenic factors may increase the effectiveness and improve the long-term outcome of vascularized bone grafting. The downside to this procedure is that it is technically difficult, time-intensive, and associated with higher donor-site morbidity. Furthermore, this procedure requires two teams: one team must prepare the femur while the other harvests the fibula.

TOTAL JOINT REPLACEMENT

Despite early operative and non-operative modalities, many patients eventually progress to advanced stages of ON. Total joint replacement remains a standard treatment for these advanced cases. Up to 10% of all total joint replacements are performed because of ON. In addition to standard total hip arthroplasty, other arthroplasty alternatives, such as limited femoral resurfacing and metal-on-metal resurfacing, exist.

Historically, the results of standard total hip arthroplasty in patients with ON have been poorer compared to those of the total hip arthroplasty population overall. Recent advances in design and surgical technique have allowed for improved survival rates. Despite these results, the downside to standard total hip arthroplasty is that it sacrifices bone and decreases the options for future operations. This is an important consideration due to the younger age of ON patients and the likelihood that they will require a revision at some point in their life.

RESURFACING ARTHROPLASTY

Limited resurfacing or hemi-resurfacing of the femoral head utilizes a cemented femoral head prosthesis that conforms to the patient's original femoral head, simulating the coupling of the native femoral head to the patient's undamaged acetabulum. By fitting the prosthesis in this manner, the chance for dislocation following surgery decreases. This procedure also conserves bone stock and readily allows for conversion to a total hip replacement in the future. Metal-on-metal resurfacings are more comprehensive than limited resurfacings, providing better functional results, more effective pain relief, and improved range of motion. First introduced in the middle of the last century, metal-on-metal resurfacings were discounted initially as a viable arthroplasty because of the unacceptably high number of cases with component loosening and failure. New technology creating improved bearing surfaces has triggered renewed interest in this technique. One recent study of 42 patients with ON reported a 5-year joint survival rate of 95% for metal-on-metal total hip resurfacing (14).

PROPOSED TREATMENT ALGORITHM AND PROGNOSIS

Many patient-specific factors must be considered when developing a treatment plan for ON, including overall health, age/life expectancy, comorbidities, and activity level. Total joint arthroplasty and other major surgical procedures are likely inappropriate for patients with chronic disease or short life expectancies. Conversely,

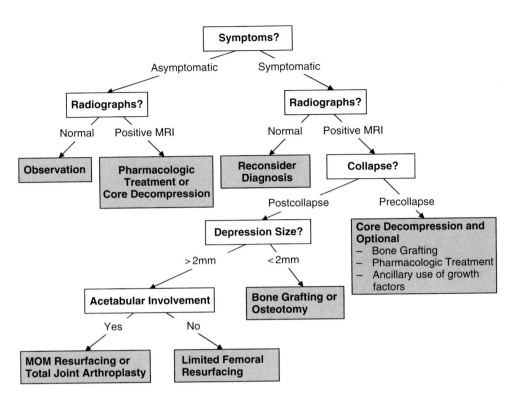

FIGURE 33-2

Proposed treatment algorithm for osteonecrosis. MOM, metal-on-metal.

young or active patients should be considered as candidates for procedures that delay total joint arthroplasty, such as bone grafts or bone preserving operations such as metal-on-metal resurfacing. Because of their increased life expectancy, younger patients are more likely to require a revision. Figure 33-2 provides a simple algorithm based on symptoms and radiographic features to determine the appropriate treatment of ON with regard to disease stage. In the future, more nonoperative methods may be available for successful hip preservation.

REFERENCES

1. Assouline-Dayan Y, Chang C, Greenspan A, Shoenfeld Y, Gershwin ME. Pathogenesis and natural history of ON. Semin Arthritis Rheum 2002;32:94–124.
2. Levin D, Norman D, Zinman C, Misselevich I, Reis DN, Boss JH. Osteoarthritis-like disorder in rats with vascular deprivation-induced necrosis of the femoral head. Pathol Res Pract 1999;195:637–647.
3. Atsumi T, Kuroki Y, Yamano K. A microangiographic study of idiopathic ON of the femoral head. Clin Orthop 1989:186–194.
4. Kikkawa M, Imai S, Hukuda S. Altered postnatal expression of insulin-like growth factor-I (IGF-I) and type X collagen preceding the Perthes' disease-like lesion of a rat model. J Bone Miner Res 2000;15:111–119.
5. Jones LC, Hungerford DS. Osteonecrosis: etiology, diagnosis, and treatment. Curr Opin Rheumatol 2004;16:443–449.
6. Mont MA, Hungerford DS. Non-traumatic avascular necrosis of the femoral head. J Bone Joint Surg Am 1995; 77:459–474.
7. Mont MA, Jones LC, Hungerford DS. Nontraumatic osteonecrosis of the femoral head: ten years later. J Bone Joint Surg Am 2006;88:1117–1132.
8. Koo KH, Kim R, Kim YS, et al. Risk period for developing osteonecrosis of the femoral head in patients on steroid treatment. Clin Rheumatol 2002;21:299–303.
9. Liu YF, et al. Type II collagen gene variants and inherited osteonecrosis of the femoral head. N Engl J Med 2005; 352:2294–2301.
10. Mont MA, Marulanda GA, Jones LC, et al. Systemic analysis of classification systems of osteonecrosis of the femoral head. J Bone Joint Surg Am. 2006;88(Suppl 3):126–130.
11. Mont MA, Carbone JJ, Fairbank AC. Core decompression versus nonoperative management for osteonecrosis of the hip. Clin Orthop 1996:169–178.
12. Mont MA, Tomek IM, Hungerford DS. Core decompression for avascular necrosis of the distal femur: long term followup. Clin Orthop 1997:124–130.
13. Mont MA, Ragland PS, Etienne G. Core decompression of the femoral head for osteonecrosis using percutaneous multiple small-diameter drilling. Clin Orthop 2004:131–138.
14. Mont MA, Seyler TM, Marker DR, Marulanda GA, Delanois RE. Use of metal-on-metal total hip resurfacing for osteonecrosis of the femoral head: an analysis of 42 hips compared to osteoarthritis. J Bone Joint Surg Am. 2006;88(Suppl 3):90–97.
15. Pritchett JW. Statin therapy decreases the risk of osteonecrosis in patients receiving steroids. Clin Orthop 2001: 173–178.

33

16. Agarwala S, Jain D, Joshi VR, et al. Efficacy of alendronate, a bisphosphonate, in the treatment of AVN of the hip. A prospective open-label study. Rheumatology (Oxford) 2005;44:352–359.

17. Lai KA, Shen WJ, Yang CY, et al. The use of alendronate to prevent early collapse of the femoral head in patients with nontraumatic osteonecrosis. A randomized clinical study. J Bone Joint Surg Am 2005;87:2155–2159.

18. Disch AC, Matziolis G, Perka C, et al. The management of necrosis-associated and idiopathic bone-marrow oedema of the proximal femur by intravenous iloprost. J Bone Joint Surg Br 2005;87:560–564.

19. Glueck CJ, Freiberg RA, Sieve L, et al. Enoxaparin prevents progression of stages I and II osteonecrosis of the hip. Clin Orthop 2005:164–170.

CHAPTER 34

Paget's Disease of Bone

Roy D. Altman, MD

- Paget's disease affects 1% of the US population over the age of 40 years and is a chronic disorder of adult skeleton characterized by increased resorption and deposition of bone resulting in replacement of the normal matrix with softened and enlarged bone.
- Most adults with Paget's disease are asymptomatic and diagnosis is found on x-ray of the bones.

- Bone pain, fracture, and nerve impingement can occur due to enlarging and poorly constructed bone matrix.
- Potent and generally safe suppressive agents have been developed and have resulted in a more aggressive approach to therapy.

Paget's disease is a chronic disorder of the adult skeleton characterized by increased resorption and deposition of bone resulting in replacement of the normal matrix with a softened and enlarged bone. Initially, there is active resorption by large and increased numbers of osteoclasts containing multiple nuclei, followed by deposition of bone by numerous osteoblasts which most often results in a weakened disorganized bony structure that is interspersed with areas of fibrosis. Although localized to isolated areas of the skeleton, there may be widespread bony distribution.

The bones most commonly affected are the pelvis, femur, skull, tibia, vertebrae, clavicle, and humerus.

Paget's disease of bone is present in approximately 1% of the US population over the age of 40 (1). Prevalence increases with age with almost a 2:1 ratio of men to women. Paget's disease is more common in Europe, particularly the United Kingdom, excluding Scandinavia, and their immigrant descendants of Australia, New Zealand, and the United States. It is rare in Africa and Asia.

The etiology of Paget's disease is unknown. It is more common among relatives of those with Paget's disease, and genetic studies have demonstrated an association to mutation variants of the Sequestrosome 1 gene on the fifth chromosome (2). There is additional evidence suggesting a virus trigger (from the paramyxovirus family) (3). There is man-to-man transmission.

SYMPTOMS

Although Paget's disease is usually asymptomatic, bone pain, bony enlargement, or bony deformity may occur. Bone pain may be deep, aching, occasionally severe, and may worsen at night. The enlarging bones may compress nerves, adding to the pain. Sometimes Paget's disease leads to the development of painful osteoarthritis in contiguous joints (4). Stiff joints and fatigue may develop slowly and subtly.

Symptoms vary, depending on degree of involvement and which bones are affected. The skull may enlarge, resulting in frontal bossing and a larger hat size. Hearing loss may be due to petrous ridge Paget's disease invasion of the cochlea. There may be headaches, dizziness, and bulging scalp veins.

Vertebrae may enlarge, weaken, and fracture, resulting in a loss in body height and a stooped forward (or simian) posturing. Involved vertebrae may compress nerves from the spinal cord, resulting in pain, dysesthesias, weakness, or even lower extremity paraparesis or paraplegia. Long bones become bowed, resulting in reduced function, abnormal gait, and contractures. The involved bone has a tendency to fracture.

There is an association with high output cardiac failure. Sarcomatous degeneration of pagetic lesions occurs in fewer than 1% of patients. Hypercalcemia can occur with/without hyperparathyroidism. The prognosis is most often good, particularly if treated. The unfortunate few who develop pagetic sarcomas have a poor prognosis.

DIAGNOSIS

Paget's disease is often discovered when x-rays or laboratory tests are performed for other reasons. The diagnosis is uncommonly suspected on the basis of symptoms and physical examination. Confirmation of the diagnosis is usually from the characteristic findings

Osteoporosis
A. Epidemiology and Clinical Assessment

KENNETH G. SAAG, MD, MSC

- More than 1.5 million osteoporosis-related fractures occur each year in the United States.
- Osteoporotic fractures most often involve the femoral neck, the vertebral bodies, or the wrist. Ninety percent (90%) of all hip and spinal fractures are related to osteoporosis.
- Among individuals now 50 years old, the lifetime risk of any fracture in the hip, spine, or distal forearm is about 40% in Caucasian women and 13% in Caucasian men.

- Two types of scores are used to quantify bone mineral density (BMD): The T score is the number of standard deviations the patient's BMD measurement is above or below the young-normal mean BMD. The Z score is the number of standard deviations the measurement is above or below the age-matched mean BMD.
- The World Health Organization (WHO) defines osteoporosis as a T score ≤ -2.5.

Epidemiology of Osteoporosis and Fractures

Over 10 million people have osteoporosis, 34 million have low bone mineral density (BMD), and over 1.5 million osteoporosis-related fractures occur each year in the United States alone (1). The 2002 year direct medical costs for osteoporotic fractures exceeded $18 billion in the United States (2).

Incidence, Prevalence, and Clinical Consequences of Common Osteoporotic Fractures

Osteoporotic fractures most often involve the femoral neck, the vertebral bodies, or the wrist. Ninety percent (90%) of all hip and spinal fractures are related to osteoporosis. Fractures of the humerus, ribs, pelvis, ankle, and clavicle also have been attributed to osteoporosis in 50% to 70% of cases.

The lifetime risk of any fracture in the hip, spine, or distal forearm is about 40% in Caucasian women 50 years of age and 13% in Caucasian men of similar age (3). The estimated lifetime risk for fracture at various sites for men and women is shown in Table 35A-1 (3–6).

The public health consequences of fractures depend not only upon fracture incidence, but also on population size. Fractures are a major international public health concern. Despite the fact that hip fractures are less common among Asians than Caucasians, 33% of all osteoporotic fractures occur in Asia. Moreover, the number of fractures is rising rapidly in Asia and in many parts of the developing world. The economic costs of osteoporotic fractures include expenses for surgery and hospitalization, rehabilitation, long-term care, medications, and loss of productivity.

Hip Fractures

In 1999, the estimated number of hip fractures among North American women was 340,000 (7). By 2050, this figure is expected to increase to >500,000 (8). Among women between the ages of 65 and 69, the incidence of hip fractures is approximately 2 per 1000 patient-years. In the 80 to 84 year old age group, however, the incidence increases 13-fold, to 26 per 1000 patient-years (9). Compared to non-nursing home residents, nursing home residents have a fourfold increased risk of hip fracture (10). Of the 300,000 annual hospitalizations resulting from hip fractures, up to 20% of patients die within 1 year of the fracture, often due to comorbidities. In addition to the increased mortality within 1 year,

TABLE 35A-1. LIFETIME RISK OF FRACTURE.

POPULATION	HIP FRACTURE (%)	DISTAL FOREARM (%)	VERTEBRAL FRACTURE CLINICAL (%)	RADIOGRAPHIC (%)
White women	14–17 (3–6)	14–16 (3–6)	16 (3, 6)	35 (4)
White men	5–6 (3–5)	2–3 (3–5)	5 (3, 6)	Unknown
Black women	6 (5)	Unknown	Unknown	Unknown
Black men	3 (5)	Unknown	Unknown	Unknown

20% require nursing home care and 50% of survivors never fully recover. The economic costs of hip fracture are similar to the costs of a stroke (11).

Vertebral Fractures

The incidence of vertebral fractures, low before age 50, rises almost exponentially thereafter. The most frequent areas of fracture are the thoracolumbar juncture (T12 and L1) and the mid-thoracic spine. Vertebral fractures are a harbinger of further osteoporosis problems: approximately half of all individuals who sustain vertebral fractures later suffer other fractures. The loss of height from vertebral fractures can lead not only to reductions in lung function, but also to depression associated with undesirable changes in physical appearance. Beyond the acute morbidity of vertebral fractures—often 6 to 8 weeks of pain that may be intense—the mortality associated with vertebral fractures is also greater than for that of the general population.

Wrist Fractures

Among American women, the incidence of wrist fractures increases rapidly at the time of menopause and plateaus after age 60. This plateau effect relates to a pattern of falling common among older individuals: the elderly are more likely to land on a hip—thereby suffering a more serious fracture—than on an outstretched hand. Women with radial fractures are more likely to be thinner and have reduced triceps strength compared to women who do not fracture.

Bone Mineral Density Criteria for Osteoporosis Diagnosis

Osteoporosis is diagnosed most definitively on the basis of an insufficiency fracture. Such injuries, often synonymously termed *fragility* or *nontraumatic* fractures, occur with falls from standing heights or even lower levels (e.g., following slipping out of a chair) or as a result of other low impact trauma. In the absence of an osteoporotic fracture of the hip, vertebral column, or wrist, bone mineral density (BMD) criteria can be used to diagnose osteoporosis. Two types of scores are used to quantify bone mineral density. First, the T score is the number of standard deviations the patient's BMD measurement is above or below the young-normal mean BMD. Second, the Z score is the number of standard deviations the measurement is above or below the age-matched mean BMD. The T and Z scores were developed because of variation in BMD measurement technology among different manufacturers.

The World Health Organization (WHO) defines osteoporosis as a T score ≤ -2.5. Severe osteoporosis is defined as a T score ≤ -2.5 *plus* the presence of at least one fracture. Osteopenia is a BMD between -1 and -2.5 standard deviations below the mean value of peak bone mass. Normal bone density is a BMD less than 1 standard deviation below the mean value of peak bone mass.

These WHO criteria are based upon epidemiological data relating fracture incidence to BMD in Caucasian women. The applicability of these BMD cutoff values to other ethnic and gender groups is not certain. For premenopausal women and men younger than age 50, a Z score—which compares BMD to age- and sex-based reference standards—may be more appropriate than a T score. Nevertheless, T scores are the standard by which fracture risk is predicted and disease status classified by the WHO. BMD criteria do not differentiate among the causes of low BMD (e.g., hyperthyroidism vs. glucocorticoid-induced osteoporosis) with regard to their relative fracture risks.

Using BMD criteria alone, one third of Caucasian women aged 60 to 70 have osteoporosis. By the age of 80, more than two thirds of these women are osteoporotic (12). Based on the femoral neck bone density in the third National Health and Nutrition Examination Survey (NHANES), an estimated 18% of Caucasian women have osteoporosis; approximately half have osteopenia (13). Using the T score cutoffs applied to women, between 1% and 4% of Caucasian men have osteoporosis and up to 33% have osteopenia (13).

35

Clinical Assessment of Osteoporosis

The clinical evaluation of osteoporosis is dedicated to identifying lifestyle risk factors for fracture (also see Chapter 35B), pertinent physical findings, and secondary causes of metabolic bone disease. Beyond bone mass measurement, typically by BMD, a medical evaluation for a patient with osteoporosis should include a comprehensive history and physical examination. The goal of the evaluation is twofold: (1) to determine consequences and complications of osteoporosis (i.e., pain and disability) and (2) to identify any coexisting conditions that could contribute to the progression or complications of osteoporosis (e.g., dietary calcium deficiency, glucocorticoid use, risk factors for low 25-hydroxy vitamin D levels, and others).

History

A careful evaluation of a person with or at risk for osteoporosis includes questions about family history of metabolic bone disease, changes in height and weight, the quantity and frequency of weight-bearing exercise, level of sun exposure, previous fractures, reproductive history (particularly for evidence of hypogonadism), endocrine disorders, dietary factors (including lifetime and current calcium consumption, vitamin D, sodium, and caffeine), tobacco smoking, alcohol intake, exercise, renal or hepatic failure, and past and current medications and supplements. In addition, factors that increase the risk of falls, such as neuromuscular disease, gait instability, and unsafe living conditions, should also be discussed. Although a history of bone pain is potentially useful if present, osteoporosis is not painful until the time of fracture (if then). Approximately two thirds of vertebral fractures, for example, are not diagnosed at the time they occur.

Physical Examination

Accurate height measurement using an instrument known as a stadiometer is a vital part of the osteoporosis physical examination (14). Comparison of a patient's current height and maximum height obtained in young adulthood (e.g., through reference to the patient's driver's license) is helpful in identifying height loss. The loss of 2 inches (5 cm) in height is a fairly sensitive indicator of vertebral compression. The spine should be examined for alignment and for spinal or paraspinal tenderness. If kyphosis is present (see Figure 35A-1), the possibility of pulmonary compromise should be considered and the patient examined for a decrease in the distance between the bottom of the ribs and the top of the iliac crest measured (the iliocostal distance). A

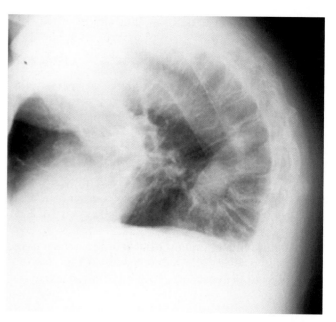

FIGURE 35A-1

Dowager's hump. Marked thoracic kyphosis in an osteoporotic patient secondary to multiple thoracic vertebral fractures as evidenced on this lateral radiograph.

"buffalo hump," easy skin bruisability, and striae suggest Cushing's syndrome. Blue sclerae could indicate osteogenesis imperfecta. The number of missing teeth has been correlated with losses in BMD. A joint assessment may suggest rheumatological causes of low BMD. A testicular exam can help identify hypogonadism. The neurological examination highlights muscular weakness or neurological compromise that could predispose to falls. Observation of the patient's gait is a critical part of the examination.

Skeletal Imaging for Osteoporosis
Conventional Radiography

Plain radiographs are inaccurate for the assessment of BMD. Bone loss must exceed 30% to 40% before it is visible by x-ray. Assessment of the trabecular pattern of the femoral neck (the Singh index) has been shown to correlate with osteoporosis. Other radiographic measurements, such as hip axis length, also correlate with fracture risk. Vertebral fractures have different patterns and can be graded semiquantitiatively on the basis of endplate deformities, anterior wedging, and crush fractures (15).

Dual-Energy X-Ray Absorptiometry

Dual-energy x-ray absorptiometry (DXA) is the most widely used bone mass measurement technique. DXA affords a fast, reliable, accurate measurement of BMD that involves low radiation exposure. DXA is currently the "gold standard" for both patient care and clinical investigation in osteoporosis (16).

Bone mineral density measurements help stratify fracture risk, guide therapy choices, and monitor response to therapy. Although bone quality and rate of bone turnover correlate independently with bone strength, BMD measured by DXA is the strongest known predictor of hip and spinal fractures. For each decline of approximately 1 standard deviation of BMD, there is a 1.3- to 3.0-fold increase in the risk of fracture. Although fracture risk at any site can be assessed accurately by DXA, BMD at the femoral neck is a better predictor of hip fracture than BMD at the spine, radius, or calcaneus. With respect to response to anti-osteoporosis therapy, increases in BMD with pharmacological therapy account for a major component of the reduction in fracture risk.

Dual-energy x-ray absorptiometry, a two-dimensional measure of BMD, does not measure true volumetric density but rather areal density. BMD is reported as an absolute value in g/cm^2; as a comparison to age-, race-, and sex-matched reference range (the Z score); and as a comparison to mean bone mass of young adult normal individuals [the T score or young adult Z score; Figure 35A-2(A,B)]. A change of 1 standard deviation in either the T or Z score correlates to a change of approximately $0.06 g/cm^2$, corresponding to a change in BMD of approximately 10%. DXAs also produce a density-based image useful in interpreting scan quality and identifying obviously compressed vertebrae and various artifacts. Some newer DXA devices also generate a higher resolution lateral spine image that can identify vertebral fractures.

Most major DXA manufacturers use the National Health and Nutrition Examination Service III (NHANES III) database to determine normal age- and sex-matched BMD parameters, particularly at the hip. DXA results vary between and within different machines, precluding comparison of results across devices without the use of conversion equations.

Dual-energy x-ray absorptiometry is used to measure bone mass at both central and peripheral sites. The central DXA sites—the hip and spine—are the optimal imaging locations for two reasons. First, measurements at these sites are associated with superior precision. Second, the quantity of trabecular bone at these sites correlates well with osteoporosis burden and fracture risk. Measurement at multiple sites increases the sensitivity for osteoporosis. For the spine, DXA reports measurements of individual vertebrae as well as total BMD of the L1 to L4 vertebrae. At the hip, BMD measurements of the femoral neck, trochanter, and total hip provide full assessment of the bones' contribution to fracture risk at that site. In contrast, Ward's triangle, an area in the wrist, has a lower predictive value and measurements at that site are less reproducible than those in the hip and spine. The clinical value of measurements of BMD at Ward's triangle is very limited. Whenever possible, decisions regarding the therapy of osteoporosis should be made on the basis of BMD measurements from central sites.

The ability to detect significant serial changes in DXA depends on the rate of change in BMD at a particular site. A 2.77% change is required between two successive DXA studies to achieve a statistically significant difference with 95% confidence. This change value is multiplied by the precision error (coefficient of variation) of the measuring device to determine the amount of BMD change that is needed to indicate a significant improvement or worsening in BMD. For example, if the device has a 2% precision error, a change in BMD of about 5.6% is needed to be confident that this is not due to chance or precision error. Controversy exists about the merit of serial DXA to monitor the response to anti-osteoporotic therapies.

Osteoporosis occurs nonhomogenously throughout the body, dependent on age and underlying cause of bone loss. Thus, discordance across measurement sites as high as 15% is not unusual, particularly in the elderly. Due to the high prevalence of spinal facet and posterior element spinal osteoarthritis among adults over 65, measurement of spinal DXA in the posterior–anterior projection may yield a falsely elevated assessment of BMD. In older adults, measurement of the hip or lateral spine imaging may circumvent this problem. Artifacts (i.e., calcium pills in the gut, metal objects on clothing, objects in pockets), positioning errors (imaging of the wrong vertebra, hip malrotation), and anatomical deformities or changes (severe scoliosis, calcified aorta, vertebral crush fractures) can limit DXA precision and accuracy (16).

Quantitative Computed Tomography and Ultrasound

Quantitative computed tomography (QCT) is similar to DXA in its ability to quantify the degree of bone loss and assess fracture risk accurately. In contrast to DXA, QCT gives a true volumetric measurement of BMD and accurately discriminates trabecular bone from cortical bone. QCT may overestimate the extent of bone loss with age and glucocorticoid use because bone marrow fat increases in these two clinical settings. In addition to a slightly higher radiation exposure (although less than on a routine CT examination), reliance on an imaging device that is heavily utilized for other clinical applications and the higher cost of QCT have limited its widespread adoption.

Quantitative ultrasound is a complementary way to measure bone mass and perhaps other properties of

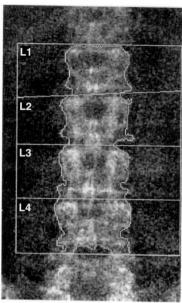

Image not for diagnostic use
k = 1.129, d0 = 44.3
116 × 145

DXA Results Summary:

Region	Area (cm²)	BMC (g)	BMD (g/cm²)	T - Score	Z - Score
L1	13.91	10.86	0.781	−1.3	0.4
L2	15.15	13.94	0.920	−1.0	0.9
L3	16.98	16.54	0.974	−1.0	1.0
L4	17.53	16.46	0.939	−1.6	0.4
Total	**63.58**	**57.80**	**0.909**	**−1.3**	**0.7**

Total BMD CV 1.0%, ACF = 1.019, BCF = 1.055, TH = 8.785
WHO Classification: Osteopenia
Fracture Risk: Increased

L1–L4

Source: Hologic

DXA Results Summary:

Scan Date	Age	BMD (g/cm²)	T - Score	BMD Change vs Baseline	BMD Change vs Previous
05/19/2004	67	0.909	−1.3	10.1%*	2.5%
05/28/2003	66	0.887	−1.5	7.4%*	−0.4%
05/22/2002	65	0.891	−1.4	7.9%*	1.7%
03/07/2001	64	0.876	−1.6	6.1%*	6.1%
10/01/1997	60	0.825	−2.0		

Total BMD CV 1.0%
A * Denotes significant change at the 95% confidence level.

FIGURE 35A-2

(A) Dual x-ray absorptiometry (DXA) report of lumbar spine. DXA of a lumbar spine showing imaging windows for vertebrae L1 to L4. Estimated vertebral areas, bone mineral content (BMC), and bone mineral density (BMD) are shown (top right). BMD is plotted against a lumbar spine reference database showing the patient's current value as well as previous readings indicated by crosses (see middle right). The dark bar of the graph (middle right) indicates 2 standard deviations above normal and the lighter bar indicates 2 standard deviations below normal for age. *T* scores indicate that the patient was initially classified as osteopenic but *T* scores have increased into the normal range following antiresorptive therapy. A 10.1% increase in BMD was noted at the lumbar spine.

bone. Compared with DXA or QCT, this method has desirable attributes of lower instrument cost, portability, and absence of ionizing radiation. Ultrasound studies are usually performed of the calcaneus, although the tibia, patella, distal radius, and proximal phalanges can also be examined. There are no universally accepted criteria for an ultrasonic diagnosis of osteoporosis and it is not possible to predict BMD by ultrasound measurements. Compared with DXA and QCT, ultrasound is relatively insensitive for osteoporosis diagnosis. Thus, even borderline abnormalities should prompt the performance of a central DXA.

Indications for Bone Mass Measurement

Bone mass testing is indicated only when the results will influence a treatment decision. Persons are more

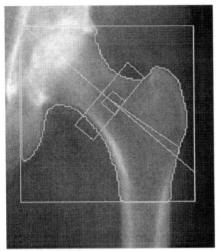

Image not for diagnostic use
k = 1.141, d0 = 51.4
106 × 105

DXA Results Summary:

Region	Area (cm²)	BMC (g)	BMD (g/cm²)	T - Score	Z - Score
Neck	5.22	3.27	0.626	−2.0	−0.4
Troch	12.52	10.13	0.809	1.1	2.2
Inter	16.30	16.99	1.042	−0.4	0.7
Total	**34.05**	**30.40**	**0.893**	**−0.4**	**0.9**
Ward's	1.11	0.46	0.419	−2.7	−0.3

Total BMD CV 1.0%, ACF = 1.019, BCF = 1.055, TH = 5.865
WHO Classification: Normal
Fracture Risk: Not Increased

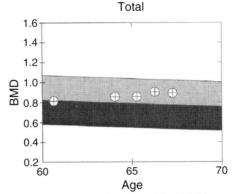

Reference curve and scores matched to White Female
Source: NHANES

Source: NHANES

DXA Results Summary:

Scan Date	Age	BMD (g/cm²)	T - Score	BMD Change vs Baseline	vs Previous
05/19/2004	67	0.893	−0.4	9.6%*	−1.4%
05/28/2003	66	0.905	−0.3	11.1%*	5.6%*
05/22/2002	65	0.857	−0.7	5.2%*	0.0%
03/07/2001	64	0.856	−0.7	5.1%*	5.1%*
10/01/1997	60	0.815	−1.0		

Total BMD CV 1.0%
B * Denotes significant change at the 95% confidence level.

FIGURE 35A-2

(B) DXA report of hip. Similar parameters as in (A) are shown for the left hip. There has been a significant increase in BMD at the hip, as was seen in the spine. The asterisk denotes a significant increase or decline between two values as determined by the precision error of the DXA machine. A 9.6% increase in BMD was noted at the total hip.

likely to initiate osteoporosis therapy if they know their BMD is below normal. The US Preventive Services Task Force has recommended that routine screening begin at age 60 for women at increased risk for osteoporotic fractures (17). The International Society for Clinical Densitometry has recommended bone density testing for all women aged 65 and over; all men aged 70 and older; anyone with a fragility fracture; anyone with a medical condition or taking medication associated with osteoporosis; anyone con-

sidering therapy for osteoporosis; and women who have been on hormone replacement therapy for prolonged periods (18).

Measurement of Bone Turnover

Biochemical markers of bone turnover are cell-based molecules that can be quantified in the urine or blood. Although bone formation and resorption are usually coupled, assays on biochemical markers of bone

35

turnover permit the evaluation of net imbalances. Table 35A-2 lists bone markers that can be classified as indices of bone formation or resorption.

Bone Formation Markers

The markers of bone formation reflect new bone synthesis by osteoblasts or the postrelease metabolism of procollagen (Table 35A-2). Bone-specific alkaline phosphatase and osteocalcin increase in the face of osteoblastic activity. Collagen precursor proteins, particularly the serum carboxyterminal and aminoterminal peptides of type I procollagen, can be measured as indicators of collagen formation.

Bone Resorption Markers

Resorptive markers reflect the activity of osteoclasts and collagen degradation (Table 35A-2). Pyridinium cross-links include pyridinoline and deoxypyridinoline. These fragments, released into the circulation, ultimately undergo renal excretion. Of the two cross-links, deoxypyridinoline is more specific for bone collagen breakdown.

Bone biomarkers provide an assessment of dynamic aspects of skeletal metabolism as opposed to the more static assessment by DXA. Bone markers are useful to categorize an individual as having fast or slow bone turnover. Fracture risk is related to faster bone turnover. A reduction in bone turnover with antiresorption therapy diminishes the risk of fracture independent of changes in BMD. Bone markers may also be helpful in the monitoring of adherence to antiresorptive therapies.

TABLE 35A-2. BIOCHEMICAL MARKERS OF BONE TURNOVER.

FORMATION	RESORPTION
Serum tests	
Bone-specific alkaline phosphatase	Aminoterminal telopeptide of type I collagen
Osteocalcin	Carboxyterminal telopeptide of type I collagen
Procollagen I carboxyterminal propeptide	
Procollagen I aminoterminal propeptide	
Urine tests	
	Amino-terminal telopeptide of type I collagen (NTX)
	Carboxy-terminal telopeptide of type I collage (CTX)
	Pyridinoline and deoxypyridinoline cross-links

TABLE 35A-3. EVALUATIONS OF SECONDARY CAUSES OF LOW BONE MASS.

Typical laboratory workup
25-hydroxy vitamin D
Serum chemistry including calcium, creatinine, albumin, phosphorous, and total protein
Complete blood count with differential
Liver function studies to include total alkaline phosphatase
Urinary calcium and creatinine (spot calcium/creatinine ratio or on 24-hour urine collection)

Additional workup to be considered as clinically indicated
Bone turnover markers (bone-specific alkaline phosphatase, osteocalcin, and/or urinary collagen cross-links)
Serum intact parathyroid hormone (iPTH)
Thyroid-stimulating hormone (TSH)
Erythrocyte sedimentation rate (ESR)
Evaluation for gonadal insufficiency
Evaluation for hypercortisolism
Acid-base evaluation
Serum and urine immunoelectrophoresis
Consider tetracycline double-labeled bone biopsy

Additional Laboratory Evaluation

The laboratory assessment seeks possible secondary causes of low BMD. Table 35A-3 lists laboratory tests that may be appropriate in certain clinical scenarios. Many of these tests will lead to a large number of false-positive results, however, if their pretest probability is low. Consequently, these tests should be ordered if the patient's historical, physical examination, and other laboratory results suggest that additional evaluation will enhance the evaluation.

One laboratory assessment currently receiving much attention is vitamin D. Measurement of the 25-OH vitamin D level is appropriate in person with osteoporosis. Levels less than 32 ng/dL (80 nmol/mL) may merit supplementation.

REFERENCES

1. National Osteoporosis Foundation. Fast facts on osteoporosis. Available at: http://www.nof.org/osteoporosis/diseasefacts.htm. Accessed July 2, 2007.
2. National Osteoporosis Foundation. Physician's guide to prevention and treatment of osteoporosis. Belle Mead, NJ: Excerpta Medica; 1998.
3. Melton III LJ, Chrischilles EA. How many women have osteoporosis? J Bone Miner Res 1992;7:1005–1010.
4. Chrischilles EA, et al. A model of lifetime osteoporosis impact. Arch Intern Med 1991;151: 2026–2032.
5. Cummings SR, Black DM, Rubin SM. Lifetime risks of hip, Colles', or vertebral fracture and coronary heart disease among white postmenopausal women. Arch Intern Med 1989;149:2445–2448.

6. National Osteoporosis Foundation. Osteoporosis: review of the evidence for prevention, diagnosis, and treatment and cost-effectiveness analysis. Status report. Osteoporos Int 1998;8(Suppl 4):S1–S88.

7. Popovic JR. 1999 National Hospital Discharge Survey: annual summary with detailed diagnosis and procedure data. Vital Health Stat 2001;13:i–v, 1–206.

8. Cooper C, Campion G, Melton LJ III. Hip fractures in the elderly: a world-wide projection. Osteoporos Int 1992;2: 285–289.

9. Farmer ME, et al. Race and sex differences in hip fracture incidence. Am J Public Health 1984;74:1374–1830.

10. Sugarman JR, et al. Hip fracture incidence in nursing home residents and community-dwelling older people, Washington State, 1993–1995. J Am Geriatr Soc 2002;50: 1638–1643.

11. Johnell O. The socioeconomic burden of fractures: today and in the 21st century. Am J Med 1997;103:20S–25S, discussion 25S–26S.

12. Ross PD. Osteoporosis: frequency, consequences, and risk factors. Arch Intern Med 1996;156:1399–1411.

13. Looker AC, et al. Prevalence of low femoral bone density in older US adults from NHANES III. J Bone Miner Res 1997;12:1761–1768.

14. Green AD, et al. Does this woman have osteoporosis? JAMA 2004;292:2890–2900.

15. Genant HK, et al. Vertebral fracture assessment using a semiquantitative technique. J Bone Miner Res 1993;8: 1137–1148.

16. Watts NB. Fundamentals and pitfalls of bone densitometry using dual-energy X-ray absorptiometry (DXA). Osteoporos Int 2004;15:847–854.

17. Nelson HD, et al. Osteoporosis and fractures in postmenopausal women using estrogen. Arch Intern Med 2002;162:2278–2284.

18. International Society for Clinical Densitometry (ISCD). Official positions of the ISCD. J Clin Densitom 2002; 5(Suppl).

35

Osteoporosis
B. Pathology and Pathophysiology

PHILIP SAMBROOK, MD, FRACP

- The pathophysiology of osteoporosis includes many genetic, hormonal, nutritional, and environmental influences. Some risk factors for this condition are well defined.
- Although genetic factors contribute strongly to determining peak bone mass, hormonal, nutritional, and environmental influences during intrauterine life, childhood, and adolescence modulate the genetically determined pattern of skeletal growth.
- The bone mass of an individual in later life is a consequence of the peak bone mass accrued in utero and during childhood and puberty, as well as the subsequent rate of bone loss.
- The high rate of hip fracture in older people is not only due to their lower bone strength but also their increased risk of falling. Established risk factors for falls and, hence, hip fracture include impaired

balance, muscle weakness, cognitive impairment, and psychotropic medication.
- Bone is continually undergoing a process of renewal called *remodeling*. In the normal adult skeleton, new bone laid down by osteoblasts exactly matches osteoclastic bone resorption; that is, bone formation and bone resorption are closely coupled.
- The principal cell types within bone are the osteoclasts, osteoblasts, and osteocytes. Osteoclasts are responsible for resorption of bone; osteoblasts are responsible directly for bone formation; osteocytes, derived from osteoblasts, appear to play a role in response to mechanical loading.
- Key regulators of osteoclastic bone resorption include RANK ligand and its two known receptors, RANK and osteoprotegerin (OPG). RANK and OPG have opposing effects on bone resorption.

The pathophysiological basis of osteoporosis is multifactorial and includes the genetic determination of peak bone mass, subtle alterations in bone remodeling due to changes in systemic and local hormones, and environmental influences. It is useful to consider these processes at multiple biological levels as well as in terms of known risk factors. Any consideration of the pathogenesis of osteoporosis requires an understanding of normal bone structure and function.

Bone Structure and Function

Bones are an extremely dense form of connective tissue made up principally of the fibrous protein collagen, impregnated with a mineral phase of calcium phosphate crystals as well as other components such as water. Although they are one of the hardest structures in the body, bones maintain a degree of elasticity due to their structure and material properties.

Types of Bone

The bone mass of an individual in later life is a consequence of the peak bone mass accrued in utero and during childhood and puberty, as well as the subsequent rate of bone loss. During development and growth, bone is produced by two main processes—intramembranous ossification, as occurs in skull bones; and endochondral ossification involving the growth plate, as occurs in limb bones. Modeling is the process that results in the achievement of bones' characteristic shape and overall structure.

Bone has a strongly hierarchical nature, from the molecular level up to the whole bone architecture. Above the level of the collagen fibril and its associated mineral, bone exists in two usually distinct forms, woven bone and lamellar bone. Woven bone is laid down quickly, most characteristically in the fetus but also in the callus that is produced during fracture repair. The collagen in woven bone is variable. Lamellar bone is laid down much more slowly and more precisely, with

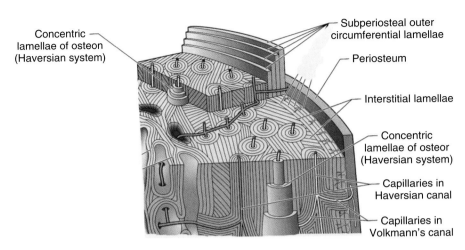

Concentric lamellae of osteon (Haversian system)

Subperiosteal outer circumferential lamellae

Periosteum

Interstitial lamellae

Concentric lamellae of osteor (Haversian system)

Capillaries in Haversian canal

Capillaries in Volkmann's canal

FIGURE 35B-1

The Haversian system. Lamellar bone comprises overlapping cylindrical units termed *Haversian systems* (osteons), each consisting of a central Haversian canal surrounded by concentric lamellae. The Haversian canals communicate directly with the medullary cavity. (From Sambrook, Schrieber, Taylor, Ellis, eds. The musculo-skeletal system. Philadelphia: Churchill Livingstone; 2001.)

the collagen fibrils and their associated mineral arranged in sheets (lamellae). Lamellar bone exists in irregularly spaced, overlapping, cylindrical units termed *Haversian systems* (Figure 35B-1). Each Haversian system consists of a central Haversian canal surrounded by concentric lamellae of bony tissue. The Haversian system is the result of the process of *remodeling*, discussed below. Remodeling differs from modeling, mentioned above, in which the gross shape of bone is altered by changes on periosteal or endosteal surfaces.

The principal cell types within bone are the osteoclasts, osteoblasts, and osteocytes. Osteoclasts, the cells responsible for resorption of bone, are derived from hematopoietic stem cells. Osteoblasts, derived from local mesenchymal cells, are the pivotal bone cell, responsible directly for bone formation. Osteoblasts also regulate osteoclastic bone resorption, through paracrine factors. Osteocytes appear to derive from osteoblasts that are "buried" during the process of remodeling that connects osteoblasts with each other via canaliculi and appears to play a role in response to mechanical loading.

At the next higher order of structure, there is the mechanically important distinction between (a) compact or cortical bone and (b) trabecular or cancellous bone. Cortical bone is found principally in the shafts (diaphyses) of long bones. Cortical bone is solid with the only spaces in it being for osteocytes, blood vessels, and erosion cavities. Trabecular bone is found principally at the ends of long bones, in vertebral bodies, and in flat bones. It has large spaces and is comprised of a meshwork of intercommunicating trabeculae. The skeleton is comprised of approximately 80% cortical bone, largely in peripheral bones, and 20% trabecular bone, mainly in the axial skeleton. These amounts vary according to site and need for mechanical support. Although trabecular bone accounts for the minority of total skeletal tissue, it is the site of greater bone turnover due to its greater surface area.

Cellular Basis of Bone Remodeling

Bone is continually undergoing renewal called *remodeling* (Figure 35B-2). In the normal adult skeleton, new bone laid down by osteoblasts exactly matches osteoclastic bone resorption; that is, bone formation and bone resorption are closely coupled. Although the skeleton contains less trabecular bone than cortical bone, trabecular bone turns over between 3 to 10 times more rapidly than cortical bone and is therefore more sensitive to changes in bone resorption and formation. Moreover, the rate of remodeling differs across anatomical sites according to physical loading, proximity to a synovial joint, or the presence of hemopoietic rather than fatty tissue in adjacent marrow.

Bone remodeling follows an ordered sequence, referred to as the *basic multicellular unit of bone turnover* or *bone remodeling unit* (BMU). In this cycle, bone resorption is initiated by the recruitment of osteoclasts, which act on matrix exposed by proteinases derived from bone lining cells. A resorptive pit (called a Howship's lacuna) is created by the osteoclasts (Figure 35B-2). This resorptive phase is then followed by a bone formation phase in which osteoblasts fill the lacuna with osteoid (unmineralized bone matrix). This cycle of coupling of bone formation and resorption is vital to the maintenance of skeletal integrity. Uncoupling of the remodeling cycle, so that either bone resorption or formation in excess of the other leads to net bone change (gain or loss).

Key regulators of osteoclastic bone resorption include RANK ligand (a member of the tumor necrosis factor ligand family) and its two known receptors, RANK and osteoprotegerin (OPG) (1). RANK and OPG have opposing effects on bone resorption. Osteoblasts express RANK ligand (RANKL) constitutively on their cell surfaces. RANKL interacts with its cognate receptor, RANK, promoting osteoclast differentiation. Interaction of RANKL with RANK on mature osteoclasts

35

FIGURE 35B-2

The bone remodeling cycle. The process of bone remodeling starts when the lining cells reveal the bone surface upon activation. Osteoclast precursors arrive at the site and become active osteoclasts as they start to dig out a resorption pit. When the osteoclasts have finished the process of resorption, osteoblasts are attracted to the site. These osteoblasts lay down the organic matrix (mainly collagen type I), which is subsequently mineralized. At the end of this process old bone has been replaced by new bone. Bone resorption and formation are coupled in this process.

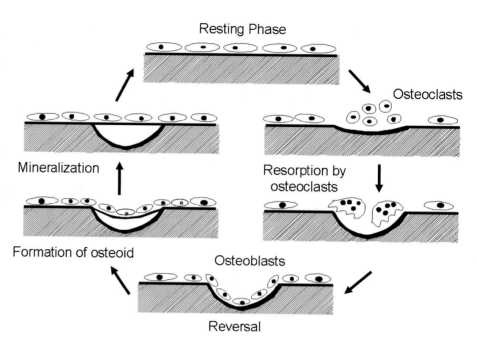

results in their activation and prolonged survival (Figure 35B-3). OPG, present in the bone microenvironment, is secreted primarily by osteoblasts and stromal cells. OPG blocks the interaction of RANKL with RANK and thus acts as a physiological regulator of bone turnover.

At the cellular level, bone loss occurs as a result of an imbalance between the activity of osteoclasts and osteoblasts. If the processes of resorption and formation are not matched, there is a remodeling imbalance; this imbalance may be magnified by an increase in the rate of initiation of new bone remodeling cycles (activation frequency). Estrogen deficiency following the menopause results in a remodeling imbalance with a substantial increase in bone turnover. Remodeling nearly doubles in the first year after menopause. This imbalance leads to a progressive loss of trabecular bone in part due to increased osteoclastogenesis. Enhanced formation of functional osteoclasts appears to be the result of increased elaboration of osteoclastogenic proinflammatory cytokines such as interleukin 1 (IL-1) and tumor necrosis factor, which are regulated in a negative fashion by estrogen (2,3).

FIGURE 35B-3

Osteoclasts are formed from macrophage, monocytic precursor cells (CFU-M). Osteoclasts express RANK, and RANKL enhances each of these steps. RANKL in bone is mainly produced in osteoblasts and stromal cells and RANKL then activates each of these steps. Osteoprotegerin (OPG) is a decoy receptor antagonist that blocks this interaction between RANKL and RANK and therefore, the formation, activation, and survival of osteoclasts leading to enhanced apoptosis. CFU, colony forming units.

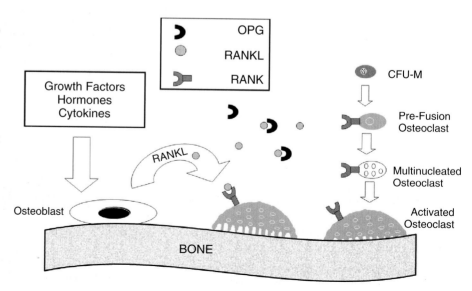

Pathophysiology

Osteoporotic fractures result from a combination of decreased bone strength and an increased incidence of falls with aging. Bone loss occurs as a consequence of estrogen deficiency in the postmenopausal women, as well as through estrogen-independent, age-related mechanisms (such as secondary hyperparathyroidism and reduced mechanical loading). Menopausal status is probably the most important risk factor of all and postmenopausal bone loss is the single most important cause of osteoporosis. The rate of loss is greatest soon after the menopause. The earlier the menopause the greater the risk. Age-related bone loss starts from 30 to 50 years of age in both men and women. Loss from different bone sites occurs at different ages and at different rates.

Although bone mineral density predicts bone strength, many other skeletal characteristics also contribute to bone strength. These include bone macroarchitecture (shape and geometry), bone microarchitecture (both trabecular and cortical), the degree of mineralization and microdamage accumulation, and the rate of bone turnover, which can affect bone's structural and material properties. These other measures are often referred to as *bone quality*. Changes in the rate of bone remodeling can also influence these material and structural properties of bone.

Calcium Homeostasis and Hormonal Control

In addition to its role as a support structure, the skeleton's other primary function is calcium homeostasis. More than 99.9% of the total body calcium resides in the skeleton. The maintenance of normal serum calcium depends on the interplay of intestinal calcium absorption, renal excretion, and skeletal mobilization or uptake of calcium. Although serum calcium represents less than 1% of total body supply, normal serum calcium levels are extremely important for normal cellular function. Serum calcium regulates and is regulated by three major hormones; parathyroid hormone (PTH), 1,25-dihydroxy vitamin D, and calcitonin. PTH and 1,25-dihydroxy vitamin D are the major regulators of calcium and bone homeostasis. PTH acts on the kidney to increase calcium reabsorption, phosphate excretion, and 1,25-dihydroxy vitamin D production. It also acts on bone to increase bone resorption. 1,25-Dihydroxy vitamin D is a potent stimulator of bone resorption and an even more potent stimulator of intestinal calcium (and phosphate) absorption. It is also necessary for bone mineralization. Intestinal calcium absorption is probably the most important calcium homeostatic pathway. Although calcitonin can directly inhibit osteoclastic bone resorption, it plays a relatively minor role in calcium homeostasis in normal adults.

A number of feedback loops operate to control the level of serum calcium, PTH, and 1,25-dihydroxy vitamin D. Low serum calcium levels stimulate 1,25-dihydroxy vitamin D synthesis directly through stimulation of PTH release (and synthesis). The physiological response to increasing levels of PTH and 1,25-dihydroxy vitamin D is a gradual rise in serum calcium level. A second set of feedback loops maintain serum calcium within a narrow physiological range. Disturbances in these control mechanisms or over/underproduction of PTH, 1,25-dihydroxy vitamin D, calcitonin occurs in various clinical states, including osteoporosis.

Mechanical Properties of Bone

The stiffness and strength of bone are dependent on two factors: its material properties and its three-dimensional architecture. In simple biomechanical terms, a bone will fracture if the load applied exceeds its strength. Bone strength is affected by changes in architecture, microdamage accumulation, mineral change, and bone turnover.

By engineering theory, the elastic modulus, also known as Young's modulus, is the ratio of stress (load) to strain (deformation) or the slope of the curve, the material stiffness. Toughness (the ability to absorb energy in impact without breaking) is the area under the curve. Increases in post–yield strain leads to tougher bone. As the mineral content increases, the stiffness (Young's modulus of elasticity) also increases but the area under the stress/strain curve, which is equivalent to toughness, decreases. Thus, bone cannot have a mineral content that makes it both very stiff and very tough (4).

In most forms of osteoporosis, the loss of bone is not distributed evenly throughout the skeleton (Figure 35B-4). For reasons that are not clear, some of the struts of

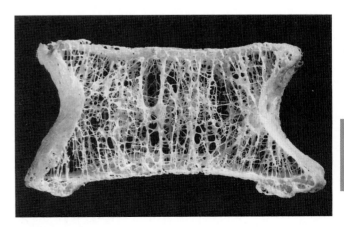

FIGURE 35B-4

Architecture of vertebral body in elderly subject. Note loss of trabecular structure with aging. (Courtesy of L. Mosekilde, Aarhus University Hospital, Denmark.)

35

trabecular bone are resorbed completely, resulting in a loss of connectivity between adjacent bone plates. This contributes markedly to decreased bone strength and increased fracture risk. Because the remodeling surface/volume ratio of trabecular bone is high, bone loss tends to affect this type of bone, such as that in the spine and hip, to a greater extent.

Changes in microarchitecture also appear to be important. Compared with normal individuals, the cortical bone of patients with hip fractures is characterized by microarchitecture showing increased porosity and decreased thickness.

Risk Factors

A number of risk factors for osteoporosis have been identified (Table 35B-1). These may be considered in relation to their underlying pathophysiological effects.

Genetic Influences

Fracture risk has a direct relationship to bone mineral density (BMD). BMD at any age is the result of the peak bone mass achieved and subsequent bone loss (postmenopausal and age-related). Although genetic factors contribute strongly to determining peak bone mass, recent studies have demonstrated that environmental influences during intrauterine life, childhood, and adolescence modulate the genetically determined pattern of skeletal growth.

There is a strong genetic contribution to skeletal size and composition. Comparisons of identical and nonidentical twins have led to estimates that more than 50% of peak bone mass is determined by genetic factors (5). A family history of a relative sustaining a fracture after age 50 should be viewed as suspicious. Genetic factors that regulate skeletal development and function including the CBFA1 gene and the RANK/RANKL system.

Genetic factors underlie racial differences in osteoporosis prevalence. Hip fractures more commonly occur in thin, frail individuals rather than those who are overweight. Low body weight is a risk factor for hip fracture. On average, African Americans have greater BMD than whites of the same age, and African Americans sustain fewer fractures. People of Asian origin have lower bone densities and higher fracture rates than whites. In the more common forms of osteoporosis, genetic factors play an important role in regulating skeletal size and geometry, bone mass, ultrasound properties of bone, and bone turnover. These phenotypes appear to be determined by the combined effects of multiple genes, environmental influences, and gene–environment interactions. Genomewide linkage studies have identified loci on chromosomes 1p36, 1q21, 2p21,

TABLE 35B-1. RISK FACTORS FOR OSTEOPOROSIS.

Established risk factors
Low bone mass/density
Advanced age
Female gender
Ethnicity (white or Asian)
Family history
High falls risk
History of low trauma fracture
Calcium intake <400 mg/day
Low body weight
Smoking

Osteoporosis associated with endocrine causes
Cushing's syndrome/corticosteroid therapy
Hyperthyroidism and thyroxine replacement therapy
Hypogonadism (see Table 35B-2)
Anorexia nervosa/exercise-induced amenorrhea
Hyperparathyroidism
Pregnancy
GNRH agonist/antagonists
Type 1 diabetes

Osteoporosis associated with altered activity
Rheumatoid arthritis
Immobilization/weightlessness
Chronic airways obstruction
Cerebovascular accident
Ankylosing spondylitis

Osteoporosis associated with "environmental" factors
Alcoholism
Celiac disease
Gastrectomy
Drugs (see Table 35B-3)
Post-transplantation bone loss
Mastocytosis

Osteoporosis associated with specific genetic conditions
Osteogenesis imperfecta
Menkes' syndrome
Ehlers–Danlos syndrome
Homocystinuria
Marfan's syndrome
Osteoporosis–pseudoglioma syndrome

5q33–35, 6p11–12, and 11q12–13 that show definite or probable linkage to BMD.

Polymorphisms of the vitamin D receptor have been associated with bone mass in several studies. This association may be modified by dietary calcium and vitamin D intake. Another important functional polymorphism affecting the transcription factor Sp1 has been identified in the collagen type I alpha 1 gene. This polymorphism predicts osteoporotic fractures independently of BMD, probably through its influence on collagen gene regulation and bone quality (6). More rarely, osteoporosis or high BMD can occur as the result of mutations in a single gene. For example, inactivating mutations in the lipoprotein receptor–related protein 5 gene cause the osteoporosis–pseudoglioma syndrome, a condition associated with low BMD. In contrast, a high bone mass syndrome is caused by activating mutations of the same gene.

Nutritional Factors

Calcium restriction in animals results in low bone mass. In humans, calcium deficiency in childhood leads to rickets. Although one might anticipate that low calcium intake would be associated with osteoporosis, therefore, the relationship between calcium intake and osteoporosis remains controversial. Calcium balance studies suggest that premenopausal women require calcium intakes in excess of 800 mg per day to avoid net bone loss. Postmenopausal women may require as much as 1500 mg per day.

Dietary calcium intake during growth may play a role in the development and maintenance of peak BMD. Various environmental and lifestyle factors, particularly physical activity, also modulate this effect. Calcium supplementation in growing children produces small increases in BMD, but these do not appear to be maintained and may represent increased mineralization of existing osteons rather than sustained increases in BMD. In many trials involving patients with osteoporosis, calcium supplementation has resulted in only modest suppression of bone turnover and small gains (if any) in bone mass.

Calcium is not the only component of diet that may affect bone. Vitamin D is vital for optimal absorption of calcium from the diet and mineralization. In many countries, vitamin D is added to food. Adequate skin exposure to ultraviolet light is also necessary for the maintenance of normal vitamin D levels.

There is little evidence that micronutrients, such as magnesium, zinc, copper, and boron have major effects on bone health. Some diets, particularly those rich in soy protein, provide significant sources of estrogens. Sodium intake may have important effects on bone and calcium metabolism. Because sodium loading results in increased renal calcium excretion, lowering dietary sodium intake may diminish age-related bone loss. Excessive protein and caffeine intakes are associated with bone loss. The effects of sodium, dietary protein, and caffeine intake on bone health are probably relatively minor compared with other environmental influences. Alcohol is another dietary component that may be quite important, with adverse effects in excess but perhaps beneficial effects at moderate levels of intake.

Physical Activity

Mechanical forces exert strong influences on bone shape and modeling. At the cellular level, it is thought that the osteocytes, which lie embedded within individual lacunae in mineralized bone, respond to mechanical deformation and loading. Early biochemical responses to mechanical loading may include induction of prostaglandin synthesis, increased nitric oxide and insulinlike growth factor preproduction, changes in amino acid transporters, and eventually increases in new bone formation. Bone is responsive to physical strain. It has been hypothesized that there exists a mechanostat that senses and responds to loading. Immobilization following major injury, illness, or space flight, for example, is associated with rapid bone loss. If sustained, as in patients with paraplegia or hemiplegia, fractures can occur. Increased bone resorption is associated with acute immobilization. Positive effects of mechanical loading on bone mass can be seen in athletes. The increase in bone density is usually site-specific and localized to the loaded limb. Physical inactivity correlates with low BMD and fractures in epidemiological studies. Although exercise programs may produce only limited changes in BMD, even small changes have been shown to reduce fractures.

Hypogonadism

Other than menopausal bone loss, any condition associated with hypogonadism may result in osteoporosis (Table 35B-2). Disorders resulting in oligo-amenorrhea are a major cause of bone loss in the younger age groups. Common causes are anorexia nervosa and primary ovarian failure associated with diseases such as Turner's syndrome and chemotherapy. Secondary ovarian failure due to pituitary disorders and functional hypogonadism caused by long-acting GnRH agonists (e.g., for endometriosis therapy) may also be associated with osteoporosis.

TABLE 35B-2. COMMON CAUSES OF "HYPOGONADAL" OSTEOPOROSIS.

In women
Bilateral oophorectomy
Chemotherapy
Aromatase inhibitors
Anorexia nervosa
Exercise-induced amenorrhea

In men
Klinefelter's syndrome
Orchidectomy
Kallman's syndrome

In men and women
Hemochromatosis
Gonadotrophin-releasing hormone analogues
Gonadal dysgenesis
Pituitary disease

Drugs and Osteoporosis

Many drugs lead to reduced BMD and therefore increase the risk of fracture (Table 35B-3). In rheumatic diseases, glucocorticoids (GC) are among the most important. Their effects are dose- and duration-dependent (7). GCs affect bone through multiple pathways, influencing both bone formation and resorption, but the most important effects appear to be a direct inhibitory effect on bone formation. For the most part, the decreased bone formation is due to direct effects on cells of the osteoblastic lineage. Enhanced osteoblast and osteocyte apoptosis has also been implicated as an important mechanism of glucocorticoid osteoporosis. GCs have been shown to reduce the birth rate of osteoblasts and osteoclasts, to cause earlier death of osteoblasts, and to reduce osteocyte viability. Changes in sex steroid production have indirect effects that also lead to decreased bone formation. GCs increase the expression of RANKL and decrease OPG expression in osteoblasts, leading to postponement of osteoclast apoptosis. Another effect of GCs is to decrease intestinal absorption of calcium. In some patients, secondary hyperparathyroidism may also increase bone turnover and expand the remodeling space, but this appears to be a temporary phenomenon. With long-term GC use, bone turnover is actually reduced.

Anticonvulsant drugs are also now recognized to result in altered bone mass and an increased risk of osteoporosis (8), as are oral anticoagulants (9). Because deficiency of estrogen and testosterone both contribute to bone loss, drugs that reduce sex hormone levels cause bone loss. Androgen deprivation therapy with agonists of gonadotropin-releasing hormone is now frequently used in the treatment of recurrent and metastatic prostate cancer because it induces medical castration, rendering patients hypogonadal. This is becoming an important iatrogenic cause of osteoporosis. Similarly, aromatase inhibitors (used to treat breast cancer) are now recognized to be associated with bone loss and fractures (10).

In contrast, some drugs may increase bone mass and reduce fractures. Thiazide diuretics decrease urinary calcium excretion and have been associated with increased BMD and reduced hip fracture rates. A variety of epidemiological studies have suggested that statin users have lower rates of hip fracture than nonusers, but large effects on bone mass and turnover have not been demonstrated in prospective clinical trials.

Bone Turnover

High rates of bone turnover predict fractures independently of other factors such as BMD. Responses to treatment may be greater in those with high turnover. The rate of bone remodeling can be assessed by serum measurements of osteocalcin and specific alkaline phosphatase (markers of bone formation) or carboxyterminal telopeptide of type I collagen (a collagen breakdown product used as a marker of bone resorption). Urinary pyridinolines can also be used for the assessment of bone resorption.

Risk Factors for Falls

The high rate of hip fracture in older people is not only due to their lower bone strength and but also their increased risk of falling. Established risk factors for falls and, hence, hip fracture include impaired balance, muscle weakness, cognitive impairment, and psychotropic medication.

REFERENCES

1. Boyle WJ, Scott Simonet W, Lacey DL. Osteoclast differentiation and activation. Nature 2003;423:337–342.
2. Cenci S, Weitzmann MN, Roggia C, et al. Estrogen deficiency induces bone loss by enhancing T-cell production of TNF-alpha. J Clin Invest 2000;106:1229–1237.
3. Pfeilschifter J, Koditz R, Pfohl M, Schatz H. Changes in proinflammatory cytokine activity after menopause. Endocr Rev 2002;23:90–119.
4. Currey JD. The mechanical properties of bone. In: Currey JD, ed. Bones: structure and mechanics. 2nd ed. Princeton, NJ: Princeton University Press; 2002:54–122.
5. Naganathan V, MacGregor A, Snieder H, Nguyen T, Spector T, Sambrook PN. Gender differences in the genetic factors responsible for variation in bone density and ultrasound. J Bone Miner Res 2002;17:725–733.
6. Mann V, Hobson EE, Li B, et al. A COL1A1 Sp1 binding site polymorphism predisposes to osteoporotic fracture by affecting bone density and quality. J Clin Invest 2001;107:899–907.
7. Van Staa TP, Leufkens HGM, Abenhaim L, Zhang B, Cooper C. Use of oral glucocorticoids and risk of fractures. J Bone Miner Res 2000;15:993–1000.

TABLE 35B-3. DRUGS ASSOCIATED WITH OSTEOPOROSIS.

Corticosteroids

Cyclosporine

Thyroxine

Heparin

Anticonvulsants

Gonadotrophin-releasing hormone agonists

Aromatse inhibitors

Cytotoxic drugs

8. Petty S, Paton LM, O'Brien TJ, et al. Effect of antiepileptic medication on bone mineral measures. Neurology 2005;65:1358–1365.

9. Gage BF, Birman-Deych E, Radford, MJ, Nilasena, DS, Binder EF. Risk of osteoporotic fracture in elderly patients taking warfarin: results from the national registry of Atrial Fibrillation 2. Arch Intern Med 2006;166:241–246.

10. Eastell R, Hannon R. Long term effects of aromatase inhibitors on bone. J Steroid Biochem Molec Biol 2005; 95:151–154.

35

Osteoporosis
C. Treatment of Postmenopausal Osteoporosis

NELSON B. WATTS, MD

- The main goal of osteoporosis treatment is the prevention of fractures.
- Increases in bone density through the use of medications explain only a small proportion of the observed reduction in fracture risk. This suggests that agents that have some additional effects on bone quality to account for the reduction in fracture risk.
- Important considerations in bone health include adequate intake of calcium and vitamin D, regular weight-bearing exercise, and avoidance of cigarette smoking and other negative factors.
- Pharmacologic intervention is indicated for women who have T scores of –2.5 and below and for women with risk factors whose T scores are –1.5 or below.
- Medications employed to treat osteoporosis include the bisphosphonates, calcitonin, selective estrogen-receptor modulators (SERMs), and parathyroid hormone.
- Pharmacologic medications for the treatment of osteoporosis are classified as either antiresorptive or anabolic agents. The only anabolic drug available currently is teriparatide (parathyroid hormone).
- Bisphosphonates work through two broad mechanisms: They reduce the ability of individual osteoclasts to resorb bone and they accelerate osteoclast apoptosis (programmed cell death).
- Calcitonin reduces bone resorption by binding to specific osteoclast receptors.
- Selective estrogen-receptor modulators produce different expression of estrogen-regulated genes in different tissues, activating some and inhibiting others. The net effect of this is a reduction in bone resorption and possibly a reduction in the risk of breast cancer.
- Teraparatide stimulates bone formation, producing gains in spine bone mineral density two to three times greater than those observed with antiresorptive drugs.
- Bisphosphonates remain the first-line therapy for most patients, but teraparatide may be preferred for higher risk patients and for those failing to achieve a desired response to treatment with antiresorptive drugs.

Osteoporosis is a silent condition characterized by reduced bone mass and microarchitectural changes leading to increased bone fragility and susceptibility to fracture. In other words, osteoporosis is a condition of reduced bone quality and quantity that predisposes to fractures under conditions of daily living.

The diagnosis of osteoporosis is made either from the results of bone density testing or because of the occurrence of a fragility fracture. The main goal of treatment of osteoporosis is prevention of fractures. For patients who have low bone mass but have not yet had fractures, the goal is prevention of the first fracture. For the patient who already has had one or more fractures, intervention is urgently needed to prevent subsequent fractures. Treatment of fractures is also important but is usually the job of the orthopedist. Management of complications of osteoporosis (physical disability, psychosocial issues) may fall to the primary care physician or osteoporosis medical specialist.

A number of pharmacological agents are approved for treatment of osteoporosis. All increase bone mineral density (BMD) and reduce the risk of fractures. However, recent studies show that the increases in bone density explain only a small proportion of the observed reduction in fracture risk. This suggests that agents must have some additional effects on bone "quality" to account for the reduction in fracture risk. However, it is not clear exactly what aspect of bone quality is improved or how to measure the change.

Lifestyle Issues

A healthful lifestyle is appropriate for everyone, whether they have osteoporosis or not. Important aspects for bone health include adequate intake of calcium and vitamin D, an active lifestyle including regular weight-bearing exercise, and avoidance of cigarette smoking and other negative factors (Table 35C-1).

The recommended intake of calcium for men and women over age 50 is 1200 mg daily. The typical post-menopausal woman gets between 500 and 600 mg of calcium daily from dietary sources, and a supplement of 500 to 700 mg of calcium daily is needed. Calcium carbonate is the least expensive supplement. For most efficient absorption, calcium carbonate should be taken in divided doses (no more than 500 mg per dose) and with food. Calcium citrate is more expensive but may cause fewer gastrointestinal problems.

Vitamin D is essential for the absorption and assimilation of calcium. Vitamin D also has direct effects on bone remodeling and either direct or indirect effects on muscle strength and balance. Vitamin D is produced in skin by ultraviolet light and some foods are fortified with vitamin D. Nevertheless, vitamin D deficiency is quite common, being present in over half of women receiving therapy for osteoporosis (1). Supplementation with 1000 to 2000 IU of vitamin D per day is often necessary to assure adequate serum levels of 25-hydroxy vitamin D (30–60 ng/mL). (Standard supplemental multivitamins contain 400 IU of vitamin D; some calcium supplements also contain 100 or 200 IU of vitamin D.) Vitamin D supplementation has been shown to reduce

TABLE 35C-1. LIFESTYLE ISSUES IMPORTANT FOR PREVENTION AND TREATMENT OF OSTEOPOROSIS.

Calcium: recommended intake is 1200 mg daily for adults over age 50
  Most women need a calcium supplement of 500 to 700 mg daily
  Calcium carbonate is inexpensive and effective
  Calcium citrate is often better tolerated for patients who have digestive distress

Vitamin D: the official recommended intake is 400 to 800 IU daily; higher doses (1000–2000 IU daily) are often required
  Standard multivitamins contain 400 IU vitamin D
  Additional vitamin D (total 800 IU daily) is advisable for persons over age 70 and can be achieved by taking calcium and vitamin D in combination in addition to a multivitamin or supplements of vitamin D

Exercise
  Weight-bearing exercise, if possible; recommend walking at least 40 minutes a session, at least 4 sessions a week
  Spinal strengthening exercises are also advisable

Avoid cigarette smoking and other possible negative factors such as high intake of caffeine, protein, phosphorus, etc.

TABLE 35C-2. ELEMENTS OF A FALL RISK-REDUCTION PROGRAM.

Use proper body mechanics and avoid pushing, pulling, bending, and lifting

Hearing and visual impairment corrected as much as possible

Flooring and carpet in good condition without uneven surfaces

No throw rugs

Lighting bright and without glare

Night lights present throughout the house

Telephones readily available

Electric cords short and *not* in walkways

Clutter does not obstruct walkways

Pets do not lie near feet or bedside

Railings in tub, shower, and toilet areas

Nonslip surfaces on floors of tub and shower

Water drainage in bathroom adequate to prevent slippery floors

Bedside table for items that might clutter floor

Kitchen cleaning and cooking supplies within easy reach

Stairs have railings on both sides, nonskid surfaces

No items stored on steps

All entry ways maintained in good condition

Shoes fit well

Be trained and use a cane if gait is unsteady

Above all, don't hurry!

the risk of falls and may have other extraskeletal benefits as well.

Calcium and vitamin D may slow bone loss in recently menopausal women but do not prevent it. In older women with established osteoporosis, however, calcium and vitamin D prevent bone loss and reduce the risk of both spinal and nonspinal fractures.

Weight-bearing exercise, such as walking or low-impact aerobics, is advisable. Patients should try to walk for 40 minutes or more, four times a week, if possible. Carrying light weights (1 or 2 lbs) when walking is desirable. Resistance exercises may be helpful.

Because most osteoporotic fractures involve some element of trauma or falling, patients should be counseled to reduce their risk of falling and to avoid activities that produce undesirable forces on the skeleton (e.g., high-impact activities, pushing, pulling, bending, and lifting). Table 35C-2 lists some elements of programs designed to reduce fall risks.

35

Possible consequences of fracture include acute and chronic pain, changes in appearance (height loss, kyphosis or "dowager's hump"), depression, dependency, and deconditioning. These problems need to be identified and treated. If the patient has pain, it is important for both the provider and the patient to understand that osteoporosis is not the cause of her pain and that treating the underlying osteoporosis is not likely to relieve it.

Pharmacologic Agents

A number of pharmacologic agents reduce the risk of osteoporotic fractures in women who have already had a fracture (prevalent fractures), in women who have low BMD (*T* score –2.5 and below), or both. Drugs have also been shown to prevent bone loss in women who have recently begun menopause. Agents approved by the US Food and Drug Administration (FDA) for treatment of osteoporosis are shown in Table 35C-3. They can be classified based on mechanism as antiresorptive (or anticatabolic) or anabolic. All but teriparatide, an anabolic drug, work by reducing bone resorption.

"Prevention" and "treatment" studies are performed in very different groups of subjects. Prevention studies are done in healthy women who are recently menopausal. A typical prevention study involves women in their early or mid-50s, 3 to 5 years postmenopause, usually with normal or borderline low BMD. In contrast, treatment studies are done in older women who have low bone mass, often after they have already had one or more fractures and are therefore at high risk for additional fractures. A typical treatment study involves women in their late 60s or early 70s, with low BMD at the spine or hip (usually both), often with one or more prevalent vertebral compression fractures. Change in BMD is an endpoint in both prevention and treatment studies. However, the most important benefit of treatment of osteoporosis is reduction of fracture risk, which can only be shown in large studies, and then only in treatment populations. Evidence for fracture risk reduction for approved agents is shown in Table 35C-3. All have been shown to reduce the risk of vertebral fractures but not all have demonstrated effectiveness for hip and nonvertebral fractures.

Bisphosphonates

Bisphosphonates share a common chemical structure (two phosphonic acids joined to a carbon) that causes them to bind avidly to hydroxyapatite crystals on the surfaces of bone. They are resistant to metabolic degradation, and work through two broad mechanisms. First, bisphosphonates reduce the ability of individual osteoclasts to resorb bone. Second, they accelerate osteoclast apoptosis (programmed cell death). Three bisphosphonates (alendronate, ibandronate, and risedronate) are approved for prevention and treatment of postmenopausal osteoporosis. Bisphosphonates are remarkably free from systemic toxicity.

Alendronate (Fosamax) was the first bisphosphonate approved by the FDA (1995) for prevention and treatment of osteoporosis. In phase III trials involving almost 1000 women in their late 60s who had established osteoporosis, alendronate 10 mg daily was shown to increase spinal bone density by almost 10% after 3 years, and, to a lesser degree, to increase BMD at other sites as well (2).

In the Vertebral Fracture Arm of the Fracture Intervention Trial (FIT), involving over 2000 older women with low femoral neck BMD and prevalent vertebral fractures, alendronate reduced the frequency of vertebral, hip, and wrist fractures by about 50% (3).

Alendronate is available in 5-mg, 10-mg, 35-mg, 40-mg, and 70-mg tablets and in unit-dose liquid of 70 mg. It is also available in a 70-mg tablet containing 2800 IU of vitamin D intended for weekly dosing. Alen-

TABLE 35C-3. FDA-APPROVED PHARMACOLOGIC AGENTS FOR TREATMENT OF POSTMENOPAUSAL OSTEOPOROSIS (IN ALPHABETICAL ORDER) AND EVIDENCE FOR FRACTURE RISK REDUCTION.

AGENT	VERTEBRAL FRACTURE	NONVERTEBRAL FRACTURE	HIP FRACTURE
Bisphosphonates			
Alendronate (Fosamax)	Yes	Yes	Yes
Ibandronate (Boniva)	Yes	No	No
Risedronate (Actonel)	Yes	Yes	Yes
Calcitonin (Miacalcin, Fortical)	Yes	No	No
Raloxifene (Evista)	Yes	No	No
Teriparatide (Forteo)	Yes	Yes	No

dronate is approved for prevention of bone loss (5 mg daily or 35 mg weekly) and treatment of osteoporosis (10 mg daily or 70 mg weekly). Alendronate is also approved for treatment of glucocorticoid-induced osteoporosis (5 mg daily for men and estrogen-replete women, 10 mg daily for estrogen-deficient women).

Risedronate (Actonel) was approved by the FDA in 2000. Its effectiveness for vertebral fracture reduction was shown in two pivotal studies of over 3600 women with low BMD and prevalent vertebral fractures (2,4). The primary endpoint in these trials was new radiographic vertebral fractures, which were reduced by 41% and 49% in these two studies. The reduction in the rate of new vertebral fractures was significant after only 1 year of treatment. Nonvertebral fractures, a secondary endpoint in these studies, were reduced by 33% to 39%, ($p = 0.02$) (4). Risedronate therapy significantly increased BMD at the spine and to a lesser degree at the hip.

In the largest trial of osteoporosis to date, involving almost 9500 women, risedronate produced a significant reduction in hip fractures in postmenopausal women who had low bone mass (5). A subset of elderly women who were enrolled in the trial because they had clinical risk factors for fractures (but not necessarily low bone mass) did not show a benefit.

Risedronate has been shown to prevent bone loss in recently menopausal women. Risedronate was well tolerated in clinical trials of almost 16,000 subjects; in aggregate, the adverse events rate has been no different from that of placebo.

Risedronate is available in 5-mg and 35-mg tablets and in a packet containing 35-mg tablets with additional tablets of calcium carbonate, to be taken separately. Risedronate is approved for the prevention and treatment of postmenopausal osteoporosis, as well as for the prevention and treatment of glucocorticoid-induced osteoporosis. The dose of risedronate is 5 mg daily or 35 mg weekly for all of these indications.

Ibandronate (Boniva) 2.5 mg daily by mouth and an intermittent regimen (20 mg orally every other day for 12 doses repeated every 3 months) was shown to reduce new vertebral fractures in a study of almost 3000 women with preexisting vertebral fractures (6). Ibandronate, approved for prevention and treatment of postmenopausal osteoporosis, can be given orally (2.5 mg daily or 150 mg monthly) or intravenously (3 mg over 15–30 seconds every 3 months). Ibandronate has not been shown to have an effect on hip fractures. Although there was no effect on nonvertebral fractures overall, a post hoc analysis of the pivotal trial data showed a significant reduction with daily oral therapy (but not an intermittent regimen) in nonvertebral fractures in women with femoral neck T scores of −3.0 or below.

Etidronate, pamidronate, and zoledronic acid are other bisphosphonates available in the United States.

Although they are not approved by the FDA for use in osteoporosis, they are sometimes used off label.

Etidronate (Didronel) has been shown to increase BMD in two prospective, randomized, controlled trials of women with postmenopausal osteoporosis. When used to treat osteoporosis, it is given in an intermittent cyclical regimen (400 mg etidronate daily for 14 days every third month). As with all bisphosphonates, etidronate must be taken on an empty stomach to be effective, but it may be taken between meals, at bedtime, or during the night.

Pamidronate (Aredia), another bisphosphonate, is not approved by the FDA for use in osteoporosis. It is given by intravenous infusion. A typical regimen is an initial dose of pamidronate 90 mg, infused over about 60 minutes, with subsequent doses of 30 mg every third month. Intravenous pamidronate is useful for patients who cannot tolerate oral bisphosphonates.

Zoledronic acid (Zometa) is approved for treatment of skeletal complications of malignancy and currently is in late phase III trials for osteoporosis. A phase II study suggested that a yearly dose of 4 mg intravenously produced changes in bone mineral density and bone turnover markers similar to other bisphosphonates (7).

Bisphosphonate Dosing, Tolerability and Adverse Effects

Bisphosphonates are poorly absorbed when taken by mouth. To assure absorption, they must be taken first thing in the morning, on an empty stomach, with nothing else but water for at least 30 minutes (in the case of monthly oral ibandronate, the wait should be at least 60 minutes). Because nitrogen-containing bisphosphonates can be irritating to the esophagus, bisphosphonates should be taken with a large glass of water (to wash the tablet down), and the patient should not lie down until after eating (to avoid reflux). Oral bisphosphonates should not be given to patients who have active upper gastrointestinal disease, and should be stopped in patients who develop upper gastrointestinal complaints or who are unable to be upright after taking it.

The most common side effect of oral bisphosphonates is esophageal irritation (heartburn, indigestion, pain on swallowing). This was seen in perhaps 10% of patients taking daily oral alendronate, but is much less common with weekly or monthly dosing. Alendronate liquid may be tolerable for patients who have side effects from tablets. Class labeling indicates that musculoskeletal complaints occur in a small number of patients and may or may not resolve when treatment is stopped; the mechanism for this is unclear. Intravenous administration of bisphosphonates is often accompanied by an acute-phase response (fever and myalgias); if this occurs, it is likely only with the first dose. Osteonecrosis of the jaw has been described, mainly in cancer

35

patients receiving high doses of intravenous pamidronate or zoledronic acid, but also in a small number of patients receiving oral bisphosphonates for treatment of osteoporosis; the mechanism for this is not clear.

How Long to Treat with Bisphosphonates

Bisphosphonates have a long residence time in bone. In theory, a reservoir of drug could accumulate to a point that treatment could be stopped with some residual antifracture benefit. Long-term data with alendronate and risedronate suggest that treatment for up to 10 years is safe but that after 3 to 5 years of treatment, a "drug holiday" of a year or two might be offered without major sacrifice of antifracture efficacy.

Calcitonin

Calcitonin is a peptide hormone secreted by specialized cells in the thyroid gland. Salmon calcitonin is used for treatment of osteoporosis because it is more potent and has a longer duration of action than human calcitonin. Calcitonin acts directly to reduce bone resorption by binding to specific receptors of the osteoclast.

Available since 1984 for subcutaneous injection (currently marketed as Calcimar, Miacalcin, Fortical), salmon calcitonin (50–100 IU daily) results in slight gains in spinal BMD—somewhat less than the gains induced by other agents. Because of the perception of limited and perhaps only transient effectiveness, the inconvenience and discomfort of injections, relatively high cost, and limited tolerance (approximately 20% of patients given subcutaneous salmon calcitonin develop nausea or flushing), subcutaneous calcitonin was not widely used.

Nasal calcitonin (Miacalcin) was introduced in 1995. Another brand, Fortical, was approved by the FDA in 2005. The nasal form is much better tolerated than the subcutaneous form. The recommended dose of nasal calcitonin is 200 IU (one spray) daily. It is approved for treatment of postmenopausal osteoporosis but not for prevention or for use in glucocorticoid-induced osteoporosis. A 5-year study of nasal calcitonin in over 1000 women with preexisting vertebral fractures showed only a modest effect on spinal bone mass, but a 33% reduction in the incidence of new vertebral fractures (8). No effect of calcitonin on nonvertebral or hip fracture was shown in this study.

Nasal calcitonin is extremely well tolerated. There are no concerns about long-term safety. Calcitonin may have an analgesic effect and is sometimes prescribed for patients who have acute painful vertebral fractures.

Estrogen

Estrogen (several oral and transdermal preparations) alone or in combination with a progestin is approved for prevention of bone loss but not for treatment of osteoporosis. Estrogen and combination hormone therapy were shown to reduce vertebral, nonvertebral, and hip fractures in the Women's Health Initiative, but hormone therapy is not recommended for the treatment of osteoporosis because of an unfavorable balance of risks and benefits (9). The main indication for estrogen or postmenopausal hormone therapy is for relief of menopausal symptoms, when it should be used in the lowest dose necessary and for the shortest period of time.

Raloxifene

Raloxifene (Evista) is a selective estrogen-receptor modulator (SERM). After binding to estrogen receptors, SERMs produce different expression of estrogen-regulated genes in different tissues, activating some and inhibiting others. Raloxifene (60 mg daily) is approved by the FDA for prevention of bone loss in recently menopausal women and for treatment of established osteoporosis. For treatment of postmenopausal osteoporosis, raloxifene was evaluated in the Multiple Outcomes of Raloxifene Evaluation (MORE) Study, which involved over 7700 women (10). The risk of new vertebral fractures was reduced by 30% to 50%. No effect of raloxifene on hip fractures or nonvertebral fractures was shown.

Raloxifene is generally well tolerated, but is associated with an increase in leg cramps and hot flashes. There is a small (~3/1000 patient-years) but significant increased risk of venous thrombosis with raloxifene, similar to what is seen with estrogen. Raloxifene produces some favorable changes in lipids [decreases in low-density lipoprotein (LDL) cholesterol, neutral for high-density lipoprotein (HDL) cholesterol and triglycerides], but appears to be neutral for cardiovascular disease. Of interest, in the osteoporosis trials, raloxifene was associated with a reduced incidence of breast cancer. Several large trials appear to confirm this effect, but as of this writing, raloxifene is not indicated for prevention of breast cancer.

Teriparatide (1–34 Recombinant Human Parathyroid Hormone)

Although continuous exposure to parathyroid hormone or its active fragments leads to increased osteoclastic bone resorption, teriparatide (rhPTH 1–34; Forteo) given by daily subcutaneous injection acts an anabolic agent. It stimulates bone formation, producing gains in spine BMD two to three times greater than those observed with antiresorptive drugs. Vertebral and nonvertebral fractures were reduced 55% to 65% over 18 to 20 months of teriparatide therapy in the pivotal Fracture Prevention Trial (11). Treatment with teriparatide should be limited to 2 years because lack of both safety and efficacy data with longer duration. It is much more expensive than other agents (~$20 per day). The dose is 20 mcg SQ daily. Side effects include nausea, dizziness, and leg cramps. Hypercalcemia may occur but is infrequent. Rats given high doses of teriparatide over most of their life span develop osteosarcomas. Thus, Forteo contains a "black box" warning that the medication is not to be used in patients at increased risk of malignant bone tumors (children, patients with prior radiation therapy, Paget's disease, or unexplained increase of serum alkaline phosphatase). Teriparatide is generally reserved for patients at very high risk of fracture or patients who seem to be failing other therapies.

Combination Therapy

Combining two antiresorptive agents (e.g., a bisphosphonate combined with estrogen or raloxifene) produces additional gains in bone mineral density; however, no studies have shown if combination therapy reduces the risk of fracture more than treatment with a single agent. Combining parathyroid hormone or teriparatide with an antiresorptive agent appears to lessen the BMD response to teriparatide (12). However, cyclic 1–34 parathyroid hormone therapy (3 months on and 3 months off) produced similar gains in BMD to daily therapy in patients receiving alendronate (13). When therapy with parathyroid hormone is stopped, BMD begins to decline, but following parathyroid hormone or teriparatide treatment with a bisphosphonate appears to produce additional gains (14).

In the Future

1–84 Parathyroid hormone has been shown to reduce new vertebral fractures in a large clinical trial. No effect on nonvertebral or hip fractures was demonstrated. In the dose of 100 mcg SQ daily, hypercalcemia appeared to be more frequent than with teriparatide. In March 2006, the sponsor received an "approvable" letter from the FDA, with concerns regarding hypercalcemia and some issues with the delivery device needing further discussion or data.

Strontium ranelate is available in other countries but not in the United States. Strontium has both antiresorptive and anabolic actions. In a dose of 2 g orally b.i.d. it has been shown to reduce the risk of vertebral and nonvertebral fractures (15,16). A post hoc analysis suggests an effect on hip fractures.

Although more data on extraskeletal effects of raloxifene are being collected, clinical trials with newer SERMs, such as droloxifene and idoxifene, have been discontinued because of adverse endometrial effects. Laxofoxifene was rejected by the FDA in 2005. Other SERMs, including arzoxifene and bazedoxifene, are being studied.

Denosumab (AMG-162) is a monoclonal antibody that is an analog of osteoprotegerin, a naturally occurring decoy receptor for RANK ligand (RANKL). RANKL is required for osteoclast differentiation. By diverting RANKL, there are fewer osteoclasts and therefore an antiresorptive effect. In a phase II trial, denosumab was shown to increase bone density in the spine, hip, and forearm at least as well as alendronate and to decrease bone turnover to a similar degree as alendronate (17). The dose of denosumab going forward in phase III trials is 60 mg given by subcutaneous injection every month. The drug seemed well tolerated in this relatively small trial.

Summary and Conclusions

Adequate calcium, vitamin D, and weight-bearing exercise are important for everyone and fundamental to any program of bone loss prevention or osteoporosis treatment. Effective pharmacologic agents are available for reducing the risk of fracture. Pharmacologic intervention is indicated for women who have T scores of −2.5 and below and for women with risk factors whose T scores are −1.5 or below. Alendronate and risedronate have the best evidence for reduction of a variety of types of fracture and are well tolerated. Teriparatide has different mechanism of action and may be preferred for higher risk patients and for those failing to achieve a desired response to treatment with antiresorptive drugs.

REFERENCES

1. Holick MF, Siris ES, Binkley N, et al. Prevalence of vitamin D inadequacy among postmenopausal North American women receiving osteoporosis therapy. J Clin Endocrinol Metab 2005;90:3215–3224.
2. Reginster J-Y, Minne HW, Sorensen OH, et al. Randomized trial of the effects of risedronate on vertebral fractures in women with established postmenopausal osteoporosis. Osteoporos Int 2000;11:83–91.
3. Black DM, Cummings SR, Karpf DB, et al. Randomised trial of effect of alendronate on risk of fracture in women with existing vertebral fractures. Lancet 1996;348:1535–1541.
4. Harris ST, Watts NB, Genant HK, et al. Effects of risedronate treatment on vertebral and nonvertebral fractures in women with postmenopausal osteoporosis—a randomized controlled trial. JAMA 1999;282:1344–1352.
5. McClung MR, Geusens P, Miller PD, et al. Effect of risedronate on the risk of hip fracture in elderly women. N Engl J Med 2001;344:333–340.
6. Chesnut CH III, Skag A, Christiansen C, et al. Effects of oral ibandronate administered daily or intermittently on

fracture risk in postmenopausal osteoporosis. J Bone Miner Res 2004;19:1241–1249.

7. Reid IR, Brown JP, Burckhardt P, et al. Intravenous zoledronic acid in postmenopausal women with low bone mineral density. N Engl J Med 2002;346:653–661.

8. Chesnut CH III, Silverman S, Andriano K, et al. A randomized trial of nasal spray salmon calcitonin in postmenopausal women with established osteoporosis: the Prevent Recurrence of Osteoporotic Fractures study. Am J Med 2000;102:267–276.

9. Writing Group for the Women's Health Initiative Investigators. Risks and benefits of estrogen plus progestin in healthy postmenopausal women. JAMA 2002;288:321–333.

10. Ettinger B, Black DM, Mitlak BH, et al. Reduction of vertebral fracture risk in postmenopausal women with osteoporosis treated with raloxifene—results from a 3-year randomized clinical trial. JAMA 1999;282:637–645.

11. Neer RM, Arnaud CD, Zanchetta JR, et al. Effect of parathyroid hormone (1–34) on fractures and bone mineral density in postmenopausal women with osteoporosis. N Engl J Med 2001;344:1434–1441.

12. Black DM, Greenspan SL, Ensrud KE, et al. The effects of parathyroid hormone and alendronate alone or in combination in postmenopausal osteoporosis. N Engl J Med 2003;349:1207–1215.

13. Cosman F, Nieves J, Zion M, Woelfert L, Luckey M, Lindsay R. Daily and cyclic parathyroid hormone in women receiving alendronate. N Engl J Med 2005;353:566–575.

14. Black DM, Bilezikian JP, Ensrud KE, et al. One year of alendronate after one year of parathyroid hormone (1–84) for osteoporosis. N Engl J Med 2005;353:555–565.

15. Meunier PJ, Roux C, Seeman E, et al. The effects of strontium ranelate on the risk of vertebral fracture in women with postmenopausal osteoporosis. N Engl J Med 2004;350:459–468.

16. Reginster J-Y, Seeman E, De Vernejoul M-C, et al. Strontium ranelate reduces the risk of nonvertebral fractures in postmenopausal women with osteoporosis: treatment of Peripheral Osteoporosis (TROPOS) Study. J Clin Endocrinol Metab 2005;90:2816–2822.

17. McClung MR, Lewiecki EM, Cohen SB, et al. Denosumab in postmenopausal women with low bone mineral density. N Engl J Med 2006;354:821–831.

Rehabilitation of Patients with Rheumatic Diseases

Thomas D. Beardmore, MD, FACP, FACR

- In the care of disabled individuals, the current system of health care delivery and education largely focuses on a disease-centered medical model that fails to consider the role of society and the interaction of the disabled individual in that society over a lifespan.
- A more holistic approach to the care of disabled individuals considers the impact of environmental factors on the patient and provides a biopsychosocial orientation rather than a purely medical one.
- Holistic health approaches promote optimal function of the disabled person by considering not only the underlying rheumatic disease but the individual as a whole functioning person. Central to this health promotion is involvement of patient responsibility for his or her health and well being, including physical, psychological, social, and societal aspects.
- Multidisciplinary efforts are important to effective rehabilitation of patients disabled by rheumatic disease. Critical members of the multidisciplinary team are the rheumatologist, orthopedist, physical and occupational therapists, rehabilitation nurse, psychologist, social worker, and vocational rehabilitation specialist.

Rehabilitation of patients with rheumatic diseases addresses activity limitation and mobility as primary factors. It utilizes all healing disciplines and technologies with an emphasis on preservation and restoration of function. Medical, surgical, psychological, and physical treatments are utilized, with the rheumatologist as leader and coordinator of the interdisciplinary team. This program can provide functional success even if control of the disease process is suboptimal.

CLASSIFICATION OF FUNCTIONING, DISABILITY, AND HEALTH

The World Health Organization (WHO) in 2001 published the International Classification of Functioning, Disability, and Health (ICF) (1). This was an attempt to understand and categorize the experiences of people living with chronic illness. Much of current health care delivery and education continues to follow the medical model and to attribute disability to a disease-related deficit that prevents normal function. This model, however, fails to consider the role of society and the interaction of the disabled individual in that society over a lifespan. The ICF approaches health and disability as an integrated model that uses neutral terminology, includes environmental factors, and provides a biopsychosocial model of orientation rather than a purely medical model.

In the ICF classification, a health condition (disease or disorder) may influence body functions (physiologic and/or psychologic) or structures (anatomic parts), an activity that an individual does (e.g., walking), and the individual's participation in his or her life and environment (e.g., job, sports, recreation). The health condition, body functions, activities, and participation all interrelate and are influenced by personal (e.g., age, coping style) and environmental (e.g., architecture, social attitudes) factors. Functioning and disability are multidimensional. Functioning can be considered the positive abilities which encompass and result from a bodily structure or function, activities, and participation. Disability would be the negative aspect of function or restriction of activity and limitation of participation. Activity occurs at the individual level and participation at the societal level. Hence, a disease (health condition) may result in impairment of a body function that has impact on activity and participation, and the latter may interrelate. Activity is functioning at the level of the person and may be limited in nature, duration, and quality. Participation is involvement in life situations in relation to impairments, activities, health conditions,

TABLE 36-1. RHEUMATIC DISEASES: EXAMPLES OF DISABILITIES.

HEALTH CONDITION	BODY FUNCTION IMPAIRMENT	ACTIVITY RESTRICTION	PARTICIPATION IMPAIRMENT
Rheumatoid arthritis	Knee pain, small flexion contracture	Unable to walk long distances	Unable to participate in recreation (e.g., golf, walking)
DLE, face and scalp	Hair loss and skin depigmentation	None	Social activity restrictions (social phobia, shyness)
Scleroderma	Raynaud's phenomenon	None	Unable to participate in winter sports
Polymyositis	Proximal muscle weakness	Limited on stairs	Unable to enter house, public buildings, curbs
SLE	Photosensitivity	None	Unable to participate in outdoor activities
Ankylosing spondylitis	Back pain and stiffness	Limited ability to lift and bend	Unable to do medium and heavy jobs, limited in recreation (e.g., bowling)

ABBREVIATIONS: DLE, discoid lupus erythematosis; SLE, systemic lupus erythematosis.

and contextual factors, and may be restricted in nature, duration, and quality. Examples of rheumatic disease disablements are illustrated in Table 36-1. In the ICF model, medical treatment would be directed toward the health condition and its influence on bodily function. Rehabilitation therapies would address limitation of activity and participation. Public education, legislation, and universal architecture design would improve limited participation by the disabled community.

REHABILITATION TEAM AND SETTING

A holistic health approach is indicated to promote optimal function. This approach deals not just with the remission or absence of the underlying rheumatic disease, but promotes consideration of the individual as a whole functioning person. Central to this health promotion is involvement of patient responsibility for his or her health and well being, including physical, psychological, social, and societal aspects.

A health team, with multidisciplinary expertise, can help achieve optimal outcomes. In the hospital, this team may consist of rheumatology as team leader, along with occupational therapy, physical therapy, psychology, social work, rehabilitation nursing, and orthopedic surgery. Integral to this rehabilitation team is the patient who must accept responsibilities for selection of realistic goals and their implementation. In early disease and in the outpatient setting, it may be unnecessary to have all disciplines assist in the rehabilitation process. In advanced complicated disease, where there are disease elements, problems with mobility, impaired activities of daily living, depression, job loss, and insurance loss, the expertise of a team is required. The team leader selects

the appropriate consultations as problems arise, assures that there is communication between team members, and that realistic achievable goals are selected.

Rehabilitation should start with the first doctor visit and extend throughout the course of the disease. During early disease, the physician can address most functional problems with attention to the medical regimen. Rehabilitation can occur in a physician's office and by selected referral to the needed discipline: mobility problems can be referred to physical therapy for outpatient treatment; activities of daily living problems can be referred to occupational therapy; and psychological problems can be referred to the psychologist, as examples. With more advanced disease, short duration inpatient rehabilitation should be considered, where more intense treatment can be provided. Daily observation of the patient will permit fine adjustments of medical and therapy programs.

In the United States, diagnostic related groups (DRGs) govern the current medical care system and reimbursement for inpatient stays. This has been designed to reduce the total cost of health care in the United States and has been successful in doing so. For acute illnesses both inpatient stays and health care costs have been reduced. Inpatient rehabilitation is not defined by the DRG system but has also responded to the trend of reduced inpatient days. Currently, inpatient care is reserved for patients who have the most advanced rheumatic disease with the most functional impairment.

The requirements for inpatient hospitalization are dictated by Medicare rules. Currently, Medicare requires that patients with rheumatic disease have reductions in activities of daily living and mobility that have not responded to outpatient treatment. The illness must be sufficiently severe to require daily monitoring by physicians and health professionals. Eighteen hours of multidisciplinary inpatient treatment from two major rehabilitative disciplines (physical therapy, occupational therapy, and speech therapy) must be provided weekly. Social work and psychological rehabilitation can be given during the hospitalization and may contribute 3 hours of adjunct therapy to the required 18 hours of treatment.

A transitional inpatient care unit or skilled nursing facility can be used for patients who have significant functional problems and do not need 3 hours of daily treatments but require at least one modality for 1 hour daily. This should be considered for patients who have less disability and require skilled nursing as well as functional training (e.g., postoperative total joint arthroplasty strengthening and gait training). The goal for both inpatient and outpatient programs is maintenance of the rehabilitative program by the patient in their environment.

Clinical trials have shown that there is a beneficial response to multidisciplinary team care when compared to regular outpatient care. For active rheumatoid arthritis, improvement from inpatient rehabilitation was maintained for up to 2 years (2). The greatest changes were seen at 2 weeks after discharge when there was statistical improvement in the Ritchie articular index, number of swollen joints, disease activity by visual analogue scale (VAS), pain by VAS, and physician global assessment. At 4 weeks, 7 of 39 patients who had received inpatient rehabilitation had achieved American College of Rheumatology ACR20 status or better compared to none receiving outpatient treatment. At 1 year, improved disease activity by VAS was still significantly greater for the inpatient group and ACR20 or better was 46% in the inpatient group compared to 23% in the outpatient group. Recent reports have shown that outpatient multidisciplinary treatment is as effective as inpatient care. Patients treated as outpatients had significant improvement over time of functional status, quality of life, health utility, and disease activity (3). Additionally coordination of this care by a clinical nurse specialist was equally effective at a reduced overall cost. The importance of multidisciplinary care is established. Additional work is needed before it can be recommended that all patients will do well with outpatient care. At this time the setting is to be determined by the skilled rheumatologist and not by economics alone. It is likely that inpatient care is best for those with the greatest disability.

In addition to rheumatoid arthritis, multidisciplinary rehabilitation treatment is efficacious in ankylosing spondylitis (4). Considering the inflammatory nature and multi-articular nature of many other rheumatic diseases, it is reasonable to think that rehabilitative medical therapies would be beneficial and should be available to all patients.

PATIENT ASSESSMENT

In addition to the usual rheumatologic history and physical, an assessment of the patient's function is needed. This is obtained most effectively by indirect questions; for example: *"How does your arthritis affect your life?"* and *"Describe to me what you do on a usual day."* This will give the patient an opportunity to relate functional impact of the rheumatic disease on activities that are important to him or her. From this information, mutually agreed upon goals formulated by the patient and health care team can be made. All team members should obtain discipline-specific history. Inquiries should be made about activities of daily living, including personal grooming and toileting, eating, transfers and ambulation, vocational activities including homemaking, and hobbies and other avocational activities. Activities of daily living are usually described as independent, supervised, assisted, or unable. Dressing is further subdivided into ability to do upper body and lower body dressing.

The occupational therapist should record specific hand and upper extremity function, including ability with power grip, power and precision pinch, pill handling, and cylindrical grasp. Physical therapy activities should be recorded, stressing trunk and lower extremity functions and mobility activities, such as being able to prone, side lie, roll from side to side, to go from supine to sitting and from sitting to standing, to ambulate, and ability to climb stairs. Ambulation can be divided into household and community, with and without aids or wheelchair assistance.

Because the rheumatic diseases affect primarily the musculoskeletal system with resultant problems related to mobility, muscular strength, and joint range of motion, the physical examination is likewise functionally oriented. Manual muscle testing is a common way of measuring strength (Table 36-2). This is graded from 0 to 5, no motor activity to normal strength. It is impor-

TABLE 36-2. GRADES OF MUSCLE STRENGTH: MANUAL MUSCLE TESTING.

GRADE	DESCRIPTION
5 (normal)	Full ROM against gravity, strong resistance
4 (good)	Full ROM against gravity, some but not full resistance
3 (fair)	Full ROM against gravity, no resistance
2 (poor)	Full ROM, gravity eliminated
1 (trace)	Slight contracture, no ROM
0 (zero)	No muscle activity demonstrable

ABBREVIATION: ROM, range of motion.

36

tant to remember that normal strength has great variability and is dependent upon sex, size, and training status, and normal individuals with normal strength can lose considerable motor function before it is detectable by an examiner. Range of motion is measured by a goniometer and deviations from normal are noted. Particular attention should be given to alignment, noting flexion contractures, instabilities, and deformities.

There are multiple ways of recording longitudinal function. The most commonly used in the rheumatologic community is the ACR Functional Classification, groups I to IV (see Appendix I). This classification is useful for broad grouping of individuals and measures normal function to incapacitation (where assistance in ambulation and activities of daily living is needed). The ACR classification has broad usage and is time-tested but insensitive to small functional changes. Other useful functional assessment tools are the Arthritis Impact Measurement Scale, the Stanford Health Assessment Questionnaire, and the Functional Impact Measure. Each of these scales relies upon self-administered reports or professional observation of functional activities. They can be used in large studies to measure functional change and have utility in both large groups and individuals in an office or hospital practice. The ICF (1) provides a framework for research into the disabling processes and has proposed comprehensive core sets that can be applied to clinical settings by defining what to measure. Those that apply to rheumatology include core sets for rheumatoid arthritis, osteoarthritis, and osteoporosis. These core sets are currently being validated.

PAIN CONTROL

Pain is a frequent chief complaint and a cause of inactivity and loss of function for patients with rheumatic disease. Patient cooperation and success with rehabilitative treatments cannot be achieved if patients have pain. Disease control through standard medical regimens is sometimes the most efficient way of controlling pain and, hence, improving activities. Supplemental use of intra-articular glucocorticoids in resistant joints can control inflammation and pain, prevent flexion contractures, and improve range of motion and function. The use of topically applied medications (e.g., capsaicin and salicylic acid cream) is also to be considered, particularly as an adjunct to physical therapy and occupational therapy treatments. Oral analgesics, including low-dose nonsteroidal anti-inflammatory drugs (NSAIDS) and narcotics, are useful adjuncts to physical therapeutic programs when given 20 to 30 minutes before the onset of the exercise program. They can be used on an occasional basis to permit normal exercise or work periods.

PHYSICAL MODALITIES

Heat and Cold

Of the physical modalities that are commonly prescribed for musculoskeletal illnesses, heat and cold have the largest body of literature to support their use. Heat and cold have been used for centuries in musculoskeletal impairments, especially in acute injuries. There is no evidence that harm is done when these modalities are applied properly, and the potential improvement in pain, muscular spasm, and ability to participate in an active exercise program all have positive benefits for patient outcome. Their low cost and ease of use permit their use in the outpatient clinic, private office, and home. Most trials in musculoskeletal disorders report beneficial effects including reduced pain and muscle spasms, increased circulation, and improved range of motion (5). Temperature change occurs in the skin, deeper tissues, and on occasion, joint cavities. In addition to beneficial effects in clinical conditions, there is experimental evidence for diminished pain response to both heat and cold in experimental animal models with induced joint inflammation. Heat or cold treatment did not change joint inflammation, but secondary pain response and behavior were improved (6).

A systematic review of the medical literature for clinical benefit from heat and cold treatment showed little controlled data with accepted quality criteria of randomization and double-blinding; however, of those studies that did meet these criteria, heat and cold had no effect on the objective measures of disease activity, including inflammation (7). All patients reported that they preferred heat or cold therapy to no treatment but there was no preference for either modality. Because there are no harmful effects from heat or cold, it should be prescribed as a home treatment as needed for pain relief.

Heat therapy is usually given as a superficial application to the skin of hot packs, electrical pads, water baths, paraffin wax, or thermal packs. The use of water baths or whirlpool can be combined with active or passive motion to improve joint range. Thermal packs contain a chemical agent which upon activation produces heat by an exothermic reaction. They have no advantages over electrical heating pads or moist heat and have the disadvantage of one-time usage and increased cost. Heat therapy is contraindicated when there is loss of normal sensation and diminished or faulty blood supply.

With thermal therapy, deeper heating of tissues can be achieved by the use of therapeutic ultrasound. There are no controlled trials to indicate its utility in the rheumatic diseases. It has the disadvantage that it cannot be performed in the usual office setting but must be in a specialist's office with the associated inconvenience and increased cost.

Cold reduces pain, muscular spasm, and circulation, causing vasospasm and associated decrease in tissue metabolism, inflammation, and edema. It is standard treatment for immediate care after musculoskeletal injury because of these effects. Cold is applied locally for up to 30 minutes and produces a cooling of the skin and subcutaneous tissues. Deep cooling does occur and is dependant on application time and soft tissue depth.

Cold is typically prescribed as ice packs, reusable gel packs, chemical packs, or by ice massage directly over the painful area. Chemical packs produce cold by an endothermic reaction, but they have little utility except on an infrequent basis because of their expense and one-time use. Cooling sprays, such as ethyl chloride, are used commonly in rheumatology in a "spray and stretch" technique especially for painful syndromes of the neck and back. The skin is superficially cooled by the spray, resulting in relief of pain and muscular spasm. Active or passive stretching can then be achieved.

Electrical Stimulation

Transcutaneous electrical nerve stimulation (TENS) may be used for outpatient treatment of pain. A low voltage electrical stimulus is delivered to the skin either intermittently or continuously by activation of a battery-operated device worn about the waist. The patient can activate and control intensity as needed. It is administered for non-inflammatory conditions, particularly chronic pain from osteoarthritis of the back, knee pain, chronic shoulder pain, or pain in other major joints of the body. TENS is usually given to patients who are resistant to heat, cold, stretching, exercise, and other modalities. A careful review of trials comparing TENS to placebo in knee osteoarthritis demonstrated superiority for TENS in pain relief and improvement of knee stiffness (8). Despite the lack of controlled trials showing efficacy in other conditions, TENS has high patient acceptance and will likely continue to be commonly prescribed.

Hydrotherapy

Hydrotherapy combines exercise therapy and warm water emersion. It may be given on an intermittent basis as an outpatient or on a sustained basis in the form of spa therapy, one of the oldest treatments for rheumatic disease. The aim is to decrease pain, relieve suffering, and promote a feeling of wellness. There are few controlled trials of this treatment. However, there is some indication that, when administered on a regular basis as an outpatient, patients who received hydrotherapy had greater benefit than those who were treated by seated emersion in water, land exercises, or relaxation therapy (9). This improvement was both physical and emotional as reflected by the AIMS-2 questionnaire. A more extensive systematic review of the pub-

lished literature for spa therapy showed many flaws in the designs of the treatments with lack of standardized treatments, infrequent comparison groups, inconsistent intention-to-treat groups, and little evidence of outcome measures such as quality-of-life measurements. The conclusion was that spa therapy could not be supported as a recommended treatment in spite of consistently positive findings in the trials and acceptance by patients (10). Positive effects from spa therapy may be influenced by environmental changes such as freedom from work and household duties, mental and physical relaxation, and pleasant spa scenery that are unrelated to the water therapy.

Rest

Rest prescription may be local or systemic. It reduces acute inflammation and pain, and promotes normal joint position. Local rest is achieved by use of splints or braces, systemic rest by bed rest. Short periods of rest as part of a comprehensive program will permit patients to participate in exercise programs and work activities. Prolonged rest is to be avoided because both local and systemic rest are associated with significant muscle loss. Only a few weeks of local immobilization can reduce muscle mass by 21% (11). About one third of patients with rheumatoid arthritis will show improvement with bed rest that is similar to that seen with activity (12). There is increasing evidence that prolonged bed rest as a primary treatment for medical conditions is not helpful and should not be prescribed routinely. This includes its use in rheumatic disease rehabilitation. Some medical conditions, including acute back pain and postoperative hip surgical patients, may worsen with bed rest (13).

Exercise Therapy

Exercise therapy must take into consideration the underlying disease activity, including degree of inflammation, joint stability, muscle atrophy, and anticipated short- and long-term functional goals. Prescribed exercise may be active or passive, assisted, resistive, or aerobic.

Passive exercises may be administered by a physical therapist in which stretch and gentle range of motion exercises are given with a goal of maintaining range and reducing contractures. They are used for conditions associated with severe pain and weakness such as acute inflammation, acute myositis, and in the postoperative period. Active exercise may be assisted in painful and weak conditions in which the person is unable to complete full range of motion. Isometric exercise, in which there is active muscle contracture without muscle shortening or joint motion, will maintain muscle strength and is prescribed as initial therapy for those unable to tolerate range of motion due to pain, for example, postoperative joint arthroplasty.

36

Most patients with rheumatic disease will benefit from a resistive and aerobic exercise program. Resistive exercises should be tailored to the individual, the area of weakness, and the underlying disorder with a goal of increased strength and endurance. Aerobic and resistive exercises are beneficial for osteoathritis (OA). Walking and resistive exercise administered for 1 hour three times a week in patients with osteoarthritis of the knee is associated with less pain, less disability, and greater flexion strength (14). Similar but lesser effects are seen with OA of the hip. Results include mild-to-moderate improvement in pain, disability outcome measures, and greater benefit on patients' global assessment (15). Exercise therapy improves aerobic capacity and motor strength for patients with rheumatoid arthritis without worsening pain or disease activity (16). In ankylosing spondylitis, recreational exercise of at least 30 minutes daily improved pain and stiffness (17). When prescribed with back exercises 5 days a week, health status improved as measured by the Health Assessment Questionnaire Disability Index (HAQ-DI). The greatest benefit was seen in those with early disease. In patients with systemic lupus erythematosis, aerobic exercises and strengthening did not worsen disease activity and were associated with decreased fatigue and improvement in functional status, strength, and cardio-vascular fitness (18).

AMBULATORY AIDS

Canes, crutches, and walkers are prescribed to improve gait, including weakness, pain, and instability of lower extremity joints. The most useful canes are those made of wood or aluminum. They should be inexpensive and lightweight, easily adjusted for height, have a comfortable grip and wide rubber tip to firmly grip smooth floor surfaces. Cane length should be fitted so that the elbow is flexed 30°. With the use of a single cane or crutch at least 25% of normal weight bearing can be shifted from a weak or painful joint to the opposite limb. With bilateral support, up to 100% of weight bearing can be unloaded from a painful lower extremity to the upper extremities. Some patients will carry a cane and not use it for support. They use it only as a signal to others that they have ambulatory problems and should be given a greater courtesy when met.

Patients should be instructed on the proper use of an ambulatory aid. Single support is carried contralateral to the painful leg. It is advanced and used to bear weight during stance on the opposite leg. Multiple tips (e.g., a quad cane) will provide increased security for those with impaired proprioception or balance problems. For patients such as those with rheumatoid arthritis who cannot bear weight on the wrist or have significant hand deformities, ambulatory aids can be modified to accommodate these problems with forearm troughs, custom hand grips, and Velcro straps. These are fitted with the elbow at 90° flexion to avoid wrist and hand stress.

Crutches are prescribed for more severe problems and provide increased support when used bilaterally. They should be adjusted so that no pressure occurs on the axillae. Instruction needs to be given about proper weight bearing on the upper extremities with the wrist and elbow in extension. With crutch use, patients may use minimal or no weight bearing on a painful or weak leg. They will be most useful in the postoperative period and for acute injuries and illnesses. Platform crutches should be prescribed for patients with significant hand and wrist arthritis and discomfort with conventional crutches.

Walkers provide a wider support base than do canes or crutches for those who need greater ambulatory stability. They must be lightweight so they can be picked up and advanced. Wheels, brakes, and seats can be attached for patient comfort and safety. They are useful in the postoperative period, and for the elderly, frail, and those who need maximum support for balance.

Wheelchairs should be prescribed when community ambulation is impaired. Patients who are limited to household ambulation will have increased independence with a wheelchair for community activities. A manual wheelchair is advised for people with normal upper extremity function and strength and endurance sufficient to propel the chair. Manual wheelchairs, which are propelled by family, can be prescribed for the postoperative period and for the frail and elderly who do not wish to travel alone. Electric wheelchairs and carts should be prescribed for those with poor upper extremity function.

UPPER EXTREMITY AIDS

There are a large variety of commercially available assistive devices to improve activities of daily living for impaired upper extremity function. Pinch and grasp can be improved by having build-up handles on tools, cookware, and eating utensils. Power equipment such as electric knives and tools can substitute for decreased power grip and poor upper extremity strength. Reachers can be used to retrieve objects from the floor and shelves. Sock cones and long handle shoehorns will facilitate donning and doffing socks and shoes. Dressing sticks can assist those with impaired shoulder mobility. Long-handled brushes, combs, and sponges can improve upper extremity grooming and perineal care.

Dressing can be facilitated by attention to detail of clothing. Problems with pinch can improve by using button hooks, zippers with tabs, and Velcro closures for clothing and shoeware. Elastic closures for trousers and V necks for pullover sweaters and blouses will also facilitate dressing.

Home safety and accessibility can be assessed via home visits by a physical and occupational therapist. Those who have mobility impairments can be aided by installation of half steps, ramps, and handrails in entryways. Doorways should be wide to permit walker or wheelchair access. Furniture placement and room size should be sufficient for easy mobility with walking aids and wheelchairs. Scatter rugs and loose electrical cords should be removed. For those with knee and hip problems including limited mobility and strength, the addition of 4-inch-thick, high density foam cushions or blocks under the chair legs can increase chair height and improve ability to rise from the seated posture. Raised toilet seats will facilitate transfer on and off of the toilet. Within the bathroom, rubber mats should be placed on tub and shower surfaces to facilitate traction and prevent falls. Grab bars and tub and shower benches should be utilized if patients have problems with balance and are at risk of falling. Handheld shower nozzles can facilitate bathing.

Orthotic Devices

Splints and braces are useful for improving stability and reducing pain and inflammation. Because effective orthoses restrict motion, short-term use is recommended to preserve muscle strength. Splints for the upper extremity are commonly used and they have general patient and physician acceptance (Table 36-3). Although pain and inflammation are reduced, there are no studies to indicate that deformities are prevented. Wrist orthoses may decrease hand function in the short term as measured by grip strength and finger and hand dexterity (19). These potential adverse effects are not an issue for patients because most will continue to wear the splints when given an option to discontinue them. Consultation with an orthotist or occupational therapist for a custom-made device is indicated for severe deformities in which immobilization is needed for pain relief and improved stability.

Orthoses that immobilizes the wrist are of value in carpal tunnel syndrome. The wrist is immobilized in a neutral position with 20° to 30° of extension of the hand at the wrist. Ring splints are useful for flexible swan neck deformities of the digits and can improve pinch strength by putting the proximal interphalangeal (PIP) joint in a slightly flexed and more functional position for precision pinch. They are not effective for fixed deformities and there are no studies to support prolonged use of ring splints for deformity prevention. Ring splints may be made of silver to enhance cosmesis and wearing compliance.

The carpometacarpal (CMC) immobilization splint (thumb post splint) is quite effective for degenerative CMC joint disease and can be used when patients have flare-ups and pain at the base of the thumb. Coupled with this, activity that increase forces across the CMC joints, such as power pinch, should be reduced. One common way of avoiding this is to increase the size of pens and pencils by using a rubber or foam grip and reminding the patient that light touch with writing instruments will prevent pain.

Casting with plaster or lightweight fiberglass can be used for immobilization as a trial to see if pain is improved before more expensive orthoses are made (e.g., ankle or foot braces) and prior to surgical arthrodesis. If cast immobilization results in pain relief, then a rigid orthosis or arthrodesis will be associated with improved pain and function.

LOWER EXTREMITY ORTHOSES

The simplest orthoses for restricting range of motion and decreasing pain would be the use of elastic bandages, elastic or neoprene sleeves, and taping. For degenerative arthritis of the knee, many patients will have improve-

TABLE 36-3. COMMON UPPER EXTREMITY ORTHOSES.

DISORDER	DEFORMITY	PROBLEM	SOLUTION
RA	Flexible swan neck deformity of fingers	None; clicking; cosmetic appearance	Ring splints (stabilizes PIP in flexion)
Carpal tunnel syndrome	None	Night pain, dysesthesias	Wrist splint, 20°–30° extension
OA of first CMC	None	CMC pain with pinch	Thumb post splint, thumb spica
RA	None	Pain; inflammation of wrist, MCPs, and PIPs	Hand-resting splint (resting posture from wrist to DIPs)
Mallet finger	Flexion of DIP	None	Rigid DIP splint, 20° hyperextension

ABBREVIATIONS: CMC, carpometacarpal; DIP, distal interphalangeal; OA, osteoarthritis; PIP, proximal interphalangeal; RA, rheumatoid arthritis.

from a multicenter study. Arthritis Rheum 1991;40:2199–2206.

25. de Buck PD, le Cessie S, van den Hout WB, et al. Randomized comparison of a multidisciplinary job-retention vocational rehabilitation program with usual care in patients with chronic arthritis at risk for job loss. Arthritis Care Res 2005;53:682–690.

26. Straaton KV, Maisiak R, Wrigley JM, Fine PR. Musculoskeletal disability, employment, and rehabilitation. J Rheumatol 1995;22:505–513.

27. Disability Evaluation Under Social Security. SSA Publication No. 64-039. ICN No. 468600, Wahington DC: US Department of Health and Human Services, Social Security Administration, Office of Disability; 2003.

CHAPTER 37

Psychosocial Factors in Arthritis

ALEX ZAUTRA, PhD
DENISE KRUSZEWSKI, MS

- Psychosocial factors are essential to a patient's vulnerability to the most important symptoms of rheumatic diseases, including pain and fatigue.
- Positive and negative emotions influence adaptation to rheumatic diseases with depression predictive of adverse outcomes.
- Cognitive factors, including a sense of control over illness, are of great importance to daily well-being.

- Interventions that improve self-efficacy improve pain and psychological functioning.
- Social factors also affect impact of diseases, with social resources and the ability to utilize them being a strong determinant of well-being among rheumatic disease patients.

Psychosocial factors play an important role in the etiology and course of rheumatic diseases. In this chapter, we introduce concepts that may aid the reader in understanding the relationship. Psychosocial challenges and physiological mechanisms involved in rheumatic disease manifestations may be best understood within the conceptual framework of stress and the individual response to stress. It has become increasingly evident that psychosocial factors are essential to understanding *who* is most affected by illness and other stressors, as well as *when* they are most vulnerable. We end the chapter with a discussion of resilience, as it important to acknowledge the capacities of individuals to cope successfully with their illness.

STRESS

Stressors can be conceptualized as initiating events that may be acute or chronic, small, or major and traumatic events, that occur from childhood through adulthood. According to the model initially proposed by Hans Seyle, illness can be considered a stressor. Stress responses can be conceptualized as reactions to these initiating events that may be measured both physiologically and psychologically. These stress responses vary between individuals, and may comprise the mechanisms underlying the link between stressors and arthritis.

The nature of a stress event may impact disease course and severity in rheumatic disease patients. For example, one study demonstrated a reduction in disease symptoms in rheumatoid arthritis (RA) patients directly following major stressful events, but increased symptoms in weeks when small stressful events had occurred (1). One explanation for this finding is that major stressful events may set into motion a physiological stress response in which some aspects of immune functioning are suppressed. In contrast, minor stressful events may enhance other aspects of immune functioning. Specifically, elevations in the immune-stimulating hormones prolactin and estradiol have been shown to mediate the association between interpersonal conflict and disease flares in RA patients (2). Thus, stressful events may induce higher levels of immune-related hormones, which results in increased disease activity.

Traumatic events, including both childhood maltreatment and adverse events later in life, have also been linked with increased disease severity in rheumatic disease patients. For example, one study showed that a higher fibromyalgia tender point count during a physical examination was associated with reports of childhood maltreatment (3). Additionally, adult traumatic events can also impact disease severity. In a study of fibromyalgia patients, post-traumatic stress disorder (PTSD) symptoms were linked with increased pain severity (4). Traumatic stressors induce psychological symptoms of PTSD, which in turn are linked with increased pain severity. Additionally, disruption in hypothalamic–pituitary–adrenal (HPA) functioning has been suggested as the physiological link between traumatic events and disease severity. In fact both hypo- and hypercortisol reactivity has been associated with traumatic experiences (5) and dysregulation of cortisol secretion has been linked with increased vulnerability to disease (6). Lower levels of cortisol may fail to check proinflammatory processes that are often elevated during stress, resulting in joint swelling and tenderness for RA patients and greater fatigue for those with fibromyalgia. These examples underscore the complexities involved in charting an association between events and disease severity, particularly when that relationship is mediated by both physiological and psychological stress responses. However, while stressors and stress responses may be factors in the experience of chronic pain, psychosocial factors also play a role in this experience. In fact, individual differences in coping responses likely play a prominent role in determining how health-related outcomes are modified by stress. Coping factors may be characterized as primarily affective, cognitive, or social, and we address each component below.

PSYCHOLOGICAL FACTORS

Affective Components

Researchers have characterized emotions as fluctuating mood states and also as stable personality traits. Both positive and negative emotions have been shown to influence adaptation among patients with rheumatic disease. One of the most frequently researched affective disorders in rheumatic disease patients is depression. Hudson and colleagues (7) have proposed that rheumatic conditions such as fibromyalgia can be classified among a spectrum of disorders that share affective disturbances, such as depression, fatigue, and allodynia. In fact, depressive symptoms can be considered part of the experience of chronic pain, rather than as a cause of the disorder. Neuroimaging studies have identified differential locations for the processing of the affective and sensory components of the pain experience (8). Studies have consistently demonstrated associations between depression and pain severity in rheumatic disease patients. RA patients exhibiting more depressive symptoms reported higher average pain across weeks, increased pain during stressful weeks, and more affective disturbance in response to pain episodes (9). Depression and stress were associated with inflammatory markers in RA patients, suggesting that these factors also increase disease activity (10). Therefore, depression appears to be key a vulnerability factor for increased pain and inflammation in patients with rheumatic diseases during times of stress. This vulnerability appears to extend beyond current depression, as recent studies have shown that RA patients with a history of depression suffer from more episodes of daily pain (11).

Other stable personality traits that are infused with affect have also been studied, such as neuroticism and extroversion. Neuroticism has been shown to increase vulnerability to stress and is linked to both pain and mood in RA patients, which suggests that this personality trait may impact both symptoms (12). On the other hand, the personality dimension of extroversion may set the stage for positive emotional experience, even during stressful times.

Thus far, the discussion has focused on differences in affective experience between individuals. However, affective experience may also vary within the individual, from day to day and even hour to hour, potentially elevating risks for illness exacerbation during those times when affective disturbance is greatest. These differences are important, addressing not *who* is most affected by stress, but *when* the person is most vulnerable. Furthermore, when thinking about how individual affective experience varies over time, it is important to examine positive as well as negative emotions because both contribute to the quality of life and adaptive capacities of rheumatic patients and do so in different ways.

Increased negative affect has been linked with increased pain, and also has been associated with greater sensitization to pain (13). Negative affect has also been linked to stress directly (14). This suggests that negative affect may be both a part of the experience of pain itself as well as a response to stress in pain patients. Conversely, positive affect may actually *decrease* vulnerability to stress in rheumatic patients. In fact, higher levels of positive affect may be particularly important during stress and pain episodes. Thus, indirectly, higher levels of positive affect may prevent the pain sensitization associated with rheumatic diseases.

As yet, little attention has been directed to other affective components that may be linked to chronic pain. Further inquiry into high and low activation states of both positive and negative affect may be fruitful. For example, anger, a high-activation negative affective state, may have different associations with stress and pain than fatigue, a low-activation negative affective state. This may also be the case for excitement, a high-activation positive affective state, versus calm, a low-activation positive affective state. Different emotional states then may lead to the construction of different types of psychosocial interventions designed to promote one or another feeling state.

Cognitive Components

It is helpful to distinguish between affective and cognitive components of stress response, even though this distinction is somewhat arbitrary. A useful way of conceptualizing cognitive stress responses is as dimensions of coping, in particular, an individual's sense of control or lack thereof. Among these cognitive processes are self-efficacy, personal mastery, and pain catastrophizing. While not considered coping, attentional deployment is also a fundamental cognitive process that has implications for the experience of pain in rheumatic disease patients.

The daily experience of rheumatic pain patients is fraught with uncertainty about when and how pain symptoms may occur. This uncertainty renders the individual's sense of control of great importance to both daily well-being as well as the response to stress. Self-efficacy is a key component that characterizes an individual's control beliefs with respect to their illness. This concept has its origins in the work of Bandura, who defined self-efficacy as a person's confidence in their ability to execute and accomplish a given task (15). The development of the Arthritis Self-Efficacy Scale by Lorig and colleagues has helped researchers to quantify this set of beliefs with respect to pain, function, and other arthritis symptoms. High scores on this scale have been linked with higher pain thresholds and tolerance for laboratory pain in arthritis patients (16). Interventions aimed at increasing self-efficacy in rheumatic disease patients have led to improvements in pain and psychological functioning (17). Thus, not only is self-efficacy a vital component of well-being in rheumatic patients, evidence suggests that individuals may be taught to improve and enhance their cognitive beliefs in this arena. Additionally, these beliefs translate into behaviors that define the daily experience of individuals. For example, a study of fibromyalgia patients showed that self-efficacy was related to decreases in pain behaviors, including grimacing and vocalizations of distress (18).

On the negative side, pain catastrophizing is characterized by beliefs in limited self-efficacy and control, particularly with regard to the experience of pain. These beliefs have been associated with increased pain severity, increased levels of pain behaviors, higher pain-related disability, and greater health care utilization in patients with a variety of rheumatic disorders (19). Neuroimaging studies have further illuminated these findings by demonstrating links between pain catastrophizing and activation in key areas of the brain associated with anticipation of pain, emotional aspects of pain, attention to pain, and motor control (20). Pain catastrophizing has also been characterized by a heightened focus on pain, which points to the importance of attentional processes for chronic pain patients.

Heightened attention to pain is related to the basic cognitive process of attentional deployment. Attentional deployment is defined as the capacity to selectively focus on, or more importantly in some cases, deflect attention away from stimuli. Deficits in this capacity have implications for rheumatic patients, including increased pain symptoms (19). Indeed, rheumatic disease patients have demonstrated decreased attentional functioning, including deficits in overall attentional deployment, selective attention, and working memory (21). These deficits have also been demonstrated in individuals who have experienced trauma, particularly childhood maltreatment (22). Additionally, just as pain may result in part from impaired attentional deployment, pain itself may serve to disrupt other attentional processes (23).

Although cognitive factors are usually studied primarily as modifiable processes that influence adaptation to chronic pain, it is important to acknowledge that there are also cognitive factors that exhibit moderate levels of stability over time. Investigators have examined factors such as internal locus of control, optimism, pessimism, and memory, to name a few. More research is needed at this point on both stable as well as more malleable cognitive contributions.

SOCIAL FACTORS

Social stressors are among the most challenging types of stressors. While this is true for even for those without illness, the consequences of social stress and associated responses may be particularly salient for individuals with rheumatic conditions. Richer formulations take into account different attachment styles as well as ramifications of lasting positive social interactions.

Social pain is an emerging concept that focuses on the interplay between social relationships and physical pain. Social pain is an emotional response to perceived exclusion from desired social relationships or perceived devaluation by significant members of an individuals' social network (24). Just as physical pain is adaptive because it signals a threat to well-being, social pain is adaptive because it motivates social connectedness. Neuroimaging studies have shown that the emotional component of physical pain and the experience of social exclusion activate the same areas in the anterior cingulate cortex (ACC) (25). This has particular ramifications for chronic pain patients, who may be subject to social exclusion due to conflict with others, including medical professionals, who do not understand their pain experience (24). This lack of understanding sometimes leads to feelings of stigmatization in rheumatic disease patients, which further adversely impacts both their disease severity and their social relations. Opportunities for social connectedness begin in the initial years of life, during interactions with family and other caregivers. It is widely believed that early attachment relationships with caregivers impact the development of self-regulation processes as well as interpersonal relationships. In particular, theories of emotion socialization postulate that children learn to modulate their own emotions based on the response of their caregivers to their emotions (26). Therefore, stable attachment relationships provide the template for effective management of emotions. Conversely, unstable caregiving relationships lay the groundwork for ineffective emotion regulation as well as difficulties forming enduring social relations. It is important to note that the type of difficulties an individual develops in these arenas may vary according to the type, severity, and chronicity of the maltreatment. Interestingly, studies have also demonstrated that many, perhaps even most, individuals who have endured childhood maltreatment are able to engage in secure adult relationships. These adult relationships are likely to influence current psychological functioning as much as childhood abuse and neglect (27).

The association between physical pain and social connectedness has been demonstrated in patients with rheumatic diseases. One study demonstrated decreased sensitivity to pain in fibromyalgia patients when in the presence of their significant other (28). Interestingly, these results were detected by decreased activity in brain areas associated with pain, as well as in decreased reports of pain, in response to thermal stimulation. However, the impact of social connectedness is more complex than it may seem. Relationships often have both beneficial and harmful aspects, and both of these dimensions impact response to stress as well as pain experience (29). Thus, while having social resources is helpful, it is not enough. Instead, the characteristics of these resources and the ability to utilize these resources, particularly during times of stress, is a strong determinant of health and well-being.

RESILIENCE

The framework of resilience provides a means of approaching the vulnerabilities and the resources of rheumatic disease patients in their adaptation to their illness and other stressors. Resilience is characterized by the presence of psychological, social, and economic resources *and* the individual's ability to access and utilize these resources. Resilience connotes both the ability to protect against the detrimental impact of stress as well as to recover from stressful events. Most importantly, resilience appears to be more the rule than an exception to the rule. In fact, Masten, in referring to how children survive the most difficult childhoods, describes resilience as "ordinary magic," involving readily accessible human adaptational systems rather than extraordinary and unusual capabilities (30). This is true for rheumatic patients as well, many of whom adapt and manage their pain expertly. For those that encounter difficulty, behavioral interventions may be most successful when assisting individuals in accessing resources that they already have rather than focusing on deficits in psychosocial functioning.

Empirical studies continue to provide strong support for research on psychosocial factors and stress to advance our understanding of the relevance of a bio-

psychosocial model of health and illness to rheumatic conditions.

REFERENCES

1. Potter PT, Zautra AJ. Stressful life events' effects on rheumatoid arthritis disease activity. J Consult Clin Psychol 1997;65:319–323.
2. Zautra AJ, Burleson MH, Matt KS, Roth S, Burrows L. Interpersonal stress, depression, and disease activity in rheumatoid arthritis and osteoarthritis patients. Health Psychol 1994;13:139–148.
3. McBeth J, MacFarlane GJ, Benjamin S, Morris S, Silman AJ. The association between tenderpoints, psychological distress, and adverse childhood experiences: a community-based study. Arthritis Rheum 1999;42:1397–1404.
4. Sherman JJ, Turk DC, Okifuji A. Prevalence and impact of posttraumatic stress disorder-like symptoms in patients with fibromyalgia syndrome. Clin J Pain 2000;16:127–134.
5. Cicchetti D, Rogosch FA. Diverse patterns of neuroendocrine activity in maltreated children. Dev Psychopathol 2001;13:677–694.
6. Heim C, Ehlert U, Hanker JP, Hellhammer DH. Abuse-related posttraumatic stress disorder and alterations of the hypothalamic-pituitary-adrenal axis in women with chronic pelvis pain. Psychosom Med 1998;60:309–318.
7. Hudson JI, Mangweth B, Pope HG, et al. (2003). Family study of affective spectrum disorder. Arch Gen Psychiatry 2003;60:170–177.
8. Rainville P, Duncan GH, Price DD, Carrier B, Bushnell MC. Pain affect encoded in human anterior cingulate but not somatosensory cortex. Science 1977;277:968–971.
9. Zautra AJ, Smith B. Depression and reactivity to stress in older women with rheumatoid arthritis and osteoarthritis. Psychosom Med 2001;63:687–696.
10. Zautra AJ, Yocum DC, Villanueva I, et al. (2003). Immune activation and depression in women with rheumatoid arthritis. J Rheumatol 2003;31:457–463.
11. Conner T, Tennen H, Zautra AJ, Affleck G, Armeli S, Fifield J. Coping with chronic arthritis pain in daily life: within-person analyses reveal hidden vulnerability for the formerly depressed. Pain 2006;128:128–135.
12. Affleck G, Tennen H, Urrows S, Higgins P. Neuroticism and the pain-mood relation in rheumatoid arthritis: insights from a prospective daily study. J Consult Clin Psychol 1992;60:119–126.
13. Janssen SA. Negative affect and sensitization to pain. Scand J Psychol 2002;43:131–137.
14. Zautra AJ, Johnson LM, Davis MC. Positive affect as a source of resilience for women in chronic pain. J Counsel Clin Psychol 2005;73:212–220.
15. Keefe FJ, Smith SJ, Buffington ALH, Gibson J, Studts JL, Caldwell DS. Recent advances and future directions in the biopsychosocial assessment and treatment of arthritis. J Consult Clin Psychol 2002;70:640–655.
16. Keefe FJ, Affleck G, Lefebvre JC, Starr K, Caldwell DS, Tennen H. Coping strategies and coping efficacy in rheu-

matoid arthritis: a daily process analysis. Pain 1997;69: 43–48.

17. Lorig KR, Mazonson PD, Holman HR. Evidence suggesting that health education for self-management in patients with chronic arthritis has sustained health benefits while reducing health care costs. Arthritis Rheum 1993;36:439–446.

18. Buckelew SP, Parker JC, Keefe FJ, et al. Self-efficacy and pain behavior among subjects with fibromyalgia. Pain 1994;59:377–384.

19. Keefe FJ, Lumley M, Anderson T, Lynch T, Carson KL. Pain and emotion: new research directions. J Clin Psychol 2001;57:587–607.

20. Gracely RH, Geisser ME, Giesecke MAB, Petzke F, Williams DA, Clauw DJ. Pain catastrophizing and neural responses to pain among persons with fibromyalgia. Brain 2004;127:835–843.

21. Dick B, Eccleston C, Crombez G. Attentional functioning in fibromyalgia, rheumatoid arthritis, and musculoskeletal pain patients. Arthritis Rheum 2002;47:634–644.

22. Perry BD, Pollard RA, Blakley TL, Baker WL, Vigilante D. Childhood trauma, the neurobiology of adaptation and use-dependent development of the brain: how states become traits. Infant Mental Health 1995;16: 271–291.

23. Eccleston C, Crombez G. Pain demands attention: a cognitive-affective model of the interruptive function of pain. Psychol Bull 1999;125:356–366.

24. MacDonald G, Leary MR. Why does social exclusion hurt? The relationship between social and physical pain. Psychol Bull 2005;131:202–223.

25. Eisenberger NI, Lieberman MD, Williams KD. Does rejection hurt? An fMRI study on social exclusion. Science 2003;302:290–292.

26. Liotti G. Disorganized/disoriented attachment in the etiology of dissociative disorders. Dissociation, 1992;4: 196–204.

27. Roche DN, Runtz MG, Hunter MA. Adult attachment: A mediator between childhood sexual abuse and later psychological adjustment. J Interpersonal Violence 1999; 14:184–207.

28. Montoya P, Larbig W, Braun C, Preissl H, Birbaumer N. Influence of social support and emotional context on pain processing and magnetic brain responses in fibromyalgia. Arthritis Rheum 2004;50:4035–4044.

29. Davis MC, Zautra AJ, Reich JW. Vulnerability to stress among women in chronic pain from fibromyalgia and osteoarthritis. Ann Behav Med 2001;23:215–226.

30. Masten AS. Ordinary magic: resilience processes in development. Am Psychol 2001;56:227–238.

CHAPTER 38

Self-Management Strategies*

Teresa J. Brady, PhD

- Self-management activities, such as participation in education programs and physical activity, are central to the nonpharmacological management of arthritis
- Self-management education, physical activity, and weight loss have all demonstrated health benefits for people with arthritis.

- Evidence suggests that very few people with arthritis participate in self-management education.

Self-management activities, such as participation in education programs and physical activity, are central to the nonpharmacological management outlined in American College of Rheumatology guidelines for arthritis management. Anything a person does to try to manage their arthritis could be considered self-management, but the Institute of Medicine (IOM) definition of self-management focuses on essential tasks. The IOM defines self-management as "the tasks that the individuals must undertake to live well with one or more chronic conditions" (1). While individuals with arthritis try a variety of strategies to live well with their disease, scientific evidence supports only a limited number of key self-management activities. This chapter reviews the evidence base for the three self-management strategies with the broadest applicability: participating in self-management education, maintaining regular, moderate intensity physical activity, and controlling weight. These three strategies also form the core public health messages for disability prevention promoted by the Centers for Disease Control and Prevention's arthritis program (see Table 38-1 for a summary of these strategies). A fourth strategy, seeking early diagnosis and appropriate medical treatment if rheumatoid arthritis is suspected, is of more targeted applicability, and will not be addressed here. This chapter will conclude with recommendations for improving the effectiveness of clinician counseling through the use of a brief behavioral counseling model to assist patients in practicing self-management.

KEY SELF-MANAGEMENT STRATEGIES

Self-Management Education—"Build Arthritis Control Skills"

The patient-oriented public health message "build your arthritis control skills" highlights the importance of self-management education. Not all patient education is designed to foster self-management. Much of the traditional patient education emphasizes providing information about the disease and its treatment, using verbal instruction supplemented by handouts and pamphlets. Self-management education is designed to build patients' confidence and skills to manage their arthritis on a day-to-day basis; it is less didactic and uses interactive methods to help patients develop the necessary skills. A meta-analysis of arthritis education trials demonstrated that education interventions that included behavioral techniques produced significantly greater improvements in pain, function, and tender joint counts than did information dissemination interventions (2). Similarly, handouts or booklets may be useful adjuncts, but do not constitute self-management education on their own. Several studies have demonstrated short-term (3–6 month) knowledge change, but no change in health status (1).

Evidence-based self-management education can be provided individually or in small groups. The most practical and economical way to provide self-management education is through referral to education programs such as the Arthritis Self-Management Program (ASMP), also known as the Arthritis Foundation Self Help Program, or the Chronic Disease Self Management Program (CDSMP). Both ASHP and CDSMP are

---

*The findings and conclusions in this book chapter are those of the author and do not necessarily represent the views of the Centers for Disease Control and Prevention.

TABLE 38-1. ARTHRITIS SELF-MANAGEMENT STRATEGIES/KEY PUBLIC HEALTH MESSAGES FOR DISABILITY PREVENTION.

STRATEGY/MESSAGE	RATIONALE	RESOURCES
Self-management education/"Build your arthritis control skills"	Research documents increases in self-efficacy and health behaviors (exercise, relaxation, cognitive symptom management) improved health outcomes (pain, disability, depression, helplessness), and reductions in health care costs (physician visits) (1)	Arthritis Self Management Program (also known as the Arthritis Foundation Self Help Program) http://www.arthritis.org/events/ Chronic Disease Self Management Program http://patienteducation.stanford.edu
Physical activity/"Be active"	Research demonstrates clinically meaningful improvements in function, flexibility, muscle strength and endurance, cardiovascular fitness, and psychological status (6)	Arthritis Foundation Exercise Program http://www.arthritis.org/events/ Arthritis Foundation Aquatic Program http://www.arthritis.org/events/ EnhanceFitness http://projectenhance.org
Weight control/"Control your weight"	Modest weight loss (10–15 pounds) can alleviate symptoms and delay progression of knee OA (13)	Analysis of weight loss programs available at http://www.consumer.gov/weightloss

38

6- to 7-week small group education programs led by trained lay and professional leaders following a structured protocol. Both programs, developed by Lorig and colleagues, were designed to enhance participants' confidence in their ability to manage their chronic disease, and to teach management skills such as problem solving, action planning, decision making, and communicating with health care professionals (1).

The arthritis-specific program, ASMP, has been disseminated by the Arthritis Foundation since 1981 and is called the Arthritis Foundation Self Help Program. Lorig and colleagues have demonstrated a 43% reduction in pain and a 19% reduction in physician visits at 4-year follow-up after participation in the ASMP. The generic chronic disease program, which was evaluated among a mix of participants with arthritis, diabetes, heart disease, and lung disease, produced significant improvements in health distress and health care utilization (physician and emergency-room visits) at 2-year follow-up. Lorig and colleagues have also developed Spanish-language versions of ASMP and CDSMP, which have similar benefits (1).

Comparisons of the relative efficacy of ASMP and CDSMP among people with arthritis have produced equivocal results. A study by Lorig and colleagues found more beneficial effects from ASMP at 4-month follow-up but this difference was largely gone at 12 months (3). In a similar study, Goeppinger and colleagues found significantly greater decreases in pain and disability at 4-month follow-up from CDSMP among their largely African-American participants (4). Both investigators concluded that both CDSMP and ASMP are beneficial for people with arthritis; Lorig concluded that the disease-specific ASMP may be preferred while

Goeppinger concluded that CDSMP may be advantageous for patients with multiple comorbidities.

Several forms of individually delivered self-management education have been developed and evaluated, but are not in widespread use. Several computer-tailored mailed education programs have shown significant benefits in health status and reductions in physician visits. Weekly educational mailings supplemented by telephone support have also demonstrated positive changes in health status. Lorig and colleagues are now testing an Internet-based version of the ASMP and CDSMP (1).

Meta-analytic reviews of arthritis self-management education studies have consistently found small but significant short-term benefits from these types of programs. For example, a recent Cochrane Collaboration review of education in rheumatoid arthritis (RA) found that behavioral interventions such as ASMP produced small-to-moderate effect sizes that equated to 10% to 12% improvements in patients' global health assessment, depression, and disability. In the same analyses, information-only interventions, such as verbal instruction or informational brochures, and social support/counseling interventions showed no significant benefits (1).

Although self-management education studies have demonstrated significant benefits in health status and cost savings, the majority of people with arthritis have not received self-management education. Only 11% of the adults with arthritis responding to a 2003 national survey reported that they had attended an educational course or class that taught them how to manage problems related to arthritis (5). Clinicians can foster participation by making specific referrals to self-management education programs such as ASMP and CDSMP. The self-management support section below will discuss strategies clinicians can use to facilitate patient participation in self-management education programs.

Physical Activity—"Be Active"

Physical activity is a core self-management activity for people with arthritis, and "be active" is a core public health message for both the general population and people with arthritis. Although early treatment recommendations cautioned patients with arthritis not to be active, a burgeoning body of research supports both professionally directed therapeutic exercise and self-directed moderate physical activity. As summarized by Westby and Minor, there is consistent evidence that people with arthritis can safely participate in moderate physical activity, such as walking, stationary bicycling, aerobic dance, aquatic exercise, and circuit training, without aggravation of their disease. This kind of regular moderate exercise can produce clinically meaningful improvements in function, flexibility, muscle strength and endurance, cardiovascular fitness, and psychological status (6).

In 2002 the American College of Rheumatology (ACR) convened a conference that developed recommendations for physical activity for people with osteoarthritis (OA) and RA; both sets of recommendations included aerobic activity (30 minutes at least 3 days per week for OA; 30–60 minutes 2–3 days per week for RA) and lower extremity strengthening programs (6). These recommendations are slightly modified from the American College of Sports Medicine recommendations for general health based on the absence of any data on physical activity programs for people with arthritis more frequent than three times per week.

In addition to the clear benefits physical activity can produce for people with arthritis, inactivity can increase disabling factors such as fatigue, low endurance, loss of strength and flexibility, and depression frequently attributed to arthritis. Inactivity also increases risks for comorbid conditions such as cardiovascular disease, diabetes, and osteoporosis among people with arthritis. However, 43% of people with self-reported arthritis say they get no leisure time physical activity, and only 32% are meeting the arthritis-specific recommendation of 30 minutes of moderate physical activity at least three times per week (7).

Research has demonstrated benefits of both group and home exercise programs (6). Arthritis-appropriate exercise programs are available through local agencies such as Young Men's Christian Association facilities (YMCAs), health or fitness clubs, senior or community centers, and parks and recreation departments. Some of these programs are disseminated and cosponsored by the Arthritis Foundation. Walking is the most widely

pursued physical activity among the general public, and people with arthritis can easily tailor walking to their abilities and current conditioning level by altering their distance or speed. The Arthritis Foundation publishes a commercially available book, *Walk with Ease*, which helps people with arthritis start a walking program.

The Arthritis Foundation has developed two community programs that provide safe physical activity options for people with arthritis: the land exercise program called the Arthritis Foundation Exercise Program and a water exercise program called the Arthritis Foundation Aquatic Program. Both programs are small group exercise programs that meet two to three times per week for flexibility and light endurance exercise. Although the current evaluation data are based on small, uncontrolled studies, preliminary results of both programs suggest both physical and psychological benefits (8).

Non–arthritis-specific physical activity programs may also help people with arthritis. For example, the EnhanceFitness program, developed by the University of Washington, uses flexibility, strengthening, endurance, and balance exercises to increase health outcomes among seniors, 60% of whom are assumed to have arthritis. EnhanceFitness has demonstrated significant improvements in most SF-36 health assessment subscales, including a 35% improvement in physical function (9).

Despite the small number of people with arthritis who are meeting arthritis-specific activity recommendations, 55% of adults with arthritis reported in 2003 that a doctor or health professional suggested increasing physical activity to help joint symptoms (5). Although studies on the results of physician counseling on physical activity are equivocal, a review by the US Preventive Services Task Force concluded that multicomponent interventions that combined provider advice with behavioral interventions such as patient goal setting, written prescriptions, and mailed or telephone follow-up appeared most promising (10). The American College of Preventive Medicine statement on physical activity counseling also recommended use of the five A's model described below (11). Linking physician counseling interventions with community-based physical activity programs may also enhance the effectiveness of physician counseling (10).

Weight Control—"Control Your Weight"

Weight loss is well recognized as a primary prevention strategy for knee OA. Felson and colleagues found that women who lost an average of 11 pounds decreased their risk of knee OA by 50% (12). Obesity is also consistently associated with progression of OA. In a review of the relationship between weight and OA, Felson and

Chaisson concluded that "a modest amount of weight loss (10–15 pounds) is likely to alleviate symptoms and delay disease progression in patients with knee OA" (13). More recently, Messier and colleagues demonstrated that each pound of weight lost resulted in a fourfold reduction in loading forces on the knee per step taken (14).

The Arthritis, Diet, and Activity Promotion Trial (ADAPT) demonstrated that a combined diet and exercise intervention was effective in improving self-reported pain and function, and physical performance measures in moderately overweight to obese adults with knee OA. Participants in the combination arm of the trial lost more weight (5.7% of body weight) and achieved greater health improvements (24% improvement in function, 30% decrease in knee pain) than the exercise-alone or diet-alone participants (15).

The ADAPT study used structured diet and exercise programs, but some commercial and mutual-support diet programs may also be effective. Although not specific to arthritis, community-based programs such as Weight Watchers combine diet modification with physical activity and have a reasonable track record for weight loss. In a large, multisite, controlled trial, Weight Watchers produced a mean weight loss of approximately 5%. In a systematic review of commercial weight loss programs, Tsai and Wadden concluded that although the evidence base is suboptimal, the health consequences of the obesity epidemic necessitate attention to weight issues and referrals to commercial and self-help programs such as Weight Watchers, TOPS, and Overeaters Anonymous (16).

However, the majority of overweight or obese patients with arthritis do not receive professional advice to lose weight. In a 2003 survey, only 37% of the overweight and obese respondents with arthritis reported that a physician or health professional suggested losing weight to help their joint symptoms (5). Mehrotra and colleagues found that receiving professional advice was the strongest predictor of weight loss attempts; obese patients who received professional advice to lose weight were three times more likely to attempt to lose weight than those who did not (17). The five A's brief counseling model described below has been applied to weight loss counseling and the Partnership for Healthy Weight Management website provides information clinicians can use to evaluate weight loss programs (http://www.consumer.gov/weightloss; 18).

PROVIDING SELF-MANAGEMENT SUPPORT IN CLINICAL PRACTICE

Self-management activities need to be, by their very nature, carried out by arthritis patients themselves. However, physicians and other clinicians play an important role in providing self-management support, defined by the IOM as "the systematic provision of education and supportive interventions by health care staff to increase patients' skill and confidence in managing their health problems" (1). Routine clinical practice does not afford the luxury of extended time to provide sophisticated behavioral interventions, but simple behavioral counseling techniques can enhance the effectiveness of provider counseling or physician advice. The five A's model, originally developed to guide smoking cessation, has been applied to self-management strategies such as physical activity and weight loss counseling and can be a useful organizing framework to guide self-management support (18–20).

The Five A's Model

The five A's model is a pragmatic sequence of steps to guide the development of realistic plans for self-management. Each of the five A's outlines a specific task the clinician needs to accomplish regardless of which self-management activity is being promoted. The five A's, as described by Glasgow and others, are summarized below (19).

Assess

Assess current behaviors and beliefs, such as current physical activity level, participation in self-management education programs, or perceived importance of weight loss. When helping patients develop an action plan for the proposed self-management activity it is also important to assess their confidence in their ability to attend class, be physically active, or lose weight, and their intention to do so.

Advise

Offer clear, specific, personalized advice such as the need to lose weight or be more physically active, the benefits of increasing activity or attending an education class, and the risk of not making the recommended change.

Agree

Using collaborative goal setting, negotiate a mutually agreeable, specific, and achievable action plan for change. Realistic self-management action plans need to focus on patients' own goals, talking into account their values, priorities, and confidence in their ability to change. A clinician may see weight loss as the most important goal, but the person with arthritis may see increasing physical activity as a more feasible first step. Written action plans facilitate success.

Assist

Help patients to develop the skills and confidence to achieve their action plan by providing educational materials and referrals to community services such as ASMP (also called the Arthritis Foundation Self Help Program), physical activity programs, or weight loss programs. Also, help them identify who can support their self-management efforts.

Arrange Follow-Up

Successful behavior change requires ongoing support and assistance. Specific referral information such as, "I want you to call the Arthritis Foundation at this number to enroll in a self-help class" or "I want you to check out these three weight loss programs" facilitate self-management activity. Follow-up telephone or e-mail contact can also provide support and reinforcement. Self-management plans should be reassessed on follow-up visits, so progress can be applauded and problems resolved.

It is important for clinicians to use all five A's of the model. In an evaluation of the five A's model in clinical practice for exercise and weight loss counseling, Flocke and colleagues found that Assess and Advise happened frequently, but Assist and Arrange Follow-Up rarely occurred (20). Clinician counseling that skips the assessment step to move right into advice, or that makes referrals without getting agreement on the self-management activity and plan, is unlikely to effectively help patients to incorporate these critical self-management activities in their daily lives.

CONCLUSION

Self-management education, physical activity, and weight loss have all demonstrated health benefits for people with arthritis. All three are embedded in ACR guidelines for arthritis management and the nation's Healthy People 2010 objectives, and are core public health messages. However, evidence suggests that very few people with arthritis attend self-management education programs. Even though the majority of people with arthritis are not sufficiently physically active, more than half of them report receiving physician counseling to increase their physical activity. While more than half the people with arthritis are overweight or obese (5), just over a third of them report receiving physician advice to lose weight to help their arthritis symptoms. These self-management activities are the responsibility of the person with arthritis, but health care providers play an essential role in providing the necessary support to facilitate patient self-management.

REFERENCES

1. Brady TJ, Boutaugh ML. Self-Management education and support. In: Bartlett S, ed. Clinical care in the rheumatic diseases. 3rd ed. Atlanta: American College of Rheumatology; 2006:203–210.
2. Superio-Cabuslay E, Ward MM, Lorig KR. Patient education interventions in osteoarthritis and rheumatoid arthritis: a meta-analytic comparison with non-steroidal anti inflammatory drug treatment. Arthritis Care Res 1996;9: 292–301.
3. Lorig K, Ritter PL, Plant K. A disease-specific self-help program compared with a generalized chronic disease self-help program for arthritis patients. Arthritis Rheum 2005;53:950–957.
4. Goeppinger J, Ensley D, Schwartz T, et al. Managing co-morbidity and eliminating health disparities: disease self-management education for persons with arthritis. Manuscript in preparation.
5. Hootman J, Langmaid G, Helmick CG, et al. Monitoring progress in arthritis management—United States and 25 states, 2003. MMWR 2005;54:484–488.
6. Westby MD, Minor MA. Exercise and physical activity. In: Bartlett S, ed. Clinical care in the rheumatic diseases. 3rd ed. Atlanta: American College of Rheumatology; 2006: 211–220.
7. Shih M, Hootman J, Krueger J, et al. Physical activity in men and women with arthritis. National Health Interview Survey, 2002. Am J Prev Med 2006;30:385–393.
8. Boutaugh ML. Arthritis Foundation community-based physical activity programs: effectiveness and implementation issues. Arthritis Rheum 2003:49:463–470.
9. Wallace JI, Buchner DM, Grothaus L, et al. Implementation and effectiveness of a community-based health promotion program for older adults. J Gerontol Med Sci 1998;53A:M301–M306.
10. Berg AO. Behavioral counseling in primary care to promote physical activity: Recommendation and rationale. Am J Nurs 2003;103:101–107.
11. Jacobson DM, Strohecker L, Comptob MT, et al. Physical activity counseling in adult primary care. Am J Prev Med 2005;29:158–162.
12. Felson DT, Lawrence RC, Dieppe PA, et al. Osteoarthritis: new insights part 1: the disease and its risk factors. Ann Intern Med 2000;133:635–646.
13. Felson DT, Chaisson CE. Understanding the relationship between body weight and osteoarthritis. Ballieres Clin Rheumatol 1997;11:671–681.
14. Messier SP, Gutekunst DJ, Davis C, et al. Weight loss reduces knee-joint load in overweight and obese older adults with osteoarthritis. Arthritis Rheum 2005;52:2026–2032.
15. Messier SP, Loeser RF, Miller GD, et al. Exercise and dietary weight loss in overweight and obese older adults with knee osteoarthritis. Arthritis Rheum 2004;50:1501–1510.
16. Tsai AG, Wadden TA. Systematic review: an evaluation of major commercial weight loss programs in the United States. Ann Intern Med 2005;142:56–66.
17. Mehrotra C, Naimi TS, Serdula M, et al. Arthritis, body mass index, and professional advice to lose weight. Impli-

cations for clinical medicine and public health. Am J Prev Med 2004;27:16–21.

18. Serdula MK, Khan LK, Dietz WH. Weight loss counseling revisited. JAMA 2003;289:1747–1750.

19. Glasgow RE, Goldstein MG, Ockene JK, Pronk NP. Translating what we have learned into practice: principles and hypotheses for interventions addressing multiple behaviors in primary care. Am J Prev Med 2004;27:88–101.

20. Flocke SA, Clark A, Schlessman K, et al. Exercise, diet and weight loss advice in the family medicine outpatient setting. Fam Med 2005:37:415–421.

38

CHAPTER 39

Pain Management

JOHN B. WINFIELD, MD

- Patients suffering with chronic diffuse pain who lack objective clinical and laboratory findings (e.g., fibromyalgia) frequently are dismissed as not having real pain, which only perpetuates their illness.
- There are four principal categories of pain: nociceptive pain, neuropathic pain, chronic pain of complex etiology, and psychogenic pain.
- Pain assessment should include attention to possible psychological and sociocultural factors that could be contributing to the pain experience.
- Diagnostic waffling, the ordering of frightening tests, excessive use of physical therapy modalities, activity limitation after minor trauma, and overly liberal work release are among the important

- factors that can convert what should be a self-limited acute pain condition into a chronic pain syndrome.
- If the clinician suspects fibromyalgia, validation of the patient's pain is important.
- Pharmacologic agents that may be useful in the management of individual pain syndromes include nonsteroidal anti-inflammatory drugs, opioids, muscle relaxants, antidepressants, antiepileptic medications, and topical agents.
- Physical therapy, cognitive–behavioral therapy, aerobic exercise, and complementary and alternative medicine approaches may all be useful in the management of pain in selected patients.

All too often in office-based practice, treatment of pain is secondary to diagnosis and treatment of the disease state. This is unfortunate because pain, especially chronic pain, is among the most disabling and costly medical problems in Western countries (1). Patients suffering with chronic diffuse pain who lack objective clinical and laboratory findings (e.g., fibromyalgia) frequently are dismissed as not having "real" pain, which only perpetuates their illness. Presence of pain should be specifically sought and evaluated in all patients and, if present, relief of pain should be a primary focus of the physician's efforts. Indeed, pain should be addressed as a *disease entity*, not as a sensory entity (2).

NATURE OF PAIN

A useful definition adopted by the International Association for the Study of Pain (IASP) defines pain as "an unpleasant sensory and emotional experience associated with actual or potential tissue damage, or described in terms of such damage" (3). Neurophysiologically, pain is a complex sensation–perception interaction involving the simultaneous processing of nociceptive input from the spinal cord. This input activates a central network that records the pain experience in multiple regions of the brain (Figure 39-1).

In addition to strictly sensory discriminative elements of nociception and afferent input from somatic reflexes, there are major contributions from pathways and regions of the brain concerned with emotional, motivational, and cognitive aspects of pain. These factors influence the subjective unpleasantness and distress associated with pain. The two principal effectors of the stress response, the hypothalamic–pituitary–adrenocortical axis and the sympathetic nervous system, are also activated. The stress response may become maladaptive in chronic pain syndromes such as fibromyalgia. Negative emotions (depression and anxiety), other negative psychological factors (loss of control, unpredictability in one's environment), and certain cognitive aspects (negative beliefs and attributions, catastrophizing) all can function as stressors with actions in these systems.

Pain Categories

There are four principal categories of pain: nociceptive pain, neuropathic pain, chronic pain of complex etiology, and psychogenic pain. *Nociceptive pain* is due to stimulation of peripheral pain receptors on thinly myelinated A delta and/or unmyelinated (C) afferents during inflammation or injury of tissues. The pain experienced generally "matches" the noxious stimulus. However, both peripheral sensitization (reduction in

What is Pain? Parallel Processing

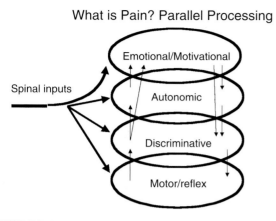

FIGURE 39-1

Pain signals from peripheral sites of tissue injury or inflammation are transmitted simultaneously to multiple areas of the brain through parallel processing. The pain *experience* derives from the combined input of these multiple brain areas. For example, a cognitive brain area gives *meaning* to the pain, which could be trivial (indigestion after eating a pizza) or very frightening (same epigastric pain input from the periphery, but unprovoked in a person recently diagnosed with stomach cancer). The latter pain experience would be much more distressing. Similarly, if a person is depressed, contributions from affective/motivational areas of the brain make the pain more distressing. (Courtesy of Alan R. Light, PhD.)

the threshold of nociceptor endings) and central sensitization [amplification of pain in the central nervous system (CNS)] can occur in "normal" nociceptive pain. These peripheral and central inputs may result in allodynia (an alteration in pain perception such that normally nonpainful stimuli, such as gentle touching, are perceived as painful) and hyperalgesia (increased pain response to a previously painful stimulus). In addition to systemic inflammatory or degenerative rheumatic diseases, nociceptive pain occurs as regional musculoskeletal pain in tenosynovitis, compressive neuropathies, nerve entrapment syndromes, bursitis, and various localized forms of arthritis. Usually self-limited with conventional treatment strategies, regional musculoskeletal pain may become chronic and disabling.

Both peripheral and central nervous system processes also play a role in *neuropathic pain*, which may follow injuries and diseases that directly affect the nervous system. There are three common types: peripheral neuropathic pain (e.g., postherpetic neuralgia, painful diabetic neuropathy, vasculitic neuropathy, radiculopathic pain due to injury to spinal nerve roots); central neuropathic pain (e.g., central poststroke pain, spinal cord injury pain); and cancer-associated neuropathic pain. Complex regional pain syndrome (reflex sympathetic dystrophy; RSD) is another neuropathic pain syndrome. Neuropathic pain may be paroxysmal, perceived as electric shock–like discomfort or burning. Neuropathic pain may be associated with hyperpathia

(persistence after the stimulus has ended, spreading or worsening in crescendo fashion with repeated touching). Central sensitization and ectopic firing of peripheral neurons, either spontaneously or through mechanical forces developed during movement, contribute to this peculiar type of pain. Management may require special pharmacologic approaches, as discussed below.

Chronic pain of complex etiology occurs in fibromyalgia and a large number of substantially overlapping regional pain syndromes, such as migraine headache, temporomandibular disorders, irritable bowel syndrome, and atypical chest pain. In practice, the diagnostic label applied to illness in a given patient often depends on which medical specialist evaluates the patient first, for example, a rheumatologist might diagnose fibromyalgia, whereas a gastroenterologist would diagnose irritable bowel syndrome. Previously termed *functional pain syndromes* on the basis of absent structural pathology, these illnesses share very close relationships in terms of etiology and pathophysiology. Recent advances in the understanding of the psychophysiologic/neurophysiologic dysregulation in such illnesses is impelling a unifying reclassification as central sensitivity syndromes (4).

Collectively, central sensitivity syndromes constitute huge personal and societal burdens, but all too frequently such illnesses are not approached effectively by traditional medicine. In fibromyalgia, the prototype of this category, pain radiates diffusely from the axial skeleton over large areas of the body, involving muscles predominately. The patient describes the symptoms as "exhausting," "miserable," or "unbearable." Altered central nociceptive processing results in a decrease in the pain perception threshold and in the threshold for pain tolerance. The hallmarks of fibromyalgia—chronic widespread pain, fatigue, and multiple somatic symptoms—have both psychological and biological bases that derive, at least in part, from chronic stress and distress. Female gender, genes (5), adverse experiences during childhood, psychological vulnerability to stress, and a stressful, often frightening environment and culture are important antecedents. Thus, fibromyalgia and related syndromes should be viewed from a biopsychosocial perspective (6). A useful guideline for the management of fibromyalgia syndrome pain in adults and children has been published recently (7).

More purely *psychogenic pain* is seen in somatoform and somatization disorders and hysteria.

MANAGEMENT OF PAIN

General Approach

The first element in management of pain is accurate assessment and diagnosis of the cause of the pain.

Assessment should include attention to possible psychological and sociocultural factors that could be contributing to the pain experience. In addition, the physician should be aware that fibromyalgia frequently coexists with inflammatory disorders, such as rheumatoid arthritis (RA) and systemic lupus erythematosus (SLE). Diagnostic "waffling," the ordering of frightening tests, excessive use of physical therapy modalities and activity limitation after minor trauma, and overly liberal work release are among the important factors that can convert what should be a self-limited acute pain condition into a chronic pain syndrome. If one suspects fibromyalgia, validation of the patient's pain is important. Comments such as "it's all in your mind" serve only to perpetuate illness. To the patient, the pain is real. On the other hand, it is important to be aware of confounders to recovery, such as pending litigation or compensation claims.

For acute nociceptive pain (< 30 days duration), pharmacological interventions should follow a stepwise approach using non-opioid and opioid analgesics either singly or in combination, as indicated by pain intensity. Depending on the specific musculoskeletal disorder, initially conservative combinations of corticosteroid injections, activity modification, splints, counterforce bracing, local heat or cold, and in some cases, surgical procedures may be indicated for pain relief and/or to preserve function. Education about the nature of the underlying problem, limitations, and prognosis should err on the side of optimism. Whenever possible, rapid return to full activity and work is best.

If there is a significant nociceptive pain element, chronic pain (>6 months duration) may be managed pharmacologically with analgesics using the same stepwise approach outlined for acute pain. Especially important is a multifaceted treatment plan that incorporates various adjuvant medicines, exercise, and psychological and behavioral approaches to reduce distress and promote self-efficacy and self-management. For many regional chronic pain syndromes, referral to an experienced specialist who advocates holistic, nonsurgical approaches is recommended.

Assessment of Pain

Assessment of pain in the physician's office should be based on a biopsychosocial perspective, that is, in addition to identification of biological variables that contribute to pain, the recognition that psychological and sociocultural factors potentially amplify or perpetuate the pain experience (see Ref. 8 for a full discussion). Pain intensity should be measured with either a verbal or numerical rating scale or a visual analog scale. In fibromyalgia, the author finds it useful to determine pain detection threshold (normal = 4 kg/cm^2) at several tender point sites by pressure algometry. Pain behav-

iors such as guarding, rubbing, grimacing, and sighing vary inversely with patients' self-efficacy for control of chronic pain. A simple self-report form that incorporates validated scales for physical and psychological health status [the modified Health Assessment Questionnaire (HAQ)], visual analog scales for pain, fatigue, patient global self-assessment, a checklist of current symptoms, and scales for helplessness and cognitive performance can be completed in just a few minutes (9). Easily adaptable to a busy practice, such information is invaluable for the psychosocial assessment of pain and in monitoring response to therapy. Marital adjustment, perceived levels of social support, and current stressors in the patient's life are important topics for evaluation. The simple inquiry "how was your childhood?" often reveals adverse childhood experiences, such as abuse, that have increased the patient's vulnerability to chronic pain (10). In multidisciplinary settings, information obtained from the Minnesota Multiphasic Personality Inventory (MMPI), the Social Support Questionnaire (SSQ), the Sickness Impact Profile (SIP), and the Multidimensional Pain Inventory (MPI) is useful for more comprehensive assessments. Subgroups of patients with chronic pain can be identified in this way that can predict response to interdisciplinary therapeutic interventions (11).

Pharmacological Management of Pain

A useful stepwise approach for pharmacological interventions based on nociceptive pain intensity [e.g., in osteoarthritis (OA)] is illustrated in Figure 39-2. Low-dose opioids for patients with OA who fail acetaminophen + nonsteriodal anti-inflammatory drugs (NSAIDs) or a cyclooxygenase-2 (COX-2) inhibitor are effective when used as part of a multimodal approach to pain control, and also may have fewer potentially life-threatening complications (12). Reasonable guidelines for use of opioids in more severe musculoskeletal pain are the exclusion of patients with histories of substance abuse, concomitant attention to psychological and social perpetuators of pain, use of an opioid treatment contract, a one physician/one dispensing pharmacy rule, and close monitoring. Drug-seeking behavior (pseudoaddiction) may indicate that pain is not being controlled adequately.

Opioid Analgesic Drugs

Opioids bind to mu, kappa, or delta opioid receptors (predominately mu for analgesic effects) in regions of the brain involved in integrating pain and to pre- and postsynaptic terminals of peripheral sensory fibers, where they inhibit release of substance P and other

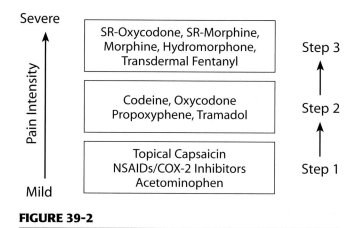

FIGURE 39-2

Stepwise approach to pharmacologic management of pain.

mediators. Tramadol also inhibits reuptake of norepinephrine and serotonin. Table 39-1 lists opioids commonly in use. The side effects of opioids include constipation, nausea and vomiting, sedation, cognitive impairment, miosis, myoclonus, urinary retention, and respiratory depression. Older persons are more sensitive to opioids with respect to both efficacy for pain relief and vulnerability to side effects; starting doses should be reduced 25% to 50%. In the great majority of patients with well-defined chronic rheumatic disease pain, opioids are effective, safe, and well tolerated. Several weeks or months are required to titrate opioid therapy in the outpatient setting. During opioid tapers, which require 2 to 3 weeks, clonidine (0.2–0.4 mg/day) is helpful in controlling withdrawal symptoms. Monitoring of patients taking analgesic medications requires

frequent re-evaluation for efficacy and side effects during initiation, titration, dose changes, and maintenance therapy.

Muscle Relaxants

Centrally acting skeletal muscle relaxants, for example, carisprodol (Soma), cyclobenzaprine (Flexeril), metaxolone (Skelaxin), methocarbamol (Robaxin, Robaxisol), tizanidine (Zanaflex), and baclofen (Lioresal, Kemstro) to list a few, have modest benefit as adjunctive therapy for nociceptive pain associated with muscle strains. Used intermittently, or as a single bedtime dose (e.g., 10 mg cyclobenzaprine), they have limited effectiveness in fibromyalgia and other chronic pain syndromes, as well. Sedation and other CNS side effects occur frequently. Abuse may occur, particularly with carisprodol, and abrupt cessation may be associated with withdrawal symptoms.

Antidepressants

Tricyclic antidepressants (TCAs) clearly are effective in neuropathic pain and may be of modest short-term benefit in diffuse and regional chronic pain syndromes, but side effects (dry mouth, drowsiness, and weight gain) limit patient acceptance. Selective serotonin reuptake inhibitors (SSRIs), for example, fluoxetine (Prozac, 10–40 mg daily) or citalopram (Celexa, 20–40 mg daily) have been shown to have limited efficacy in randomized, controlled trials in fibromyalgia; the combination of a TCA with an SSRI in this disorder typically produces greater improvement in pain, sleep, and overall well-being than either drug used alone.

TABLE 39-1. OPIOID ANALGESIC DRUGS.

DRUGS	ORAL EQUIVALENT	STARTING DOSE	COMMENT
Short-acting			
Morphine sulfate (Roxanol)	30 mg	15–30 mg every 4 hours	For all, start low and titrate; begin bowel program early; most of these opioids are available in combination with acetaminophen or aspirin (do not exceed maximum dose). For all, short-acting opioid often is needed for breakthrough pain.
Codeine (Fiornal)	120 mg	30–60 mg every 4–6 hours	
Hydrocodone (Lortab)	30 mg	5–10 mg every 3–4 hours	
Oxycodone (Percodan)	20–30 mg	5–10 mg every 3–4 hours	
Hydromorphone (Dilaudid)	7.5 mg	1.5 mg every 3–4 hours	
Propoxyphene (Darvon)	100 mg	100 mg every 4 hours	
Tramadol (Ultram)	120 mg	50–100 mg every 6 hours	
Methadone (Dolophine)	–	15–60 mg every 8 hours	
Long-acting			
SR-Morphine (MS Contin)	30 mg	5–10 mg every 3–4 hours	
SR-Oxycodone (Oxycontin)	20–30 mg	10–20 mg every 12 hours	
Transdermal fentanyl (Duragesic)	Not available	See package insert	

Dual-action (serotonin/noradrenaline) reuptake inhibitors (SNRIs) such as venlafaxine (Effexor, 150–225 mg daily or duloxetine (Cymbalta, 30–60 mg daily) (13) are superior to SSRIs for pain control and improve many symptoms in fibromyalgia irrespective of comorbid depression. When concomitant depression is present in a chronic pain syndrome, it is essential that depression be treated aggressively. SSRIs and SNRIs must be tapered gradually upon discontinuation. Following the institution of therapy, patients should be observed for worsening of depression and the emergence of suicidal thoughts.

Antiepileptic Drugs

Carbamazepine (Tegretol) and a series of other new antiepileptic drugs have become first-line agents for neuropathic pain (14). Gabapentin (Neurontin, 900–1800 mg daily in three divided doses), a 3-alkylated gamma-amino butyric acid (GABA) analog originally introduced as an anticonvulsant and more recently released pregabalin (Lyrica, 150–425 mg daily in divided doses) (15) are useful in chronic pain states, including fibromyalgia, related syndromes, and various types of neuropathic pain. These agents may ameliorate associated depressed mood and anxiety, as well. The dose of these agents should be escalated slowly over weeks; discontinuance of these agents should likewise be done gradually.

Topical Agents

Obtained from red chili peppers, topical capsaicin binds to vanilloid receptors on peripheral terminals of nociceptive neurons, thereby inhibiting activation of the pain pathway by noxious stimuli. Essentially free of toxicity other than mild burning at the site of application, capsaicin is useful as adjunctive therapy in diffuse and regional musculoskeletal pain syndromes, joint pain in arthritis, and in neuropathic pain disorders. Up to three 5% lidocaine patches (Lidoderm) may be applied to localized painful areas for 12 to 18 hours in a 24-hour period with good efficacy and safety.

Other Pharmacological Agents

Anxiolytics, for example, clonazepam (Klonopin), lorazepam (Ativan), temazepam (Restoril), alprazolam (Xanax), and buspirone (Buspar) have antinociceptive effects in chronic pain and are often used in combination with antidepressants and antiepileptic drugs. Pramipexole (Mirapex, dopamine 3 receptor agonist) has been shown to improve pain scores, fatigue, and function in patients requiring opioids for pain control.

Pharmacologic Management of Fibromyalgia

Low-dose amitriptyline at bedtime, perhaps in combination with cyclobenzaprine (Flexeril), is a well-established therapy for fibromyalgia and related chronic pain syndromes. SNRIs in combination with gabapentin (Neurontin) or pregabalin (Lyrica) are very useful in patients with severe allodynia and hyperalgesia. Corticosteroids and NSAIDs are of no benefit in fibromyalgia pain per se, but are useful treatments for coexisting inflammatory processes ("pain generators"). Opioids should be avoided if at all possible for fibromyalgia pain. However, certain patients with extreme pain unresponsive to other agents will require opioids to improve quality of life and maintain function. If used, opioids should be combined with multidisciplinary approaches, psychotherapeutic interventions, and the cautions mentioned above.

Pharmacological and nonpharmacological treatment of poor sleep is crucial for improving overall sense of well-being. Sleep disturbances should be managed aggressively, beginning with instruction in the elements of good sleep hygiene, such as avoidance of daytime naps and caffeine. Most patients require medication, and many nonbenzodiazepine hypnotics, for example, zolpidem (Ambien), zaleplon (Sonata, 1-hour half-life, useful with mid-sleep awakenings), or eszopiclone (Lunesta) are now available in addition to traditional hypnotics. Oxybate (Xyrem) also is very promising. A formal sleep assessment may be required for patients who do not respond to the above measures.

Fatigue, often a dominant complaint in fibromyalgia, generally improves with effective treatment of pain, depression, and sleep disturbances in combination with a graded aerobic exercise program. Modafinil (Provigil, 100–200 mg q.a.m.) is beneficial in patients for whom overwhelming fatigue is a persistent complaint, and may be useful as a bridge therapy during the early phase of an aerobic exercise program.

Psychological and Behavioral Approaches

The importance of strategies in this area has been emphasized recently (8,16). Depression, anxiety, stress, sleep disturbance, pain beliefs and coping strategies, and self-efficacy all are central to the pain experience in many patients, and frequently determine the outcome of chronic pain. Unless psychosocial and behavioral variables are recognized and approached, strictly pharmacological interventions to reduce nociceptive pain from inflammation or the diffuse pain in fibromyalgia and related syndromes are of limited benefit. Established behavioral treatments in RA and OA that improve ratings of pain or pain behavior are the Arthritis Self-Management Program (17) and cognitive–behavioral therapy (cognitive–behavioral therapy includes components for education, training in relaxation and coping skills, rehearsals of the skills learned, and relapse prevention). Self-care education and telephone counseling are probably efficacious in OA, but have not been studied in RA. The role of cognitive–behavioral therapy for the diffuse pain of fibromyalgia and related regional pain syndromes remains to be clarified.

Physical Therapy/ Physical Modalities

The objectives here are to diminish pain, improve function, minimize disability, and promote self-efficacy. Although certain strategies and modalities are clearly beneficial, this area needs properly designed trials to establish efficacy.

Exercise

In addition to positive effects on underlying pathological processes in bones, joints, and muscles, exercise is essential to the treatment of fibromyalgia and related chronic pain syndromes. The benefits of exercise, in addition to gains in cardiovascular fitness, muscle tone, and strength, include improvements in both subjective and objective measures of pain and in the overall sense of well-being. Many patients with chronic pain perceive their muscles to be weak and easily fatigued, and bear the negative belief (fear) that activity will exacerbate their condition. Consequently, exercise is avoided and their muscles become deconditioned. Normal activities become challenging. Excessive activity "on a good day" induces a major flare of pain and fatigue, possibly due, in part, to the peripheral and central effects of proinflammatory cytokines (tumor necrosis factor, interleukins 1 and 6) released in response to exercise-damaged myofibers. Ideally, exercise should be low-impact (walking, water aerobics, stationary bicycle, rather than running), beginning very gently and progressing gradually to endurance and strength training. Encouragement and positive reinforcement can reduce the virtually universal problem of poor compliance. Obesity, poor posture, and overloading activities at work and home also contribute to muscle pain and fatigue and should be addressed. Daily stretching exercises after hot showers are very helpful.

Heat and Cold

Heat (hot packs, paraffin, hydrotherapy in its many forms) is of proven benefit in nociceptive pain, especially when combined with exercise (range of motion, stretching, strengthening). Diffuse and regional pain is improved by such strategies as sauna, hot baths and showers, and hot mud. While not superior to superficial heat, cold (cold packs, immersion, or vapocoolant sprays) may provide more immediate analgesic benefit, particularly when applied soon after an injury.

Massage, Trigger Point Injections, Acupuncture, and Transcutaneous Electrical Nerve Stimulation

Gentle massage is well received by patients with diffuse pain syndromes, but as a totally passive modality it fails to promote self-efficacy for control of pain. Injection of "trigger points" is of short-term benefit only and should generally be avoided. Neurophysiologic effects of acupuncture and electroacupuncture include release of opioids and other mediators in the nervous system. Several randomized, controlled trials have shown acupuncture to improve subjective pain and to raise pain thresholds, but its long-term benefit in chronic pain syndromes remains unclear. An advantage of transcutaneous electrical nerve stimulation (TENS) for localized musculoskeletal pain is that the patient can apply this modality at home.

Complementary and Alternative Medicine

The immense popularity of complementary and alternative medicine (CAM) today contrasts with the current paucity of data regarding the biochemical nature and mechanism of action of most alternative remedies and the lack of rigorous studies addressing efficacy, safety, and cost-effectiveness of these strategies. Many physicians lack knowledge in this area and may be overtly hostile toward CAM. Consequently, patients are reluctant to inform their physicians about CAM they are using for self-management. This can be dangerous because of unsuspected drug interactions. Patients with chronic pain and fatigue, for example, fibromyalgia, are the largest users of CAM, often because of frustration with the inefficacy of traditional medicine and lack of empathy and understanding on the part of many physicians. Until neuroscience, behavioral science, and health care systems advance to such a point that effective biopsychosocial treatment strategies are applied in most patients with chronic pain, CAM approaches will continue to proliferate. In the meantime, a practical approach is to inquire about CAM usage, refrain from expression of negative opinions if a particular CAM treatment is relatively inexpensive and appears to be safe, and to encourage "whatever works" in the context of the power of the placebo effect and the promotion of self-efficacy for control of pain.

Pain in Children

Except for children less than 1 year of age, the approach to the management of pain in children is similar to that in adults. Issues meriting particular attention include the young child's inability to report pain and fear (e.g., of doctors and needles), age-related pharmacological factors, and psychosocial variables that differ from those in adults (e.g., school absenteeism). Although clinically significant pain often is not fully recognized and treated, recurrent complaints of pain all over the body are common in otherwise healthy children. In such cases, the physician must be sensitive and wise, avoid unnecessary testing, and emphasize lifestyle interventions, reduction of school stressors, and aerobic exercise (see Ref. 18 for a useful review).

Pain in Older Persons

Pain, particularly musculoskeletal pain, is very common in older persons and is neither part of normal aging nor better tolerated than in younger persons. Those misconceptions contribute importantly to the unfortunate undertreatment (or lack of treatment!) of chronic pain in the elderly in both community and institutional settings. Indeed, in a study of nursing-home residents, 71% had at least one pain complaint and two thirds had constant or daily pain, but only 15% had received analgesic medication in the previous 24 hours (19). The experience of pain in older persons differs somewhat from that in young and middle-aged individuals: higher pain thresholds, less frequent self-report of pain, atypical presentation of pain (e.g., as confusion, restlessness, or other behavioral change), less prominent anxiety associated with the pain, and frequent coexisting depression. Older persons exhibit lower self-efficacy and tend to use passive coping strategies (e.g., praying and hoping) rather than cognitive coping methods. Their susceptibility to associated impairments is greater.

The American Geriatrics Society has published clinical practice guidelines for the management of chronic pain in older persons (20). Special barriers to accurate pain assessment in this population include reluctance to report pain, use of atypical descriptors of pain, fear of diagnostic tests and medications, and communication difficulties due to sensory and cognitive impairments. With respect to pharmacologic therapy in the elderly, goals, hopes, and tradeoffs should be discussed openly. For mild pain, acetaminophen alone or

in combination with celecoxib (Celebrex) is useful. The use of opioids for moderate or severe pain is appropriate, but dosing should follow the "start low, go slow" maxim. The health care provider must be aware of economic barriers that some elderly patients confront in obtaining medications. Nonpharmacologic treatment of pain in older persons should be an integral part of care plans.

Procedure-Based Pain Management

Injection of local anesthetics, epidural techniques, and radiofrequency ablation procedures all have a place in certain cases, but not infrequently are used inappropriately in anesthesia pain clinics. Furthermore, risk–benefit and long-term efficacy of such approaches in chronic diffuse pain have not been fully established.

REFERENCES

1. Koleva D, Krulichova I, Bertolini G, Caimi V, Garattini L. Pain in primary care: an Italian survey. Eur J Public Health 2005;15:475–479.
2. Siddall PJ, Cousins MJ. Persistent pain as a disease entity: implications for clinical management. Anesth Analg 2004;99:510–520, table.
3. International Association for the Study of Pain. Classification of chronic pain. Description of chronic pain syndromes and definitions of pain terms. New York: Elsevier; 1994.
4. Yunus MB. Fibromyalgia and overlapping disorders: the unifying concept of central sensitivity syndromes and the issue of nosology. Semin Arthritis Rheum 2007;36:339–356.
5. Diatchenko L, Slade GD, Nackley AG, et al. Genetic basis for individual variations in pain perception and the development of a chronic pain condition. Hum Mol Genet 2005;14:135–143.
6. Winfield JB. Pain in fibromyalgia. Rheum Dis Clin North Am 1999;25:55–79.
7. Burckhardt C, Goldenberg D, Crofford LJ, et al. Guideline for the management of fibromyalgia syndrome pain in adults and children. APS clinical practice guidelines series, no. 4. Glenview, IL: American Pain Society; 2005:1–109.
8. Keefe FJ, Bonk V. Psychosocial assessment of pain in patients having rheumatic diseases. Rheum Dis Clin North Am 1999;25:81–103.
9. Pincus T, Swearingen C, Wolfe F. Toward a multidimensional Health Assessment Questionnaire (MDHAQ): assessment of advanced activities of daily living and psychological status in the patient-friendly health assessment questionnaire format. Arthritis Rheum 1999;42:2220–2230.
10. Winfield JB. Psychological determinants of fibromyalgia and related syndromes. Curr Rev Pain 2000;4:276–286.
11. Turk DC. The potential of treatment matching for subgroups of patients with chronic pain: lumping versus splitting. Clin J Pain 2005;21:44–55.

12. Goodwin JL, Kraemer JJ, Bajwa ZH. The use of opioids in the treatment of osteoarthritis: when, why, and how? Curr Pain Headache Rep 2005;9:390–398.

13. Arnold LM, Lu Y, Crofford LJ, et al. A double-blind, multicenter trial comparing duloxetine with placebo in the treatment of fibromyalgia patients with or without major depressive disorder. Arthritis Rheum 2004;50:2974–2984.

14. Sindrup SH, Jensen TS. Efficacy of pharmacological treatments of neuropathic pain: an update and effect related to mechanism of drug action. Pain 1999;83:389–400.

15. Crofford LJ, Rowbotham MC, Mease PJ, et al. Pregabalin for the treatment of fibromyalgia syndrome: results of a randomized, double-blind, placebo-controlled trial. Arthritis Rheum 2005;52:1264–1273.

16. Bradley LA, Alberts KR. Psychosocial and behavioral approaches to pain management for patients with rheumatic disease. Rheum Dis Clin North Am 1999;25:215–232.

17. Lorig KR, Mazonson PD, Holman HR. Evidence suggesting that health education for self-management in patients with chronic arthritis has sustained health benefits while reducing health care costs. Arthritis Rheum 1993;36:439–446.

18. Zempsky WT, Schechter NL. Office-based pain management. The 15-minute consultation [review; 65 refs]. Pediatr Clin North Am 2000;47:601–615.

19. Ferrell BA, et al. Pain in the nursing home. J Am Geriatr Soc 1990;38:409–414.

20. AGS panel on Chronic Pain in Older Persons. The management of chronic pain in older persons. J Am Geriatrics Soc 1998;46:635–651.

39

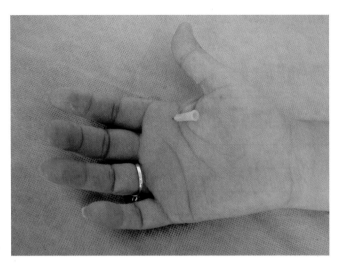

FIGURE 40-1

Trigger finger injection. In the second finger, needle entry is just distal to the proximal palmar crease.

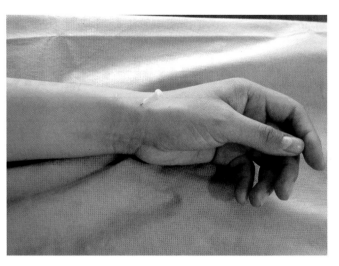

FIGURE 40-3

de Quervain´s tenosinovitis injection. The needle is aimed at the distended tendon sheath.

disease, carpal tunnel syndrome, tennis elbow, and wrist and elbow (radiocapitular) injections. Shoulder and knee injections require a 35- or 38-mm, 21-gauge needle. In obese people, a trochanteric injection may call for the use of a spinal needle.

- **To dilute or not to dilute.** I am often asked: "Do you mix the steroid with a local anesthetic?" If one wants to limit the spread of the injection, such as in a trigger finger or thumb, tennis elbow, and retrocalcaneal

bursa, the straight steroid should be used. If a larger tissue volume needs to be infiltrated, such as in the trochanteric syndrome, adding a local anesthetic is advantageous.

- **Prepping the skin.** Alcohol or an iodopovidone solution may be used for antisepsis. Both are effective against bacteria, fungi, and viruses. Alcohol (70%–92%) acts by 1 minute and iodopovidone 10% by 2 minutes. I rub the skin three times and wait for the appropriate time. The last word on skin prepping has not been said (31).
- **Gloves.** Postinjection infection occurs irrespective of the use of sterile gloves (30). I believe the use of

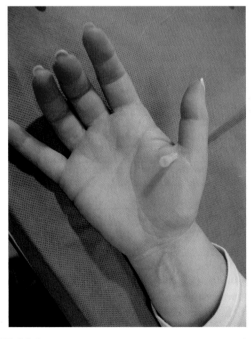

FIGURE 40-2

Trigger thumb injection. The needle is aimed at the thumb sesamoids.

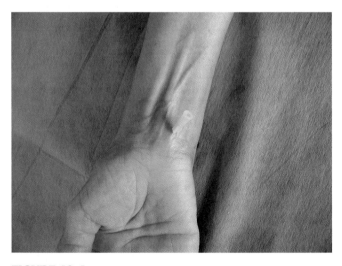

FIGURE 40-4

Carpal tunnel syndrome injection. Note the needle entry 1.5 cm proximal to the distal wrist crease and ulnar to palmaris longus tendon.

gloves is desirable, at the very least in the operator´s nondominant hand, to avoid inadvertent contamination by leaking fluid when the syringe used to drain the joint is replaced by the one containing the steroid (32).

- **Local anesthesia.** Some clinicians spare the use of local anesthesia because they rely on a quick, almost painless, effective thrust which brings the needle into the desired place. I use lidocaine 2% without epinephrine because my entries are often inaccurate and need to be retried.
- **Should a synovial effusion be drained prior to the injection?** In patients with RA, removal of a knee effusion prior to injecting the steroid improves outcome (33).
- **To avoid sudden disconnection of the needle while injecting a thick steroid suspension.** Hold the needle between index and thumb (of the nondominant hand) while you depress the plunger with the other hand´s thumb.
- **Is it possible to inject an anticoagulated patient?** There is evidence that anticoagulated patients with an international normalized ratio (INR) in the therapeutic range can have the joints and soft tissues safely injected (34). Firm pressure should be exerted at the site for several minutes. Beware of carpal tunnel injections in this setting because a bleed, however small, could be disastrous.
- **Hemostasis in hand and wrist injections.** In hand and wrist injections, including carpal tunnel injections, raising the extremity straight up prevents venous bleed.
- **Should the injected structure be rested?** In knee synovitis, resting the joint for 24 hours following the steroid injection leads to a better outcome (35).

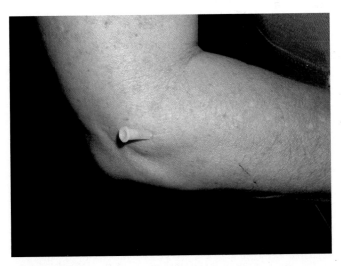

FIGURE 40-5

Tennis elbow injection. Needle entry is 2 to 3 mm distal to the lateral epicondyle.

TABLE 40-2. LOCAL AND SYSTEMIC REACTIONS TO THE INJECTED MATERIAL.
Facial flushing and palpitations
Skin atrophy
Fat atrophy
Hypopigmentation
Postinjection flare
Infection
Tendon rupture
Corticosteroid arthropathy
Osteonecrosis
Hyperglycemia
Pituitary inhibition
Anaphylaxis

- **How many injections are allowed in a given structure?** Three times total (not per year) appears to me to be the right answer. Realities of life dictate many exceptions to this rule.
- **Complications** (Table 40-2). A frequent untoward reaction is facial flushing with palpitations. This reaction seldom lasts more than 4 hours. In diabetics, depending on the steroid dose (consider, e.g., a diabetic patient with three trigger fingers plus a bilateral carpal tunnel syndrome) a transient elevation of serum glucose should be expected. Skin hypopigmentation at the injection site occurs frequently in dark skinned individuals after injecting a superficial structure, such as in de Quervain tenosynovitis.

INTRA-ARTICULAR HYALURONATES (VISCOSUPPLEMENTATION)

Intra-articular hyaluronates are often used for the treatment of pain in osteoarthritic joints (36). The beneficial effect of viscosupplementation has a delayed action but it lasts longer than intra-articular corticosteroids (37). Two types of agents are available. One is Hylan G-F 20, a high-molecular-weight preparation (MW 6,000,000). There are also lower molecular weight hyaluronan preparations in the range of MW 800,000 to 2,000,000. Viscosupplementation was initially used in the knee. However, other joints such as the shoulder, the hip, and the ankle have all been treated with benefit. The usual treatment course includes three weekly intra-articular injections. Several untoward reactions may occur. Postinjection pain, with or without a joint effusion, is common. Another complication is a pseudo–septic synovitis. This worrisome reaction requires hospital admission and parenteral antibiotics pending culture results. A granulomatous reaction has also been reported. Finally, allergic reactions may occur in patients with avian protein allergy. Indications of viscosupplementation include (a) patients who cannot take anti-inflammatory medications and whose pain is unrelieved by analgesics and (b) patients with advanced osteoarthritis who refuse or are not candidates for surgery. Viscosupplementation is expensive. However, a recent cost analysis has shown superiority of viscosupplementation over appropriate care without viscosupplementation (38).

REFERENCES

1. Naredo E, Cabero F, Beneyto P, et al. A randomized comparative study of short term response to blind injection versus sonographic-guided injection of local corticosteroids in patients with painful shoulder. J Rheumatol 2004;31:308–314.
2. Murphy D, Failla JM, Koniuch MP. Steroid versus placebo injection for trigger finger. J Hand Surg [Am] 1995;20:628–631.
3. Maneerit J, Sriworakun C, Budhraja N, et al. Trigger thumb: results of a prospective randomised study of percutaneous release with steroid injection versus steroid injection alone. J Hand Surg [Br] 2003;28:586–589.
4. Zingas C, Failla JM, Van Holsbeeck M. Injection accuracy and clinical relief of de Quervain's tendinitis. J Hand Surg [Am] 1998;23:89–96.
5. McCarty DJ, Marman JG, Grassanovich JL, et al. Treatment of rheumatoid joint inflammation with intrasynovial triamcinolone hexacetonide. J Rheumatol 1995;22:1631–1635.
6. Rizzo M, Beckenbaugh RD. Treatment of mucous cysts of the fingers: review of 134 cases with minimum 2-year follow-up evaluation. J Hand Surg [Am] 2003;28:519–524.
7. Meenagh GK, Patton J, Kynes C, et al. A randomised controlled trial of intra-articular corticosteroid injection of the carpometacarpal joint of the thumb in osteoarthritis. Ann Rheum Dis 2004;63:1260–1263.
8. Hui AC, Wong S, Leung CH, et al. A randomized controlled trial of surgery vs steroid injection for carpal tunnel syndrome. Neurology 2005;64:2074–2078.
9. Smith DL, McAfee JH, Lucas LM, et al. Treatment of nonseptic olecranon bursitis. A controlled, blinded prospective trial. Arch Intern Med 1989;149:2527–2530.
10. Smidt N, Lewis M, Hay EM, et al. A comparison of two primary care trials on tennis elbow: issues of external validity. Ann Rheum Dis 2005;64:1406–1409.
11. Stahl S, Kaufman T. The efficacy of an injection of steroids for medial epicondylitis. A prospective study of sixty elbows. J Bone Joint Surg Am 1997;79:1648–1652.
12. Akgun K, Birtane M, Akarirmak U. Is local subacromial corticosteroid injection beneficial in subacromial impingement syndrome? Clin Rheum 2004;23:496–500.
13. Carette S, Moffet H, Tardif J, et al. Intraarticular corticosteroids, supervised physiotherapy, or a combination of the two in the treatment of adhesive capsulitis of the shoulder: a placebo-controlled trial. Arthritis Rheum 2003;48:829–838.
14. Vecchio PC, Adebajo AO, Hazleman BL. Suprascapular nerve block for persistent rotator cuff lesions. J Rheumatol 1993;20:453–455.
15. Jacob AK. Sallay PI. Therapeutic efficacy of corticosteroid injections in the acromioclavicular joint. Biomed Sci Instrum 1997;34:380–385.
16. Carette S, Fehlings MG. Clinical practice. Cervical radiculopathy. N Engl J Med 2005;353:392–399.
17. Carette S, Leclaire R, Marcoux S, et al. Epidural corticosteroid injections for sciatica due to herniated nucleus pulposus. N Engl J Med 1997;336:1634–1640.
18. Carette S, Marcoux S, Truchon R, et al. A controlled trial of corticosteroid injections into facet joints for chronic low back pain. N Engl J Med 1991;325:1002–1007.
19. Zelle BA, Gruen GS, Brown S, et al. Sacroiliac joint dysfunction: evaluation and management. Clin J Pain 2005;21:446–455.
20. Kullenberg B, Runesson R, Tuvhag R, et al. Intraarticular corticosteroid injection: pain relief in osteoarthritis of the hip? J Rheumatol 2004;31:2265–2268.
21. Godwin M, Dawes M. Intra-articular steroid injections for painful knees. Systematic review with meta-analysis. Can Fam Physician 2004;50:241–248.
22. Weitoft T, Larsson A, Saxne T, et al. Changes of cartilage and bone markers after intra-articular glucocorticoid treatment with and without postinjection rest in patients with rheumatoid arthritis. Ann Rheum Dis 2005;64:1750–1753.
23. Calvo-Alén J, Rua-Figueroa I, Erausquin C. Treatment of anserine bursitis. Local corticosteroid injection vs. a NSAID. A prospective study. Rev Esp Reumatol 1993;20:13–15.
24. Canoso JJ, Wohlgethan JR, Newberg AH, et al. Aspiration of the retrocalcaneal bursa. Ann Rheum Dis 1984;43:308–312.
25. Genc H, Saracoglu M, Nacir B, et al. Long-term ultrasonographic follow-up of plantar fasciitis patients treated with steroid injection. Joint Bone Spine 2005;72:61–65.
26. Thomson CE, Gibson JN, Martin D. Interventions for the treatment of Morton's neuroma. Cochrane Database Syst Rev 2004:CD003118.
27. Ching DW, Petrie JP, Klemp P, et al. Injection therapy of superficial rheumatoid nodules. Br J Rheumatol 1992;31:775–777.
28. Kamanli A, Kaya A, Ardicoglu O, et al. Comparison of lidocaine injection, botulinum toxin injection, and dry needling to trigger points in myofascial pain syndrome. Rheumatol Int 2005;25:604–611.
29. Eberhard BA, Sison MC, Gottlieb BS, et al. Comparison of the intraarticular effectiveness of triamcinolone hexacetonide and triamcinolone acetonide in treatment of juvenile rheumatoid arthritis. J Rheumatol 2004;31:2507–2512.

30. Seror P, Pluvinage P, d'Andre FL, et al. Frequency of sepsis after local corticosteroid injection (an inquiry on 1160000 injections in rheumatological private practice in France). Rheumatology 1999;38:1272–1274.

31. Edwards PS, Lipp A, Holmes A. Preoperative skin antiseptics for preventing surgical wound infections after clean surgery [review]. Cochrane Database Syst Rev 2004: CD003949.

32. Yood RA. Use of gloves for rheumatology procedures. Arthritis Rheum 1993;36:575.

33. Weitoft T, Uddenfeldt P. Importance of synovial fluid aspiration when injecting intra-articular corticosteroids. Ann Rheum Dis 2000;59:233–235.

34. Thumboo J, O'Duffy JD. A prospective study of the safety of joint and soft tissue aspirations and injections in patients taking warfarin sodium. Arthritis Rheum 1998; 41:736–739.

35. Chakravarty K, Pharoah PD, Scott DG. A randomized controlled study of post-injection rest following intra-articular steroid therapy for knee synovitis. Br J Rheumatol 1994;33:464–468.

36. Bellamy N, Campbell J, Robinson V. Viscosupplementation for the treatment of osteoarthritis of the knee. Cochrane Database Syst Rev 2005:CD005321.

37. Caborn D, Rush J, Lanzer W, et al. Synvisc 901 Study Group. A randomized, single-blind comparison of the efficacy and tolerability of hylan G-F 20 and triamcinolone hexacetonide in patients with osteoarthritis of the knee. J Rheumatol 2004;31:333–343.

38. Torrance GW, Raynauld JP, Walker V. Canadian Knee OA Study Group. A prospective, randomized, pragmatic, health outcomes trial evaluating the incorporation of hylan G-F 20 into the treatment paradigm for patients with knee osteoarthritis (part 2 of 2): economic results. Osteoarthr Cartil 2002;10:518–527.

40

CHAPTER 41

Nonsteroidal Anti-Inflammatory Drugs

LESLIE J. CROFFORD, MD

- Nonsteriodal anti-inflammatory drugs (NSAIDs) relieve inflammation and pain by inhibiting the production of prostaglandins.
- Prostaglandin (PG) biosynthesis occurs via a three-enzyme cascade. Current NSAIDs inhibit the enzyme cyclooxygenase (COX), accounting for their efficacy and toxicity.
- Pharmacologic properties of the different NSAIDs, including specificity for COX-1 or -2 and drug half-life, influence the toxicity profile.

- The most important NSAID toxicities include gastro-intestinal ulceration, asthma and allergic reactions, and effects on the kidneys, liver, and cardiovascular system.
- Safe use of NSAIDs requires consideration of individual comorbidities to choose the best agent, appropriate monitoring for toxicity, and use of appropriate gastroprotective agents.

Pain (dolor), swelling (tumor), erythema (rubor), and warmth (calor), the cardinal features of inflammation, are present in most patients with rheumatic diseases. Therapeutic strategies to reduce inflammation have been used for centuries, beginning with botanical treatments in both Western and Eastern medical traditions (1). The first isolated plant constituent to be tested as an anti-inflammatory drug was salicylic acid from willow bark, which was chemically altered to acetyl salicylic acid to improve its pharmacologic properties. Acetyl salicylic acid became "aspirin" in 1899, one of the first drugs to be widely marketed, and aspirin remains one of the most widely used drugs today. Other drugs that share the anti-inflammatory, analgesic, and antipyretic properties of aspirin are termed *nonsteroidal anti-inflammatory drugs* (NSAIDs), and are a chemically diverse group of compounds (Table 41-1). It was established in 1971 that salicylates and other NSAIDs act by blocking the synthesis of prostaglandins (PGs), products of the metabolism of the membrane-associated fatty acid arachidonic acid. This finding demonstrated conclusively that PGs play an important role in mediating symptoms and signs of inflammation. However, PGs play a role in normal physiology as well as in disease. As a consequence, all NSAIDs possess predictable therapeutic and adverse effects that must be understood in order to use these drugs safely.

Prostaglandins are synthesized by the action of at least three biosynthetic enzymes, one of which, cyclo-oxygenase (COX), is the target of all currently available NSAIDs. In recent years, important progress has been made towards understanding the action of NSAIDs by clarifying the biology of PG production. This advance came with the discovery of COX-2, the isoform whose expression is increased during inflammation. Specific inhibition of COX-2 blocks production of high levels of PGs at sites of inflammation while preserving PG production mediated by COX-1 in certain other tissues. Nonspecific NSAIDs, which inhibit both COX-1 and COX-2, have some differences when compared with COX-2–specific NSAIDs with regard to their adverse-event profiles. Comparative studies, however, find equal efficacy demonstrating that COX-2–derived PGs are responsible for the inflammation and pain of arthritis. Other important differences between these NSAIDs are related to their chemical class and pharmacologic properties other than the specificity for COX isoforms. All these factors are involved in the relative efficacy and safety of NSAIDs for patients with rheumatic diseases. It should be emphasized that advances in the understanding of PG biology may lead to other targets that would further advance anti-inflammatory therapy.

PROSTAGLANDIN BIOLOGY

The diversity of PG functions is achieved by cell- and tissue-specific generation of different stable PGs, multiple PG receptors linked to different intracellular

TABLE 41-1. NONSTERIODAL ANTI-INFLAMMATORY DRUGS AND SALICYLATES.

CHEMICAL CLASS	GENERIC NAME	BRAND NAME(S)
Carboxylic acids: salicylic acids and esters	Aspirin Diflunisal	Anacin,[a] Ascriptin,[a] Bayer,[a] Bufferin,[a] Easprin, Ecotrin,[a] Empirin,[a] Midol,[a] others Dolobid
Carboxylic acids: phenyl acetic acid	Diclofenac potassium Diclofenac sodium Diclofenac sodium + misoprostol	Cataflam Voltaren, Voltaren XR Arthrotec
Carboxylic acids: carbo- and heterocyclic acids	Etodolac Indomethacin Ketorolac Sulindac Tolmetin sodium	Lodine, Lodine XL Indocin, Indocin SR Toradol Clinoril Tolectin
Proprionic acids	Flurbiprofen Ketoprofen Oxaprozin Naproxen Naproxen sodium Ibuprofen	Ansaid Odudis, Oruvail, Actron,[a] Orudis KT[a] Daypro Naprosyn, Naprelan Anaprox, Aleve[a] Motrin, Dolgesic, Advil,[a] Motrin IB,[a] Excedrin IB, Genpril,[a] Nuprin,[a] others
Fenamic acids	Meclofenamate sodium	Meclomen
Enolic acids	Piroxicam Meloxicam	Feldene Mobic
Nonacidic	Nabumetone	Relafen
Sulfonamide	Celecoxib	Celebrex
Nonacetylated salicylates	Choline salicylate Magnesium salicylate Choline magnesium trisalicylate Salsalate Sodium salicylate	Arthrotec Bayer Select,[a] Doan's Pills[a] Trilisate, tricosal Amigesic, Disalcid, others

[a] Available over-the-counter.
Not intended to be an exhaustive list.

signaling pathways, and PG production pathways involving enzymes that are induced to dramatically increase local PG production. Biosynthesis of PGs involves a three-step sequence including (i) hydrolysis of the 20 carbon-containing polyunsaturated fatty acid, arachidonic acid, from cell membranes; (ii) oxygenation to the endoperoxide PGH_2 by COX; and (iii) conversion to the biologically active end products via specific PG synthases (Figure 41-1). The first step in PG synthesis is mediated by a phospholipase A_2 (PLA_2). Although the synthesis of PGs is regulated acutely by activation of phospholipases and release of arachidonate, the net level of prostanoid production is determined by the level of COX expression (2).

Cyclooxygenase-1 and COX-2 are homodimers that insert into one half of the lipid bilayer of the nuclear envelope and endoplasmic reticulum. They are bifunctional enzymes that catalyze both cyclooxygenation and peroxidation reactions. Although structurally similar,

there are important differences in a small number of amino acids that lead to important biologic differences. For example, COX-2 is more easily "primed" by intracellular hydroperoxides and is active at lower concentrations of arachidonic acid. In addition, amino acid changes in the hydrophobic core of the enzymes lead to differences in "shape" of the COX active site that has been exploited to develop drugs that specifically inhibit COX-2 (2).

The most striking difference between the COX isoforms, however, is at the level of expression and regulation of mRNA and protein levels. These differences lead directly to the differing biological roles of COX-1 and COX-2. COX-1 is expressed in most tissues and levels do not vary greatly. COX-1–derived PGs mediate important physiologic processes in many tissues and COX-1 is available to increase PG production acutely when an abrupt increase in levels of arachidonic acid occurs following cell stimulation. However, COX-1

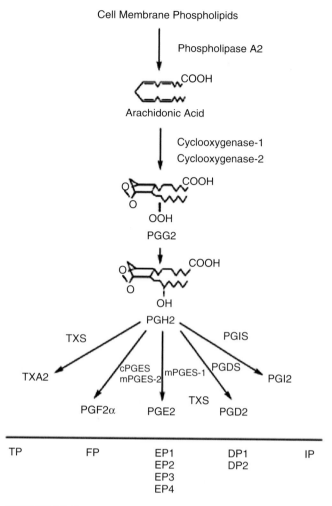

FIGURE 41-1

Prostaglandin biosynthetic pathway. The first step in prostaglandin (PG) biosynthesis is the release of arachidonic acid from cell membrane phospholipids by phospholipase A2. Cyclooxygenase (COX)-1 and COX-2 then adds two molecules of oxygen followed by a hydroperoxidase reaction to create first PGG_2 and then PGH_2. PGH_2 is an unstable intermediate rapidly converted to stable PGs by the respective PG synthases in a cell- and tissue-specific manner. PGE_2 has three different synthase enzymes, one of which (mPGES-1) is inducible by proinflammatory signals similar to COX-2. Stable PGs act in an autocrine or paracrine manner on cell surface receptors.

does not contribute substantially to the large increases in PG production that occur during inflammation. COX-1 is the only isoform expressed in mature platelets and is the dominant isoform in normal gastric mucosa (3).

Cyclooxygenase-2 expression is restricted to a few tissues, notably the kidney and brain, under basal conditions. COX-2 also plays an important role in normal reproductive, cardiovascular, and skeletal physiology. Most important for rheumatic diseases is the fact that COX-2 expression is highly induced and accounts for the large increase in PG levels produced locally during inflammation. COX-2 expression is increased by a number of cytokines, including interleukin 1 (IL-1) and tumor necrosis factor alpha (TNF-alpha), and other mediators associated with inflammation (3). COX-2 expression is inhibited by glucocorticoids, accounting for some of their anti-inflammatory properties (see Chapter 42).

The product of the COX enzymes, PGH_2, is an unstable intermediate that is rapidly converted to one of several possible prostanoids by terminal synthases. In general, this process is cell-specific with differentiated cells producing only one or two PGs in abundance (2). The most important stable prostanoids include PGD_2, PGE_2, $PGF_{2\alpha}$, prostacyclin (PGI_2), and thromboxane A_2 (TXA_2). All have different biological roles that are important to the understanding of NSAID efficacy and safety.

PGE_2 is thought to be the most important mediator of inflammation (4). There are several forms of PGE synthase enzymes, including the microsomal PGE synthase-1 (mPGES-1) which, like COX-2, is highly induced during inflammation. mPGES-1 expression is increased by proinflammatory cytokines and inhibited by glucocorticoids. mPGES-1 acts in concert with COX-2 to generate locally high levels of PGE_2 during inflammation. There are four receptors for PGE_2 (EP receptors) with different signaling pathways. Molecular evolution studies demonstrate several receptor clusters, all containing receptors for PGE_2 (5). The earliest divergence is between clusters associated with either an increase of cAMP (EP2, EP4, IP–prostacyclin receptor, and DP–PGD_2 receptor) or decrease of cAMP (one isoform of EP3, TP–thromboxane receptor). The ancestral EP1 receptor diverged from the EP3 receptors and functions to increase intracellular Ca^{2+} along with the FP ($PGF_{2\alpha}$) and TP receptors.

There is considerable interest in potential nuclear actions of PGs. This may occur by interaction with nuclear receptors or by interaction with intracellular proteins. In biological fluids, PGD_2 is slowly dehydrated to yield the cyclopentanone PGs, PGJ_2 (6). PGJ_2 and other cyclopentanone PGs contain a highly reactive alpha beta-unsaturated ketone moiety that allows adduct formation with other proteins. It is thought that the cyclopentanone PGs play a role in the resolution of inflammation by acting as ligands for peroxisome proliferator-activated receptors (PPARs). It has also been suggested that covalent modification of certain transcription factors may lead to modulation of immune and inflammatory responses (7).

MECHANISM OF ACTION

The most important mechanism of NSAID action is to inhibit production of PGs by competing with arachidonic acid for binding in the COX catalytic site. NSAIDs have little effect on peroxidase activity (2). It should be noted here that acetaminophen, while not classified as an NSAID, inhibits COX activity in vitro. It is thought that acetaminophen acts by inhibiting the peroxidase activity of the COX enzymes. Failure of acetaminophen to act as an anti-inflammatory agent may be related to its lack of effect under conditions of high hydroperoxide tone such as is found in inflammatory sites (8). NSAIDs may exhibit different kinetic modes of inhibition including (i) rapid, reversible binding (e.g., ibuprofen); (ii) rapid, lower affinity reversible binding followed by time-dependent, higher affinity, slowly reversible binding (e.g., naproxen, celecoxib); or (iii) rapid, reversible binding followed by covalent modification (e.g., aspirin) (2). From a clinical perspective, it is important to characterize NSAIDs according to specificity for inhibition of COX-1 or COX-2 (9). All NSAIDs currently in clinical use that inhibit COX-1 also inhibit COX-2 at therapeutic concentrations. However, at low doses (81 mg) aspirin acts as a specific inhibitor of COX-1. The specificity for COX-2 is based on the structural difference between the hydrophobic channels resulting in an NSAID binding site about 20% larger than COX-1 and including a side pocket.

Very high doses of NSAIDs have been shown to have COX-independent activities on cellular processes that could contribute to some of their actions. The practical importance of these mechanisms is unknown. Sodium salicylate and aspirin were shown to inhibit activation of the transcription factor NF-κB, leading some to suggest that this could be an important anti-inflammatory mechanism. Similar to some PGs, certain NSAIDs bind to and activate members of the PPAR family and other intracellular receptors. Another potential mechanism is induction of endogenous anti-inflammatory mechanisms. It was shown that the anti-inflammatory effect of salicylate can be inhibited by an adenosine A2 receptor antagonist in a murine model of inflammation, suggesting that salicylate may stimulate adenosine release. Specific COX-2 inhibitors may have unique structural features that promote COX-independent apoptosis of some cancer cells and angiogenesis (10).

CLINICAL PHARMACOLOGY

The chemical class and pharmacologic properties of various salicylates and other NSAIDs is listed in Table 41-1. Most NSAIDs are weak organic acids completely absorbed from the gastrointestinal (GI) tract. Once absorbed, NSAIDs are highly (> 95%) bound to plasma proteins, and the amount of free drug is relatively small. However, clinically significant reductions in albumin, such as occur in patients with active rheumatoid arthritis (RA), the elderly, and those with other chronic illnesses, can lead to an increase in free drug and an increased risk for toxicity. Due to increased vascular permeability in local sites of inflammation, the high degree of protein binding may result in delivery of higher levels of NSAIDs.

Nonsteriodal anti-inflammatory drugs with a longer half-life take a longer time to reach steady state concentrations. This can have consequences for the time to reach full therapeutic effect. The clearance of NSAIDs is usually by hepatic metabolism with production of inactive metabolites that are excreted in the bile and urine. Most NSAIDs are metabolized through the microsomal cytochrome P450-containing mixed-function oxidase system. Drugs metabolized through this pathway are expected to have drug interactions. Furthermore, there is genetic variation in enzyme activity such that some groups may metabolize drugs more slowly. The pharmacokinetics of some NSAIDs can be affected by liver disease, renal disease, or old age (11).

Salicylates are acetylated (e.g., aspirin) or nonacetylated (e.g., sodium salicylate, choline salicylate, choline magnesium trisalicylate, salicysalicylic acid). Aspirin and salicylates are readily absorbed in the acidic or neutralized stomach and intestine. The formulation of these agents affects the absorption properties, but not bioavailability. Buffered aspirin tablets contain antacids that increase the pH of the microenvironment, while enteric coating slows absorption. The bioavailability of rectal aspirin suppositories increases with retention time. Aspirin is rapidly deacetylated to salicylate either spontaneously or enzymatically. Albumin is the dominant protein to which salicylates bind, and in conditions where albumin concentrations are low, including active RA, the pharmacologic and toxic effects of an increment in dose are more pronounced. Salicylate is metabolized principally by the liver and excreted primarily by the kidney. The serum levels of salicylate bear only a modest relationship to the dose ingested and a small increment in dose may lead to a profound increment in serum level.

THERAPEUTIC ACTIONS

Nonsteriodal anti-inflammatory drugs have antipyretic, analgesic, and anti-inflammatory properties. The majority of evidence suggests that most of these properties are mediated by inhibition of COX-2 (3). Fever occurs in response to inflammation and induction of cytokines that function as endogenous pyrogens. PGs have long been known to mediate the fever response. COX-2 expression is induced in the brain vasculature with temporal correlation to the development of fever. In the absence of COX-2, fever fails to develop. PGs produced locally at the site of inflammation sensitize

41

peripheral nociceptors. PGs also prolong proinflammatory actions of bradykinin, histamine, nitric oxide, and other pain mediators. Recent studies have also demonstrated a role for PGs in central sensitization at the spinal level, resulting in hyperalgesia (increased pain to a normally painful stimulus) and allodynia (pain to a normally innocuous stimulus). There is constitutive expression of COX-2 in the dorsal horn of the spinal cord that is increased during inflammation, and inhibition of COX-2, but not COX-1, reduces spinal PG production (12).

Nonsteriodal anti-inflammatory drugs are used in virtually all rheumatic diseases associated with pain and inflammation. Their efficacy is best studied in osteoarthritis (OA), RA, gout, and acute pain. The question of whether an individual NSAID provides improved efficacy for a particular indication has been difficult to discern in randomized, controlled trials. However, historical preference for some agents in some conditions (e.g., indomethacin for gout or ankylosing spondylitis) continues, and a mechanistic basis for this preference may yet be identified. The utility of NSAIDs is limited chiefly by their adverse-effect profile and, in general, NSAIDs should be used for the shortest time possible and at the lowest dose that controls symptoms.

Aspirin is indicated for secondary prevention of cardiovascular disease. The use of aspirin to prevent cardiovascular disease events in patients without a prior history of cardiovascular disease is controversial. However, recent recommendations from the US Preventive Services Task Force suggest that those patients with an increased (3%–5%) risk for coronary heart disease events over 5 years may receive greater benefit than harm from aspirin chemoprophylaxis (13). There is no data to suggest that NSAIDs other than aspirin are effective agents for prophylaxis of cardiovascular thrombotic events, therefore NSAIDs are commonly used in combination with low-dose aspirin. Care should be taken to illicit the history of aspirin use and to consider drug interactions. There is recent data to suggest that some NSAIDs may reduce the ability of aspirin to exert its antithrombotic effect (14,15).

ADVERSE EFFECTS

Nonsteriodal anti-inflammatory drugs produce toxic effects in many organ systems (Table 41-2). Most of these adverse effects are related to inhibition of PGs mediating important physiologic functions. Because the therapeutic and adverse effects are related to the same mechanism of action, the therapeutic window for these medications is relatively narrow. Of course, there are adverse effects related to specific drugs and unrelated to inhibition of PGs.

TABLE 41-2. ADVERSE EFFECTS OF NONSPECIFIC AND COX-2–SPECIFIC NONSTERIODAL ANTI-INFLAMMATORY DRUGS.

ORGAN SYSTEM	NONSPECIFIC NSAIDS	DIFFERENCES WITH COX-2–SPECIFIC NSAIDs
Gastrointestinal	Dyspepsia Gastroduodenal ulceration Bleeding (all levels) Colitis	Decreased UGI ulceration Decreased bleeding
Renal	Hypertension Edema Acute renal failure Interstitial nephritis Papillary necrosis	
Hepatic	Elevated transaminases Rare severe hepatic reactions	
Asthma	Exacerbation of AERD	No cross-reactivity in AERD
Allergic reactions	Hypersensitivity reactions	Celecoxib contraindicated in patients with sulfonamide allergies
Cardiovascular	Platelet dysfunction	Arterial thrombosis in high-risk patients with high-dose, long-acting, highly specific inhibitors (rofecoxib)
Central nervous system	Dizziness Somnolence Cognitive dysfunction Aseptic meningitis	

ABBREVIATIONS: AERD, aspirin-exacerbated respiratory disease; NSAIDs, nonsteriodal anti-inflammatory drugs; UGI, upper gastrointestinal tract.

Gastrointestinal

Injury to the upper gastrointestinal tract in the form of ulcers and their complications are the most important toxicity associated with aspirin and nonspecific NSAIDs. Millions of individuals regularly use aspirin and NSAIDs, magnifying the overall importance of NSAID gastroenteropathy from a public health standpoint. It was the expectation of reduced gastroduodenal injury that drove development of specific COX-2 inhibitors. The risk profile for gastric injury is reduced for those agents with the lowest potential for COX-1 inhibition.

Prospective data derived from Arthritis, Rheumatism, and Aging Medical Information System (ARAMIS) showed that 13 of every 1000 patients with RA that take nonspecific NSAIDs for 1 year have a serious gastrointestinal complication (16). Although the rate of NSAID-related serious gastrointestinal complications has decreased, in part due to use of protective strategies and COX-2–specific NSAIDs, no protective strategy has eliminated the risk of NSAID use. Unfortunately, despite a number of strategies available for risk reduction, there is a high level of failure to adequately protect patients using NSAIDs. The mortality rate among patients who are hospitalized for NSAID-induced upper gastrointestinal bleeding is 5% to 10%. Bleeding is by far the most common ulcer complication, but obstruction and perforation may also occur (17).

Epidemiological studies have shown that the use of nonspecific NSAIDs increases the risk of ulcer complications by a factor of 4 compared with nonusers, and even low-dose aspirin ($\leq$325 mg) doubles the risk of bleeding ulcers (18). The absolute risk of serious GI complications (bleeding, perforation, or obstruction) in a patient with no other risk factors is about 0.5% per year and the risk in RA patients is about 2% to 4% per year (16).

In addition to injury of the gastroduodenal mucosa, NSAID use is associated with symptoms of dyspepsia and damage to other regions of the gastrointestinal tract. At least 10% to 20% of patients taking NSAIDs experience dyspepsia (17). Symptoms or the lack thereof are not good predictors of NSAID-related GI complications because only a minority of patients with serious GI events report antecedent dyspepsia (16). Other adverse GI events include pill esophagitis, small bowel ulceration, small bowel strictures, colonic strictures, diverticular disease, and exacerbation of inflammatory bowel disease (17). Patients admitted to the hospital with large or small bowel perforations or bleeding are twice as likely to be taking NSAIDs. In an autopsy series of over 700 patients, 8% of patients taking NSAIDs or low-dose aspirin compared with 0.6% of those not taking NSAIDs revealed small intestinal ulceration, while 24% of NSAID users had gastroduodenal ulcers (19). COX-2 expression is higher in the colon than in more proximal portions of the GI tract under basal conditions and increases markedly if colonic inflammation is present. COX-2 inhibition or genetic deficiency markedly exacerbates experimental colitis, suggesting that COX-2–derived PGs may be a protective mechanism for mucosal defense (20).

Mucosal damage associated with inhibiting PG synthesis is associated with a decrease in epithelial mucus, secretion of bicarbonate, mucosal blood flow, epithelial proliferation, and mucosal resistance to injury. Impaired mucosal resistance permits injury by endogenous factors (e.g., acid, pepsin, and bile salts) and exogenous factors (e.g., NSAIDs), thereby amplifying bleeding risk by causing new mucosal lesions. Topical mucosal injury is initiated by the acidic properties of aspirin and many other NSAIDs. In addition, topical injury may occur as a result of indirect mechanisms, mediated through the biliary excretion and subsequent duodenogastric reflux of active NSAID metabolites (e.g., sulindac). Inhibition of prostaglandins, however, is the principal mechanism underlying development of gastroduodenal ulceration. This is most graphically illustrated by the fact that enteric coating and parenteral or rectal administration fails to reduce ulcer risk. In addition, platelet dysfunction can increase the risk of bleeding associated with damaged gastrointestinal mucosa (17).

In the normal gastroduodenal mucosa and in platelets, COX-1 is the isoform responsible for PG production. However, inhibition of COX-2 may contribute to risk in situations where damage is present. During injury of the GI tract, as in other tissues, COX-2 is induced. PGs derived from COX-2 would normally exert suppressive effects on inflammatory cells, notably neutrophils, that contribute to damage. These findings are perhaps relevant to the high risk of recurrence ($\sim$ 25%) in patients with previous ulcers even when protective strategies are used (21).

Not all patients are at similar risk for NSAID-related GI bleeding. Factors consistently associated with increased risk for developing NSAID-associated gastroduodenal ulcers are shown in Table 41-3 (17). These risk factors can be identified in prospective clinical trials of gastroprotective strategies and risk reduction is higher in those at greatest risk (22). The only way to completely prevent NSAID-associated GI injury is not to use them; however, using the lowest effective dose of an NSAID for the shortest time required may reduce risk. There are several other strategies available to reduce the risks of upper GI complications due to aspirin and NSAID use (Table 41-3).

Several large randomized, controlled clinical trails have been performed to evaluated the occurrence of clinical significant ulcers and ulcer complications in patients treated with specific COX-2 inhibitors compared to nonspecific NSAIDs (23–25). Data from these randomized controlled trials and other studies suggest that drugs that are more specific towards the COX-2

has also been shown that chronic dosing of certain NSAIDs (e.g., ibuprofen, but not diclofenac or celecoxib) can prevent aspirin from blocking platelet COX-1 and inhibiting the antiplatelet effect of aspirin (14).

Antihypertensives

Nonsteriodal anti-inflammatory drugs reduce the response to diuretics, particularly loop diuretics. This effect is due to inhibition of PG synthesis as opposed to a pharmacokinetic interaction. NSAIDs also inhibit the effectiveness of angiotensin-converting enzyme inhibitors, perhaps due to increased sodium retention (28).

Anticoagulants

Clinically significant increases in prothrombin times can be seen in patients taking virtually any NSAID with warfarin. This can occur either due to protein binding displacement or due to altered metabolism of warfarin and prothrombin. Coagulation time should be monitored more closely than usual in patients starting NSAIDs.

Methotrexate

Aspirin reduces clearance of methotrexate and this effect is shared by some other NSAIDs (35). Celecoxib did not alter methotrexate pharmacokinetics in patients with rheumatoid arthritis (36).

SUMMARY AND CONCLUSIONS

Nonsteriodal anti-inflammatory drugs are an important part of the therapeutic armamentarium in patients with rheumatic diseases, but as with all drugs their benefit/risk ratio should be evaluated carefully. NSAIDs are effective anti-inflammatory and analgesic agents that allow many patients to achieve improved health-related quality of life. These very important beneficial effects should be weighted against the potential for adverse effects in an individual patient. It is of particular importance to evaluate risk in the elderly, those with multiple concomitant illnesses, and patients with multiple coprescriptions. In general, caution should be used in these patients and careful attention should be paid to using the lowest dose, shortest acting NSAIDs with care; to discontinuing these medications when not needed (e.g., use on an as-needed basis); using appropriate protective strategies for those with risk factors for GI toxicity is essential. In those at particular risk, acetaminophen and non-aspirin salicylates may provide viable alternatives. Although not currently available, strategies for reducing proinflammatory PGs by inhibiting other biosynthetic enzymes or PG receptors may prove fruitful.

REFERENCES

1. Vane JR, Botting RM. The history of anti-inflammatory drugs and their mechanism of action. In: Bazan N, Botting J, Vane J, eds. New targets in inflammation: inhibitors of COX-2 or adhesion molecules. London: Kluwer Academic Publishers and William Harvey Press; 1996:1–12.
2. Smith WL, DeWitt DL, Garavito RM. Cyclooxygenases: structural, cellular, and molecular biology. Ann Rev Biochem 2000;69:145–182.
3. Crofford LJ, Lipsky PE, Brooks P, Abramson SB, Simon LS, van de Putte LBA. Basic biology and clinical application of specific COX-2 inhibitors. Arthritis Rheum 2000; 43:4–13.
4. Stichtenoth DO, Thoren S, Bian H, Peters-Golden M, Jakobsson P-J, Crofford LJ. Microsomal prostaglandin E synthase is regulated by pro-inflammatory cytokines and glucocorticoids in primary rheumatoid synovial cells. J Immunol 2001;167:469–474.
5. Toh H, Ichikawa A, Narumiya S. Molecular evolution of receptors for eicosanoids. FEBS Lett 1995;361:17–21.
6. Narumiya S, FitzGerald GA. Genetic and pharmacological analysis of prostanoid receptor function. J Clin Invest 2001;108:25–30.
7. Tilley SL, Coffman TM, Koller BH. Mixed messages: modulation of inflammation and immune responses by prostaglandins and thromboxanes. J Clin Invest 2001;108: 15–23.
8. Boutaud O, Aronoff DM, Richardson JH, Marnett LJ, Oates JA. Determinants of the cellular specificity of acetaminophen as an inhibitor of prostaglandin H2 synthases. Proc Natl Acad Sci U S A 2002;99:7130–7135.
9. Lipsky PE, Abramson SB, Crofford L, DuBois RN, Simon L, van de Putte LBA. The classification of cyclooxygenase inhibitors [editorial]. J Rheumatol 1998;25: 2298–2303.
10. Tegeder I, Pfeilschifter J, Geisslinger G. Cyclooxygenase-independent actions of cyclooxygenase inhibitors. FASEB J 2001;15:2057–2072.
11. Verbeek RK. Pathophysiologic factors affecting the pharmacokinetics of non-steroidal anti-inflammatory drugs. J Rheumatol 1988;15:44–57.
12. Yaksh TL, Dirig DM, Conway CM, Svensson C, Luo ZD, Isakson PC. The acute antihyperalgesic action of non-steroidal, anti-inflammatory drugs and release of spinal prostglandin E2 is mediated by inhibition of constitutive spinal cyclooxygenase-2 (COX-2) but not COX-1. J Neurosci 2001;21:5847–5853.
13. Hayden M, Pignone M, Phillips C, Mulrow C. Aspirin for the primary prevention of cardiovascular events: a summary of the evidence for the U.S. Preventive Services Task Force. Ann Intern Med 2002;136:161–172.
14. Catella-Lawson F, Reilly M, Kapoor SC, et al. Cyclooxygenase inhibitors and the antiplatelet effects of aspirin. N Engl J Med 2001;345:1809–1817.
15. MacDonald TM, Wei L. Effect of ibuprofen on cardioprotective effect of aspirin. Lancet 2003;361:573–574.
16. Singh G, Ramey DR, Morfeld D, Shi H, Hatoum HT, Fries JF. Gatrointestinal tract complications of nonsteroidal anti-inflammatory drug treatment in rheumatoid

arthritis: a prospective observational cohort study. Arch Intern Med 1996;156:1530–1536.

17. Wolfe MM, Lichtenstein DR, Singh G. Gastrointestinal toxicity of nonsteroidal antiinflammatory drugs. N Engl J Med 1999;340:1888–1899.

18. Garcia Rodriguez LA, Hernandez-Diaz S. Relative risk of upper gastrointestinal complications among users of acetaminophen and nonsteroidal anti-inflammatory drugs. Epidemiology 2001;12:570–576.

19. Allison MC, Howatson AG, Torrance CJ, Lee FD, Russell RI. Gastrointestinal damage associated with the use of nonsteroidal aniinflammatory drugs. N Engl J Med 1992; 327:749–754.

20. Wallace JL. Prostaglandin biology in inflammatory bowel disease. Gastroenterol Clin North Am 2001;30: 971–980.

21. Chan FKL, Hung LCT, Suen BY, et al. Celecoxib versus diclofenac and omeprazole in reducing the risk of recurrent ulcer bleeding in patients with arthritis. N Engl J Med 2002;347:2104–2110.

22. Laine L, Bombardier C, Hawkey CJ, et al. Stratifying the risk of NSAID-related upper gastrointestinal clinical events: results of a double-blind outcomes study in patients with rheumatoid arthritis. Gastroenterology 2002;123: 1006–1012.

23. Bombardier C, Laine L, Reicin A, et al. Comparison of upper gastrointestinal toxicity of rofecoxib and naproxen in patients with rheumatoid arthritis. N Engl J Med 2000; 343:1520–1528.

24. Silverstein FE, Faich G, Goldstein JL, et al. Gastrointestinal toxicity with celecoxib vs nonsteroidal anti-inflammatory drugs for osteoarthritis and rheumatoid arthritis. The CLASS study: a randomized controlled trial. JAMA 2000;284:1247–1255.

25. Schnitzer TJ, Burmester GR, Mysler E, et al. Comparison of lumiracoxib with naproxen and ibuprofen in the Therapeutic Arthritis Research and Gastrointestinal Event Trial (TARGET), reduction in ulcer complications: randomised controlled trial. Lancet 2004;364: 665–674.

26. Chan FKL, Chung SCS, Suen BY, et al. Preventing recurrent upper gastrointestinal bleeding in patients with helicobacter pylori infection who are taking low-dose aspirin or naproxen. N Engl J Med 2001;344:967–973.

27. Graham DY, Agrawal NM, Campbell DR, et al. Ulcer prevention in long-term users of nonsteroidal anti-inflammatory drugs. Arch Intern Med 2002;162:169–175.

28. Brater DC, Harris C, Redfern JS, Gertz BJ. Renal effects of COX-2 selective inhibitors. Am J Nephrol 2001;21: 1–15.

29. Qi Z, Hao C-M, Langenbach RI, et al. Opposite effects of cyclooxygenase-1 and -2 activity on the pressor response to angiotensin II. J Clin Invest 2002;110:61–69.

30. Belay ED, Bresee JS, Holman RC, Kahn AD, Sharhriai A, Schonberger LB. Reye's syndrome in the United States from 1981 through 1997. N Engl J Med 1999;340:1377–1382.

31. Crofford LJ. COX-2: where are we in 2003? Specific cyclooxygenase-2 inhibitors and aspirin-exacerbated respiratory disease. Arthritis Res Ther 2003;5:25–27.

32. FitzGerald GA, Patrono C. The coxibs, selective inhibitors of cyclooxygenase-2. N Engl J Med 2001;345:433–442.

33. McGettigan P, Henry D. Cardiovascular risk and inhibition of cyclooxygenase: a systematic review of the observational studies of selective and nonselective inhibitors of cyclooxygenase 2. JAMA 2006;296:1633–1644.

34. Hudson M, Richard H, Pilote L. Differences in outcomes of patients with congestive heart failure prescribed celecoxib, rofecoxib, or non-steroidal anti-inflammatory drugs: population based study. BMJ 2005;330:1370.

35. Furst DE, Hillson J. Aspirin and other nonsteroidal anti-inflammatory drugs. In: Koopman WJ, ed. Arthritis and allied conditions. Philadelphia: Lippincott Williams & Wilkins; 2001:665–716.

36. Karim A, Tolbert DS, Hunt TL, Hubbard RC, Harper KM, Geis GS. Celecoxib, a specific COX-2 inhibitor, has no significant effect on methotrexate pharmacokinetics in patients with rheumatoid arthritis. J Rheumatol 1999; 26:2539–2543.

41

CHAPTER 42

Glucocorticoids

FRANK BUTTGEREIT, MD
GERD-RÜDIGER BURMESTER, MD

- Glucocorticoids (GCs) have powerful anti-inflammatory and immunomodulatory effects and are useful for treating many rheumatic diseases.
- Glucocorticoids work by inhibiting leukocyte access to inflamed tissues, interfering with the function of cells involved in the inflammatory process, and suppressing the production of humoral factors such as cytokines and prostaglandins involved in immune inflammatory processes.
- Glucocorticoids accomplish their effects by several mechanisms, including altering synthesis of proteins, releasing proteins from intracellular protein complexes that include GC receptors, and changing the properties of biological membranes.
- Initial GC dosage should be determined by the type and severity of the disease manifestation under treatment.
- Because of significant toxicity associated with long-term GC use, doses of <7.5 mg daily are recommended only if required to control symptoms.

Glucocorticoids (GCs) have been in use for more than 50 years. They are powerful and cost-effective drugs with strong anti-inflammatory and immunomodulatory effects that are used to treat rheumatic and other diseases. Their therapeutic use has increased continuously in recent years (1,2). Furthermore, our understanding of the action of glucocorticoids has advanced in recent years, especially with regard to mechanisms of action, clinical usage, side-effect potential, and the development of new glucocorticoid drugs (2–5). GCs are the subject of this chapter as the terms *corticosteroids* or *corticoids* do not precisely designate these compounds. The adrenal cortex indeed synthesizes glucocorticoids, but also mineralocorticoids and androgens. The term *steroids*, although often used (e.g., in steroid-induced osteoporosis), is similarly incorrect because it simply describes chemical compounds characterized by a common multiple-ring structure which include cholesterol and sex hormones.

MECHANISMS OF ACTION

Cellular Effects on Immune Cells

Glucocorticoids mediate important anti-inflammatory and immunomodulatory effects when used therapeutically. There are many specific effects of the commonly used GC drugs, which include prednisone, predniso-lone, methylprednisolone, and dexamethasone. However, for daily practice we can summarize their clinical actions as follows:

- Inhibit leukocyte traffic and access of leukocytes to the site of inflammation
- Interfere with functions of leukocytes, fibroblasts, and endothelial cells
- Suppress the production and actions of humoral factors involved in the inflammatory process

Virtually all primary and secondary immune cells are more or less affected. The most important effects on the different cell types are listed in Table 42-1.

Molecular Mechanisms

Four different mechanisms have been identified to date. The interested reader can find more details in recent reviews (2,3). Cytosolic GC receptor (*cGCR*)-*mediated genomic effects* refers to the classical mechanism by which GCs up- or downregulate the synthesis of specific regulatory proteins. The GC molecules bind to the cGCR alpha. The activated GC/cGCR complex in turn binds to specific DNA-binding sites called *glucocorticoid responsive elements*. In some cases, this results in upregulated synthesis of certain proteins. This process, called *transactivation*, affects between 10 and 100 genes per cell that are regulated in this way (6). There are also

TABLE 42-1. IMPORTANT EFFECTS OF
GLUCOCORTICOIDS ON PRIMARY AND SECONDARY
IMMUNE CELLS.

Monocytes/macrophages
  ↓ number of circulating cells (↓ myelopoiesis, ↓ release)
  ↓ expression of MHC class II molecules and Fc receptors
  ↓ synthesis of proinflammatory cytokines (e.g., IL-2, IL-6, TNF-
    alpha) and prostaglandins

T cells
  ↓ number of circulating cells (redistribution effects)
  ↓ production and action of IL-2 (most important)

Granulocytes
  ↓ number of eosinophil and basophil granulocytes
  ↑ number of circulating neutrophils

Endothelial cells
  ↓ vessel permeability
  ↓ expression of adhesion molecules
  ↓ production of IL-1 and prostaglandins

Fibroblasts
  ↓ proliferation
  ↓ production of fibronectin and prostaglandins

SOURCE: From Buttgereit F, Saag K, Cutolo M, et al. Scand J Rheum 2005;34:14–21, by permission of *Scandinavian Journal of Rheumatology* (www.tandf.no/rheumatology) and Taylor & Francis.
ABBREVIATIONS: IL, interleukin; MHC, major histocompatibility complex; TNF, tumor necrosis factor.

negative glucocorticoid responsive elements, but inhibitory effects are typically mediated instead by negative interference of the GC/cGCR complex with transcription factors such as NF-κB and activator protein 1 (AP-1). Via this latter mechanism, GCs downregulate the synthesis of proinflammatory cytokines, such as interleukin 1 (IL-1), interleukin 6 (IL-6), and tumor necrosis factor alpha (TNF-alpha). Many genes are regulated via this mode of action, which is termed *transrepression*. Altogether, it is estimated that GCs influence the transcription of approximately 1% of the entire genome (7).

With respect to the regulation of genomic GC actions, it must be mentioned that an alternative splice variant of the cGCR alpha exists, the cGCR beta isoform. This isoform does not bind ligand and may inhibit classic cGCR alpha–mediated transactivation of target genes (2,8).

Recently, it became evident that GCs also mediate effects via so called *cGCR-mediated nongenomic effects*. Croxtall and colleagues have suggested that following GC binding the GC/cGCR complex mediates not only classical genomic actions, but ligand binding also initiates a rapid release of proteins (chaperones and co-chaperones such as Src) from the multiprotein complex that includes the cGCR. These (co-)chaperones are considered to be responsible for producing measurable

effects within a few minutes, far more rapidly than genomic effects (9).

Glucocorticoids also mediate rapid and therapeutic relevant effects via membrane-bound GCR (mGCR) termed *mGCR-mediated nongenomic effects* (2). mGCRs have been recently identified on human PBMC from healthy controls. A strong positive correlation between the frequency of mGCR-positive monocytes and various parameters of disease activity was found in patients with rheumatoid arthritis (RA). One of the suggested functions of mGCR is to mediate cell lysis by inducing apoptosis. Therefore, it is currently assumed that mGCR mediates a negative feedback regulation as follows: Immunostimulation (or high disease activity) induces mGCR expression on immune cells, such as monocytes. This in turn leads to a significantly higher percentage of cells undergoing GC-induced apoptosis, which ameliorates the activity of the immune system. This mechanism remains speculative and further experiments are needed to confirm the functional activity of mGCR (2).

Finally, GCs at high concentrations are able to intercalate into cellular membranes, such as plasma and mitochondrial membrane, and change their properties. This is the basis for *nonspecific nongenomic effects*, possibly mediated by changes in the cation transport through the plasma membrane and in the proton leak of the mitochondria. These physicochemical interactions with biological membranes are very likely to be the key to the very rapid immunosuppressive and anti-inflammatory effects of high dose GCs. Very high GC concentrations are achieved by intra-articular GC injections or intravenous GC pulse therapy.

THERAPEUTIC USE

Most of the desired clinical effects of GC treatment in rheumatic patients are mediated by transrepression. These include the reduction of clinical signs and symptoms of inflammation and the retardation of the radiological progression in rheumatoid arthritis.

Inhibition of Inflammation

An inflammatory process (e.g., arthritis, myositis) is usually characterized by upregulated synthesis of inflammatory mediators, such as prostaglandin E_2 (PGE_2) and cytokines. Among the most important clinical effects of GCs are reduced synthesis of enymes involved in the biosynthesis of PGE_2 (see Chapter 41) and proinflammatory cytokines, such as IL-1 and TNF-alpha. This is accomplished by transrepression that finally leads, usually within hours or a few days depending on the dosage applied, to the well-known and striking relief from signs and symptoms of inflammation, including pain.

Retardation of Radiographic Progression

The ability of GC to retard radiological progression in RA was first demonstrated by Kirwan (10). In 1997, Boers and colleagues published a multicenter, double-blind, randomized trial (COBRA), in which patients with early RA were randomized to either step-down therapy with two disease-modifying antirheumatic drugs (DMARDs; sulfasalazine and methotrexate) and prednisolone (start 60 mg/day, tapered in 6 weekly steps to 7.5 mg/day and stopped at 28 weeks), or sulfasalazine alone. In the combined drug strategy group, a statistically significant and clinically relevant effect in retarding joint damage was shown compared with the effect of sulfasalazine alone (11). In an extension of this study, long-term (4–5 years) beneficial benefits were also shown regarding radiological damage following the combination strategy (12). These data were later supported by other studies, with some of them very recently published (13–15).

Proinflammatory cytokines such as IL-1 and TNF-alpha are key players in the process of joint damage in RA. They stimulate osteoblasts and T cells to produce RANKL which bind to RANK on osteoclast precursor cells and on mature osteoblasts. This finally leads to more activated osteoclasts, which are responsible for bone resorption/erosions in RA. The ability of GCs to reduce the synthesis of these proinflammatory cytokines via transrepression may contribute to their effects on radiological progression in RA.

Glucocorticoid Use in Daily Practice

The basis for the use of different GC dosages in different clinical conditions is essentially empirical, as the evidence to support preferences in specific clinical settings is remarkably scarce (5). It is clear, however, that the GC dosages used are proportionately higher in patients with increased clinical activity and with increased severity of the disease under treatment. The rationale for this (mostly successful) clinical decision is the following: (i) Higher dosages increase cGCR saturation in a dose-dependent manner which intensifies the therapeutically relevant, *genomic* GC actions discussed above; (ii) it is assumed that with increasing dosages the *nongenomic* actions of GCs increasingly come into play (2).

Over the last few decades, clinicians in their daily practice had already created landmark GC doses that were still cloudy in their definition but clearly grouped around 7.5, 30, and 100 mg prednisolone equivalent per day. As a result of a consensus conference, in 2002 recommendations on standardized nomenclature for GC doses and GC treatment regimens were published (Table 42-2) (5).

TABLE 42-2. STANDARDIZED NOMENCLATURE FOR GLUCOCORTICOID DOSES AND GLUCOCORTICOID TREATMENT REGIMENS.

TERMINOLOGY	DOSAGE[a]	CLINICAL APPLICATION	GENOMIC ACTIONS (RECEPTOR SATURATION)	NONGENOMIC ACTIONS	ADVERSE EFFECTS
Low dose	≤7.5	Maintenance therapy for many rheumatic diseases	+ (<50%)	?	Relatively few
Medium dose	>7.5 to ≤30	Initially given in primary chronic rheumatic diseases	++ (>50% to <100%)	(+)	Dose-dependent and considerable if treatment is given for longer periods
High dose	>30 to ≤100	Initially given in subacute rheumatic diseases	++ (+) (almost 100%)	+	Cannot be administered for long-term therapy because of severe side effects
Very high dose	>100	Initially given in acute and/or potentially life-threatening exacerbations of rheumatic diseases	+++ ([almost] 100%)	++	Cannot be administered for long-term therapy because of dramatic side effects
Pulse therapy	≥250 for one or a few days	Particularly severe and/or potentially life-threatening forms of rheumatic diseases	+++ (100%)	+++	High proportion of cases with a relatively low incidence of side effects

[a] Dosage is given in milligrams of prednisone equivalent per day.
Data from references 2 and 5.

TABLE 42-3. SUGGESTED MECHANISMS MEDIATING GLUCOCORTICOID RESISTANCE IN RHEUMATIC DISEASES (SELECTION).

Reduced number of GCR and/or reduced affinity of the ligand

Polymorphic changes and/or overexpression of chaperones/co-chaperones

Increased expression of inflammatory transcription factors

Changes in the phosphorylation status of the GCR

Overexpression of GCR beta

Multidrug resistance gene MDR1

Alteration in the expression of membrane bound GCRs (mGCRs)

SOURCE: From Buttgereit F, Saag K, Cutolo M, et al. Scand J Rheum 2005;34:14–21, by permission of *Scandinavian Journal of Rheumatology* (www.tandf.no/rheumatology) and Taylor & Francis.
ABBREVIATIONS: GCR, glucocorticoid receptor.

Glucocorticoid Resistance

Glucocorticoid resistance in RA is not well defined. However, in routine daily practice the loss of symptomatic relief over time is considered to be a sign of GC resistance (6). By this definition, over 30% of patients with RA become resistant after 3 to 6 months. The current knowledge of the molecular basis for GC resistance in the rheumatic diseases is summarized in Table 42-3. It should be noted that GC resistance in the sense defined above is different from a specific disease entity, called familial/sporadic GC resistance, a rare condition defined as generalized, partial target-tissue resistance to GCs. In this disease, several different hereditary mutations in the GCR gene have been identified which impair normal signal transduction (6).

ADVERSE EFFECTS

Apart from their desired clinical actions, GCs unfortunately also have pleiotropic effects causing a number of adverse reactions which limit their clinical use, especially at higher dosages and for longer time periods (Table 42-2). A critical and pragmatic overview of scientific evidence on the adverse effects of GCs given at lower dosages (≤10mg/day prednisolone equivalent) in RA has been recently published (16). As one key message, safety data from recent randomized, controlled clinical trials of low-dose glucocorticoid treatment in RA suggest that adverse effects associated with these lower GC dosages are modest, and are often not statistically different from those of placebo.

Musculoskeletal Adverse Effects

Glucocorticoids are the most common cause of secondary *osteoporosis*. The incidence of osteoporosis is time-and dose-dependent, but there is no consensus about a safe dose. Although some studies suggest that doses of 7.5mg of prednisone a day or less are relatively safe, a longitudinal study observed an average loss of 9.5% from spinal trabecular bone over 20 weeks in patients exposed to 7.5mg of prednisolone per day. It should be noted, however, that in cases of inflammatory diseases, such as RA, osteoporosis is multifactorial. Beside the use of GCs, there are other factors that promote the development of osteoporosis, including decreased physical activity, duration of disease, and disease activity (1,17). In parallel, disease-independent risk factors such as age, gender, genetic predisposition, nutritional factors, endocrine changes, or body weight must be considered (1). Nonetheless, osteoporosis is probably the most common adverse effect of chronic low-dose GC therapy. Strategies for the prevention and treatment of GC-induced osteoporosis are well established (see Chapter 35).

In patients treated with low doses of GCs, *osteonecrosis* is uncommon. For GCs at higher dosages it is still a matter of debate to what extent GCs and/or the underlying disease, respectively, contribute to the pathogenesis of osteonecrosis. Although quite often suspected, *myopathy* is currently believed to be exceedingly rare with GC doses of <7.5mg prednisolone equivalent daily.

Endocrine and Metabolic Adverse Effects

In patients without preexisting abnormalities of glucose tolerance, GC dose-dependently cause increased fasting glucose levels and a more pronounced increase of postprandial values. Patients with risk factors for the development of diabetes mellitus, including family history, increased age, obesity, and previous gestational diabetes mellitus, are at increased risk of developing new-onset hyperglycemia during GC treatment. This is usually rapidly reversible when GCs are stopped, but some patients will go on to develop persistent diabetes.

One of the most notable effects of chronic endogenous and exogenous GC excess is the *redistribution of body fat* and the *increase of body weight*. Centripetal fat accumulation with sparing of the extremities is a characteristic feature of patients exposed to long-term therapy with GCs.

Cardiovascular Adverse Effects

Glucocorticoids induce *dyslipidemia,* whereas their role in *atherosclerosis* is controversial. Higher dosages of GCs are considered to contribute to the development of *cardiovascular disease,* but evidence is currently lacking to show that low-dose GCs significantly increase the incidence of *cardiovascular disease* in RA. Because

42

synthetic GCs have little mineralocorticoid effects, their potential to induce *hypernatraemia, hypokalaemia,* and *sodium and water retention* is low at low doses. Nonetheless, induction of *hypertension* is seen in about 20% of patients exposed to exogenous GC. The mechanisms involved have not been fully elucidated, but it is suggested that GC-induced hypertension is dose-related and is less likely with medium or low-dose treatment. Incidences of *arrhythmia* and *sudden death* are rare and mostly limited to patients receiving high-dose pulse GC.

Dermatological Adverse Effects

Clinically relevant adverse effects on the skin include iatrogenic *Cushing's syndrome, catabolic effects* (cutaneous atrophy, purpura, striae, easy bruisability, and impaired wound healing), *steroid acne,* and *hair effects.* Cushingoid appearance, purpura, and easy bruisability is seen in over 5% of the patients exposed to ≥5 mg prednisone equivalent for ≥1 year.

Ophthalmological Adverse Effects

Long-term use of systemic GCs may induce formation of posterior subcapsular *cataract* attributed to GCs. In a group of patients with RA treated with 5 to 15 mg/day prednisone for a mean of 6 years, 15% were found to have cataracts, compared with 4.5% of matched RA controls not using prednisone. Systemic GCs also increase the risk of *glaucoma.* In the general population, 18% to 36% of those exposed to GCs had an increase in intraocular pressure. The incidence of this adverse effect tends to be higher in families, suggesting a genetic basis. Patients with preexisting glaucoma are especially sensitive and will have this condition aggravated upon exposure to GCs.

Gastrointestinal Adverse Effects

The overall estimated relative risk for *gastrointestinal ulcer disease* among current GCs users has been reported to be 2.0. However, the increased risk was almost completely due to cotreatment with nonsteroidal anti-inflammatory drugs (NSAIDs; see Chapter 41). The relative risk for patients comedicated with NSAIDs was 4.4, but for those receiving GCs alone there was no significantly increased risk (1.1).

Infectious Adverse Effects

The use of GCs is associated with increased susceptibility to various viral, bacterial, fungal, and parasitic infections. In a meta-analysis of 71 trials involving over 2000 patients with different diseases and different dosages of GCs, a relative risk of infection was found to be 2.0.

Therefore, physicians should anticipate the risk of infections with both usual and unusual organisms, realizing that GCs may blunt the classic clinical features and delay the diagnosis.

Psychological and Behavioral Disturbances

It has become consensus in the literature that the overall incidence of GC-induced *psychosis* is 5% to 6%. However, most cases are associated with high doses of GCs and an influence of the underlying disease, such as systemic lupus erythematosus (SLE), is often difficult to rule out. GC treatment has been associated with a variety of *minor mood disturbances* such as depressed or elated mood, irritability or emotional lability, anxiety and insomnia, and memory and cognition impairments. The exact incidence of such symptoms in rheumatic patients exposed to common doses of GCs is not known, but doses of < 20 to 25 mg prednisone equivalent per day are associated with few or no significant disturbances.

NEW GLUCOCORTICOID RECEPTOR LIGANDS IN THE PIPELINE

Over the last five decades, strategies such as intra-articular injections or optimized dosing regimens have been developed to improve the benefit/risk ratio (4). A new approach is the targeted delivery of conventional glucocorticoids using liposomes. Liposomes are small vesicles approximately 100 nm in size, which are used as a carrier system for GC drugs. These liposomes have been reported to accumulate selectively at the site of inflammation (18). Consequently, very high local concentrations of GCs are achieved, as, for example, in the inflamed joint. It has been recently shown in mice that liposomal prednisolone phosphate is able to produce a strong and sustained resolution of joint inflammation (18). Other current approaches to optimize the therapy with conventional GC drugs are formulations to change the timing of glucocorticoid delivery ("timed-release tablet formulation"). Also, the investigation of glycyrrhetinic acid as a potential drug needs to be mentioned here. This substance inhibits 11-beta-hydroxysteroid dehydrogenase and increases the levels and thus the action of endogenous glucocorticoids.

It seems, however, that efforts with conventional GC drugs have almost reached their limits (4). Further improvement will require qualitatively new drugs, which are currently under development. The intensive research to develop innovative novel GC receptor ligands with a clearly improved therapeutic ratio has yielded at least two promising developments to date. The first development concerns the so-called nitrosteroids. These agents are structurally characterized by an aliphatic or aromatic molecule which links a conventional GC drug with nitric oxide (NO). Drugs such as NO-prednisolone or NO-hydrocortisone slowly release NO which synergistically enhances anti-inflammatory effects and induces less osteoporosis than prednisolone in animal models (19). The second group of new agents are the selective glucocorticoid receptor agonists (SEGRAs) or "dissociating glucocorticoids." As a background, it has become evident over the last few years that many adverse effects of GCs are predominantly caused by the transactivation mechanism (e.g., diabetes, glaucoma), whereas anti-inflammatory effects are mediated mostly by transrepression mechanisms (e.g., inhibition of the synthesis of proinflammatory cytokines and prostaglandin biosynthetic enzymes) (2,20,21). SEGRAs induce predominantly the desired transrepression effects while having reduced undesirable transactivation activity as compared with conventional GC drugs (22,23). A recent report showed a drug of this class to have effective anti-inflammatory actions but to be accompanied by reduced adverse effects, such as increased body weight and skin atrophy, in animal experiments (21).

In summary, results of research over the past few years have greatly increased our knowledge of GCs as the most effective anti-inflammatory agents available. In particular, novel findings on mechanisms of action and new information on dose/effect relationships have stimulated intensive research activity with the aim of bringing increased knowledge from scientific research into clinical use as quickly as possible. There are promising approaches aimed at developing new GC receptor ligands that may improve the benefit/risk ratio and well-being of patients with rheumatic diseases.

REFERENCES

1. Thiele K, Buttgereit F, Zink A. Current use of glucocorticoids in patients with rheumatoid arthritis in Germany. Arthritis Rheum 2005;53:740–747.
2. Buttgereit F, Straub RH, Wehling M, Burmester GR. Glucocorticoids in the treatment of rheumatic diseases. An update on mechanisms of action. Arthritis Rheum 2004;50:3408–3417.
3. Rhen T, Cidlowski JA. Antiinflammatory action of glucocorticoids – new mechanisms for old drugs. N Engl J Med 2005;353:1711–1723.
4. Buttgereit F, Burmester GR, Lipworth BJ. Optimised glucocorticoid therapy: the sharpening of an old spear. Lancet 2005;375:801–803.
5. Buttgereit F, da Silva JA, Boers M, et al. Standardised nomenclature for glucocorticoid dosages and glucocorticoid treatment regimens: current questions and tentative answers in rheumatology. Ann Rheum Dis 2002;61:718–722.
6. Adcock IM, Lane SJ. Mechanisms of steroid action and resistance in inflammation. Corticosteroid-insensitive asthma: molecular mechanisms. J Endocrinol 2003;178:347–355.
7. Goulding NJ, Flower RJ. Glucocorticoid biology – a molecular maze and clinical challenge. In: Goulding NJ, Flower RJ, eds. Milestones in drug therapy: glucocorticoids. Basel: Birkhäuser Verlag; 2001:5.
8. Buttgereit F, Saag K, Cutolo M, da Silva JAP, Bijlsma JWJ. The molecular basis for the effectiveness, toxicity, and resistance to glucocorticoids: focus on the treatment of rheumatoid arthritis. Scand J Rheum 2005;34:14–21.
9. Croxtall JD, Choudhury Q, Flower RJ. Glucocorticoids act within minutes to inhibit recruitment of signalling factors to activated EGF receptors through a receptor-dependent, transcription-independent mechanism. Br J Pharmacol 2000;130:289–298.
10. Kirwan JR. The effect of glucocorticoids on joint destruction in rheumatoid arthritis. The Arthritis and Rheumatism Council Low-Dose Glucocorticoid Study Group. N Engl J Med 1995;333:142–146.
11. Boers M, Verhoeven AC, Markusse HM, et al. Randomised comparison of combined step-down prednisolone, methotrexate and sulfasalazine with sulfasalazine alone in early rheumatoid arthritis. Lancet 1997;350:309–318.
12. Landewe RB, Boers M, Verhoeven AC, et al. COBRA combination therapy in patients with early rheumatoid arthritis: long-term structural benefits of a brief intervention. Arthritis Rheum 2002;46:347–356.
13. Van Everdingen AA, Jacobs JW, Siewertsz Van Reesema DR, Bijlsma JW. Low-dose prednisone therapy for patients with early active rheumatoid arthritis: clinical efficacy, disease-modifying properties, and side effects: a randomized, double-blind, placebo-controlled clinical trial. Ann Intern Med 2002;136:1–12.
14. Wassenberg S, Rau R, Steinfeld P, Zeidler H. Very low-dose prednisolone in early rheumatoid arthritis retards radiographic progression over two years: a multicenter, double-blind, placebo-controlled trial. Arthritis Rheum 2005;52:3371–3380.
15. Svensson B, Boonen A, Albertsson K, van der Heijde D, Keller C, Hafstrom I. Low-dose prednisolone in addition to the initial disease-modifying antirheumatic drug in patients with early active rheumatoid arthritis reduces joint destruction and increases the remission rate: a two-year randomized trial. Arthritis Rheum 2005;52:3360–3370.
16. Da Silva JA, Jacobs JW, Kirwan JR, et al. Safety of low dose glucocorticoid treatment in rheumatoid arthritis: published evidence and prospective trial data. Ann Rheum Dis 2006;65:285–293.
17. Iwamoto J, Takeda T, Ichimura S. Forearm bone mineral density in postmenopausal women with rheumatoid arthritis. Calcif Tissue Int 2002;70:1–8.
18. Metselaar JM, Wauben MH, Wagenaar-Hilbers JP, Boerman OC, Storm G. Complete remission of experimental arthritis by joint targeting of glucocorticoids with long-circulating liposomes. Arthritis Rheum 2003;48:2059–2066.

19. Paul-Clark MJ, Mancini L, Del Soldato P, Flower RJ, Perretti, M. Potent antiarthritic properties of a glucocorticoid derivative, NCX-1015, in an experimental model of arthritis. Proc Natl Acad Sci U S A 2002;99:1677–1682.

20. Schacke H, Döcke WD, Asadullah K. Mechanisms involved in the side effects of glucocorticoids. Pharm Ther 2002;96:23–43.

21. Schacke H, Schottelius A, Döcke W, et al. Dissociation of transactivation from transrepression by a selective glucocorticoid receptor agonist leads to separation of therapeutic effects from side effects. Proc Natl Acad Sci U S A. 2004;101:227–232.

22. Miner JN. Designer glucocorticoids. Biochem Pharmacol 2002;64:355–361.

23. Coghlan MJ, Jacobson PB, Lane B, et al. A novel anti-inflammatory maintains glucocorticoid efficacy with reduced side effects. Mol Endocrinol 2003;17:860–869.

CHAPTER 43

Operative Treatment of Arthritis

JOSEPH A. BUCKWALTER, MS, MD
W. TIMOTHY BALLARD, MD

- Surgical treatments of arthritis and musculoskeletal diseases may be used to prevent progression, relieve pain, and/or improve joint function.
- The success of surgical interventions is dependent on careful considerations of pre-, intra-, and postoperative aspects of the surgery.

- Total joint replacements are now possible for most of the major joints affected and damaged by arthritis.

Pain not relieved by other treatments is the most common indication for operative treatment of arthritis. Loss of joint function is a less common indication for surgical treatment because function restoration is usually less predictable than pain relief. Operative treatments include joint debridement, synovectomy, osteotomy, soft tissue arthroplasty, resection arthroplasty, fusion, and joint replacement. In addition, people with rheumatoid arthritis (RA) may benefit from tenosynovectomy and repair or reconstruction of ruptured tendons.

Although operative treatments can produce excellent results, they also expose patients to serious risks. Potential operative and perioperative complications include extensive blood loss, cardiac arrhythmia and arrest, nerve and blood vessel injury, infection, venous thrombosis, and pulmonary embolism. Late postoperative complications include delayed infection and loosening and wear of implants. Even in the absence of complications, the results of surgical procedures such as joint debridements, synovectomies, and osteotomies may deteriorate with time. For these reasons, the potential risks and expected short-term and long-term outcomes of operative treatment must be carefully considered for each patient. Nonetheless, individuals who fail to gain satisfactory results from nonsurgical therapy or who have progressive disease should be evaluated by a surgeon before they develop deformity, joint instability, contractures, or advanced muscle atrophy. Delaying surgery until these problems develop can compromise the results and increase the risk of complications.

PREOPERATIVE EVALUATION

With the exception of people in whom arthritic disorders have caused or may cause spinal instability and neurologic damage, operative treatment is elective. Patients should have an extensive preoperative evaluation and should understand the full range of therapeutic options. The physician needs a thorough understanding of the degree of pain and functional limitation and an understanding of the patient's social and occupational needs and expectations. Before planning surgery, patients should understand the potential benefits and risks. In general, the patients most likely to notice significant lasting benefit from operative treatment are those with joint pain unrelieved by nonsurgical treatment. Patient age, overall health status, and capacity to adhere to postoperative rehabilitation and precautions also help determine the outcome.

Even in people with obvious joint disease, pain, and loss of function, failure to carefully evaluate the cause of the symptoms can lead to disappointing results. Common diagnostic dilemmas include differentiating hip joint pain from lumbar radicular pain and shoulder joint pain from cervical radicular pain. Rheumatoid arthritis and other types of inflammatory arthritis may cause such severe joint deformity that detecting neurologic involvement becomes difficult. Patients may develop joint sepsis that is not readily apparent because of the inflammatory nature of their underlying disease and the use of medications that suppress the inflammatory response to infection. A careful history, physical examination, and plain radiographs are sufficient to define the cause of symptoms for most, but in some cases, joint aspiration, electrodiagnostic studies, and additional imaging studies are needed to clarify the cause of pain and loss of function.

Before considering surgical intervention, patients should first be treated with nonoperative interventions including medications, ambulatory aides, activity modification, physical therapy, and orthoses. Braces may control instability and decrease pain in the spine, knee, ankle, wrist, or thumb. A cane may be considered for patients with lower extremity arthritis. In addition to reducing the body weight load to the joints of the lower extremity, a cane reduces the hip abductor forces required to keep the pelvis level during gait, thereby reducing hip joint reactive forces by up to 20% in the contralateral hip.

Weight reduction for obese patients can decrease symptoms and increase the probability of successful operative treatment. There is some evidence of an increased incidence of infection in obese patients following total joint arthroplasty (1), as well as increased intraoperative blood loss (2). It is not clear whether or not obesity increases the risk of implant loosening, but this may be because heavier patients are less active. For some overweight patients, the pain and loss of mobility caused by arthritis makes it more difficult to reduce their weight or avoid gaining weight. In these individuals, surgeons may recommend proceeding with operative treatment despite the increased risks associated with obesity.

The importance of a thorough preoperative history and physical examination, as well as careful perioperative medical management, cannot be overemphasized. Many patients who could benefit from surgical treatment, especially people with osteoarthritis (OA), are elderly and may have decreased cardiac, pulmonary, renal, or peripheral vascular function. These conditions require evaluation and, in some cases, treatment before surgery. Carious teeth, pharyngitis, cystitis, and other potential sources of infection should be treated prior to surgery. Men with symptoms of prostatic hypertrophy need a urologic evaluation before surgery and women should be evaluated for asymptomatic urinary tract infections. Preoperative laboratory evaluation should include a measure of hemoglobin and hematocrit, urinalysis, and other diagnostic tests as indicated by the individual's medical history.

PREPARATION FOR OPERATIVE TREATMENT

All patients should receive instruction concerning the planned procedure, the risks and common complications, the type and extent of postoperative rehabilitation, and expectations for postoperative pain relief and

function. To reduce the risks of operative and postoperative complications, including excessive bleeding and compromised healing, doses of nonsteroidal anti-inflammatory drugs (NSAIDs) and corticosteroids should be decreased before surgery when possible. Preoperative evaluation and instruction by physical and occupational therapists facilitate rehabilitation for some patients. In selected patients, delaying surgery will make it possible to achieve optimal management of cardiovascular or other systemic disorders, allow them to improve their nutritional status and muscle strength, or reduce their weight.

DISEASE-RELATED FACTORS

Options and indications for surgical treatment vary considerably among the arthritic diseases. Thus, the physician must consider the unique features of each disease in making decisions or advising patients concerning operative treatment.

Osteoarthritis

A number of surgical procedures have the intent of decreasing symptoms for people with OA while preserving or restoring a cartilaginous articular surface. These include arthroscopic joint debridement, resection or perforation of subchondral bone to stimulate formation of cartilaginous tissue, and use of grafts to replace degenerated articular cartilage. By removing loose fragments of cartilage, bone, and meniscus (and, in some instances, osteophytes), joint debridement may improve joint mechanical function and may decrease pain. Penetration of subchondral bone in regions of advanced cartilage degeneration stimulates formation of cartilaginous repair tissue, but because it lacks the properties of normal articular cartilage, this tissue frequently degenerates. Replacing localized regions of degenerated cartilage with osteochondral, perichondral, periosteal, and chondrocyte grafts has produced promising short-term results in small series of patients. Overall, current procedures performed with the intent of preserving or restoring a cartilaginous articular surface and decreasing symptoms are not likely to be beneficial in people with advanced joint degeneration, but they may be helpful in selected people with less severe disease.

Osteotomies correct malalignment and shift loads from severely degenerated regions of the articular surface to regions that have remaining articular cartilage. In selected patients with OA, osteotomies of the hip and knee decrease pain, but in general the results are less predictable than joint replacement. For these reasons, surgeons most commonly recommend osteotomies for young active people who have a stable joint with a functional range of motion, good muscle function, and some remaining articular cartilage.

Joint fusion (i.e., arthrodesis) can relieve pain and restore skeletal stability and alignment in people with advanced OA. Because this procedure eliminates joint motion, it has limited application. Furthermore, fusion of one joint increases the loading and motion of other joints, perhaps accelerating degeneration. For example, fusion of the hip increases the probability of developing degenerative disease in the lumbar spine and ipsilateral knee joints. Currently, surgeons most commonly perform fusions for treating degeneration of cervical and lumbar spine, hand interphalangeal, first metatarsophalangeal, wrist, and ankle joints.

For selected joints, resection of degenerated articular surfaces and replacement with implants fabricated from polyethylene, metal, or other synthetic materials can relieve pain and allow the patient to maintain joint mobility (Figure 43-1). Over the past several decades, replacing the hip and knee have proven to be effective methods of relieving pain and maintaining or improving function. Recent advances have led to better methods and implants for replacement of the hip, knee, shoulder, and elbow. Unfortunately, joint replacements have limitations, primarily because the new surface lacks the mechanical properties and durability of articular cartilage and because the prostheses must be fixed to the patients' bones. None of the currently available synthetic materials duplicates the ability of articular cartilage to provide a painless, low friction gliding surface and to distribute loads across the synovial joint, nor can current implants achieve the stability and durability of the bond between articular cartilage and bone. Thus, wear of implants limits their life span, and loosening can lead to failure. For these reasons, current joint replacements cannot be expected to provide a lifetime of normal function for young active patients.

Rheumatoid Arthritis

People with RA require careful evaluation to prevent operative and perioperative neurologic injury, establish the sequence and timing of joints to be treated surgically, and reduce the risks of infection and other complications.

People with RA commonly have cervical spine involvement that can lead to spinal instability and increased risk of neurologic deficits. Neurologic changes may be difficult to recognize due to limited joint motion and associated disuse muscle atrophy. To evaluate the risk of neurologic injury, people with RA should have active flexion and extension lateral cervical radiographs within 1 year before surgery. In a retrospective review of 113 patients with RA who underwent total hip or knee arthroplasty, Collins and colleagues (3) reported significant atlantoaxial subluxation, atlantoaxial impaction, and/or subaxial subluxation in 69 patients (61%). Thirty-five of these 69 patients (50%) had no clinical signs or symptoms of instability at the time of admission for joint replacement arthroplasty. Instability of greater than 7 to 10 mm at the atlantoaxial joint or greater than 4 mm at subaxial levels on flexion and extension lateral radiographs generally requires stabilization prior to other elective surgery. Patients with lesser degrees of atlantoaxial and subaxial involvement should be evaluated by the anesthesiologist preoperatively and consideration given to an awake intubation.

Patients with multiple joint involvement require careful planning and timing of various joint procedures to allow optimal rehabilitation. Patients undergoing

43

FIGURE 43-1

(A) Anteroposterior radiograph of the pelvis of a 61-year-old female showing a normal left hip and severe osteoarthritis of the right hip. Note that the x-rays are turned as though the patient was facing the reader. (B) The same patient after an uncemented total hip arthroplasty. (C) Photograph of an uncemented total hip arthroplasty like that used in this patient.

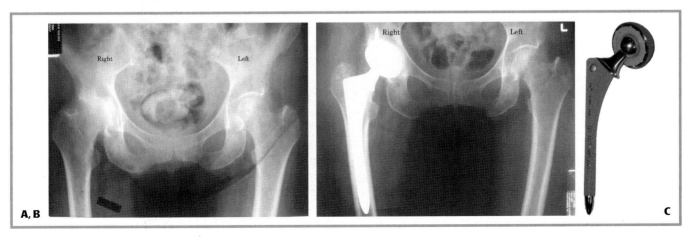

lower extremity surgery may require surgical stabilization of the upper extremity first to allow crutch ambulation and use of the upper extremities to assist with transfers, rising from a chair, and stair climbing. For example, a person with severe wrist involvement as well as hip involvement may benefit from wrist arthrodesis prior to total hip arthroplasty. The patient with multiple lower extremity joint involvement may benefit from treating joints either sequentially or simultaneously, depending on the joints involved and the severity of the disease. The patient with severe disease and contractures of both knees, for example, may benefit from having both knees replaced at the same time. In that situation, if only one knee is replaced, a flexion contracture in the untreated knee will cause the patient to keep the operatively treated knee flexed when standing and thereby compromise rehabilitation following surgery. Foot and ankle disease are generally addressed prior to hip and knee arthroplasty to provide the patient a stable lower extremity on which to stand and rehabilitate the hip and knee.

Long-term use of corticosteroids increases the complexity of surgical treatment of people with RA. In general, these patients will require "stress dose" steroids perioperatively due to inhibition of their adrenal function. Long-term corticosteroid use combined with the effects of the disease can cause connective tissue changes that make the skin and superficial blood vessels friable. Extreme caution must be used in physically handling such a patient. For example, in severely affected patients, mild pressure can cause a hematoma or skin ulceration and adhesive tape can tear the skin. In addition, chronic low-dose corticosteroid use in patients with RA has been correlated with an increased incidence of fracture, infection, and gastrointestinal hemorrhage or ulcer. People with RA treated with total joint arthroplasties demonstrated a higher incidence of infection than patients with OA treated with total joint arthroplasties (1). Patients with RA frequently have more than one joint arthroplasty, and infection of one arthroplasty is associated with an increased incidence of subsequent infection of another replaced joint (4).

Many people with RA are treated with NSAIDs and/or methotrexate preoperatively. A review of 165 patients undergoing total hip arthroplasty found a higher incidence of gastrointestinal bleeding and/or hypotension in patients receiving NSAIDs at the time of hospital admission (5). Several studies have demonstrated that there is no increase in wound or other postoperative complications in patients who continue methotrexate therapy perioperatively. Perhala and colleagues (6) compared 60 patients with RA who underwent a total of 92 joint arthroplasties without interruption of methotrexate therapy to a group of 61 patients not receiving methotrexate who underwent a total of 110 joint arthro-

plasties. Eight patients on methotrexate had a total of eight wound complications (8.7%) versus five patients with a total of six wound complications in the non-methotrexate group (5.5%, $p = 0.366$). In a randomized, nonblinded prospective study of 64 patients with RA on methotrexate therapy, Sany and coworkers (7) reported no infections and no difference in wound healing between patients whose therapy was discontinued 7 days before an orthopedic procedure and those whose therapy was continued perioperatively.

Tumor necrosis factor (TNF) inhibitors are an exciting class of agents which are relatively new to the treatment of inflammatory arthritis. Tumor necrosis factor alpha (TNF-alpha) is one of the cytokines which stimulates cartilage matrix degradation via metalloproteinases. Whereas these medications have offered decreased pain and increased function to many patients with inflammatory arthritis, they are also now known to be associated with an increased incidence of various infections. Strict guidelines for their perioperative utilization have not been established. Nonetheless, it is currently not advisable to treat patients in the perioperative period with TNF inhibitors, particularly when an implant such as a total joint replacement is being placed.

Juvenile Inflammatory Arthritis

Joint replacement arthroplasty in children with juvenile inflammatory arthritis (JIA) is reserved for patients who are debilitated by pain and/or decreased function, and is generally delayed until patients are skeletally mature. Joint replacement is also delayed because the life expectancy of the young patient is greater than that of current prostheses. Moreover, each subsequent revision surgery necessarily involves greater periprosthetic bone loss and less predictable long-term results. People with JIA are often candidates for tendon lengthening to correct contractures, and prophylactic procedures, such as synovectomy, to alleviate symptoms and possibly delay articular destruction.

Patients with JIA present important anesthetic risks. Although they do not develop cervical spine involvement and accompanying neurologic deficits as commonly as adults with RA, these problems do occur in association with JIA. Therefore, people with JIA require preoperative screening radiographs as described for patients with RA. Unilateral collapse of the lateral mass of the atlas, with or without axis involvement, may result in a fixed rotational head tilt deformity that makes it difficult to establish an airway for general anesthesia. Micrognathia associated with temporomandibular joint involvement can also make endotracheal intubation difficult. Restricted motion of the axial and appendicular skeleton can make regional anesthesia difficult as well.

Osteonecrosis

Treatment of osteonecrosis remains controversial, partially because the natural history of the disorder remains unknown. Nonsteroidal anti-inflammatory agents and decreased joint loading are commonly employed for temporary symptomatic relief, though neither has been shown to affect the long-term results. Electromagnetic stimulation has also been employed on an experimental basis. Most surgical treatments of osteonecrosis have been developed for treatment of the hip. Core decompression (i.e., drilling a channel from the lateral surface of the femur into the necrotic region of the femoral head), with or without bone grafting, has been advocated for patients who have femoral osteonecrosis without collapse or acetabular changes. In most series, these procedures have decreased pain in a high percentage of the patients. This treatment is generally considered ineffective in people whose femoral head shows any signs of collapse; however, for these patients, various other surgical options exist. These options include femoral osteotomies, designed to place an intact segment of the femoral head in a weight-bearing position, and hip arthrodesis. Replacement of the femoral head or total hip have met with excellent results in this population, but prosthesis durability is a concern, particularly in young patients.

Ankylosing Spondylitis

Joint replacements decrease pain and improve function for people with advanced joint disease due to ankylosing spondylitis (AS). Osteotomies that correct spinal deformities can also be of benefit for some. Spinal involvement can lead to extensive ligamentous calcification and heterotopic ossification that make regional anesthesia difficult, if not impossible. Patients with prolonged disease also develop severe kyphotic deformities of the cervical, thoracic, and lumbar spine that impede endotracheal intubation. Restricted chest excursion may further complicate intraoperative and postoperative care. Patients with AS tend to bleed more during and after surgery than similar, otherwise healthy individuals. The explanation for this bleeding tendency appears to be that compared with normal tissues, the ossified soft tissues are less capable of contracting to assist in hemostasis. There does not appear to be an associated defect in blood coagulation or platelet function.

People with AS, diffuse idiopathic skeletal hyperostosis, or post-traumatic osteoarthrosis are at increased risk for postoperative heterotopic ossification. Although patients with AS have excellent pain relief after total hip arthroplasty, gains in total range of motion are often limited due to periarticular heterotopic ossification, as well as longstanding soft tissue contractures and muscle atrophy. Various regimens have been tried to prevent postoperative soft tissue ossification, but radiation therapy delivered locally appears to be the most effective means of preventing heterotopic bone formation after surgery. Fractionated and single low-dose radiation therapy to the hip and abductor musculature have been effective when begun early in the postoperative period.

Psoriatic Arthritis

The perioperative concerns with NSAIDs and methotrexate discussed with RA apply to psoriatic arthritis as well. A unique perioperative risk in people with psoriatic arthritis is the development of a flare of psoriasis at the operative site due to the physiologic and/or psychological stress of surgery. Also known as isomorphic or Koebner's phenomenon, this process may predispose the patient to a generalized flare of psoriasis as well. People with psoriatic arthritis may have an increased incidence of postoperative infections. Menon and Wroblewski (8) reported superficial wound infection in 9.1% and deep wound infections in 5.5% of their 38 patients with psoriasis treated with total hip arthroplasty.

Hemophilic Arthropathy

Despite the risk of excessive bleeding, operative treatment can produce good results in people with hemophilic arthropathy. Synovectomy is commonly performed in the knee and elbow, and gives improved range of motion and decreased pain to the majority of patients. Total knee and total hip replacements can improve function and relieve pain in hemophilic patients with advanced joint degeneration (9).

Hemophilic arthropathy may be particularly difficult to manage perioperatively. Factor replacement has important risks and must be carefully monitored. A thrombotic event may be precipitated by repeated factor infusions, and resultant disseminated intravascular coagulation after elective surgery has been reported. The subgroup of patients with high levels of factor antibody are generally contraindicated for major elective surgery.

Whether or not people with well-controlled hemophilia without acquired immunodeficiency syndrome (AIDS) are at increased risk for non–transfusion-related infection is unclear. Septic arthritis has been reported as a rare complication of hemophilia, but one that must be promptly diagnosed and definitively treated. Human immunodeficiency virus (HIV)-1–infected hemophilia patients who have not developed AIDS do not appear to have an increased incidence of infection after surgery when compared with patients who are seronegative for HIV-1.

43

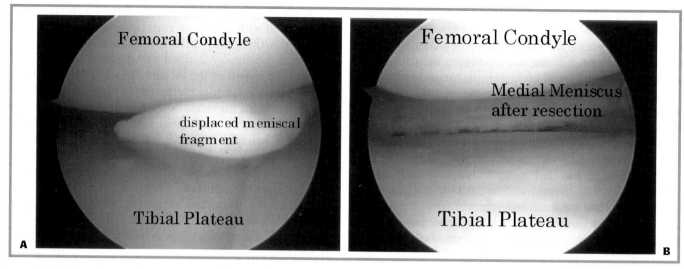

FIGURE 43-3

(A) Arthroscopic view of the medial knee compartment of a 35-year-old male showing a displaced medial meniscal tear. The fragment is between the medial femoral condyle and the medial tibial plateau. (B) The same medial compartment after removal of the meniscal fragment.

preserved lateral compartment. Femoral osteotomies are preferred for valgus and excessive varus deformities of the knee. Osteotomies generally are chosen over total knee arthroplasties for young, heavy, active patients, and should be reserved for patients with non-inflammatory disease. Appropriate candidates have <50° of flexion contracture, >90° of flexion, and isolated medial or lateral tibiofemoral arthritis without significant patellofemoral involvement. Good results have been reported in 80% to 90% of patients for 6 to 9 years postosteotomy, with 60% to 70% good results at 10 to 15 years follow-up (14). It is difficult to compare these results with those of total knee arthroplasty, where the patients are generally older and less active.

Total knee arthroplasty, similar to total hip arthroplasty, may be performed with cement or bone ingrowth as the means of fixation (Figure 43-4). Several large series reveal that tibial and femoral results are excellent regardless of the type of fixation, with 97% survivorship of prostheses at 10- and 12-year analyses (15). Despite

FIGURE 43-4

(A) Anteroposterior radiograph of both knees in a 74-year-old patient with severe osteoarthritis. (B) Acute postoperative radiograph showing bilateral cemented posterior stabilized total knee arthroplasties. Note the staples from surgical repair of the skin.

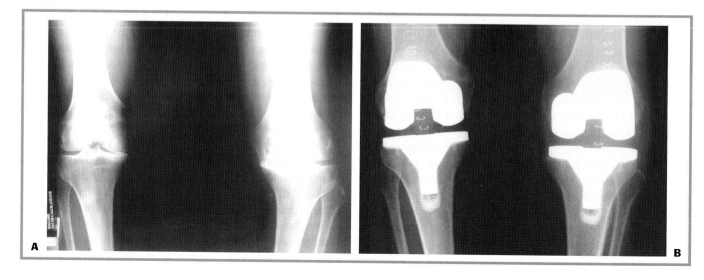

excellent results with cement fixation, some surgeons reserve cemented tibial and femoral components for patients older than 50 or 60, or patients with poor bone stock, based on the assumption that uncemented components will last longer for young patients and preserve their bone stock. Patellar problems are the leading cause of failure after total knee arthroplasty. Unlike tibial and femoral results, results of uncemented patellar components, which require a metal backing for bone ingrowth, are substantially inferior to results of cemented all-polyethylene patellar components, and have thus fallen out of favor in recent years.

Unicompartmental arthroplasty is a type of knee arthroplasty wherein the femoral condyle and adjacent proximal tibial plateau in either the medial or lateral compartment is replaced while the opposite side is left with native cartilage. Although these devices have been available for several decades, there has been a resurgence of interest in their utilization due to the fact that they require removal of less bone and allow preservation of more of the native joint. In addition, they may offer appropriately selected patients less blood loss and quicker recovery than total knee arthroplasty. However, these devices are not recommended for patients with substantial deformity or tricompartmental osteoarthritis.

Knee arthrodesis is an option for patients with recalcitrant infection or failed total knee arthroplasty that cannot be revised effectively. Despite loss of knee motion, a functional lower extremity that permits painless weight bearing can be expected using current techniques. Resection arthroplasty has also been used for patients with failed total knee arthroplasty.

Foot and Ankle

Surgical options for arthritis of the foot and ankle include cheilectomy (resection of an osteophyte), arthroscopic debridement, osteotomy, arthrodesis, and replacement arthroplasty.

Osteophytes may develop at the periphery of a joint and cause symptoms related to impingement during normal walking. These are not uncommon on the dorsum of the first metatarsophalangeal joint and the anterior aspect of the tibiotalar joint. Although it does not cure the underlying disease, cheilectomy often provides relief of mechanical symptoms and associated pain. Loose bodies may also be a source of mechanical symptoms and are amenable to arthroscopic removal.

Supramalleolar tibial osteotomy allows realignment of the weight-bearing axis through the tibiotalar joint. This can help to preserve the joint in various congenital and post-traumatic degenerative conditions of the ankle. Low tibial osteotomy has been shown to be particularly effective in long-term relief of symptoms with intermediate-stage primary OA. Osteotomy is generally reserved for non-inflammatory arthritides, but it may also provide relief of pain and decreased frequency of intra-articular bleeding in patients with hemophilic arthropathy.

Arthrodeses of the foot and ankle offer pain relief and stability to people with severe arthritis. Fusions of these joints are well tolerated, even by children, despite some restriction of stressful activities such as hill climbing and running. Although the vast majority of patients with ankle and/or peritalar arthrodeses obtain excellent relief of pain and increased function, initial nonunion of the arthrodesis occurs in 5% to 30% of cases. Infection and delayed wound healing have been reported in 25% to 40% of patients with RA who undergo tibiotalar arthrodesis, yet the majority have an excellent long-term result.

Unlike total replacement arthroplasty of the hip and knee, ankle replacement arthroplasties have not produced predictable results. By 5 to 10 years after surgery, 60% to 90% of these prostheses have failed. Most surgeons now limit the use of this procedure to treatment of inflammatory arthritis in minimally active elderly patients who have multiple joint involvement.

Hand and Wrist

The distal interphalangeal joints and thumb carpometacarpal joints are the most commonly involved joints in OA of the hand, while proximal interphalangeal, metacarpophalangeal, carpometacarpal, radiocarpal, and distal radioulnar joints are more commonly involved in inflammatory arthropathy. Surgeons use a variety of joint and soft tissue procedures to treat these disorders.

When evaluating the wrist and hand in people with RA, it is imperative to obtain a history of the patient's functional abilities, carefully noting any recent changes. Inability to actively flex or extend interphalangeal and/or metacarpophalangeal joints with preservation of passive motion usually signals a ruptured tendon. Flexor and extensor tendons in patients with rheumatoid disease are more susceptible to rupture than normal tendons. Underlying ultrastructural changes associated with the inflammatory process weaken the tendons, and abnormal bony prominences, particularly at the distal radioulnar joint, abrade the weakened tendons, making them prone to rupture. Tenosynovectomy not only provides decreased pain with increased range of motion and grip strength, but also appears to protect the tendons, particularly when combined with resection of abnormal bony prominences. Acute tendon ruptures should be evaluated early by a surgeon for consideration of reconstruction prior to the development of fibrosis and contractures. In the rheumatoid hand, the metacarpophalangeal joints of the fingers are generally reconstructed with silicone implants that function as

43

flexible spacers. Ulnar drift of the digits with resultant ulnar subluxation of the extensor tendons may be at least partially corrected by surgical centralization of the extensor tendons and transfer of the intrinsic hand muscle insertions from one digit to the adjacent digit on the ulnar side.

Arthrodesis is commonly employed in the interphalangeal joints, carpus, and wrist for end-stage joint degeneration due to most arthritic disorders. Interphalangeal joints are best managed with arthrodesis in a partially flexed position. Solid fusion can be reliably obtained in more than 95% of cases using various techniques. Arthrodesis may also be performed at the radiocarpal joint or selectively at diseased intercarpal joints. Although some reduction in wrist motion and grip strength are commonly noted with limited intercarpal arthrodeses, long-term pain relief and stability are excellent.

Surgeons rarely recommend arthrodesis of arthritic thumb carpometacarpal joints, because motion of these joints is particularly important for overall hand function. The degenerative thumb carpometacarpal joint is amenable to interposition arthroplasty (resection of the joint surfaces and interposition of soft tissue, usually a portion of the abductor pollicis longus or flexor carpi radialis tendons), which yields excellent pain relief and increased grip strength. Experience with arthroplasty of the wrist is limited, partially due to the predictable results obtained with wrist fusion. Intermediate-term results have been mixed. Silicone spacer implants yielded a high incidence of failure with poor pain relief in approximately 50% of patients an average of 5 to 6 years after the procedure. Wrist arthroplasty designs have yielded improved clinical outcome, but component failure remains a problem. In selected patients with degenerative disease of the radiocarpal joint, resection of the proximal row of carpal bones (i.e., proximal row carpectomy) can reduce pain.

Elbow

Routine activities of daily living require a wide range of elbow flexion and extension as well as pronation and supination. Although elbow fusion can be reliably obtained with internal fixation, this results in substantial impairment because shoulder and wrist motion cannot adequately compensate for loss of elbow motion. Fortunately, radial head excision, synovectomy, arthroscopy, and arthroplasty are alternatives that have yielded good results.

Arthritis involving primarily the radiohumeral articulation is not uncommon with rheumatoid and post-traumatic joint disease. Radial head resection offers increased range of motion and decreased pain in appropriately selected patients. Resultant proximal migration

of the radius is minimal after this procedure, and elbow instability is seldom a concern if the medial collateral ligament complex is intact. Patients generally have good intermediate-term relief of pain with increased range of motion. In one series, 84% of people with RA reported good pain relief 6 months after the procedure (16). Synovectomy may be performed alone or in conjunction with other procedures, such as radial head resection. Patients with hemophilia likewise have decreased pain and swelling following synovectomy, as well as a decreased incidence of hemarthrosis. Arthroscopy has been used effectively to perform synovectomies as well as remove loose bodies and osteophytes from arthritic elbows.

Elbow joint replacement arthroplasty, while newer than hip and knee arthroplasty, has developed rapidly. The rate of loosening in young active patients with post-traumatic arthropathy approaches 50% at 5- to 8-year follow-up. However, intermediate-term results in low-demand patients with inflammatory disease are promising, with survival of the components and good or excellent results reported in more than 90% of RA patients at 3- to 8-year follow-up (17). Motion was reportedly improved to a functional range and pain relief was substantial for >90% of these patients.

Shoulder

The high degree of compensatory movement in the scapulothoracic articulation, as well as elsewhere throughout the upper extremity, may be responsible for the relatively low incidence of patients requiring operative treatment of arthritic glenohumeral joints. Nonetheless, some patients will be debilitated by an arthritic shoulder, fail nonoperative treatment, and present for consideration of surgical intervention.

Shoulder arthrodesis yields excellent pain relief and provides a stable upper extremity with long-term durability for young patients with severe glenohumeral arthritis. Fusion is reliably obtained in the majority of patients with relatively few complications. Despite rigid fusion of the glenohumeral joint, abduction of 50° and flexion of 40″ in the shoulder girdle is possible via scapulothoracic motion.

Total shoulder arthroplasty has recently become increasingly used for the treatment of severe glenohumeral arthritis (Figure 43-5). The majority are performed for RA of the glenohumeral joint. Pain relief and improved general functions of daily living are reported in the majority of patients; the most common long-term complication reported is glenoid component loosening (18). To this end, recent efforts have explored the use of hemiarthroplasty, which is the replacement of the humeral head without resurfacing the glenoid. This method has proven effective in selected patients including those with cuff tear arthropathy—chronic,

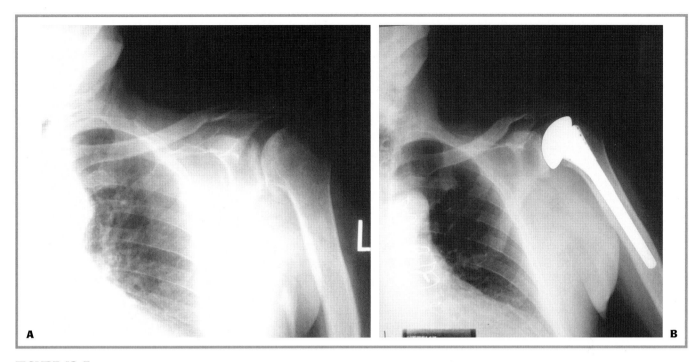

FIGURE 43-5

(A) Radiograph of an 80-year-old male with severe glenohumeral arthritis of the left shoulder.
(B) Same patient after a shoulder arthroplasty.

massive rotator cuff tears with secondary superior migration of the humeral head and resultant erosive changes of the glenohumeral joint and inferior surface of the acromion.

Cervical Spine

The clinical problems caused by arthritis of the cervical spine are pain, compromised neurologic function, and mechanical instability that causes or has the potential to cause pain and neurologic deficits. Spinal fusions can decrease pain, restore stability, and, in some instances, prevent development of neurologic deficits. Surgical decompression of the spinal cord and nerve roots can relieve pain and improve neurologic function in selected patients.

Generally accepted indications for surgical intervention in people with RA with cervical spine involvement are pain refractory to nonoperative modalities, neurologic deterioration, and radiographic evidence of impending spinal cord compression. Whereas the anterior atlantodental interval has been traditionally used to determine the degree of atlantoaxial instability, the posterior atlantodental interval has been shown to be an important predictor of the potential for postoperative neurologic improvement (19). The available evidence also suggests that patients who undergo cervical arthrodesis earlier in the course of their disease have more satisfactory results than those in whom arthrodesis is delayed. Some authors have recommended that patients with atlantoaxial subluxation and a posterior atlanto-odontoid interval of 14 mm or less, patients who have atlantoaxial subluxation and at least 5 mm of basilar invagination, and patients who have subaxial subluxation and a sagittal spinal canal diameter of 14 mm or less, even in the absence of neurologic findings, undergo posterior surgical fusion at the involved levels. Pain is relieved in the majority of patients, but neurologic improvement is variable and closely related to preoperative radiographic instability and neurologic status.

Radiographic evidence of OA in the cervical spine occurs in about 50% of people older than 50 years and 75% of people older than 65. In contrast to people with RA, these patients rarely have instability. However, they may develop pain and neurologic signs as a result of degenerative stenosis. Posterior decompression may be accomplished via laminectomy or laminaplasty. Laminectomy, or removal of part or all of one or more cervical laminae, allows excellent visualization and decompression at the expense of potentially destabilizing the spine with resultant kyphosis. Laminaplasty may be performed by one of many techniques, but in general involves cutting through the laminae completely on one side at the involved levels of the spine and cutting 80% of the way through the contralateral laminae at those same levels. The cervical spinal canal may then be opened on the hinge of the partially cut laminae. This allows excellent multilevel decompression at the expense of decreased cervical motion. The choice between these two procedures remains controversial.

PERIOPERATIVE MANAGEMENT

The goals of perioperative management include restoration of motion and function, relief of pain, and prevention of complications. To obtain optimal surgical results, joint replacement patients must participate in a physical therapy regimen directed at improving range of motion and restoring function. Physical therapy typically starts within 24 hours after a joint replacement and is generally continued for 6 or more weeks through a combination of inpatient rehabilitation, home health care, and outpatient services. Newer rehabilitation protocols have led to a dramatic increase in the number of patients who are discharged from the hospital after 48 to 72 hours and follow-up with outpatient physical therapy services. In general, inpatient rehabilitation is now reserved for the postoperative care of patients with slow progress or multiple comorbid factors. Whereas continuous passive motion (CPM) machines were previously routinely used in the early phases of rehabilitation, they are now infrequently used except with extenuating circumstances.

Narcotic analgesics are generally required in the acute postoperative period, and are tapered off during the ensuing weeks. Patient-controlled analgesia (PCA) pumps provide effective and efficient delivery of narcotics through a combination of basal infusion rate and intermittent dosing, which the patient dictates as needed by pressing a button. The maximum dose per hour is preset by the physician. As an alternative, spinal and epidural infusions have become increasingly popular for total hip and knee arthroplasty patients. Each not only may be used for surgical anesthesia, but also can provide postoperative analgesia. An indwelling epidural catheter can be left in place for 2 to 3 days postoperatively and titrated to provide pain relief while sparing motor control for ambulation and other exercises. As an added benefit, the vasodilation associated with epidural anesthesia may further decrease the risk of thromboembolus.

Thromboembolic disease is a potential complication after any spine or lower extremity procedure. This complication is particularly common among unprophylaxed hip arthroplasty patients. In the absence of prophylaxis, the incidence of deep venous thrombosis has been reported as high as 74% and the incidence of symptomatic pulmonary embolism as high as 3.4% (20). A recent meta-analysis of thromboembolic prophylactic agents has shown a significantly lower risk of deep venous thrombosis and symptomatic pulmonary embolism with warfarin, pneumatic compression, and low-molecular-weight heparins (20). Of these, warfarin was thought to be the safest and most effective. Low-molecular-weight

heparins were associated with a risk of postoperative bleeding.

Patients undergoing major joint reconstruction commonly require perioperative blood transfusion. Concern regarding the associated risks of blood-borne disease, anaphylaxis, and transfusion reaction has given rise to improved techniques for postoperative blood management. For many years, preoperative autologous donation has provided a relatively safe, albeit expensive and time-consuming, alternative to allogeneic transfusion. More recent advances have seen the advent of perioperative blood salvage and erythropoietin analogs. Blood-salvage devices that reinfuse blood from the operative site are an effective means of reducing allogeneic transfusion after arthroplasty (21). Erythropoietin analogs may further reduce the risk by stimulating the patient's marrow to increase erythrocyte production prior to elective surgery.

POSTOPERATIVE COMPLICATIONS

The majority of serious postoperative complications, including infection, nerve and blood vessel injury, pulmonary embolus, and joint dislocation, occur within the first postoperative weeks; however, complications may occur at any time after surgery. Arthroplasty patients in particular must be monitored indefinitely for subtle radiographic evidence of periprosthetic osteolysis, which, when treated early, may halt progression to massive bone loss and catastrophic failure (see Figure 43-2) (10). The vast majority of failures among lower extremity total joint prostheses occur after the first decade postoperatively, and most patients remain asymptomatic until substantial bone loss, subsidence, and even fracture have occurred. It is therefore imperative that routine follow-up, including careful standardized clinical and comparative radiographic evaluation, be obtained on a regular basis throughout the patient's life.

In addition, patients must be carefully monitored for early signs of infection. Early detection of infection in a prosthetic joint may make it possible to save the implants. However, successful treatment of chronic joint infections without removal of the implants occurs rarely. Patients with multiple joint arthroplasties who develop sepsis in one prosthetic joint should be treated aggressively and observed closely because they have a substantial risk of developing a metachronous infection in another artificial joint.

The relationship between bacteremias caused by diagnostic and surgical procedures and subsequent infection of a total joint arthroplasty remain uncertain. However, several reports suggest that bacteremias associated with dental procedures can seed total joint arthroplasties. For this reason, 2g of penicillin 1 hour prior to dental manipulation and 1g 6 hours after the first dose have been recommended for patients with total joint arthroplasties (22). One gram of erythromycin 1 hour prior to dental manipulation and 500 mg 6 hours after the first dose may be utilized for penicillin-sensitive patients. Oral antibiotic prophylaxis appropriate for the regional flora has also been recommended prior to and following urologic, gastrointestinal, and other bacteremia-evoking manipulations.

NEW OPERATIVE TREATMENTS

Replacements of the hip and knee predictably relieve pain and provide stability and motion for large numbers of patients. Unfortunately, wear and loosening can cause failure of these implants. Other current operative treatments also relieve or reduce pain for many patients with arthritis: however, they are generally less successful in restoring joint function. Joint fusions and even joint replacements place important limits on function and other current treatments do not reliably arrest or reverse joint degeneration. Thus, there is a clear need for new therapeutic approaches. New articular bearing surfaces, including highly polished metallic alloys, highly cross-linked polyethylene, and ceramic surfaces are under investigation. Improved results of wrist and ankle joint replacement may be possible with new implant designs.

Although they have not yet been shown to be effective in arthritic joints, operative approaches intended to preserve or restore cartilaginous articular surfaces that include surgical debridement of degenerated tissue and correction of mechanical abnormalities combined with implantation of artificial matrices, growth factors, and transplanted chondrocytes or mesenchymal stem cells have the potential to restore a joint surface.

REFERENCES

1. Wymenga AB, Horn JRY, Theeuwes A, Muyfiens HL, Siootl TJ. Perioperative factors associated with septic arthritis after arthroplasty. Prospective multicenter study of 362 knee and 2,651 hip operations. Acta Orthop Scand 1992;63:665–671.
2. Lehman DE, Capello WN, Feinberg JR. Total hip arthroplasty without cement in obese patients. J Bone Joint Surg Am 1994;76:854–862.
3. Collins DN, Barnes CL, FitzRandolph RL. Cervical spine instability in rheumatoid patients having total hip or knee arthroplasty. Clin Orthop 1991;272:127–135.
4. Murray RP, Bourne MH, Fitzgerald RH. Metachronous infections in patients who have had more than one total joint arthroplasty. J Bone Joint Surg Am 1991;73;1469–1474.
5. Connelly CS, Panush RS. Should nonsteroidal anti-inflammatory drugs be stopped before elective surgery? Arch Intern Med 1991;151:1963–1966.
6. Perhala RS, Wilke WS, Clough JD, Segal AM. Local infections complications following large joint replacement in rheumatoid arthritis patients treated with methotrexate versus those not treated with methotrexate. Arthritis Rheum 1991:34:146–152.
7. Sany J, Anaya JM, Canovas F, et al. Influence of methotrexate on the frequency of postoperative infectious complications in patients with rheumatoid arthritis. J Rheumatol 1993:20:1129–1132.
8. Menon TJ, Wroblewski BM. Charnley low-friction arthroplasty in patients with psoriasis. Clin Orthop 1983;300:127–128.
9. Kelly SS, Lachiewicz PE, Gilbert MS, Bolander ME, Jankiewicz JJ. Hip arthroplasty in hemophilic arthropathy. J Bone Joint Surg Am 1995;67:828–834.
10. Total Hip Replacement. NIH Consensus Statement 1994;12:1–31. Available at: http://consensus.nih.gov/1994/1994HipReplacement098html.htm.
11. Callagham JJ, Albright JC, Goetz DD, Olejniczak JP, Johnston RG. Charnley total hip arthroplasty. Minimum twenty-five-year follow-up. J Bone Joint Surg Am 2000;82:487–497.
12. Fitzgerald RH. Total hip arthroplasty sepsis. Prevention and diagnosis. Orthop Clin North Am 1992;23:259–264.
13. Sullivan PM, MacKenzie JR, Callaghan JJ, Johnston RG. Total hip arthroplasty with cement in patients who are less than fifty years old. J Bone Joint Surg Am 1994;76:863–869.
14. Insall IN, Joseph DM, Msika G. High tibial osteotomy for varus gonarthrosis. A long-term follow-up study. J Bone Joint Surg Am 1984;66:1040–1048.
15. Rand JA, Ilstrup DM. Survivorship analysis of total knee arthroplasty. Cumulative rates of survival of 9200 total knee arthroplasties. J Bone Joint Surg Am 1991;73:397–409.
16. Summers GD, Talor AR, Webley M. Elbow synovectomy and excision of the radial head in rheumatoid arthritis: a short term palliative procedure. J Rheumatol 1988;15:566–569.
17. Kraay MJ, Figgie MP, Inglis AE, Wolfe SW, Ranawat CS. Primary semiconstrained total elbow arthroplasty. Survival analysis of l13 consecutive cases. J Bone Joint Surg Br 1994;76:636–640.
18. Brostrom LA, Wallensten R, Olsson E, Anderson D. The Kessel prosthesis in total shoulder arthroplasty. A five-year experience. Clin Orthop 1992;277:155–160.
19. Boden SD, Dodge LD, Bohlman HH, Rechtine GR. Rheumatoid arthritis of the cervical spine. J Bone Joint Surg Am 1993;75:1282–1297.
20. Freedman KB, Brookenthal KR, Fitzgerald RH, Williams S, Lonner JH. A meta-analysis of thromboembolic prophylaxis following elective total hip arthroplasty. J Bone Joint Surg Am 2000;82:929–938.
21. Grosvenor D, Goyal V, Goodman S. Efficacy of postoperative blood salvage following total hip arthroplasty in patients with and without deposited autologous units. J Bone Joint Surg Am 2000;82:951–954.
22. Nelson JP, Fitzgerald RH, Jaspers MT, Little JW. Prophylactic antimicrobial coverage in arthroplasty patients. J Bone Joint Surg Am 1990;72:1–2.

43

CHAPTER 44

Complementary and Alternative Therapies

ERIN L. ARNOLD, MD
WILLIAM J. ARNOLD, MD

■ Complementary and alternative therapies are popular and widely used among patients with rheumatic and musculoskeletal diseases.

■ Marketing and word of mouth, ready availability, and interest in "natural" treatments contribute to their popularity.

■ Scientific basis and clinical trails of most therapies is limited or lacking.

More and more people are employing complementary and alternative medicine (CAM) to treat their illnesses. A survey of English-speaking patients found that 42.1% used at least 1 of 16 specific CAM therapies during a 12-month period (1). In this study population, visits to CAM practitioners exceeded total visits to primary care physicians, and more than 50% of the patients had a musculoskeletal disease (arthritis, back, or neck pain). Total out-of-pocket expenditures for CAM treatments were estimated to be $27 billion, similar to out-of-pocket expenditures for all US physician services. The study found that patients were most likely to use CAM therapies in conjunction with, rather than in place of, conventional therapies.

Most rheumatic conditions are characterized by chronic pain, an unpredictable disease course, and often without satisfactory response to therapy. As a consequence, patients with rheumatic diseases, in particular osteoarthritis (OA) and fibromyalgia, often seek out CAM therapies in addition to the conventional treatment their doctors recommend (2).

Patients are often reluctant to discuss CAM therapies with their physicians. To protect patients from dangerous drug interactions and treatment modalities known to be harmful, use of CAM therapies must be elicited as a part of the comprehensive history and physical examination (3). Between 38.5% and 55% of patients do not disclose use of CAM therapies to their physicians (1,2) simply because their physicians fail to ask. The fear of physician disapproval of CAM therapies accounts for only 15% of patient nondisclosure (2).

As the medical community awaits more rigorous assessment of CAM therapies, physicians should be motivated by existing evidence (1–3) to ask patients about their use of CAM therapies.

MEDITATION, BIOFEEDBACK, AND STRESS REDUCTION

Meditation, biofeedback, and stress reduction are used widely for the treatment of pain, depression, and anxiety. These therapeutic modalities are especially popular with people who have fibromyalgia.

Meditation teaches the patient to develop concentration, calmness, and insight as a way of treating symptoms (4). A prospective, observational, case-control study found that people with fibromyalgia were more likely than control patients in a rheumatology practice ($p < 0.01$) to use CAM (5). People with fibromyalgia perceived spiritual practices (meditation, relaxation, self-help groups, prayer) as more beneficial than over-the-counter products, use of other health care practitioners, and dietary modifications. In an uncontrolled study of 225 patients with chronic pain enrolled in a meditation program, 60% showed continued improvement of pain at 4 years follow-up (4).

Biofeedback, with the assistance of electronic monitors, teaches people how to use their mind to affect body functions (e.g., circulation and pain sensation). In people with RA, biofeedback has been shown to decrease clinic visits, hospitalization days, and medical costs (6). In a review of 23 people with Raynaud's phenomenon using biofeedback therapy, Yocum and colleagues (7) found that at 18 months, patients continued to be able to raise baseline finger temperatures and that the greatest temperature increase was observed in patients with connective tissue disorders, including lupus and scleroderma.

Relaxation techniques focus on the reduction of stress by using such tactics as breathing exercises to help provide relief. In a randomized, controlled trial of people with RA, relaxation techniques were shown to significantly reduce pain, disease activity, and anxiety (8).

PRAYER AND SPIRITUALITY

A majority of Americans believe in the healing power of prayer. Seven percent of patients surveyed by Eisenberg and colleagues (1) reported using some form of spiritual healing in conjunction with conventional therapies, and 35% reported using prayer to address health-related problems. Patients with chronic illnesses seek treatment that includes attention to the mind and spirit as well as the body.

A number of studies have shown an association between spiritual involvement and positive health outcomes. Distant healing is considered to be a conscious, dedicated act directed at benefiting another person's physical or emotional well-being at a distance. It includes prayer, therapeutic touch, Reiki, and LeShane healing. A systematic review of randomized trials of distant healing found that 13 of 23 studies (57%) that met inclusion criteria yielded statistically significant, positive treatment effects of distant healing (9). Nine of the 23 studies showed no effect and one showed a negative effect, making it difficult to draw definitive conclusions about efficacy, but also difficult to simply dismiss the power of distant healing.

EXERCISE

Strengthening, stretching, general conditioning exercises, and yoga have been shown to provide symptomatic relief for various forms of arthritis.. In older adults a regular exercise program was shown to result in a 32% reduction in functional decline (10). The lack of regular exercise almost doubled the odds of functional decline [adjusted odds ratio (OR) 1.5; 95% confidence interval (CI), 1.5–2.]. In a randomized, controlled trial, people with OA of the knee who were enrolled in a program of physical therapy combined with supervised and unsupervised exercise were found to have clinically and statistically significant improvement (11). The benefits attained in the treatment group continued to be apparent at 1 year, with fewer patients requiring knee surgery than did patients in the control group. In a separate study, patients with carpal tunnel syndrome experienced a statistically significant improvement in grip strength and pain reduction with a yoga program based on upper body postures; flexibility exercises; correct alignment of hands, wrists, arms, and shoulders; stretching; and increased awareness of optimal joint position (12).

ACUPUNCTURE

Based on the belief that there are patterns of energy flow (Qi) that are essential for health, acupuncture is a procedure that treats illness by correcting Qi imbalances. Solid, sterile metal needles are used to penetrate the skin and manually or electrically stimulate known flow patterns. Acupuncture frequently is used to treat pain and is considered a useful therapy for such conditions as OA, Raynaud's phenomenon, fibromyalgia, and low back pain (13). A meta-analysis of randomized, controlled trials of acupuncture for the treatment of back pain found that acupuncture was superior to other control interventions (14). A randomized, controlled trial of acupuncture in people with OA of the knee found statistically significant reductions of pain in patients treated with acupuncture (15). Chronic low back pain was effectively relieved by acupuncture in a meta-analysis of randomized, controlled trials (16).

MASSAGE

Massage is one of the CAM interventions used most frequently and is, in general, risk-free. Various massage techniques can be used (Table 44-1), and patients need

44

TABLE 44-1.   MASSAGE AND BODYWORK.

Western massage
Swedish massage: full-body stroking and kneading of the
    superficial muscle layers, using oil or lotion
Deep tissue massage: strong pressure on deep muscles or tissue
    layers
Trigger point therapy: deep finger pressure on trigger points
Myofascial release: steady pressure to stretch fascia

Oriental bodywork and massage
Acupressure (i.e., Shiatsu): finger and hand pressure used at
    acupuncture points
Structural integration bodywork
Chiropractic adjustment: short-level, high velocity thrust directed
    specifically at a "manipulable lesion"
Osteopathic manipulation: thrust, muscle energy, counterstrain,
    articulation, and myofascial release directed at a specific lesion
Rolfing: release of muscles and tissue layers from surrounding
    fascia using deep pressure and fascia release techniques
Reflexology: stimulation of massage points in the feet, hands,
    and ears that correspond to organs and body parts
Craniosacral therapy: gentle manipulation of the skull bones to
    balance the fluids in the craniosacral system

to be encouraged to discuss their medical conditions with the massage therapist. With this information, therapists can devise a plan for massage that will achieve the desired outcome and avoid negative experiences. For example, people at risk for fracture because of known osteoporosis or chronic corticosteroid use should avoid deep pressure. In a randomized, placebo-controlled trial comparing Swedish massage, transcutaneous electrical nerve stimulation (TENS), and sham TENS therapy in people with fibromyalgia, patients in the massage group showed decreases in insomnia, pain, fatigue, anxiety, and depression as well as decreased cortisol production (17).

HERBS, SUPPLEMENTS, AND VITAMINS

Herbal remedies are the fastest-growing form of CAM therapy in the United States. Viewed as "natural," and therefore safe, herbs actually are potent medications. Potential benefits of herbal therapy must be balanced against the possible harmful side effects from interactions with other prescription medications or the presence of illicit constituents or contaminants. Because most herbs used to relieve pain affect eicosanoid metabolism, the side effects may be similar to those of nonsteroidal anti-inflammatory drugs (NSAIDs). Many commonly used herbs and supplements affect the clotting system and preoperative assessments must include questions concerning herbal intake.

Neither herbal nor supplement preparations undergo strict production inspection or quality control under the 1994 Dietary Supplement Health Education Act. *Contaminants* such as lead and arsenic as well as NSAIDs and steroids have been found in herbal preparations. Supplement preparations may or may not contain specified amounts or even any of the advertised supplement. Besides presenting a patient safety issue, this variability also makes any studies of these supplements difficult to interpret.

The best-studied nutritional supplements to date have been glucosamine sulfate and chondroitin sulfate. The Glucosamine–Chondroitin Arthritis Intervention Trial (GAIT) measured the effects of glucosamine alone, chondroitin alone, a glucosamine–chondroitin combination, and celecoxib alone against placebo in 1583 people with either mild or moderate-to-severe pain from knee osteoarthritis (18). In moderate-to-severe pain, 79% who took the glucosamine–chondroitin combination reported pain relief compared to 54% in people who took placebo. Patients with mild pain responded similarly to the glucosamine–chondroitin combination and placebo (63% and 62%, respectively). Because neither of these supplements have significant

side effects, most clinicians have accepted or even encourage their use in people with OA of the knee.

Evidence from studies in an animal model of inflammatory arthritis suggests a protective effect of polyphenols contained in green tea (*Camelia senensis*) (19). The equivalent of three to four daily cups of green tea prevented or ameliorated the development of arthritis. Methylsulfonyl methane (MSM) has been shown to reduce WOMAC pain scores and improve functional scores in patients with knee pain and osteoarthritis when compared to placebo (20).

In symptomatic patients with systemic lupus erythematosus (SLE), omega 3 fish oil supplements significantly reduced disease activity (measured with SLAM-R) compared to placebo (21).

Vitamins C and D have been hypothesized to benefit patients with OA. Low levels of vitamin D have been found in people with OA of the hip and knee (22). Hypovitaminosis D is an established risk factor for fractures in patients with OA. Low serum 25-hydroxy vitamin D [25(OH)D] levels, have been found to correlate with low bone mineral density (BMD) and the presence of primary knee OA (23). Greater intake of vitamin D has been found to be associated with a lower risk of developing RA [relative risk (RR) 0.66; 95% CI, 0.42–1.01; $p = 0.06$) in older women (55–69 years old) (24). Patients with higher levels of vitamin C intake appear to have a lower incidence of OA. Theoretically, antioxidant supplements could help to prevent the progression of OA of the knee (25).

DIET AND ARTHRITIS

Except for prevention and treatment of gout, there is no definitive scientific evidence that what an individual eats can cause or cure arthritis. However, an increasing amount of literature suggests that a change in diet may relieve some symptoms and even impact the progression of disease. For example, oleocanthal, a component of extra virgin olive oil can cause a dose-dependent inhibition of both cyclooxygenase (COX)-1 and COX-2, therefore inhibiting inflammation (26) and, in some studies, reduce the risk of developing RA (27). Unfortunately one would have to consume about a half liter of oil to obtain the effects of two ibuprofen tablets. The lack of consistency among findings limits the ability to make specific dietary recommendations for the prevention or treatment of arthritis. However, encouraging patients to modify their diets may result in beneficial weight loss as well as an overall improvement in health. A weight loss of as little as 5 kg may reduce the incidence of OA of the knees by 50% in women, particularly women who are more than 10% over their ideal body weight (28).

Red meat and certain vegetable oils (corn, sunflower, and safflower) contain omega 6 fatty acids, which are synthesized into arachidonic acid, the building blocks for prostaglandins and leukotrienes. Eliminating or reducing the amount of omega 6 while substituting omega 3 oils may help reduce pain and inflammation. Omega 3 fatty acids are eicosapentaenoic acid (EPA) and docosahexaenoic acid (DHA), fatty acids that compete with omega 6 fatty acids to form arachidonic acid. In fact, diets high in omega 3 fatty acids appear to have a protective effect against rheumatoid arthritis onset (27). Good sources for omega 3 fatty acids are fresh cold-water fish, sardines in their own oil, flaxseed, green soybeans and tofu, and canola and olive oils. Patients also can take food supplements to get more omega 3 fatty acids.

MISCELLANEOUS THERAPIES

Wearing copper bracelets is believed to ease arthritis pain. In a placebo-controlled trial, Walker and Keats demonstrated that a significant number of patients assigned to wear copper bracelets experienced arthritis pain relief, compared with little relief reported by individuals assigned to wear bracelets that were painted to look like copper (29). These investigators also reported that the copper bracelets were lighter at the end of the study period and suggested that copper was absorbed by the skin. While the concept of absorbing copper through the skin is controversial, it is worthwhile to recommend that patients who are interested in trying this alternative therapy buy a bracelet that has not been treated to prevent tarnishing.

Static magnet therapy, as opposed to pulsed electromagnetic therapy (the use of pulsed electric current in combination with a permanent magnet, a medically accepted therapy) is believed to relieve pain by increasing circulation, suppressing inflammation, affecting C-fibers, and changing the polarization of cells. Two scientific trials (30,31) have suggested that static magnetic therapy may relieve arthritis symptoms. However, the short follow-up periods and the small sample sizes limit the results' applicability and emphasize the need for more studies.

Bee stings or injections are believed by some to reduce arthritis symptoms. Applied at painful areas or trigger points, the known anti-inflammatory chemicals in bee venom are thought to relieve inflammation. Animal studies have shown that bee venom reduces inflammation (32) and prevents rats from getting an induced form of arthritis (33). However, no human studies have been done, and it is felt that the risk of an anaphylactic reaction outweighs the unproven benefit of symptom relief.

AVAILABLE RESOURCES

Internet sites to help physicians assist their patients in making educated decisions about the use of CAM therapies can be found in Table 44-2 and Appendix IV.

TABLE 44-2. RESOURCES AVAILABLE ON THE INTERNET.

Alternative medicine
Altmednet.com: http://www.altmednet.com (many CAM links)
Arthritis Foundation: http://www.arthritis.org
Cochrane Collaboration: http://www.cochrane.org/index.htm (systematic review)
National Center for Complementary and Alternative Medicine: http://nccam.nih.gov (affiliated with NIH, conducts and supports research as well as providing information about CAM)

Healing systems
Ayurvedic medicine: http://ayurvedahc.com
Chinese medicine: http://acupuncture.com
Naturopathic medicine: The American Association of Naturopathic Physicians http://www.naturopathic.org
Homeopathic medicine: National Center for Homeopathy: http://www.homeopathic.org
Chiropractic medicine: American Chiropractic Association: http://www.amerchiro.org
Osteopathic medicine: American Osteopathic Association: http://www.aoa-net.org

Meditation, biofeedback, stress reduction
The Mind–Body Medical Institute: http://www.mindbody.harvard.edu (information and referrals)
Insight Meditation Society: http://www.dharma.org (information and links)

Prayer and spirituality
National Institute for Healthcare Research: http://www.nihr.org

Yoga
The American Yoga Association: http://www.americanyogaassociation.org/

Massage
The National Certification Board for Therapeutic Massage and Bodywork: http://www.ncbtmb.com (referral list)
The American Massage Therapy Association: http://www.amtamassage.org (information about massage as well as locator service for therapists)

Herbs, supplements, vitamins
US Food and Drug Administration: http://www.fda.gov (access to MEDWATCH as well as warnings on herbal products)
American Botanical Council: http://www.herbs.org (factual information about herbs)
HerbMed: http://www.amfoundation.org/ (herbal database)
NIH Office of Dietary Supplements: http://dietary-supplements.info.nih.gov
American Dietetic Association: http://www.eatright.org (referrals to registered dietitians)
American Herbalists Guild: http://www.americanherbalistsguild.com (referrals to herbal practitioners)

ABBREVIATIONS: CMA, complementary and alternative medicine; NIH, National Institutes of Health.

44

REFERENCES

1. Eisenberg DM, Davis RB, Ettner SL, et al. Trends in alternative medicine use in the United States. 1990–1997. JAMA 1998;280:1569–1575.
2. Rao JK, Miboliak K, Kroenke K, Bradley J, Tierney WM, Weinberger M. Use of complementary therapies for arthritis among patients of rheumatologists. Ann Intern Med 1999:131:409–416.
3. Sugarman J, Burk L. Physicians' ethical obligations regarding alternative medicine. JAMA 1998;280:1623–1625.
4. Kabat-Zinn J, Lipworth L, Burney R, Sellers W. Four year follow-up of a meditation-based program for the self-regulation of chronic pain: treatment outcomes and compliance. Clin J Pain 1986;2:159–171.
5. Pioro-Boisset M, Esdaile JM, Fitzcharles MA. Alternative medicine use in fibromyalgia syndrome. Arthritis Care Res 1996;9:13–17.
6. Young LD, Bradley LA, Tllmer RA. Decreases in health care resource utilization in patients with rheumatoid arthritis following a cognitive behavioral intervention. Biofeedback Self Regul 1995;259–268.
7. Yocum DE, Hodes R, Sundstrom WK, Cleeland CS. Use of biofeedback training in treatment of Raynaud's disease and phenomenon. Rheumatology 1985;12:90–93.
8. Bradley LA, Young LD, Anderson KO, et al. Effects of psychological therapy on pain behavior of rheumatoid arthritis patients. Treatment outcome and six-month followup. Arthritis Rheum 1987;30:1105–1114.
9. Astin LA, Harkness E, Ernst E. The efficacy of distant healing: a systematic review of randomised trials. Ann Intern Med 2000;132:903–910.
10. Dunlop DD, Selmanik P, Song J, et al. Risk factors for functional decline in older adults with arthritis. Arthritis Rheum 2005;52:1274–1282.
11. Deyle D, Henderson NE, Matekel RL, Ryder MG, Garber MB, Allison SC. Effectiveness of manual physical therapy and exercise in osteoarthritis of the knee. Ann Intern Med 2000;132:173–181.
12. Garfinkel MS, Singhal A, Katz WA, Allan DA, Reshetar R, Schumacher HR. Yoga-based intervention of carpal tunnel syndrome: a randomized trial. JAMA 1998;280:1601–1603.
13. NIH Consensus Development Panel on Acupuncture. Acupuncture. JAMA 1998;280:1518–1524.
14. Ernst E, White AR. Acupuncture for back pain: a meta-analysis of randomized controlled trials. Arch Intern Med 1998;158:2235–2241.
15. Berman BM, Lao L, Langenberg P, Lee WL, Gilpin AM, Hochberg M. Effectiveness of acupuncture as adjunctive therapy in osteoarthritis of the knee; a randomized, controlled trial. Ann Intern Med 2004;141:901–910.
16. Manheimer E, White A, Berman B, Forys K, Ernst E. Meta-analysis: acupuncture for low back pain. Ann Intern Med 2005;142:651–663.
17. Sunshine WI, Field TM, Quintino O, et al. Fibromyalgia benefits from massage therapy and transcutaneous electrical stimulation. J Pain Rheumatol 1996;2:18–22.
18. Clegg DO, Reda DJ, et al. Glucosamine, chondroitin sulfate, and the two in combination for painful knee osteoarthritis. N Engl J Med 2006;354:858–860.
19. Haqqui TM, Anthony DD, Gupta S, et al. Prevention of collagen-induced arthritis in mice by polyphenolic fraction from green tea. Proc Natl Acad Sci U S A 1999;96:4524–4529.
20. Kim L, Axelrod L, Howard P, et al. Efficacy of methylsulfonylmethane (MSM) in knee osteoarthritis pain; a pilot clinical trial. Paper presented at: American Association of Naturopathic Physicians 20th annual meeting; August 24–27, 2005; Phoenix, AZ.
21. Duffy EM, Meenagh GK, McMillan SA, et al. The clinical effect of dietary supplementation with omega-3 fish oils and or copper in systemic lupus erythematosus. J Rheumatol 2004;31:1551–1556.
22. McAlindon TE. Influence of vitamin D status on the incidence of progression of knee osteoarthritis. Ann Intern Med 1996;125:353–361.
23. Bischoff-Ferrari HA, Zhang Y, Kiel DP, Felson DT. Positive association between serum 25-hydroxyvitamin D level and bone density in osteoarthritis. Arthritis Rheum 2005;53:821–826.
24. Merlino LA, Curtis J, Mikuls TR, Cerhan JR, Criswell LA, Saag KG, Iowa Women's Health Study. Vitamin D intake is inversely associated with rheumatoid arthritis: results from the Iowa Women's Health Study. Arthritis Rheum 2004;50:72–77.
25. McAlindon TE, Jacques P, Zhang Y, et al. Do antioxidant micronutrients protect against the development of knee osteoarthritis? Arthritis Rheum 1996;39:648–656.
26. Beauchamp GK, Keast RSJ, Morel D, et al. Ibuprofen-like activity in extra-virgin olive oil. Nature 2005;437:45–46.
27. Pattison DJ, Harrison RA, Symmons DPM. The role of diet in susceptibility to rheumatoid arthritis: a systematic review. J Rheumatol 2004;31:1310–1319.
28. Felson DT. Weight loss reduces the risk for symptomatic knee OA in women: the Framingham study. Ann Intern Med 1992;116:535–542.
29. Walker WK, Keats DM. An investigation of the therapeutic value of the "copper bracelet" - dermal assimilation of copper in arthritic/rheumatoid conditions. Agents Actions 1976;6:454–459.
30. Valbona C, Hazlewood CF, Jurida G. Response of pain to static magnetic fields in postpolio patients: a double-blind pilot study. Arch Phys Med Rehab 1997;78:1200–1203.
31. Weintraub MI. Magnetic biostimulation in painful diabetic peripheral neuropathy: a novel intervention. Am J Pain Manage 1999;9:9–18.
32. Chang YR, Bliven ML. Anti-arthritic effect of bee venom. Agents Actions 1979;9:205–211.
33. Eiseman JL, Von Bredow J, Alvar AP. Effect of honeybee (Apis mellifera) venom on the course of adjuvant-induced arthritis and depression of drug metabolism in the rat. Biochem Pharmacol 1982;31:1139–1146.

Criteria for the Classification and Diagnosis of the Rheumatic Diseases

The criteria presented in the following section have been developed with several different purposes in mind. For a given disorder, one may have criteria for (1) classification of groups of patients (e.g., for population surveys, selection of patients for therapeutic trials, or analysis of results on interinstitutional patient comparisons); (2) diagnosis of individual patients; and (3) estimations of disease frequency, severity, and outcome.

The original intention was to propose criteria as guidelines for classification of disease syndromes for the purpose of assuring correctness of diagnosis in patients taking part in clinical investigation rather than for individual patient diagnosis. However, the proposed criteria have in fact been used as guidelines for patient diagnosis as well as for research classification. One must be cautious in such application because the various criteria are derived from the use of analytic techniques that allow the minimum number of variables to achieve the best group discrimination, rather than to attempt to arrive at a diagnosis in an individual patient.

The proposed criteria are empiric and not intended to include or exclude a particular diagnosis in any individual patient. They are valuable in offering a standard to permit comparison of groups of patients from different centers that take part in various clinical investigations, including therapeutic trials.

The ideal criterion is absolutely sensitive (i.e., all patients with the disorder show this physical finding or the positive laboratory test) and absolutely specific (i.e., the positive finding or test is never present in any other disease). Unfortunately, few such criteria or sets of criteria exist. Usually, the greater the sensitivity of a finding, the lower its specificity, and vice versa. When criteria are established attempts are made to select reasonable combinations of sensitivity and specificity.

An updated listing of additional criteria sets for rheumatic and musculoskeletal disorders is available on the American College of Rheumatology website (http://www.rheumatology.org/publications/classification/index.asp?aud=mem).

CRITERIA FOR THE CLASSIFICATION Of FIBROMYALGIA[a]

1. History of widespread pain
   Definition. Pain is considered widespread when all of the following are present: pain in the left side of the body, pain in the right side of the body, pain above the waist, and pain below the waist. In addition, axial skeletal pain (cervical spine or anterior chest or thoracic spine or low back) must be present. In this definition, shoulder and buttock pain is considered as pain for each involved side. "Low back" pain is considered lower segment pain.

2. Pain in 11 of 18 tender point sites on digital palpation.[b]
   Definition. Pain, on digital palpation, must be present in at least 11 of the following 18 tender point sites:
   Occiput: bilateral, at the suboccipital muscle insertions.
   Low cervical: bilateral, at the anterior aspects of the intertransverse spaces at C5–C7.
   Trapezius: bilateral, at the midpoint of the upper border.
   Supraspinatus: bilateral, at origins, above the scapula spine near the medial border.
   Second rib: bilateral, at the second costochondral junctions, just lateral to the junctions on upper surfaces.
   Lateral epicondyle: bilateral, 2 cm distal to the epicondyles.
   Gluteal: bilateral, in upper outer quadrants of buttocks in anterior fold of muscle.
   Greater trochanter: bilateral, posterior to the trochanteric prominence.
   Knee: bilateral, at the medial fat pad proximal to the joint line.

SOURCE: Adapted from Wolfe F, Smythe HA, Yunus MS, et al. The American College of Rheumatology 1990 criteria for the classification of fibromyalgia. Report of the multicenter criteria committee. Arthritis Rheum 1990;33:100–172, with permission of the American College of Rheumatology.
[a] For classification purposes, patients will be said to have fibromyalgia if both criteria are satisfied. Widespread pain must have been present at least 3 months. The presence of a second clinical disorder does not exclude the diagnosis of fibromyalgia.
[b] Digital palpation should be performed with an approximate force of 4 kg. For a tender point to be considered "positive" the subject must state that the palpation was painful. "Tender" is not to be considered "painful."

CRITERIA FOR THE CLASSIFICATION OF RHEUMATOID ARTHRITIS[a]

CRITERION	DEFINITION
1. Morning stiffness	Morning stiffness in and around the joints, lasting at least 1 hour before maximal improvement
2. Arthritis of three or more joint areas	At least three joint areas simultaneously have had soft tissue swelling or fluid (not bony overgrowth alone) observed by a physician. The 14 possible areas are right or left PIP, MCP, wrist, elbow, knee, ankle, and MTP joints
3. Arthritis of hand joints	At least one area swollen (as defined above) in a wrist, MCP, or PIP joint
4. Symmetric arthritis	Simultaneous involvement of the same joint areas (as defined in 2) on both sides of the body (bilateral involvement of PIPs, MCPs, or MTPs is acceptable without absolute symmetry)
5. Rheumatoid nodules	Subcutaneous nodules, over bony prominences, or extensor surfaces, or in juxta-articular regions, observed by a physician
6. Serum rheumatoid factor	Demonstration of abnormal amounts of serum rheumatoid factor by any method for which the result has been positive in ≤ 5% of normal control subjects
7. Radiographic changes	Radiographic changes typical of rheumatoid arthritis on posteroanterior hand and wrist radiographs, which must include erosions or unequivocal bony decalcification localized in or most marked adjacent to the involved joints (osteoarthritis changes alone do not qualify)

SOURCE: Reprinted from Arnett FC, Edworthy SM, Bloch DA. et al. The American Rheumatism Association 1987 revised criteria for the classification of rheumatoid arthritis. Arthritis Rheum 1988;31:315−324, with permission of the American College of Rheumatology.
ABBREVIATIONS: MCP, metacarpophalangeal; MTP, metatarsophalangeal; PIP, proxomal interphalangeal.
[a] For classification purposes, a patient shall be said to have rheumatoid arthritis if he/she has satisfied at least four of these seven criteria. Criteria 1 through 4 must have been present for at least 6 weeks. Patients with two clinical diagnoses are not excluded. Designation as classic, definite, or probable rheumatoid arthritis is *not* to be made.

CLASSIFICATION OF PROGRESSION OF RHEUMATOID ARTHRITIS

Stage I, Early
*1. No destructive changes on roentgenographic examination
2. Radiographic evidence of osteoporosis may be present

Stage II, Moderate
*1. Radiographic evidence of osteoporosis, with or without slight subchondral bone destruction; slight cartilage destruction may be present
*2. No joint deformities, although limitation of joint mobility may be present
3. Adjacent muscle atrophy
4. Extra-articular soft tissue lesions, such as nodules and tenosynovitis may be present

Stage III, Severe
*1. Radiographic evidence of cartilage and bone destruction, in addition to osteoporosis
*2. Joint deformity, such as subluxation, ulnar deviation, or hyperextension, without fibrous or bony ankylosis
3. Extensive muscle atrophy
4. Extra-articular soft tissue lesions, such as nodules and tenosynovitis may be present

Stage IV, Terminal
*1. Fibrous or bony ankylosis
2. Criteria of stage III

SOURCE: Reprinted from Steinbrocker O, Traeger CH. Batterman RC. Therapeutic criteria in rheumatoid arthritis. JAMA 1949;140:659−662, with permission.
*The criteria prefaced by an asterisk are those that must be present to permit classification of a patient in any particular stage or grade.

CRITERIA FOR CLINICAL REMISSION IN RHEUMATOID ARTHRITIS[a]

Five or more of the following requirements must be fulfilled for at least 2 consecutive months:

1. Duration of morning stiffness not exceeding 15 minutes
2. No fatigue
3. No joint pain (by history)
4. No joint tenderness or pain on motion
5. No soft tissue swelling in joints or tendon sheaths
6. Erythrocyte sedimentation rate (Westergren method) less than 30 mm/hour for a female or 20 mm/hour for a male

SOURCE: Reprinted from Pinals RS, Masi AT, Larsen RA. et al. Preliminary criteria for clinical remission in rheumatoid arthritis. Arthritis Rheum 1981;24:1308–1315, with permission of the American College of Rheumatology.
[a] These criteria are intended to describe either spontaneous remission or a state of drug-induced disease suppression, which simulates spontaneous remission. No alternative explanation may be invoked to account for the failure to meet a particular requirement. For instance, in the presence of knee pain, which might be related to degenerative arthritis, a point for "no joint pain" may not be awarded. Exclusions: Clinical manifestations of active vasculitis, pericarditis, pleuritis or myositis, and unexplained recent weight loss or fever attributable to rheumatoid arthritis will prohibit a designation of complete clinical remission.

CRITERIA FOR CLASSIFICATION OF FUNCTIONAL STATUS IN RHEUMATOID ARTHRITIS[a]

Class I	Completely able to perform usual activities of daily living (self-care, vocational, and avocational)
Class II	Able to perform usual self-care and vocational activities, but limited in avocational activities
Class III	Able to perform usual self-care activities, but limited in vocational and avocational activities
Class IV	Limited in ability to perform usual self-care, vocational, and avocational activities

SOURCE: Reprinted from Hochberg MC, Chang RW, Dwosh I. et al. The American College of Rheumatology 1991 revised criteria for the classification of global functional status in rheumatoid arthritis. Arthritis Rheum 1992;35;498–502, with permission of the American College of Rheumatology.
[a] Usual self-care activities include dressing, feeding, bathing, grooming, and toileting. Avocational (recreational and/or leisure) and vocational (work, school, homemaking) activities are patient-desired and age- and sex-specific.

AMERICAN COLLEGE OF RHEUMATOLOGY PRELIMINARY DEFINITION OF IMPROVEMENT IN RHEUMATOID ARTHRITIS (ACR20)

Required $\begin{cases} \geq 20\% \text{ improvement in tender joint count} \\ \geq 20\% \text{ improvement in swollen joint count} \end{cases}$

+

≥ 20% improvement in three of the following five:
Patient pain assessment
Patient global assessment
Physician global assessment
Patient self-assessed disability
Acute-phase reactant (ESR or CRP)

DISEASE ACTIVITY MEASURE	METHOD OF ASSESSMENT
1. Tender joint count	ACR tender joint count, an assessment of 28 or more joints. The joint count should be done by scoring several different aspects of tenderness, as assessed by pressure and joint manipulation on physical examination. The information on various types of tenderness should then be collapsed into a single tender-versus-nontender dichotomy.
2. Swollen joint count	ACR swollen joint count, an assessment of 28 or more joints. Joints are classified as either swollen or not swollen.
3. Patient's assessment of pain	A horizontal visual analog scale (usually 10 cm) or Likert scale assessment of the patient's current level of pain.
4. Patient's global assessment of disease activity	The patient's overall assessment of how the arthritis is doing. One acceptable method for determining this is the question from the AIMS instrument: "Considering all the ways your arthritis affects you, mark 'X' on the scale for how well you are doing." An anchored, horizontal, visual analog scale (usually 10 cm) should be provided. A Likert scale response is also acceptable.

APPENDIX I

(continued)

AMERICAN COLLEGE OF RHEUMATOLOGY PRELIMINARY DEFINITION OF IMPROVEMENT IN RHEUMATOID ARTHRITIS (ACR20) (continued)

DISEASE ACTIVITY MEASURE	METHOD OF ASSESSMENT
5. Physician's global assessment of disease activity	A horizontal visual analog scale (usually 10 cm) or Likert scale measure of the physician's assessment of the patient's current disease activity.
6. Patient's assessment of physical function	Any patient self-assessment instrument which has been validated, has reliability, has been proven in RA trials to be sensitive to change, and which measures physical function in RA patients is acceptable. Instruments which have been demonstrated to be sensitive in RA trials include the AIMS, the HAQ, the Quality (or Index) of Well Being, the MHIQ, and the MACTAR.
7. Acute-phase reactant value	A Westergren ESR or a CRP level.

SOURCE: Reprinted from Felson DT, Anderson JJ, Boers M, et al. American College of Rheumatology preliminary definition of improvement in rheumatoid arthritis. Arthritis Rheum 1995;38:727–735, with permission of the American College of Rheumatology.
ABBREVIATIONS: ACR, American College of Rheumatology; AIMS, Arthritis Impact Measurement Scales; CRP, C-reactive protein; ESR, erythrocyte sedimentation rate; HAQ, Health Assessment Questionnaire; MACTAR, McMaster Toronto Arthritis Patient Preference Disability Questionnaire; MHIQ, McMaster Health Index Questionnaire; RA, rheumatoid arthritis.

CRITERIA FOR THE CLASSIFICATION OF SPONDYLOARTHROPATHY[a]

Inflammatory spinal pain or
Synovitis
    Asymmetric or
    Predominantly in the lower limbs and one or more of the following
    Positive family history
    Psoriasis

Inflammatory bowel disease

Urethritis, cervicitis, or acute diarrhea within 1 month before arthritis

Buttock pain alternating between right and left gluteal areas

Enthesopathy

Sacroiliitis

VARIABLE	DEFINITION
Inflammatory spinal pain	History or present symptoms of spinal pain in back, dorsal, or cervical region, with at least four of the following: (a) onset before age 45, (b) insidious onset, (c) improved by exercise, (d) associated with morning stiffness, (e) at least 3 months' duration
Synovitis	Past or present asymmetric arthritis or arthritis predominantly in the lower limbs
Family history	Presence in first-degree or second-degree relatives of any of the following: (a) ankylosing spondylitis, (b) psoriasis, (c) acute uveitis, (d) reactive arthritis, (e) inflammatory bowel disease
Psoriasis	Past or present psoriasis diagnosed by a physician
Inflammatory bowel disease	Past or present Crohn's disease or ulcerative colitis diagnosed by a physician and confirmed by radiographic examination or endoscopy
Alternating buttock pain	Past or present pain alternating between the right and left gluteal regions
Enthesopathy	Past or present spontaneous pain or tenderness at examination of the site of the insertion of the Achilles tendon or plantar fascia
Acute diarrhea	Episode of diarrhea occurring within 1 month before arthritis

CRITERIA FOR THE CLASSIFICATION OF SPONDYLOARTHROPATHY[a] (continued)

VARIABLE	DEFINITION
Urethritis	Nongonococcal urethritis or cervicitis occurring within 1 month before arthritis
Sacroiliitis	Bilateral grade 2−4 or unilateral grade 3−4, according to the following radiographic grading system: 0 = normal, 1 = possible, 2 = minimal, 3 = moderate, and 4 = ankylosis

SOURCE: Reprinted from Dougados M, Van Der linden S, Juhlin R, et al. The European Spondylarthropathy Study Group preliminary criteria for the classification of spondylarthropathy. Arthritis Rheum 1991;34:1218−1227, with permission of the American College of Rheumatology.
[a] This classification method yields a sensitivity of 78.4% and a specificity of 89.6%. When radiographic evidence of sacroiliitis was included, the sensitivity improved to 87.0% with a minor decrease in specificity to 86.7%. Definition of the variables used in classification criteria follow.

CRITERIA FOR THE DIAGNOSIS OF RHEUMATIC FEVER[a]

MAJOR MANIFESTATIONS	MINOR MANIFESTATIONS	SUPPORTING EVIDENCE OF PRECEDING STREPTOCOCCAL INFECTION
Carditis	Clinical findings	Positive throat culture or rapid streptococcal antigen test
Polyarthritis	Arthralgia	Elevated or rising streptococcal antibody titer
Chorea	Fever	
Erythema marginatum	Laboratory findings	
Subcutaneous nodules	Elevated acute phase reactants Erythrocyte sedimentation rate C-reactive protein Prolonged PR interval	

SOURCE: Reprinted from Special Writing Group of the Committee on Rheumatic Fever, Endocarditis, and Kawasaki Disease of the Council on Cardiovascular Disease in the Young, American Heart Association: guidelines for the diagnosis of rheumatic fever: Jones criteria, updated 1992. JAMA 1992;268:2069−2073, with permission.
[a] If supported by evidence of preceding group A streptococcal infection, the presence of two major manifestations, or of one major and two minor manifestations indicates a high probability of acute rheumatic fever.

CRITERIA FOR THE CLASSIFICATION AND REPORTING OF OSTEOARTHRITIS OF THE HAND, HIP, AND KNEE

CLASSIFICATION CRITERIA FOR OSTEOARTHRITIS OF THE HAND, TRADITIONAL FORMAT[a]

Hand pain, aching, or stiffness and

Three or four of the following features:
  Hard tissue enlargement of 2 or more of 10 selected joints
  Hard tissue enlargement of 2 or more DIP joints
  Fewer than three swollen MCP joints
  Deformity of at least 1 of 10 selected joints

SOURCE: Reprinted from Altman R, Alarcon G, Appelrouth D, et al. The American College of Rheumatology criteria for the classification and reporting of osteoarthritis of the hand. Arthritis Rheum 1990;33:1601−1610, with permission of the American College of Rheumatology.
ABBREVIATION: MCP, metacarpophalangeal.
[a] The 10 selected joints are the second and third distal interphalangeal (DIP), the second and third proximal interphalangeal (PIP), and the first carpometacarpal (CMC) joints of both hands. This classification method yields a sensitivity of 94% and a specificity of 87%.

CLASSIFICATION CRITERIA FOR OSTEOARTHRITIS OF THE HIP, TRADITIONAL FORMAT[a]

Hip pain
and

At least two of the following three features:
  ESR ≤ 20 mm/hour
  Radiographic femoral or acetabular osteophytes
  Radiographic joint space narrowing (superior, axial, and/or medial)

SOURCE: Reprinted from Altman R, Alarcon G, Appelrouth D, et al. The American College of Rheumatology criteria for the classification and reporting of osteoarthritis of the hip. Arthritis Rheum 1991;34:505−514, with permission of the American College of Rheumatology.
ABBREVIATION: ESR, erythrocyte sedimentation rate (Westergren).
[a] This classification method yields a sensitivity of 89% and a specificity of 91%.

APPENDIX I

(continued)

CRITERIA FOR THE CLASSIFICATION AND REPORTING OF OSTEOARTHRITIS OF THE HAND, HIP, AND KNEE (*continued*)

CRITERIA FOR CLASSIFICATION OF OSTEOARTHRITIS (OA) OF THE KNEE

Clinical and laboratory
Knee pain plus at least five of nine:
  Age >50 years
  Stiffness <30 minutes
  Crepitus
  Bony tenderness
  Bony enlargement
  No palpable warmth
  ESR <40 mm/hour
  RF <1:40
  SF OA
92% sensitive
75% specific

Clinical and radiographic
Knee pain plus at least one of three:
  Age >50 years
  Stiffness <30 minutes
  Crepitus
+
Osteophytes
91% sensitive
86% specific

Clinical[a]
Knee pain plus at least three of six:
  Age >50 years
  Stiffness <30 minutes
  Crepitus
  Bony tenderness
  Bony enlargement
  No palpable warmth
95% sensitive
69% specific

SOURCE: Reprinted from Altman R, Asch E, Bloch G, et al. Development of criteria for the classification and reporting of osteoarthritis: classification of osteoarthritis of the knee. Arthritis Rheum 1986;29:1039–1049, with permission of the American College of Rheumatology.
ABBREVIATIONS: ESR, erythrocyte sedimentation rate (Westergren); RF, rheumatoid factor; SF OA, synovial fluid signs of OA (clear, viscous, or white blood cell count <2000/mm³).
[a] Alternative for the clinical category would be four of six, which is 84% sensitive and 89% specific.

CRITERIA FOR THE CLASSIFICATION OF ACUTE GOUTY ARTHRITIS

A. The presence of characteristic urate crystals in the joint fluid, or

B. A tophus proved to contain urate crystals by chemical means or polarized light microscopy or the presence of 6 of the following 12 clinical, laboratory, and x-ray phenomena listed below:

1. More than one attack of acute arthritis
2. Maximal inflammation developed within 1 day
3. Attack of monarticular arthritis
4. Joint redness observed
5. First metatarsophalangeal joint painful or swollen
6. Unilateral attack involving first metatarsophalangeal joint
7. Unilateral attack involving tarsal joint
8. Suspected tophus
9. Hyperuricemia
10. Asymmetric swelling within a joint (radiograph)
11. Subcortical cysts without erosions (radiograph)
12. Negative culture of joint fluid for microorganisms during attack of joint inflammation

SOURCE: Adapted from Wallace SL, Robinson H, Masi AT, et al. Preliminary criteria for the classification of the acute arthritis of primary gout. Arthritis Rheum 1977;20:895–900, with permission of the American College of Rheumatology.

CRITERIA FOR THE CLASSIFICATION OF SYSTEMIC LUPUS ERYTHEMATOSUS[a]

CRITERION	DEFINITION
1. Malar rash	Fixed erythema, flat or raised, over the malar eminences, tending to spare the nasolabial folds
2. Discoid rash	Erythematous raised patches with adherent keratotic scaling and follicular plugging; atrophic scarring may occur in older lesions
3. Photosensitivity	Skin rash as a result of unusual reaction to sunlight, by patient history or physician observation
4. Oral ulcers	Oral or nasopharyngeal ulceration, usually painless, observed by a physician
5. Arthritis	Nonerosive arthritis involving two or more peripheral joints, characterized by tenderness, swelling, or effusion
6. Serositis	(a) Pleuritis-convincing history of pleuritic pain or rub heard by a physician or evidence of pleural effusion OR (b) Pericarditis-documented by ECG or rub or evidence of pericardial effusion
7. Renal disorder	(a) Persistent proteinuria greater than 0.5 g per day or greater than 3+ if quantitation not performed OR (b) Cellular casts—may be red cell, hemoglobin, granular, tubular, or mixed
8. Neurologic disorder	(a) Seizures—in the absence of offending drugs or known metabolic derangements; e.g., uremia, ketoacidosis, or electrolyte imbalance OR (b) Psychosis—in the absence of offending drugs or known metabolic derangements; e.g., uremia, ketoacidosis, or electrolyte imbalance
9. Hematologic disorder	(a) Hemolytic anemia with reticulocytosis OR (b) Leukopenia, less than 4000/mm^3 total on two or more occasions OR (c) Lymphopenia, less than 1500/mm^3 on two or more occasions OR (d) Thrombocytopenia, less than l00,000/mm^3 in the absence of offending drugs
10. Immunologic disorder[b]	(a) Anti-DNA: antibody to native DNA in abnormal titer OR (b) Anti-SM: presence of antibody to SM nuclear antigen OR (c) Positive finding of antiphospholipid antibodies based on (1) an abnormal serum level of IgG or IgM anticardiolipin antibodies, (2) a positive test result for lupus anticoagulant using a standard method, or (3) a false-positive serologic test for syphilis known to be positive for at least 6 months and confirmed by *Treponema pallidum* immobilization or fluorescent treponemal antibody absorption test
11. Antinuclear antibody	An abnormal titer of antinuclear antibody by immunofluorescence or an equivalent assay at any point in time and in the absence of drugs known to be associated with "drug-induced lupus" syndrome

SOURCE: Adapted from Tan EM, Cohen AS, Fries JF, et al. The 1982 revised criteria for the classification of systemic lupus erythematosus (SLE). Arthritis Rheum 1982;25:1271–1277, with permission of the American College of Rheumatology.
SOURCE: Adapted from Hochberg ME. Updating the American College of Rheumatology revised criteria for the classification of systemic lupus erythematosus [letter]. Arthritis Rheum 1997;40:1725, with permission of the American College of Rheumatology.
[a] This classification is based on 11 criteria. For the purpose of identifying patients in clinical studies, a person must have SLE if any 4 or more of the 11 criteria are present, serially or simultaneously, during any interval of observation.
[b] The modifications to criterion number 10 were made in 1997.

CRITERIA FOR THE CLASSIFICATION OF SYSTEMIC SCLEROSIS (SCLERODERMA)[a]

A. Major criterion

Proximal scleroderma: Symmetric thickening, tightening, and induration of the skin of the fingers and the skin proximal to the metacarpophalangeal or metatarsophalangeal joints. The changes may affect the entire extremity, face, neck, and trunk (thorax and abdomen).

B. Minor criteria

1. *Sclerodactyly:* Above-indicated skin changes limited to the fingers
2. *Digital pitting scars* or *loss of substance from the finger pad:* Depressed areas at tips of fingers or loss of digital pad tissue as a result of ischemia
3. *Bibasilar pulmonary fibrosis:* Bilateral reticular pattern of linear or lineonodular densities most pronounced in basilar portions of the lungs on standard chest roentgenogram; may assume appearance of diffuse mottling or "honeycomb lung." These changes should not be attributable to primary lung disease.

SOURCE: Adapted from Subcommittee for Scleroderma Criteria of the American Rheumatism Association Diagnostic and Therapeutic Criteria Committee. Preliminary criteria for the classification of systemic sclerosis (scleroderma). Arthritis Rheum 1980;23:581–590, with permission of the American College of Rheumatology.
[a] For the purposes of classifying patients in clinical trials, population surveys, and other studies, a person shall be said to have systemic sclerosis (scleroderma) if the one major or two or more minor criteria are present. Localized forms of scleroderma, eosinophilic fasciitis, and the various forms of pseudoscleroderma are excluded from these criteria.

CRITERIA FOR THE DIAGNOSIS OF POLYMYOSITIS AND DERMATOMYOSITIS[a]

CRITERION	DEFINITION
1. Symmetrical weakness	Weakness of limb-girdle muscles and anterior neck flexors, progressing over weeks to months, with or without dysphagia or respiratory muscle involvement
2. Muscle biopsy evidence	Evidence of necrosis of type I and n fibers, phagocytosis, regeneration with basophilia, large vesicular sarcolemmal nuclei and prominent nucleoli, atrophy in a perifascicular distribution, variation in fiber size, and an inflammatory exudate, often perivascular
3. Elevation of muscle enzymes	Elevation in serum of skeletal muscle enzymes, particularly creatine phosphokinase and often aldolase, serum glutamate oxaloacetate, and pyruvate transaminases, and lactate dehydrogenase
4. Electromyographic evidence	Electromyographic triad of short, small, polyphasic motor units, fibrillations, positive sharp waves, and insertional irritability, and bizarre, high-frequency repetitive discharges
5. Dermatologic features	A lilac discoloration of the eyelids (heliotrope) with periorbital edema, a scaly, erythematous dermatitis over the dorsum of the hands (especially the metacarpophalangeal and proximal interphalangeal joints, Gottron's sign), and involvement of the knees, elbows, and medial malleoli, as well as the face, neck, and upper torso

Data from Bohan A, Peter JB. Polymyositis and dermatomyositis (first of two parts). N Engl J Med 1975;292:344–347, with permission.

[a] Confidence limits can be defined as follows: For a definite diagnosis of dermatomyositis, three of four criteria plus the rash must be present. For a definite diagnosis of polymyositis, four criteria must be present without the rash. For a probable diagnosis of dermatomyositis, two criteria plus the rash must be present. For a probable diagnosis of polymyositis, three criteria must be present without the rash. For a possible diagnosis of dermatomyositis, one criterion plus the rash must be present. For a possible diagnosis of polymyositis, two criteria must be present without the rash.

The following findings exclude a diagnosis of dermatomyositis or polymyositis.

- Evidence of central or peripheral neurologic disease, including motor-neuron disorders with fasciculations or long-tract signs, sensory changes, decreased nerve conduction times, and fiber-type atrophy and grouping on muscle biopsy.
- Muscle weakness with a slowly progressive, unremitting course and a positive family history or calf enlargement to suggest a muscular dystrophy.
- Biopsy evidence of granulomatous myositis such as with sarcoidosis.
- Infections, including trichinosis, schistosomiasis, trypanosomiasis, staphylococcosis, and toxoplasmosis.
- Recent use of various drugs and toxins, such as clofibrate and alcohol.
- Rhabdomyolysis as manifested by gross myoglobinuria related to strenuous exercise, infections, crush injuries, occlusions of major limb arteries, prolonged coma or convulsions, high-voltage accidents, heat stroke, the malignant-hyperpyrexia syndrome, and envenomation by certain sea snakes.
- Metabolic disorders such as McArdle's syndrome.
- Endocrinopathies such as thyrotoxicosis, myxedema, hyperparathyroidism, hypoparathyroidism, diabetes mellitus, or Cushing's syndrome.
- Myasthenia gravis with response to cholinergics, sensitivity to d-tubocurarine, and decremental response to repetitive nerve stimulation.

CRITERIA FOR THE CLASSIFICATION OF SJÖGREN'S SYNDROME[a]

1. Ocular symptoms

   Definition. A positive response to at least one of the following three questions:
   (a) Have you had daily, persistent, troublesome dry eyes for more than 3 months?
   (b) Do you have a recurrent sensation of sand or gravel in the eyes?
   (c) Do you use tear substitutes more than three times a day?

2. Oral symptoms

   Definition. A positive response to at least one of the following three questions:
   (a) Have you had a daily feeling of dry mouth for more than 3 months?
   (b) Have you had recurrent or persistently swollen salivary glands as an adult?
   (c) Do you frequently drink liquids to aid in swallowing dry foods?

3. Ocular signs

   Definition. Objective evidence of ocular involvement, determined on the basis of a positive result on at least one of the following two tests:
   (a) Schirmer-I test (≤5 mm in 5 minutes)
   (b) Rose bengal score (~ 4, according to the van Bijsterveld scoring system)

4. Histopathologic features

   Definition. Focus score ~ 1 on minor salivary gland biopsy (focus defined as an agglomeration of at least 50 mononuclear cells; focus score defined as the number of foci per 4 mm^2 of glandular tissue)

CRITERIA FOR THE CLASSIFICATION OF SJÖGREN'S SYNDROME[a] (continued)

5. Salivary gland involvement
   Definition. Objective evidence of salivary gland involvement, determined on the basis of a positive result on at least one of the following three tests:
   (a) Salivary scintigraphy
   (b) Parotid sialography
   (c) Unstimulated salivary flow ($\leq$ 1.5 mL in 15 minutes)

6. Autoantibodies
   Definition. Presence of at least one of the following serum autoantibodies:
   (a) Antibodies to Ro/SS-A or La/SS-B antigens
   (b) Antinuclear antibodies
   (c) Rheumatoid factor

Exclusion criteria: preexisting lymphoma, acquired immunodeficiency syndrome, sarcoidosis, or graft-versus-host disease

SOURCE: Reprinted from Vitali C, Bombardieri S, Moutsopoulos HM, et al. Preliminary criteria for the classification of Sjögren's syndrome. Arthritis Rheum 1993;36:340–347, with permission of the American College of Rheumatology.
[a] For primary Sjögren's syndrome, the presence of three of six items showed a very high sensitivity (99.1%), but insufficient specificity (57.8%). Thus, this combination could be accepted as the basis for a diagnosis of probable primary Sjögren's syndrome. However, the presence of four of six items (accepting as serologic parameters only positive anti–Ro/SS-A and anti–La/SS-B antibodies) had a good sensitivity (93.5%) and specificity (94.0%), and therefore may be used to establish a definitive diagnosis of primary Sjögren's syndrome.

CRITERIA FOR THE CLASSIFICATION OF POLYARTERITIS NODOSA[a]

CRITERION	DEFINITION
1. Weight loss $\geq$4 kg	Loss of 4 kg or more of body weight since illness began, not due to dieting or other factors
2. Livedo reticularis	Mottled reticular pattern over the skin of portions of the extremities or torso
3. Testicular pain or tenderness	Pain or tenderness of the testicles, not due to infection, trauma, or other causes
4. Myalgias, weakness, or leg tenderness	Diffuse myalgias (excluding shoulder and hip girdle) or weakness of muscles or tenderness of leg muscles
5. Mononeuropathy or polyneuropathy	Development of mononeuropathy, multiple mononeuropathies, or polyneuropathy
6. Diastolic BP >90 mm Hg	Development of hypertension with the diastolic BP higher than 90 mm Hg
7. Elevated BUN or creatinine	Elevation of BUN >40 mg/dL or creatinine >1.5 mg/dL, not due to dehydration or obstruction
8. Hepatitis B virus	Presence of hepatitis B surface antigen or antibody in serum
9. Arteriographic abnormality	Arteriogram showing aneurysms or occlusions of the visceral arteries, not due to arteriosclerosis, fibromuscular dysplasia, or other non-inflammatory causes
10. Biopsy of small or medium-sized	Histologic changes showing the presence of granulocytes or artery containing polymorphonuclear leukocytes and mononuclear leukocytes in the artery wall

SOURCE: Reprinted from Lightfoot RW Jr, Michel BA, Bloch DA, et al. The American College of Rheumatology 1990 criteria for the classification of polyarteritis nodosa. Arthritis Rheum 1990;33:1088–1093, with permission of the American College of Rheumatology.
ABBREVIATIONS: BP, blood pressure; BUN, blood urea nitrogen.
[a] For classification purposes, a patient shall be said to have polyarteritis nodosa if at least 3 of these 10 criteria are present. The presence of any three or more criteria yields a sensitivity of 82.2% and a specificity of 86.6%.

APPENDIX I

CRITERIA FOR THE CLASSIFICATION OF HENOCH–SCHONLEIN PURPURA[a]

CRITERION	DEFINITION
1. Palpable purpura	Slightly raised "palpable" hemorrhagic skin lesions, not related to thrombocytopenia
2. Age at disease onset	Patient 20 years or younger at onset of first symptoms
3. Bowel angina	Diffuse abdominal pain, worse after meals, or the diagnosis of bowel ischemia, usually including bloody diarrhea
4. Wall granulocytes on biopsy	Histologic changes showing granulocytes in the walls of arterioles or venules

SOURCE: Reprinted from Mills JA, Michel BA, Bloch DA, et al. The American College of Rheumatology 1990 criteria for the classification of Henoch–Schonlein purpura. Arthritis Rheum 1990;33:1114–1121, with permission of the American College of Rheumatology.
[a]For purposes of classification, a patient shall be said to have Henoch–Schonlein purpura if at least two of these four criteria are present. The presence of any two or more criteria yields a sensitivity of 87.1% and a specificity of 87.7%.

CRITERIA FOR THE CLASSIFICATION OF CHURG–STRAUSS SYNDROME[a]

CRITERION	DEFINITION
1. Asthma	History of wheezing or diffuse high-pitched rales on expiration
2. Eosinophilia	Eosinophilia >10% on white blood cell differential count
3. Mononeuropathy or polyneuropathy	Development of mononeuropathy, multiple mononeuropathies, or polyneuropathy (i.e., glove/stocking distribution) attributable to a systemic vasculitis
4. Pulmonary infiltrates, nonfixed	Migratory or transitory pulmonary infiltrates on radiographs (not including fixed infiltrates), attributable to a systemic vasculitis
5. Paranasal sinus abnormality	History of acute or chronic paranasal sinus pain or tenderness or radiographic opacification of the paranasal sinuses
6. Extravascular eosinophils	Biopsy including artery, arteriole, or venule, showing accumulations of eosinophils in extravascular areas

SOURCE: Adapted from Masi AT, Hunder GG, Lie JT, et al. The American College of Rheumatology 1990 criteria for the classification of Churg–Strauss syndrome (allergic granulomatosis and angiitis). Arthritis Rheum 1990;33:1094–1100, with permission of the American College of Rheumatology.
[a]For classification purposes, a patient shall be said to have Churg–Strauss syndrome if at least four of these six criteria are positive. The presence of any four or more of the six criteria yields a sensitivity of 85% and a specificity of 99.7%.

CRITERIA FOR THE CLASSIFICATION OF WEGENER'S GRANULOMATOSIS[a]

CRITERION	DEFINITION
1. Nasal or oral inflammation	Development of painful or painless oral ulcers or purulent or bloody nasal discharge
2. Abnormal chest radiograph	Chest radiograph showing the presence of nodules, fixed infiltrates, or cavities
3. Urinary sediment	Microhematuria (> 5 red blood cells per high power field) or red cell casts in urine sediment
4. Granulomatous inflammation on biopsy	Histologic changes showing granulomatous inflammation within the wall of an artery or in the perivascular or extravascular area (artery or arteriole)

SOURCE: Reprinted from Leavitt RY, Fauci AS, Bloch DA, et al. The American College of Rheumatology 1990 criteria for the classification of Wegener's granulomatosis. Arthritis Rheum 1990;33:1101–1107, with permission of the American College of Rheumatology.
[a]For purposes of classification, a patient shall be said to have Wegener's granulomatosis if at least two of these four criteria are present. The presence of any two or more criteria yields a sensitivity of 88.2% and a specificity of 92.0%.

CRITERIA FOR THE CLASSIFICATION OF GIANT CELL ARTERITIS[a]

CRITERION	DEFINITION
1. Age at disease onset ≥50 years	Development of symptoms or findings beginning at age 50 or older
2. New headache	New onset of or new type of localized pain in the head
3. Temporal artery abnormality	Temporal artery tenderness to palpation or decreased pulsation, unrelated to arteriosclerosis of cervical arteries
4. Elevated erythrocyte sedimentation rate	Erythrocyte sedimentation rate ≥ 50 mm/hour by the Westergren method
5. Abnormal artery biopsy	Biopsy specimen with artery showing vasculitis characterized by a predominance of mononuclear cell infiltration or granulomatous inflammation, usually with multinucleated giant cells

SOURCE: Reprinted from Hunder GG, Bloch DA, Michel BA, et al. The American College of Rheumatology 1990 criteria for the classification of giant cell arteritis. Arthritis Rheum 1990;33:1122–1128, with permission of the American College of Rheumatology.
[a] For purposes of classification, a patient shall be said to have giant cell (temporal) arteritis if at least three of these five criteria are present. The presence of any three or more criteria yields a sensitivity of 93.5% and a specificity of 91.2%.

CRITERIA FOR THE CLASSIFICATION OF TAKAYASU ARTERITIS[a]

CRITERION	DEFINITION
1. Age at disease onset ≤40 years	Development of symptoms or findings related to Takayasu arteritis at age ≤ 40 years
2. Claudication of extremities	Development and worsening of fatigue and discomfort in muscles of one or more extremity while in use, especially the upper extremities
3. Decreased brachial artery pulse	Decreased pulsation of one or both brachial arteries
4. BP difference >10 mm Hg	Difference of >10 mm Hg in systolic blood pressure between arms
5. Bruit over subclavian arteries or aorta	Bruit audible on auscultation over one or both subclavian arteries or abdominal aorta
6. Arteriogram abnormality	Arteriographic narrowing or occlusion of the entire aorta, its primary branches, or large arteries in the proximal upper or lower extremities, not due to arteriosclerosis, fibromuscular dysplasia, or similar causes; changes usually focal or segmental

SOURCE: Reprinted from Arend WP, Michel BA, Bloch DA, et al. The American College of Rheumatology 1990 criteria for the classification of Takayasu arteritis. Arthritis Rheum 1990;33:1129–1132, with permission of the American College of Rheumatology.
ABBREVIATIONS: BP, blood pressure (systolic; difference between arms).
[a] For purposes of classification, a patient shall be said to have Takayasu arteritis if at least three of these six criteria are present. The presence of any three or more criteria yields a sensitivity of 90.5% and a specificity of 97.8%.

APPENDIX I

CRITERIA FOR THE CLASSIFICATION OF HYPERSENSITIVITY VASCULITIS.[a]

CRITERION	DEFINITION
1. Age at disease onset >16 years	Development of symptoms after age 16
2. Medication at disease onset	Medication was taken at the onset of symptoms that may have been a precipitating factor
3. Palpable purpura	Slightly elevated purpuric rash over one or more areas of the skin; does not blanch with pressure and is not related to thrombocytopenia
4. Maculopapular rash	Flat and raised lesions of various sizes over one or more areas of the skin
5. Biopsy including arteriole and venule	Histologic changes showing granulocytes in a perivascular or extravascular location

SOURCE: Reprinted from Calabrese LH, Michel BA, Bloch DA, et al. The American College of Rheumatology 1990 criteria for the classification of hypersensitivity vasculitis. Arthritis Rheum 1990;33:1108–1113, with permission of the American College of Rheumatology.
[a] For purposes of classification, a patient shall be said to have hypersensitivity vasculitis if at least three of these five criteria are present. The presence of any three or more criteria yields a sensitivity of 71.0% and a specificity of 83.9%.

DIAGNOSTIC GUIDELINES FOR KAWASAKI SYNDROME.[a]

1. Fever lasting >5 days:

Plus four of the following criteria:

2. Polymorphous rash

3. Bilateral conjunctival injection

4. One or more of the following mucous membrane changes:
   Diffuse injection of oral and pharyngeal mucosa
   Erythema or fissuring of the lips
   Strawberry tongue

5. Acute, nonpurulent cervical lymphadenopathy (one lymph node must be >1.5 cm)

6. One or more of the following extremity changes:
   Erythema of palms and/or soles
   Indurative edema of hands and/or feet
   Membranous desquamation of the fingertips

SOURCE: Reprinted from Kawasaki T, Kosaki T, Okawa S, et al. A new infantile acute febrile mucocutaneous lymph node syndrome (MLNS) prevailing in Japan. Pediatrics 1974;54:271–276, with permission.
[a] Other illnesses with similar clinical signs must be excluded.

CRITERIA FOR THE DIAGNOSIS OF BEHÇET'S DISEASE.[a]

CRITERION	DEFINITION
1. Recurrent oral ulceration	Minor aphthous, major aphthous, or herpetiform ulceration observed by physician or patient, which recurred at least three times in one 12-month period
Plus two of	
2. Recurrent genital ulceration	Aphthous ulceration or scarring, observed by physician or patient
3. Eye lesions	Anterior uveitis, posterior uveitis, or cells in vitreous on slit lamp examination; or retinal vasculitis observed by ophthalmologist
4. Skin lesions	Erythema nodosum observed by physician or patient, pseudofolliculitis, or papulopustular lesions; or acneiform nodules observed by physician in postadolescent patients not on corticosteroid treatment
5. Positive pathergy test	Read by physician at 24–48 hours

SOURCE: Reprinted from International Study Group for Behçet's Disease. Criteria for diagnosis of Behçet's disease. Lancet 1990;335:1078–1080, with permission.
[a] Findings applicable only in the absence of other clinical explanations. The presence of recurrent oral ulceration and any two of the remaining criteria yields a sensitivity of 91% and a specificity of 96%.

PRELIMINARY CLASSIFICATION CRITERIA FOR ANTIPHOSPHOLIPID SYNDROME.[a]

Vascular thrombosis
(a) One or more clinical episodes of arterial, venous, or small vessel thrombosis in any tissue or organ *and*
(b) Thrombosis confirmed by imaging or Doppler studies or histopathology, with the exception of superficial venous thrombosis *and*
(c) For histopathologic confirmation, thrombosis present without significant evidence of inflammation in the vessel wall.

Pregnancy morbidity
(a) One or more unexplained deaths of a morphologically normal fetus at or beyond the 10th week of gestation, with normal fetal morphology documented by ultrasound or by direct examination of the fetus *or*
(b) One or more premature births of a morphologically normal neonate at or before the 34th week of gestation because of severe pre-eclampsia or severe placental insufficiency *or*
(c) Three or more unexplained consecutive spontaneous abortions before the 10th week of gestation, with maternal anatomic or hormonal abnormalities and paternal and maternal chromosomal causes excluded.

Laboratory criteria
(a) Anticardiolipin antibody of IgG and/or IgM isotype in blood, present in medium or high titer on two or more occasions at least 6 weeks apart, measured by standard enzyme-linked immunosorbent assay for beta$_2$ glycoprotein I–dependent anticardiolipin antibodies *or*
(b) Lupus anticoagulant present in plasma on two or more occasions at least 6 weeks apart, detected according to the guidelines of the International Society on Thrombosis and Hemostasis.

SOURCE: Adapted from Wilson WA, Gharavi AE. Koike T, et al. International consensus statement on preliminary classification criteria for definite antiphospholipid syndrome. Report of an International Workshop. Arthritis Rheum 1999;42:1309–1311 with permission of the American College of Rheumatology.
[a] Definite APS is considered to be present if at least one of the clinical and one of the laboratory criteria are met.

WORLD HEALTH ORGANIZATION CRITERIA FOR THE DIAGNOSIS OF OSTEOPENIA AND OSTEOPOROSIS.

Normal	BMC or BMD not more than 1 standard deviation below peak adult bone mass T score >-1
Osteopenia	BMC or BMD that lies between 1 and 2.5 standard deviations below peak adult bone mass T score between -1 and -2.5
Osteoporosis	BMC or BMD value more than 2.5 standard deviations below peak adult bone mass T score $\leq$-2.5
Severe Osteoporosis	BMC or BMD value more than 2.5 standard deviations below peak adult bone mass and the presence of one or more fragility fractures T score $\leq$-2.5 plus fragility fracture

SOURCE: Adapted from Assessment of fracture risk and its application to screening for postmenopausal osteoporosis. Report of a WHO study group. World Health Organ Techn Rep Ser 1994;843:1–129.
[a]World Health Organization criteria for the diagnosis of osteoporosis based on bone mineral content (BMC) or bone mineral density (BMD) measurements. These criteria can be applied to either the central or peripheral skeletal measurement sites.

CRITERIA FOR THE DIAGNOSIS OF JUVENILE RHEUMATOID ARTHRITIS (JRA).

I. General

The JRA Criteria Subcommittee in 1982 reviewed the 1977 Criteria (1) and recommended that *juvenile rheumatoid arthritis* be the name for the principal form of chronic arthritic disease in children and that this general class should be classified into three onset subtypes: systemic, polyarticular, and pauciarticular. The onset subtypes may be further subclassified into subsets as indicated below. The following classification enumerates the requirements for the diagnosis of JRA and the three clinical onset subtypes and lists subsets of each subtype that may be useful in further classification.

II. General criteria for the diagnosis of juvenile rheumatoid arthritis
   A. Persistent arthritis of at least 6 weeks' duration in one or more joints
   B. Exclusion of other causes of arthritis (see list of exclusions)

III. JRA onset subtypes

The onset subtype is determined by manifestations during the first 6 months of disease and remains the principal classification, although manifestations more closely resembling another subtype may appear later.
   A. Systemic onset JRA: This subtype is defined as JRA with persistent intermittent fever (daily intermittent temperatures to 103°F or more) with or without rheumatoid rash or other organ involvement. Typical fever and rash will be considered probable systemic onset JRA if not associated with arthritis. Before a definite diagnosis can be made, arthritis, as defined, must be present.
   B. Pauciarticular onset JRA: This subtype is defined as JRA with arthritis in four or fewer joints during the first 6 months of disease. Patients with systemic onset JRA are excluded from this onset subtype.
   C. Polyarticular JRA: This subtype is defined as JRA with arthritis in five or more joints during the first 6 months of disease. Patients with systemic JRA onset are excluded from this subtype.
   D. The onset subtypes may include the following subsets:
      1. Systemic onset
         a. Polyarthritis
         b. Oligoarthritis
      2. Oligoarthritis (pauciarticular onset)
         a. Antinuclear antibody (ANA)–positive chronic uveitis
         b. Rheumatoid factor (RF) positive
         c. Seronegative, B27 positive
         d. Not otherwise classified
      3. Polyarthritis
         a. RF positivity
         b. Not otherwise classified

IV. Exclusions
   A. Other rheumatic diseases
      1. Rheumatic fever
      2. Systemic lupus erythematosus
      3. Ankylosing spondylitis
      4. Polymyositis or dermatomyositis
      5. Vasculitic syndromes
      6. Scleroderma
      7. Psoriatic arthritis
      8. Reiter's syndrome
      9. Sjögren's syndrome
      10. Mixed connective tissue disease
      11. Behçet's syndrome

(continued)

CRITERIA FOR THE DIAGNOSIS OF JUVENILE RHEUMATOID ARTHRITIS (JRA). (*continued*)

IV. Exclusions
- B. Infectious arthritis
- C. Inflammatory bowel disease
- D. Neoplastic diseases including leukemia
- E. Nonrheumatic conditions of bones and joints
- F. Hematologic diseases
- G. Psychogenic arthralgia
- H. Miscellaneous
    1. Sarcoidosis
    2. Hypertrophic osteoarthropathy
    3. Villonodular synovitis
    4. Chronic active hepatitis
    5. Familial Mediterranean fever

V. Other proposed terminology

Juvenile chronic arthritis (JCA) and juvenile arthritis (JA) are new diagnostic terms currently in use in some places for the arthritides of childhood. The diagnoses of JCA and JA are not equivalent to each other, nor to the older diagnosis of juvenile rheumatoid arthritis or Still's disease. Hence reports of studies of JCA or JA cannot be directly compared with one another nor to reports of JRA or Still's disease. Juvenile chronic arthritis is described in more detail in a report of the European Conference on the Rheumatic Diseases of Children (2) and juvenile arthritis in the report of the Ross Conference (3).

1. JRA Criteria Subcommittee of the Diagnostic and Therapeutic Criteria Committee of the American Rheumatism Association. Current proposed revisions of the JRA criteria. Arthritis Rheum 1977;20(Suppl):195–199.
2. Ansell BW. Chronic arthritis in childhood. Ann Rheum Dis 1978;37:107–120.
3. Fink CW. Keynote address: Arthritis in childhood. Report of the 80th Ross Conference in Pediatric Research. Columbus, OH: Ross Laboratories; 1979:1–2.

Guidelines for the Management of Rheumatic Diseases

Practice guidelines represent a recent and important development in rheumatology. Guidelines, which are developed by a panel of experts, address a broad range of clinical issues from the approach to diagnosis of musculoskeletal signs and symptoms to patient management. Guidelines provide a framework for clinical practice and serve a valuable educational function for students of the rheumatic diseases. Moreover, because in very few instances have guidelines been tested in clinical settings, they present an opportunity to study whether they result in efficiencies or improvements in diagnosis and patient management.

INITIAL EVALUATION OF THE ADULT PATIENT WITH ACUTE MUSCULOSKELETAL SYMPTOMS.

FEATURE	DIFFERENTIAL DIAGNOSIS
History of significant trauma	Soft tissue injury, internal derangement, or fracture
Hot, swollen joint	Infection, systemic rheumatic disease, gout, pseudogout
Constitutional signs and symptoms (e.g., fever, weight loss, malaise)	Infection, sepsis, systemic rheumatic disease
Weakness	
Focal	Focal nerve lesion (compartment syndrome, entrapment neuropathy, mononeuritis multiplex, motor neuron disease, radiculopathy[a])
Diffuse	Myositis, metabolic myopathy, paraneoplastic syndrome, degenerative neuromuscular disorder, toxin, myelopathy,[a] transverse myelitis
Neurogenic pain (burning, numbness, paresthesia)	
Asymmetric	Radiculopathy,[a] reflex sympathetic dystrophy, entrapment neuropathy
Symmetric	Myelopathy,[a] peripheral neuropathy
Claudication pain pattern	Peripheral vascular disease, giant cell arteritis (jaw pain), lumbar spinal stenosis

SOURCE: Reprinted from American College of Rheumatology Ad Hoc Committee on Clinical Guidelines: guidelines for the initial evaluation of the adult patient with acute musculoskeletal symptoms. Arthritis Rheum 1996;39:1–8, with permission of the American College of Rheumatology.
[a] Radiculopathy and myelopathy may be due to infectious, neoplastic, or mechanical processes.

RECOMMENDED MONITORING STRATEGIES FOR DRUG TREATMENT OF RHEUMATOID ARTHRITIS.[a]

DRUGS	TOXICITIES REQUIRING MONITORING[b]	MONITORING BASELINE EVALUATION	SYSTEM REVIEW/EXAMINATION	LABORATORY
Salicylates, nonsteroidal anti-inflammatory drugs	Gastrointestinal ulceration and bleeding	CBC, creatinine, AST, ALT	Dark/black stool, dyspepsia, nausea or vomiting, abdominal pain, edema, shortness of breath	CBC yearly, LFTs, creatinine testing may be required[c]
Hydroxychloroquine	Macular damage	None unless patient is over age 40 or has previous eye disease	Visual changes, funduscopic and visual fields every 6–12 months	–

(continued)

RECOMMENDED MONITORING STRATEGIES FOR DRUG TREATMENT OF RHEUMATOID ARTHRITIS.[a] (*continued*)

DRUGS	TOXICITIES REQUIRING MONITORING[b]	MONITORING BASELINE EVALUATION	SYSTEM REVIEW/EXAMINATION	LABORATORY
Sulfasalazine	Myelosuppression	CBC, and AST or ALT in patients at risk, G6PD	Symptoms of myelosuppression,[d] photosensitivity, rash	CBC every 2–4 weeks for first 3 months, then every 3 months
Methotrexate	Myelosuppression, hepatic fibrosis, cirrhosis, pulmonary infiltrates or fibrosis	CBC, chest radiography within past year, hepatitis B and C serology in high-risk patients, AST or ALT, albumin, alkaline phosphatase, and creatinine	Symptoms of myelosuppression,[d] shortness of breath, nausea/vomiting, lymph node swelling	CBC, platelet count, AST, albumin, creatinine every 4–8 weeks
Gold, intramuscular	Myelosuppression, proteinuria	CBC, platelet count, creatinine, urine dipstick for protein	Symptoms of myelosuppression,[d] edema, rash, oral ulcers, diarrhea	CBC, platelet count, urine dipstick every 1–2 weeks for first 20 weeks, then at the time of each (or every other) injection
Gold, oral	Myelosuppression, proteinuria	CBC, platelet count, urine dipstick for protein	Symptoms of myelosuppression,[d] edema, rash, diarrhea	CBC platelet count, urine dipstick for protein every 4–12 weeks
D-penicillamine	Myelosuppression, proteinuria	CBC, platelet count, creatinine, urine dipstick for protein	Symptoms of myelosuppression[d], edema, rash	CBC, urine dipstick for protein every 2 weeks until dosage stable, then every 1–3 months
Azathioprine	Myelosuppression, hepatotoxicity, lymphoproliferative disorders	CBC, platelet count, creatinine, AST or ALT	Symptoms of myelosuppression[d]	CBC and platelet count every 1–2 weeks with changes in dosage, and every 1–3 months thereafter
Corticosteroids (oral ≤ 10 mg of prednisone or equivalent)	Hypertension, hyperglycemia	BP, chemistry panel, bone densitometry in high-risk patients	BP at each visit, polyuria, polydipsia, edema, shortness of breath, visual changes, weight gain	Urinalysis for glucose yearly

Agents for refractory RA or severe extra-articular complications

DRUGS	TOXICITIES REQUIRING MONITORING[b]	MONITORING BASELINE EVALUATION	SYSTEM REVIEW/EXAMINATION	LABORATORY
Cyclophosphamide	Myelosuppression, myeloproliferative disorders, malignancy, hemorrhagic cystitis	CBC, platelet count, urinalysis, creatinine, AST or ALT	Symptoms of myelosuppression,[d] hematuria	CBC and platelet count every 1–2 weeks with changes in dosage, and every 1–3 months thereafter, urinalysis and urine cytology every 6–12 months after cessation
Chlorambucil	Myelosuppression, myeloproliferative disorders, malignancy	CBC, urinalysis, creatinine, AST or ALT	Symptoms of myelosuppression[d]	CBC and platelet count every 1–2 weeks with changes in dosage, and every 1–3 months thereafter
Cyclosporin A	Renal insufficiency, anemia, hypertension	CBC, creatinine, uric acid, LFTs, BP	Edema, BP every 2 weeks until dosage stable, then monthly	Creatinine every 2 weeks until dose is stable, then monthly; periodic CBC, potassium, and LFTs

ANTIRHEUMATIC DRUG THERAPY IN PREGNANCY AND LACTATION, AND EFFECTS ON FERTILITY.

DRUG	FDA USE-IN-PREGNANCY RATING[a]	CROSSES PLACENTA	MAJOR MATERNAL TOXICITIES	FETAL TOXICITIES	LACTATION	FERTILITY
Aspirin	C; D in third trimester	Yes	Anemia, peripartum hemorrhage, prolonged labor	Premature closure of ductus, pulmonary hypertension, ICH	Use cautiously; excreted at low concentration; doses >1 tablet (325 mg) result in high concentration in infant plasma	No data
NSAIDs	B; D in third trimester	Yes	As for aspirin	As for aspirin	Compatible according to AAP	No data
Corticosteroids Prednisone	B	Dexamethasone and beta-methasone	Exacerbation of diabetes and hypertension, PROM	IUGR	5% to 20% of maternal dose excreted in breast milk; compatible, but wait 4 hours if dose >20 mg	
Dexamethasone	C	As above				
Hydroxychloroquine	C	Yes: fetal concentration 50% of maternal	Few	Few	Contraindicated (slow elimination rate, potential for accumulation)	No data
Gold	C	Yes	No data	1 report of cleft palate and severe CNS abnormalities	Excreted into breast milk (20% of maternal dose); rash, hepatitis, and hematologic abnormalities reported, but AAP considers it compatible	No data
D-penicillamine	D	Yes	No data	Cutis laxa connective tissue abnormalities	No data	No data
Sulfasalazine	B; D if near term	Yes	No data	No increase in congenital malformation, kernicterus if administered near term	Excreted into breast milk (40% to 60% maternal dose); bloody diarrhea in 1 infant; AAP recommends caution	Females: no effect; males: significant oligospermia (2 months to return to normal)
Azathioprine	D	Yes	No data	IUGR (rate up to 40%) and prematurity, transient immunosuppression in neonate, possible effect on germlines of offspring	No data; hypothetical risk of immunosuppression outweighs benefit	Not studied; can interfere with effectiveness of IUD

(continued)

APPENDIX II

ANTIRHEUMATIC DRUG THERAPY IN PREGNANCY AND LACTATION, AND EFFECTS ON FERTILITY. (*continued*)

DRUG	FDA USE-IN-PREGNANCY RATING[a]	CROSSES PLACENTA	MAJOR MATERNAL TOXICITIES	FETAL TOXICITIES	LACTATION	FERTILITY
Chlorambucil	D	Teratogenic effects potentiated by caffeine	No data	Renal angiogenesis	Contraindicated	No data
Methotrexate	X	No data	Spontaneous abortion	Fetal abnormalities (including cleft palate and hydrocephalus)	Contraindicated; small amounts excreted with potential to accumulate in fetal tissues	Females: Infrequent long-term effect; males: reversible oligospermia
Cyclophosphamide	D	Yes: 25% of maternal level	No data	Severe abnor- malities; case report: male twin devel- oped papillary cancer at 11 years and neuroblas- toma at 14 years	Contraindicated; has caused bone marrow depression	Females: age >25 years, concurrent radiation, and prolonged exposure increase risk of infertility; males: dose- dependent oligospermia and azoosper- mia regardless of age or exposure
Cyclosporin A	C	Yes	No data	IUGR and prematurity; 1 case report: hypoplasia of right leg; not an animal teratogen and unlikely to be a human one	Contraindicated due to potential for immunosuppression	No data

SOURCE: Reprinted from American College of Rheumatology Ad Hoc Committee on Clinical Guidelines. Guidelines for monitoring drug therapy in rheumatoid arthritis. Arthritis Rheum 1996;39:723–731, with permission of the American College of Rheumatology.

ABBREVIATIONS: AAP, American Academy of Pediatrics; CNS, central nervous system; ICH, intracranial hemorrhage; IUD, intrauterine device; IUGR, intrauterine growth retardation; PROM, premature rupture of membranes.

[a] Food and Drug Administration (FDA) use-in-pregnancy ratings are as follows: A, controlled studies show no risk. Adequate, well-controlled studies in pregnant women have failed to demonstrate risk to the fetus. B, No evidence of risk in humans. Either animal findings show risk but human findings do not, or, if no adequate human studies have been performed, animal findings are negative. C, Risk cannot be ruled out. Human studies are lacking and results of animal studies are either positive for fetal risk or lacking as well. However, potential benefits may justify the potential risk. D, Positive evidence of risk. Investigational or post-marketing data show risk to the fetus. Nevertheless, potential benefits may outweigh the potential risk. X, Contraindicated in pregnancy. Studies in animals or humans, or investigational or postmarketing reports, have shown fetal risk which clearly outweighs any possible benefit to the patient.

MONITORING DRUG THERAPY IN SYSTEMIC LUPUS ERYTHEMATOSUS.

DRUG	TOXICITIES REQUIRING MONITORING	MONITORING		
		Baseline evaluation	System review	Laboratory
Salicylates, NSAIDs	Gastrointestinal bleeding, hepatic toxicity, renal toxicity, hypertension	CBC, creatinine, urinalysis, AST, ALT	Dark/black stool, dyspepsia, nausea/vomiting, abdominal pain, shortness of breath, edema	CBC yearly, creatinine yearly
Glucocorticoids	Hypertension, hyperglycemia, hyperlipidemia, hypokalemia, osteoporosis, avascular necrosis, cataract, weight gain, infections, fluid retention	BP, bone densitometry, glucose, potassium, cholesterol, triglycerides (HDL, LDL)	Polyuria, polydipsia, edema, shortness of breath, BP at each visit, visual changes, bone pain	Urinary dipstick for glucose every 3–6 months, total cholesterol yearly, bone densitometry yearly to assess osteoporosis
Hydroxychloroquine	Macular damage	None unless patient is over 40 years of age or has previous eye disease	Visual changes	Fundoscopic and visual fields every 6–12 months
Azathioprine	Myelosuppression, hepatotoxicity, lymphoproliferative disorders	CBC, platelet count, creatinine, AST or ALT	Symptoms of myelosuppression	CBC and platelet count every 1–2 weeks with changes in dose (every 1–3 months thereafter), AST yearly, Pap test at regular intervals
Cyclophosphamide	Myelosuppression, myeloproliferative disorders, malignancy, immunosuppression, hemorrhagic cystitis, secondary infertility	CBC and differential and platelet count, urinalysis	Symptoms of myelosuppression, hematuria, infertility	CBC and urinalysis monthly, urine cytology and Pap test yearly for life
Methotrexate	Myelosuppression, hepatic fibrosis, cirrhosis, pulmonary infiltrates, fibrosis	CBC, chest radiograph within past year, hepatitis B and C serology in high-risk patients, AST, albumin, bilirubin, creatinine	Symptoms of myelosuppression, shortness of breath, nausea/vomiting, oral ulcer	CBC and platelet count, AST or ALT, and albumin every 4–8 weeks, serum creatinine, urinalysis

SOURCE: Reproduced from Guidelines for referral and management of systemic lupus erythematosus in adults. Arthritis Rheum 1999;42:1785–1796, with permission of the American College of Rheumatology.
ABBREVIATIONS: ALT, alanine transaminase; AST, aspartate transaminase; BP, blood pressure; CBC, complete blood cell count; HDL, high-density lipoprotein; LDL, low-density lipoprotein; Pap, Papanicolaou.

APPENDIX II

GUIDELINES FOR CLINICAL USE OF THE ANTINUCLEAR ANTIBODY TEST: CONDITIONS ASSOCIATED WITH POSITIVE IF-ANA TEST RESULTS.[a]

DISEASE	FREQUENCY OF POSITIVE ANA RESULT (%)
Diseases for which an ANA test is very useful for diagnosis	
SLE	95–100
Systemic sclerosis (scleroderma)	60–80
Diseases for which an ANA test is somewhat useful for diagnosis	
Sjögren's syndrome	40–70
Idiopathic inflammatory myositis (dermatomyositis or polymyositis)	30–80
Diseases for which an ANA test is useful for monitoring or prognosis	
Juvenile chronic oligoarticular arthritis with uveitis	20–50
Raynaud's phenomenon	20–60
Conditions in which a positive ANA test result is an intrinsic part of the diagnostic criteria	
Drug-induced SLE	~100
Autoimmune hepatic disease	~100
MCTD	~100
Diseases for which an ANA test is not useful in diagnosis	
Rheumatoid arthritis	30–50
Multiple sclerosis	25
Idiopathic thrombocytopenic purpura	10–30
Thyroid disease	30–50
Discoid lupus	5–25
Infectious diseases	Varies widely
Malignancies	Varies widely
Patients with silicone breast implants	15–25
Fibromyalgia	15–25
Relatives of patients with autoimmune diseases (SLE or scleroderma)	5–25
Normal persons[a]	
≥1:40	20–30
≥1:80	10–12
≥1:160	5
≥1:320	3

ABBREVIATIONS: ANA, antinuclear antibody; IF, immunofluorescent; MCTD, mixed connective tissue disease; SLE, systemic lupus erythematosus.
[a] Values are titers. Prevalence of positive ANA test result varies with titer. Female sex and increasing age tend to be more commonly associated with positive ANA.

FLOW CHART FOR CLINICAL ANTINUCLEAR ANTIBODY TESTING.

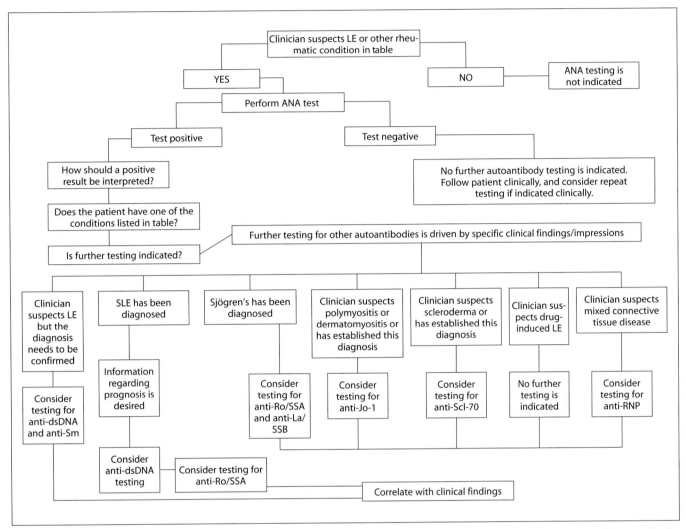

SOURCE: Reprinted from Kavanaugh A, Tomar R, Reveille J, et al. Guidelines for clinical use of the antinuclear antibody test and tests for specific autoantibodies to nuclear antigens. Arch Pathol Lab Med 2000;124:71–81, with permission of the College of American Pathologists.
ABBREVIATIONS: LE, lupus erythematosus; RNP, ribonucleoprotein.

RECOMMENDATIONS FOR THE MEDICAL MANAGEMENT OF OSTEOARTHRITIS OF THE HIP AND KNEE.

Nonpharmacologic therapy for patients with osteoarthritis
Patient education
Self-management programs (e.g., Arthritis Foundation Self-Management Program)
Personalized social support through telephone contact
Weight loss (if overweight)
Aerobic exercise programs
Physical therapy
Range-of-motion exercises
Muscle-strengthening exercises
Assistive devices for ambulation
Patellar taping
Appropriate footwear
Lateral-wedged insoles (for genu varum)
Bracing
Occupational therapy
Joint protection and energy conservation
Assistive devices for activities of daily living

Pharmacologic therapy for patients with osteoarthritis[a]
ORAL
   Acetaminophen
   COX-2–specific inhibitor
   Nonselective NSAID plus misoprostol or a proton pump inhibitor[b]
   Nonacetylated salicylate
   Other pure analgesics
      Tramadol
      Opioids
INTRA-ARTICULAR
   Glucocorticoids
   Hyaluronan
   Topical
      Capsaicin
      Methylsalicylate

SOURCE: Reprinted from American College of Rheumatology Subcommittee on Osteoarthritis Guidelines. Recommendations for the medical management of osteoarthritis of the hip and knee. Arthritis Rheum 2000;43:1905–1915, with permission of the American College of Rheumatology.
ABBREVIATIONS: COX-2, cyclooxygenase-2; NSAID, nonsteroidal anti-inflammatory drug.
[a] The choice of agent(s) should be individualized for each patient.
[b] Misoprostol and proton pump inhibitors are recommended in patients who are at increased risk for upper gastrointestinal adverse events.

RECOMMENDATIONS FOR THE PREVENTION AND TREATMENT OF GLUCOCORTICOID-INDUCED OSTEOPOROSIS.

Patient beginning therapy with glucocortocoid (prednisone equivalents of ≥5 mg/day) with plans for treatment duration of ≥3 months
Modify lifestyle risk factors for osteoporosis
   Smoking cessation or avoidance
   Reduction of alcohol consumption if excessive
Instruct in weight-bearing physical exercise
Initiate calcium supplementation
Initiate supplementation with vitamin D (plain or activated form)
Prescribe bisphosphonate (use with caution in premenopausal women)

Patient receiving long-term glucocorticoid therapy (prednisone equivalent of ≥5 mg/day)
Modify lifestyle risk factors for osteoporosis
   Smoking cessation or avoidance
   Reduction of alcohol consumption if excessive
Instruct in weight-bearing physical exercise
Initiate calcium supplementation
Initiate supplementation with vitamin D (plain or activated form)
Prescribe treatment to replace gonadal sex hormones if deficient or otherwise clinically indicated
Measure bone mineral density (BMD) at lumbar spine and/or hip
If BMD is not normal (i.e., T score below −1), then
   Prescribe bisphosphonate (use with caution in premenopausal women)
   Consider calcitonin as second-line agent if patient has contraindication to or does not tolerate bisphosphonate therapy
If BMD is normal, follow-up and repeat BMD measurement either annually or biannually.

SOURCE: Reprinted from American College of Rheumatology Ad Hoc Committee on Glucocorticoid-Induced Osteoporosis. Recommendations for the prevention and treatment of glucocorticoid-induced osteoporosis. 2001 update. Arthritis Rheum 2001;44:1496–1503, with permission of the American College of Rheumatology.

Supplement and Vitamin and Mineral Guide

SUPPLEMENTS

Originally published in *Arthritis Today*, September–October 2006, reprinted by permission of the Arthritis Foundation.

Supplements by Condition or Symptom

Cartilage Degeneration: ASU, Chondroitin, Glucosamine, SAM-e

Decreased Mobility: Chondroitin, DMSO, Flax, GLA, Glucosamine, Indian frankincense, MSM, SAM-e

Depression: St. John's wort, SAM-e

Inflammation: Bromelain, Cat's claw, Chondroitin, Devil's claw, DMSO, Fish oil, Flax, Ginger; GLA, MSM, SAM-e, Stinging nettle, Thunder god vine, Turmeric

Pain: Bromelain, Chondroitin, Devil's claw, DMSO, Ginger, GLA, Glucosamine, Indian frankincense, MSM, SAM-e, Stinging nettle, Thunder god vine, Turmeric

Sleep Difficulties: Melatonin, Valerian

Ankylosing spondylitis: DHEA, Melatonin

Fibromyalgia: SAM-e, St. John's wort, Valerian

Gout: Devil's claw, Stinging nettle

Lupus: DHEA, Fish oil, Flax, Thunder god vine

Osteoarthritis (OA): ASU, Bromelain, Cat's claw, Chondroitin, Devil's claw, DMSO, Ginger; Glucosamine, Indian frankincense, MSM, SAM-e, Stinging nettle, Turmeric

Psoriasis: Fish oil

Raynaud's phenomenon: Evening primrose, Flax, Ginger, Ginkgo, GLA

Rheumatoid arthritis (RA): Black currant oil (or seed), Borage oil (or seed), Bromelain, DMSO, Evening primrose, Fish oil, Flax oil (or seed), Ginger, GLA, Indian frankincense/boswellia, Thunder god vine, Turmeric

Scleroderma: DMSO

Sjögren's Syndrome: GLA

ASU (Avocado Soybean Unsaponifiables)

Origin: A natural vegetable extract made from avocado and soybean oils.
Dosage: Softgel; take 300 mg daily.
Claims: Slows the progression of osteoarthritis (OA).

Black Currant Oil (*Ribes nigrum*; see GLA)

Origin: Black currant seed oil is obtained from seeds of the black currant. Black currant seed oil contains 15% to 20% gamma-linolenic acid (GLA). Do not confuse with black currant berry.
Dosage: Liquid and capsules; typical dosage ranges from 360 mg to 3000 mg daily.

Caution: Black currant oil may increase immune response in elderly.

Borage Oil (*Borago officinalis*; see GLA)

Origin: Oil from the seeds of the borage plant. Borage seed oil contains about 20% to 26% GLA.
Dosage: Liquid and capsules; take 1300 mg (oil) daily.

Boswellia

See Indian Frankincense

Bromelain (Pineapple, *Ananas comosus*)

Origin: Group of enzymes found in pineapple that break down protein.
Dosage: Capsules and tablets; take 500 to 2000 mg three times a day between meals.
Claims: Decreases pain and swelling of rheumatoid arthritis (RA) and OA, and increases mobility.

Caution: Bromelain can cause stomach upset and diarrhea and should be avoided if the patient is allergic to pineapples. It can also increase the effect of blood-thinning medicine.

Cat's Claw (*Uncaria tomentosa*)

Origin: Dried root bark of a woody vine that grows in the Amazon rain forests in Peru and other South American countries.

Dosage: Capsules, tablets, liquid, and tea bags; 250 to 1000 mg daily. Buy only products that contain *Uncaria tomentosa*. Another plant (*Acacia greggi*), which also has the name cat's claw, is highly toxic.

Claims: Believed to have anti-inflammatory properties; may stimulate immune system.

Caution: Cat's claw can cause headache, dizziness, and vomiting, and can lower blood pressure, should be avoided with anti-hypertensive medications or blood thinners.

Chondroitin Sulfate

Origin: Chondroitin is a component of human connective tissues found in cartilage and bone. In supplements, chondroitin sulfate usually comes from bovine trachea or pork byproducts.

Dosage: Capsules, tablets, and powder; 800 to 1200 mg daily in two to four divided doses. Often combined with glucosamine. Allow up to 1 month to notice effect.

Claims: Reduces pain and inflammation, improves joint function and slows progression of OA.

Caution: Some chondroitin tablets may contain high levels of manganese, which may be problematic with long-term use. Because chondroitin is made from bovine products, there is the remote possibility of contamination associated with mad cow disease. Chondroitin taken with blood-thinning medications or NSAIDs may increase the risk of bleeding. In patients who are allergic to sulfonamides, start with a low dose of chondroitin sulfate and watch for any side effects. Other side effects include diarrhea, constipation, and abdominal pain.

Curcumin

See Turmeric

Devil's Claw (Also known as Devil's Claw Root, Grapple Plant or Wood Spider; *Harpagophytum procumbens*)

Origin: A traditional herb used in South Africa.

Dosage: Capsules, tincture, powder, and liquid; take 750 to 1000 mg three times a day.

Claims: Relieves pain and inflammation. May help lower uric acid levels in people with gout. Acts as a digestive aid and appetite stimulant.

Caution: Devil's claw should not be taken in patients who are pregnant, have gallstones or ulcers, or are taking an antacid or blood thinners. It can affect heart rate and may interfere with cardiac, blood-thinning, and diabetes medications. It may also cause diarrhea.

DHEA (Dehydroepiandrosterone)

Origin: An androgen steroid hormone naturally produced in the body by the adrenal glands. Do not confuse 7-Keto DHEA with DHEA.

Dosage: Capsule and tablets available both as prescription (200 mg) and nonprescription (10, 15, or 25 mg) products; typically 200 mg for lupus. Effects of long-term use are unknown.

Claims: Helps control lupus flares; increases the blood level of DHEA.

Caution: DHEA side effects include stomach upset, abdominal pain, and high blood pressure, as well as acne. It also decreases levels of good cholesterol (high-density lipoprotein, or HDL) and may cause facial hair growth, voice deepening, and changes in menstrual pattern. DHEA can also increase insulin resistance for people with diabetes, and exacerbate liver disease. Use is contraindicated in men with prostate cancer and women with uterine fibroids.

DMSO (Dimethyl Sulfoxide; see MSM)

Origin: A colorless, sulfur-containing organic byproduct of wood pulp processing.

Dosage: Cream, gel; topically, 25% DMSO solution; take internally, only if prescribed by a physician.

Claims: Relieves pain and inflammation, improves joint mobility in OA, RA, juvenile rheumatoid arthritis (JRA), and scleroderma, and manages amyloidosis. Increases blood flow to skin.

Studies: Controlled studies as a topical application for DMSO and OA have yielded conflicting results. Few human studies.

Caution: Side effects of DMSO taken internally include headache, dizziness, drowsiness, nausea, vomiting, diarrhea, constipation, and anorexia. Topical DMSO also can cause skin irritation and dermatitis. Avoid in patients with diabetes, asthma, or liver, kidney, or heart conditions. Never take industrial-grade DMSO. Wash off any lotions or skin products before applying DMSO.

Evening Primrose (Also known as Evening Primrose Oil or Primrose; *Oenothera biennis* and other *Oenothera* species; see GLA)

Origin: The seeds of a native American wildflower, containing 7% to 10% gamma-linolenic acid (GLA).

Dosage: Capsules, oil, and softgel; generally five 500-mg capsules per day. For RA, 540 mg daily to 2.8 g daily in divided doses. Evening primrose oil may take up to 6 months to work.

Fish Oil

Origin: Oil from cold-water fish such as mackerel, salmon, herring, tuna, halibut, and cod.

Dosage: Fish, capsules, or chewable tablets. For general health, two 3-ounce servings of fish a week are recommended. However, it's difficult to get a therapeutic dose of fish oil from food alone. To treat arthritis-related conditions, use fish oil capsules with at least 30% EPA/DHA, the active ingredients. For lupus and psoriasis, 2 g EPA/DHA three times a day. For Raynaud's phenomenon, 1 g four times a day. For RA, up to 2.6 g fish oil (1 .6 g EPA) twice a day.

Claims: Reduces inflammation and morning stiffness. Treats RA, lupus, psoriasis, depression, and Raynaud's phenomenon. Important for brain function and may inhibit RA development.

Studies: An analysis of nine studies of people with RA taking omega 3 showed a reduction in the number of tender joints but no reduction in joint damage. In six studies, people with RA were able to reduce their dosages of NSAIDs or corticosteroids. A 2005 study of people with RA showed enhanced positive effects when fish oil supplements were used in combination with olive oil.

Caution: Women who are pregnant or hoping to conceive should avoid shark, swordfish, king mackerel, and tilefish, and should eat no more than 8 ounces of albacore tuna each month, due to potentially dangerous levels of mercury. Fish oil supplements at normal doses are safe. Look for brands that follow good manufacturing practices and contain fish oils without mercury.

Flaxseed (Flax, Raxseed Oil, Linseed Oil; *Linum usitatissimum*)

Origin: Seed of the flax plant, containing omega 3 and omega 6 fatty acids and lignans (beneficial plant compounds, similar to fiber).

Dosage: Whole seeds, ground meal or flour, capsules, or oil. Whole seeds must be ground into meal or flour; 30 g (1 ounce) daily. Capsules, available in 1000 mg to 1300 mg, no typical dosage. Oil, 1 to 3 tablespoons daily.

Claims: Eases symptoms of RA, lupus, and Raynaud's phenomenon. Lubricates joints and lessens stiffness and joint pain. Lowers total cholesterol and reduces risk of heart disease and some types of cancer. Improves hot flashes and dry skin.

Caution: Fiber in flaxseed can impair absorption of some medications, and as flaxseed acts as a blood thinner, should be avoided in patients taking blood thinners, aspirin, or other NSAIDs. Flaxseed should be avoided in hormone-sensitive breast or uterine cancer, and used with caution with the use of hypercholesterolemia and cholesterol-lowering drugs.

Ginger (*Zingiber officinale*)

Origin: The dried or fresh root of the ginger plant.

Dosage: Powder, extract, tincture, capsules, and oils; up to 2 g in three divided doses per day or up to 4 cups of tea daily.

Claims: Decreases joint pain and reduces inflammation in people with OA and RA. Increases circulation in people with Raynaud's phenomenon.

Studies: A recent study showed that ginger extract inhibited inflammatory molecules, including TNF-alpha and cyclooxygenase-2 (COX-2). A 2005 study reinforced the anti-inflammatory effects of ginger. Another 2005 study showed ginger killed *Helicobacter pylori*, a bacterium that causes stomach ulcers.

Caution: Ginger can interfere with medications for blood thinning and should be avoided in the presence of gallstones.

Ginkgo (*Ginkgo biloba*)

Origin: Leaf of the ginkgo biloba tree, native to East Asia.

Dosage: Liquid, tablet, softgel, capsule, and extract; typically 120 mg to 240 mg extract daily. Choose supplements standardized to 5% to 7% terpene lactones and 24% flavonol glycosides, the active ingredients in ginkgo.

Claims: Increases blood flow and circulation in Raynaud's phenomenon and claudication.

Caution: Ginkgo's side effects include stomach upset, dizziness, or headaches. Avoid ginkgo with blood-thinning medication like aspirin, epilepsy, diabetes, or prior to surgery.

GLA (Gamma-Linolenic Acid)

Origin: A type of omega 6 fatty acid found in evening primrose oil, black currant oil, and borage oil.

Dosage: Capsules or oil; 2 g to 3 g daily.

Claims: Lessens joint pain, stiffness, and swelling associated with RA. Eases symptoms of Raynaud's phenomenon and Sjögren's syndromes.

Studies: One of the most promising studies was a placebo-controlled trial of 56 patients with active RA who received 2.8 g GLA for 6 months. Participants showed significant improvements related to joint pain, stiffness, and grip strength. GLA doses at this level were found to be safe and effective for RA. A 2005 study showed that people with Sjögren's syndrome who took GLA and linolenic acid had significant improvement in eye discomfort and tear production.

Glucosamine (Glucosamine sulfate, glucosamine hydrochloride, N-acetyl glucosamine)

Origin: Major component of joint cartilage. Supplements are derived from the shells of shellfish such as shrimp, lobster, and crab.

Dosage: Capsules, tablets, liquid, or powder (to be mixed into a drink); 1500 mg per day for all forms. Often combined with chondroitin. May take 1 month to notice effect.

Claims: Slows deterioration of cartilage, relieves OA pain, and improves joint mobility.

Studies: The NIH Glucosamine/Chondroitin Arthritis Intervention Trail (GAIT) concluded that glucosamine may be beneficial. The study of 1583 people with knee OA showed that the supplements were more effective when combined, but that they did not work significantly better than placebo or the NSAID celecoxib in people with mild pain. However, a subgroup of people in the study who had moderate-to-severe pain did show significant benefit, even more than with the NSAID. Half of the study participants will continue to be evaluated for 18 months to see if glucosamine and chondroitin can slow or stop the progression of knee OA. A 2005 Cochrane review of glucosamine analyzed the outcomes of 20 studies comprising 2570 patients. Glucosamine was found to be safe, but not superior to placebo in reducing pain and stiffness and improving function.

Caution: Glucosamine may cause mild stomach upset, nausea, heartburn, diarrhea, and constipation, as well as increased blood glucose, cholesterol, triglyceride, and blood pressure. Glucosamine should be avoided in individuals allergic to shellfish.

Indian Frankincense (Frankincense, Boswellia, Boswellin, Salai Guggal; *Boswellia serrata*)

Origin: Gum resin from the bark of the Boswellia tree found in India.

Dosage: Capsule or pill; typically 300 mg to 400 mg three times per day. Look for products with 60% boswellic acids, the active ingredient.

Claims: Reduces inflammation and treats RA, OA, and bursitis symptoms. Indian frankincense may treat symptoms of ulcerative colitis and Crohn's disease.

Studies: In a 2004 study, Indian frankincense was tested as a treatment for knee OA. Researchers recruited 30 people with knee OA and gave half the group a daily supplement containing 333 mg of Indian frankincense; others got placebo. People who took Indian frankincense reported less knee pain, better mobility, and an ability to walk longer distances than those taking placebo.

Melatonin

Origin: A hormone produced by the pineal gland, which is located at the base of the brain.

Dosage: Capsules or tablets; 1 mg to 5 mg at bedtime for insomnia, for no longer than 2 weeks.

Claims: Aids sleep and treats jet lag.

Studies: A systematic review of studies shows no evidence that melatonin effectively treats sleep disorders or is useful for altered sleep patterns, such as from shift work or jet lag. However, there is evidence that it is safe with short-term use. Another review of studies showed that melatonin reduced the onset of sleep by 4 minutes and increased the duration of sleep by nearly 13 minutes; another showed that people taking melatonin slept almost 30 minutes longer than people taking placebo.

Caution: Certain medications interact with melatonin, including NSAIDs, beta-blockers, antidepressants, diuretics, and vitamin B12 supplements. Melatonin should be avoided in patients with autoimmune disease, depression, kidney disease, epilepsy, heart disease, or leukemia.

MSM (Methylsulfonyfmethane)

Origin: Organic sulfur compound found naturally in fruits, vegetables, grains, animals, and humans.

Dosage: Tablets, liquid, capsule, or powder, topical and oral. Typically 1000 mg to 3000 mg daily with meals.

Claims: Reduces pain and inflammation.

Studies: A 2006 pilot study of 50 men and women with knee OA showed that 6000 mg of MSM improved symptoms of pain and physical function without major side effects. No large, well-controlled human studies have been performed.

Caution: MSM may cause stomach upset or diarrhea and should be avoided in patients taking blood thinners.

SAM-e (S-adenosyl-L-methionine)

Origin: A naturally occurring chemical in the body.
Dosage: Tablets; 600 mg to 1200 mg daily for OA; 1600 mg daily for depression. Because of possible interactions, SAM-e should not be taken without doctor's supervision.
Claims: Treats pain, stiffness, and joint swelling; improves mobility; rebuilds cartilage and eases symptoms of OA, fibromyalgia, bursitis, tendinitis, chronic low back pain, and depression.
Studies: Over the last two decades, multiple clinical trials involving thousands of people have shown SAM-e to improve joint health and treat OA. It has been found to be equal to NSAIDs in clinical studies. Most of this research has been done in Europe, where SAM-e is sold as a drug. A double-blind study of 61 adults with knee OA done in the United States shows that SAM-e had a slower onset of action but was as effective as celecoxib in reducing pain and improving joint function. A 2002 analysis of 14 SAM-e studies showed it is effective for reducing pain and improving mobility in people with OA.

Caution: High doses of SAM-e can cause flatulence, vomiting, diarrhea, headache, and nausea. SAM-e may interact with antidepressive medications and should be avoided in patients with bipolar disorder or who are taking monoamine oxidase inhibitors (MAOIs). It may also worsen Parkinson's disease.

St. John's Wort (*Hypericum perforatum*)

Origin: The yellow flower, leaves, and stem of the St. John's wort plant is native to Europe and grows wild in the United States.
Dosage: Extract in the form of powder (dried), liquid (10 to 60 drops one to four times per day) or tablet, capsules, and tea; extract, typically 900 mg daily.
Claims: Acts as an antidepressant drug and reduces inflammation and pain.
Studies: No scientific evidence shows that St. John's wort is effective for reducing inflammation. A Cochrane review of studies on St. John's wort for depression showed that current evidence is inconsistent. A study also found that the herb is not effective for social anxiety disorder.

Caution: Although St. John's wort taken alone is considered safe, it is potentially dangerous if taken with prescription antidepressants. St. John's wort can cause insomnia, restlessness, anxiety, irritability, stomach upset, fatigue, dry mouth, dizziness, or increased sensitivity to sunlight. It should be avoided in patients with Alzheimer's disease, human immunodeficiency (HIV) infection, depression, schizophrenia, infertility, or bipolar disorder. It may also reduce effectiveness of oral contraceptives.

Stinging Nettle (*Urtica dioica*)

Origin: The leaves and stem of the stinging nettle plant, a stalk-like plant found in the United States, Canada, and Europe.
Dosage: Tea, capsule, tablet, tincture, extract, or whole leaf; capsules, up to 1300 mg daily; tea, 1 cup, three times a day; tincture, 1 mL to 4 mL three times a day; nettle leaf applied directly to the skin.
Claims: Reduces inflammation, aches, and pains of OA.
Studies: A German study shows that hox alpha, a new extract of stinging nettle leaf, contains an anti-inflammatory substance that suppressed several cytokines in inflammatory joint diseases. In a Turkish study, stinging nettle extract showed antimicrobial effects against nine microorganisms, as well as anti-ulcer and analgesic activity. Stinging nettle root extract combined with sabal fruit extract was shown to be superior to placebo for treating prostate hyperplasia (a precancerous condition), and was well tolerated.

Caution: Nettle may interfere with blood thinners, diabetes, and heart medications, and lower blood pressure.

Thunder God Vine (*Tripterygium wilfordii*)

Origin: Root of a vinelike plant from Asia.
Dosage: Extract; 30 mg daily.
Claims: Reduces pain and inflammation and treats symptoms of RA, lupus, and other autoimmune diseases.
Studies: A 2006 review of randomized clinical trials shows that thunder god vine improved symptoms of RA but serious side effects occurred.

Caution: This root can cause stomach upset, skin reactions, temporary infertility in men, and amenorrhea in women. It should not be used in patients taking immunosuppressive drugs or prednisone.

Tumeric (*Curcuma longa, Curcuma domestica*)

Origin: A yellow-colored powder ground from the roots of the lilylike turmeric plant. It is a common ingredient in curry powder. The turmeric plant grows in India and Indonesia and is related to the ginger family.

APPENDIX III

Dosage: Capsules or spice. Capsule, typically 400 mg to 600 mg three times per day; or 0.5 g to 1 g of powdered root up to 3 g per day.
Claims: Reduces pain, inflammation, and stiffness related to RA and OA; treats bursitis. Known as a cleansing agent, tumeric often is used as a digestive aid in India.
Studies: Several recent studies show that curcumin or turmeric has anti-inflammatory properties and modifies immune system responses. A 2006 study showed turmeric was more effective at preventing joint inflammation than reducing joint inflammation.

Caution: High doses of turmeric can act as a blood thinner and cause stomach upset. It should be avoided in patients with gallstones or who are taking blood-thinning medications.

Valerian (*Valeriana officianalis*)

Origin: The dried root of the perennial herb valerian.
Dosage: Capsules, tablets, tincture, softgel, or tea; 300 mg to 500 mg of valerian extract daily (maximum dose is 15 g of root per day). For insomnia and muscle soreness, take 1 teaspoon of liquid extract diluted in water or a 400-mg to 450-mg capsule, tablet, or softgel 30 to 45 minutes before bedtime or as needed. For a milder effect, drink a cup of valerian tea before bed. Avoid powdered valerian root.
Claims: Treats insomnia and eases pain; has antispasmodic and sedative effects.
Studies: A randomized, placebo-controlled trial of 184 adults showed two tablets per night for 28 nights produced significant improvements in sleep and quality of life.

Caution: Valerian may cause headache, excitability, uneasiness, and insomnia. Patients should be advised to limit driving or operating machinery while taking it. Patients should avoid or limit alcohol, barbiturates, tranquilizers, or other sedative-type drugs or herbs. Valerian should not be used longer than 1 month, or in patients with liver disease.

VITAMIN AND MINERAL GUIDE

Originally published in *Arthritis Today*, September–October 2005, reprinted by permission of the Arthritis Foundation.

Fat-Soluble Vitamins

Getting sufficient doses of vitamins is important, but make sure diet and supplements don't exceed recommendations. Excesses of these vitamins are stored, rather than excreted.

Vitamin A

Other names: Beta-carotene, retinal, retinol, and retinoic acid. Vitamin A palmitate and vitamin A acetate are retinol forms. "Retinoids" collectively refers to different forms of vitamin A.
Why: Maintains the immune system; protects eyesight; keeps skin and tissues of the mouth, stomach, intestine, and respiratory system healthy; acts as an antioxidant.
How much: RDA = 3000 IU for men; 2333 IU for women.
Too much: UL = 10,000 IU from retinol.

High levels are associated with bone fractures, liver abnormalities, and birth defects. Other signs: headaches; dry, itchy skin; hair loss; bone and joint pain; and vomiting and appetite loss.

Too little: Rare; symptoms include night blindness and weakened immune system.
Foods: Beta-carotene: apricots, cantaloupe, carrots, dark leafy greens, and sweet potato. Retinol: cheese, liver, eggs, and fortified milk.
Supplements: Supplements often contain vitamin A.
Interactions: Cholestyramine (Questran), colestipol, and mineral oil can reduce vitamin A absorption, while oral contraceptives can increase levels. Supplements combined with isotretinoin (Accutane) can increase drug's toxicity.
Research note: Researchers found that high levels of vitamin A from retinol (not beta-carotene) significantly increased bone fractures among men, confirming research showing that high levels of vitamin A from retinol raised the risk of hip fractures in women.

Vitamin D

Other names: Cholecalciferol, calciferol, ergocalciferol, dihydroxy vitamin D-2 or D-3.
Why: Builds and maintains strong teeth and bones; protects against osteoporosis; aids in calcium absorption; helps utilize phosphorus. Both calcium and phosphorus are important for bone mineralization.
How much: RDA = 200 IU for adults through age 50; 400 IU from 51 to 70 years of age; 600 IU over age 70.
Too much: UL = 2000 IU: nausea, vomiting, poor appetite, constipation, weakness, and weight loss; increases blood levels of calcium, causing confusion, heart rhythm abnormalities, or calcinosis and deposits of calcium in soft tissues.
Too little: A high risk of osteoporosis. Low levels lead to muscle weakness.

Why: Builds and m
tissue; enhances i
as an antioxidant;
How much: RDA =
women; smokers
aim for an additio
Too much: UL of vit
to diarrhea, nause
Too little: Weight l
gums; slower heali
colds.
Foods: Peppers, oran
fruits, strawberri
sprouts, cabbage, c
destroys vitamin C
Supplements: Daily in
recommended for
think the RDA for
suggest nearly 1000
levels at high conc
vitamin C react th
ingredients, such as
not been shown to
Interactions: Regular u
tory drugs (NSAID
oral contraceptives,
need for vitamin C.
Research note: In a rec
tion and arthritis, p
least amount of the
likely to be diagnos
ate the most fruits a

Folate

Other names: Folic acid
Why: Promotes healthy
formation of DNA;
How much: RDA = 4
pregnant women. At l
should come from t
foods and supplemen
Too much: UL = 1000 m
than 1500 mcg (1.5 m
such as nausea, appet
a vitamin B$_{12}$ deficien
damage. Folic acid ma
than the UL for peop
Too little: Increases the
can increase homocys
nant women increase
in their babies. Incre
depression, heart dise
Foods: Spinach, kale, co
garbanzo beans, lentil
liver, and fortified bre

Foods: Fortified milk and breakfast cereals are good sources of vitamin D; small amounts also are in egg yolks, butter, salmon, tuna, and sardines.
Supplements: Because vitamin D needs increase with age, many experts recommend as much as 800 IU for seniors. Just 10 to 15 minutes of sun exposure two to three times a week (without sunscreen) is sufficient to meet daily requirements.
Interactions: Corticosteroids, such as prednisone, antacids that contain magnesium, cholestyramine (Questran), and mineral oil can interfere with vitamin D absorption.
Research note: In a study of 221 people with knee osteoarthritis (OA), those who increased their daily vitamin D intake gained muscle strength and improved physical function.

Vitamin E

Other names: Alpha-tocopherol, gamma-tocopherol, tocopherol acetate, and tocopherol succinate.
Why: Acts as a scavenger, cleaning up free radicals; also aids in the formation of red blood cells, reproduction, and growth.
How much: RDA = 15 mg for adults.
Too much: UL = 1000 mg daily. May cause increased bleeding time.
Too little: Associated with fat malabsorption diseases like Crohn's disease.
Foods: Peanut butter, almonds, sunflower seeds, margarine, wheat germ, corn oil, soybean oil, and turnip greens.
Supplements: Supplements should include mixed tocopherols, natural vitamin E, generally labeled "D." The synthetic form "D,L" is only half as active.
Interactions: Blood-thinning medications, aspirin, NSAIDs, and drugs for schizophrenia or chemotherapy.
Research note: A 2004 review of 19 clinical studies sparked a debate about the safety of vitamin E supplementation. However, a closer look showed most of the people who experienced negative effects were elderly and had chronic illnesses. A study of 136 people with knee OA found that supplemental vitamin E didn't have any beneficial effect.

Vitamin K

Other names: Phylloquinone (K-1), menaquinone (K-2), menadione (K-3) and dihydophylloquinone.
Why: Aids blood clotting and activates osteocalcin, a protein that builds and strengthens bones.
How much: RDA for vitamin K = 90 mcg for women; 120 mcg for men.
Too much: No UL set.

Too little: Too little vitamin K increases blood clotting time and can cause bruises beneath skin and bleeding gums.
Foods: Leafy greens.
Supplements: Multivitamins often contain amounts lower than the RDA because vitamin K may have a blood-clotting effect.
Interactions: Antibiotics can decrease vitamin K production. Excess vitamin K intake may decrease effectiveness of blood-thinning drugs.
Research note: A study of more than 72,000 women found a link between low dietary vitamin K intake and an increased risk of hip fracture. Women who ate iceberg or romaine lettuce one or more times daily were 45% less likely to break a hip than those who ate lettuce once a week or less.

Water-Soluble Vitamins

During digestion, these vitamins are absorbed into the blood and transported around the body. The body uses them quickly, however, and excretes—rather than stores—what it doesn't need.

Vitamin B$_1$

Other names: Thiamine and thiamin.
Why: Converts glucose to energy; essential for normal functioning of the heart, brain, nervous system, and muscles.
How much: RDA = 1.2 mg for men; 1.1 mg for women.
Too much: No known symptoms, but an allergic reaction may result in flushing, itching, or swelling.
Too little: Deficiency is associated with abnormal carbohydrate metabolism. Prolonged deficiency can affect the nervous and cardiovascular systems.
Foods: All plant and animal foods contain thiamine, especially whole wheat, brown rice, fish, and lentils. Enriched pasta, bread, cereals, and rice.
Supplements: Multivitamins generally provide 100% or more of the daily requirements.
Interactions: Research links long-term use of the diuretic furosemid (Lasix) to vitamin B$_1$ deficiency. Regular use of antacids also may interfere with thiamine's absorption.

Vitamin B$_2$

Other names: Riboflavin.
Why: Promotes healthy development; helps produce skin and red blood cells; helps convert glucose to energy.
How much: RDA = 1.3 mg daily for men; 1.1 mg daily for women.
Too much: UL not determined. High doses are believed harmless, but may turn urine orange or yellow.

Too little: Absorpti...
  thyroidism. Symp...
  and sensitivity to...
Foods: Organ mea...
  grains. Riboflavi...
Supplements: Gene...
  multivitamins, w...
  DV for riboflavir...
Interactions: None k...
Research note: A di...
  off or slow the pr...
  prevent migraine...

Vitamin B₃

Other names: Niacin...
Why: Helps with pr...
  and fats); keeps ...
  healthy.
How much: RDA = ...
Too much: UL = 35 r...
  higher doses as a t...
  triglyceride levels...
  ears; itching, nau...
  gout. More seriou...
  tions, and liver da...
Too little: Rare; symp...
  and dementia.
Foods: Chicken, tuna...
  peanut butter, and...
Supplements: Typicall...
  which generally pr...
  requirements.
Interactions: Taking ...
  may interfere with...
  lesterol medication...
  Pregnant women s...
  RDA. Take with fo...
Research note: Studies...
  a decreased risk of...

Vitamin B₆

Other names: Pyridoxi...
  pyridoxine hydroch...
Why: Needed in more...
  the body and for f...
  cells, and antibodie...
  function and energy...
How much: RDA = 1....
  over age 50, 1.7 mg ...
Too much: UL = 100 r...
  can lead to nerve ...
  numbness of the ext...
Too little: Rare; sympt...
  sore tongue, depress...

Supplements: Inflammatory arthritis accelerates bone loss, so getting the optimal intake daily is critical. Supplement with 500-mg doses one or more times a day with meals but avoid taking after eating foods containing oxalic or phytic acid, such as spinach, parsley, beans, and whole cereals. Calcium may interfere with absorption of iron, magnesium, and zinc, so take it separate from a multivitamin. Avoid supplements containing coral calcium, bone meal, oyster shell, or dolomite; they may be contaminated with lead.

Interactions: Calcium may decrease absorption or effectiveness of some bone drugs, antibiotics, and calcium channel blockers. Aluminum-containing antacids, anticonvulsants, corticosteroids, diuretics and laxatives may reduce calcium levels.

Research note: A review of five studies shows the combination of calcium and vitamin D supplements significantly prevented bone loss in people taking corticosteroids. In another study of 65 people with RA, those who took calcium (1000 mg) and vitamin D (500 IU) supplements not only reversed steroid-induced bone loss but also gained bone mass.

Chromium

Why: Helps body use insulin, protein, fat, and carbohydrates.
How much: AI = 35 mcg for men age 14 to 50; 30 mcg for men over age 50; 25 mcg for women age 14 to 50; 20 mcg for women over age 50.
Too much: No known symptoms.
Too little: Impaired glucose utilization.
Food: Black pepper, brewer's yeast, brown sugar, mushrooms, whole grains, and wheat germ.
Supplements: Not necessary or recommended.
Research note: There is no conclusive evidence that chromium supplements can prevent or treat diabetes, but research continues. Using chromium and beta-blockers modestly increases levels of high-density lipoprotein (HDL) levels. Chromium may add to effects of diabetes medications. Antacids, corticosteroids, H2-blockers, and proton pump inhibitors may decrease chromium levels.

Copper

Other names: Cupric oxide, copper gluconate, copper sulfate, and copper citrate.
Why: Helps build red blood cells, transport iron, and make connective tissue; keeps immune system, nerves, and blood vessels healthy; and removes free radicals.
How much: RDA = 900 mcg daily for adults.
Too much: UL = 10,000 mcg: nausea, vomiting, diarrhea, abdominal pain, headache, or death.

Too little: Rare; anemia and osteoporosis.
Foods: Organ meats, seafood, cashews, semisweet chocolate, peanut butter, lentils, and mushrooms.
Supplements: Not necessary or recommended; a multivitamin, typically provides the RDA.
Interactions: High levels of zinc, iron, and possibly vitamin C can block copper absorption.
Research note: Although copper does have anti-inflammatory properties, there currently is no research to support dietary copper or supplementation as a treatment for arthritis.

Fluoride

Why: Necessary for strong bones and teeth (especially tooth enamel).
How much: AI = 4 mg for men; 3 mg for women.
Too much: UL = 10 mg daily: mottled and brown teeth.
Too little: Tooth decay.
Foods: Fluoridated water, tea, and canned salmon and sardines (with bones).
Supplements: By prescription only for infants and children without access to fluoridated water.
Interactions: Calcium supplements and calcium- and aluminum-containing antacids.
Research note: Doesn't prevent osteoporosis. Safety concerns related to joint pain and stress fractures from taking extremely high doses.

Iron

Other names: Ferrous fumarate, ferrous gluconate, and ferrous sulfate.
Why: Necessary for production of hemoglobin.
How much: RDA = 8 mg daily for men; 18 mg daily for women until menopause; 8 mg daily for women after menopause.
Too much: UL = 45 mg per day: nausea, vomiting, diarrhea or constipation, and dark-colored stools. Iron builds up in body tissues and vital organs, leading to cirrhosis, diabetes, heart disease, and arthritis (particularly in the knuckles). High levels also lower zinc absorption.
Too little: The most common form of nutritional deficiency, mostly affecting young children, female teenagers, and women of childbearing years. Symptoms of mild deficiency include tiredness, shortness of breath, decreased mental performance, poor appetite, unstable body temperature, and decreased immunity.
Foods: Heme iron comes from beef, lamb, chicken, turkey, veal liver, ham, bologna or tuna, and is well absorbed by the body. Non-heme iron comes from plant sources and fortified grains, such as raisins,

peas, lentils, figs, oatmeal, and grits, and is not as well absorbed.

Supplements: Men and postmenopausal women should take multivitamins or other supplements with little or no iron.

Interactions: Calcium. High doses of vitamin C, meat, fish, poultry, citric acid, and cream of tartar enhance absorption of iron from plant sources. Coffee, tea, wine, tofu, legumes, grains, and rice inhibit absorption of iron from plant sources.

Magnesium

Other names: Magnesium chloride, gluconate, oxide, citrate (supplement forms); magnesium hydroxide (antacid) and magnesium sulfate (Epsom salt).

Why: Needed for more than 300 biochemical reactions in the body. Maintains muscle and nerve function, keeps heart rhythm regular, strengthens teeth and bones.

How much: RDA = 420 mg for men older than 31; 320 mg for women older than 31.

Too much: UL = 350 mg, supplements only; no upper limit via diet. Too much causes diarrhea, confusion, muscle weakness, nausea, irregular heartbeat, and low blood pressure.

Too little: Symptoms include loss of appetite, nausea, vomiting, fatigue, and weakness.

Foods: Kelp, wheat germ, soy beans, almonds, cashews, sunflower seeds, beans, potatoes, peanut butter, and hard (high mineral) water.

Supplements: Diet usually adequate, but supplementing is OK.

Interactions: May reduce effects or absorption of some diuretics, bone drugs, antibiotics, and iron. Chemotherapy may decrease magnesium level. Fiber may increase absorption.

Phosphorus

Why: Strengthens teeth and bones; also involved in energy production.

How much: RDA = 700 mg.

Too much: UL = 4000 mg daily before age 70; 3000 mg daily after age 70. Too much may cause diarrhea and upset stomach. Chronic overdose may cause kidney damage.

Too little: Rare; symptoms could include weak bones and muscles, fatigue, loss of appetite, bone pain, and increased susceptibility to infection.

Foods: Milk, yogurt, cheese, eggs, whole wheat bread, soft drinks, turkey, salmon, halibut, peanuts, almonds, and lentils.

Supplements: Not necessary or recommended.

Interactions: Aluminum-containing antacids, potassium supplements, and potassium-sparing diuretics.

Research note: There is no scientific evidence showing that phosphorus, namely in soft drinks, contributes to bone loss. However, drinking soft drinks in lieu of milk may contribute to osteopenia or osteoporosis.

Selenium

Other names: Sodium selenite (inorganic, supplement form) and selenomethionine (organic form found in food).

Why: Works with vitamins C and E as an antioxidant; essential for proper function of immune system and thyroid gland.

How much: RDA = 55 mcg daily.

Too much: UL = 400 mcg daily. Too much may cause hair and nail loss, fatigue, and mild nerve damage.

Too little: Rare; impaired immunity and heart damage.

Foods: Brazil nuts, walnuts, wheat germ, organ meats, shrimp, crab, tuna, turkey, and garlic.

Supplements: Not recommended beyond a multivitamin unless under a doctor's supervision.

Research note: Supplementation of 200 mcg daily may lower the risk of prostate cancer in men, but further studies must be done before scientists make any recommendations. Although people with RA tend to have low selenium levels, there is no evidence that selenium supplements are beneficial.

Sodium

Other names: Sodium chloride (table salt), sodium citrate, monosodium glutamate (MSG), sodium nitrate, sodium bicarbonate (baking soda), sodium phosphate (baking powder), and sodium saccharin.

Why: Regulates body fluids and blood pressure and helps nerve impulse function and muscle contraction.

How much: AI = 1.5 g for adults 19 to 50; 1.3 g for adults 51 to 70. DV is 2.4 g (2 g sodium = 1 teaspoon table salt). Average daily intake in the United States is 5 g.

Too much: No UL determined; excess may cause high blood pressure, stomach cancer, kidney stones, and osteoporosis.

Too little: Less than 0.5 g daily leads to headache, nausea, dizziness, fatigue, muscle cramps, and fainting.

Foods: Salt (75% percent of our salt intake comes from sodium added to seasonings or processed foods).

Supplements: Not necessary or recommended.

Interactions: Diuretics, NSAIDs, opiates, and tricyclic antidepressants. People taking corticosteroids should stay below 3 g daily.

Research note: One study found women who consumed a high salt diet (9 g daily) lost 33% more calcium and

APPENDIX III

23% more of a bone protein than those on a low salt diet (2 g/day).

Zinc

Other names: Zinc gluconate and zinc acetate.

Why: Involved in wound healing, cell reproduction, tissue growth, sexual maturation, and taste and smell; also associated with more than 100 enzymatic reactions in the body.

How much: RDA = 11 mg daily for men; 8 mg daily for women.

Too much: UL = 40 mg daily: immune suppression (same as deficiency), diarrhea, abdominal cramps and vomiting, and copper deficiency.

Too little: Mild deficiency impairs immunity, leading to poor wound healing and infection.

Foods: Oysters, mussels, lobster, beef, pork, lamb, chicken, turkey, milk, cheese, yogurt, maple syrup, peanuts, peanut butter, beans, and lentils.

Supplements: Multivitamins with no more than 100% DV recommended.

Interactions: Antibiotics may bind with zinc, decreasing both drug and nutrient absorption. Take multivitamins and antibiotics separately. Calcium can decrease absorption of zinc supplements.

Research note: Zinc may protect against age-related macular degeneration.

INDEX